Oncology Nursing

FIFTH EDITION

Martha E. Langhorne, MSN, RN, FNP, AOCN®

Advanced Practice Nurse, Oncology/Nursing Education and Research
United Health Services Hospitals
Johnson City, New York
Nurse Practitioner
United Medical Associates Gastroenterology
Binghamton, New York

Janet S. Fulton, PhD, RN, APRN-BC

Associate Professor
Indiana University
School of Nursing
Indianapolis, Indiana

Shirley E. Otto, MSN, CRNI, AOCN®

Oncology Consultant
Wichita, Kansas

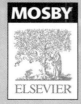

MOSBY

ELSEVIER

MOSBY
ELSEVIER

11830 Westline Industrial Drive
St. Louis, Missouri 63146

ONCOLOGY NURSING

ISBN: 978-0-323-04185-0

**Copyright © 2007, 2001, 1997, 1994, 1991 by Mosby, Inc.,
an affiliate of Elsevier Inc**.

Notice

Knowledge and best practice in this field are constantly changing. As new research and experience broaden our knowledge, changes in practice, treatment and drug therapy may become necessary or appropriate. Readers are advised to check the most current information provided (i) on procedures featured or (ii) by the manufacturer of each product to be administered, to verify the recommended dose or formula, the method and duration of administration, and contraindications. It is the responsibility of the practitioner, relying on their own experience and knowledge of the patient, to make diagnoses, to determine dosages and the best treatment for each individual patient, and to take all appropriate safety precautions. To the fullest extent of the law, neither the Publisher nor the [Editors/Authors] assumes any liability for any injury and/or damage to persons or property arising out or related to any use of the material contained in this book.

The Publisher

Previous editions copyrighted 2001, 1997, 1994, 1991

Library of Congress Cataloging-in-Publication Data

Library of Congress Control Number: 2007921395

Senior Acquisitions Editor: Sandra Clark Brown
Senior Developmental Editor: Cindi Anderson
Publishing Services Manager: Jeff Patterson
Project Manager: Amy Rickles
Design Direction: Amy Buxton

This book is lovingly dedicated to the memory of
Joseph Francis Ciesielski and Teresa C. Langsner,
my father and sister, respectively; and also to my mother, Eleanor Ciesielski, age 87,
who lives with us and reminds me every day to be grateful.

MARTHA E. LANGHORNE

Contributors

PATRICIA AGRE RN, EdD
Director
Patient/Family Education
Memorial Sloan-Kettering Cancer Center
New York, New York
Chapter 33. Patient Education

JULI AISTARS, RN, MS, AOCN®
Clinical Nurse Specialist
Radiation Oncology
Northwest Community Hospital
Arlington Heights, Illinois
Chapter 20. Radiation Therapy

REBECCA A. ALLAN, MSN, RN
Clinical Nurse Specialist
Gynecology/Urology
Karmanos Cancer Center
Detroit, Michigan
Chapter 11. Gynecologic Cancers

CAROL PAPPAS APPEL, MSN, RN, AOCNP
Oncology Nurse Practitioner
Cancer Care Associates
Royal Oak, Michigan
Chapter 22. Biotherapy

DEBRA BARTON, RN, PhD, AOCN®
Assistant Professor, Oncology
Mayo Clinic College of Medicine
Rochester, Minnesota
Chapter 42. Hot Flashes

EILEEN BOHAN, RN, BSN, CNRN
Senior Program Coordinator, Neurosurgical Oncology
Department of Neurosurgery
Johns Hopkins University
Baltimore, Maryland
Chapter 6. Cancer of the Brain and Central Nervous System

VIRGINIA BRADEN BOWMAN, RN, MSN, AOCNS
Head and Neck Reconstructive Surgery Unit
The University of Texas MD Anderson Cancer Center
Houston, Texas
Chapter 12. Head and Neck Cancers

PATRICIA A. CARTER, PhD, RN, CNS
Associate Professor
School of Nursing
The University of Texas at Austin
Austin, Texas
Chapter 40. Sleep Disturbance

RUTH A. CHAPLEN, RN, MSN, APRN-BC, AOCN®
Nurse Practitioner
Karmanos Cancer Institute
Clinical Instructor
Wayne State University
Detroit, Michigan
Chapter 9. Gastrointestinal Cancers

MELISSA CHRISTENSEN, RN, MSN, CPNP
Certified Pediatric Nurse Practitioner
Center for Cancer and Blood Disorders
The Children's Hospital
University of Colorado at Denver and Health Sciences Center
Denver, Colorado
Chapter 18. Pediatric Oncology

ROBIN L. COYNE, APRN, BC
Family Nurse Practitioner
Cancer Prevention Center
The University of Texas MD Anderson Cancer Center
Houston, Texas
Chapter 4. Prevention, Screening, and Detection

REBECCA CRANE-OKADA, PhD, RN, AOCN®
Clinical Nurse Researcher
Oncology Clinical Nurse Specialist
Joyce Eisenberg Keefer Breast Center
John Wayne Cancer Institute, Saint John's Health Center
Santa Monica, California
Chapter 7. Breast Cancers

MEI R. FU, PhD, RN, CNS
Assistant Professor
College of Nursing
New York University
New York, New York
Chapter 41. Nausea

JANET S. FULTON, PhD, RN, APRN-BC
Associate Professor
Indiana University
School of Nursing
Indianapolis, Indiana
Chapter 29. Oral Mucositis

AUDREY G. GIFT, PhD, RN, FAAN
Professor
College of Nursing
Michigan State University
East Lansing, Michigan
Chapter 14. Lung Cancer; Chapter 38. Dyspnea

JACQUELINE J. GLOVER, PhD
Associate Professor
Pediatrics and the Center for Bioethics and Humanities
University of Colorado at Denver and Health Sciences Center
Denver, Colorado
Chapter 36. Ethical Considerations

BARBARA HOLMES GOBEL, RN, MS, AOCN®
Oncology Clinical Nurse Specialist
Northwestern Memorial Hospital
Chicago, Illinois
Chapter 28. Bone Marrow Suppression

DEBRA E. HEIDRICH, MSN, RN, CHPN, AOCN®
Consultant
Pain and Palliative Care
West Chester, Ohio
Chapter 34. Palliative Care

MOLLY S. HEMENWAY, RN, MS, CPNP
Senior Instructor, Pediatric Nurse Practitioner
Center for Cancer and Blood Disorders
The Children's Hospital
University of Colorado at Denver and Health Sciences Center
Denver, Colorado
Chapter 18. Pediatric Oncology

AMY J. HOFFMAN, PhD(c), MSN, RN
Doctoral Candidate
College of Nursing
Michigan State University
East Lansing, Michigan
Chapter 14. Lung Cancer; Chapter 38. Dyspnea

GAIL B. JOHNSON, MSN, RN, CNS, AOCN®
Clinical Nurse Specialist
Department of Surgical Oncology
The University Hospital of Cincinnati—Barrett Cancer Center
Cincinnati, Ohio
Chapter 5. Cancer Diagnosis and Staging

MARY PAT JOHNSTON, RN, BSN, MS, AOCN®
Oncology Clinical Nurse Specialist
Regional Cancer Center
Pro Health Care, Waukesha Memorial Hospital
Waukesha, Wisconsin
Chapter 39. Pain

CLAIRE A. KELLER, RN, MN, CPNP, OCN®, CPON®
Pediatric Nurse Practitioner
Department of Pediatric Hematology/Oncology
University of Minnesota Medical Center, Fairview
Minneapolis, Minnesota
Chapter 23. Bone Marrow and Stem Cell Transplant

NANCY A. KING, MSN, RN, CPNP
APN Inpatient Oncology/Hematology Unit and Butterfly
Program Coordinator
The Children's Hospital Center for Cancer and Blood Disorders
The Children's Hospital
University of Colorado at Denver and Health Sciences Center
Denver, Colorado
Chapter 18. Pediatric Oncology

JOANNE LESTER, PhD, C, CNP, AOCN®
Oncology Nurse Practitioner, Nurse Researcher
Division of Surgical Oncology, Comprehensive
    Breast Health Center
The Ohio State University/James Cancer Hospital and Solove
    Research Institute
Columbus, Ohio
Chapter 19. Surgery

MOLLY LONEY, RN, MSN
Oncology Clinical Nurse Specialist
Hirsch Cancer Center
Hillcrest Hospital
Mayfield Heights, Ohio
Chapter 7. Breast Cancers

JENNIFER R. MADDEN, RN, MSN, CPNP
Assistant Professor, Department of Pediatrics
Pediatric Nurse Practitioner, Department of Neuro-oncology
Center for Cancer and Blood Disorders
The Children's Hospital
University of Colorado at Denver and Health Sciences Center
Denver, Colorado
Chapter 18. Pediatric Oncology

LISA MALBURG, RN, MSN, APRN, BC, AOCN®
Nurse Practitioner
Phase I Program
Karmanos Cancer Institute
Detroit, Michigan
Chapter 9. Gastrointestinal Cancers

ELLYN E. MATTHEWS, PhD, RN, AOCN®, CRNI®
Assistant Professor
School of Nursing
University of Colorado at Denver and Health Sciences Center
Denver, Colorado
Chapter 35. Family Caregiving

ROXANNE W. McDANIEL, PhD, RN
Associate Dean
Sinclair School of Nursing
University of Missouri-Columbia
Columbia, Missouri
Chapter 41. Nausea

SANDRA A. MITCHELL, CRNP, MScN, AOCN®
Predoctoral Fellow
Clinical Center
National Institutes of Health
Bethesda, Maryland
Doctoral Candidate
University of Utah College of Nursing
Salt Lake City, Utah
Chapter 32. Functional Status in the Patient with Cancer

HELENE MOHAMED, BSN, RN
Cancer Prevention Center
The University of Texas MD Anderson Cancer Center
Houston, Texas
Chapter 4. Prevention, Screening and Detection

MARY E. MURPHY, RN, MS, AOCN®, CHPN
Director of Clinical Systems
Advanced Practice Nurse, Focused Care Program
Department of Nursing
Hospice of Dayton, Inc.
Dayton, Ohio
Chapter 8. Colorectal Cancers

JAMIE S. MYERS, RN, MN, AOCN®
Regional Scientific Associate Director
Department of Scientific Operations
Novartis Oncology
East Hanover, New Jersey
Chapter 24. Complications of Cancer and Cancer Treatment

PAULA NELSON-MARTEN, RN, PhD
Associate Professor
School of Nursing
University of Colorado at Denver and Health Sciences Center
Denver, Colorado
Chapter 36. Ethical Considerations

KIM O'RILEY, RN, MN
Nurse Practitioner, Leukemia/Lymphoma
Barbara Ann Karmanos Cancer Center
Detroit, Michigan
Chapter 13. Leukemia

MAUREEN E. O'ROURKE, RN, PhD
Associate Clinical Professor of Nursing
Department of Adult Health
University of North Carolina Greensboro
Greensboro, North Carolina
Adjunct Assistant Professor of Medicine
Department of Hematology/Oncology
Wake Forest University School of Medicine
Winston-Salem, North Carolina
Chapter 10. Genitourinary Cancers

COLLEEN O'LEARY, RN, BSN, OCN®
Staff Educator Medical Oncology
Northwestern Memorial Hospital
Chicago, Illinois
Chapter 28. Bone Marrow Suppression

ROSANNE ELBE OSOSKI, RN, MSN
Nurse Practitioner
Walt Comprehensive Breast Center
Karmanos Cancer Center
Detroit, Michigan
Chapter 13. Leukemia

SHIRLEY E. OTTO, MSN, CRNI, AOCN®
Oncology Consultant
Wichita, Kansas
Chapter 16. Multiple Myeloma; Chapter 21. Chemotherapy

JUDITH K. PAYNE, PhD, RN, AOCN®
Assistant Professor
Department of Oncology
Duke University School of Nursing
Durham, North Carolina
Chapter 25. Cancer Clinical Trials

ANGELA CARRIE PELTZ, PA-C, MPAS
Bone Marrow Transplant Physician Assistant
Instructor, School of Medicine
Center for Cancers and Blood Disorders
The Children's Hospital
University of Colorado at Denver and Health Sciences Center
Denver, Colorado
Chapter 18. Pediatric Oncology

KATHLEEN PERANSKI, RN, MSN, OCN®
Nurse Manager
Inpatient Oncology Unit/Cardiac Stepdown Unit
United Health Services Hospitals
Johnson City, New York
Chapter 15. Malignant Lymphoma

JULIE PONTO, RN, PhD(c), APRN-BC, AOCN®
Associate Professor
Master's Program in Nursing
Winona State University
Rochester, Minnesota
Chapter 2. Genetics

ELIZABETH POUNDER, MS, PA-C
Senior Instructor
Center for Cancer and Blood Disorders
The Children's Hospital
University of Colorado at Denver and Health Sciences Center
Denver, Colorado
Chapter 18. Pediatric Oncology

VERNA A. RHODES, RN, EdS, FAAN
Associate Professor Emeritus
Sinclair School of Nursing
University of Missouri—Columbia
Columbia, Missouri
Chapter 41. Nausea

LISA SCHULMEISTER, RN, MN, CS, OCN®
Oncology Nursing Consultant
New Orleans, Louisiana
Chapter 3. Epidemiology; Chapter 26. Nutrition

ANNE MARIE SHAFTIC, MSN, RN,C, NP-C, AOCNP
Nurse Practitioner
Department of Oncology
Holy Name Hospital
Teaneck, New Jersey
Chapter 33. Patient Education

JUDITH A. SHELL, PhD, LMFT, RN
Medical Family Therapist
Marriage and Family Therapist
Osceola Cancer Center
Kissimmee, Florida
Chapter 30. Psychosocial Care; Chapter 31. Sexuality

NORMA SHERIDAN-LEOS, RN, MSN, AOCN®, CPHQ
Clinical Quality Improvement Analyst
Department of Quality Improvement
The University of Texas MD Anderson Cancer Center
Houston, Texas
Chapter 17. Skin Cancers

MICHELLE L. TREON, BSN, RN, OCN®
Oncology Clinical Nurse Coordinator
Adult Cancer Center
Clarian Health Partners, Indiana University Hospital
Indianapolis, Indiana
Chapter 29. Oral Mucositis

RUTH VAN GERPEN, RN, MS, OCN®
Clinical Nurse Specialist
Department of Oncology
BryanLGH Medical Center
Lincoln, Nebraska
Chapter 1. Pathophysiology

SARAH R. WILSON, RN, BSN, OCN®
Manager
Department of Multidisciplinary Oncology Care
Presbyterian Cancer Center
Charlotte, North Carolina
Chapter 37. Fatigue

KATHLEEN D. WRIGHT, MS, CWOCN, APRN
Clinical Leader
Wound Ostomy Continence Nursing
Nanticoke Health Services
Seaford, Delaware
Chapter 27. Skin Integrity

Reviewers

CATHY FORTENBAUGH, BSN, MSN, AOCN®, APN, C
Clinical Nurse Specialist
Pennsylvania Oncology Hematology Associates
Philadelphia, Pennsylvania

EMILY HAOZOUS, BA, MSN, APRN, BC
Doctoral Student
Yale University School of Nursing
New Haven, Connecticut

SUSAN K. STEELE, DNS, APRN, CNS, AOCN®
Assistant Professor of Nursing
Louisiana State Health Sciences Center
School of Nursing
New Orleans, Louisiana

JANET H. VAN CLEAVE, AOCN®, ACNP, MSN, BSN, MBA
Nurse Practitioner
The Mount Sinai Medical Center
New York, New York

Preface

We, Martha Langhorne and Janet Fulton, would like the first message to the readers of this 5th edition of *Oncology Nursing* to be an expression of gratitude, praise, and thanks to Shirley Otto MSN, CRNI, AOCN®, the creator and original editor of this text. *Oncology Nursing* is one of the most popular hands-on oncology nursing text available in the United States, and through four previous editions it has offered to its readers updated, cutting-edge knowledge and insight into the care of oncology patients. The book has been used by nurses and other health care providers in a wide variety of settings, both nationally and internationally. Educators have relied on *Oncology Nursing* as a resource for students and new oncology staff. It is not clear that Shirley is aware of the enormity of her contribution to oncology care and oncology nursing practice. As she plans for retirement, it is her intent to see the book continue. Following Shirley's footsteps, we as new editors are accepting the challenge of continuing a legacy of excellence. Shirley has been extremely supportive and respectful of our ideas for evolving this next edition, encouraging us to put "our mark on the book."

We also benefited from the collegial relationships that Shirley fostered over the years. Many previous authors were again eager to contribute while new authors were pleased to have the opportunity to write for the "Otto text." We are privileged to have so many knowledgeable and experienced chapter contributors. The unique mix of clinicians and researchers gives the book its practical yet cutting-edge approach. We are appreciative of the considerable talent of our contributors and their willingness to share their time to make this edition possible. We value their efforts, as we believe readers will also.

Every chapter has undergone major revisions with an emphasis on evidence for practice. To address our increasingly aging population, each chapter contributor added a section on geriatric considerations. A case study has also been added to each chapter along with review questions. The study questions provide excellent review for nurses preparing for oncology certification. We have included the most recent updated staging information available at the time of publication as well as creative graphs, tables, and charts where appropriate.

Units 1 through 3 are similar to previous editions. They describe oncology diseases and include epidemiology, diagnosis, prognosis, medical treatments, and nursing care considerations. Unit 4 is redesigned, and Unit 5 is new. These units address supportive care and symptom management with an emphasis on autonomous nursing interventions—those interventions that patients, families, and the public expect from nurses to help prevent and manage cancer-related concerns.

As new editors for this book, it is worth noting that our collaboration began not with this book but years ago while working together on a committee of the Oncology Nursing Society. Our many years of collegial relationship made the task of revising and updating the book easy. Martha's clinical expertise and Janet's academic and editorial experience were a perfect blend of strengths. We believe the book is now, as in the past, an essential supportive work for the oncology nurse in an easy to use format.

Many thanks to the Elsevier staff—Sandra Clark Brown, Cindi Anderson, and Amy Rickles—who have been kind, gracious, patient, and helpful during this process. Producing a book, we now know, is no easy undertaking, and the guiding hand of the publisher is essential.

We cannot end without thanking our families. Thomas, Timothy, and Eliot Langhorne and Morgan, Alexander, and David Fulton have been patient, supportive, and humorous when needed across the many months it took to create the 5th edition of *Oncology Nursing*. They are "our boys" and we are ever so thankful they are part of our lives.

With a measure of pride and humility we present to you the 5th edition of *Oncology Nursing*!

MARTHA E. LANGHORNE MSN, RN, FNP, AOCN®
JANET S. FULTON PhD, RN, APRN-BC

Contents in Brief

Contents

Clinical Aspects of Cancer Diagnosis

CHAPTER 1

Pathophysiology

Ruth Van Gerpen

Cancer, as a single word, incorporates a vast diversity of diseases since there are as many tumor types as there are cell types in the human body. Therefore cancer is not a single disease, but a group of heterogeneous diseases that share common biologic properties (e.g., clonal cell growth and invasive ability). The cancer research revolution has also demonstrated that all cancers are genetic and share common molecular pathogeneses. All cancers are the result of mutations in oncogenes and tumor suppressor genes. Each specific cancer occurs through mutations in specific genes.[1,2]

Proliferative Growth Patterns

Cell proliferation is the process by which cells divide and reproduce. In normal tissue, cell proliferation is regulated so that the number of cells actively dividing is equal to the number of cells dying or being shed. Abnormal cell differentiation and growth results in an abnormal mass of tissue, called a neoplasm. Neoplasia means "new growth" and refers to an abnormal mass of tissue characterized by autonomous, excessive, and uncoordinated growth.[3-5] Although they are not synonymous, the terms neoplasm and tumor are often used interchangeably. Neoplasms are classified as benign or malignant. Cancer is the common term for all malignant tumors.

BENIGN GROWTH PATTERNS

The most significant benign growth patterns are *hypertrophy, hyperplasia, metaplasia,* and *dysplasia.* **Hypertrophy** is an increase in cell size resulting in an increase in organ size. It commonly results from increased workload, hormonal stimulation, or compensation directly related to the functional loss of other tissue. **Hyperplasia** is a reversible increase in the number of cells in an organ or a tissue in response to a specific growth stimulus. For example, endometrial hyperplasia and benign prostatic hyperplasia are the result of excessive hormonal stimulation. However, cancer can develop if the growth control mechanisms become defective.[3,5]

Metaplasia is the conversion of one cell type to another cell type not usually found in the involved tissue. Metaplasia can be induced by inflammation, vitamin deficiencies, chronic irritation, or various chemical agents. An example of metaplasia is substitution of columnar epithelial cells of the respiratory tract by squamous epithelial cells in response to inhaled irritants such as cigarette smoke. The process is reversible if the stimulus is removed, or metaplasia may progress to dysplasia if the stimulus persists. **Dysplasia** is characterized by abnormal changes in the size, shape, or organization of cells. The common stimulus creating a dysplasia is usually an external one such as radiation, inflammation, toxic chemicals, or chronic irritation. For example, dysplasia is associated with the chronic bronchitis commonly seen in smokers, and also in prolonged inflammation of the uterine cervix. Dysplasia is also reversible if the stimulus is removed.

Dysplasia often precedes a tissue's becoming cancerous, and some forms of dysplasia are known as precancerous lesions.[5,6]

Benign neoplasms contain well-differentiated cells that are clustered together in a single mass. These tumors usually do not cause death unless their location or size interferes with vital functions. In contrast, malignant neoplasms are less well-differentiated and have the ability to spread to other sites. If untreated or uncontrolled, malignant neoplasms usually cause death.

Benign and malignant neoplasms are usually differentiated by their cell characteristics, manner of growth, rate of growth, potential for metastases or spreading to other parts of the body, ability to produce systemic effects, tendency to cause tissue destruction, and capacity to cause death.[5,6] Table 1-1 summarizes the characteristics of benign and malignant neoplasms.

Tumor Terminology

Neoplasms are composed of two types of tissue: parenchymal tissue and the supportive stroma of connective tissue and blood vessels. Tumors are identified according to the tissue of origin and the benign or malignant character of the tumor (Table 1-2). Benign tumors are designated by attaching the suffix -*oma*, the Greek root for tumor, to the parenchymal tissue of origin. For example, a benign tumor of fibrous tissue is called a fibroma, and a benign tumor of glandular tissue is an adenoma. Exceptions to this rule include hepatomas, lymphomas, and melanomas. By name, these cancers should be benign. However, they are all malignant. The more accurate terms are hepatocellular carcinoma, lymphosarcoma, and malignant melanoma.[3,7]

Malignant tumors also use the suffix -*oma* to designate the presence of a tumor. In addition, malignant tumors of epithelial origin are designated by the root *carcin*, crablike, or carcinoma. Certain prefixes are added to describe the type of epithelial tissue from which the carcinoma originates. For example, adenocarcinoma describes tumors originating from glandular (columnar) epithelium. Squamous cell carcinoma describes tumors arising from squamous epithelial tissue. Carcinoma in situ refers to preinvasive epithelial tumors of glandular or squamous cell origin such as carcinoma in situ of the endometrium or cervix.

Malignant tumors arising from mesenchymal cells (connective tissue, muscle, blood vessels) are designated by the root *sarc*, meaning fleshy. For example, liposarcoma describes tumors arising from fat, tumors arising from bone are described as osteosarcoma, and leiomyosarcoma describes tumors arising from smooth muscle.[3,7,8]

Characteristics of Cancer Cells

ALTERED CELL DIFFERENTIATION

In normal cell growth, cells become more specialized and acquire specific structural and functional characteristics as they mature, a process called differentiation. During transformation

TABLE 1-1	Comparison of Benign and Malignant Tumors	
CHARACTERISTIC	**BENIGN**	**MALIGNANT**
Differentiation/anaplasia	Well-differentiated; structure may be typical of tissue of origin	Some lack of differentiation with anaplasia; structure is often atypical
Rate of growth	Usually progressive and slow; may come to a standstill or regress; mitotic figures are rare and normal	Erratic and may be slow to rapid; mitotic figures may be numerous and abnormal
Local invasion	Usually cohesive and expansile; well-demarcated masses that do not invade or infiltrate surrounding normal tissues	Locally invasive, infiltrating the surrounding normal tissues; sometimes may be seemingly cohesive and expansile
Metastasis	Absent	Frequently present; the larger and more undifferentiated the primary, the more likely are metastases

From Kumar V, Fausto N, Abbas A, editors: *Robbins & Cotran pathologic basis of disease,* ed 7, Philadelphia, 2004, Saunders.

TABLE 1-2	Classification of Human Tumors		
TUMOR TYPE	**CELL/TISSUE OF ORIGIN**	**BENIGN TUMORS**	**MALIGNANT TUMORS**
Mesenchymal tumors	Fibroblast	Fibroma	Fibrosarcoma
	Fat cell	Lipoma	Liposarcoma
	Blood vessels	Hemangioma	Angiosarcoma
	Smooth muscle cell	Leiomyoma	Leiomyosarcoma
	Striated muscle cell	Rhabdomyosarcoma	Rhabdomyosarcoma
	Cartilage	Chondroma	Chondrosarcoma
	Bone cell	Osteoma	Osteosarcoma
Epithelial tumors	Squamous epithelium	Epithelioma (papilloma)	Squamous cell carcinoma
	Transitional epithelium	Transitional cell papilloma	Transitional cell carcinoma
	Glandular/ductal epithelium	Adenoma	Adenocarcinoma
	Neuroendocrine cells	Carcinoid	Oat cell carcinoma
Internal organ-specific	Liver cell	Liver cell adenoma	Liver cell carcinoma
	Kidney cell	Renal cell adenoma	Renal cell carcinoma
Tumors of blood cell and lymphocytes	White blood stem cells	–	Leukemia
	Lymphoid cells	–	Lymphoma
	Plasma cells	–	Multiple myeloma
Tumors of neural cell precursors	Neuroblast	Ganglioneuroma	Neuroblastoma
Tumors of glial cells and neural supporting cells	Glial cells	–	Glioma
	Meningial cells	Meningioma	–
	Schwann cells	Schwannoma	Malignant schwannoma
Germ cell tumors	Embryonic cells	Teratoma	Embryonal carcinoma Teratocarcinoma Seminoma/dysgerminoma

From Damjanov, I: *Pathology for the health-related professions,* ed 2, Philadelphia, 2000, Saunders.

from a normal cell to a malignant cell, altered differentiation can result from changes in the appearance and metabolism of the cell, the presence of tumor-specific antigens, and the loss of normal function.[6,9-11]

Appearance Changes. Cancer cells vary in size and shape, a feature called pleomorphism. Some are unusually large, whereas others are extremely small. Nuclei may be disproportionately large, or there may be multiple nuclei. A variety of abnormal mitotic features may be present. There may be an abnormal number of chromosomes, called aneuploidy, or abnormal arrangements of chromosomes.[4,11,12]

In cancer, differentiation refers to the extent to which cancer cells resemble similar normal cells. Cancer cells vary in their ability to retain the morphologic and functional traits of the original tissue. Cells that are more mature in appearance and closely resemble the normal cell are well differentiated. Cells that grow rapidly and do not have the original tissue's morphologic characteristics and specialized cell functions are termed undifferentiated. Anaplastic or undifferentiated cells appear cytologically disorganized and have no resemblance to the tissue of origin. The more undifferentiated a malignant cell, the more aggressive it is believed to be.[3,9,11]

TABLE 1-3 **Paraneoplastic Syndromes**		
CLINICAL SYNDROMES	**MAJOR FORMS OF UNDERLYING CANCER**	**CAUSAL MECHANISM**
Endocrinopathies		
Cushing syndrome	Small cell carcinoma of lung	ACTH or ACTH-like substance
	Pancreatic carcinoma	
	Neural tumors	
Syndrome of inappropriate antidiuretic hormone secretion	Small cell carcinoma of lung; intracranial neoplasms	Antidiuretic hormone or atrial natriuretic hormones
Hypercalcemia	Squamous cell carcinoma of lung	Parathyroid hormone-related peptide, TGF-α, TNF-α, IL-1
	Breast carcinoma	
	Renal carcinoma	
	Adult T-cell leukemia/lymphoma	
	Ovarian carcinoma	
Hypoglycemia	Fibrosarcoma	Insulin or insulin-like substance
	Other mesenchymal sarcomas	
	Hepatocellular carcinoma	
Carcinoid syndrome	Bronchial adenoma (carcinoid)	Serotonin, bradykinin
	Pancreatic carcinoma	
	Gastric carcinoma	
Polycythemia	Renal carcinoma	Erythropoietin
	Cerebellar hemangioma	
	Hepatocellular carcinoma	
Nerve and Muscle Syndromes		
Myasthenia	Bronchogenic carcinoma	Immunologic
Disorders of the central and peripheral nervous systems	Breast carcinoma	
Dermatologic Disorders		
Acanthosis nigricans	Gastric carcinoma	Immunologic, secretion of epidermal growth factor
	Lung carcinoma	
	Uterine carcinoma	
Dermatomyositis	Bronchogenic, breast carcinoma	Immunologic
Osseous, Articular, and Soft Tissue Changes		
Hypertrophic osteoarthropathy and clubbing of the fingers	Bronchogenic carcinoma	Unknown
Vascular and Hematologic Changes		
Venous thrombosis (Trousseau phenomenon)	Pancreatic carcinoma	Tumor products (mucins that activate clotting)
	Bronchogenic carcinoma	
	Other cancers	
Nonbacterial thrombotic endocarditis	Advanced cancers	Hypercoagulability
Anemia	Thymic neoplasms	Unknown
Others		
Nephrotic syndrome	Various cancers	Tumor antigens, immune complexes

ACTH, Adrenocorticotropic hormone; *TGF*, transforming growth factor; *TNF*, tumor necrosis factor; *IL*, interleukin.
From Kumar V, Fausto N, Abbas A, editors: *Robbins & Cotran pathologic basis of disease*, ed 7. Philadelphia, 2004, Saunders.

Altered Metabolism. Cell membrane changes may result in the production of surface enzymes that aid invasion and metastasis. In addition, a loss of glycoproteins that normally assist in cellular adhesion and organization results in a loss of cell-to-cell adhesion and increases cell mobility. Higher rates of anaerobic glycolysis in the cancer cell also make the cell less dependent on oxygen. Production of abnormal growth factor receptors may independently signal the cell to grow and may increase sensitivity to normal growth factors.

Cancer cells may inappropriately secrete hormones or hormone-like substances in an organ or tissue that does not normally produce or release those hormones, resulting in paraneoplastic syndromes or signs and symptoms not directly related to the local effects of the tumor. For example, in small cell carcinoma of the lung, antidiuretic hormone (ADH) is produced, resulting in hyponatremia (Table 1-3).[3,5,11,12]

Tumor-Specific Antigens. Some tumors produce an excess of specific antigens or produce new tumor-associated

TABLE 1-4	Selected Tumors Markers
MARKERS	**ASSOCIATED CANCERS**
Hormones	
Human chorionic gonadotropin	Trophoblastic tumors, nonseminomatous testicular tumor
Calcitonin	Medullary carcinoma of thyroid
Catecholamine and metabolites	Pheochromocytoma and related tumors
Ectopic hormones	Refer to Table 1-3
Oncofetal Antigens	
α-Fetoprotein	Liver cell cancer, nonseminomatous germ cell tumors of testis
Carcinoembryonic	Carcinomas of the colon, pancreas, antigen lung, stomach, and heart
Isoenzymes	
Prostatic acid phosphatase	Prostate cancer
Neuron-specific enolase	Small cell cancer of lung, neuroblastoma
Specific Proteins	
Immunoglobulins	Multiple myeloma and other gammopathies
Prostate-specific antigen and prostate-specific membrane antigen	Prostate cancer
Mucins and Others Glycoproteins	
CA-125	Ovarian cancer
CA-19-9	Colon cancer, pancreatic cancer
CA-15-3	Breast cancer
New Molecular Markers	
p53, APC, and RAS mutations in stool and serum	Colon cancer
p53 and RAS mutations in stool and serum	Pancreatic cancer
p53 and RAS mutations in sputum and serum	Lung cancer
p53 mutations in urine	Bladder cancer

From Kumar V, Fausto N, Abbas A, editors: *Robbins & Cotran pathologic basis of disease*, ed 7, Philadelphia, 2004, Saunders.

antigens marking the cancer cell as "non-self." An example is the prostate-specific antigen (PSA) which is a protein produced by prostate gland cells. An elevation in PSA may indicate prostate cancer. Certain tumor antigens may be useful as tumor markers and can be used as a diagnostic tool or in monitoring the effectiveness of cancer treatment (Table 1-4).[5,11,12]

Altered Cellular Function. The need for cell renewal or replacement is the usual stimulus for cell proliferation. Cell production stops when the stimulus is gone, producing a balance between cell production and cell loss. The rate of normal cellular proliferation differs in each tissue. In some tissues, such as bone marrow, hair follicles, or epithelial lining of the gastrointestinal tract, the rate of cellular proliferation is rapid. In other tissues, such as the myocardium, neurons, and cartilage, cellular proliferation does not occur. In cancer, proliferation continues once the stimulus initiates the process, and cancer cells progress in continued, uncontrolled growth. Normal control mechanisms fail to stop this proliferation.

Cancer cells also demonstrate a loss of contact inhibition. Normal cells cease movement when they come in contact with another cell and symmetrically arrange themselves around each other. Cancer cells invade others without respect to these constraints. In addition, when normal cells are surrounded by other cells, they simply stop dividing. Cancer cells lack or exhibit decreased contact inhibition of growth, continuing to divide and even piling atop one another.

Cancer cells are less genetically stable than normal cells because of the development of abnormal chromosome arrangements. Chromosomal instability results in new, increasingly malignant mutants as cancer cells proliferate. These mutant cells can create a surviving subpopulation of advanced neoplasms with unique biologic and cytogenetic characteristics that are highly resistant to therapy.[3,7,12]

Cancer cells also possess the capacity to metastasize, the hallmark of a malignant neoplasm. **Metastasis,** the spread of cancer cells from a primary site to distant secondary sites, is aided by the production of enzymes on the surface of the cancer cell.

Tumor Growth

The rate of tissue growth in normal and cancerous tissue depends on three factors: the duration of the cell cycle, the number of cells that are actively dividing, and the cell loss.[3,6]

CELL CYCLE

The *cell cycle* is a coordinated sequence of events resulting in duplication of DNA and division into two daughter cells. The four phases of the cell cycle are G_1, S, G_2, and M (Fig. 1-1).[12-14]

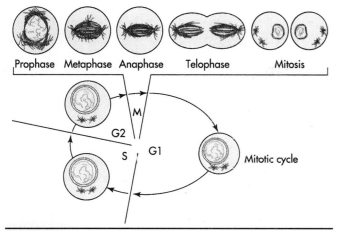

FIG. 1-1   The cell cycle. (Adapted from Phipps WJ, Sands JK, Marek JF, editors: *Medical-surgical nursing: concepts and clinical practice*, ed 6, St Louis, 1999, Mosby.)

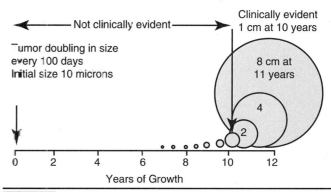

FIG. 1-2   Tumor growth, showing doubling time related to tumor size. (From Meier P: Perspectives in oncology. In Black JM, Hawks JH: *Medical-surgical nursing: clinical management for positive outcomes*, ed 7, Philadelphia, 2005, Saunders.)

G_1 or Gap 1. In the G_1 phase, which lasts from hours to days or longer, RNA and protein synthesis occurs in preparation for DNA replication.

S Phase or Synthesis. In the S phase, which lasts approximately 10 to 20 hours, DNA replication occurs in preparation for division.

G_2 or Gap 2. During the G_2 phase, which ranges from 2 to 10 hours, DNA synthesis ceases while RNA and protein synthesis continues. In addition, precursors of the mitotic spindle apparatus are produced.

M Phase or Mitosis. In the M phase, which lasts from 30 to 60 minutes, cell division occurs. This phase is further subdivided into five stages: prophase, prometaphase, metaphase, anaphase, and telophase. After mitosis the daughter cells enter the G_1 phase and begin the cell reproductive cycle again or redirect themselves into a resting phase, called G_0.

G_0 or Resting Phase. In the G_0 phase, cells perform all functions other than those related to proliferation. Nondividing cells are not considered to be in the cell cycle. Cells in the G_0 phase are activated to reenter the cell cycle in response to various stimuli that signal for cell renewal.

The duration of the cell cycle varies depending on the cell type, the frequency in which the cells divide, and other characteristics such as appropriate growth factors. Very rapidly dividing cells can complete the cell cycle in less than 8 hours, whereas other cells can take longer than 1 year. The variability primarily occurs in the G_0 and G_1 phases.[6,14-16]

Proteins called cyclins control entry and progression of cells through the cell cycle. The cyclins (D, E, A, B) combine with and activate enzymes called cyclin-dependent kinases (CDKs). Once activated, the cyclin-CDK complexes allow the cell to progress through each stage of the cell cycle and serve as checkpoints or monitors of the cell cycle. Two critical checkpoints occur in the cell cycle. The first, called the restriction point, occurs at the G_1-S transition when the cell checks for DNA damage and decides whether to proceed with replication. If DNA damage is present, repair mechanisms are activated and progress through the cell cycle is delayed. The second checkpoint occurs at the G_2-M transition, where the cell verifies accurate DNA replication and determines if mitosis can safely occur. Defects in cell-cycle checkpoint components, such as the p53 protein, are a major cause of genetic instability in cancer cells.[3,6,10,14,16]

CELL-CYCLE TIME

Cell-cycle time is the amount of time required for a cell to move from one mitosis to another mitosis, or the sum of M, G_1, S, and G_2. The length of the total cell cycle varies with the specific type of cell. A common misconception is that the rate of cancer cell proliferation is faster than that of a normal cell. Usually cancer cells proliferate at the same rate as the normal cells of the tissue of origin. The difference is that the proliferation of cancer cells is continuous. The length of the G_0 phase is the major factor in determining the cell-cycle time.[10,15]

DOUBLING TIME

In the simplest model for cell growth, a cell divides to produce two daughter cells, each of which then divides, producing four cells, eight cells, and so on. Thus, cell numbers increase in powers of two, called exponential growth. The growth rate of tumors is expressed in doubling time. *Doubling time* is the length of time it takes for a tumor to double its volume. Tumor cells undergo a series of doublings as the tumor increases in size. The average doubling time for most primary solid tumors is approximately 2 months. Rapidly growing tumors such as testicular cancer may double every month, whereas slow-growing tumors such as prostate cancer may double every year. As shown in Fig. 1-2, it may take 10 years for a tumor to reach 1 cm in size. In only another year, that same tumor may grow to 8 cm.[11] Factors that affect doubling time are cell-cycle time, growth fraction, and cell loss by either cell death, differentiation, or metastasis.[15,17]

A tumor is usually clinically undetectable until it has doubled 30 times and contains more than 1 billion cells. At this point, it is approximately 1 cm in size and equals 1 gm in weight. With only 10 more doublings, the tumor contains more than 1 trillion cells or weighs 1 kg, which is enough to cause death.[3]

GROWTH FRACTION

Because not all tumor cells divide simultaneously, growth fraction is an important concept in the determination of doubling time. Growth fraction is the ratio of the total number of cells to the number of dividing cells. Tumors with larger growth fractions increase their tumor volume more quickly. As tumor volume increases, growth fraction decreases as a result of hypoxia, decreased nutrient availability, and toxins. In the later stages of tumor growth, only a small portion of cells are actively dividing. Cell growth usually continues only at the periphery of the tumor, with the center becoming increasingly dormant and eventually becoming necrotic. The tumor eventually reaches a point where cell death approximates cell birth, and a plateau is reached. The rapid proliferation of tumor cells followed by the continuous, but slower growth is called the Gompertzian growth curve. The growth curve (Fig. 1-3) illustrates the initial exponential growth of cancer cells, followed by the steady and progressive decrease in the fraction of proliferating cells and an increase in the rate of cell death.[3,6,15]

Molecular Pathogenesis of Cancer

Cancer cells differ from their normal counterparts in that they have abnormal regulation. Cells lose their normal characteristics and acquire abnormal characteristics that affect the appearance of the cells, the expression of proteins on the cell surface, cell growth, cell reproduction, and cell death. Seven fundamental changes in cell physiology have been proposed that collectively determine malignant cell growth (Fig. 1-4).[3,18,19]

1. *Self-sufficiency in growth signals.* Tumors possess the capability to proliferate without external stimuli, usually resulting from oncogene activation. Proto-oncogenes are normal genes that regulate normal cell growth and repair. Oncogenes are altered proto-oncogenes that promote autonomous cell growth in cancer cells. Oncogenes are like the accelerator of an automobile, resulting in increased cell birth or decreased cell death when expressed. Many cancer cells develop growth self-sufficiency by acquiring the ability to produce the necessary growth factors to which they respond (Table 1-5).[3,12,18]
2. *Insensitivity to growth-inhibitory signals.* Tumor suppressor genes, or the brakes of the cell, inhibit cell growth through cell-cycle control and regulation of apoptosis. Alterations in tumor suppressor genes resulting in failure to inhibit tumor cell growth are a key event in many cancers (Table 1-6).

Tumor suppressor genes are categorized as either gatekeepers or caretakers. Gatekeepers are genes that directly control the growth of tumors by inhibiting cell proliferation and/or promoting cell death. In contrast to gatekeepers, caretaker genes do not directly regulate cell proliferation, but control the rate of mutation. Therefore mutation of a caretaker gene leads to genetic instability that indirectly promotes growth and accelerates conversion of a normal cell to a neoplastic cell.[2,16,20]

3. *Evasion of apoptosis.* The proliferation of cancer cells may occur not only by the activation of oncogenes or inactivation of tumor suppressor genes, but also by mutations in the genes that regulate apoptosis, or programmed cell death.[21]
4. *Defects in DNA repair.* The DNA of normal dividing cells is susceptible to damage from environmental agents and to alterations resulting from errors that occur spontaneously during DNA replication. If DNA repair does not occur promptly, malignant transformation of the cell can occur. Individuals born with an inherited mutation of DNA repair genes are at a significantly increased risk of developing cancer.[3,18]
5. *Limitless replication potential.* Telomeres are structures at the end of each chromosome that shorten with each cell division. Once the telomeres are shortened beyond a certain point, proliferation ceases or apoptosis occurs. In germ cells, telomere shortening is prevented by the enzyme telomerase, thus enabling these cells to self-replicate extensively. Maintenance of telomere length and telomerase activity is essential for cancer cells to maintain unlimited replication potential and attain immortality.[3,9,22]
6. *Sustained angiogenesis.* Tumors stimulate the formation of a vascular supply, a process called angiogenesis, which is essential for continued tumor growth and metastasis. Tumor cells produce angiogenic factors such as vascular endothelial growth factor (VEGF) to stimulate and sustain blood vessel growth.[3,5]
7. *Ability to invade and metastasize.* Metastasis is the spread of cancer cells from a primary tumor to distant sites in the body. It is a complex process requiring tumor cells to break loose from the primary tumor, enter the blood vessels or lymphatic system, and produce a secondary tumor at a distant location.[3,6,11]

Carcinogenesis

Carcinogenesis is the process by which normal cells are transformed into cancer cells. The process begins with a single cell—the clonal cell—that has sustained genetic change.[23] Recent evidence suggests that carcinogenesis is a multistep process and involves a number of genetic mutations that cause progressive transformation of normal cells into highly malignant derivatives.[19]

THEORIES OF CARCINOGENESIS

In 1941, Rous and Kidd proposed a two-stage theory for the development of cancer involving an initiation stage brought about by a mutagen, followed by a promotion stage mediated by another agent. In 1947, Berenblum and Shubik developed a series of experiments that demonstrated the two-stage theory for skin cancer. The initiating agent was methylcholanthrene, and the promoting agent was croton oil. Over the years, the two-stage theory has evolved into the three-stage theory of carcinogenesis. This theory proposes that the process of transforming a normal cell into a cancer cell consists of three stages: initiation, promotion, and progression (Fig. 1-5).[5,7,9]

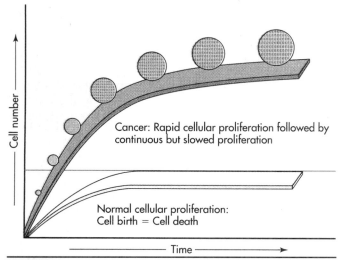

FIG. 1-3   Gompertzian function. (From Phipps WJ, Sands JK, Marek JF, editors: *Medical-surgical nursing: concepts and clinical practice*, ed 6, St Louis, 1999, Mosby.)

In the first stage, *initiation*, cells are exposed to an initiating agent or carcinogen that makes them susceptible to malignant transformation. An initiating agent is a chemical, biologic, or physical agent capable of producing irreversible changes in the DNA of a cell. Viral, environmental or lifestyle, and genetic factors have all been identified as initiators of carcinogenesis.[5,7-9]

In the second stage, *promotion*, promoting agents or cocarcinogens cause unregulated accelerated growth in previously initiated cells. Promotion is reversible if the promoting agents are removed during the early stages of carcinogenesis. Cells that have been irreversibly initiated may be promoted even after long latency periods ranging from 1 to 40 years. Examples of promoting agents include hormones, plant products, chemicals, and drugs. Many chemical carcinogens are called complete carcinogens because they can initiate and promote malignant transformation. Cigarette smoke is an example of a complete carcinogen. The effects of cocarcinogens may be inhibited by certain cancer-reversing or cancer-suppressing agents (e.g., vitamins, minerals, carotenoids, flavonoids) or certain host characteristics (e.g., immune function, age, hormonal factors) or both.[5,7,9]

In the final stage, *progression*, the tumor cells acquire malignant characteristics that include changes in growth rate, invasive potential, metastatic frequency, morphologic traits, and responsiveness to therapy. By the time a malignant tumor is clinically evident, differences among individual cells within the tumor are apparent, resulting in heterogeneity within a tumor. Cells within a tumor can be heterogeneous with respect to the ability to invade surrounding tissue, genetic composition, growth rate, metastatic potential, hormone receptors, and susceptibility to antineoplastic therapy. The degree of heterogeneity increases as the tumor increases in size.[3,7,9]

With an increased understanding of oncogenes and tumor suppressor genes, a solid foundation for the concept of multistep carcinogenesis has developed. Most human cancers that have been studied reveal multiple genetic alterations involving activation of several oncogenes and a loss of two or more tumor suppressor genes. It is believed that each of these alterations represents a vital step in the progression from a normal cell to a malignant tumor. A striking example of multistep carcinogenesis has been documented in colon cancer. APC gene mutations are the first step in the classical "adenoma-carcinoma" pathway for developing colorectal cancer, causing adenomatous polyp development. Additional mutations in other genes, such as K-*ras* and p53, cause the polyps to become abnormal and eventually malignant.[3]

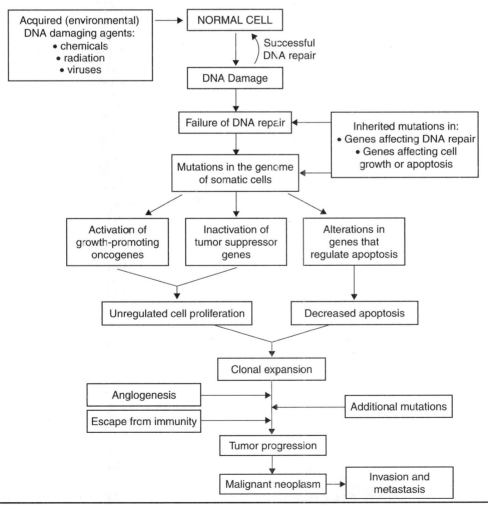

FIG. 1-4   The molecular basis of cancer. (From Kumar V, Fausto N, Abbas A, editors: *Robbins & Cotran pathologic basis of disease*, ed 7, Philadelphia, 2004, Saunders.)

TABLE 1-5	Selected Oncogenes, Their Mode of Activation, and Associated Human Tumors		
CATEGORY	**PROTO-ONCOGENES**	**MODE OF ACTIVATION**	**ASSOCIATED HUMAN TUMOR**
Growth Factors			
PDGF-β chain	*sis*	Overexpression	Astrocytoma
			Osteosarcoma
Fibroblast growth factors	*hst-1*	Overexpression	Stomach cancer
	int-2	Amplification	Bladder cancer
			Breast cancer
			Melanoma
TGF-α	TGF-α	Overexpression	Astrocytomas
			Hepatocellular carcinomas
HGF	HGF	Overexpression	Thyroid cancer
Growth Factor Receptors			
EGF-receptor family	*erb*-β1 (EGFR)	Overexpression	Squamous cell carcinomas of lung, gliomas
	erb-β2	Amplification	Breast and ovarian cancers
CSF-1 receptor	*fms*	Point mutation	Leukemia
Receptor for	RET	Point mutation	Multiple endocrine neoplasia 2A and 2B,
neurotrophic factors			familial medullary thyroid carcinomas
PDGF receptor	PDGF-R	Overexpression	Gliomas
Receptor for stem cell	*kit*	Point mutation	Gastrointestinal stromal tumors and other
(steel) factor			soft tissue tumors
Proteins Involved in Signal Transduction			
GTP-binding	K-*ras*	Point mutation	Colon, lung, and pancreatic tumors
	H-*ras*	Point mutation	Bladder and kidney tumors
	N-*ras*	Point mutation	Melanomas, hematologic malignancies
Nonreceptor tyrosine	*abl*	Translocation	Chronic myeloid leukemia
kinase			Acute lymphoblastic leukemia
Ras signal transduction	β-*raf*	Point mutation	Melanomas
Wnt signal transduction	β-catenin	Point mutation	Hepatoblastomas, hepatocellular carcinoma
		Overexpression	
Nuclear Regulatory Proteins			
Transcriptional activators	c-*myc*	Translocation	Burkitt's lymphoma
	n-*myc*	Amplification	Neuroblastoma, small cell carcinoma
	1-*myc*	Amplification	of lung
			Small cell carcinoma of lung
Cell-Cycle Regulators			
Cyclins	CYCLIN D	Translocation	Mantle cell lymphoma
		Amplification	Breast and esophageal cancers
	CYCLIN E	Overexpression	Breast cancer
Cyclin-dependent kinase	CDK4	Amplification or	Glioblastoma, melanoma, sarcoma
		point mutation	

CSF, Colony-stimulating factor; *ECFR*, epidermal growth factor receptor; *EGF*, epidermal growth factor; *GTP*, guanosine triphosphate; *HGF*, hepatocyte growth factor; *PDGF-R*, platelet-derived growth factor receptor; *TGF*, transforming growth factor.
From Kumar V, Fausto N, Abbas A, editors: *Robbins & Cotran pathologic basis of disease*, ed 7, Philadelphia, 2004, Saunders.

CARCINOGENIC FACTORS

It is becoming increasingly evident that cancer occurs because of interactions among multiple risk factors or repeated exposure to a single carcinogenic agent. Risk factors that have been linked to cancer are heredity; hormonal factors; environmental agents including chemicals, radiation, and cancer-causing viruses and bacteria; and the immune response.

Heredity. It is estimated that 5% to 10% of all cancers result from hereditary or genetic predisposition, and the frequency is even lower (around 0.1%) for certain types of tumors. Hereditary cancer

syndromes are characterized by the same or related cancer in multiple family members in multiple generations, an earlier age of onset than expected, unique tumor site combinations, bilateral cancers in paired organs, and the presence of rare cancers.[2,24]

Hormonal Factors. Hormones are important regulators of growth. By stimulating proliferation, hormones may increase the risk of mutation and at the same time stimulate the replication of the mutated cell. Thus hormones are complete carcinogens. For example, a direct carcinogenic effect of estrogen is known from the occurrence of vaginal and cervical clear cell carcinomas

TABLE 1-6	Selected Tumor Suppressor Genes Involved in Human Neoplasms			
SUBCELLULAR LOCATION	**GENE**	**FUNCTION**	**TUMORS ASSOCIATED WITH SOMATIC MUTATIONS**	**TUMORS ASSOCIATED WITH INHERITED MUTATIONS**
Cell surface	TGF-β receptor	Growth inhibition	Carcinomas of colon	Unknown
	E-cadherin	Cell adhesion	Carcinomas of stomach	Familial gastric cancer
Inner aspect of plasma membrane	NF-1	Inhibition of RAS signal induction and of p12 cell-cycle inhibitor	Neuroblastomas	Neurofibromatosis type 1 and sarcomas
Cytoskeleton	NF-2	Cytoskeletal stability	Schwannomas and meningiomas	Neurofibromatosis type 2, acoustic schwannomas and meningiomas
Cytosol	APC/β-catenin	Inhibition of signal transduction	Carcinomas of stomach, colon, pancreas; melanoma	Familial adenomatous polyposis colorectal/colon cancer
	PTEN	PI-3 kinase signal transduction	Endometrial and prostate cancers	Unknown
	SMAD2 and SMAD4	TGF-β signal transduction	Colon, pancreas tumors	Unknown
Nucleus	RB	Regulation of cell cycle	Retinoblastoma, osteosarcoma, carcinomas of breast, colon, lung	Retinoblastoma, osteosarcomas
	p53	Cell-cycle arrest and apoptosis in response to DNA damage	Most human cancers	Li-Fraumeni syndrome, multiple carcinomas and sarcomas
	WT-1	Nuclear transcription	Wilms tumor	Wilms tumor
	p16 (INK4a)	Regulation of cell cycle by inhibition of cyclin-dependent kinases	Pancreatic, breast, and esophageal cancers	Malignant melanoma
	BRCA1 and BRCA2	DNA repair	Unknown	Carcinomas of female breast and ovary; carcincomas of male breast
	KLF6	Transcription factor	Prostate	Unknown

From Kumar V, Fausto N, Abbas A, editors: *Robbins & Cotran pathologic basis of disease*, ed 7, Philadelphia, 2004. Saunders.

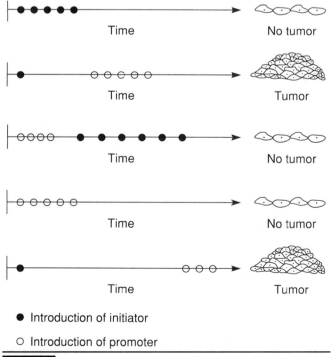

● Introduction of initiator

○ Introduction of promoter

FIG. 1-5 Interactions of initiation and promotion.

in girls born of mothers having been treated with diethylstilbesterol during pregnancy. In addition, the administration of estrogens to women is associated with an increased incidence of endometrial cancer. Cancers in hormone-responsive tissues—breast, endometrium, ovary, and prostate—are responsible for 35% of all newly diagnosed tumors in men and 40% of all newly diagnosed cancers in women in the United States.[6,25]

Environmental Agents. It is estimated that more than 75% of cancers occur as the result of environmental exposures.[25]

Chemicals. In 1775, an English physician named Percival Pott observed that the high incidence of cancer of the scrotum in chimney sweeps was due to their exposure to coal tars. A century later, scientists in Germany found a high incidence of bladder cancer among workers exposed to aromatic amines (chemicals used in the dyeing and pigment industry). Since then, more than 6 million chemicals have been identified and registered with the Chemical Abstracts Service; however, fewer than 1000 of these chemicals have been examined for their potential to cause cancer. Some have been found to cause cancer in animals, and others are known to cause cancer in humans. These agents include both natural products such as aflatoxin B_1 and artificial products such as vinyl chloride.[6,7,26] Box 1-1 provides examples of known chemicals that act as carcinogens.

BOX 1-1   Major Chemical Carcinogens

Direct-Acting Carcinogens

Alkylating Agents
β-Propiolactone
Dimethyl sulfate
Diepoxybutane
Anticancer drugs (cyclophosphamide, chlorambucil, nitrosoureas, and others)

Acylating Agents
1-Acetyl-imidazole
Dimethylcarbamyl chloride

Procarcinogens that Require Metabolic Activation

Polycyclic and Heterocyclic Aromatic Hydrocarbons
Benz(a)anthracene
Benzo(a)pyrene
Dibenz(a,h)anthracene
3-Methylcholanthrene
7,12-Dimethylbenz(a)anthracene

Aromatic Amines, Amides, Azo Dyes
2-Naphthylamine (β-naphthylamine)
Benzidine
2-Acetylaminofluorene
Dimethylaminoazobenzene (butter yellow)

Natural Plant and Microbial Products
Aflatoxin B_1
Griseofulvin
Cycasin
Safrole
Betel nuts

Others
Nitrosamine and amides
Vinyl chloride, nickel, chromium
Insecticides, fungicides
Polychlorinated biphenyls

From Kumar V, Fausto N, Abbas A, editors: *Robbins & Cotran Pathologic Basis of Disease*, ed 7, Philadelphia, 2004, Saunders.

Chemical carcinogens may be divided into two categories: direct-acting chemical carcinogens, which do not require activation to become carcinogenic, such as busulfan and nitrogen mustard; and procarcinogens or initiators, which become carcinogenic only after metabolic activation. Most chemical carcinogens are procarcinogens. Examples include soot, coal tar products, and cigarette smoke. The exposure to many chemical carcinogens is associated with lifestyle risk factors such as smoking, diet, and alcohol consumption.[6,7,27]

Radiation. Radiation was recognized as a carcinogen only 4 years after Roentgen's discovery of x-rays. Since then, the carcinogenic effects of radiation have been well documented including those on atomic bomb survivors, industrial workers, and miners. Radiation appears to initiate carcinogenesis by damaging susceptible DNA and thus producing changes in the DNA structure.

There are two forms of radiation that induce cancer: ultraviolet radiation and ionizing radiation.

Sources of ultraviolet radiation include the sun and certain industrial sources (e.g., welding arcs, germicidal lights). The risk of developing skin cancer from sunlight has been reported for more than 100 years. Ultraviolet radiation from the sun induces a change in DNA, and if the damaged DNA is not properly repaired, malignant transformation occurs resulting in basal and squamous cell carcinomas of the exposed areas of the skin. The risk of carcinogenesis by ultraviolet radiation is increased by prolonged exposure resulting from occupational or recreational activities, lighter skin pigmentation, greater intensity and duration of exposure, and proximity to the equator. The most dramatic example is in individuals with xeroderma pigmentosum, a hereditary disease in which DNA repair of ultraviolet radiation is damaged. These individuals are extremely sensitive to sunlight and have a high incidence of skin cancer, including melanoma.[5-7,27]

The majority of ionizing radiation exposure is from natural sources such as cosmic rays, radioactive ground minerals, and gases such as radon, radium, and uranium. Exposure can also occur from diagnostic and therapeutic sources, which include x-rays, radiation therapy, and radioisotopes used in diagnostic imaging. The period of time between radiation exposure and the appearance of a radiation-induced tumor is known as the latent period. The latent period for radiation-induced leukemias is generally shorter than for solid tumors. Factors that influence the latent period and the risk of carcinogenesis by ionizing radiation include the following:[7,27]

- *Host characteristics*—includes level of tissue oxygenation, genetic composition, and age
- *Cell-cycle phase*—cells in G_2 phase are more sensitive than cells in S or G_1 phase.
- *Degree of differentiation*—immature cells are the most vulnerable
- *Cellular proliferation rate*—cells with high mitotic rates are most vulnerable
- *Tissue type*—bone marrow, thyroid, breast, lung, and salivary glands are the most sensitive
- *Rate of dose and total dose*—the higher the dose rate and total dose, the greater the chance for mutation

Oncogenic Viruses. An oncogenic virus is one that can induce or cause cancer. Viruses are thought to contribute to human carcinogenesis by infecting the host DNA or RNA, resulting in proto-oncogenic changes and cell mutation. Age and immunocompetence are believed to interact with and affect a person's vulnerability to viral carcinogens. Five DNA viruses have been linked to cancer in humans:[4,28]

1. *Human papillomavirus (HPV)*—cervical carcinoma, anal carcinoma
2. *Epstein-Barr virus (EBV)*—Burkitt's lymphoma, B-cell lymphoma in immunosuppressed individuals, nasopharyngeal carcinoma
3. *Hepatitis B virus (HBV)*—hepatocellular carcinoma
4. *Hepatitis C virus (HCV)*—hepatocellular carcinoma
5. *Human herpesvirus-8 (HHV-8)*—Kaposi's sarcoma

Although there are a number of retroviruses (RNA viruses) that cause cancer in animals, human T-cell leukemia virus-1 (HTLV-1) is the only one directly linked to cancer in humans. HTLV-1 is associated with a form of T-cell leukemia. The human immunodeficiency virus (HIV) is an important cofactor in many human cancers because of its immunosuppressive effects.[4,29]

Bacteria and Parasites. Significant evidence exists linking gastric infection with the *Helicobacter pylori* bacteria to the development of gastric lymphoma and gastric carcinoma. Gastric lymphomas occur in mucosa-associated lymphoid tissue (MALT) and are sometimes called MALTomas. Chronic infection with *H. pylori* leads to proliferation of B cells and potential acquisition of genetic mutations. Tumor growth initially requires immune stimulation by *H. pylori*, but at later stages the bacteria is no longer required.[3,5] Infection with the *Schistosoma hematobium* parasite has been linked to bladder cancer and liver cancer. In addition, infestation with the *Opisthorchis viverrini* parasite has been found to cause hepatic cholangiocarcinoma.[4,25]

Immune System Deficiencies. Cancer cells express tumor-associated antigens that are not found on normal cells. When a developing tumor expresses a tumor-associated antigen, the immune system recognizes these antigens as foreign and destroys the cancer cells or immunologic surveillance. These cells are killed by cytotoxic T cells that have receptors for specific tumor antigens and natural killer (NK) lymphocytes, macrophages, and B lymphocytes, thus preventing the malignant cells from developing into clinically detectable tumors. In spite of the immune system's ability to identify and destroy cancer cells, some cancer cells are capable of bypassing surveillance, thus escaping and causing cancer.[30,31] Possible explanations for immunologic escape include the following:[5,11,30,31]

- *Tumor cell camouflage*—In the early phase of growth, the tumor antigens may be weak and thus do not promote an immune response until the cancer is too large for the immune system to destroy.
- *Antigenic modulation*—Cancer cells may change or lose antigens in response to recognition by the immune system.
- *Overwhelming antigen exposure*—Cancer cells may express an excess of tumor-associated antigens. The antigens bind to specific antibodies or to lymphocyte receptors.
- *Blocking agents*—Blocking antibodies may bind with tumor-associated antigens to prevent recognition by T cells, or free antigen produced by the cancer cell binds with T cells to prevent recognition of the cancer cell.

Routes of Tumor Spread

Tumor spread throughout the body can occur by direct extension or local invasion of adjacent organs, metastases by implantation or serosal seeding, and metastases to distant organs by the lymph or circulatory system. Factors affecting tumor spread include the rate of cell growth, the degree of differentiation, and the location. Local invasion is the first step in the metastatic process and may occur as a function of direct tumor extension. Mechanisms important in local invasion include tumor growth, mechanical pressure, tumor-secreted enzymes, decreased cellular adhesion, and increased motility.[32] Serosal seeding occurs when tumors, which have invaded a body cavity from surrounding tissue, attach to the surface of an organ within the cavity. Most often, the peritoneal cavity is involved; other spaces such as the pleural cavity, the pericardial cavity, or the joint spaces may be affected.[6]

The most common route for metastases is via the lymphatic system. Tumor cells entering the lymphatic vessels are carried to regional lymph nodes. Entrapment of the tumor cells may occur in the first lymph node encountered, or the cell may bypass the first node and spread to more distant sites, called skip metastasis.[12] For many types of cancer, the first indication of spread is a mass in the regional lymph nodes. For example, an enlarged axillary lymph node may signal breast cancer. A significant feature of the lymphatic system is that the main lymphatic trunk enters the venous system just before the veins enter the heart. Therefore the lymphatic and circulatory systems are interconnected, and cancer cells that enter the lymphatic system are also able to enter the bloodstream.[5]

In tumor spread via the circulatory system, the tumor cells usually follow the venous flow that drains the site of the neoplasm. Venous blood from the gastrointestinal tract, pancreas, and spleen is routed through the portal vein of the liver before entering the circulation. Therefore the liver is a common metastatic site for cancers that originate in these organs.[5,6] Other common sites of metastases in addition to the liver include the lung, bone, and the central nervous system.[12]

METASTASIS

Metastasis, derived from the Greek prefix *meta-*, or beyond, is the spread of cancer cells from a primary tumor to organs and distant sites in the body. A cancer cell's ability to invade adjacent tissues and metastasize to distant sites is its most virulent property and is a distinguishing characteristic of cancer. Approximately 60% of patients with invasive cancer have overt or occult metastases at diagnosis. The process of metastasis is a cascade of linked sequential steps.[2,3,32,33] All of these steps must be completed for a metastatic lesion to develop (see Fig. 1-6).

- *Growth and progression of the primary tumor.* The first requirement for metastasis is rapid growth of the primary tumor. Most tumors must reach 1 billion cells or 1 cm in size before metastasis is possible.[3,32,33]
- *Angiogenesis at the primary site.* Extensive vascularization, or angiogenesis, is necessary for the tumor to exceed 1 mm in diameter. The release of angiogenic factors by tumor cells is necessary to stimulate new capillary formation. The growth of the tumor and the rate of spread are correlated with tumor vascularity.[3,5,32-34]
- *Local invasion.* To reach blood vessels or the lymphatic system, tumor cells must break down the tissue stroma and the basement membrane. Several factors are involved in tumor cell invasion. First, rapid tumor growth creates a mechanical pressure that forces finger-like projections of cancer cells into adjacent tissue. Second, increased cell motility can contribute to tumor cell invasion. The lack of adhesion among tumor cells increases the ability of the cancer cells to escape and invade. Third, tumor cells secrete enzymes such as the matrix metalloproteinases that are capable of destroying the basement membrane.[3,32-34]
- *Detachment and embolization.* Millions of cells are shed into the circulation daily from locally invasive cancer, but fewer than 0.01% successfully survive to grow into a metastatic lesion.[32] Once in the circulation, tumor cells are vulnerable to destruction by the host immune cells. For protection, tumor cells aggregate with blood cells, primarily platelets, and form fibrin-platelet emboli. This protects the tumor cells and promotes metastasis by enhancing their ability to adhere to the capillary walls of the target organ.[34]

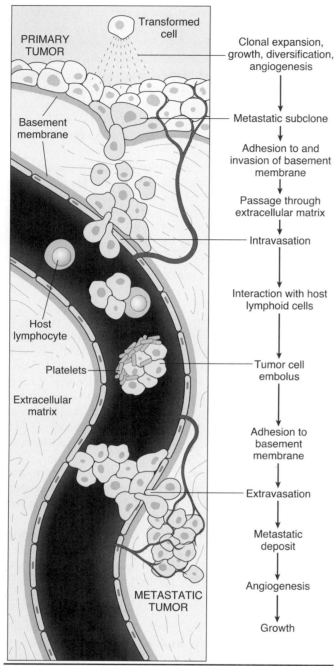

PRIMARY TUMOR

Transformed cell

Clonal expansion, growth, diversification, angiogenesis

Basement membrane

Metastatic subclone

Adhesion to and invasion of basement membrane

Passage through extracellular matrix

Intravasation

Host lymphocyte

Interaction with host lymphoid cells

Platelets

Tumor cell embolus

Extracellular matrix

Adhesion to basement membrane

Extravasation

Metastatic deposit

Angiogenesis

METASTATIC TUMOR

Growth

FIG. 1-6 The metastatic cascade. (From Kumar V, Fausto N, Abbas A, editors: *Robbins & Cotran pathologic basis of disease*, ed 7, Philadelphia, 2005, Saunders.)

- *Arrest in distant organ capillary beds.* In many types of cancers, the most frequent location of metastases is the first capillary bed or lymphatic tissue in an organ adjacent to the tumor site. This explains why lung and liver metastases are the first parenchymal metastases seen from most cancers. Others show preference for specific organs, known as organ tropism. For example, ocular melanoma frequently metastasizes to the liver, and prostate carcinoma often spreads to the bone. Factors that may influence certain tumors to metastasize to specific sites include patterns of blood flow or tumor-cell expression of specific surface molecules that prefer specific organs; organs may also attract circulating tumor cells through specific receptors or growth factors. These factors may be the outcome of "cross-talk" between cancer cells and normal cells, which results in cancer cells releasing cytokines that cause the normal cells to produce substances that recognize receptors on the cancer cells.[3,9,12,32-34]

- *Extravasation.* After the tumor cells have arrested or firmly attached themselves to the endothelial cells of a vessel, the tumor cells must penetrate or extravasate through the vessel wall to grow into the extravascular tissue. Arrested tumor cells use the same process to gain entrance through the endothelial basement membrane that was used to gain initial access to the vascular system. Once the endothelium is damaged, tumor cells escape through the vessel wall and invade the organ tissue.[3,10,34]

- *Proliferation.* Once tumor cells arrive in the extravascular tissue, a blood supply and nutrients must be acquired for continued growth. The new environment may differ considerably from the original site. In general, more poorly differentiated cancer cells are better able to adapt to foreign tissues and survive.[3,10,34]

Conclusion

The essential features of the cancer cell that distinguish it from the normal cell are its ability to reproduce uncontrollably, resist growth-inhibitory signals, develop necessary vasculature, invade normal tissue, spread to distant body sites, and destroy the host. These factors constitute the essence of the transformed cell. It is now understood that the transformation occurs as a result of multiple genetic mutations occurring over years.

The oncology nurse involved in the care of patients with cancer needs a strong foundation in the pathophysiology and the genetics of cancer. Nurses will be on the forefront of teaching individuals about health promotion, prevention, and risk reduction; educating patients about the new treatment modalities; assisting them with managing the diverse side effects; and providing follow-up.

REVIEW QUESTIONS

✓ Case Study

Your patient, Mrs. W., a 65-year-old white woman, is admitted with complaints of back pain that has responded to chiropractic treatment or analgesics. During evaluation, lesions on her thoracic spine were identified as suspicious for metastatic disease. In pursuing a primary site of origin, a mass in her lung is discovered on the x-ray film. A biopsy was performed and revealed a poorly differentiated adenocarcinoma of the lung. Mrs. W. has never smoked in her life. She did, however, work as a waitress in various diners during the 1960s and 1970s, and her husband has smoked two packs of cigarettes per day for 40 years (80 pack-years). Mrs. W. does not have a family history of lung cancer. While being cared for, Mrs. W. asks, "Why has this happened to me? I never smoked a day in my life!" Discuss how you would respond to her question and statement.

DISCUSSION

Exposure to secondhand smoke is a known risk factor for the development of cancer. Evidence has primarily come from comparing lung cancer rates (mostly in women) in nonsmokers married to smokers to rates of nonsmokers married to nonsmokers. Tobacco smoke contains more than 40 carcinogenic chemicals, many of which can initiate the carcinogenic process by causing mutations in genes such as p53.[25]

Cells that have been initiated may be promoted even after long latency periods, ranging from 1 to 40 years. Cigarette smoke is a complete carcinogen—it can initiate and promote malignant transformation. In reference to your patient, her continued exposure to secondhand smoke at work and at home likely contributed to her cancer.

QUESTIONS

1. In teaching a class of graduates nurses who will care for Mrs. W. you emphasize that an adenocarcinoma arises from which of the following?
   a. Bone
   b. Glandular epithelium
   c. Smooth muscle
   d. Cartilage
2. In a review of Mrs. W's chart, the pathology reports dysplasia. What does this refer to?
   a. An increase in cell size
   b. An increase in the number of cells
   c. Abnormal changes in cell size, shape, and organization
   d. Replacement of one cell type for another cell type
3. In explaining to the family the probable cause of Mrs. W.'s back pain, which difference between malignant and benign tumors is most relevant?
   a. The ability to produce pain
   b. The ability to cause death
   c. The ability to metastasize
   d. The ability to impair function
4. In preparing a pathophysiology lecture, you specify at which time during the cell cycle the cell verifies accurate DNA replication:
   a. The S phase
   b. The restriction point
   c. The M phase
   d. The G_2-M transition
5. When Mrs. W.'s family inquires as to how long ago her current cancer may have begun, you try to explain tumor growth fraction. What is this?
   a. The ratio of the total number of cells in a tumor to the number of dividing cells
   b. The time needed for a tumor mass to double its volume
   c. The minimum clinically detectable burden of tumor
   d. Cell numbers increasing in powers of two
6. How are proto-oncogenes best described?
   a. Genes that inhibit cell growth
   b. Genes that regulate normal cell growth and repair
   c. Genes that control the rate of mutation
   d. Genes that promote cell death
7. Which of the following is among the most common sites of metastasis?
   a. Kidney
   b. Liver
   c. Breast
   d. Spleen
8. In order for metastasis to occur, a sequence of steps must occur. What is the initial step?
   a. Development of new blood vessels
   b. Local invasion
   c. Formation of fibrin-platelet emboli
   d. Rapid growth of the primary tumor
9. During a community education program on cancer risk reduction, the nurse teaches that the risk of cancer from smoking can be reversed if a person stops smoking. This information is based on what understanding of carcinogenesis?
   a. The initiation stage
   b. The promotion stage
   c. The progression stage
   d. The transformation stage
10. JW, a 45-year-old nephew of Mrs. W., is admitted and examined as potentially having hepatocellular carcinoma. While obtaining a personal health history, what would staff ask about?
   a. Gastric infection with *H. pylori*
   b. Hepatitis B virus (HBV)
   c. Human papillomavirus (HPV)
   d. Epstein-Barr virus (EBV)

ANSWERS

1. **B.** *Rationale:* A tumor arising from glandular epithelium is an adenocarcinoma. Tumors arising from bone, smooth muscle, or cartilage are identified as sarcomas. A tumor from the bone is an osteosarcoma, a tumor from smooth muscle is a leiomyosarcoma, and a tumor from cartilage is a chrondosarcoma.
2. **C.** *Rationale:* Dysplasia is characterized by abnormal changes in the size, shape, or organization of cells. An increase in cell size is hypertrophy. An increase in the number of cells is hyperplasia, and metaplasia is the replacement of one cell type for another cell type.
3. **C.** *Rationale:* The ability to metastasize is a hallmark characteristic of malignant tumors since benign tumors do not spread. Both benign and malignant tumors can produce pain, cause death, and impair function if their location or size interferes with vital structures.
4. **D.** *Rationale:* During the G_2-M transition, the cell verifies accurate DNA replication and determines if mitosis can safely progress. DNA replication occurs in the S phase, the cell checks for DNA damage at the restriction point (G_1-S transition), and cell division occurs in the M phase.
5. **A.** *Rationale:* The time needed for a tumor mass to double its volume is the doubling time of a tumor. Doubling occurs in powers of two or exponential growth. The minimum clinically detectable burden of tumor is 30 doublings or more than 1 billion cells.
6. **B.** *Rationale:* Proto-oncogenes are normal genes that regulate normal cell growth and repair. Functions of tumor suppressor genes include inhibiting cell growth, controlling the rate of mutation, and promoting cell death.

Continued

REVIEW QUESTIONS—CONT'D

7. **B.** *Rationale:* The most common sites of metastasis are the liver, the lung, bone, and the central nervous system.

8. **D.** *Rationale:* The first requirement for metastasis is the rapid growth of the primary tumor. Subsequent steps include angiogenesis (development of new blood vessels), local invasion, and detachment and tumor-cell embolization.

9. **B.** *Rationale:* During the initiation stage, changes to the DNA of a cell are irreversible. However, promotion is reversible if the promoting agent, such as cigarette smoke, is removed

during the early stages of carcinogenesis. Progression is the acquisition of malignant characteristics by the tumor cells. Transformation of a normal cell to a malignant cell is the process proposed by the theory of carcinogensis.

10. **B.** *Rationale:* The hepatitis B virus is associated with hepatocellular carcinoma. Infection with *H. pylori* is associated with gastric lymphomas, human papillomavirus is linked to cervical and anal carcinoma, and the Epstein-Barr virus is associated with Burkitt's lymphoma.

REFERENCES

1. Holland JF: Cardinal manifestations of cancer. In Kufe DW, Pollock RE, Weichselbaum RR et al, editors: *Holland-Frei cancer medicine 6*, Hamilton Ontario, 2003, BC Decker.

2. Kinzler KW, Vogelstein B: Introduction. In Vogelstein B, Kinzler KW, editors: *The genetic basis of human cancer*, ed 2, New York, 2002, McGraw-Hill.

3. Kumar V, Fausto N, Abbas A, editors: *Robbins & Cotran pathologic basis of disease*, ed 7, Philadelphia, 2004, Saunders.

4. Damjanov I: *Pathology for the health-related professions*, ed 2, Philadelphia, 2000, Saunders.

5. McCance KL, Roberts LK: Biology of cancer. In McCance KL, Huether SE, editors: *Pathophysiology: the biologic basis for disease in adults and children*, ed 14, St. Louis, 2002, Mosby.

6. Twite K: Neoplasia. In Porth CM, editor: *Pathophysiology: concepts of altered health states*, Philadelphia, 2005, Lippincott Williams & Wilkins.

7. Caudell KA: Alterations in cell differentiation: neoplasia. In Porth CM, Kunert MP, editors: *Pathophysiology: concepts of altered health states*, ed 6, Philadelphia, 2002, Lippincott Williams & Wilkins.

8. Pitot HC. *Fundamentals of oncology*, ed 4, New York, 2002, Marcel Dekker.

9. Banasik JL: Neoplasia. In Copstead LC, Banasik JL, editors: *Pathophysiology*, St. Louis, 2003, Elsevier.

10. Merkle CJ, Loescher LJ: The cancer problem. In Yarbro CH, Goodman M, Hansen Frogge M, editors: *Cancer nursing: principles and practice*, ed 6, Sudbury, MA, 2005, Jones and Bartlett.

11. Meier P: Perspectives in oncology. In Black JM, Hawks JH, Keene A, editors: *Medical-surgical nursing: clinical management for positive outcomes*, ed 6, Philadelphia, 2001, Saunders.

12. Volker DL: Biology of cancer and carcinogenesis. In Itano JK, Taoka KN, editors: *core curriculum for oncology nursing*, ed 4, St. Louis, 2005, Saunders.

13. Clurman BE, Roberts JM: Cell cycle control: an overview, In Vogelstein B, Kinzler KW, editors: *The genetic basis of human cancer*, ed 2, New York, 2002, McGraw-Hill.

14. Reed SI: Cell cycle. In Devita VT, Devita VT Jr, Hellman S et al, editors: In *Cancer: principles and practice of oncology*, ed 7, Philadelphia, 2004, Lippincott Williams & Wilkins.

15. Temple SV, Poniatowski BC: Nursing implications of antineoplastic therapy. In Itano JK, Taoka KN, editors: *Core curriculum for oncology nursing*, ed 4, St. Louis, 2005, Saunders.

16. Rieger PT: The biology of cancer genetics, *Semin Oncol Nurs* 20(3): 145-154, 2004.

17. Fidler IJ, Langley RR, Kerbel RS et al: Angiogenesis. In Devita VT, Devita VT Jr, Hellman S et al, editors: *Cancer: principles and practice of oncology*, ed 7, Philadelphia, 2004, Lippincott Williams & Wilkins.

18. Hahn WC, Weinberg RA: Rules for making human tumor cells, *N Engl J Med* 347:1593-1603, 2003.

19. Hanahan D, Weinberg RA: The hallmarks of cancer. *Cell* 100(1):7, 57-70, 2000.

20. Kinzler KW, Vogelstein B: Familial cancer syndromes: the role of caretakers and gatekeepers. In Vogelstein B, Kinzler KW, editors: *The genetic basis of human cancer*, ed 2, New York, 2002, McGraw-Hill.

21. Rudin CM, Thompson CB: Apoptosis and cancer. In Vogelstein B, Kinzler KW, editors: *The genetic basis of human cancer*, ed 2, New York, 2002, McGraw-Hill.

22. Hahn WC: Role of telomeres and telomerase in the pathogenesis of human cancer, *J Clin Oncol* 21:2034-2043, 2003.

23. Nowell P: The clonal evolution of tumor cell populations, *Science* 194:23-28, 1976.

24. Tranin AS, Masny A, Jenkins J, editors. *Genetics in oncology practice: cancer risk assessment*, Pittsburgh, 2003, Oncology Nursing Society.

25. Heath CW, Fontham ETH: Cancer Etiology. In Lenhard RE, Osteen RT, Gansler T, editors: *Clinical oncology*, Atlanta, 2001, American Cancer Society.

26. Yuspa SH, Shields PG: Etiology of cancer: Chemical factors. In Devita VT, Devita VT Jr, Hellman S et al, editors: *Cancer: principles and practice of oncology*, ed 7, Philadelphia, 2004, Lippincott Williams & Wilkins.

27. Ullrich RL: Etiology of cancer: Physical factors. In Devita VT, Devita VT Jr, Hellman S et al, editors: *Cancer: principles and practice of oncology*, ed 7, Philadelphia, 2004, Lippincott Williams & Wilkins.

28. Howley PM, Ganem D, Kieff E: DNA Viruses. In Devita VT, Devita VT Jr, Hellman S et al, editors: *Cancer: principles and practice of oncology*, ed 7, Philadelphia, 2004, Lippincott Williams & Wilkins.

29. Buchschacher GL, Wong-Staal F: RNA Viruses. In Devita VT, Devita VT Jr, Hellman S et al, editors: *Cancer: principles and practice of oncology*, ed 7, Philadelphia, 2004, Lippincott Williams & Wilkins.

30. Bender CM, Yasko JM, Strohl RA: Nursing management: Cancer. In *Medical-surgical nursing: assessment and management of clinical problems*, ed 5, St. Louis, 2000, Mosby.

31. Pardoll DM: Immunology and cancer. In Abelhoff M, Armitage J, Niederhuber J et al, editors: *Clinical oncology*, ed 3, Philadelphia, 2004, Churchill Livingston.

32. Liotta LA, Kohn EC: Invasion and metastases. In Kufe DW et al, editors: *Holland-Frei cancer medicine 6*, Hamilton, Ontario, 2003, BC Decker.

33. Stetler-Stevenson WG: Invasion and metastases. In Devita VT, Devita VT Jr, Hellman S et al, editors: *Cancer: principles and practice of oncology*, ed 7, Philadelphia, 2004, Lippincott Williams & Wilkins.

34. Fidler IJ: Biology of cancer metastasis. In Abelhoff M, Armitage J, Niederhuber J et al, editors: *Clinical oncology*, ed 3, Philadelphia, 2004, Churchill Livingston.

CHAPTER 2

Genetics

Julie Ponto

Overview of Genetics

The field of cancer genetics has grown tremendously in the past several years, significantly influencing what is known and understood about cancer development. These discoveries about genetics and cancer have important implications for cancer prevention, screening, and treatment. A basic understanding of human genetics is necessary in order to understand the relationship between genetics and cancer.

Chromosomes are the inherited material that determines human characteristics. Chromosomes consist of DNA, the double-stranded helix made known by Watson and Crick. Chromosomes are found within the nucleus of every cell. Humans have 46 chromosomes, which form 23 chromosome pairs. One chromosome of each pair is inherited from each parent at the time of conception.[1] Twenty-two of the chromosome pairs are called autosomes and exist in both males and females.[1] The twenty-third chromosome pair are the sex chromosomes, which determine a person's gender: males have an X chromosome and a Y chromosome, and females have two X chromosomes.[1]

Chromosomes are separated into two arms by the centromere; the long arm of each chromosome is known as the q arm, and the shorter arm is the p arm. The number of the chromosome and the long or short arm are used to identify areas of the chromosome for purposes of locating genes along the chromosome.[1] For example, *chromosome 22q* indicates the long arm of chromosome 22.

Chromosomes consist of long, tightly wound strands of DNA, which house the genes (Fig. 2-1). Each chromosome contains hundreds to thousands of genes, which are the instructional units of the DNA.[1] Genes contain the instructional code for making specific proteins. The genes that generate instructions for the production of protein are called coding genes, or exons. In addition, chromosomes contain noncoding genes, called introns, whose function is not well understood.

The genes are composed of chemical bases whose order and pairing determine which protein is coded by the gene. Four chemical bases exist in human genes; adenine, thymine, cytosine, and guanine. Adenine and thymine pair together, as do cytosine and guanine; these couplets are called base pairs. The order of these base pairs determines which amino acids are produced, which in turn combine to form various proteins. These four chemical bases result in the stepwise production of the hundreds of different proteins that the body uses.

Variations and alterations may occur in the base pair sequencing, which can lead to significant or insignificant coding changes. Alterations in the genetic sequence are called *mutations*. Mutations may occur during DNA synthesis or replication, and may be inherited or induced by external influences from a person's environment (e.g., cigarette smoke).

Under normal circumstances, cells have the capability to correct these mistakes or to program cell death (a process known as apoptosis) in the event that the errors cannot be corrected. Some mutations have no significant effect on protein function. Disease-associated mutations do alter protein function and can result in genetic instability, unregulated cell growth, and tumorigenesis.

There are numerous types of mutation. The most frequent mutation is the misspelling of a single DNA base. This *missense mutation* occurs when the wrong base is substituted. A *nonsense mutation* occurs when a base pair is completely lost. A *frameshift mutation* can result when one base is lost (frameshift deletion) or added (frameshift insertion), shifting the reading of subsequent bases. This causes a change in amino acid coding and thus, a change in the protein formed. Mutations may be inherited or acquired. Inherited, or *"germline," mutations* occur in germ cells (ova and sperm). The mutation is then passed on to offspring in all the body cells. Disease resulting from germline mutations accounts for a small percentage of all cancer occurrence.

Acquired or *somatic mutations* are not inherited but occur sometime after birth. An alteration in DNA occurs as a result of chance or exposure to cancer-causing agents. The mutations are found in the tumor cells of the affected organ, not in all body cells as is seen with germline mutations. Most cancers are thought to occur in this manner. A single exposure or genetic change is usually not sufficient to cause a cancer to occur. Rather, multiple changes and multiple exposures over many years result in the development of cancer.

Knudsen's *two-hit hypothesis* describes a model for carcinogenesis in which two genetic events occur, resulting in the loss of both copies of a tumor suppressor gene. Without this "off switch," unregulated cell growth leads to cancer. For example, in the individual who has inherited a mutated copy of a tumor suppressor gene (the first "hit"), there is only one functional copy remaining. This individual is at greater risk of developing a cancer than someone without an inherited mutation. Only one additional genetic event or somatic mutation (the second hit) is needed to eliminate the remaining functional copy of the tumor suppressor gene and result in tumorigenesis.

Mutations are inherited in a dominant or recessive pattern. With *autosomal dominant inheritance*, only one parent is needed to donate a copy of a mutated gene for a disease to be expressed. The disease is seen in males and females, over several generations (a vertical pattern of inheritance), and is usually considered highly penetrant (the frequency of disease occurrence), meaning the risk of developing cancer is high. There is a 50% chance that each offspring of a mutation carrier will inherit a copy of the mutated gene.

Autosomal recessive inheritance occurs when two mutated genes are necessary for disease. Both parents would have to carry

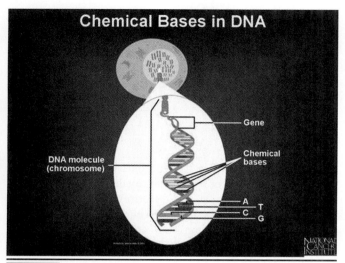

FIG. 2-1 Structure of a chromosome. (Courtesy of the National Cancer Institute.)

the same gene mutation and both pass the mutation on to an offspring. As carriers, the parents do not actually have the disease. Their offspring have a 50% chance of inheriting a single copy of the mutated gene and thus becoming a carrier, a 25% chance of inheriting a copy of the mutated gene from each parent and expressing the disease, and a 25% chance of not inheriting a mutated gene copy from either parent, thus neither becoming a carrier nor expressing the disease. Often several members of the same generation are affected (horizontal pattern of inheritance), and both genders can be affected.

X-linked inheritance is caused by genetic mutations on the X chromosome. The mutations are passed through the mother and can be either dominant or recessive. With X-linked dominant inheritance, both genders have a 50% chance of inheriting a copy of the mutated gene and expressing the disease and a 50% chance of inheriting neither the mutation nor the disease. With X-linked recessive inheritance, there is a 50% chance of a woman passing a mutation to a son (who would express the disease) or a daughter (who would be a carrier) and a 50% chance of passing a normal copy of the gene to her offspring.

Genetics and Cancer Development

Cancer develops as a result of mutations in DNA, therefore all cancer is genetic. However, not all cancer is caused by inherited genetic mutations. Most cancer develops as a result of acquired mutations, which alter the genes that control cell growth. Under normal conditions, cell growth is regulated by a balance between growth-promoting genes and growth-suppressing genes. However, mutations in these genes result in unregulated cell growth, and cancer. Most likely, multiple genetic mutations are necessary to result in the unregulated cell growth that becomes a malignancy.

The normal, growth-promoting genes are called proto-oncogenes. Mutated proto-oncogenes are called oncogenes and are responsible for unregulated cell growth and the development of cancer. Oncogenes act like the accelerator of a car in that they accelerate or speed up the cellular growth process. Oncogenes have been associated with the development of leukemias, lymphomas, and various solid tumors.[2]

Cellular growth is also regulated by growth-suppressing genes called tumor suppressor genes. These genes act to slow down the cellular growth process. When mutated, tumor suppressor genes no longer slow down or stop the cell growth process that allows cells to grow in an uncontrolled fashion and develop into a malignancy. One of the most common tumor suppressor genes, p53, has been associated with the development of up to 50% of all cancers.

The human body is able to repair gene defects through mismatch repair genes. However, when mismatch repair genes are mutated, the ability to repair defects is lost. The cancer syndrome hereditary nonpolyposis colorectal cancer (HNPCC) occurs as a result of a mutation in mismatch repair genes and results in the development of a constellation of cancers including colorectal, endometrial, and ovarian cancer.

Normally, cells that are old and perhaps defective may also be eliminated through apoptosis, or programmed cell death. This is the body's way of eliminating defective cells that may lead to the development of cancer. Mutations in apoptosis genes prevent this normal culling from occurring, allowing old and damaged cells to continue living and reproducing and thus allowing the development of a malignancy.

The Human Genome Project

The Human Genome Project (HGP) was an international, collaborative project in which the entire human genome was mapped and sequenced. Although many discoveries laid the foundation for the HGP, the project began in earnest as a coordinated effort in 1990 with the publication of the initial 5-year research plan. By 2001, 90% of the project was complete and published.[3] In April 2003, the completion of the full sequencing was announced. The human genome was found to have almost 3 billion base pairs, and 30,000 to 35,000 human genes, surprisingly fewer than anticipated.[4] Although the location of these 30,000 to 35,000 genes is known, their function and structure have yet to be determined.[4]

Sequencing the HGP represented a significant step forward in our understanding of genetic components of human disease and illness; however, much more work is still needed. Scientists are now applying the information from the HGP in a variety of ways to better understand the role of genes in health and illness. Dr. Frances Collins, director of the National Human Genome Research Institute, identified the next steps necessary in human genome research, including characterizing the protein-coding sequences, determining the structural and functional components of the human genome, exploring the role of genome variations, and further elucidating the role of human genetics in diseases such as cancer.[5]

Sporadic versus Familial versus Inherited Risk

The lifetime risk of developing cancer is approximately 1 in 2 for men and 1 in 3 for women.[6] This risk of cancer in the general population is not attributable to any known factors and is therefore called the *sporadic risk* of developing cancer. No matter what our inherited or environmental risks, every individual possesses a risk of cancer because of the sporadic incidence of cancer in the population.

Some families have a higher than sporadic incidence of cancer in the family, but it is a pattern of cancer that does not appear to fit any known inherited cancer syndromes. This type of cancer risk is termed a *familial risk* or a *familial cancer syndrome.* Families share multiple cancer risk factors such as secondary smoke inhalation and shared environmental or dietary factors that may account for the higher than sporadic risk of cancer in the family. In addition, some familial cancer syndromes may be due to as yet unidentified inherited factors.

A risk for cancer is considered *inherited* or *potentially inherited* when the family has a pattern of cancer that is consistent with known inherited cancer syndromes, such as breast-ovarian syndrome or HNPCC. Less than 10% of all cancers occur because of an inherited susceptibility. Cancers due to an inherited susceptibility typically occur at a younger age than expected for that type of cancer, bilaterally in paired organs, and in a larger number of family members than would be expected as a result of sporadic risk.

Cancer Risk Assessment

A family suspected of having an inherited susceptibility to cancer requires a cancer risk assessment in which their cancer risk is thoroughly evaluated. Many cancer risk assessment programs exist; a list of such programs can be found at *http://www.cancer.gov/search/geneticsservices.* An interdisciplinary team of health care providers may be involved in the cancer risk assessment process, sharing responsibility for a comprehensive risk assessment.

The individual undergoing evaluation through a cancer risk assessment program is called the **proband.** This individual could be already diagnosed with cancer or could be a person without cancer but concerned about his or her cancer risk because of a high incidence of cancer in the family.

A thorough medical and family history is necessary for a cancer risk assessment. A family history assessment begins with the construction of a pedigree or family tree (Figs. 2-2 and 2-3). The pedigree can assist in determining the number and percentage of family members affected, the likelihood of an inherited syndrome, and the pattern of inheritance.[1] Ideally, information is collected on a minimum of three generations. The pedigree includes the identification of the proband's first-, second-, and third-degree relatives from both the maternal and paternal sides of the family. First-degree relatives include siblings, children, and parents. Second-degree relatives include grandparents, aunts and uncles, and nieces and nephews on both the maternal and paternal sides of the family. Third-degree relatives include maternal and paternal great-grandparents, great-aunts and great-uncles, and cousins. Health information is collected on all relatives including their date of birth, date and cause of death (if applicable), and whether or not each individual has had cancer. If a relative has had cancer, additional information is collected such as the type of cancer, age at diagnosis, and known cancer risk factors (e.g., tobacco use or asbestos exposure). Interventions undertaken to reduce the risk of cancer, such as cancer prevention surgeries and chemoprevention strategies, should also be collected on all relatives.

Records on family members who are suspected of having had a cancer diagnosis are obtained so that cancer diagnoses can be confirmed. Sometimes a relative was presumed to have had a particular cancer, when in fact he or she did not, or their cancer was in situ as opposed to invasive disease. Ideally, diagnoses are verified by pathology reports, but death certificates or hospital records may be informative.

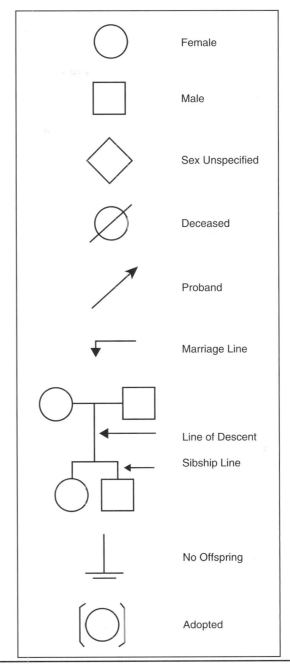

FIG. 2-2   Common pedigree symbols. (Courtesy of the National Cancer Institute.)

Maternal and paternal ethnicity of the family is collected because of the higher prevalence of cancer-causing mutations in some ethnic groups (e.g., Ashkenazi Jewish families). This information may direct genetic testing toward those mutations. The proband is asked if any family member has undergone genetic testing for cancer and, if so, the results of that testing.

Once a comprehensive family history has been obtained, the personal medical history of the proband is obtained. Cancer risk factor information is collected, for instance, chemical exposures and behaviors that increase cancer risk, such as smoking and alcohol consumption. In addition, past cancer screening activities, including mammography, colonoscopy, and others, are determined and records are obtained to verify screening results. History of

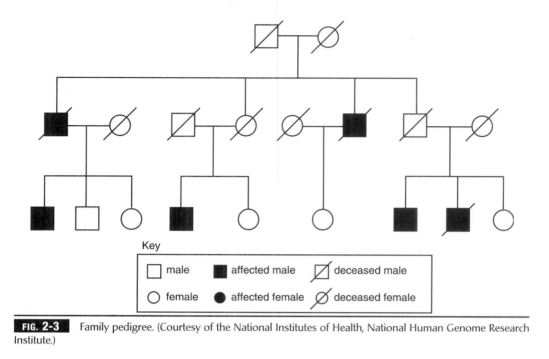

FIG. 2-3 Family pedigree. (Courtesy of the National Institutes of Health, National Human Genome Research Institute.)

cancer, precancerous lesions, and/or biopsies is obtained. Pathology records are obtained to verify all positive history.

A physical examination that focuses on signs, symptoms, or indications of cancer is performed. Any cancer screening examinations that are due, such as a Pap smear or prostate examination, can be performed at this time. Medical history and past physical examination information can be combined with family history information to provide a comprehensive cancer risk evaluation.

Cancer Genetic Counseling

Genetic counseling is a critical component of a cancer genetic evaluation process. Genetic counseling is comprehensive in its approach to provide education, health promotion, informed consent, and support to individuals and families facing the uncertainty of hereditary cancer and cancer syndromes.

The education component of genetic counseling is accomplished using a variety of teaching methods, including one-on-one discussions, videotapes, and educational booklets and articles. Whatever method is used, it is imperative that there is ample opportunity for questions to be answered. Genetic information is complex and technical in nature. Basic principles of medical genetics, patterns of heredity, and risk calculations are presented in a clear and concise manner. Basic information about cancer epidemiology, carcinogenesis, disease presentation, diagnosis, and treatment is also provided. All information is tailored to the specific cancer risks of the individual and family. The education component lays the foundation for decision making regarding genetic testing, surveillance, and treatment options.

Genetic counseling is the term used to describe the process of psychosocial assessment, anxiety reduction, grief counseling, and decision making about genetic testing.[2] Information about benefits, risks, and limitations of testing are discussed in detail. It is crucial to the process that the counselor understands the person's perception of risk and cancer development. The person's

fears, experiences with family members with cancer, and individual coping abilities shape the ability to process the information and make an informed decision. Having family members present for the education and counseling can assist in supporting the person's decisions. However, it is important to be sure that the person is truly making his or her own decisions and not being coerced by the family. This can be challenging, because testing an individual has implications for the entire family. The counselor discusses with the proband whether or not he or she plans to inform the family members of the test results and how to deal with potential reactions. Genetic counseling is an ongoing process provided before and after genetic testing is offered, whether or not the person chooses to undergo genetic testing. Providing genetic counseling has been associated with a decreased level of cancer anxiety.[7]

In October 2004, the Oncology Nursing Society revised and approved its position statement on the role of the oncology nurse in cancer genetic counseling (Fig. 2-4). This position identifies the growing importance of genetics in cancer care and the significant role oncology nurses have in providing comprehensive cancer genetic counseling.

Cancer Genetic Testing

Genetic testing is offered to persons who are likely to carry a mutation in a cancer-susceptibility gene for which a test exists to identify the mutation. The results of testing must be interpretable and must affect medical management.[8] Genetic testing is not a screening method for people with the general population risk of developing cancer.

Testing is done through DNA analysis of a blood specimen. Although several methods of testing or gene mutations exist, DNA sequencing is the gold standard and is the most sensitive method for identifying mutations. It looks at every nucleotide base pair on both copies of the gene being tested to determine whether mutations exist.

The Role of the Oncology Nurse in Cancer Genetic Counseling

The identification of genes that, when altered (mutated), are associated with cancer development is transforming the understanding of and approach to the detection and management of cancer. Genetic information is being used to understand the biology of disease, characterize malignancies, develop new therapeutic modalities, and identify individuals at increased risk of developing cancer. As genetic technology evolves and knowledge of cancer genetics expands, healthcare providers must respond by informing patients, families, and the public about the implications of these developments for cancer prevention and risk reduction, early detection, and treatment. Ultimately, the genetic revolution will have an impact on the entire specialty of oncology nursing. Oncology nurses in all settings will be expected to supply patients, families, and the public with information about genetics related to cancer prevention, risk management, and early detection along with providing resources, education, psychosocial support, and counseling or referrals related to hereditary cancers. Additionally, a percentage of advanced practice nurses with specialized training will be involved in the clinical application of cancer genetics, including counseling and education regarding cancer predisposition genetic testing. Oncology nurses with appropriate education and experience are ideal for providing comprehensive care in the area of cancer genetics and for meeting the needs of the increased number of individuals requiring cancer genetic risk counseling.

It Is the Position of ONS That

- The rapid integration of advances in cancer genetics will require increased numbers of individuals to be educated in genetics and cancer care.
- Cancer genetics information must be integrated into relevant curriculum content and taught at all levels of nursing education. Oncology nurses at both the general and advanced practice levels must have educational preparation in the principles of human genetics and in the critical evaluation of ethical, legal, and social implications of the use of genetic technology in cancer care.
- Oncology nursing practice related to cancer genetics includes three levels of practice—the general oncology nurse, the advanced practice oncology nurse, and the advanced practice oncology nurse with specialty training in cancer genetics. Nurses providing comprehensive cancer genetic risk counseling must be advanced practice oncology nurses with specialized education in hereditary cancer genetics.
- Continuing education and specialized educational programs must be developed and provided to practicing oncology nurses.
- Partnering with healthcare providers and specialty organizations with a focus in genetics is essential for providing comprehensive care to high-risk individuals.
- Comprehensive cancer genetic risk counseling includes cancer risk assessment and education, facilitation of genetic testing, pre- and post-test counseling and follow-up, provision of personally tailored cancer risk management options and recommendations, and psychosocial counseling and support services. Practice must be consistent with guidelines defined by an individual's state nurse practice act, the nurse's educational preparation, the scope of the nurse's role, and standards of oncology nursing practice.

Bibliography

Calzone, K.A., Jenkins, J., & Masny, A. (2002). Core competencies in cancer genetics for advanced practice oncology nurses. *Oncology Nursing Forum, 29,* 1327–1333.

Calzone, K.A., & Masny, A. (2004). Genetics and oncology nursing. *Seminars in Oncology Nursing, 20,* 178–185.

Calzone, K.A., & Tranin, A.S. (2003). The scope of cancer genetics nursing practice. In A.S. Tranin, A. Masny, & J. Jenkins (Eds.), *Genetics in oncology practice: Cancer risk assessment* (pp. 13–22). Pittsburgh, PA: Oncology Nursing Society.

International Society of Nurses in Genetics, Inc. (1998). *Statement on the scope and standards of genetics clinical nursing practice.* Washington, DC: American Nurses Publishing.

Approved by the ONS Board of Directors, 8/97; revised 8/00, 7/02, 10/04.

To obtain copies of this or any ONS position, contact the Customer Service Center at the ONS National Office at 125 Enterprise Drive, Pittsburgh, PA 15275-1214 (866-257-4ONS; customer.service@ons.org). Positions also may be downloaded from the ONS Web site (www.ons.org).

FIG. 2-4 ONS Position Statement. (From Oncology Nursing Society Position: The role of the oncology nurse in cancer genetic counseling. *Oncol Nurs Forum* 27(9):1348, 2000.)

Informed consent is a mandatory component of genetic testing. There are a number of ramifications to genetic testing, and it is imperative that a person be made aware of the issues before undergoing it. In addition to the psychosocial issues already addressed, a detailed discussion regarding the benefits, risks, and limitations of testing must be provided. The potential benefits to testing include the following:

- Identifying persons with mutations in cancer susceptibility genes so they may take advantage of more intensive screening programs and prevention options
- Identifying persons who do not carry mutations so that they are not put through unnecessary intensive surveillance and surgeries
- Relieving uncertainty
- Determining a more accurate risk status of individuals and family members[9]

The potential risks of genetic testing include the following:

- *Severe psychologic reactions.* People who learn they carry a mutation in a cancer-susceptibility gene may experience anger, fear, guilt, and depression. Persons who learn they do not carry a mutation may experience "survivor guilt," particularly if they are the only member of their family who is not a mutation carrier.
- *Interpreting a negative test result as having no risk of developing cancer.* People may use this as a rationale not to undergo regular population screening recommendations.
- *Workplace or insurance discrimination.* However, as a result of the 1997 enactment of the Health Insurance Portability Accountability Act, group health plans cannot consider genetic information a preexisting condition.
- *Family disruptions.* Not all family members want to know test results. In some instances, test results could confirm that the person is not biologically related to other "family" members. The knowledge of having a mutation in a cancer-susceptibility gene could deter a person from having children or even getting married.[2]

The limitations of genetic testing include the following:

- *Accuracy of the test.* A mutation may be present but technology may not exist to identify it. Therefore, the test is negative for known mutations, but inconclusive for unknown mutations. Testing can reveal the presence of a variant in a gene, the significance of which is unknown at this time.
- *Applicability of the information obtained.* A negative test result is only informative if a mutation has been identified in the family and it is not found in the person tested. This is why an affected family member is the ideal candidate to be tested first.
- *Availability of medical management strategies.* There are no effective screening or cancer prevention measures for many cancers, so why do testing if there is no proven screening or prevention available? In most instances, a positive test result only indicates a *probability* of developing cancer; it does not indicate a *certainty.*

Informed consent must also include a discussion regarding the cost of testing, how the test is to be performed, and who in the family is the most appropriate member to test first. The cost of testing varies. Some insurance plans pay for testing, others pay a portion of the cost, and some pay nothing at all. Some people wish to self-pay for testing to avoid alerting their insurance company to their mutation status, for fear of discrimination.

In determining the most appropriate person in the family to test first, generally it is most informative to test a family member who has cancer and is most likely to carry a mutation, if a mutation exists in the family (i.e., diagnosed at a young age, has had more than one primary cancer). If a mutation is identified in a person with cancer, the likelihood that the mutation caused the cancer is greater. Then, subsequent family members can be tested for the specific mutation, and testing is most informative.

In October 2004, the Oncology Nursing Society revised and approved its position on cancer predisposition genetic testing and risk assessment (Fig. 2-5). It outlines the necessary ethical, legal, and social components to genetic testing and risk assessment counseling.

Inherited Genetic Syndromes

HEREDITARY BREAST AND OVARIAN CANCER (HBOC)

Approximately 5% to 10% of all breast and ovarian cancer is thought to be due to mutations in the *BRCA1* or *BRCA2* genes. *BRCA1* and *BRCA2* are most likely tumor suppressor genes, but may also have a role in DNA repair. When mutated, *BRCA1* and *BRCA2* result in unregulated and abnormal cell growth and malignancies primarily of the breast and ovary. Other cancers have been associated with *BRCA1* and *BRCA2*.[10] Indications of the presence of *BRCA1* or *BRCA2* in a family include the early onset of breast cancer (before menopause), ovarian cancer, bilateral breast cancer, male breast cancer, breast and ovarian cancer in the same person, Ashkenazi Jewish ethnicity, and a known *BRCA1* or *BRCA2* mutation in the family.[11]

BRCA1 was identified in 1990 and found to be a large gene located on chromosome 17, specifically 17q12-21.[12] Hundreds of different mutations have been identified in *BRCA1* and linked to cancer susceptibility. *BRCA1* may be responsible for as much as 90% of hereditary breast and ovarian cancer.[10] Persons carrying a *BRCA1* mutation have up to a 85% lifetime risk of developing breast cancer, compared to a 12% risk in the general population, and a 40% lifetime risk of developing ovarian cancer, compared to a 1% to 2% risk in the general population. *BRCA1* may also raise a carrier's risk of developing prostate cancer.

Founder mutations are mutations seen with high frequency in a population founded by a small ancestral group, where one or more of the founders were carriers of the mutation. Two *BRCA1* founder mutations were identified in the Ashkenazi Jewish population, 185delAG and 5382insC mutations. These two founder mutations, along with a third on *BRCA2*, occur in approximately 1 of 40 women of Ashkenazi Jewish decent. Additional founder mutations have been identified in the Netherlands, Sweden, and Iceland.

The *BRCA2* gene was isolated in 1995 and localized to the long arm of chromosome 13 (13q). Hundreds of different *BRCA2* mutations have been identified on this very large gene. As with *BRCA1*, *BRCA2* is a tumor suppressor gene and is inherited in an autosomal dominant fashion. *BRCA2* mutations are responsible for about 35% of all inherited breast cancers. The lifetime risk of developing breast cancer in a woman with a *BRCA2* mutation is 50% to 85%. However, the lifetime risk of developing ovarian cancer is 10% to 20%, somewhat lower than with *BRCA1* mutations. *BRCA2* mutations are associated with male breast

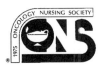

Cancer Predisposition Genetic Testing and Risk Assessment Counseling

The ability to identify individuals who are at increased risk for developing cancer because of an inherited altered (mutated) cancer predisposition gene is possible through cancer predisposition genetic testing. However, while providing the capability to target high-risk individuals who might benefit from specific strategies for medical management, genetic testing also raises ethical, legal, and social issues associated with revealing a person's genetic makeup.

It Is the Position of ONS That

- Risk assessment counseling and cancer predisposition genetic testing are components of comprehensive cancer care and should be available despite the cost to the healthcare system.
- All healthcare providers offering these services to patients and family members must have educational preparation in both human genetic principles and oncology.
- Cancer predisposition genetic testing requires informed consent and must include pre- and post-test counseling and follow-up by qualified individuals (e.g., advanced practice oncology nurses, oncologists with specialized education in hereditary cancer genetics, certified genetic counselors with specialized training in oncology).
- Ethical principles of beneficence, nonmaleficence, respect for autonomy, and justice must form the foundation for counseling services, guide the development of standards of care in cancer genetic counseling, and be included in criteria used to identify potential problems arising from cancer predisposition genetic testing and the counseling process.
- Comprehensive cancer genetic counseling must occur in a manner consistent with individual cultural and healthcare beliefs.
- Efforts must be made to include family members in the counseling process and to seek ways to address barriers to genetic testing and risk assessment in diverse populations.
- Legislation that provides protection from genetic

discrimination in both employment and insurance arenas and reimbursement for and access to genetic counseling, cancer predisposition genetic testing services, and appropriate medical management must be implemented and monitored.
- Ongoing educational resources for healthcare providers, individuals at increased risk, and the lay public must be developed, evaluated, and disseminated.
- A research plan related to all aspects of cancer genetics, including the efficacy of programs for prevention and early detection, the psychological impact of cancer predisposition genetic testing, and long-term outcomes of testing and risk management strategies, must be developed and evaluated.
- Efforts to improve the standardization and regulation of laboratories that provide cancer predisposition genetic testing must be evaluated and monitored.

Bibliography

Lowrey, K.M. (2004). Legal and ethical issues in cancer genetics nursing. *Seminars in Oncology Nursing, 20,* 203–208.

Mahon, S.M. (1998). Cancer risk assessment: Conceptual considerations for clinical practice. *Oncology Nursing Forum, 25,* 1535–1547.

Tranin, A.S., Masny, A., & Jenkins, J. (Eds.). (2003). *Genetics in oncology practice: Cancer risk assessment.* Pittsburgh, PA: Oncology Nursing Society.

Approved by the ONS Board of Directors, 8/97; revised 8/00, 7/02, 10/04.

To obtain copies of this or any ONS position, contact the Customer Service Center at the ONS National Office at 125 Enterprise Drive, Pittsburgh, PA 15275-1214 (866-257-4ONS; customer.service@ons.org). Positions also may be downloaded from the ONS Web site (www.ons.org).

FIG. 2-5 ONS Position Statement. (From Oncology Nursing Society Position: Cancer predisposition genetic testing and risk assessment counseling, *Oncol Nurs Forum* 27(9):1349, 2000.)

cancer, prostate, pancreatic, and stomach cancers, and melanoma.[10]

There are two known *BRCA2* founder mutations, 6174delT and 999del5. The first of these mutations was identified in 8% of Ashkenazi Jewish women diagnosed with breast cancer before age 42 and in 1.5% of all Ashkenazi Jews. The 999del5 founder mutation appears to be responsible for more than 50% of all inherited breast and ovarian cancer in Iceland.

Risk Prediction Models for Hereditary Breast and Ovarian Cancers. Several models are available to assess the breast and ovarian cancer risk among individuals based on their family and personal histories. These models are used to predict the risk of developing breast and ovarian cancer and the risk of having a mutation in a breast cancer susceptibility gene. The most commonly used models include the Gail model, the Claus model, and the Couch and the Frank tables. A statistical program, BRCAPRO, is another option for determining breast and ovarian cancer risk.

Gail Model. The Gail model is based on data from the Breast Cancer Detection and Demonstration Project (BCDDP) and was used in the National Surgical Adjuvant Breast and Bowel Project (NSABP) Breast Cancer Prevention Trials (BCPT) and Study of Tamoxifen and Raloxifene (STAR) to estimate breast cancer risk.[13] This model is available online at *http://brca. nic.nih.gov*. The calculation of risk is based on several personal and family history factors including current age, age at menarche, age at first live birth, number of maternal first-degree relatives with breast cancer, race, number of breast biopsies, and whether atypical hyperplasia was present in any biopsy specimen. The Gail model calculates the 5-year and lifetime risks of developing breast cancer. According to the Gail model, a 45-year-old nulliparous white woman who had menarche at age 11 and two breast biopsies, with a mother and sister with breast cancer, would have an 8.8% risk of developing breast cancer within the next 5 years and a 47.8% chance of developing breast cancer in her lifetime.

The Gail model is limited in its ability to estimate risk in hereditary breast cancer and most often underestimates risk. Because of the autosomal dominant pattern of inheritance of hereditary breast cancers, both the maternal and paternal family history must be considered when calculating risk. The Gail model calculates risk based on maternal family history only. In addition, it does not factor in the age at diagnosis, a significant factor in hereditary breast and ovarian cancers. Also, only first-degree relatives with breast cancer are included in the Gail model, leaving significant second-degree relatives with breast cancer out of the calculation.

Moreover, the Gail model does not account for male breast cancers or ovarian cancers in the family history. Using our previous example, if the same woman had a paternal grandmother and a paternal aunt with breast cancer instead of a mother and sister with breast cancer, the Gail model would calculate her 5-year risk as 2.9%, with a 19% lifetime risk. This would clearly underestimate her risk of hereditary breast and ovarian cancers by not incorporating the risk she has on the paternal side of her family.

Claus Model. The Claus model was developed based on data from the CASH (Cancer and Steroid Hormone) Study evaluating 4730 breast cancer patients, aged 20 to 54, and 4688 age-matched controls.[14] This model calculates the predicted cumulative probability of developing breast cancer using the current age and the age at onset of various first- and second-degree relatives with either breast or ovarian cancer. The model predicts that although most individuals with breast cancer are not mutation carriers, the likelihood of having a mutation increases by the number of relatives with the disease, especially when these relatives were diagnosed at an early age. The Claus model considers both maternal and paternal family history.[14] Using the Claus model, our earlier example of the 45-year-old woman with the mother (diagnosed at age 39) and sister (diagnosed at age 27) with breast cancer, her lifetime risk of developing breast cancer is 46%. With the paternal grandmother and aunt diagnosed at the same ages (39 and 27), her lifetime risk of breast cancer is 26%.

Although the Claus model has greater applicability with inherited breast and ovarian cancers than the Gail model, it too has limitations. It is more likely to underestimate the risk of developing breast cancer among individuals with gene mutations, whereas it overestimates the risk in those who do not have mutations in cancer-susceptibility genes. Also, because this model was developed before the knowledge that Ashkenazi Jewish heritage significantly increased the risk of hereditary breast cancer, this population's risk would be underestimated using the Claus model.

Couch Tables. The Couch tables were developed from a study of women with breast cancer and a strong family history of breast cancer, who were evaluated both in breast cancer clinics for high-risk women and in general practice clinics.[15] The 263 women were tested for *BRCA1* mutations, and the resultant tables predict the probability of detecting a *BRCA1* mutation in families with breast and ovarian cancer. These tables are useful in families that have multiple members with breast and ovarian cancer. The Couch tables consider the average age at diagnosis of breast cancer among all affected relatives, and both breast and ovarian cancer, as well as breast and ovarian cancer in a single family member. There are separate tables for persons of Ashkenazi Jewish heritage. To continue with our example of the 45-year-old woman, according to the Couch tables, her probability of having a *BRCA1* mutation with either maternal or paternal affected relatives is 17.4% (the average age of diagnosis is 33) if she is not Ashkenazi Jewish, and 48% if she is Ashkenazi Jewish.

Limitations of the Couch tables include small sample size, lack of ethnic diversity in the sample and, because the average age of diagnosis is used, it may underestimate risk in families with sporadic cases of breast cancer (over age 60) among inherited cases. In this same example, if the woman also had a grandmother with breast cancer diagnosed at 80, the average age at diagnosis in her family would be 49 and her probability would fall to 5% if she is not Ashkenazi Jewish, and 19% if she is Ashkenazi Jewish. If the grandmother's breast cancer was sporadic, the woman's probability of mutation is clearly underestimated.

Frank Table. The Frank table was developed from a study of 238 women with early onset of either breast cancer or ovarian cancer (at any age), with at least one first- or second-degree relative with either breast or ovarian cancer.[16] It predicts the probability of carrying a *BRCA1* or *BRCA2* mutation. This table accounts for early age of onset and the presence of both breast and ovarian cancer in the family. Bilateral breast or ovarian cancer is also a factor in the risk analysis, as is male breast cancer. Using the Frank table, the 45-year-old woman's probability of having a *BRCA1* or *BRCA2* mutation is 20% (her mother and sister have a 40% probability of mutation in either *BRCA1* or *BRCA2*). The limitations include the small sample size and the lack of ethnic diversity among study participants.

BRCAPRO. A computerized risk calculation model, BRCAPRO, is the most comprehensive risk calculation model currently available.[17] BRCAPRO is a statistical model that provides an estimate of *BRCA1* and *BRCA2* mutation carrier status. The model takes into consideration breast and ovarian cancer, current age or age at death of affected family members, unaffected family members, male breast cancer, Ashkenazi Jewish ancestry, and *BRCA1 and BRCA2* mutation status. BRCAPRO has been validated in a clinical population.[18] Drawbacks of BRCAPRO include the following: the task of entering family data is time consuming, data are limited to first- and second-degree relatives, and the applicability to moderate risk families is unknown.

Persons undergoing cancer risk assessment and genetic counseling, who have a greater than 10% calculated probability of having a mutation in *BRCA1* or *BRCA2*, would be considered eligible for genetic testing. Even when eligible for testing, the decision to have genetic testing ultimately lies with the individual.

Genetic Testing for *BRCA1* and *BRCA2* Mutations. *BRCA1* and *BRCA2* mutation testing has been commercially available since 1996. Results are usually available in 3 to 4 weeks. Insurance plans may pay all or part of the cost of testing. Genetic testing may also be available to eligible individuals in the research setting. There is usually no cost for research testing; however, results may not be available for years, if ever. The purpose of research testing is less for clinical management than it is for furthering knowledge about mutations and mutation carriers in families.

Complete gene sequencing is most commonly undertaken. An affected member of the family is tested first, preferably the most likely candidate for having a mutation (e.g. youngest age of onset, bilateral breast cancer or both breast and ovarian cancer). If a mutation is identified, testing of other family members can be limited to the previously identified mutation. This is much less labor intensive and, consequently, less costly than complete gene sequencing.

Persons of Ashkenazi Jewish heritage may undergo direct testing of the three common Ashkenazi mutations (185delAG, 5582insC, and 6174delT) as an alternative to full gene sequencing. If one of these three mutations is not identified, complete sequencing of *BRCA1* and *BRCA2* may then be carried out, if the person so chooses.

Genetic testing is recommended only when the results will affect the medical management of the patient. A negative test result in a family with a known *BRCA1* or *BRCA2* mutation is considered confirmatory. This person would not be at high risk for breast or ovarian cancer and would not require heightened surveillance or other strategies used to manage high-risk individuals. It is very important to remember that a negative test result does not completely eliminate the risk of breast or ovarian cancer. Rather, the individual has the population risk for these diseases due to sporadic cancers and would still need to undergo age-appropriate screening according to American Cancer Society guidelines. A positive result in a family with a known mutation would identify that individual as someone in need of heightened surveillance. A negative test result in a family with no known *BRCA1* or *BRCA2* mutation is not informative, because there could be an undetected mutation in *BRCA1* or *BRCA2*, or they may have a mutation in another cancer-susceptibility gene.

Financial expense is not the only "cost" of *BRCA1* or *BRCA2* testing. The psychologic costs must be considered. In families in which all but one sibling is found to carry a mutation, the survivor guilt experienced by some noncarriers can be as difficult to handle as the news of being positive for the mutation. It can be devastating for a parent to learn that he or she passed a mutation to a child, especially if the child (as an adult) develops breast or ovarian cancer and the parent does not. *For these reasons as well as others, it is critical that people receive genetic counseling before having genetic testing.* The psychologic risks and benefits of genetic testing are thoroughly discussed with individuals and families as part of the genetic counseling process.[2]

Clinical Management of the *BRCA* Mutation–Positive Patient. Individuals who have a mutation in *BRCA1* or *BRCA2*, or individuals who have not been tested but are from a family in which a mutation in *BRCA1* or *BRCA2* has been identified, are provided a number of options for management. These options include chemoprevention, prophylactic surgery, and close surveillance.

Chemoprevention of breast cancer became an option after results of the BCPT demonstrated a 49% reduction in incidence of invasive breast cancers among high-risk women with the use of tamoxifen.[19] It is likely that some mutation carriers were among the high-risk women in the trial. A subanalysis of *BRCA1* and/or *BRCA2* mutation carriers in the BCPT showed tamoxifen to be equally efficacious in mutation carriers.[20] However, these data must be interpreted cautiously, given the relatively few mutation carriers in the study sample. STAR, a second study comparing the breast cancer–reducing effects of tamoxifen and raloxifene, is underway. It was recently closed to accrual, and results should be forthcoming.

Chemoprevention in ovarian cancer is limited to the use of oral contraceptives (OCP). Although OCP use reduces the risk of ovarian cancer in the general population, studies in women with *BRCA1* and/or *BRCA2* mutations are less conclusive. Several small case-control studies have shown a reduction in ovarian cancer risk (up to 60%) whereas one large population-based study did not.[21-23] OCPs may be a favorable option for women with *BRCA1* mutations who are not interested in a surgical approach to risk reduction. However, there may also be an increased risk of breast cancer among this subset of women.[24] More research is needed in this area to effectively answer the questions about chemoprevention of both breast and ovarian cancers.

Prophylactic surgical procedures, including mastectomy and oophorectomy, significantly reduce the incidence of breast and ovarian cancers, respectively. Studies have shown a reduction of breast cancer risk of up to 90% in women undergoing prophylactic mastectomy, and these results appear to apply to *BRCA1* and/or *BRCA2* mutation carriers also.[25-28] Results are limited by the retrospective study design and/or the relatively short time of follow-up. Even though some breast tissue remains after prophylactic mastectomy, this procedure is a reasonable option for women at high risk, such as mutation carriers.

Select studies have shown a reduction in ovarian cancer risk following prophylactic oophorectomy.[29-30] These studies are also limited by a retrospective design or small sample size. Additional studies are ongoing to help clarify the role of prophylactic oophorectomy; in the meantime, prophylactic oophorectomy may be a reasonable option for mutation carriers who have completed childbearing.

Increased surveillance is an option for *BRCA1* and/or *BRCA2* mutation carriers as an alternative to chemoprevention or prophylactic surgeries. Frequent surveillance may also be initiated during the time a mutation carrier is deciding on other prevention strategies. The Cancer Genetics Studies Consortium recommends monthly breast self-exam beginning in young adulthood, annual or semiannual clinical breast examination beginning at ages 25 to 35, and annual mammography beginning at ages 25 to 35.[31] Other screening techniques, such as magnetic resonance imaging and whole breast ultrasound, are being evaluated for efficacy in *BRCA1* and/or *BRCA2* mutation carriers. Current recommendations regarding screening for ovarian cancer include annual or semiannual CA-125 and transvaginal ultrasound.[31]

BREAST CANCER ONLY

Some families exhibit an inherited cancer syndrome consisting of breast cancer exclusively. *BRCA1* may be responsible for up to 45% of these hereditary breast cancer–only families, and *BRCA2* mutations may be responsible for up to 35% of breast cancer families. Careful genetic assessment of these families is particularly important to determine whether a small family size or other issues may be accounting for the lack of other cancers. Mutation testing can be informative in these families and guide cancer screening recommendations.

OVARIAN CANCER ONLY

Similar to breast cancer–only families, some families with a known or presumed inherited syndrome exhibit ovarian cancer only. These families likely have a *BRCA1* mutation or a mutation as yet unidentified. Certain gene mutations have been associated with a higher incidence of ovarian cancer, but further research in this area is necessary to determine appropriate screening and management approaches.

HEREDITARY COLORECTAL CANCER SYNDROMES

Hereditary colorectal cancers are the result of germline mutations in specific cancer-susceptibility genes. They are responsible for approximately 5% to 6% of all colorectal cancers.[32,33] There are a number of well-characterized inherited predisposition syndromes to colorectal cancer, most commonly HNPCC and familial adenomatous polyposis (FAP). A person with a mutation in the mismatch repair genes that lead to HNPCC has an 80% lifetime risk of developing colorectal cancer.[34] In FAP, the lifetime risk approaches 100%.[32,35] When compared to the population risk of 5%, the hereditary colorectal cancer syndromes confer a significantly increased risk of colorectal cancer.[6]

Hereditary Nonpolyposis Colorectal Cancer (HNPCC). HNPCC, or Lynch syndrome, is one of the most common of the hereditary colorectal cancer syndromes. It accounts for approximately 5% of all colorectal cancers, or about 7200 cases annually.[36] Lynch syndrome was described in the 1960s, before the discovery of the genetic mutations responsible for its manifestation. In 1993, the first mismatch repair gene, *MSH2*, was associated with HNPCC and localized on the short arm of chromosome 2. Four additional genetic mutations in mismatch repair genes are associated with HNPCC: these include *MLH1* (located on chromosome 3), *MSH6* (on chromosome 2), *PMS1* (also found on chromosome 2), and *PMS2* (located on chromosome 7).[32,34,35,37] They are transmitted via an autosomal dominant pattern of inheritance and confer a risk of developing colorectal cancer of about 80%.

Approximately 90% of all HNPCC cases are due to *MSH2* and *MLH1* gene mutations.[35]

Mismatch repair genes are responsible for making corrections in the nucleotide sequences. Mutations in mismatch repair genes allow mistakes to propagate, resulting in genetic instability at repeat sequences (*microsatellites*) within the gene. This is known as *microsatellite instability* (MSI) and leads to an accumulation of additional mutations, unregulated cell growth and, eventually, cancer. High-frequency microsatellite instability has been found in 95% of HNPCC cases and in approximately 15% of sporadic cases of colorectal cancer.[32]

Clinical features of HNPCC include early age of onset, with the average age at diagnosis of 44 to 45 years.[33,35] Affected persons have few polyps and only one or two adenomas.[34] In HNPCC cases, the progression from adenoma to carcinoma is accelerated over that of sporadic cancers.[35] At least 70% of the cancers involve the right colon, proximal to the splenic flexure.[34] The presence of synchronous and metachronous colorectal cancers is not uncommon. A number of extracolonic cancers are associated with HNPCC, leading some to consider the term HNPCC a misnomer.[36] Extracolonic cancers associated with HNPCC include endometrial, ovarian, urinary tract, stomach, small bowel, and bile duct cancers.[33,35,36] Therefore, one mutation can put a person at risk for six cancers. These occur more frequently in HNPCC families than within the general population. Endometrial cancer is the most common extracolonic cancer among HNPCC mutation carriers, with a lifetime risk of 40% to 60%, whereas the lifetime risk of the other extracolonic cancers in HNPCC is less than 15%.[35,38]

In 1991, the International Collaborative Group on HNPCC published the Amsterdam Criteria for identifying HNPCC families. The criteria include that there are three or more relatives with colorectal cancer, one case being a first-degree relative of the others. The cancers must occur within two or more generations and have one diagnosis by the age of 50. In addition, FAP should be excluded as a cause of the colorectal cancer cases. The Amsterdam criteria were modified to include the extracolonic cancers so often seen in HNPCC families.[39] Further modifications in the diagnostic criteria for HNPCC have corresponded to developments in the field; the most recent revisions, published in 2004, are known as the Revised Bethesda Criteria.[40] (Box 2-1).

Genetic Testing for HNPCC. The ideal genetic testing approach for HNPCC has yet to be established. One approach to testing individuals who meet the Revised Bethesda Criteria is to conduct MSI or immunohistochemistry (IHC) analysis on tumor tissue with germline mutation testing on individuals with deficits.[40] If a mutation is detected with germline testing, family members may then be tested for that mutation. If a family member tests negative for that mutation, he or she can resume population screening, since the general population risk of developing colorectal cancer would still be present. In a situation where a deficit has been detected by MSI or IHC but no germline mutation is found, the results are considered noninformative, and the proband and family members should be counseled as though a mutation had been found.[40]

As an alternative to tumor tissue screening, people may receive germline mutation testing directly. Full gene sequencing is currently available for *MSH2*, *MLH1*, and *MSH6* genes.[40]

Issues complicating genetic testing using MSI or IHC screening are that (1) *MSH6* mutations are often MSI/IHC negative,

Revised Bethesda Guidelines for HNPCC

1. Colorectal cancer diagnosed in a patient who is less than 50 years of age.
2. Presence of synchronous, metachronous colorectal, or other HNPCC-associated tumors, regardless of age.
3. Colorectal cancer with the MSI-H (microsatellite instability–high) histology diagnosed in a patient who is less than 60 years of age.
4. Colorectal cancer diagnosed in one or more first-degree relatives with an HNPCC-related tumor, with one of the cancers being diagnosed under age 50 years.
5. Colorectal cancer diagnosed in two or more first- or second-degree relatives with HNPCC-related tumors, regardless of age.

HNPCC, Hereditary nonpolyposis colorectal cancer.
Adapted from Umar A, Boland CR, Terdiman JP et al: Revised Bethesda Guidelines for hereditary nonpolyposis colorectal cancer (Lynch syndrome) and microsatellite instability, *J Natl Cancer Inst* 96:261-268, 2004.

(2) some individuals with germline mutations have negative MSI and/or IHC screening, and (3) tumor tissue isn't always available for testing.[37,41] More research is necessary to determine the ideal method of testing families with a suspected predisposition for HNPCC.

Clinical Management of HNPCC. Persons with a known HNPCC mutation or who are suspected to carry such a mutation are at significantly increased risk of developing colorectal and other cancers. These individuals require close and careful follow-up to increase the likelihood of finding a cancer early. Current screening guidelines recommend that these high-risk individuals begin colorectal cancer screening between ages 20 and 25.[32,35] Colonoscopy is the necessary screening examination, given the increased occurrence of cancer in the right colon.[33,35] Colonoscopy should be performed more frequently than in the general population because of the increased speed of carcinogenesis in HNPCC; therefore colonoscopy is recommended every 1 to 2 years until age 40, and annually thereafter.[35,42,43]

Because of the increased incidence, endometrial cancer screening is also recommended. Annual transvaginal ultrasound and/or endometrial aspiration has been recommended beginning between ages 25 and 35.[32,35,43] Screening for ovarian and urinary cancers remains controversial; suggested screening strategies include transvaginal ultrasound and CA-125 annually, beginning at age 30, and urinalysis for renal tumors.[32,35] Individual counseling regarding the potential risks, benefits, and controversies associated with screening extracolonic malignancies is warranted.

The efficacy of prophylactic surgeries in persons with HNPCC has not been established. Prophylactic surgery for colorectal, endometrial, and ovarian cancers may be discussed as options with patients on an individual basis.[35,43]

Familial Adenomatous Polyposis (FAP). FAP is a hereditary colorectal cancer syndrome that is responsible for up to 1% of all colorectal cancers.[32,36] The lifetime risk of developing colorectal cancer in FAP families is greater than 95% (compared to the population risk of about 5% to 6%).[44] FAP results from germline mutations in the adenomatous polyposis coli (*APC*) gene located at 5q21. The *APC* gene functions as a tumor suppressor and requires both alleles to be mutated before function is lost.

In most FAP families, there appear to be separate, distinct mutations of the *APC* gene. There are over 300 known *APC* gene mutations, most leading to truncation of the APC protein.[45] Nonsense and frameshift mutations are the most common types of mutations seen in FAP. *APC* gene mutations are also seen in 30% of persons with no family history of colorectal cancer. This is known as a *de novo mutation* and arises in the sperm or ovum of an unaffected person. It is then passed on to their offspring who, with no family history of colorectal cancer, develop FAP and colorectal cancer.

A founder mutation in the *APC* gene has been identified in persons of Ashkenazi Jewish heritage.[46] The mutation, I1307K, is a missense mutation that, unlike other FAP mutations that truncate the APC protein, instead causes the creation of an unstable DNA sequence. This leads to the development of somatic mutations that result in familial colorectal cancer.[32] The I1307K mutation has been associated with a twofold risk of colorectal cancer among Ashkenazi Jews; however, one recent study found no increased cancer risk.[47]

A number of clinical features are associated with FAP, none more impressive than the hundreds to thousands of adenomatous polyps found in the colon of affected persons, usually at a very young age. The diagnosis of FAP is made on the basis of having at least 100 adenomatous polyps throughout the colon. These polyps can be found in children as young as 10 years of age.

Another clinical feature associated with FAP is congenital hypertrophy of the retinal pigment epithelium (CHRPE). These pigmented lesions are visible on funduscopic examination of the retina. CHRPE is a benign finding and was used as a marker for FAP before genetic testing was available. Individuals with mutations in the *APC* gene are also at risk for extracolonic tumors such as upper gastrointestinal, brain, and thyroid carcinomas, desmoid tumors, osteomas, hepatoblastomas, and hepatopancreatic tumors.[33]

There is a variant of FAP, Gardner's syndrome, in which a person exhibits the same clinical features common to persons with FAP along with additional distinct features, including epidermal cysts, osteomas, desmoid tumors, and jaw cysts.

Attenuated FAP is another variation of FAP. This syndrome is characterized by a smaller number of adenomas throughout the colon, usually fewer than 100. Attenuated FAP occurs later in life, usually over the age of 50, but is still associated with a high risk of colorectal cancer, as well as a higher risk of upper gastrointestinal polyps and cancers. Persons with attenuated FAP rarely exhibit CHRPE. Mutations associated with attenuated FAP are found on the same *APC* gene, but appear to be located at either end of the gene.

Genetic Testing for FAP. Genetic testing for *APC* gene mutations is commercially available and is indicated in persons who have known polyposis or the presence of over 100 adenomatous polyps throughout the colon. There need not be a family history of colorectal cancer because of the incidence of de novo mutations in FAP. Testing is also indicated for relatives of known *APC* gene mutation carriers, as well as persons suspected of having attenuated FAP.

There are a number of benefits to testing for FAP. First, identification of individuals with a mutation before the development of colorectal cancer can improve morbidity and mortality from colorectal cancer. These individuals would be screened more diligently than the general population. Secondly, by identifying individuals in the family who are not mutation carriers, heightened surveillance is made unnecessary.

The psychologic impact of genetic testing and prophylactic surgery are important considerations in FAP, given its very early onset. With FAP, there is almost certainty regarding the development of cancer, particularly at a young age. Adolescents and young adults are going through developmental stages in which body image is important. Reluctance to undergo colonoscopic surveillance because of embarrassment and fear is not uncommon. Also, the fear of undergoing colectomy and possibly colostomy is very real to these individuals. Despite these concerns, adolescents experienced no greater anxiety following genetic test results than adults.[48] This area of research warrants further attention.

Unfortunately, there remain certain limitations to testing for FAP. Testing unaffected persons with no prior knowledge of an identified mutation in the family could result in uninformative results. For persons suspected of having attenuated FAP, mutations on the extreme ends of the gene can go undetected, leading to false-negative test results.

Clinical Management of FAP. The clinical management options for persons with FAP include screening, prophylactic surgery, and chemoprevention.

Colonoscopic and endoscopic examination with polypectomy is recommended until too many polyps exist to allow safe removal.[35] Prophylactic subtotal colectomy is then recommended, followed by annual endoscopic evaluation of the remaining rectum.[35] Given the very early onset of FAP, prophylactic surgery is delayed until absolutely necessary, at least until puberty.

Chemoprevention is an option for persons with FAP who have undergone prophylactic surgery. COX-2 inhibitors such as celecoxib, rofecoxib, and sulindac, reduce the size and number of polyps in individuals after subtotal colectomy by up to 28%.[49-52] Whether this reduction in polyps will translate to a reduction in mortality is not yet known. In addition, the role of COX-2 inhibitors before prophylactic surgery has yet to be determined.

MULTIPLE ENDOCRINE NEOPLASIA

Multiple endocrine neoplasia (MEN) is a hereditary disorder characterized by the occurrence of tumors involving endocrine glands. MEN can be further divided into clinically and genetically distinct syndromes known as MEN1 and MEN2.
- *MEN1*. MEN1 is an autosomal dominant inherited syndrome associated with germline mutations in the *MEN1* gene located on the long arm of chromosome 11 (11q13). The syndrome is characterized by tumors of the pituitary and parathyroid glands, as well as the pancreatic islet cells. Tumors can also involve the adrenal cortex.
- *MEN2*. MEN2 is also an autosomal dominant inherited syndrome associated with germline mutations of the *RET* gene, located on the long arm of chromosome 10 (10q11.2). MEN2 is subdivided into three subtypes known as MEN2A, MEN2B, and familial medullary thyroid carcinoma (FMTC). Each of these syndromes has its own distinct features, but the feature common to all three is the presence of medullary thyroid carcinoma (MTC).

Hereditary MTC affects the C cells, which are responsible for the production of calcitonin. These cells develop hyperplasia, which is the precursor for the hereditary form of MTC. An abnormally elevated calcitonin level can be identified as early as 5 years of age. MTC accounts for 3% to 9% of all thyroid cancers.[53] Of all MTCs, 75% are sporadic and the remaining 25% are due to MEN2. Hereditary MTC is distinctly different from sporadic MTC in that most hereditary cases are bilateral,

with an earlier age of onset than sporadic cases. Of all hereditary MTC cases, approximately 70% are due to MEN2A, 22% to 25% are due to FMTC, and 5% to 9% are due to MEN2B.[53]

MEN2A is an autosomal inherited disorder that is comprised of MTC, pheochromocytoma, and parathyroid hyperplasia. Distinct skin lesions, known as cutaneous lichen amyloidosis, may also be associated with this disorder in some families. Persons who develop clinical manifestations of MEN2A have a 100% lifetime risk of developing MTC and a 50% risk of developing pheochromocytoma, of which only about 4% are malignant. There is also a 20% to 25% risk of developing hyperparathyroidism, which is usually not symptomatic.[53] In MEN2A families, the diagnosis of MTC is made early in life. The average age of diagnosis is 15 years of age.

MEN2B is also an autosomal dominant inherited disorder characterized by MTCs diagnosed at an earlier age than seen with MEN2A. This is a more aggressive form of MTC, with an average age of diagnosis of 5 years. Pheochromocytoma is also present, but hyperparathyroidism is not. MEN2B is also characterized by developmental abnormalities including mucosal neuromas, ganglioneuromatosis, Marfan-like features, and the presence of megacolon. Persons with MEN2B have a number of clinical features including thick lips, lumpy tongues, elongated faces, and thick eyelids.[54]

Familial MTC is an autosomal dominant inherited disorder characterized by the diagnosis of MTC in four or more family members. Pheochromocytoma and hyperparathyroidism are not associated with FMTC. The cases of MTC in this syndrome are usually of later age of onset and are slower-growing than those associated with MEN2A and MEN2B.[54]

Genetic Testing for MEN2 Syndromes. The MEN2 syndromes are all associated with germline mutations in the *RET* gene on chromosome 10. The *RET* (rearranged during transfection) gene is a proto-oncogene that encodes a cell surface glycoprotein within the receptor tyrosine kinase family. These receptor tyrosine kinases transduce signals for cell growth and differentiation. When there is a mutation in the *RET* proto-oncogene, it remains activated, leading to unchecked cell growth and tumorigenesis.

Testing for the *RET* mutation has become a standard of care and is recommended for all persons with MTC and at-risk family members. Even though approximately 75% of all MTC is considered sporadic, at least 50% of all MEN2B cases have no family history and most likely have de novo mutations.[55] If germline mutations are found in persons with suspected sporadic MTC, the diagnosis of MEN2 is made and the patient and family are managed accordingly.

There are definite benefits to *RET* mutation testing. By identifying mutation carriers very early, before the development of MTC, there is a substantial reduction in morbidity and mortality from the disease.[55] Also, by identifying mutation-negative individuals, they are spared unnecessary screening and evaluation. Testing is very reliable in MEN2A and MEN2B families.[53] Unfortunately, some families have no detectable mutation, despite the presence of clinical features of MEN2. This is most likely due to FMTC, but occasionally it is due to MEN2A or MEN2B.

Clinical Management of the RET Mutation Carrier. Persons with known *RET* mutations have a 100% risk of developing MTC. Therefore prophylactic thyroidectomy is recommended for all mutation carriers. This is usually done between the ages of 5 and 10 years in MEN2A families and in as early as infancy in MEN2B families. Surgery can be delayed in FMTC families, because the onset of disease is later and the course often less aggressive.

Postoperatively, the patient is placed on thyroid replacement hormone. Biochemical screening can be done to monitor for residual or metastatic MTC and for the development of pheochromocytoma or hyperparathyroidism. Blood and urine screening is done annually or biannually.

OTHER HEREDITARY CANCER SYNDROMES

Other hereditary cancer syndromes continue to be described in the literature as health care providers and researchers develop greater awareness of clustering of cancers in families. One such syndrome receiving attention is hereditary prostate cancer.

Prostate Cancer. The lifetime risk of prostate cancer for men in the United States is 1 in 6, making it the most common cancer in men.[6] Family history of cancer is among the top three known risk factors for prostate cancer, along with age and race. In fact, familial clustering of prostate cancer has been identified for some time, with first-degree relatives of affected men having a two- to threefold risk for prostate cancer. Although no single gene mutations have been definitively identified with prostate cancer, several genes have been implicated in prostate cancer susceptibility, including genes on chromosomes 1, 8, 17, 20 and X.[56] In addition, hereditary prostate cancer has been associated with a variety of cancer syndromes including those associated with *BRCA1* and *BRCA2*.

Although criteria for families at high risk of having an inherited predisposition have not been confirmed through gene linkage, some have been suggested. These criteria include one or more of the following: (1) three or more first-degree relatives with prostate cancer, (2) three sequential generations on either the maternal or the paternal lineage, or (3) two or more men affected by age 55.[57]

Since no inherited prostate cancer–specific genetic locus has been identified for hereditary prostate cancer, no genetic testing for prostate cancer currently exists. However, male carriers of a *BRCA1* or *BRCA2* gene mutation have an increased risk of developing prostate cancer.[58,59]

Little information currently exists regarding primary or secondary prevention of prostate cancer in men at increased risk of prostate cancer. The recently published results of the Prostate Cancer Prevention Trial (PCPT) comparing finasteride to placebo showed a 25% reduction in prostate cancer among those receiving finasteride and appeared to be equally efficacious in persons with and without a positive family history of prostate cancer.[60] Randomized clinical trials evaluating screening methods in men at increased risk of prostate cancer are lacking in the literature. Case-control studies have been inconclusive regarding the recommended frequency of serum prostate-specific antigen (PSA) testing and digital rectal examination in high-risk individuals.[61,62]

Future Directions

Genetics will continue to play a pivotal role in the detection and prevention of cancer in the future. As additional gene mutations are identified and linked to various cancers, targeted cancer screening will be available. Greater understanding of the genetic pathogenesis of cancer will improve our ability to treat and ultimately prevent the development of cancer.

Oncology nurses have an important role in identifying persons at increased risk of cancer, counseling individuals and families regarding their cancer risk and management strategies, and conducting research related to the implications of genetic susceptibility, genetic testing, and cancer risk–reduction strategies. In their roles as educators, advocates, researchers, clinicians, and leaders, oncology nurses can inform and support individuals with known or suspected hereditary cancer syndromes.

Acknowledgement

The author would like to acknowledge Carol Pappas Appel for her authorship of an earlier version of this chapter.

REVIEW QUESTIONS

✓ Case Study

A 45-year-old Caucasian woman, PL, has expressed concern about the cancers in her family and what her cancer risks might be. Her family history of cancer includes a sister diagnosed with ovarian cancer at 48, mother with breast cancer at age 50, a maternal aunt with ovarian cancer at age 54, a second maternal aunt without cancer, and a paternal aunt with breast cancer at age 55. In addition, her father was diagnosed with prostate cancer at age 64, and a paternal aunt was diagnosed with breast cancer at age 62. There is no known cancer in the remaining two paternal aunts or one paternal uncle.

PL's personal history includes menarche at age 15 and the birth of two daughters, now aged 22 and 20. PL was 23 and 25 when they were born, and she states that she breastfed them

for approximately 8 months each. PL has had regular mammograms for the past 4 years and one previous breast biopsy, which she says was 2 years ago and showed a fibroadenoma. Her most recent mammogram was approximately 14 months ago. PL has had annual gynecologic exams, which she reports have been normal. PL is premenopausal; her last menstrual period was 2 weeks ago. Menses occur about every 30 days. PL took oral contraceptives for a total of approximately 10 years following the birth of her children.

PL is married to her children's father, who accompanies her to this visit. PL smokes 1 pack of cigarettes per day and drinks one to two glasses of wine each week.

On physical examination, no breast or gynecologic abnormalities were detected.

Continued

REVIEW QUESTIONS—CONT'D

PL is concerned about her family history of cancer, the implications for her, and what options are recommended for her to reduce her risk of cancer.

DISCUSSION

PL's history of cancer raises concern that there might be an inherited predisposition to cancer. PL requires a comprehensive genetic risk evaluation including a complete pedigree consultation, medical record confirmation of the cancers in her family and her own medical history, and genetic counseling regarding her options.

At minimum, PL requires annual gynecologic examinations, annual mammography, annual clinical breast examination, and breast self-examination, given her age. Of particular concern is her smoking behavior. PL requires smoking cessation counseling and education about reducing her cancer risk by quitting smoking.

A comprehensive genetic cancer risk evaluation will help identify her specific cancer risks and the potential benefits and risks of undergoing genetic testing.

QUESTIONS

1. Which of the following is an example of a second-degree relative in PL's family pedigree?
   a. Sister
   b. Cousin
   c. Uncle
   d. Daughter
2. What in this family history raises the greatest concern regarding a possibly inherited syndrome?
   a. Father with prostate cancer at age 64
   b. Sister with ovarian cancer at age 48
   c. Paternal aunt with breast cancer at age 62
   d. Two ovarian cancers in maternal history
3. The most comprehensive gene mutation calculation method best suited for this family is which of the following?
   a. The Gail model
   b. The Claus model
   c. The couch tables
   d. BRCAPRO
4. Which of the following gene mutations is suggested in this family history?
   a. *APC*
   b. *RET*
   c. *BRCA*
   d. *MSH2*
5. Testing for a gene mutation is most conclusive if it
   a. Has been done through full gene sequencing.
   b. Is negative in an unaffected individual tested first in the family.
   c. Is positive in an individual when a family mutation is known.
   d. Is negative in an affected individual tested last in the family.

6. If PL is found to have a gene mutation predisposing to cancer, this is the probability that her daughter has inherited the mutation:
   a. 10%
   b. 25%
   c. 50%
   d. 100%
7. If this family carries the suspected mutation, its members may be at risk for these cancers:
   a. Ovarian, endometrial, colon
   b. Prostate, pancreatic, melanoma
   c. Ovarian, kidney, pancreatic
   d. Endometrial, colon, melanoma
8. Which of the following is included in the breast cancer screening guidelines for mutation carriers?
   a. Annual breast magnetic resonance imaging (MRI)
   b. Prophylactic mastectomy
   c. Semiannual mammography
   d. Annual clinical breast exam
9. Research has shown that chemoprevention for breast cancer is possible with which of the following?
   a. Raloxifene
   b. Tamoxifen
   c. Oral contraceptives
   d. Celecoxib
10. Effective prevention for ovarian cancer includes
    a. One to two glasses of wine per week.
    b. An annual gynecologic exam.
    c. A CA-125 blood test.
    d. Oral contraceptives.

ANSWERS

1. **C.** *Rationale:* An uncle is a second-degree relative, a sister or daughter is a first-degree relative, and a cousin is a third-degree relative.
2. **D.** *Rationale:* The family history of greatest concern in PL's family is the two maternal relatives with ovarian cancer, including PL's sister and maternal aunt. The two ovarian cancers are of greater concern than one ovarian cancer alone, and are of greater concern than either of the other cancers, which are more common cancers and have occurred at common ages for those cancers.
3. **D.** *Rationale:* BRCAPRO is the most comprehensive mutation calculation model because it provides an estimate of both *BRCA1* and *BRCA2* risk and accounts for multiple family factors including Ashkenazi descent.
4. **C.** *Rationale:* This family history is suggestive of a *BRCA* mutation, which is associated with breast and ovarian cancer. An *APC* mutation is associated with FAP, a *RET* gene mutation is associated with MEN 2, and a *MSH2* gene mutation is associated with hereditary nonpolyposis colon cancer.
5. **C.** *Rationale:* Gene mutation testing is most conclusive if it is negative when a known mutation exists in the family. Gene sequencing, though the gold standard method for testing, may identify genetic variants with unknown significance. A negative test in an unaffected

individual in the absence of a known mutation in the family is inconclusive.

6. C. *Rationale:* Parents pass one copy of each of their two gene pairs to their children. If PL carries a gene mutation in one of her two BRCA gene pairs, her daughter would have 1 out of 2, or 50%, chance of inheriting the mutated gene.

7. B. *Rationale:* Persons with *BRCA* mutations—particularly *BRCA2*, which has a higher likelihood of ovarian cancer—are at risk for prostate and pancreatic cancers and melanoma. Endometrial and kidney cancers are not particularly associated with *BRCA* mutations.

8. D. *Rationale:* Mammography is recommended for breast cancer screening; however, semiannual mammography has

not yet been shown to be of greater benefit. Prophylactic mastectomy is a cancer prevention strategy. Breast MRI is being evaluated in clinical trials. Annual (or semiannual) breast exam is recommended for mutation carriers.

9. B. *Rationale:* Tamixofen has been shown to reduce the incidence of breast cancer by 49%. Raloxifene is stillbeing evaluated. Oral contraceptives may reduce the risk of ovarian cancer. Celecoxib reduces the number of colon polyps.

10. D. *Rationale:* Ovarian cancer incidence may be reduced through the use of oral contraceptives. There is no evidence to suggest alcohol consumption lowers ovarian cancer incidence. Annual gynecologic exams and CA-125 assessment are screening techniques; they do not prevent ovarian cancer.

REFERENCES

1. Lessick M, Middelton LA: Perspectives in genetics. In Black JM, Hawks JH, editors: *Medical-surgical nursing: clinical management for positive outcomes*, ed 7, St Louis, 2005, Saunders.
2. Lea DH, Jenkins JF, Francomano CA: *Genetics in clinical practice: new directions for nursing and health care*, Boston, 1998, Jones & Bartlett.
3. International Human Genome Sequencing Consortium: Initial sequencing and analysis of the human genome, *Nature* 409:860-921, 2001.
4. National Human Genome Research Institute: An overview of the human genome project, retrieved August 21, 2005 from http://www.genome.gov/12011238.
5. Collins FS, Green ED, Guttmacher AE et al: A vision for the future of genomics research, *Nature* 422:835-847, 2003.
6. Jemal A, Murray T, Ward E: Cancer statistics 2005, *CA Cancer J Clin* 55:10-30, 2005.
7. Meiser B: Long-term outcomes of genetic counseling in women at increased risk of developing hereditary breast cancer, *Patient Educ Couns* 44(3):215-225, 2001.
8. American Society of Clinical Oncology Policy Statement Update: genetic testing for cancer susceptibility, *J Clin Oncol* 21(12):2397-2406, 2003.
9. Li FP: Cancer control in susceptible groups: opportunities and challenges, *J Clin Oncol* 17(2):719, 1999.
10. Carter RF: BRCA1, BRCA2 and breast cancer: a concise clinical review, *Clin Invest Med* 24(3):147-157, 2001.
11. Frank TS, Deffenbaugh AM, Reld JE et al: Clinical characteristics of individuals with germline mutations in BRCA1 and BRCA1: analysis of 10,000 individuals, *J Clin Oncol* 20:1480-1490, 2002.
12. Narod SA, Feunteun J, Lynch HT et al: Familial breast-ovarian cancer locus on chromosome 17q12-q23, *Lancet* 338(8759):82-83, 1991.
13. Gail MH, Brinton LA, Byar DP et al: Projecting individualized probabilities of developing breast cancer for white females who are being examined annually, *J Natl Cancer Inst* 81(24):1879-1886, 1989.
14. Claus EB, Risch N, Thompson WD: Autosomal dominant inheritance of early-onset breast cancer. Implications for risk prediction, *Cancer* 73(3):643-651, 1994.
15. Couch FJ, DeShano ML, Blackwood MA et al: BRCA1 mutations in women attending clinics that evaluate the risk of breast cancer, *N Engl J Med* 336(20):1409-1415, 1997.
16. Frank TS, Manley SA, Olopade OI et al: Sequence analysis of BRCA1 and BRCA2: correlation of mutations with family history and ovarian cancer risk, *J Clin Oncol* 16(7):2417-2425, 1998.
17. Parmigiani G, Berry D, Aguilar O: Determining carrier probabilities for breast cancer-susceptibility genes BRCA1 and BRCA2, *Am J Hum Genet* 62(1):145-158, 1998.
18. Berry DA, Iversen ES Jr, Gudbjartsson DF et al: BRCAPRO validation, sensitivity of genetic testing of BRCA1/BRCA2, and prevalence of other breast cancer susceptibility genes, *J Clin Oncol* 20(11):2701-2712, 2002.
19. Fisher B, Costantino JP, Wickerham DL et al: Tamoxifen for prevention of breast cancer: report of the National Surgical Adjuvant Breast and Bowel Project P-1 Study, *J Natl Cancer Inst* 90(18):1371-1388, 1998.
20. King MC, Wieand S, Hale K et al: Tamoxifen and breast cancer incidence among women with inherited mutations in BRCA1 and BRCA2: National Surgical Adjuvant Breast and Bowel Project (NSABP-P1) Breast Cancer Prevention Trial, *JAMA* 286(18):2251-2256, 2001.
21. Whittemore AS, Balise RR, Pharoah PD et al: Oral contraceptive use and ovarian cancer risk among carriers of BRCA1 or BRCA2 mutations, *Br J Cancer* 91(11):1911-1915, 2004.
22. McGuire V, Felberg A, Mills M et al: Relation of contraceptive and reproductive history to ovarian cancer risk in carriers and noncarriers of BRCA1 gene mutations, *Am J Epidemiol* 160(7):613-618, 2004.
23. Modan B, Hartge P, Hirsh-Yechezkel G et al: Parity, oral contraceptives, and the risk of ovarian cancer among carriers and noncarriers of a BRCA1 or BRCA2 mutation, *N Engl J Med* 345(4):235-240, 2001.
24. Narod SA, Dubé MP, Klijn J et al: Oral contraceptives and the risk of breast cancer in BRCA1 and BRCA2 mutation carriers, *J Natl Cancer Inst* 94(23):1773-1779, 2002.
25. Hartmann LC, Schaid DJ, Woods JE et al: Efficacy of bilateral prophylactic mastectomy in women with a family history of breast cancer, *N Engl J Med* 34(2):77-84, 1999.
26. Hartmann LC, Sellers TA, Schaid DJ et al: Efficacy of bilateral prophylactic mastectomy in BRCA1 and BRCA2 gene mutation carriers, *J Natl Cancer Inst* 93(21):1633-1637, 2001.
27. Meijers-Heijboer H, van Geel B, van Putten WL et al: Breast cancer after prophylactic bilateral mastectomy in women with a BRCA1 or BRCA2 mutation, *N Engl J Med* 345(3):159-154, 2001.
28. Rebbeck TR, Friebel T, Lynch HT et al: Bilateral prophylactic mastectomy reduces breast cancer risk in BRCA1 and BRCA2 mutation carriers: the PROSE Study Group, *J Clin Oncol* 22(6):1055-1062, 2004.
29. Rebbeck TR, Lynch HT, Neuhausen SL et al: Prophylactic oophorectomy in carriers of BRCA1 or BRCA2 mutations, *N Engl J Med* 346(21):1616-1622, 2002.
30. Kauff ND, Satagopan JM, Robson ME et al: Risk-reducing salpingo-oophorectomy in women with a BRCA1 or BRCA2 mutation, *N Engl J Med* 346(21):1609-1615, 2002.
31. Burke W, Daly M, Garber J et al: Recommendations for follow-up care of individuals with an inherited predisposition to cancer. II. BRCA1 and BRCA2. Cancer Genetics Studies Consortium, *JAMA* 277(12):997-1003, 1997.
32. Trimbath JD, Giardiello FM: Review article: genetic testing and counseling for hereditary colorectal cancer, *Aliment Pharmacol Ther* 16:1843-1857, 2002.
33. Abdel-Rahman WM, Peltomaki P: Molecular basis and diagnostics of hereditary colorectal cancers, *Ann Med* 36:379-388, 2004.
34. Calvert P, Frucht H: The genetics of colorectal cancer, *Ann Intern Med* 137:603-612, 2002.
35. Lynch HT, de la Chapelle A: Hereditary colorectal cancer, *N Engl J Med* 348(10):919-932, 2003.
36. de la Chapelle A: Genetic predisposition to colorectal cancer, *Nat Rev* 4:769-780, 2004.
37. Matloff ET, Brierley KL, Chimera CM: A clinician's guide to hereditary colon cancer, *Cancer J* 10:280-287, 2004.
38. Brown G, St. John D, Macrae F: Cancer risk in young women at risk of hereditary nonpolyposis colorectal cancer: implications for gynecologic surveillance, *Gynecol Oncol* 80:346-349, 2001.
39. Vasen H, Watson P, Mecklin J et al: New criteria for hereditary nonpolyposis colorectal cancer (HNPCC, Lynch syndrome) predisposed by the International Collaborative Group on HNPCC (ICG-HNPCC), *Gastroenterology* 116:1453-1456, 1999.

40. Umar A, Boland CR, Terdiman JP et al: Revised Bethesda Guidelines for hereditary nonpolyposis colorectal cancer (Lynch syndrome) and microsatellite instability, *J Natl Cancer Inst* 96:261-268, 2004.

41. Scartozzi M, Bianchi F, Rosati S: Mutations of hMLH1 and hMSH2 in patients with suspected hereditary nonpolyposis colorectal cancer: correlation with microsatellite instability and abnormalities of mismatch repair protein expression, *J Clin Oncol* 20:1203-1208, 2002.

42. Levin B, Barthel JS, Burt RW et al: Colorectal cancer screening clinical practice guidelines, *J Natl Compr Canc Netw* 4(4):384, 2006.

43. Burke W, Petersen G, Lynch P et al: Recommendations for follow-up care of individuals with an inherited predisposition to cancer. I. Hereditary nonpolyposis colon cancer. Cancer Genetics Studies Consortium, *JAMA* 277(11):915-9, 1997.

44. Fearnhead N, Britton M, Bodmer W: The ABC of APC, *Hum Mol Genet* 10:721-733, 2001.

45. Laurent-Puig P, Beroud C, Soussi T: APC gene: database of germline and somatic mutations in human tumors and cell lines, *Nucl Acids Res* 26:269-270, 1998.

46. Laken SJ, Petersen GM, Gruber SB et al: Familial colorectal cancer in Ashkenazim due to a hypermutable tract in APC, *Nat Genet* 17(1):79-83, 1997.

47. Strul H, Barenboim E, Leshno M et al: The I1307K adenomatous polyposis coli gene variant does not contribute in the assessment of the risk for colorectal cancer in Ashkenazi Jews, *Cancer Epidemiol Biomarkers Prev* 12(10):1012-1015, 2003.

48. Michie S, Bobrow M, Marteau TM: Predictive genetic testing in children and adults: a study of emotional impact, *J Med Genet* 38(8):519-526, 2001.

49. U.S. Food and Drug Administration (April 7, 2005). Patient information sheet celecoxib (marketed as Celebrex). Retrieved September 4, 2006, from http://www.fda.gov/cder/drug/infopage/celebrex/celebrex-ptsk.htm

50. Steinbach G, Lynch PM, Phillips RK et al: The effect of celecoxib, a cyclooxygenase-2 inhibitor, in familial adenomatous polyposis, *N Engl J Med* 342(26):1946-1952, 2000.

51. Giardiello FM, Yang VW, Hylind LM et al: Primary chemoprevention of familial adenomatous polyposis with sulindac, *N Engl J Med* 346(14): 1054-1059, 2002.

52. Higuchi T, Iwama T, Yoshinaga K et al: A randomized, double-blind, placebo-controlled trial of the effects of rofecoxib, a selective cyclooxygenase-2 inhibitor, on rectal polyps in familial adenomatous polyposis patients, *Clin Cancer Res* 9(13):4756-4760, 2003.

53. Cohen EG, Shaha AR, Rinaldo A et al: Medullary thyroid carcinoma, *Acta Otolaryngol* 124:544-557, 2004.

54. Leboulleux S, Baudin E, Travagli J et al: Medullary thyroid carcinoma, *Clin Endocrin* 61:299-310, 2004.

55. Hansford JR, Mulligan LM: Multiple endocrine neoplasia type 2 and RET: from neoplasia to neurogenesis, *J Med Genet* 37:817-827, 2000.

56. Cunningham JM, McDonnell SK, Marks A et al: Genome linkage screen for prostate cancer susceptibility loci: results from the Mayo Clinic familial prostate cancer study, *Prostate* 57(4):335-346, 2003.

57. Carter BS, Bova GS, Beaty TH et al: Hereditary prostate cancer: epidemiologic and clinical features, *J Urol* 150(3):797-802, 1993.

58. Thompson D, Easton DF, Breast Cancer Linkage Consortium: Cancer incidence in BRCA1 mutation carriers. *J Natl Cancer Inst* 94(18): 1358-1365, 2002.

59. Breast Cancer Linkage Consortium: Cancer risks in BRCA2 mutation carriers, *J Natl Cancer Inst* 91(15):1310-1316, 1999.

60. Thompson IM, Goodman PJ, Tangen CM et al: The influence of finasteride on the development of prostate cancer, *N Engl J Med* 349(3): 215-224, 2003.

61. Catalona WJ, Antenor JA, Roehl KA et al: Screening for prostate cancer in high risk populations, *J Urol* 168(5):1980-1983; discussion 1983-1984, 2002.

62. Valeri A, Cormier L, Moineau MP et al: Targeted screening for prostate cancer in high risk families: early onset is a significant risk factor for disease in first degree relatives, *J Urol* 168(2):483-487, 2002.

CHAPTER 3

Epidemiology

Lisa Schulmeister

The science of *epidemiology* studies the variations in disease frequencies among human population groups and the factors influencing these variations. The goal of epidemiology is to identify the cause of disease so that the causative agent may be removed and, ultimately, the disease can be prevented. Unlike basic research, the emphasis of epidemiology is on humans rather than animals, and unlike clinical medicine, epidemiology studies groups or populations rather than individuals. In addition, epidemiology focuses on the events occurring before the illness rather than the treatment after disease diagnosis. The endpoint of therapeutic research is to discover effective cancer treatments; the endpoint of epidemiologic research is to prevent cancer.[1]

Epidemiology was initially associated with the study of infectious diseases. In the 1940s, however, scientists began to notice an increasing number of deaths from chronic causes, such as cancer and heart disease. One of the earliest and best-known epidemiologic studies was performed by the British surgeon Percival Pott in 1775.[2] Pott first described occupational carcinogens by noting the high incidence of scrotal cancer in chimneysweeps. The astute observation of Dr. Pott preceded the laboratory discovery of the carcinogenic properties of polycyclic hydrocarbons, such as coal and soot, by decades.

In addition to epidemiologic principles, population demographics and the natural and social sciences are used to help determine what causes cancer. Examples of how these fields are applied in epidemiology include studies of geographic variations in occurrence and types of cancer, the relationship of cancer incidence to social habits and environmental agents, the comparison of populations with and without cancer, and the impact of the removal of suspected cancer-causing agents on cancer incidence.

A basic understanding of epidemiologic terminology and techniques assists oncology nurses to interpret research study findings about cancer patterns and causation. This knowledge is useful in delivering evidence-based care and targeting populations for education, prevention, and screening programs.

Terminology

Although many terms are used in epidemiology, the four terms most applicable to oncology are incidence, prevalence, mortality, and survival.

INCIDENCE

The number of newly diagnosed cases of cancer in a specified period of time in a defined population is called the cancer *incidence*. It is defined as follows:

$$\frac{\text{Number of persons developing cancer in a specified period of time}}{\text{Total population living at that time}} = \text{Incidence}$$

The specified time period usually is 1 year, and the rates are expressed per 100,000 persons. The advantage of expressing incidence as a rate is that it allows comparison of rates among different populations. In the United States in 2005, there were 211,240 newly diagnosed cases of breast cancer in women, and the incidence rate was 132.5/100,000. The fact that in 2005 Utah had 1150 new cases of breast cancer and California had 21,170 new cases of breast cancer has little meaning because of their population differences. In Utah, the incidence rate of breast cancer was 115.7, and in California it was 139.6. Examining incidence rate, rather than overall numbers of cases, allows more accurate comparison of incidence by state, and also allows comparison with the overall U.S. incidence of breast cancer. At first glance, it appears that California has a much higher breast cancer incidence than Utah; however, the California incidence rate is only slightly higher than the overall rate of breast cancer in the United States. When large differences in cancer incidence exist, epidemiologists design studies to determine why the incidence varies. In addition, epidemiologic data allow comparison of U.S. cancer incidence with that of other countries around the world. In 2005, the estimated new cancer cases in the United States was 1,372,910.[3,4] The most recent global cancer statistics, from 2002, indicate 10.9 million new cases of cancer diagnosed worldwide.[5]

The longest ongoing population-based resource is the Connecticut Tumor Registry, which has been collecting incidence data since 1935. Before 1973, cancer incidence data were collected through several periodic surveys in selected U.S. areas. These surveys, coordinated by the National Cancer Institute (NCI), were conducted in 1937-1939, 1947-1948, and 1969-1971. In 1973 the NCI established and funded the Surveillance, Epidemiology, and End-Results (SEER) program to gather information on cancer incidence, mortality, and survival. The SEER program currently collects and publishes cancer incidence and survival data from 14 population-based cancer registries and three supplemental registries covering approximately 26% of the U.S. population. Information on more than 3 million in situ and invasive cancer cases is included in the SEER database, and approximately 170,000 new cases are added each year within the SEER coverage areas. The SEER registries routinely collect data on patient demographics, primary tumor site, morphology, stage at diagnosis, first course of treatment, and follow-up for vital status. The SEER program is the only comprehensive source of population-based information in the United States that includes stage of cancer at the time of diagnosis and survival rates within each stage.[6]

In addition to SEER data, incidence information is also collected in individual hospital cancer registries. Individual tumor registries, certified by the American College of Surgeons (ACS), abstract demographic and disease-related information from the charts of patients with newly diagnosed cancer, and all patients are followed for survival data. The registries also conduct disease-specific studies as requested by the ACS. Incidence data collection focuses on two specific areas: demographic and medical. *Demographic* information extrapolates age, gender, race, marital status, and place of residence. *Medical* data on the same individual report onset of illness, location of tumor, stage, histology, treatment, and survival over time. These data assist epidemiologists in describing the current cancer problem in terms of geographic distribution, age and race of patients, and increase or decrease in specific types of cancer.[7]

PREVALENCE

The measurement of all cancer cases, both old and new, at a *designated point in time,* is called cancer *prevalence.*[1] The prevalence rate is defined as follows:

$$\frac{\text{Number of persons with cancer at a given point in time}}{\text{Total population living at that time}} = \text{Prevalence}$$

Prevalence is a statistic of primary interest in public health because it identifies the level of burden of disease or health-related events on the population and health care system. Prevalence represents new and preexisting cases in persons alive on a certain date, in contrast to incidence, which reflects new cases of a condition diagnosed during a given period of time. Prevalence therefore is a function of both the incidence of the disease and survival. The prevalence rate provides useful information for health care planning, including physical facilities, staffing needs, and the design and implementation of screening programs.[8]

MORTALITY

The number of deaths attributed to cancer in a specified time period and in a defined population is the cancer *mortality.*[1] The mortality rate is defined as follows:

$$\frac{\text{Number of persons dying of cancer in a specified period of time}}{\text{Total population living at that time}} = \text{Mortality}$$

The 2005 estimated number of cancer deaths in the United States is 570,280 persons.[3] Unlike incidence data, mortality data have routinely been collected in the United States since 1930. The National Center for Health Statistics provides the mortality data reported by the SEER Program.[9] Cancer mortality data, for specific racial or ethnic populations at the national and state levels, are essential for developing cancer prevention and control programs. These data provide valuable information for identifying where to enhance screening efforts, for increasing access to health care, for assessing the quality of health care, and for developing research plans.[10]

SURVIVAL

The link between incidence and mortality data is *survival analysis,* the observation over time of persons with cancer and the calculation of their probability of dying over several time periods.[1] The most commonly reported measures of patient survival by cancer registries are 5- and 10-year cumulative survival rates. Cumulative survival data often are outdated at the time they are derived (i.e., after a follow-up of at least 5 or 10 years), are cohort-based (give equal emphasis to data about people diagnosed today and many years ago), and do not take into account the impact of recent advances in cancer detection and treatment

on survival. A newer method of survival analysis, *period analysis,* gives more weight to recent data in calculating survival rates, thus taking into account newer, more successful diagnostic and treatment methods.[11]

Relative survival is the observed survival (the proportion of patients with cancer surviving for a specified time period) adjusted for expected mortality. Relative survival provides an estimate of the likelihood that patients with cancer will not die from causes associated with their cancer. The relative survival rate measures the survival of the patient cohort compared with the component of the general population having the same characteristics as the patient cohort with respect to age, race, sex, and calendar period. Generally, this means that the relative survival rate measures the effect of the cancer alone, because it is usually the only factor that makes the patient cohort different from the general population. However, sometimes the patients in a cohort may have some other factor that places them at a greater risk for dying compared with the general population. For example, there is a higher percentage of smokers among patients with lung cancer than among the general population. Smokers tend to be at greater risk for other diseases, such as heart disease. Relative survival cannot separate the risk of death from lung cancer from the risk of dying of noncancer causes due to smoking. Therefore, the relative survival rate for lung cancer is an underestimate of the effect of lung cancer alone.[12]

Conditional median survival is another epidemiologic technique that has been used as a tool to examine and estimate the survival of patients with advanced cancers. Researchers found that the longer patients with a poor prognosis survived, the longer they could be expected to survive. In other words, the prognosis of patients with advanced disease changes as a result of their continued survival, and conditional median survival calculation factors into this continued survival.[13]

Children have the highest cancer survival rate. From 1980 to 2005, the 5-year survival rate of childhood cancer climbed from 37% to 70% to 77% in the United States and Europe. This significant increase is due to high enrollment of children in clinical trials, accessibility of specialized pediatric oncology care, and advances in the treatment of childhood cancers.[14-16] The survival rate for adults varies greatly by cancer site and stage at diagnosis; however, the overall relative 5-year survival rate is 62.7%.[17]

IDENTIFICATION OF TRENDS

Incidence, prevalence, mortality, and survival data aid in the identification of trends, which leads to questions of causation. For instance, the age-adjusted incidence rates of cutaneous melanoma almost tripled among males, from 6.7 in 1973 to 19.3 in 1997, and more than doubled among females, from 5.9 to 13.8 during the same time period. Researchers sought to determine if these trends reflected real changes in incidence rates or if these trends were due to increased screening for melanoma. They concluded that the increase in melanoma incidence is real, and is likely due to increased sunlight exposure. This finding has significant implications in terms of cancer prevention and public education.[18] Box 3-1 lists additional examples of current trends in cancer incidence, mortality, and survival.

Types of Studies

The epidemiologic method is composed of an orderly progression of three types of studies: descriptive, analytic,

Current Trends in Cancer Incidence, Mortality, and Survival

Incidence

Approximately 1,372,910 new cases of invasive cancer were diagnosed in the United States in 2005.

More than 1 million cases of basal and squamous cell skin cancer were diagnosed in 2005.

Overall incidence is highest in African Americans (544.5) and lowest in Native Americans (242).

Prostate cancer incidence rates are 62% higher for African American men than white men.

Leading sites of incidence in men are prostate, lung and bronchus, and colon and rectum.

Leading sites of incidence in women are breast, lung and bronchus, and colon and rectum.

Melanoma incidence has increased 1000% in the past 50 years.

Mortality

More than 570,280 cancer-related deaths occurred in the United States in 2005.

Cancer has surpassed heart disease as the leading cause of death for people younger than 85 years.

Leading cause of death from cancer in men are cancers of the lung and bronchus, the prostate, and the colon.

Leading causes of death from cancer in women are cancers of the lung and bronchus, the breast, and the colon.

Lung cancer accounts for 31% of male cancer deaths.

Lung cancer accounts for 27% of female cancer deaths.

Risk of dying of lung cancer is 22 times higher for male smokers and 12 times higher for female smokers.

Leukemia is the leading cause of cancer death before age 20 among women, whereas breast cancer ranks first from ages 20 to 59, and lung cancer ranks first at age 60 and older.

Leukemia is the most common fatal cancer among men under age 40, whereas cancer of the lung and bronchus is the most common fatal cancer among men over the age of 40.

Cancer is the second most common cause of death among children under the age of 15.

African Americans men have a 40% higher death rate and African American women have a 20% higher death rate from all cancers combined when compared to white men and women.

Mortality rates have continued to decrease for major cancer sites in men and women except for female lung cancer, in which rates have leveled off for the first time after increasing for many decades.

Survival

Overall 5-year relative cancer survival rate is 62.7%.

Data from Jemal A, Murray T, Ward E et al: Cancer statistics, 2005, *CA Cancer J Clin* 55:10, 2005; National Cancer Institute: Surveillance, epidemiology, and end results program, retrieved May 17, 2005, from http://seer.cancer/gov/about; and Smith M, Hare ML: An overview of progress in childhood cancer survival, *J Pediatr Oncol Nurs* 21:160, 2004.

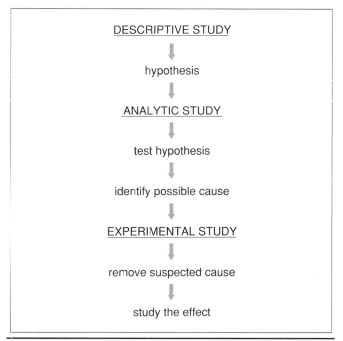

FIG. 3-1   The epidemiologic method.

experimental study, removes the suspected cause and evaluates the effect on the population (Fig. 3-1).

DESCRIPTIVE STUDIES

Descriptive studies form the body of data within which the hypothesis may be sought. The disease of cancer can be described in many ways. One method of description might be evaluating the *frequency* of a cancer. This is the purpose of keeping incidence, prevalence, and mortality data. Specific methods are available to describe the *classification* of the cancer: site of the tumor, morphology and grade, and the stage of the disease. This information is found in the patient's medical record at the time of diagnosis and can be extrapolated by the epidemiologist. Person, place, and time are classic descriptive epidemiologic variables that serve as a major source of clues to cancer etiology.

Person. Age, gender, and racial differences account for fundamental differences in cancer rates.

Age. With a few exceptions, cancer becomes more prevalent in older persons. Over half of all cancers occur in persons age 65 or older.[19] In 2005, cancer surpassed heart disease as the leading cause of death for older adults aged 60 to 80 years and was the second most common cause of death in persons older than age 80.[20] Researchers in both gerontology and oncology continue to explore the relationship between the aging process and the development of cancer. Research in the areas of genetics, carcinogenesis at the cellular level, and immunology, and epidemiologic studies of the association of type and duration of carcinogen exposures and cancer incidence are being conducted to better understand why cancer occurs most often in older people.[21-23]

Demographic predictions indicate that the older population is the fastest growing segment of the population and that by 2020, 1 in 5 Americans will be 65 years old or older, and by 2050, one fourth will be over the age of 65.[24] A corresponding rise in cancer incidence among the elderly is expected. Also, with further

and experimental. *Descriptive studies* are observational in nature and record the existing patterns of disease. Identified trends generate a hypothesis as to the possible cause of the cancer trend. The intermediate step, the *analytic study*, tests the hypothesis and tries to identify the causal relationship. The final step, the decline in deaths from heart disease, cancer will become an even more prominent cause of death in the older population.

Gender. More men develop cancer than women, and more men die from cancer than women. In 2005, 710,040 men and 662,870 women were diagnosed with cancer and 295,280 men and 275,000 women died of the disesase.[3] Gender differences are apparent for certain cancers, such as breast cancer. Breast cancer is common among women and is rare among men, accounting for less than 1% of all breast cancers.[25]

Race and Ethnicity. Cancer incidence and mortality vary among racial and ethnic groups. For all cancer sites combined, African American men have a 24% higher incidence rate and a 40% higher death rate than white men. African American women have a lower incidence rate but a nearly 20% higher death rate than white women for all cancer sites combined. For common cancer sites, incidence and death rates are consistently higher in African Americans than in whites, except for breast cancer (incidence) and lung cancer (mortality) among women. Death rates from prostate, stomach, and cervical cancers among African Americans are more than twice the rates in whites. Factors that contribute to these mortality differences include differences in exposure (e.g. *Helicobacter pylori* for stomach cancer), access to regular screening (breast, cervical, and colorectal cancers), and timely, high quality treatments (many cancers). The higher breast cancer incidence rate of white women is thought to reflect a combination of more frequent mammography, which makes diagnosis more likely, delayed age at first birth, and historically greater use of hormone replacement therapy.[3,26] The higher breast cancer mortality of African American women may be related to a difference in cell cycle–regulatory protein expression[27] or cell cycle abnormalities[28] that have been observed in African American women with breast cancer that cause them to have unfavorable prognostic indicators. Only 10% of white women with breast cancer have high-grade tumors that are estrogen receptor–negative. In comparison, 32% of African American women with breast cancer have tumors with these unfavorable characteristics.[29]

Although racial and ethnic populations present unique opportunities for studying environmental and host differences, there also are many limitations of this type of research. First, racial or ethnic classification has historically been limited to general terms with several ethnic populations grouped together. Newer classifications used by the U.S. Census bureau and the SEER program will provide a better understanding of ethnic differences. However, the problem remains of how people classify themselves by race and/or ethnicity, or are so classified, since many people in the United States are of mixed heritage. In addition, racial and ethnic disparities in cancer incidence and mortality are embedded in larger historical, geographic, sociocultural, economic, and political contexts. For example, a higher mortality rate of a certain ethnic group may be related to socioeconomic circumstances and lack of access to specialized medical care rather than ethnicity.[30]

Other factors. Other "person" or host factors such as general health and wellness status—including nutritional status, cultural and socioeconomic variables, marital status, psychologic factors, and susceptibility factors—help to describe the cancer situation. These variables add to the body of information and may help define the hypothesis of a particular cancer cause.

Place. The evaluation of incidence and mortality statistics for various geographic locales has led to the identification of international similarities and differences in the cancer burden. Cancer is no longer a rare disease in developing countries of the world. The majority of cancers in developed countries are those associated with affluence, such as cancers of the colon and rectum, the breast, and the prostate gland, and these cancers have a good prognosis. In developing countries, cancers of the liver, the stomach, and the esophagus are more common, and all have a poor prognosis. Overall, cancer prognosis is poorer in developing countries, and estimated survival rates there are lower than those for developed countries.[5]

Japan exemplifies a unique cancer spectrum when compared with other countries. The Japanese population has a low international incidence rate of breast cancer and the highest international incidence of stomach cancer. Differing genetic constitutions and social habits may be possible explanations. Japanese women who migrate to Hawaii or California and adopt new habits develop cancer risks similar to American women, with an increase in their breast cancer incidence and a decrease in stomach cancers.[31]

In addition to a specific location, the category of place in descriptive studies also involves physical and biologic environmental variables such as geologic structure, water sources, flora, weather, climate, plants, and animals. Temperature, water consumption, and latitude have been correlated with cancer incidence rates. There is an inverse correlation between cancer incidence rates and temperature and fluoride concentrations in water, and a positive correlation between latitude and cancer incidence rates.[32] Exposure to ultraviolet radiation (sunlight) at higher latitudes is associated with an increased cutaneous melanoma incidence.[33,34]

Time. Evaluating the incidence of cancer over time may indicate significant trends. The increased incidence of mesothelioma throughout the 1970s and early 1980s has been attributed to occupational exposure to asbestos during World War II.[35] Similarly, the well-recognized time trend of mounting lung cancer deaths led to the extensive series of studies that ultimately incriminated cigarette smoking as a principal cause of death for both men and women.[36,37]

Studying descriptive data and incidence trends raises many questions about environmental, geographic, dietary, and sociocultural variables of affected populations. Sources of variability and even sources of nonvariability may serve as an element of hypothesis formulation. Box 3-2 lists factors used in descriptive epidemiologic studies.

ANALYTIC STUDIES

Descriptive epidemiologic studies generate possible causes of disease. These etiologic hypotheses are then tested in the second investigative phase, the analytic study. Analytic epidemiology also assists in further defining risk factors. This type of study is observational in nature, and its purpose is to elucidate which type of exposure causes which kind(s) of cancer.[1] The three types of analytic studies are cross-sectional studies, case-control studies, and cohort studies. The element of *time* distinguishes these types of studies. A cross-sectional study occurs in the present, case-control studies are based on subjects with past exposure (*retrospective*), and cohort studies examine populations who have been exposed to see if they develop the disease in the future (*prospective*).

Cross-Sectional Studies. These studies may also be called *prevalence surveys*. The purpose is to canvas a population of subjects to ascertain a relationship between the disease and variables of interest as they exist in the group at a specific time. The drawback of such a survey is that the causal nature of a relationship

| BOX 3-2 | **Descriptive Epidemiology Factors** |

Frequency
Incidence
Prevalence
Mortality

Disease
Site
Morphology
Grade
Stage

Person
Age
Gender
Race/ethnicity
Relationship status
Nutritional status
Socioeconomic variables
Psychologic factors
Susceptibility factors

Place
Physical environment
Biologic environment
Geographic location

Time
Changes in frequency patterns over specified periods of time

cannot be established, because the design does not allow accounting for the time sequence of events.[1,38,39]

Cohort Design. This type of study examines over time a population or group of individuals with or without a specific exposure to determine their disease incident rate or health outcome or both. When the study is conducted prospectively, it may also be referred to as a *concurrent study.* People selected for a cohort study all have been exposed to the suspected cancer-causing factor. These subjects are followed into the future to evaluate the possible development of cancer.[38,39] For example, to test the hypothesis that tanning in a tanning salon causes skin cancer, two groups of people are followed: a group who tanned in parlors and a group who did not. All subjects are followed over a period of years to determine if the exposed group had a higher incidence of skin cancer. The disease incidence or mortality rates for various levels of exposure (high, medium, low, none) are then compared. If a causal relationship exists between tanning booths and skin cancer, one would expect to see the highest incidence of skin cancer in the sample with the most frequent exposure to tanning beds.

A second type of cohort study is the *historical cohort design,* also called the *historical prospective study.* This design is frequently used in occupational studies because both the exposure and the onset of cancer have already occurred. Information is collected by reviewing records of the sample under study and reconstructing the disease history. It is important in a cohort or prospective study that the time the study begins is clearly identified, that all of the participants are free of cancer when enrolled

in the study, and that all participants are followed the same way. Complete long-term follow-up of all the participants in a cohort study, using medical records, death certificates, and other available resources, is crucial. Prospective studies have the disadvantage of being very large and expensive trials that take an extended period of time to complete.[38,39]

A third type of cohort study is a *migrant study.* Migrant studies take advantage of the wide geographic variation in cancer risk and incidence. Cancer rates from migrants, obtained from routinely collected incidence and mortality statistics, are compared with those in the host country or country of origin; the rate of change with time since migration (or age at migration) and in subsequent generations is assessed, and the results are interpreted in the light of differences in socioeconomic status and degree of cultural assimilation. Rapid changes in cancer risk and incidence following migration imply that lifestyle or environmental factors are of overriding importance in cancer etiology.[1]

Case-Control Design. This method evaluates a case group of persons diagnosed with the cancer under study who have exposure to the suspected cancer-causing agent. This group is compared with a control group chosen from the general population. The case-control design is a retrospective study that evaluates the outcome of past events. This type of study is frequently used because it is quickly implemented and can be performed with even small numbers of cases.[39]

An example of a case-control study is the evaluation of two groups of women—one group with a diagnosis of endometrial cancer and one group without. Both groups are interviewed to determine prior use of estrogens to test the hypothesis that estrogen use causes endometrial cancer. The percentage of women with endometrial cancer who used estrogens is referred to as the exposure frequency. If the exposure frequency is greater in the case group than the control group, the incidence of endometrial cancer after estrogen use is greater than the incidence of endometrial cancer without estrogen use.

Study Analysis. The endpoint of an analytic study is the determination of risk. *Risk* refers to the likelihood that people who are without a disease but who come in contact with certain factors thought to increase the disease risk will acquire the disease.[1] Factors associated with an increased risk of acquiring cancer are *risk factors.* Risk factors may be associated with the environment (e.g., ultraviolet radiation, toxins), personal behavior (e.g., tobacco and alcohol use, sexual practices), or personal history (e.g., genetic changes).

Risk can be calculated as either relative or attributable. *Relative risk* estimates how much the risk of acquiring cancer increases with exposure to a risk factor.[1] Relative risk can also be thought of as the ratio of the rate of cancer between exposed and unexposed persons—the higher the relative risk, the stronger the association between the risk factor and the cancer. A relative risk of 1 means the risk is the same for both groups. Thus a relative risk factor of 10 implies that the risk of acquiring cancer is 10 times greater for an exposed person than an unexposed person. Relative risk ratios are a useful tool for identifying factors that increase risk for developing a particular kind of cancer. Early age of sexual intercourse, multiple sexual partners, and cigarette smoking are known risk factors for developing cervical cancer; women with these behaviors show several times the rate of cervical cancer than women without these behaviors.[40]

Attributable risk describes the expected or normal number of unexposed people who acquire cancer, such as the number of nonsmokers expected to develop lung cancer in a year. Attributable risk is calculated by simply subtracting the rate of incidence in the exposed population from the rate of incidence in the nonexposed population. If a nonsmoking population develops lung cancer at a rate of 200/100,000 and a smoking population develops lung cancer at a rate of 543/100,000, then 343 cases of lung cancer per 100,000 population were caused by smoking and could have been prevented.

EXPERIMENTAL STUDIES

An experimental study modifies host characteristics, makes lifestyle changes, or uses screening to prevent disease. Experimental studies are prospective and often take the form of a randomized clinical trial. Experimental studies may also be called *intervention studies, clinical trials,* or *prophylactic studies.* A *randomized clinical trial* is an experiment involving volunteers that determines which intervention is superior among various alternatives. An example of the experimental study design is the chemoprevention trial, in which an agent is given to achieve regression of a precursor lesion, to prevent cancer recurrence, or to prevent the development of cancer in a high-risk population. An example of a chemoprevention trial is the Breast Cancer Prevention Trial, initiated in 1992 by the NCI and the National Surgical Adjuvant Breast and Bowel Project (NSABP), which found that tamoxifen was effective in significantly reducing the incidence of both invasive and noninvasive breast cancer in women at high risk for the disease.[41]

Causes of Cancer

Because one of the primary purposes of epidemiology is to discover the causes of cancer, the concept of "cause" must be understood. *Sufficient cause* is one that produces the effect. In other words, if sufficient cause existed and were removed, the event would not occur. Since cancer is a complex and multifactorial disease, there is no single sufficient cause whose removal will prevent the disease. What must be examined, then, are various components of sufficient causes. The presence of a component increases the probability of the effect, but other components are required to produce it. Components may be active or passive. Personal susceptibility factors (e.g., genetics, environment, immunity) are *passive components;* carcinogens are *active components.* Each of these component causes is not "complete"; blocking the action of a component cause can make an otherwise sufficient cause become insufficient to produce the effect.[1] Table 3-1 lists a number of environmental causes of cancer, the type of exposure, and the kind of resulting cancer.[42-62] Some of these carcinogenic agents were identified by laboratory research; others were identified by the epidemiologic methods detailed in this chapter.

Conclusion

Examples of cancer-causing agents highlight the role of epidemiology in the cancer problem. Once a cancer-causing agent is identified, steps must be taken to eliminate or limit exposure. This involves public health and government agencies at the local, state, and national levels. Nurses must be knowledgeable about environmental carcinogens not only to answer patients' questions but also to take more accurate health histories and adequately assess high-risk exposures. Oncology nurses can use their knowledge of epidemiology, cancer patterns, and trends to develop educational programs to increase awareness and prevention activity. Screening and detection efforts can be targeted to populations that are at great risk for specific cancers. Familiarity with terminology and epidemiologic methods enables the nurse to interpret medical literature more accurately; new information can be more easily understood and therefore integrated into the personal knowledge base. Nurses can develop a more acute awareness in their practice setting, allowing possible observations of clusters or trends. Curiosity and observation may lead to nursing research questions.

TABLE 3-1	**Environmental Causes of Human Cancer**	
AGENT	**TYPE OF EXPOSURE**	**SITE OF CANCER**
Aflatoxin	Contaminated foodstuffs	Liver
Alkylating agents (melphalan, cyclophosphamide, chlorambucil, semustine)	Medication	Leukemia
Androgen–anabolic steroids	Medication	Liver
Aromatic amines (benzidine, 2-naphthylamine, 4-aminobiphenyl)	Manufacturing of dyes and other chemicals	Bladder
Arsenic (inorganic)	Mining and smelting of certain ores, pesticide manufacturing and use, medication, drinking water	Bladder, lung, skin, liver (angiosarcoma), soft tissue sarcoma
Arylamines	Manufacturing	Bladder
Asbestos	Manufacturing and use	Lung, pleura, peritoneum, renal cell
Benzene	Leather, petroleum, rubber and other industries	Leukemia, lip, lung and bronchus
Bis(chloromethyl)ether	Manufacturing	Lung (small cell)
Chlornaphazine	Medication	Bladder
Chromium compounds	Manufacturing	Lung
Dioxin	Leather industry	Soft tissue sarcoma
Ionizing radiation	Atomic bomb explosions, treatment and diagnosis, radium dial painting, uranium and metal mining	Most sites
Isopropyl alcohol production	Manufacturing by strong acid process	Nasal sinuses
Mustard gas	Manufacturing	Lung, larynx, nasal sinuses

TABLE 3-1	Environmental Causes of Human Cancer—cont'd	
AGENT	**TYPE OF EXPOSURE**	**SITE OF CANCER**
Nickel dust	Refining	Lung, nasal sinuses
Parasites	Infection	
Schistosoma haematobium		Bladder (squamous carcinoma)
Clonorchis (Opisthorchis) sinensis		Liver (cholangiocarcinoma)
Pesticides	Application	Non-Hodgkin's lymphoma, lung
Phenacetin-containing analgesics	Medication	Renal pelvis
Phenoxyherbicides	Application	Soft-tissue sarcoma, non-Hodgkin's lymphoma
Polycyclic hydrocarbons	Coal carbonization products and some mineral oils	Lung, skin (squamous carcinoma)
Radon	Inhalation	Lung
Silica	Manufacturing	Lung
Tobacco smoke	Secondhand ("passive smoking")	Lung
Ultraviolet radiation	Sunlight, sunlamps, tanning beds	Skin (including melanoma), lip
Viruses	Infection	
• Epstein-Barr virus		Burkitt's lymphoma, nasopharyngeal carcinoma, Hodgkin's disease
• Hepatitis B and C viruses		Hepatocellular carcinoma
• Human immunodeficiency virus		Kaposi's sarcoma, non-Hodgkin's lymphoma, Hodgkin's disease, squamous cell carcinoma of conjunctiva, small bowel lymphoma, leiomyosarcoma
• Human papillomavirus		Cervix, other anogenital tumors
• Human T-cell leukemia and/or lymphoma (lymphotrophic) virus type I		T-cell leukemia and/or lymphoma
Vinyl chloride	Manufacturing of polyvinyl chloride	Liver (angiosarcoma), soft tissue sarcoma
Wood dusts	Furniture manufacturing (hardwood)	Nasal sinuses (adenocarcinoma)

Data from references 1, 32, 34–36, 40, 42–62.

REVIEW QUESTIONS

✓ Case Study

Mrs. Smith, age 51, was diagnosed with lung cancer last week. She arrives for her first appointment with her oncologist and is accompanied by her husband and college-aged son and daughter. The oncologist is participating in an epidemiologic study of lung cancer in nonsmokers and informs Mrs. Smith that she is eligible to participate in the study, since she has never smoked.

QUESTIONS

1. The nurse reviews the information about the epidemiology study with Mrs. Smith and her family and explains the endpoint of epidemiologic research:
   a. To prevent cancer
   b. To detect cancer
   c. To cure cancer
   d. To delay the development of cancer
2. Mrs. Smith states that she is the fourth person in her neighborhood to be diagnosed with lung cancer and asks how the National Cancer Institute computes lung cancer incidence. The nurse explains how to calculate cancer incidence:
   a. Divide the number of persons with lung cancer at a given point in time by the total population living at that time.

   b. Divide the number of persons dying of lung cancer in a specified period of time by the total population living at that time.
   c. Divide the number of persons developing lung cancer in a specified period of time by the total population living at that time.
   d. Divide the number of persons developing lung cancer in a specified time by the total population dying of lung cancer a specified period of time.

3. Mrs. Smith's daughter states that she recently saw a newspaper article that stated that over 16,000 cases of lung cancer had been diagnosed in New York City during the past year whereas only 130 had been diagnosed in the rural county where her mother lives. To what can this large difference in number of people diagnosed with lung cancer be attributed?
   a. Differences in lifestyle
   b. Differences in population
   c. Differences in environment
   d. Differences in screening programs
4. Mrs. Smith's son asks, "What is the overall 5-year survival rate for all cancers combined?" The nurse responds by informing the Smith family that the survival rate for adults

Continued

REVIEW QUESTIONS

varies greatly by cancer site and stage at diagnosis, and that current data indicate that the overall relative 5-year survival is the following:
   a. 13%
   b. 21.5%
   c. 46.2%
   d. 62.7%

5. The nurse provides information about lung cancer statistics and tells the Smith family,
   a. "Lung cancer is the most common cancer diagnosed in women."
   b. "Lung cancer is the most common cause of death from cancer in women."
   c. "Lung cancer is the most common cause of death from cancer for women in Mrs. Smith's age group."
   d. "Lung cancer is second to heart disease in causing death in Mrs. Smith age group."

6. Mrs. Smith mentions that her father died from mesothelioma of the lung and asks if her lung cancer is hereditary. To which of the following can the nurse link mesothelioma of the lung, in response?
   a. Smoking
   b. A high-fat diet
   c. Residing in higher latitudes
   d. Occupational exposure to asbestos

7. The nurse explains that the epidemiologic study that Mrs. Smith is eligible for is a case-control study and describes this type of study as the following:
   a. Retrospective
   b. Concurrent
   c. Prospective
   d. Historical

8. The nurse informs the Smith family that the epidemiologic study survey asks questions about passive and active components that influence cancer risk, and gives an example of an active component:
   a. Genetics
   b. Immunity
   c. Environment
   d. Carcinogens

9. The epidemiologic study of lung cancer in nonsmokers that Mrs. Smith is eligible to participate in will obtain information about her exposure to which of the following?
   a. Radon
   b. Dioxin
   c. Aflatoxin
   d. Arylamines

10. The development of lung cancer is associated with which of the following environmental agents?
   a. Wood dust
   b. Phenoxyherbicides
   c. Ultraviolet radiation
   d. Secondhand smoke

ANSWERS

1. **A.** *Rationale:* The goal of cancer epidemiology is to identify causes of cancer so that causative agents may be removed, and ultimately prevent cancer. Early detection studies identify the ways to best detect cancer. Curing cancer is the goal of therapeutic research. Delaying the development of cancer is the goal of chemoprevention and other similar strategies, rather than the goal of epidemiology.

2. **C.** *Rationale:* Cancer incidence is determined by dividing the number of persons developing lung cancer in a specified period of time by the total population living at that time. Dividing the number of persons with lung cancer at a given point in time by the total population living at that time is the calculation used to determine lung cancer prevalence. Dividing the number of persons dying of lung cancer in a specified period of time by the total population living at that time is the calculation used to determine cancer mortality. Dividing the number of persons developing lung cancer in a specified time by the total population dying of lung cancer in a specified period of time is a calculation of lung cancer survival.

3. **B.** *Rationale:* New York City has a much larger population than rural areas; consequently, it has a larger total number of people who have been diagnosed with lung cancer. To determine if the incidence of cancer differs in these areas, the total number of cancers per 100,000 people is examined. Although lifestyle and environmental factors influence cancer incidence, in this case, the reason for the large difference in overall number of lung cancer cases is because of the population differences between the urban and rural areas. Screening programs help detect cancer; they do not influence how many people will develop cancer in a specified period of time.

4. **D.** *Rationale:* The overall relative 5-year survival rate for all types of cancer currently is 62.7%.

5. **B.** *Rationale:* Lung cancer is the most common cause of death from cancer in women. Breast cancer is the most common cancer diagnosed in women. Breast cancer causes the most deaths from cancer in women aged 20 to 59 years. Cancer has surpassed heart disease as the leading cause of death for people younger than 85 years of age.

6. **D.** *Rationale:* Mesothelioma of the lung is linked to occupational exposure to asbestos. Smoking, high-fat diets, and residing in higher latitude areas have been linked to various types of cancer; however, exposure to asbestos is the most common cause of mesothelioma.

7. **A.** *Rationale:* Case-control studies are retrospective. Cross-sectional and cohort studies are concurrent studies. Cohort studies also may be prospective, so choice C also is incorrect. Historical designs are used with cohort studies.

8. **D.** *Rationale:* Carcinogens is an example of an active component. The other choices are all examples of passive components.

9. **A.** *Rationale:* Radon is associated with the development of lung cancer. Dioxin exposure is associated with the development of soft tissue sarcoma. Aflatoxin is associated with cancer of the liver. Arylamines are associated with bladder cancer.

10. **D.** *Rationale:* The development of lung cancer is associated with exposure to secondhand smoke, also known as passive smoking. Wood dust is associated with the development of cancer of the nasal sinuses. Phenoxyherbicides are associated with the development of sarcoma and non-Hodgkin's lymphoma. Ultraviolet radiation is associated with cancers of the skin and lip.

REFERENCES

1. Trichopoulous D, Lipworth L, Petridou E: Epidemiology of cancer. In DeVita VT, Hellman S, Rosenberg SA, editors: *Cancer principles and practice of oncology,* ed 6, Philadelphia, 2001, Lippincott-Raven.
2. Young RH: A brief history of the pathology of the gonads, *Mod Pathol* 18 Suppl 2:S3, 2005.
3. Jemal A, Murray T, Ward E et al: Cancer statistics, 2005, *CA Cancer J Clin* 55:10, 2005.
4. Ries LAG, Eisner MP, Kosary CL et al, editors: *SEER cancer statistics review, 1975-2002,* National Cancer Institute. Bethesda, MD, http://seer.cancer.gov/csr/1975_2002/, based on November 2004 SEER data submission, posted to the SEER website 2005.
5. Parkin DM, Bray F, Ferlay J et al: Global cancer statistics, 2002, *CA Cancer J Clin* 55:74, 2005.
6. National Cancer Institute: Surveillance, epidemiology, and end results program, retrieved May 17, 2005, from http://seer.cancer/gov/about.
7. American College of Surgeons: National cancer database (NCDB) benchmark and survival reports, retrieved May 17, 2005, from http://www.facs.org/cancer/databases.html.
8. National Cancer Institute Statistical Research and Applications Branch: Overview of cancer prevalence statistics, retrieved May 17, 2005, from http://srab.cancer.gov/prevalence/.
9. National Center for Health Statistics: Mortality data from the national vital statistics system, retrieved May 17, 2005, from http://www.cdc.gov/nchs/about/dvs/mortdata.htm.
10. Stewart SL, King JB, Thompson TD et al: Cancer mortality surveillance—United States, 1999-2000, *MMWR Surveill Summ* 53:1, 2004.
11. Brenner H, Hakulinen T: Up-to-date long-term survival curves of patients with cancer by period analysis, *J Clin Oncol* 20:826, 2002.
12. National Cancer Institute: Relative survival, retrieved May 17, 2005, from http://seer.cancer.gov/seerstat/WebHelp/Relative_Survival.htm.
13. Kato I, Severson RK, Schwartz AG: Conditional median survival of patients with advanced carcinoma: surveillance, epidemiology, and end results data, *Cancer* 92:2211, 2001.
14. Gatta G, Capocaccia R, Coleman MP et al: Childhood cancer survival in Europe and the United States, *Cancer* 95:1767, 2002.
15. Smith M, Hare ML: An overview of progress in childhood cancer survival, *J Pediatr Oncol Nurs* 21:160, 2004.
16. National Cancer Institute: National Cancer Institute research on childhood cancers, retrieved May 17, 2005, from http://cis.nci.nih.gov/fact/6_40.htm.
17. Gloeckler Ries LA, Reichman ME, Lewis DR et al: Cancer survival and incidence from the Surveillance, Epidemiology, and End Results (SEER) program, *Oncologist* 8:539, 2003.
18. Jemal A, Devesa SS, Hartge P et al: Recent trends in cutaneous melanoma incidence among whites in the United States, *J Natl Cancer Inst* 93:678, 2001.
19. Denduluri N, Ershler WB: Aging biology and cancer, *Semin Oncol* 31:137, 2004.
20. Twombly R: Cancer surpasses heart disease as leading cause of death for all but the very elderly, *J Natl Cancer Inst* 97:330, 2005.
21. Anisimov VN: Biological interactions of aging and carcinogenesis, *Cancer Treat Res* 124:17, 2005.
22. Ershler WB: The influence of advanced age on cancer occurrence and growth, *Cancer Treat Res* 124:75, 2005.
23. Nejako A, Aranton B, Dix D: Carcinogenesis: a cellular model for age-dependence, *Anticancer Res* 25:1385, 2005.
24. United States Census Bureau: Projected population of the United States, by age and sex: 2000 to 2050, retrieved May 18, 2005, from http://www.census.gov/ipc/www/usinterimproj/natprojtab02a.pdf.
25. Weiss JR, Moysich KB, Swede H: Epidemiology of male breast cancer, *Cancer Epidemiol Biomarkers Prev* 14:20, 2005.
26. Bernstein L, Teal CR, Joslyn S et al: Ethnicity-related variation in breast cancer risk factors, *Cancer* 97(1 Suppl):222, 2003.
27. Porter PL, Lund MJ, Lin MG et al: Racial differences in the expression of cell cycle-regulatory proteins in breast carcinoma. *Cancer* 100:2533, 2004.
28. Cell cycle abnormalities may be key to aggressive breast cancer in African-American women, *Cancer Biol Ther* 3:585, 2004.
29. Chlebowski RT, Chen Z, Anderson GL et al: Ethnicity and breast cancer: factors influencing differences in incidence and outcome, *J Natl Cancer Inst* 97:439, 2005.
30. Williams DR, Jackson PB: Social sources of racial disparities in health, *Health Aff* 24:325, 2005.
31. Imamura Y, Yoshimi I: Comparison of cancer mortality (stomach cancer) in five countries: France, Italy, Japan, UK and USA from the WHO mortality database (1960-2000), *Jpn J Clin Oncol* 35:103, 2005.
32. Steiner GG: Cancer incidence rates and environmental factors: an ecological study, *J Environ Pathol Toxicol Oncol* 21:205, 2002.
33. Eide MJ, Weinstock MA: Association of UV index, latitude, and melanoma incidence in nonwhite populations—US Surveillance, Epidemiology, and End Results (SEER) program, 1992-2001, *Arch Dermatol* 141:477, 2005.
34. Gandini S, Sera F, Cattaruzza MS et al: Meta-analysis of risk factors for cutaneous melanoma: II. Sun exposure, *Eur J Cancer* 41:45, 2005.
35. Jaurand MC, Fleury-Feith J: Pathogenesis of malignant pleural mesothelioma, *Respirology* 10:2, 2005.
36. Ezzati M, Henley SJ, Lopez AD et al: Role of smoking in global and regional epidemiology: current patterns and data needs, *Int J Cancer* early view (articles online in advance of print), retrieved May 18, 2005, from http://www3.interscience.wiley.com/cgi-bin/abstract/110489172/ABSTRACT, published online May 4, 2005.
37. Jemal A, Ward E, Thun MJ: Contemporary lung cancer trends among U.S. women, *Cancer Epidemiol Biomarkers Prev* 14:582, 2005.
38. Diomidus M: Epidemiological study designs, *Stud Health Technol Inform* 65:126, 2002.
39. Enarson DA, Kennedy SM, Miller DL: Choosing a research study design and selecting a population to study, *Int J Tuberc Lung Dis* 8:1151, 2004.
40. Benard VB, Eheman CR, Lawson HW et al: Cervical screening in the National Breast and Cervical Cancer Early Detection Program, *Obstet Gynecol* 103:564, 2004.
41. Wickerham DL: Tamoxifen's impact as a preventive agent in clinical practice and an update on the STAR trial. *Recent Results Cancer Res* 163:37, 2003.
42. Alberg AJ, Brock MV, Samet J.: Epidemiology of lung cancer: looking to the future, *J Clin Oncol* 23:3175, 2005.
43. Baseman JG, Koutsky LA: The epidemiology of human papillomavirus infections, *J Clin Virol* 32(Suppl 1):S16, 2005.
44. Baxter NN, Tepper JE, Durham SB et al: Increased risk of rectal cancer after prostate radiation: a population-based study, *Gastroenterology* 128:319, 2005.
45. Bosch FX, Ribes J, Cleries R et al: Epidemiology of hepatocellular carcinoma, *Clin Liver Dis* 9:191, 2005.
46. Chen J: Estimated risks of radon-induced lung cancer for different exposure profiles based on the new EPA model, *Health Phys* 88:323, 2005.
47. Colditz GA: Epidemiology and prevention of breast cancer, *Cancer Epidemiol Biomarkers Prev* 14:768, 2005.
48. Dobrossy L: Epidemiology of head and neck cancer: magnitude of the problem, *Cancer Metastasis Rev* 24:9, 2005.
49. Dumitrescu RG, Cotarla I: Understanding breast cancer risk—where do we stand in 2005? *J Cell Mol Med* 9:208, 2005.
40. Eide MJ, Weinstock MA: Association of UV index, latitude, and melanoma incidence in nonwhite populations—US Surveillance, Epidemiology, and End Results (SEER) program, 1992-2001, *Arch Dermatol* 141:477, 2005.
51. Gallagher RP, Spinelli JJ, Lee TK: Tanning beds, sunlamps, and risk of cutaneous malignant melanoma, *Cancer Epidemiol Biomarkers Prev* 14:562, 2005.
52. Garner MJ, Turner MC, Ghadirian P et al: Epidemiology of testicular cancer: an overview. *Int J Cancer*, early view (articles online in advance of print), retrieved May 16, 2005, from http://www3.interscience.wiley.com/cgi-bin/abstract/110438953/ABSTRACT, published online April 7, 2005.
53. Hessel PA, Gamble JF, McDonald JC: Asbestos, asbestosis, and lung cancer: a critical assessment of the epidemiological evidence, *Thorax* 60:433, 2005.
54. Jaga K, Dharmani C: The epidemiology of pesticide exposure and cancer: a review, *Rev Environ Health* 20:15, 2005.
55. Krewski D, Lubin JH, Zielinski JM et al: Residential radon and risk of lung cancer: a combined analysis of 7 North American case-control studies, *Epidemiology* 16:137, 2005.
56. McGlynn KA, London WT: Epidemiology and natural history of hepatocellular carcinoma, *Best Pract Res Clin Gastroenterol* 19:3, 2005.
57. Papapolychroniadis C: Environmental and other risk factors for colorectal carcinogenesis, *Tech Coloproctol* 8(Suppl 1):S7, 2004.
58. Polednak AP: Recent trends in the incidence rates for selected alcohol-related cancers in the United States, *Alcohol Alcohol* 40:234, 2005.
59. Saladi RN, Persaud AN: The causes of skin cancer: a comprehensive review, *Drugs Today* 41:37, 2005.

60. Sorahan T, Kinlen LJ, Doll R: Cancer risks in a historical UK cohort of benzene exposed workers, *Occup Environ Med* 62:231, 2005.

61. Vasn Maele-Fabry G, Willems JL: Prostate cancer among pesticide applicators: a meta-analysis, *Int Arch Occup Environ Health* 77:559, 2004.

62. Vineis P, Airoldi L, Veglia P et al: Environmental tobacco smoke and risk of respiratory cancer and chronic obstructive pulmonary disease in former smokers and never smokers in the EPIC prospective study, *BMJ* 330:277, 2005.

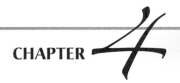

CHAPTER 4

Prevention, Screening, and Detection

Robin L. Coyne and Helene Mohamed

Cancer continues to be second only to cardiovascular disease as a leading cause of death in the United States. The American Cancer Society (ACS) estimates that 1,399,790, new cancer cases will be diagnosed in 2006. This figure excludes more than 1 million basal and squamous cell carcinoma of the skin and all carcinoma in situ diagnoses, with the exception of carcinoma in situ of the bladder. Approximately 564,830 Americans, or 1,500 individuals per day, are expected to die of cancer this year. One in 4 deaths is cancer related.[1,2] The ACS estimates of cancer incidence and mortality for 2006 are outlined in Fig. 4-1.

Prevention of human cancers is a major focus in education and research as America forges through the new millennium. Despite advances in cancer screening techniques and treatment of cancers, overall mortality statistics exceed desired outcomes. A number of health care agencies have an interest in cancer control and promoting healthy lifestyle. The U.S. Department of Health and Human Services (DHHS) *Healthy People 2010* objectives identified two overarching goals: increase quality and years of healthy life, and eliminate health disparities.[3] Within the context of these goals, DHHS has identified 28 health and illness focus areas, which are outlined in Box 4-1. Cancer is the third focus area; the goal is to reduce the number of cancer cases as well as illness, disability, and death caused by cancer. These reductions can be achieved by smoking cessation, diet modification, early detection of cancer through screening, use of chemoprevention agents, and state-of-the art cancer treatments. In 2004, the ACS, the American Heart Association, and the American Diabetes Association collaborated to promote a preventive health agenda designed to reduce morbidity and mortality associated with cancer, heart disease, and diabetes. Together the agencies seek to reduce the prevalence of tobacco use, poor nutrition, and sedentary lifestyle. These risk factors negatively affect Americans by increasing disease burden and mortality related to cancer, heart disease, and diabetes. Together these agencies lobby for federal funding to support primary prevention programs and clinical interventions designed to meet their goals.[4]

Cancer Prevention Guidelines

Primary prevention is aimed at measures to ensure that the cancer never develops, whereas secondary prevention is aimed at detecting and treating the cancer early, during the most curable stage. Neoplastic transformation in the development of human cancers is a multistep process involving three sequences of events: initiation, promotion, and progression. Prevention, screening, and early detection are among the best strategies available to interrupt the multistep neoplastic process in an effort to conquer cancer. Regularly scheduled cancer screenings by health care professionals can result in detection of cancers of the breast, the colon, the rectum, the cervix, the prostate, the testis, the oral cavity, and the skin at an early stage when the outcomes are likely to be most positive for the patient. Several chemopreventive agents have been found to effectively reduce cancer risk and are currently in use. Research on nutritional supplements and pharmaceutical agents with potential cancer prevention benefits is ongoing and promising. Vaccines are being designed to prevent cancer. Immunization may, one day, result in the elimination of certain cancers. Further reductions in cancer incidence may be achieved through elimination of occupational and environmental risks and changes in lifestyle, focusing on healthy choices in diet and exercise. Early diagnosis is crucial to reducing the morbidity and mortality associated with cancer. Table 4-1 shows trends in 5-year survival rates for multiple cancer sites. Data from 1995-2000 reveal a statistically significant ($p < 0.05\%$) improvement in 5-year survival for all cancer sites as compared to the proceeding 20 years. Mortality rates for lung, colon and rectal, female breast, and prostate cancer continue to decrease over time.[1]

The majority of risk factors that place humans at risk for developing cancer are modifiable. The ACS estimates that 80% of all cancers may be associated with environmental exposures and are potentially preventable, and that one third of all cancer deaths in 2006 will be directly related to tobacco use, poor nutrition, and physical inactivity resulting in obesity.[5] Table 4-2 presents site-specific guidelines related to cancer risk factors, signs and symptoms, screening, and early detection.

Socioeconomic Factors, Diversity, and Cancer Disparities

Disparity in cancer incidence and mortality exist among racial and ethnic groups in the United States. African Americans suffer a disproportionate rate of cancer and cancer-related death. African Americans have the highest mortality rate for all cancer sites relative to all other ethnic groups.[7,15] Differences in cancer incidence, mortality, and survival among minority Americans are disproportionately high for most cancer sites when compared with the majority of Americans. Table 4-3 describes cancer incidence and mortality rates by race and ethnic group.[2] Barriers to primary prevention and health care are reported as major factors in the differences in cancer incidence, delayed diagnosis, poor survival statistics, and increased mortality from cancer in minority and socioeconomically disadvantaged (SED) populations.

Poverty is the leading predictor of cancer disparities. Socioeconomic status has a greater influence on cancer rates and mortality than biologic or inherited characteristics related to race.[16] Minority groups are more likely than whites to be of a

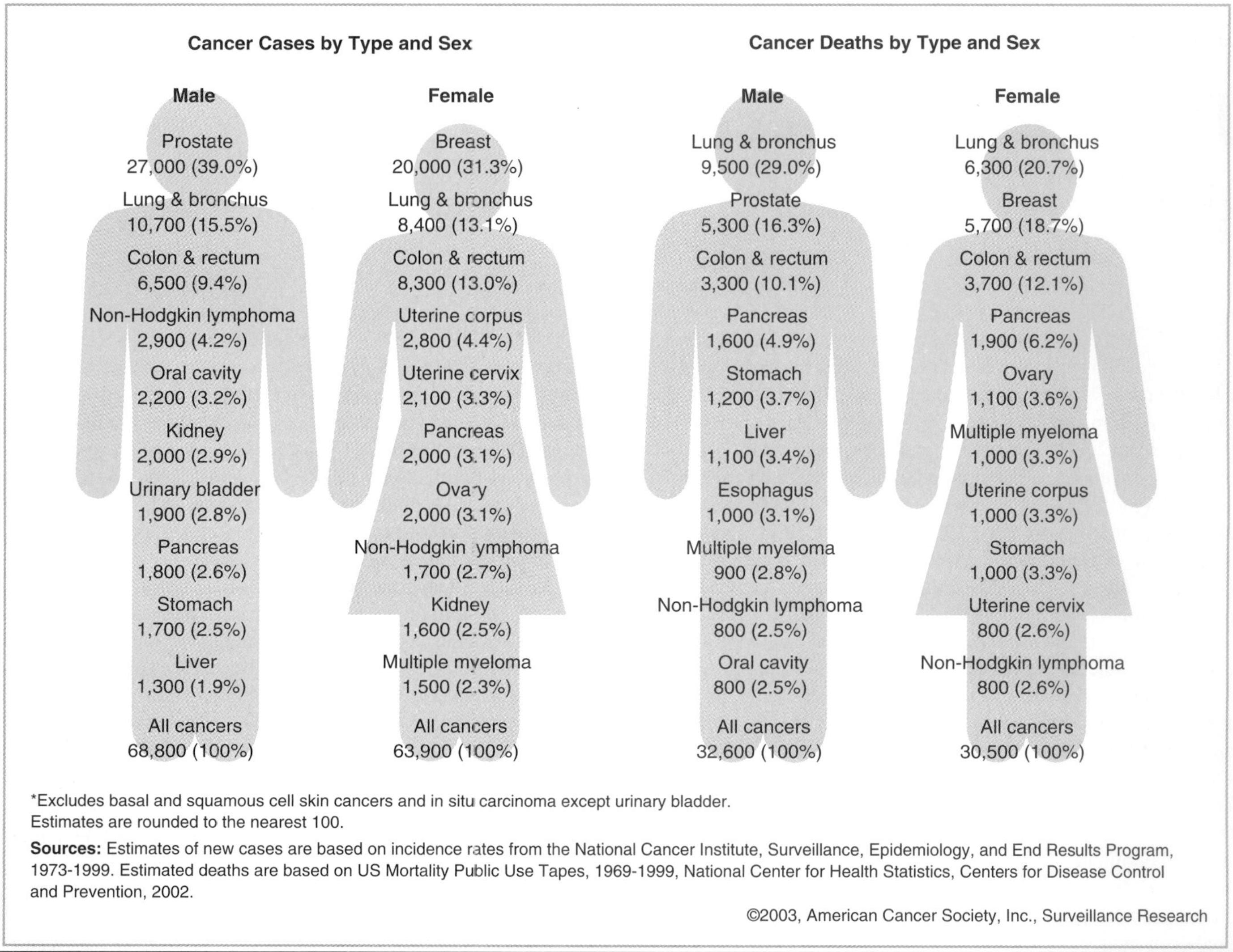

Cancer Cases by Type and Sex

Male	Female
Prostate 27,000 (39.0%)	Breast 20,000 (31.3%)
Lung & bronchus 10,700 (15.5%)	Lung & bronchus 8,400 (13.1%)
Colon & rectum 6,500 (9.4%)	Colon & rectum 8,300 (13.0%)
Non-Hodgkin lymphoma 2,900 (4.2%)	Uterine corpus 2,800 (4.4%)
Oral cavity 2,200 (3.2%)	Uterine cervix 2,100 (3.3%)
Kidney 2,000 (2.9%)	Pancreas 2,000 (3.1%)
Urinary bladder 1,900 (2.8%)	Ovary 2,000 (3.1%)
Pancreas 1,800 (2.6%)	Non-Hodgkin lymphoma 1,700 (2.7%)
Stomach 1,700 (2.5%)	Kidney 1,600 (2.5%)
Liver 1,300 (1.9%)	Multiple myeloma 1,500 (2.3%)
All cancers 68,800 (100%)	All cancers 63,900 (100%)

Cancer Deaths by Type and Sex

Male	Female
Lung & bronchus 9,500 (29.0%)	Lung & bronchus 6,300 (20.7%)
Prostate 5,300 (16.3%)	Breast 5,700 (18.7%)
Colon & rectum 3,300 (10.1%)	Colon & rectum 3,700 (12.1%)
Pancreas 1,600 (4.9%)	Pancreas 1,900 (6.2%)
Stomach 1,200 (3.7%)	Ovary 1,100 (3.6%)
Liver 1,100 (3.4%)	Multiple myeloma 1,000 (3.3%)
Esophagus 1,000 (3.1%)	Uterine corpus 1,000 (3.3%)
Multiple myeloma 900 (2.8%)	Stomach 1,000 (3.3%)
Non-Hodgkin lymphoma 800 (2.5%)	Uterine cervix 800 (2.6%)
Oral cavity 800 (2.5%)	Non-Hodgkin lymphoma 800 (2.6%)
All cancers 32,600 (100%)	All cancers 30,500 (100%)

*Excludes basal and squamous cell skin cancers and in situ carcinoma except urinary bladder. Estimates are rounded to the nearest 100.

Sources: Estimates of new cases are based on incidence rates from the National Cancer Institute, Surveillance, Epidemiology, and End Results Program, 1973-1999. Estimated deaths are based on US Mortality Public Use Tapes, 1969-1999, National Center for Health Statistics, Centers for Disease Control and Prevention, 2002.

FIG. 4-1   Leading site of new cancer cases and deaths—2006. (From American Cancer Society: *Cancer facts and figures, 2006* Atlanta, 2006, Author. Copyright 2006 American Cancer Society, Inc. Reprinted with permission.)

lower educational level and live in poverty. Poverty is a proxy for other elements of living, including lack of education, unemployment, substandard housing, inadequate nutrition, risk-promoting behaviors and life-style, and limited or no access to health care.[2,3,7,17-18] Differences in survival for African American and SED (poor) populations largely result from the late stage of cancer diagnosis. The disproportionate distribution of African Americans at lower socioeconomic levels accounts for a large percentage of their excess cancer burden. It is, therefore, imperative for health care professionals to target SED and minority populations with culturally sensitive and relevant educational information on cancer prevention, risk reduction, and early detection and to legislate for changes in health care policies to facilitate access to health care for all Americans.

Secondary prevention activities serve to identify cancers at an early stage, reduce cancer burden, and improve survival outcomes. Limited access to cancer screening tests has a negative impact on stage of diagnosis, morbidity, and mortality rates. While cancer screening is widely recommended for colorectal, female breast,

cervix, and prostate cancer, the proportion of cancers in these sites identified in an early stage is significantly lower in high-poverty areas. Table 4-4 summarizes the differences in stage of diagnosis among ethnic groups. In 2000, the National Health Interview Survey examined trends in cancer control and cancer screening activities among ethnic and socioeconomic groups, examining data collected between 1987 and 2000. A twofold increase in "recent use" of mammogram was reported during the late 1980s and early 1990s. Almost 80% of women in the United States reported having a Pap smear performed at least once in the previous 3 years. Colorectal cancer screening by fecal occult blood testing (FOBT), sigmoidoscopy, or digital rectal examination increased modestly through 1998. Fecal occult blood testing use increased from 18% to 29% for men and 21% to 26% for women in 1987 as compared to 1998.[19]

Despite increased mammogram screening, chronic disparity in utilization continues to separate ethnic groups. In 2000, 72% of white women, 68.2% of African Americans, 62.6% of Hispanic or Latinas, 52.4% of American Indians or Alaska Natives, and

Healthy People 2010 Focus Areas

1. Access to quality health services
2. Arthritis, osteoporosis, and chronic back conditions
3. Cancer
4. Chronic kidney disease
5. Diabetes
6. Disability and secondary conditions
7. Educational and community-based programs
8. Environmental health
9. Family planning
10. Food safety
11. Health communication
12. Heart disease and stroke
13. Human immunodeficiency virus (HIV)
14. Immunization and infectious diseases
15. Injury and violence prevention
16. Maternal, infant, and child health
17. Medical product safety
18. Mental health and mental disorders
19. Nutrition and overweight
20. Occupational safety and health
21. Oral health
22. Physical activity and fitness
23. Public health infrastructure
24. Respiratory diseases
25. Sexually transmitted diseases
26. Substance abuse
27. Tobacco use
28. Vision and hearing

From U.S. Department of Health and Human Services: *Healthy people 2010: understanding and improving health*, Washington, DC, 2000, U.S. Government Printing Office, No. 012-00-00543-6, www.health.gov/healthypeople.

57.0% of Asian Americans ages 40 years and older received a screening mammogram within the last 2 years. The greatest disparity in mammogram screening for breast cancer occurred in women who lacked health insurance (39.5%) and in immigrant women (41.4%). These same trends were evident for cervical cancer screening, prostate-specific antigen (PSA) testing, and colorectal cancer screening.[5]

The Institute of Medicine (IOM) was charged by Congress in 1999 to assess racial and ethnic inequalities in health care when factors such as health insurance and ability to pay for health care were comparable. Over 100 research studies were reviewed. Ethnic groups were found to differ in their response to medical interventions and help-seeking behavior. Minorities were more likely to delay health care than whites. Approximately 3% to 6% of all African Americans were likely to reject medical recommendations for treatment. Conversely, overt and subtle biases among health care providers were shown to negatively affect the quality of health care received by minorities. Cultural and linguistic barriers to health care exist. Some clinicians may find it difficult to effectively relate to minority clients. Clinical encounters may be further clouded by stereotypes and beliefs about ethnic behavior. Diagnostic and treatment recommendations made by health care providers often differed by the race or ethnicity of the client.[20] The IOM recommends strategies to

reduce health care disparities among ethnic groups. Health care education should foster awareness of prejudices and cultural and social factors that contribute to health care disparities. Standardized data on ethnic and racial health care practices would also improve research capabilities and outcomes.[21]

The ACS and National Cancer Institute (NCI) are promoting nationwide cancer education, screening, and early detection initiatives, targeting African Americans, Hispanic/Latinos, Asian Americans, and Pacific Islanders, as well as American Indians and the underserved or SED populations. The second goal of *Healthy People 2010* is to eliminate health disparities for the population as a whole.[3] The ACS challenge for 2015 is to eliminate cancer disparities through equal access to cancer prevention and education, early detection, diagnosis, and treatment of cancer despite race, gender, or ethnic background.[16] Research endeavors, advocacy, education, and community involvement are considered key components to success. Table 4-5 outlines selected programs and resources targeting cancer disparities.[16]

Environmental Risks

The U.S. Food and Drug Administration (FDA), the Environmental Protection Agency (EPA), the Nuclear Regulatory Commission, and the Occupational Safety and Health Administration (OSHA) are responsible for setting public safety standards. To protect the public from unnecessary cancer risk, carcinogen exposure in the general population is limited to levels that do not increase the risk for cancer by greater than one case per 1 million persons over a lifetime. Chemicals such as benzene, asbestos, vinyl chloride, and arsenic are known carcinogens in humans. Arsenic and benzene are considered carcinogens for leukemia, respiratory, and gastrointestinal cancers. Mesothelioma, a rare lung cancer, is typically related to occupational asbestos exposure. Vinyl chloride is a known liver carcinogen.[2,22]

Cancer risks associated with certain pesticides have been unproven. In high doses, certain chemicals used in the agricultural industry have been shown to cause cancer in animals. Low doses found on fruits and vegetables have not been associated with increased cancer risk. Consumption of these food products does not increase the risk for cancer development in the general population, although industrial farm workers exposed to greater concentrations of pesticides may be at higher risk for certain cancers.[2]

Recent immigrants to the United States have a higher prevalence of *Helicobacter pylori* infections and chronic hepatitis B that results in higher rates of stomach and liver cancer, respectively, in Hispanic/Latinos and Asian Americans.[7,16] Gastric infection with *H. pylori* may result in chronic inflammation or atrophy of gastric cells that can lead to gastric adenocarcinoma.[23,24] Risk factors for primary liver cancer include infection with the hepatitis B and C viruses as well as exposure to aflatoxin, heavy alcohol consumption, and use of oral contraception and anabolic steroids.[23] Human papilloma virus (HPV) DNA has been isolated in cervical cancers. High-risk HPV strains 16, 18, 31, and 45 are strongly associated with cervical cancer development. Of all women with squamous cell carcinoma of the cervix, 90% to 95% were found to have been infected with HPV, type 16 being the most common.[23]

There are three types of radiation: high-frequency ionizing radiation (IR), ultraviolet (UV) radiation, and nonionizing radiation. Both IR and UV radiation cause cancer in humans. Exposure to moderate- or high-dose IR radiation, radon gas, and atomic energy can result in increased risk for leukemia, thyroid, breast,

| TABLE 4-1 | Trends in 5-Year Relative Survival Rates*(%) by Race and Year of Diagnosis, United States, 1974-2001 |

	RELATIVE 5-YEAR SURVIVAL RATE (%)								
	WHITE			AFRICAN AMERICAN			ALL RACES		
Site	1974-76	1983-85	1995-2001	1974-76	1983-85	1995-2001	1974-76	1983-85	1995-2001
All cancers	51	54	66†	39	40	56†	50	53	65†
Brain	22	26	33†	26	32	38†	22	27	33†
Breast (female)	75	79	90†	63	64	76†	75	78	88†
Colon	51	58	65†	46	49	55†	50	58	64†
Esophagus	5	9	16†	4	6	10†	5	8	15†
Hodgkin lymphoma	72	79	86†	69	78	80†	71	79	85†
Kidney	52	56	65†	49	55	64†	52	56	65†
Larynx	66	68	68	60	55	51	66	67	66
Leukemia	35	42	49†	31	34	38	34	41	48†
Liver#	4	6	9†	1	4	5†	4	6	9†
Lung and bronchus	13	14	16†	11	11	13†	12	14	15†
Melanoma of the skin	81	85	92†	67‡	74§	76‡	80	85	92†
Multiple myeloma	24	27	32†	28	31	33	25	28	32†
Non-Hodgkin lymphoma	48	54	61†	48	45	52	47	54	60†
Oral cavity	55	56	62†	36	35	40	54	54	59†
Ovary¶	37	40	44†	41	42	38	37	41	45†
Pancreas	3	3	4†	3	5	4†	3	3	4†
Prostate	68	76	100†	58	64	97†	67	75	100†
Rectum	49	56	65†	42	44	56†	49	55	65†
Stomach	15	16	21†	16	19	23†	15	17	23†
Testis	79	91	96†	76‡	88‡	88	79	91	96†
Thyroid	92	93	97†	88	91	95	92	93	97†
Urinary bladder	74	78	83†	48	60	64†	73	78	82†
Uterine cervix	70	71	75†	64	61	66	69	69	73†
Uterine corpus	89	85	86†	62	55	62	88	83	84†

*Survival rates are adjusted for normal life expectancy and are based on cases diagnosed 1974-1976, 1983-1985, and 1995-2001, and followed through 2002.
†The difference in rates between 1974-1976 and 1995-2001 is statistically significant ($p < 0.05$).
‡The standard error of the survival rate is between 5 and 10 percentage points.
§The standard error of the survival rate is greater than 10 percentage points.
¶Recent changes in classification of ovarian cancer, namely excluding borderline tumors, have affected 1995-2001 survival rates.
#Includes intrahepatic bile duct.
Source: Surveillance, Epidemiology, and End Results Program, 1975-2002, Division of Cancer Control and Population Sciences, Bethesda, MD, 2005, National Cancer Institute.
From American Cancer Society, *Cancer Facts and Figures, 2006*, Atlanta, 2006, Author.
Copyright 2006 American Cancer Society, Inc. Reprinted with permission.

and lung cancer, especially when exposure occurs at a young age. High-energy IR creates an electrically charged ion that damages DNA at the cellular level, through either direct interaction between radiation and DNA or by creating reactive free radicals. Poorly repaired DNA or cell death may result. Modifications in DNA cells that result in irreversible damage, without cell death, ultimately lead to malignancy.[25,26]

The sun is the primary source of natural UV light exposure that is known to cause skin cancer. The three types of skin cancers are basal cell, squamous cell, and melanoma.[25] Melanoma is the most potentially lethal of the three. Since the 1970s, the incidence of melanoma has been increasing by 6% per year. The ACS estimates that 62,190 new cases of melanoma and more than 1 million cases of basal or squamous cell cancers will occur in 2006. Approximately, 10,710 deaths are expected, 7910 from melanoma and 2280 from nonepithelial skin cancer.[2]

Skin cancer rates are 10 times higher in whites than in African Americans.[2] At greatest risk for developing skin cancer are persons with a history or a family history of melanoma, or persons who are naturally blond or red-headed with fair skin, making them susceptible to severe sunburn. Persons working outdoors or experiencing occupational exposure to coal tar, arsenic compounds, and radium are more likely to develop melanoma.[22] Among African Americans the incidence of skin cancer development is low because of heavier skin pigmentation.

The UV rays of the sun are strongest between 10 AM and 4 PM. Sun exposure should be limited during those hours and protective clothing (i.e., hats, scarves, long sleeves) worn to offer some protection from the UV rays. Children should be especially protected because of the link between severe sunburn in childhood and greatly increased risk of melanoma in later life.[2] Sunscreens should be worn when deliberate sun exposure is expected (i.e., when poolside or on the beach). A sunscreen with a sun protection factor (SPF) of 15 or higher should be worn on all sun-exposed skin surfaces. Sunscreens protect against a spectrum of UV rays and should be applied before sun exposure and

Text continued on page 52

TABLE 4-2   Site-Specific Cancer Risk, Screening, and Early Detection Guidelines

SITE	ASSOCIATED RISK FACTORS	SIGNS AND SYMPTOMS	SCREENING AND DETECTION
Biliary tract (gallbladder and bile ducts)	Older Americans (ages 60s to 70s) Female predominance Higher in white women than African American women Chronic infection with liver parasites (*Clonorchis sinensis*) Eating raw or pickled freshwater fish from Southeast Asia Chronic ulcerative colitis	Pruritus Jaundice Abdominal pain Nausea and vomiting Fever Malaise Enlarged liver Palpable mass in upper right quadrant Lower extremity edema Ascites	Physical examination Ultrasound
Bladder	Occupational exposure (e.g., textiles, rubber) Cigarette smoking Chronic bladder infections	Microscopic or gross hematuria Dysuria Bladder irritability Urinary urgency, frequency, and hesitancy	Urinalysis Urine cytology Physical examination Cystoscopy
Brain	Environmental exposures (e.g., vinyl chlorides) Epstein-Barr virus	Persistent generalized headache Vomiting Seizures Loss of fine motor control Unsteady gait Change in personality Lethargy Slurring of speech Loss of memory Impaired vision	Physical examination Prompt follow-up with onset of signs and symptoms
Breast	Previous history of cancer (colon, thyroid, endometrial, ovary, breast) Obesity High fat intake Family history of breast cancer Exposure to ionizing radiation before age 35 Early menarche Late menopause Nulliparity First pregnancy after age 30	Painless mass or thickening in breast or axilla Skin dimpling, puckering, or nipple retraction Nipple discharge or scaliness Edema (peau d'orange) Erythema ulceration Change in size, contour, or shape of breast	Consist of three modalities[21]: 1. Breast self awareness. 2. Clinical examination ages 20-40: every 3 years; over 40: every year 3. Annual mammography: over 40. Baseline mammogram at age 25 recommended for genetically predisposed women Ultrasound Magnetic resonance imaging Image guided fine-needle aspiration or core needle biopsy Genetic testing: *BRCA* genes
Central nervous system	Unknown etiology Speculated to be related to genetic disorders	Headache Nausea and vomiting Edema Loss of fine motor coordination Unsteady gait Seizures Vision and speech problems	No effective screening measures Family history Computed tomography scan of brain Magnetic resonance imaging Cerebrospinal fluid analysis Tumor markers α-Fetoprotein β-Human chorionic gonadotropin
Cervix	Early age at first intercourse (before age 20) Multiple sex partners Smoking Human papillomavirus infection (condylomata acuminata, warts) Herpes simplex virus type 2 Diet	Abnormal vaginal bleeding Persistent postcoital spotting	Papanicolaou (Pap) test Pelvic examination Colposcopy

Continued

TABLE 4-2   Site-Specific Cancer Risk, Screening, and Early Detection Guidelines—cont'd

SITE	ASSOCIATED RISK FACTORS	SIGNS AND SYMPTOMS	SCREENING AND DETECTION
Colon and rectum	Colorectal polyps(s) Diets high in fat Diets low in fiber Genetic component: • Familial polyposis • Gardner's syndrome • Peutz–Jeghers syndrome • Inflammatory bowel disease • Crohn's disease • Ulcerative colitis	Depend on location of tumor: Right colon • Anemia • Gastrointestinal bleeding • Persistent lower abdominal pain • Right lower quadrant mass Left colon • Gross blood in stool • Decrease in stool caliber • Change in bowel habits, constipation, diarrhea Rectum • Hematochezia • Tenesmus • Feeling of incomplete evacuation • Rectal pain (late sign) • Prolapse of tumor	Digital rectal examination (DRE), annually after age 40 Stool occult blood testing, annually from age 50 Flexible sigmoidoscopy Double-contrast barium enema Colonoscopy (See Table 4-8 for frequency of these tests/procedures)
Endometrium	Postmenopause High socioeconomic status Nulliparity Obesity: >50 pounds over ideal body weight Prolonged use of exogenous estrogen without supplemental progesterone Tamoxifen citrate High fat intake Diabetes Hypertension Stein–Leventhal syndrome (failure to ovulate and infertility–polycystic ovaries) Menstrual aberration	Early sign • Abnormal vaginal bleeding Late signs • Pain in pelvis, legs, or back • General weakness • Weight loss	Endometrial biopsy
Esophagus	Men (50-70 years old) Nitrosamines and ethanol consumption Cigarette smoking Precancerous lesions Achalasia (failure of lower esophagus to relax with swallowing) Combined smoking and drinking Barrett's esophagus (chronic gastric reflux)	Early • Dysphagia • Weight loss • Regurgitation • Aspiration • Odynophagia (pain on swallowing) • Gastroesophageal reflux Advanced • Left supraclavicular adenopathy • Chronic cough • Choking after eating • Massive hemoptysis • Hematemesis • Hoarseness	Double-contrast barium swallow Esophagoscopy with staining techniques Brush biopsy Radioisotopes in tumor scanning
Head and neck	Tobacco (inhaled or chewed) Ethyl alcohol Combination of tobacco and alcohol	Mouth and oral cavity • Swelling • Ulcer that does not heal	Semiannual dental/oral examination Awareness of signs and symptoms

TABLE 4-2	Site-Specific Cancer Risk, Screening, and Early Detection Guidelines—cont'd		
SITE	**ASSOCIATED RISK FACTORS**	**SIGNS AND SYMPTOMS**	**SCREENING AND DETECTION**
	Poor oral hygiene Wood dust inhalation Nickel exposure Leukoplakia	Nose and sinuses • Pain • Swelling • Bloody nasal discharge • Nasal obstruction • Salivary glands • Painless swelling • Unilateral facial paralysis Hypopharynx • Dysphagia • Persistent earache • Lymphadenopathy Nasopharynx • Double vision • Hearing loss • Loss of smell • Hoarseness • Adenopathy Larynx • Hoarseness • Difficulty breathing	CAUTION—Seven warning signs: Change in bowel or bladder habits A sore that does not heal Unusual bleeding or discharge Thickening or lump in the breast or elsewhere Indigestion or difficulty in swallowing Obvious change in wart or mole Nagging cough or hoarseness
Human immunodeficiency virus/acquired immunodeficiency syndrome (HIV/AIDS)–related (Kaposi's sarcoma [KS])	All age-groups Homosexual or bisexual men highest risk Intravenous drug users Unprotected sexual contact Multiple sex partners	Multifocal, widespread lesions on skin (face, extremities, torso) Persistent intermittent fever Weight loss, diarrhea Malaise, fatigue Severe cellular immune deficiency Generalized lymphadenopathy Respiratory infections: • *Pneumocystis carinii* • Tuberculosis Difficulty breathing Oral lesions Enlarged liver and spleen	High-risk group Appearance of skin lesions HIV serum testing Oral examination
Leukemia • Acute	Men at higher risk than women Whites at higher risk than African Americans Exposure to radiation Exposure to toxic organic chemicals (e.g., benzene) Drugs (e.g., alkylating agents, chloramphenicol)	Low-grade fever Anemia, pallor Lymphadenopathy Generalized weakness Frequent infections Easy bruising Bleeding (nose, gums) Petechiae on lower extremities Bone and joint pain	Complete blood count Platelet count Physical examination
• Chronic	Benzene exposure High-dose radiation Philadelphia chromosome	Lymphadenopathy Splenomegaly Weight loss Night sweats Malaise, weakness Recurrent infections, fever Early satiety	
Liver	Exposure to aflatoxin Environmental exposures Viral hepatitis More frequent in males	Early • Bloating • Abdominal pain • Fever • Weight loss • Decreased appetite • Nausea	Annual physical examination Awareness of risk factors Ultrasound Computed tomography scan Magnetic resonance imaging

Continued

TABLE 4-2	Site-Specific Cancer Risk, Screening, and Early Detection Guidelines—cont'd		
SITE	**ASSOCIATED RISK FACTORS**	**SIGNS AND SYMPTOMS**	**SCREENING AND DETECTION**
	Alcoholic cirrhosis Parasitic infestation Chronic venous obstruction Paraneoplastic syndromes Anabolic steroid use	Advanced • Jaundice • Ascites • Extreme weight loss • Anorexia	
Lung	Cigarette smoking (active, passive) Increase in age Asbestos Occupational exposure among miners Air pollution (e.g., benzopyrenes, hydrocarbons) Genetic predisposition Vitamin A deficiency	Nagging cough Dull ache in the chest Recurrent or persistent upper respiratory infection Wheezing Dyspnea Hemoptysis Change in volume, color, and odor of sputum	Chest x-ray Computed tomography scan Positron emission tomography scan
Lymphoma • Hodgkin's	Epstein-Barr virus Higher socioeconomic status Small family	Persistent swelling or painless lymph nodes (neck, axilla) Recurrent fevers Night sweats Weight loss Pruritus Cough, shortness of breath Leukocytosis	Physical examination Complete blood count
• Non-Hodgkin's	Occupational exposure (flour and agricultural industries) Abnormalities of immune system HIV Exposure to radiation or chemotherapy	Lymphadenopathy Fatigue Fever, chills Night sweats Decreased appetite Weight loss	
Multiple myeloma	Older Americans (sixth and seventh generation) High levels of immunoglobulin (B cells) African Americans at significantly increased risk than whites (14:1)	Early • Anemia • Fatigue • Bone pain (back, legs) • Weakness • Unexplained bleeding (nose, gums) • Recurrent upper respiratory infection Advanced • Hypercalcemia • Pathologic fractures	Annual physical examination Radiologic tests

Ovary	Familial disposition
	Late menopause
	Nulliparity
	First pregnancy after age 30
		Early
		• Vague abdominal discomfort
		• Dyspepsia
		• Flatulence
		• Bloating
		• Digestive disturbance
		Advanced
		• Abdominal distention
		• Pain
		• Abdominal and pelvic masses
		• Ascites
		• Lower extremity edema
			Pelvic ultrasonography (with vaginal probe)
			Elevated serum markers:
			  Carcinoembryonic antigen (CEA)
			  CA-125 antigen
			
			Genetic testing: *BRCA* genes

Pancreas	Older men Smoking Chronic pancreatitis	Early • Hypoglycemia • Weight loss, anorexia	Blood glucose test Physical examination Abdominal ultrasound

TABLE 4-2   Site-Specific Cancer Risk, Screening, and Early Detection Guidelines—cont'd

SITE	ASSOCIATED RISK FACTORS	SIGNS AND SYMPTOMS	SCREENING AND DETECTION
	Ethanol consumption	• Abdominal pain • Cramping pain associated with diarrhea • Pruritus	Abdominal CT c/FNA Endoscopic retrograde cholangionpancreatography (ERCP)
	Diabetes	Advanced • Jaundice • Ascites • Lower extremity edema	
Prostate	Occupational exposure Cadmium, heavy metals, chemicals Age (median age of incidence, 70 years) Increased fat intake African American median age 45	Early • Difficult starting urinary stream • Unexplained cystitis • Urinary bleeding • Dribbling • Bladder retention Advanced • Bladder outlet obstruction • Urinary retention • Ureteral obstruction with anuria • Azotemia • Uremia • Anorexia • Hematuria • Bone pain	DRE Prostate-specific antigen (PSA) Biochemical markers Transrectal ultrasound (TRUS)
Skin (nonmelanoma)	Fair-skinned, freckles Blonde hair, blue eyes Sun exposure Severe sunburn in childhood Familial conditions Previous skin cancers History of dysplastic nevi	Changes in wart or mole Sore that does not heal ABCDs of skin cancer: • A—Asymmetry (change in size and shape) • B—Border irregularity • C—Color (change in color) • D—Diameter (> than 6 mm)	Extensive skin examination Mole mapping
Soft-tissue sarcoma (bone or muscle)	Familial and genetic syndromes (e.g., von Recklinghausen's disease) High-dose radiation Toxic chemical exposure (e.g., Agent Orange)	Swelling of extremity Painless mass Fever Malaise Weight loss Occasionally hypoglycemia Functional difficulty or pain in joints Pathologic fractures	Annual physical examination Awareness of cancer's early warning signs
Stomach	Dietary carcinogens (e.g., smoked, salt-cured and charcoal-cooked foods) Familial and genetic disposition Persons with type A blood (15% to 20% increase incidence) Benign gastric ulcers Tobacco Alcohol	Feeling of fullness Weight loss Loss of appetite Anemia (iron deficiency) Malaise Complaints of indigestion Gastrointestinal bleeding Abdominal pain Persistent epigastric distress	Occult blood testing Complete blood count Endoscopy
Testis	Cryptorchid testes Young white men have rate 4 times that of African Americans	Early • Painless mass • Gynecomastia • Heavy sensation in scrotum	Testicular self-examination (monthly) beginning in adolescence Testicular ultrasound

Continued

TABLE 4-2	Site-Specific Cancer Risk, Screening, and Early Detection Guidelines—cont'd		
SITE	ASSOCIATED RISK FACTORS	SIGNS AND SYMPTOMS	SCREENING AND DETECTION
		Advanced • Ureteral obstruction • Abdominal mass • Pulmonary symptoms • Elevated human chorionic gonadotropin	
Vulva	Postmenopausal History of genital warts Human papillomavirus Other sexually transmitted diseases Lower socioeconomic status Multiple sex partners Precancerous or cancerous lesions of cervix	Lump or ulcer Itching Pain Burning Bleeding Discharge	Visual and manual inspection of external genitalia Colposcopic exam Vulvar biopsy

Data from references 2, 6-14.

reapplied after being in the water. Suntanning parlors, which are increasing in popularity among Americans, should be avoided.

Early detection of skin cancers is crucial to saving lives and reducing the extent of surgical intervention needed. Basal and squamous cell cancers of the skin usually appear over areas of the body chronically exposed to the sun, including the nose, the cheeks, and the ears. These cancers appear as pale, waxlike nodules or a red, scaly patch that tends to bleed. Melanomas are small, molelike eruptions on the skin that can appear anywhere on the body, including the soles of the feet and the palms of the hands. Melanomas change in color, shape, and size and can ulcerate and bleed.

A simple "ABCD" rule outlines the warning signs of melanoma: A is for asymmetry; B is for border irregularity; C is for change in color or pigmentation; and D is for diameter greater than 6 mm. Adults should practice skin self-examination monthly and report any suspicious indicators to a member of the health care team.[2]

The public continues to express concern about cancer risk and exposure to electromagnetic radiation or nonionizing radiation. The presence of electric power lines, running through and surrounding residential and industrial areas where one lives and works, is the basis of this growing concern. Epidemiologic studies have been in progress since the late 1970s, attempting to document a possible link between electromagnetic radiation exposure over time and the development of certain cancers in humans. In a review of the literature by Heath,[27] at present no form of electromagnetic energy at frequency levels below those of ionizing radiation (x-rays) and ultraviolet (UV) radiation has been shown to cause cancer.[2,25]

Tobacco

Overwhelming evidence exists that tobacco use is the single greatest cause of preventable morbidity and mortality in the United States. According to the surgeon general, there is sufficient evidence to infer a causal relationship between smoking and cancers of the bladder, the cervix, the oral cavity, the esophagus,

the larynx, the kidney, the lung, the pancreas, and the stomach. A causal relationship has also been established for tobacco use and leukemia.[28]

A reported 90% of all lung cancer is caused by tobacco smoke from pipes, cigarettes, cigars, and sidestream or secondhand smoke.[29-31] It is important to understand that light or low-tar cigarettes are not significantly safer than regular cigarettes, nor is smokeless tobacco a safe alternative to smoking. The ACS estimates that cigarette smoking is responsible for 87% of all lung cancer deaths.[2] Passive exposure to cigarette smoke (sidestream and exhaled smoke) appears to increase the risk of lung cancer in nonsmokers who live with smokers.[32]

The United States has an undeniable need to eliminate tobacco use. A multifaceted effort has been proposed to implement effective, evidence-based interventions and programs to prevent tobacco use among children, promote smoking cessation, and reduce exposure to secondhand smoke. One of the national health objectives for the year 2010 is to reduce the initiation of cigarette smoking among adolescents and adults.[3] In 2003, 27.5% of high-school students reported using tobacco in various forms: cigarettes, cigars, pipes, and smokeless tobacco. Fortunately, the prevalence of current cigarette use has decreased among whites, African Americans, and Hispanic/Latino twelfth-graders between 1997 and 2003, as depicted in Fig. 4-2. The overall trend in teen cigarette smoking over the past 20 years is illustrated in Fig. 4-3. Despite the tobacco industry's attempts to market their products to children and adolescents, increased public awareness and education regarding tobacco risks are making a positive impact. Practices that have proven effective in reducing adolescent smoking include implementation of tobacco excise taxes, school-based smoking prevention programs beginning at or before sixth grade, antismoking media campaigns, and smoking cessation support. Ongoing education regarding avoidance of smokeless tobacco products, cigars, and pipe use is equally as important.

| TABLE 4-3 | Incidence and Mortality Rates: by Site, Race and Ethnicity, US, 1998-2002 |

INCIDENCE*	WHITE	AFRICAN AMERICAN	ASIAN AMERICAN AND PACIFIC ISLANDER	AMERICAN INDIAN AND ALASKA NATIVE	HISPANIC/LATINO†
All sites					
Males	55.64	682.6	383.3	255.4	420.7
Females	429.3	398.5	303.5	220.5	310.9
Breast (female)	141.1	119.4	96.5	54.8	89.9
Colon and rectum					
Males	61.7	72.5	56.0	36.7	48.3
Females	45.3	56.0	39.7	32.2	32.3
Lung and bronchus					
Males	76.7	113.9	59.4	42.6	44.6
Females	51.1	55.2	28.3	23.6	23.3
Prostate	169.0	272.0	101.4	50.3	141.9
Stomach					
Males	10.7	17.7	21.0	15.9	17.2
Females	5.0	9.6	12.0	9.1	10.1
Liver and bile duct					
Males	7.4	12.1	21.4	8.7	14.1
Females	2.9	3.7	7.9	5.2	6.1
Uterine cervix	8.7	11.1	8.9	4.9	15.8

MORTALITY	WHITE	AFRICAN AMERICAN	ASIAN AMERICAN AND PACIFIC ISLANDER	AMERICAN INDIAN AND ALASKA NATIVE	HISPANIC/LATINO†
All sites					
Male	242.5	339.4	148.0	159.7	171.4
Female	164.5	194.3	99.4	113.8	111.0
Breast (female)	25.9	34.7	12.7	13.8	16.7
Colon and rectum					
Males	24.3	34.0	15.8	16.2	17.7
Females	16.8	24.1	10.6	11.8	11.6
Lung and bronchus					
Males	75.2	101.3	39.4	47.0	38.7
Females	41.8	39.9	18.8	27.1	14.8
Prostate	27.7	68.1	12.1	18.3	23.0
Stomach					
Males	5.6	12.8	11.2	7.3	9.5
Females	2.8	6.3	6.8	4.1	5.3
Liver and bile duct					
Males	6.2	9.5	15.4	7.9	10.7
Females	2.7	3.8	6.5	4.3	5.1
Uterine cervix	2.5	5.3	2.7	2.6	3.5

*Per 100,000, age-adjusted to the 2000 U.S. standard population.
†Hispanic/Latinos are not mutually exclusive from whites, African Americans, Asian Americans and Pacific Islanders, and American Indians and Alaska Natives.
From Ries LG, Eisner MP, Kosary CL et al, editors: *SEER Cancer Statistics Review*, 975-2002, Bethesda, Maryland, 2005. National Cancer Institute, http://seer.cancer.ov/csr/1975_2002/.

TABLE 4-4   **Stage at Diagnosis of Colorectal, Breast, Prostate, and Cervical Cancer, by Race and Ethnicity, 1996–2000**

	LOCALIZED		REGIONAL		DISTANT	
	RATE*	%	RATE*	%	RATE*	%
Colorectal						
White	21.4	42	19.7	39	9.6	19
African American	22.4	39	21.0	36	14.2	25
Hispanic/Latino†	14.6	39	14.4	39	7.9	22
American Indian and Alaska Native	11.8	35	13.2	40	8.5	25
Asian American and Pacific Islander	18.9	42	17.9	40	7.7	18
Breast (female)						
White	90.2	66	39.8	29	7.5	5
African American	65.6	55	40.6	36	10.6	9
Hispanic/Latino†	50.7	57	29.2	35	6.2	7
American Indian and Alaska Native	32.4	56	19.9	36	4.8	8
Asian American and Pacific Islander	63.1	65	28.2	30	4.3	5
Prostate‡						
White	145.2	95			8.2	5
African American	225.9	93			20.0	7
Hispanic/Latino†	112.1	93			9.7	7
American Indian and Alaska Native	42.6	88			7.2	12
Asian American and Pacific Islander	84.9	92			8.0	8
Uterine cervix						
White	5.0	58	2.9	33	0.8	9
African American	5.5	51	4.4	39	1.2	10
Hispanic/Latino†	8.1	57	5.8	34	1.6	9
American Indian and Alaska Native	3.3	57	2.5	36	0.5	
Asian American and Pacific Islander	5.0	54	3.8	38	0.9	8

*Per 100,000, age-adjusted to the 2000 US population.
†Hispanics/Latinos are not mutually exclusive from whites, African Americans, Asian Americans and Pacific Islanders, and American Indians and Alaska Natives.
‡The rate and percent for localized stage represents local and regional stages combined.
From Ries LAG, Eisner MP, Kosary CL et al, editors: *SEER Cancer Statistics Review, 1975-2000*, Bethesda, Maryland, 2003. National Cancer Institute, http://seer.cancer.gov/csr/1975_2000,2003.
Copyright 2004 American Cancer Society, Inc. Reprinted with permission.

Among current smokers, more than 80% started smoking before age 21, and about half started before age 18.[7,33] Currently, an estimated 25% of men and 20% of women smoke cigarettes on a daily basis. Smoking prevalence varies by educational background and socioeconomic and ethnic group. Of college graduates, 9.9% were current smokers in 2002, compared with 31% of high-school graduates.[5]

Smoking cessation reduces the risk of death from lung cancer; after 15 years, former smokers have lung cancer death rates only about 2 times greater than nonsmokers.[34] A variety of programs are available through state and national organizations to assist people in quitting. Smokers interested in quitting may obtain education materials and support by calling 1-800-QUIT-NOW or accessing *www.smokefree.gov*. Clinical practice guidelines for health care providers have been developed through a collaborative effort of the NCI, the Agency for Health Care Policy Research, and the American Psychiatric Association.[35] Clinicians should assess individuals for current or prior tobacco dependence. Current smokers should always be encouraged to quit, and former smokers should be assessed for relapse potential. Desire to quit should be established. Interest in smoking cessation would lead the clinician through the process of reviewing the "5 As": *a*sk about ongoing tobacco use at each visit, *a*dvise the user to quit, *a*ssess motivation or willingness to attempt quitting, *a*ssist the person in quitting, and *a*rrange follow-up support. Regular advice to stop smoking was shown to increase the rates of smoking cessation by up to 30% in randomized controlled trials.[35]

Smokers motivated to quit benefit from medication and psychosocial therapies to assist them with established goals. Five medications are currently approved by the FDA to treat nicotine dependence. First-line smoking cessation aids such as bupropion, an atypical antidepressant, and nicotine replacement therapies in the form of gum, patches, nasal sprays, and inhalers double the abstinent rate in randomized double-blind trials when compared to placebo.[36,37] Behavioral therapy alone produced a similar result. Combining medications approved for smoking cessation with behavioral therapy has proven even more effective.

The clinical practice guidelines recommend that persons lacking the motivation to quit smoking receive ongoing education and assistance from their clinician. The "5 *R*s" are recommended: identify personal *r*elevance for quitting (i.e., family history of cancer, heart disease), educate on *r*isks associated with tobacco

TABLE 4-5	Selected Programs and Resources Targeting Cancer Disparities	
NAME OF PROGRAM AND WEB SITE	SPONSORS/PARTNERS	DESCRIPTION
Intercultural Cancer Council (ICC) http://iccnetwork.org	Baylor College of Medicine	The ICC promotes policies, programs, partnerships, and research to eliminate the unequal cancer burden among racial and ethnic minorities and medically underserved populations in the United States and its associated territories. Prepares *Cancer Fact Sheets* that provide detailed information on cancer occurrence and risk factors among racial and ethnic minorities and the medically underserved.
Center to Reduce Cancer Health Disparities (CRCHD) http://crchd.nci.nih.gov	National Cancer Institute	The CRCHD was created in 2001 to carry out NCI's Strategic Plan for Reducing Cancer Health Disparities. NCI's goal is to nearly triple the funding for cancer health disparities in four years. Research will investigate social, cultural, environmental, biological, and behavioral determinants of cancer disparities across the cancer control continuum from prevention to end-of-life care.
Special Populations Networks for Cancer Awareness, Research, and Training http://crchd.nci.nih.gov/spn	National Cancer Institute	The purpose of the special populations networks is to build relationships between large research institutions and community based programs and to find ways of addressing important questions about the burden of cancer in minority communities. The major goal is to build infrastructure to promote cancer awareness within minority and medically underserved communities and to launch from these communities more research and cancer control activities aimed at specific population subgroups. Currently the special populations networks consists of 18 projects in 15 states.
Racial and Ethnic Approaches to Community Health (REACH) http://www.cdc.gov/reach2010	Centers for Disease Control and Prevention	The REACH program funds community coalitions to develop and implement activities to reduce the level of disparities in one or more of six priority areas, which include breast and cervical cancer screening. The program emphasizes the importance of working more closely with communities to identify culturally sensitive implementation strategies.
National Breast and Cervical Cancer Early Detection Program (NBCCEDP) http://www.cdc.gov/cancer/nbccedp	Centers for Disease Control and Prevention	The NBCCEDP was created by Congress in 1990 to help improve access to breast and cervical cancer screening among underserved women. This program, funded at $200.6 million or fiscal year 2003, provides both screening and diagnostic services and has been implemented in all 50 states, 5 U.S. territories, the District of Columbia, and 15 American Indian and Alaskan Native organizations.

From American Cancer Society: *Cancer facts and figures*, Atlanta, 2004, Author.
Copyright 2004 American Cancer Society, Inc. Reprinted with permission.

use, emphasize potential rewards of smoking cessation (i.e., foods taste better, save money), and help identify personal roadblocks and determine interventions to overcome them. Because tobacco addiction is a chronic condition, relapse is common and long-term abstinence is difficult. Repetition (the final "r") is critical to produce long-term results.[35] Nurses in all settings may support smoking cessation efforts by reminding patients of the dangers of tobacco use and the means available to assist them in quitting.

Alcohol

Excessive consumption of ethyl alcohol can lead to cancers in the head and neck, the larynx, the liver, the colon, the pancreas, and the breast.[2,5,14] The exact mechanisms by which chronic alcohol ingestion stimulates carcinogenesis are unknown. Studies in animals support the concept that ethanol does not act independently as a carcinogen, but instead is a cocarcinogen and/or tumor promoter. The metabolism of ethanol produces acetaldehyde (AA), which is a known carcinogen.[38] Acetaldehyde is mutagenic; it attaches to DNA and may trigger the replication errors and/or mutation in oncogenes or tumor suppressor genes.[38,39] Acetaldehyde interferes with DNA synthesis and repair, which can result in tumor development.[38]

Moderate alcohol consumption increases the risk for colon and breast cancer.[38] Alcohol intake has been positively associated with an increased risk of postmenopausal breast cancer in epidemiologic studies.[40-43] Nearly 60% of all breast cancers are hormone dependent, with overstimulation of the estrogen receptor (ER).[40,44] The precise mechanism of alcohol-induced mammary cancer is unknown; however, there are various theories in the field of research. Some findings suggest that ethanol inactivates *BRCA1*, a potent inhibitor of ER activity. Not only does ethanol suppress *BRCA1*, it also directly stimulates ER activity.[45] Other studies have shown that alcohol increases the production of estrogen or decreases metabolic estradiol clearance, which could increase the cumulative level of estrogen.[40,46-48] Numerous in vitro studies

have revealed that ethanol directly stimulates the proliferation of ER-positive human breast cancer cells. Alcohol consumption does not affect the ER-negative cells.[40,45,49] The combination of alcohol consumption and postmenopausal estrogen replacement therapy synergistically enhances the risk of breast cancer.[45,48,50] Suzuki and colleagues suggest the risk is 3.5 times higher in women with these two risk factors.[40]

Epidemiologic studies have shown that alcohol consumption increases the risk of colorectal polyps.[51-54] Compared with total abstainers, persons who consume alcohol and smoke have 12 times the risk for developing colorectal polyps. For drinkers who did not smoke the risk was threefold that of abstainers.[53] For women, the risk of developing colorectal adenomas increased with 10 or more alcoholic beverages a week. Among men, the risk was increased with a consumption of 21 or more alcoholic beverages a week.[52] The exact mechanism of how alcohol promotes colorectal cancer is still controversial.[55] A variety of experimental studies have shown that chronic ethanol consumption increased mucosal cell regeneration in the rectum, possibly a result of AA toxicity. Acetaldehyde can react with various intracellular and extracellular proteins to form both stable and unstable products, which may lead to cellular damage or dysfunction through alteration of protein functions.[55] Chronic regeneration of mucosal cells associated with prolonged alcohol consumption predisposes people to the development of colorectal cancer.[51,56]

The public has long been advised to consume alcohol in moderation. The U.S. Department of Agriculture (USDA) defines moderate drinking as one alcoholic beverage daily for women and two for men. Twelve ounces of beer, 5 ounces of wine, and 1.5 ounces of 80-proof distilled spirits are considered the standard portions of each type of drink.[57]

Diet and Obesity

According to the World Health Organization (WHO), there are more than 1 billion overweight adults worldwide, 300 million of whom are classified as clinically obese. The number of overweight

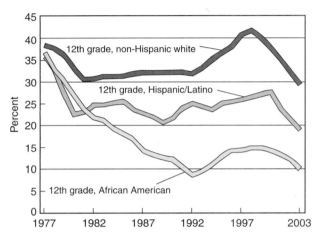

*Used cigarettes in the last 30 days

Source: Monitoring the Future Survey, 1975-2003, National Institute on Drug Abuse

American Cancer Society, Surveillance Research

FIG. 4-2 Current* cigarette smoking among twelfth-graders, by race/ethnicity, 1997-2003. *Use cigarettes within the last 30 days. (From American Cancer Society: *Cancer prevention and early detection facts and figures, 2005*, Atlanta, 2005, Author. Copyright 2005 American Cancer Society, Inc. Reprinted with permission.)

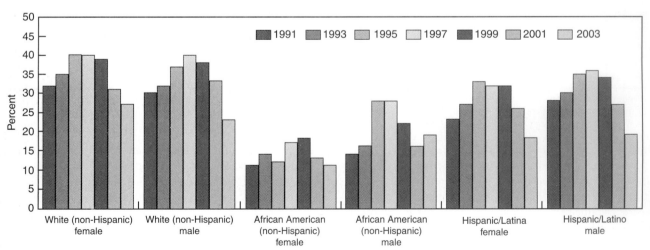

*Smoked cigarettes on one or more of the 30 days preceding the survey.

Source: Youth Risk Behavior Surveillance System. *MMWR Morb Mortal Wkly Rep.* 2004;53(23):499-502.

American Cancer Society, Surveillance Research

FIG. 4-3 Current* cigarette smoking among high school students, by race/ethnicity, 1991-2003. *Use cigarettes within the last 30 days. (From American Cancer Society: *Cancer prevention and early detection facts and figures, 2005.* Atlanta, 2005, Author. Copyright 2005 American Cancer Society, Inc. Reprinted with permission.)

children and adolescents has also doubled in the last 2 decades. There are approximately 22 million children under the age of 5 who are overweight. A key predictor for adulthood obesity is adolescent obesity.[58] The ACS reports that approximately one half of overweight children and 70% of overweight adolescents continue to be overweight into adulthood.[2] Adolescents and adults from poor households are twice as likely to be overweight than those from middle- and high-income households.[3,34]

Increased consumption of high-energy, dense foods and inactivity are the major contributing factors of obesity. For adults 20 years of age and older, obesity is measured by body mass index (BMI), which is a formula based on kilograms of weight divided by height in meters squared. Table 4-6 defines the BMI weight classifications. Adults with a BMI greater than or equal to 30 are considered obese. For children, obesity is measured by BMI greater than the 95th percentile for age and sex.[59] BMI measurement in children is not as accurate compared to BMI for adults, because children continue to grow.[60]

Healthy People 2010 includes nutrition and overweight objectives aimed at reducing the proportion of children, adolescents, and adults who are overweight or obese. These conditions substantially increase the risk of illness from hypertension, cardiovascular disease, diabetes, arthritis, gallbladder disease, sleep disturbances, and breathing problems, as well as cancers of the endometrium, the breast, the prostate, and the colon.[3] Scientific evidence suggests that one third of the 564,830 estimated cancer deaths in 2006 will be related to poor nutrition, sedentary lifestyle, and obesity.[2,61]

Obesity increases colorectal cancer risk; a stronger association is seen in men than women. Men are more likely to deposit body fat centrally than women, which makes BMI a more accurate measurement of the relevant exposure. High BMI measurement means a linear increase in circulating levels of insulin in the body.[62] Increased numbers of fat cells affect insulin production, which may negatively impact cellular glucose consumption. With inactivity and excessive calorie consumption, body tissues become resistant to insulin, and the body compensates by producing more insulin. High insulin levels promote the growth of colonic mucosal cells and colonic carcinoma cells in vitro studies.[62-64] Postmenopausal women who are obese have high levels of circulating estrogen that may diminish the obesity-associated risk of colorectal cancer.[62]

There is a 30% to 50% increased risk for breast cancer in postmenopausal women who are obese. Obese women with a BMI greater than 40 are 3 times more likely to die from breast cancer than lean women with a BMI of less than 20.[5] Adipose tissues produce estrogen, which contributes to increased risk for breast cancer in postmenopausal women. Conversely, reduction of breast cancer risk in premenopausal women with a BMI greater than 28 is likely due to an increased propensity for young,

these women to have anovulatory menstrual cycles and reduced levels of circulating steroid hormones.[62]

High levels of insulin increase the risk for endometrial cancer. Insulin resistance stimulates the pathophysiology of anovulation in premenopausal women. With normal menstrual cycles, progesterone is released to reduce endometrial cell proliferation. Without progesterone, estrogen promotes endometrial cell proliferation. The same mechanism and increased risk applies to obese adolescents. In obese postmenopausal women, adipose tissue continues to produce estrogen. Many postmenopausal women also consume estrogen to alleviate postmenopausal symptoms. Escalating levels of insulin also lead to elevated androgens, a male hormone that has been associated with hyperplasia of the endometrium. Endometrial hyperplasia may progress to endometrial cancer.[65] As with breast cancer, higher concentrations of estrogen in obese women increase the risk for endometrial cancer.[62]

Even though there is no direct causation between obesity and prostate cancer risk, diets high in animal fats have been associated with an increase risk of prostate cancer in men. It has been suggested that diet can influence androgen levels, and changes in endogenous hormones may affect prostate cancer growth.[66,67] Obese men tend to have lower testosterone levels and higher estradiol levels, which may predispose them to developing more poorly differentiated, advanced prostate cancers, and may explain the higher mortality rate associated with prostate cancer.[68] In several studies, obese men who developed prostate cancer were at significantly greater risk for fatal prostate cancer.[69] Multiple cohort studies suggests obese men with a BMI between 30-34.9 were 20% more likely to die from prostate cancer than normal weight men with a BMI between 18.5-24.9.[68-70]

Increased mortality among obese men with prostate cancer may be influenced by prostate cancer screening, detection, and treatment. Obese men tend to have larger prostates than men of ideal body weight. It may be more difficult to perform a proper digital rectal examination, feel an abnormality, and identify cancer on biopsy when obesity is a factor.[68,71] Obese men may have lower serum PSA values as a result of lower testosterone and higher estradiol levels.[68,72,73] Potential inaccuracy of the PSA in obese men may delay cancer diagnosis and lead to advanced disease.

At this time, the only consensus recommendations related to cancer, diet, and nutrition are to reduce the intake of fat, both saturated and unsaturated, to increase the amount of daily intake of natural fiber in the diet, and to increase physical activity. Specific dietary recommendations, related to macronutrients and micronutrients, chemoprevention, and sources of mutagenic and carcinogenic chemicals used to preserve, protect, or cultivate food sources, remain clouded in uncertainty. The DHHS estimates that as much as 40% of a family's food budget is spent in restaurants and take-out meals. Foods eaten away from home are usually higher in fat, cholesterol, and sodium and lower in fiber (containing fewer vegetables and fruits) than meals prepared at home. Compared to men and women of normal weight, men with a BMI of 40 or greater have a 52% increase in cancer mortality, and women with a BMI of 40 or greater have a 62% increase in mortality from all cancer combined.[74] Healthy eating habits and physical activity should start in childhood, since the majority of overweight children will develop into overweight adults. The ACS recommends that children and adults reduce consumption of fast food, make healthier food choices, and increase physical activity.

TABLE 4-6	BMI Classifications
BMI	**WEIGHT CLASSIFICATION**
<18.5	Underweight
18.5–24.9	Normal weight
25–29.9	Overweight
>30	Obesity

Dietary fat acts as a cancer promoter. From 1909 through 2000, there was a 39% increase in fat distributed in the U.S. food supply.[75] Fat and oils composed 22% of all food energy in the U.S. food supply in the year 2000. The Dietary Guidelines for Americans 2005 recommends that fat consumption be limited to 20% to 35% of daily calorie intake.

Dietary fiber found in fresh fruits, vegetables, legumes, whole-grain breads, and cereals protect against cancer development by clearing hormones and fats from the body.[67] Fiber reduces the concentration of fecal bile acids, dilutes colonic content, reduces the level of fecal mutagens, and decreases transient time of fecal material in the gut.[76-78] Cruciferous vegetables such as broccoli, brussels sprouts, and cabbage, among others, contain sulforaphane, which increases the activity of enzymes that inactivate cancer-causing chemicals. Other compounds found in these vegetables also interfere with estrogen metabolism, which disturbs carcinogen activity.[67] Several micronutrients have been profiled as having protective effects in reducing cancer risk. Naturally occurring vitamin A in the form of β-carotene, found in yellow and green vegetables and fruits, and retinol, occurring in foods of animal origin such as dairy products, eggs, and liver are associated with a protective effect against cancer. Inverse associations have been found in studies relating vitamin A precursors and cancers of the lung, the larynx, the esophagus, the stomach, and the prostate.[79-81]

The majority of Americans eat an average of 10 grams of fiber a day. The recommendation for dietary intake of fiber is 25 to 35 grams per day.[67] The DHHS, the NIH, and the NCI agree to the "eat 5 to 9 a day" initiative to change eating habits and behaviors of Americans by including at least five to nine servings of fruits and vegetables a day in the diet. Children ages 2 to 6 should eat a minimum of 5 serving of fruits and vegetables every day. Women should aim for 7 servings, and men should aim for 9 servings in a day. Research shows that cancer rates could be reduced by more than 20% by people consuming at least 5 servings of fruit and vegetables daily. More information can be accessed on the Web via *www.5aday.gov*. My Pyramid (Fig. 4-4) is a personalized food pyramid that takes physical activity into account. The personalized food pyramid can be accessed on the Web at *www.MyPyramid.gov*. The pyramid reinforces the principles of good nutrition as well as balance and variety in daily food choices and physical activity. My Pyramid is also consistent with the dietary guidelines from both the ACS and NCI.[82]

The ACS, the NCI, and other organizations with an interest in health promotion through dietary modifications have developed dietary guidelines to reduce cancer and other health risks. The ACS has identified the four nutrition and physical activity guidelines:

1. Choose most of the foods you eat from plant sources. Restrict consumption of red meats that are excessive in fat.
2. Engage in a physically active lifestyle. Adults should commit to moderate activity for 30 minutes or more on 5 or more days of the week. Children and adolescents should commit to moderate activity for at least 60 minutes or more.
3. Maintain a healthy weight by balancing caloric consumption with physical activity.
4. Limit consumption of alcoholic beverages.[2]

The *Healthy People 2010* objectives for physical activity and fitness are aimed at increasing the proportion of adolescents who engage in vigorous physical activity that promotes cardiorespiratory fitness 3 or more days per week for 20 minutes or more per occasion, and increasing the proportion of adults who engage regularly, preferably daily, in moderate physical activity at least 30 minutes per day. Regular physical activity is associated with a decreased risk of colon cancer.[2,83]

Chemoprevention

The NCI continues to sponsor human chemoprevention, diet, and nutrition trials in an effort to answer questions and update earlier studies related to diet, medications, and the cancer connection. Cancer prevention trials are aimed at behavior modification or deliberate and planned intervention designed to interfere with carcinogenesis. Hormonal agents, nutritional supplements, non-steroidal antiinflammatory agents (NSAIDs), and statins are just a few of the agents being evaluated in clinical trials.

Tamoxifen citrate (Nolvadex), a selective estrogen-receptor modulator drug (SERM), has been studied as an adjuvant therapy following conventional treatment of breast cancer, thereby establishing extensive knowledge of the pharmacokinetics, the metabolic activity, and the risk-benefit profile of the medication. During breast cancer clinical trials, it became apparent that woman receiving tamoxifen as adjuvant therapy benefited from a significant reduction in the risk for developing contralateral breast cancers.[84,85] In the early 1990s it was hypothesized that tamoxifen could reduce the risk of breast cancer in women at increased risk for breast cancer but with no prior history of the disease.

The National Surgical Adjuvant Breast and Bowel Project (NSABP) P-1 Breast Cancer Prevention Trial (BCPT) was designed to compare 5 years of tamoxifen therapy to placebo in a prospective, randomized double-blind trial. A total of 13,388 participants were randomized to either tamoxifen, 20 mg, or placebo daily. Women ages 35 to 59 years with a 5-year predicted risk for breast cancer equal to or greater than 1.66%, using the GAIL Model Risk Assessment, were eligible for participation. The GAIL Model estimates a woman's 5-year and lifetime risk for breast cancer by assessing breast cancer risk factors: age, age at menarche, age at first live birth, number of previous breast biopsies, history of atypical hyperplasia, and number of first-degree relatives with breast cancer. Women with a history of atypical hyperplasia or lobular carcinoma in situ and all women 60 years of age or older were also considered candidates for the BCPT.

Tamoxifen, which acts as an estrogen antagonist in breast tissue, conversely acts as an estrogen agonist in the endometrium and bones. Five years of tamoxifen therapy was shown to reduce the risk for ER-positive breast cancers by 49% (p < 0.0001). Women with a history of lobular carcinoma in situ or atypical hyperplasia realized a 56% and 86% reduction in breast cancer risk, respectively.[86] Woman randomized to tamoxifen were less likely to fracture the hip, the spine, or the radius than women randomized to placebo, although the reduction in fracture risk was not statistically significant. Health risks associated with the medication include a two- to threefold increased risk of thromboembolic events and endometrial cancer. Cataracts were more prevalent in the tamoxifen group, as evidenced by a risk ratio of 1:21. Vasomotor symptoms were a common, and sometimes dose-limiting, side effect of tamoxifen.[86]

The BCPT trial closed early in 1998 because of overwhelming evidence that tamoxifen significantly reduced the risk for ER-positive breast cancers. In a landmark decision, which helped to validate the science of cancer chemoprevention, the FDA

Anatomy of MyPyramid

One size doesn't fit all
USDA's new MyPyramid symbolizes a personalized approach to healthy eating and physical activity. The symbol has been designed to be simple. It has been developed to remind consumers to make healthy food choices and to be active every day. The different parts of the symbol are described below.

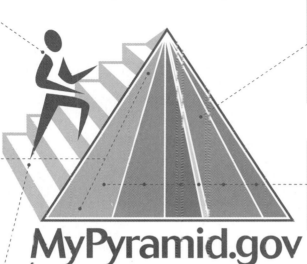

Activity
Activity is represented by the steps and the person climbing them, as a reminder of the importance of daily physical activity.

Moderation
Moderation is represented by the narrowing of each food group from bottom to top. The wider base stands for foods with little or no solid fats or added sugars. These should be selected more often. The narrower top area stands for foods containing more added sugars and solid fats. The more active you are, the more of these foods can fit into your diet.

Personalization
Personalization is shown by the person on the steps, the slogan, and the URL. Find the kinds and amounts of food to eat each day at MyPyramid.gov.

Proportionality
Proportionality is shown by the different widths of the food group bands. The widths suggest how much food a person should choose from each group. The widths are just a general guide, not exact proportions. Check the Web site for how much is right for you.

Variety
Variety is symbolized by the 6 color bands representing the 5 food groups of the Pyramid and oils. This illustrates that foods from all groups are needed each day for good health.

Gradual Improvement
Gradual improvement is encouraged by the slogan. It suggests that individuals can benefit from taking small steps to improve their diet and lifestyle each day.

MyPyramid.gov
STEPS TO A HEALTHIER YOU

USDA   U.S. Department of Agriculture
Center for Nutrition Policy and Promotion
April 2005 CNPP-16
USDA is an equal opportunity provider and employer.

GRAINS   VEGETABLES   FRUITS   OILS   MILK   MEAT & BEANS

FIG. 4-4   Anatomy of MyPyramid. (From U.S. Department of Agriculture Center for Nutrition Policy and Promotion, April 2005, CNPP-16.)

approved tamoxifen citrate for the indication of breast cancer risk reduction. Tamoxifen was the first drug to be approved as a chemopreventive agent.

In 2005, Fisher and colleagues published 7 additional years of data obtained from the BCPT participants.[87] Ongoing risk reduction was confirmed well beyond 5 years of tamoxifen therapy. Table 4-7 compares the risk ratio for breast cancer, osteoporotic fractures, thromboembolic events, endometrial cancer, and cataract development, as determined by the BCPT trial through study closure in 1998 and long-term follow-up documented in 2005.

Despite evidence that tamoxifen reduces the risk for breast cancer, many risk-eligible women are hesitant to take the medication. It is estimated that 2.5 million American women between the ages of 35 and 70 years are at increased risk for breast cancer and would benefit from tamoxifen.[87] In several studies, only a small portion of women receiving risk-reduction counseling and education on the risk and benefits of tamoxifen initiate the medication. In a study conducted by Melnikow and colleagues, less than 20% of women were interested in tamoxifen despite a high self-perceived breast cancer risk.[88] Port and others concluded

that woman at increased risk for breast cancer often perceived that the risks of taking tamoxifen outweigh the benefit of risk reduction.[89] Of 43 eligible candidates, only 2 women (4.7%) initiated tamoxifen. Side effect profiles and the health risks of the tamoxifen, particularly the increased risk of thromboembolic events and endometrial cancers, are often the reasons risk eligible women decline.

The NSABP P-2 Study of Tamoxifen and Raloxifene (STAR) trial is under way to evaluate the efficacy of tamoxifen versus raloxifene in reducing the risk for breast cancer in postmenopausal women at increased risk for the disease.[90] Secondary endpoint data from the Multiple Outcomes of Raloxifene (MORE) trial suggested a reduction in the incidence of breast cancer in women randomized to raloxifene to treat osteoporosis.[91] Although raloxifene has a similar risk profile to tamoxifen, when thromboembolic events are considered, this SERM does not increase the risk for endometrial cancer. The study has accrued 19,747 postmenopausal women nationwide. Each participant was randomized to either tamoxifen, 20 mg, or raloxifene, 60 mg, daily for 5 years. Data analysis and outcomes are expected

TABLE 4-7 Risk Ratios		
BREAST CANCER PREVENTION TRIAL–TAMOXIFEN ARM	**RISK RATIO: STUDY CLOSURE 1998**	**RISK RATIO: LONG-TERM FOLLOW-UP**
Breast cancer	0.51	0.57
Osteoporotic fracture	0.81	0.68
Endometrial cancer	2.53	3.28
Pulmonary embolism	3.01	2.15
Deep vein thrombosis	1.60	2.16
Cataracts	1.14	1.21

Data from Fisher B, Costantino JP, Wickerham L et al: Tamoxifen for prevention of breast cancer: report of the National Surgical Adjuvant Breast and Bowel Project P-1 Study, *J Natl Cancer Inst* 90:1371, 1998; and Fisher B, Costantino JP, Wickerham L et al: Tamoxifen for the prevention of breast cancer: current status of the National Surgical Adjuvant Breast and Bowel Project P-1 Study, *J Natl Cancer Inst* 97:1652, 2005.

within the next year to 18 months. The safest, most effective medication for reducing breast cancer risk, as determined by the STAR trial, is likely to be compared to an aromatase inhibitor in future breast cancer chemoprevention clinical trials.

Aromatase inhibitors prevent the conversion of androgens to estrogen in the body. The Arimidex, Tamoxifen Alone or in Combination (ATAC) trial compared the efficacy and safety profile of anastrozole (Arimidex), a nonsteroidal aromatase inhibitor, to tamoxifen in the adjuvant setting. Anastrozole was more effective in increasing disease-free survival (p = 0.03) and time to recurrence (p = 0.015), while reducing the incidence of contralateral breast cancers (p = 0.042) in postmenopausal women. There was also a decreased incidence of endometrial cancer (p = 0.007) and thromboembolic events (p = 0.001). Conversely, there were a greater number of musculoskeletal disorders and fractures (p = 0.001) in the anastrozole arm as compared to tamoxifen.[92] In four separate adjuvant trials, the efficacy of three aromatase inhibitors (anastrozole, exemestane and letrozole) was reported to be significantly better than tamoxifen, particularly in reducing the incidence of contralateral breast cancer.[93] The risk-benefit profile of aromatase inhibitors is favorable for breast cancer chemoprevention endeavors. The NCI is currently sponsoring Phase II and Phase III trials to evaluate the safety and efficacy of exemestane and letrozole in preventing breast cancer in postmenopausal women meeting certain criteria for increased risk.[94]

Colorectal cancer is the third leading cause of cancer-related death in both men and women.[2] Stepwise histologic changes occur in the colon mucosa that result in colorectal cancer. The progression of normal mucosa to adenomatous polyp to adenoma allows for a biologic marker by which to study chemopreventive properties of medications and nutrients.[95] Calcium and NSAIDs such as celecoxib, aspirin, and sulindac show promise in preventing colorectal cancer.

Familial adenomatous polyposis (FAP) is a genetic condition that carries a 100% lifetime risk of colon cancer. The condition is characterized by more than 100 colon polyps in an individual. A study conducted by Steinbach and colleagues examined the efficacy of celecoxib, a COX-2 inhibitor, in reducing polyp development in persons with FAP.[96] Celecoxib was administered in 100 mg and 400 mg doses twice daily, versus placebo, for 6 months. Celecoxib, 400 mg, twice daily proved to be most effective in reducing polyp incidence and burden (sum of polyp diameters). The mean number of colon polyps was reduced by 28%, and the polyp burden was reduced by 30.7%, which was significantly more effective (p = 0.003) when compared to placebo. Celexocib, 100 mg, twice daily was somewhat less effective, with an 11.9% reduction in polyp development and a 14.6% reduction in polyp burden. As a result of this study the FDA approved celecoxib in the management of patients with FAP.[95]

Prostate cancer is the most common cancer among U.S. males.[2] Epidemiology studies suggest certain nutrients and hormonal therapies may reduce the risk for prostate cancer. Vitamins A, D, and E and selenium are just a few supplements being pursued.

Finasteride is a steroidal analogue of testosterone. As a 5-alpha-reductase inhibitor, finasteride blocks the conversion of testosterone to the androgen dihydrotestosterone that is active within the prostate and may be associated with prostate cancer risk.[95,97] The primary endpoint of the Prostate Cancer Prevention trial (PCPT) was to determine the prevalence of prostate cancer following 7 years of finasteride therapy versus placebo in disease-free men. Upon completing therapy, prostate biopsies were performed to determine the incidence of prostate cancer between the two groups. Of the 4368 men in the finasteride group undergoing biopsy for final analysis, 803 (18.4%) were diagnosed with prostate cancer. In the placebo group, 4692 men were biopsied and 1147 (24.4%) had evidence of disease. Although the prevalence of prostate cancer was significantly reduced in the finasteride group, (p < 0.0001), high-grade tumors, Gleason grades 7 through 10, were more common. Experts recognize the chemopreventive properties of finasteride but caution clinicians on its use to reduce the risk for prostate cancer secondary to the prevalence of high-grade tumors and sexual side effects. Men should not be given finasteride to reduce the risk of prostate cancer development without extensive counseling regarding the potential risks of the drug.[98]

Selenium, an essential trace element, and alpha-tocopherol (vitamin E), a fat-soluble vitamin, show promise in preventing prostate cancer in both epidemiology studies and clinical trials designed to examine the safety and efficacy of the supplements. Secondary endpoint analysis from the Nutritional Prevention of Cancer (NPC) trial and the Alpha-Tocopherol, Beta-Carotene Cancer Prevention (ATBC) study revealed a reduction in prostate cancer incidence with selenium and vitamin E.[99,100] As a follow-up chemoprevention trial to PCPT, the Selenium and Vitamin E Cancer Prevention Trial (SELECT) opened in July 2001. This Phase III randomized double-blind trial is designed to evaluate the incidence of prostate cancer in men when selenium (200 mcg daily from L-selenomethionine) alone, vitamin E (400 international units daily of all-rac-alpha-tocopheryl acetate) alone, selenium and vitamin E in combination, or placebo is administered over a minimum of 7 years. Across the United States and Puerto Rico, 32,400 participants have been enlisted and recruitment has closed. In an effort to learn more about the increased burden of prostate cancer in African American men, SELECT investigators were challenged to enroll minority participants. Twenty four percent of all participants were to be minority; 20% African Americans, 3% Hispanics and 1% Asians. Although SELECT recruited more African Americans than any other chemoprevention trial to date, the goal fell short by 5%. Non–African American men at least 55 years of age and African American men 50 years and older with a serum PSA level less than 4.0 ng/ml and normal digital rectal exam (DRE) were eligible for the clinical trial. Final analysis is anticipated in 2013.[101,102]

Genetic Risk and Testing

Although the vast majority of cancer occurs sporadically, an estimated 5% to 10% of all cancer may be associated with the 200 hereditary cancer susceptibility syndromes identified to date.[103,104] FAP is characterized by greater than 100 colorectal adenomas in one individual and a 90% risk for developing colon cancer by the age of 50 if the polyps go untreated. Hereditary nonpolyposis colon cancer (HNPCC), or Lynch syndrome, describes a form of autosomal dominant hereditary cancers of the colon, stomach and endometrium. Li-Fraumeni syndrome is a hereditary cancer susceptibility syndrome associated with a germline mutation in the *TP53* tumor suppression gene that results in early-onset sarcomas, brain tumors, breast cancer, and leukemia.[103-105] Multiple endocrine neoplasia (MEN) types 1 and 2, Cowden disease, and Bloom's syndrome are other inherited cancer syndromes that have been recognized through years of genetic research.[104]

Hereditary breast and ovarian cancer syndrome is probably the genetic syndrome most commonly recognized by lay persons and health care providers. The development of breast and ovarian cancer is the result of changes in certain genes and mutations. Family history is an important, but not an exclusive, risk factor for breast cancer. Women with at least one first-degree relative with breast cancer have a two- to fourfold risk for developing the disease.[106] Hereditary genetic mutations account for about 5% of breast cancer. The associated increased risk of breast and ovarian cancer is caused by an alteration or mutation of two genes— *BRCA1* and *BRCA2*. Women with a mutation of either the *BRCA1* or *BRCA2* gene carry a 36% to 85% risk of developing breast cancer and a 16% to 60% risk of developing ovarian cancer over their lifetime.[105]

A thorough and complete family history can be invaluable in identifying relative risks and traits within a family aggregate. The relative risk measures the strength of the relationship between risk factors and the specific cancer. In 2002, the American Society of Clinical Oncology (ASCO) updated its policy statement on genetic testing for cancer susceptibility and recommended that genetic testing be offered to persons with a strong family history of cancer.[107] The National Comprehensive Cancer Network (NCCN) has developed practice guidelines to assist clinicians in identifying persons who would benefit from genetic risk assessment counseling.[105] The NCCN suggests that clinicians obtain a thorough family history and be alert to patterns

such as premenopausal breast cancer, bilateral breast cancer, or ovarian cancer in a single individual, and clustering of breast cancer with male breast cancer, thyroid cancer, endometrial cancer, pancreatic cancer, or sarcoma. Any male breast cancer or ovarian cancer should be a red flag for potential hereditary susceptibility syndrome. Two breast primaries or breast and ovarian cancers in close family members on the same side of the family should be of concern.[105] Both ASCO and the NCCN agree that extensive counseling must occur before a person consents to genetic testing. Persons testing positive for a genetic mutation, particularly the *BRCA1* or *BRCA2* gene, will need extensive education and counseling regarding cancer prevention and early detection activities. Routine screening tests such as mammogram, biannual breast examination, biannual CA-125, and transvaginal ultrasound may be used to help to identify cancer in an early stage. Tamoxifen citrate may be an option for reducing ER positive breast cancer risk.[105,108] Breast magnetic resonance imaging (MRI), as compared with annual screening mammogram, or mammogram with breast ultrasound, may yield an early-stage breast cancer diagnosis in women with familial or hereditary risk for breast cancer.[109] Even more deliberate decision making may be necessary when considering surgical intervention for risk reduction such as prophylactic mastectomy or prophylactic oopherectomy.[105,108] Risks, benefits, and limitations of each preventive practice should be reviewed in detail with the patient.

The risk of losing insurance coverage and other financial risks are part of individual counseling. Although the Health Insurance Portability and Accountability Act passed by Congress in 1996 was designed to improve protection against discrimination by employment-based health insurance carriers, no previsions were made for individual health insurance coverage.[107] The average cost of the genetic assessment ranges from $200 for counseling only to over $2000 for counseling, testing, and results. In many instances, health insurance will not cover the expense.[110]

The science and application of genetic testing is still in the developmental stage. Although the role of genetics is not completely clear in human oncogenesis, it is certain that the environmental carcinogens in the tissue are modified by the host genetic makeup.[33] No known genetic basis exists to explain the major racial differences in cancer incidence and outcome.[111,112] Continued research into the genetic-hereditary factor in the development of human cancers represents another edge in the fight toward cancer prevention and risk reduction.

Early Detection and Screening Recommendations

Many Americans are adopting more health-conscious behaviors, including diet modification, physical fitness, smoking cessation, and overall healthier lifestyles. Heightened awareness of health-promoting activities and early detection techniques related to cancer continue to be a focus of many cancer information agencies (e.g., ACS, NCI) and professional organizations (e.g., Oncology Nursing Society). Overall cancer survival can be increased through early detection. Regular breast, cervical, colorectal, and prostate screening techniques are validated by scientific evidence of their effectiveness in detecting cancers early. The ACS has updated the screening and early detection guidelines for average-risk persons as outlined in Table 4-8.[2]

The ACS last updated breast cancer screening guidelines in 2003. The ACS recommends that women be counseled regarding breast cancer risk. Breast self-examination (BSE) is no longer recommended, yet open dialogue between clinician and patient regarding potential benefits and limitations of the activity is essential.[113] In a large, randomized clinical trial conducted in Shanghai, China, evaluation of breast abnormalities identified during BSE often resulted in false-positive results. Neither stage of diagnosis nor breast cancer survival rates were improved in women taught BSE when compared to a group of women with no formal training or access to breast cancer screening.[114] Annual screening mammograms should begin at age 40. Despite debate regarding the efficacy of screening mammography, the U.S. Preventive Services Task Force (USPSTF) examined evidence from multiple randomized controlled trials, concluding that there is fair evidence that screening mammography reduces breast cancer deaths in women ages 40 to 74.[115,116] The ACS now recommends that women younger than age 40, at increased risk for breast cancer, be counseled regarding the potential benefits, harms, and limitations of beginning screening mammogram at a younger age. Studies suggest that breast imaging modalities such as breast ultrasound and breast MRI may be considered valuable for screening women meeting criteria for increased risk.[113]

The ACS guidelines for cervical cancer screening were last updated in 2002. Significant changes were made, incorporating new technologies such as human papilloma virus testing and liquid-based cytology Pap smears. It is recommended that cervical cancer screening begin 3 years following initiation of vaginal intercourse, or no later than age 21. Screening should continue annually with conventional Pap smear, or every 2 years with liquid-based cytology, until the age of 30. Without any history of abnormal Pap smear or cervical dysplasia, women over 30 may defer Pap testing for 2 to 3 years using either cytologic technique. Human papilloma virus (HPV) DNA testing may be added to either the conventional or liquid-based Pap smear every 3 years as well. Women at high risk for cervical cancer, that is, history of in utero diethylstilbestrol (DES) exposure, personal history of treated cervical cancer, or immunocompromised women such as those who are HIV positive, should continue annual screening. Women with a history of CIN 2 or CIN 3 who have undergone subtotal or total hysterectomy should continue Pap smear screening until 3 consecutive normal Pap smears are obtained and there are no abnormal results over a period of 10 years. Women with a history of subtotal hysterectomy for benign disease should continue cervical cancer screening as recommended for women of average risk. Cervical cancer screening can be discontinued in women who have a history of total hysterectomy for a benign condition.[113]

According to the ACS, there is insufficient evidence to recommend screening for endometrial cancer in women of average risk. Women at increased risk for endometrial cancer because of strong family history of endometrial or colorectal cancers, tamoxifen therapy, or history of unopposed estrogen therapy should be counseled on signs and symptoms of the disease, and screening should be considered.[113]

The ACS updated guidelines for screening and early detection of adenomatous polyps in 2001. Average-risk persons ages 50 years and older have several options for colorectal cancer screening. The FOBT or fecal immunochemical test (FIT) is recommended annually, alone or in combination with flexible sigmoidoscopy or double-contrast barium enema every 5 years. Colonoscopy is recommended every 10 years.[2,113] These recommendations mirror colorectal cancer screening guidelines issued in 2002 by the USPSTF. The USPSTF found good evidence that routine use of FOBT and fair evidence that flexible sigmoidoscopy alone or in combination with FOBT reduced mortality from colorectal cancer. Three randomized controlled trial utilizing FOBT revealed a reduction in mortality, whereas only outcomes from case-control studies on colorectal cancer screening with flexible sigmoidoscopy are available.[117] Although a highly sensitive technique for identifying adenomatous polyps, there was no evidence that colonoscopy reduced colorectal cancer mortality.[118]

Prostate cancer screening remains controversial. Shortly after the induction of PSA testing in 1986, the incidence of prostate cancer increased significantly, and mortality rates increased by 1% through 1992. This surge in prostate cancer detection was directly associated with PSA screening. In 1993, prostate cancer mortality rates began to decline by 1% per year.[117] Despite some evidence of risk reduction, there have been no randomized clinical trials to date on the efficacy of PSA in screening for prostate cancer. After reviewing the data, the USPSTF concluded that there was no strong evidence that screening for prostate cancer reduces mortality.[119] Despite the lack of clear benefit, the ACS updated guidelines on prostate cancer screening in 2001, recommending that non–African American men with a life expectancy of at least 10 years be offered prostate cancer screening with PSA and DRE annually by the age of 50. African American men are considered at high risk for developing prostate cancer, so annual PSA and DRE screening should begin at the age of 45. Men referred for prostate cancer screening should be counseled on the potential risks, benefits, and harms related to testing.[113]

Future Directions in Cancer Prevention and Early Detection

The science of cancer prevention continues to escalate and move rapidly forward. More is being understood regarding primary prevention in the realms of nutrition, exercise, tobacco control, and environmental factors. The quality of secondary prevention strategies continues to improve. Conventional and innovative screening tests are being examined.

New agents are being developed to treat nicotine dependence. Rimonabant (Acomplia) is a selective antagonist of the cannabinoid type 1 receptor in the central nervous system. The medication acts on the endocannabinoid (EC) system that helps to regulate behaviors associated with eating, fear, and anxiety. In the 1990s, researchers became familiar with the process by which substances such as marijuana may activate the EC system.[120] Increased food intake and desire to smoke may be the result. Rimonabant is being studied as a smoking cessation and weight loss agent. Two Phase III clinical trials have been conducted. The RIO-lipid study enrolled obese individuals with dyslipidemia to determine the efficacy of rimonabant in stimulating weight loss. The STRATUS-US study enrolled 787 smokers randomized to either rimonabant, 5 mg or 20 mg, versus placebo daily for 10 weeks. The percentage of participants who abstained from tobacco use in the last 4 weeks of treatment was 36.2% in the rimonabant, 20 mg, group, 20.2% for rimonabant, 5 mg, and 20.6% in the placebo group (p < 0.002).[121] Rimonabant has low risk profile. The most common side effects associated with rimonabant were nausea and upper respiratory tract infection. FDA approval is being sought by the maker of rimonabant, Sanofi-Aventis, for the indication of treating nicotine dependence.[120,122,123]

TABLE 4-8	Screening Guidelines for the Early Detection of Cancer in Asymptomatic People
SITE	**RECOMMENDATION**
Breast	• Yearly mammograms are recommended starting at age 40. The age at which screening should be stopped should be individualized by considering the potential risks and benefits of screening in the context of overall health status and longevity. • Clinical breast exam should be part of a periodic health exam, about every 3 years for women in their 20s and 30s, and every year for women 40 and older. • Women should know how their breasts normally feel and report any breast change promptly to their health care providers. Breast self-exam is an option for women starting in their 20s. • Women at increased risk (e.g., family history, genetic tendency, past breast cancer) should talk with their doctors about the benefits and limitations of starting mammography screening earlier, having additional tests (i.e., breast ultrasound and MRI), or having more frequent exams.
Colon & rectum	Beginning at age 50, men and women should begin screening with 1 of the examination schedules below: • A fecal occult blood test (FOBT) or fecal immunochemical test (FIT) every year • A flexible sigmoidoscopy (FSIG) every 5 years • Annual FOBT or FIT and flexible sigmoidoscopy every 5 years* • A double-contrast barium enema every 5 years • A colonoscopy every 10 years *Combined testing is preferred over either annual FOBT or FIT, or FSIG every 5 years, alone. People who are at moderate or high risk for colorectal cancer should talk with a doctor about a different testing schedule.
Prostate	The PSA test and the digital rectal examination should be offered annually, beginning at age 50, to men who have a life expectancy of at least 10 years. Men at high risk (African American men and men with a strong family history of 1 or more first-degree relatives diagnosed with prostate cancer at an early age) should begin testing at age 45. For both men at average risk and high risk, information should be provided about what is known and what is uncertain about the benefits and limitations of early detection and treatment of prostate cancer so that they can make an informed decision about testing.
Uterus	**Cervix:** Screening should begin approximately 3 years after a woman begins having vaginal intercourse, but no later than 21 years of age. Screening should be done every year with regular Pap tests or every 2 years using liquid-based tests. At or after age 30, women who have had 3 normal test results in a row may get screened every 2 to 3 years. Alternatively, cervical cancer screening with HPV DNA testing and conventional or liquid-based cytology could be performed every 3 years. However, doctors may suggest a woman get screened more often if she has certain risk factors, such as HIV infection or a weak immune system. Women 70 years and older who have had 3 or more consecutive normal Pap tests in the last 10 years may choose to stop cervical cancer screening. Screening after total hysterectomy (with removal of the cervix) is not necessary unless the surgery was done as a treatment for cervical cancer. **Endometrium:** The American Cancer Society recommends that at the time of menopause all women should be informed about the risks and symptoms of endometrial cancer, and strongly encouraged to report any unexpected bleeding or spotting to their physicians. Annual screening for endometrial cancer with endometrial biopsy beginning at age 35 should be offered to women with or at risk for hereditary nonpolyposis colon cancer (HNPCC).
Cancer-related checkup	For individuals undergoing periodic health examinations, a cancer-related checkup should include health counseling, and, depending on a person's age and gender, might include examinations for cancers of the thyroid, oral cavity, skin, lymph nodes, testes, and ovaries, as well as for some nonmalignant diseases.

American Cancer Society guidelines for early cancer detection are assessed annually in order to identify whether there is new scientific evidence sufficient to warrant a reevaluation of current recommendations. If evidence is sufficiently compelling to consider a change or clarification in a current guideline or the development of a new guideline, a formal procedure is initiated. Guidelines are formally evaluated every 5 years regardless of whether new evidence suggests a change in the existing recommendations. There are 9 steps in this procedure, and these "guidelines for guideline development" were formally established to provide a specific methodology for science and expert judgment to form the underpinnings of specific statements and recommendations from the Society. These procedures constitute a deliberate process to ensure that all Society recommendations have the same methodological and evidence-based process at their core. This process also employs a system for rating strength and consistency of evidence that is similar to that employed by the Agency for Health Care Research and Quality (AHCRQ) and the U.S. Preventive Services Task Force (USPSTF).
Copyright 2006 American Cancer Society, Inc. Reprinted with permission.

Varenicline, a drug that selectively binds to the alpha-4 beta-2 nicotine receptor, has been studied in Phase II trials. There is preliminary evidence that varenicline may be effective in promoting smoke cessation without significant side effects.[123]

Three nicotine vaccines are being developed to promote smoking cessation and long-term abstinence. TA-NIC, NicVAX, and Nicotine Obeta may potentially improve smoking cessation by prolonging periods of abstinence, prevent relapse in former smokers, and prevent adolescents from initiating tobacco use. The theory is that the vaccine stimulates the body to produce antibodies against nicotine, blocking the uptake of nicotine in the brain. The result is a reduction in positive reinforcement and the stimulation of pleasure centers that can be associated with chronic nicotine use.[123,124] In a study examining the safety and immunogenicity of NicVAX, doses from 50 mg to 200 mg were considered safe and well tolerated by study participants. Although smoking cessation was not an endpoint of the study, data suggested that 30-day abstinence rates were greater in persons treated with NicVAX, 200 mg, than those treated with lower doses of vaccine or placebo.[125]

HPV is a highly infectious disease that affects approximately 70% of all women. High-risk strains of HPV such as 16, 18, 33, and 45 have been implicated in cervical cancer.[126-129] Two pharmaceutical companies, Merck & Co. and GlaxoSmithKline, have developed cervical cancer vaccines. GlaxoSmithKline plans to market the Cervarix vaccine that provides immunity against HPV types 16 and 18, high-risk strains of HPV associated with up to 70% of all cervical cancer. Merck's Gardasil vaccine will protect against HPV 16 and 18 as well as HPV 6 and 11, lower-risk strains of the virus that cause 90% of all cases of genital warts.[126,130] In clinical trials, vaccines against HPV have been found to be both safe and effective in reducing the incidence of infection from HPV 6, 11, 16, and 18.[128,129,131-133] Questions remain regarding long-term immunity from the virus. The efficacy of vaccination in preventing cervical cancer and reducing mortality has not yet been proven. There will certainly be a debate regarding the appropriate age at which to vaccinate against HPV. Because the HPV vaccines provide immunity prophylactically it would be best administered before the onset of sexual activity. In a society where teenagers often initiate sexual activity as early as 13, preadolescent vaccination will have to be considered. HPV vaccine studies to date have been performed in young women; the question arises about considering vaccination of young men, as well.[126]

Diagnostic tests such as mammogram, PSA, FOBT, flexible sigmoidoscopy, and colonoscopy are the mainstay for cancer screening and early detection. MRI, positron emission tomography (PET) scans, and computed tomography (CT) scans are also being considered for cancer screening. Although the ACS does not currently recommend lung cancer screening in asymptomatic, average-risk persons, consideration is being given to screening former or current smokers using standard chest films or spiral CT. There is some evidence that spiral CT, which creates a 3-dimensional image of the lungs, is more sensitive for detecting small pulmonary tumors that may represent early-stage lung cancer.[113,134,135] As a result, the National Lung Cancer Screening Trial is being sponsored by the NCI. Approximately 50,000 current or former smokers were randomized to either spiral CT or chest x-ray to determine if there is a significant reduction of lung cancer deaths in either group. Screening will be performed annually for 3 years with follow-up through 2009.[134,136,137]

Conclusion

Cancer mortality will not be reduced without continued public awareness and a multidisciplinary approach involving health care professionals, epidemiologists, and researchers. Agencies such as the ACS, Leukemia Society, and NCI play a vital role in cancer control efforts through funding and support of all aspects of cancer research and public and professional education. These agencies and organizations also must increase activity and involvement in social and political decisions influencing health care policy, cancer research, and treatment.

Nurses can play a vital role in cancer prevention, screening, and risk reduction by identifying high-risk individuals and assessing lifestyle, personal and family history, and occupational or environmental exposure to carcinogens. Nurses may recognize individuals eligible for approved chemopreventive agents and those persons who meet inclusion criteria for cancer prevention clinical trials. Nurses should promote follow-up and surveillance for those persons at high risk. We can act as advocates for tobacco control by serving as nonsmoking role models and counseling patients and families on the risks of tobacco use. As clinicians, we are able to educate patients on available smoking cessation interventions.

Minority and underserved Americans offer the greatest challenge to nurses and other health care professionals. The underserved and SED populations make up a significant percentage of the American public and often bear the greatest burden of cancer risk and mortality. This is reflected in poorer overall survival, most frequently because of the later stage at which the cancer is detected. Barriers for this population include limited access to health care because of lack of health insurance, unemployment, homelessness, transportation issues, and inability to wait 6 to 8 hours in an overcrowded health care facility because of family and job responsibilities.

To offer public health teaching and support, the nurse and other health care professionals must be sensitive to social, cultural, ethnic, and religious beliefs, values, and attitudes that can affect a person's receptivity to health promotion and disease prevention strategies. Nurses can best prepare to meet public education needs through sensitivity-training sessions, development of printed materials that reflect cultural diversity and are at an appropriate literacy level, and thorough "train-the-trainer" programs for volunteers. Train-the-trainer programs facilitate contact with previously difficult-to-reach groups by training a volunteer from within the community or group to deliver the message of cancer prevention, risk reduction, and health promotion. Cancer prevention efforts should be aimed at safe sexual practices, reduced occupational and environmental exposure to carcinogens, health promotion activities, and education.[138,139]

REVIEW QUESTIONS

✔ Case Study

Mary, a 42-year-old Caucasian woman, is seen by the nurse practitioner in the wellness clinic for an annual well-woman exam. Her last mammogram was 1 year ago. She does not perform monthly breast self-examination. Mary's last Pap smear was several years ago; it was normal, and she denies any prior history of abnormal Pap smears. Her last menstrual period was 2 weeks ago, she reports; her age of menarche was 11, and she is nulliparous. The patient has had three sexual partners in the past and is currently single, not engaging in sexual intercourse. She denies any gynecologic concerns such as irregular vaginal bleeding, spotting, pelvic pressure, or pelvic bloating. Mary denies any history of medical problems, has never had surgery, and takes no medications, but she is allergic to penicillin.

Mary started smoking at the age of 15. She smokes one pack of cigarettes a day and drinks approximately 3 beers per week.

She voices a desire to stop smoking. Mary tried to stop smoking "cold turkey" several times but was only able to quit for 2 to 3 weeks at a time. Her family history is as follows: maternal aunt with breast cancer at the age of 44, younger sister with breast cancer diagnosed at 41, maternal grandmother with ovarian cancer at age 58, maternal great-grandmother with breast cancer at 54, paternal uncle with lung cancer at 76, and her father was diagnosed with colon cancer at the age of 67. She has two older brothers, ages 46 and 48, who are alive and well.

On physical examination Mary is in no acute distress and is pleasant and alert. Vital signs are blood pressure = 138/72, pulse = 88, respirations = 20. Weight = 201 lbs, and height is 5 feet 4 inches with calculated BMI = 34.5. Eyes, ears, nose, and throat are essentially negative. Inspection of the oral cavity reveals no suspicious lesions of the tongue or buccal mucosa; tongue is free of masses on palpation. Neck supple without cervical lymphadenopathy; no thyroid masses. Heart with regular rate and rhythm. Lungs clear to auscultation. Breasts symmetrical without skin or contour changes; no palpable breast masses or lympadenopathy of the axillary regions. Abdomen soft, round, nontender; no masses or hepatosplenomegaly. External genitals without lesions; bartholins, urethra and skenes gland (BUS) in normal limits, and cervix is pink without visible lesions. Pap smear was obtained from the cervical os and liquid-based sample sent to cytology. Bimanual examination reveals the uterus is mobile and antiverted and the adnexa are without masses. The Gail Model Risk Assessment was calculated. Mary's estimated 5-year risk for developing breast cancer = 1.4%. Both the screening mammogram and Pap smear were normal.

The nurse practitioner's assessment of Mary is that she is a healthy young woman without physical abnormalities but at risk for developing tobacco-related cancers, breast cancer, or ovarian cancer over her lifetime. In light of a negative exam the primary goal is to educate Mary on modifiable risk factors associated with cancer, counsel her regarding her personal risk for developing cancer, and refer the patient for further cancer screening that may be deemed appropriate. Mary is encouraged to follow up annually for mammogram, Pap smear, and general cancer screening examination. She is instructed that after 3 consecutive Pap smears at our facility she may defer annual cervical cancer screening and have her Pap smear performed every 2 years. Mary was reminded to use condoms routinely if she becomes sexually active to prevent HIV infection and other sexually transmitted diseases.

Breast self-awareness is reviewed with Mary. Although the nurse practitioner did not formally teach Mary BSE, signs and symptoms of breast cancer such as a mass, skin change, dimpling, and nipple retraction were reviewed with the patient. The Gail Model Risk Assessment was reviewed with the patient. Because her 5-year risk for developing breast cancer was less than 1.66%, she is not a candidate for tamoxifen therapy to reduce the risk of estrogen receptor–positive breast cancers. However, she reports multiple maternal relatives with breast cancer and a maternal grandmother with ovarian cancer. Breast cancer in second and third generations are not included in the Gail Model, so the tool is likely to underestimate Mary's risk for breast cancer. Mary may be at increased risk for breast

and ovarian cancer because of a hereditary susceptibility. A referral is made to the genetic counselor.

Mary is strongly encouraged to stop smoking. The strong association between tobacco use and oral, larynx, throat, lung, and bladder cancer were reviewed with the patient. She is given information regarding behavioral therapy, nicotine replacement, and buproprion. The patient is counseled on diet, nutrition, and the impact of obesity on cancer risk. She is encouraged to eat 5 to 9 fruits and vegetables daily, obtain a healthy weight, and incorporate physical activity into her daily activities. Although she does not consume alcohol in excess, Mary is reminded that alcohol may increase the risk for breast, endometrial, and colon cancer.

QUESTIONS

1. Neoplastic transformation in human cancers involves the following sequence of events:
   a. Stimulus, response, and initiation
   b. Risk, exposure, and progression
   c. Initiation, promotion, and progression
   d. Irritation, promotion, and susceptibility
2. According to the American Cancer Society guidelines, for optimal breast health, asymptomatic women should do which of the following?
   a. Annual breast self-examination (BSE) and mammography starting at age 50
   b. Clinical breast examination (CBE) and BSE, annual, starting at age 40
   c. Annual CBE and mammogram starting at age 40
   d. Annual CBE and mammogram every 3 years starting at age 50
3. Human papilloma virus (HPV) is a precursor to genital condyloma, cervical dysplasia, and cervical cancer. Which high-risk HPV strains are among those being targeted by new cervical cancer vaccines?
   a. 16 and 18
   b. 31 and 52
   c. 33 and 45
   d. 6 and 11
4. The nurse practitioner sees a 45-year-old African American male for an annual physical exam. Which of the following would be the most appropriate screening test for his race and age?
   a. DRE and PSA
   b. Colonoscopy
   c. Ultrasound of the bladder
   d. Stool for occult blood
5. The overall incidence of cancers can best be reduced by which of the following?
   a. Early detection
   b. Screening
   c. Prevention
   d. Early treatment
6. The American Cancer Society estimates that 80% of all cancers are associated with which of the following?
   a. Genetic predisposition
   b. Racial and ethnic factors
   c. Socioeconomic factors
   d. Environmental exposures

Continued

REVIEW QUESTIONS—CONT'D

7. Mary is not a good candidate for tamoxifen because
   a. She is not yet postmenopausal.
   b. She has never had children.
   c. Her risk for cervical cancer would increase exponentially with tamoxifen because of her history of multiple sexual partners.
   d. Her estimated 5-year risk for breast cancer is 1.4%.
8. What is the single most effective means by which Mary can reduce her risk for cancer?
   a. Stop smoking
   b. Stop drinking alcohol
   c. Undergo genetic testing
   d. Continue to abstain from intercourse
9. The nurse practitioner prescribes the following medication for Mary to use in combination with a nicotine replacement therapy and behavioral therapy for smoking cessation:
   a. Rimonabant
   b. Buproprion
   c. TA-NIC
   d. Varenicline
10. According to the ACS cervical cancer screening guidelines, by what schedule might Mary be screened for cervical cancer after three consecutive, negative Pap smears?
    a. Every 5 years with conventional Pap smears
    b. Every 5 years with liquid-based Pap smears
    c. Every 2 to 3 years with liquid-based Pap smears
    d. Mary may discontinue cervical cancer screening unless she develops bloody vaginal discharge

ANSWERS

1. **C.** *Rationale:* Neoplastic transformation involves initiation, promotion and progression, the multistep cellular change that results in malignancy if the process is not stopped. Stimulation of the neoplastic process, risk factors, carcinogens or irritant exposure, and cancer susceptibility may contribute to the development of malignancy, but none describes the pathologic changes that occur at the cellular level.

2. **C.** *Rationale:* The ACS recommends that women at average risk for breast cancer begin annual CBE and mammogram at the age of 40. Breast self-awareness rather than formalized monthly BSE is now the standard. Delaying mammography to the age of 50 may result in later-stage breast cancer diagnoses, and deferring CBE and mammogram every 3 years after age 50 may result in delay of breast cancer diagnosis. Several studies have shown a reduction in breast cancer mortality when mammograms begin at age 40.

3. **A.** *Rationale:* Two vaccines have proven efficacy for providing immunity for high-risk HPV strains that are implicated in cervical cancer development. Cervarix provides immunity against HPV 16 and 18. Gardasil is effective in providing immunity against HPV 16, 18, 6, and 11. HPV 6 and 11 are low-risk HPV strains that do not contribute to cervical cancer development but cause genital condyloma. HPV 31, 33, 45, and 52 are considered high-risk strains for cervical cancer, but neither vaccine provides protection against these virus subtypes.

4. **A.** *Rationale:* The ACS recommends African American men begin annual prostate cancer screening at age 45 because they are at higher risk for prostate cancer than men of other ethnic backgrounds. African American men at average risk for colon cancer should begin colorectal cancer screening with either colonoscopy, flexible sigmoidoscopy, barium enema, or fecal occult blood testing at the age of 50. Bladder ultrasound is a diagnostic test and not a recognized screening test for bladder cancer. This test would not be indicated in an asymptomatic person.

5. **C.** *Rationale:* Cancer prevention activities targeting modifiable risk factors (i.e., tobacco control, diet, healthy lifestyle) will reduce the incidence of cancer. Cancer screening, early detection, and treatment will reduce cancer mortality, but these activities will not reduce cancer occurrence.

6. **D.** *Rationale:* The ACS estimates that 80% of all cancers are associated with environmental exposures and are preventable. Genetic predispositions account for only 5% to 10% of cancer. Cancer incidence and mortality varies among ethnic groups, but it is unclear how biologic differences affect cancer development. Persons of lower socioeconomic status are more likely to be diagnosed with later-stage cancer that results in poorer survival than for persons of high socioeconomic status.

7. **D.** *Rationale:* Mary is not a candidate for tamoxifen because her 5-year risk for breast cancer is only 1.4%. Tamoxifen is available to women who have a 5-year risk for breast cancer greater than 1.66% as calculated by the Gail Model Risk Assessment. Premenopausal women age 35 and older with an increased risk for breast cancer per the Gail Model are eligible for the medication. Nulliparity is not a contraindication to tamoxifen use. Tamoxifen increases the risk for uterine cancer, not cervical cancer. Multiple sexual partners increase the risk for cervical cancer, not uterine cancer.

8. **A.** *Rationale:* Smoking cessation would significantly reduce Mary's lifetime risk for a number of tobacco-induced cancers. Alcohol consumption, although a risk factor for certain cancer development, is not as significantly a risk for Mary since she drinks in moderation. Genetic testing will help Mary to assess her risk for cancer development and provide her with a means by which to manage her risk. Abstaining from intercourse will reduce her risk for cervical cancer.

9. **B.** *Rationale:* Buproprion is an antidepressant medication approved by the FDA for smoking cessation. Rimonabant, varenicline, and TA-NIC are promising new agents for smoking cessation, but they are not yet approved by the FDA.

10. **C.** *Rationale:* The ACS recommends that women older than 30 with three consecutively negative Pap smears may delay cervical cancer screening by either conventional or liquid-based cytology to every 2 to 3 years. Five years would be considered too lengthy an interval, and the ACS does not recommend discontinuation of Pap smears unless the woman is at least 70 years of age or has undergone a hysterectomy for a benign condition.

REFERENCES

1. Jemal A, Murray T, Ward E et al: Cancer Statistics 2005, *CA Cancer J Clin* 55:10, 2005.
2. American Cancer Society: *Cancer facts and figures*, 2006. Atlanta, 2005, Author.
3. U.S. Department of Health and Human Services. *Healthy people 2010: understanding and improving health.* US Government Printing Office, Washington, DC, 2000, No. 012-00-00543-6, www.health.gov/healthypeople.
4. Eyre H, Kahn R, Robertson RM et al, Preventing cancer, cardiovascular disease, and diabetes: a common agenda for the American Cancer Society, the American Diabetes Association, and the American Heart Association, *CA Cancer J Clin* 54:190, 2004.
5. American Cancer Society: *Cancer prevention and early detection facts and figures 2005*, Atlanta, 2005, Author.
6. Burke W, Daly M, Garber J, Botkin J: Recommendations for follow-up care of individuals with an inherited predisposition to cancer. II. BRCA1 and BRCA2. Cancer genetics cancer consortium, *JAMA* 277:997, 1997.
7. American Cancer Society: *Cancer facts and figures for African Americans 2005-2006*, Atlanta, 2005, Author.
8. Cookson MS, Smith JA: PSA testing: to screen or not to screen? *Primary Care Consultant* 40:4, 670, 2000.
9. Cuzick J: Human papillomavirus testing for primary cervical cancer screening, *JAMA*, 283:108, 2000.
10. Fink DJ, Mettlin CJ: Cancer detection: the cancer related checkup guidelines. In Murphy G, Lawrence W, Lenhard R, editors: *ACS textbook of clinical oncology,* ed 2, Atlanta, 1995, American Cancer Society.
11. Boyer KL, Ford MB, Judkins AF et al: *Primary care oncology,* Philadelphia, 1999, W.B. Saunders Company.
12. Heusinkveld KB: Cancer prevention and risk assessment. In Varricchio C, editor: *A cancer source book for nurses,* Atlanta, 1997, American Cancer Society.
13. Murphy GP, Lawrence W, Lenhard RE: *ACS textbook of clinical oncology,* ed 2, Atlanta, 1995, American Cancer Society.
14. Gullatte MM: Prevention, screening, and detection. In Otto S, editor: *Oncology nursing,* ed 3, St. Louis, 1997, Mosby.
15. Bradley CJ, Given CW, Roberts C: Disparities in cancer diagnosis and survival, *Cancer* 91:178, 2001.
16. American Cancer Society: *Cancer facts and figures, 2004*, Atlanta, 2004, Author.
17. Baquet CR, Horm, JW, Gibbs, T: Socioeconomic factors and cancer incidence among blacks and whites, *J Natl Cancer Inst* 83:551, 1991.
18. Noe LL, Becker RV, Gradishar MD et al: The cost effectiveness of tamoxifen in the prevention of breast cancer, *Am J Managed Care* 5:5393, 1999.
19. Hiatt RA, Kabunde C, Breen N et al: Cancer screening practices from national health interview surveys: past, present and future, *J Natl Cancer Inst* 94:1837, 2002.
20. Institute of Medicine: *Unequal treatment: what healthcare providers need to know about racial and ethnic disparities in healthcare,* Washington, DC, 2002, National Academy of Sciences.
21. Shinagawa SM: The excess burden of breast carcinoma in minority and medically underserved communities, application, research and redressing institutional racism, *Cancer* 88(Suppl):1218, 2000.
22. Steenland K, Burnett C, Lalich N et al: Dying for work: the magnitude of US mortality from selected causes of death associated with occupation, *Am J Indust Med* 43:461, 2003.
23. Haverkos HW: Viruses, chemicals and co-carcinogenesis, *Oncogene* 23:6492, 2004.
24. Parsonnet J, Friedman GD, Vandersteen DP et al: *Helicobacter pylori* infection and the risk of gastric carcinoma, *New Engl J Med* 325:1127, 1991.
25. Wakeford, R: The cancer epidemiology of radiation, *Oncogene* 23:6404, 2004.
26. Ron E, Ikeda T, Preston DL et al: Male breast cancer incidence among atomic bomb survivors, *J Natl Cancer Inst* 90:603, 2005.
27. Heath CW: Electromagnetic field exposure and cancer: a review of epidemiologic evidence, *CA Cancer J Clin* 46:29, 1996.
28. Executive Summary: *The health consequences of smoking*, Surgeon General Report, 2004. retrieved January, 27, 2006, from www.surgeon-general.gov/tobacco/.
29. Iribarren C and others: Effect of cigar smoking on the risk of cardiovascular diseases, chronic obstructive pulmonary disease and cancer in men, *N Engl J Med* 340:1773, 1999.
30. Satcher D: Cigars and public health, *N Engl J Med* 340:1829, 1999.
31. Wingo PA, Ries LAG, Giovino GA et al: Annual report on the status of cancer, 1973–1996, *J Natl Cancer Inst* 91:675, 1999.
32. Heath CW: Cancer prevention. In Holleb AI, Fink DJ, Murphy GP, editors: *ACS textbook of clinical oncology,* Atlanta, 1991, American Cancer Society.
33. Ruckdeschel JC: *Myths and facts about lung cancer: what you need to know,* New York, 1999, PRR.
34. *Cancer risk report: prevention and control,* Atlanta, 1998, American Cancer Society.
35. Fiore MC, Bailey WC, Cohen SJ, et al: *Treating tobacco use and dependence. Quick reference guide for clinicians.* Rockville, MD, 2000, U.S. Department of Health and Human Services, Public Health Service.
36. Rigotti NA: Treatment of tobacco use and dependence, *New Engl J Med* 346:506 2002.
37. Hughes JR: New treatments for smoking cessation, *CA Cancer J Clin* 50:143, 2000.
38. Poschl G, Seitz HK: Alcohol and cancer, *Alcohol Alcohol* 39:155, 2004.
39. Fang JL and Vaca CE: Detection of DNA adducts of acetaldehyde in peripheral white blood cells of alcohol abusers, *Carcinogenesis* 18:627, 1997.
40. Suzuki R, Ye W, Rylander-Rudqvist T et al: Alcohol and postmenopausal breast cancer risk defined by estrogen and progesterone receptor status: a prospective cohort study, *J Natl Cancer Inst* 97:1601, 2005.
41. Longnecker MP: Alcoholic beverage consumption in relation to risk of breast cancer: meta-analysis and review, *Cancer Causes Control* 5:73, 1994.
42. World Cancer Research Fund: *Food, nutrition and prevention of cancer: a global perspective,* Washington, DC, 1997, American Institute for Cancer Research.
43. Hamajima N, Hirose K, Tajima K, et al: Alcohol, tobacco and breast cancer in women, *Br J Cancer* 87:1234, 2002.
44. Clark R, Dickson RB, Lippman ME: Hormonal aspects of breast cancer. Growth factors, drugs and stromal interactions, *Crit Rev Oncol Hematol* 12:1, 1992.
45. Fan S, Meng Q, Gao B et al: Alcohol stimulates estrogen receptor signaling in human breast cancer cells lines, *Cancer Res* 60:5635, 2000.
46. Dorgan JF, Baer DJ, Albert PS et al: Serum hormones and the alcohol-breast cancer association in postmenopausal women, *J Natl Cancer Inst* 93:710, 2001.
47. Gavaler JS, Rosenblum E: Exposure-dependent effects of ethanol on serum estradiol and uterus mass in sexually mature oophorectomized rates: a model for bilaterally ovariectomized-postmenopausal women, *J Stud Alcohol* 48:295, 1987.
48. Ginsburg E: Estrogen, alcohol and breast cancer risk, *J Steroid Biochem Mol Biol* 69:299, 1999.
49. Singletary KW, Frey RS, Yan W: Effect of ethanol on proliferation and estrogen receptor-alpha expression in human breast cancer cells, *Cancer Lett* 165:131, 2001.
50. Zumoff B, The critical role of alcohol consumption in determining the risk of breast cancer with postmenopausal estrogen administration, *J Clin Endocrinol Metabol* 82:1656, 1997.
51. Simanowski UA, Homann N, Knuhl M et al: Increased rectal cell proliferation following alcohol abuse, *Gut* 49:418, 2001.
52. Tiemersma E, Wark P, Ocke M et al: Alcohol consumption, alcohol dehydrogenase 3 polymorphism, and colorectal adenomas, *Cancer Epidemiol Biomarker Prev* 12:419, 2003.
53. Cope GF, Wyatt JI, Pinder IF et al: Alcohol consumption in patients with colorectal adenomatous polyps, *Gut* 32:70, 1991.
54. Kikendall J, Bowen P, Burgess M, et al: Cigarettes and alcohol as independent risk factors for colonic adenomas, *Gastroenterology,* 97:660, 1989.
55. Bardou M, Montembault S, Giraud V et al: Excessive alcohol consumption favors high-risk polyp or colorectal cancer occurrence among patients with adenomas: a case control study, *Gut* 50:38, 2002.
56. Seitz HK, Simanowski UA, Garzon FT et al: Possible role of acetaldehyde in ethanol-related rectal cocarcinogenesis in the rat, *Gastroenterology* 98:406, 1990.
57. The U.S. Department of Agriculture: Does alcohol have a place in a healthy diet? *Nutrit Insights*, retrieved January, 27, 2006, from www.usda.gov/fcs/cnpp.htm.

58. Deckelbaum R, Williams C: Childhood obesity: the health issue, *Obesity Res* 9:S239, 2001.

59. Strauss RS, Pollack HA: Epidemic increase in childhood overweight, 1986-1998, *JAMA* 22:2845, 2001.

60. Troiano R, Flegal K: Overweight children and adolescents: description, epidemiology, and demographics, *Pediatrics* 101:497, 1998.

61. Gorman C: Colon cancer: Katie's crusade, *Time* 70, 2000.

62. Calle E, Thun M: Obesity and cancer, *Oncogene* 23:6365, 2004.

63. Macauly VM: Insulin-like growth factors and cancer, *Br J Cancer* 65:311, 1992.

64. LeRoith D: Seminars in medicine of the Beth Israel Deaconess Medical Center. Insulin-like growth factors, *New Engl J Med* 336:633, 1997.

65. Kaaks R, Lukanova A, Kurzer M: Obesity, endogenous hormones, and endometrial cancer risk, *Cancer Epidemiol Biomarkers Prev* 11:1531, 2002.

66. Kolonel L, Nomura A, Cooney R: Dietary fat and prostate cancer: current status, *J Natl Cancer Inst* 91:414, 1999.

67. Heber D, Fair WR, Ornish D: The Association for the Cure of Cancer of the Prostate: *Nutrition and prostate cancer: a monograph from the CaP CURE Nutrition Project,* 2nd ed, Santa Monica, 1998, Cap CURE.

68. Freedland S: The biology behind obesity and prostate cancer: a growing problem, *Clin Cancer Res* 11:6763, 2005.

69. Snowdon DA, Phillips RL, Choi W: Diet, obesity and risk of fatal prostate cancer, *Am J Epidemiol* 120:244, 1984.

70. Rodriquez C, Patel AV, Calle EE et al: Body mass index, height, and prostate cancer mortality in two large cohorts of adult men in the United States, *Cancer Epidemiol Biomarkers Prev* 10:345, 2001.

71. Dahle SE, Chokkalingam AP, Gao YYT et al: Body size and serum levels of insulin and leptin in relation to the risk of benign prostatic hyperplasia, *J Urol* 168:599, 2002.

72. Barqawi A, Golden B, O'Donnell C et al: Observed effect of age and body mass index on total and complexed PSA: analysis from a national screening program, *Urology* 65:708, 2005.

73. Baillargeon J, Pollock B, Kristal et al: The association of body mass index and prostate-specific antigen in a population-based study, *Cancer* 103:1092, 2005.

74. Calle E, Rodriquez C, Walker-Thurmond K et al: Overweight, obesity and mortality from cancer in a prospectively studied cohort of U.S. adults, *New Engl J Med* 348:1625, 2003.

75. USDA Nutrient content of the U.S. food supply, 1909-2000, retrieved December 20, 2005, from http://www.cnpp.usda.gov/Pubs/Food%20 Supply/FoodSupply2003Rpt/FoodSupply1909-2000.pdf.

76. Griffiths EK, Schapira DV: Serum ferritin and stool occult blood and colon cancer screening, *Cancer Detect Prev* 15:303, 1991.

77. Gullatte MM: Cancer prevention and early detection in black Americans: colon and rectum, *J Natl Black Nurses Assoc* 3:49, 1989.

78. Ziegler RG, Devesa SS, Fravmeni JF Jr: Epidemiologic patterns of colorectal cancer. In DeVita VT Jr, Hellman S, Rosenberg SA, editors: *Important advances in oncology,* Philadelphia, 1991, Lippincott.

79. Drago JR: The role of new modalities in the early detection and diagnosis of prostate cancer, *CA Cancer J Clin* 39:326, 1989.

80. Gullatte MM: Cancer prevention and early detection in black Americans: prostate, *In Touch* 9:4, 1988.

81. *Nutrition and cancer prevention: guidelines on diet, nutrition, and cancer prevention: reducing the risk of cancer with healthy food choices and physical activity,* Atlanta, 1999, American Cancer Society.

82. Bal DG, Nixon DW, Foerster SB et al: Cancer prevention. In Murphy G, Lawrence W, Lenhard R, editors: *ACS textbook of clinical oncology,* ed 2, Atlanta, 1995, American Cancer Society.

83. Pate RR, Pratt M, Blair SN et al: Physical activity and public health: a recommendation from the Centers for Disease Control and Prevention and the American College of Sports Medicine, *JAMA* 273:402, 1995.

84. Rutqvist LE, Cedermark B, Glas U et al: Contralateral primary tumors in breast cancer patients in a randomized trial of adjuvant tamoxifen therapy, *J Natl Cancer Inst* 83:18, 1991.

85. Fisher B, Redmond C: New perspective on cancer of the contralateral breast: a marker for assessing tamoxifen as a preventive agent, *J Natl Cancer Inst* 83:1278, 1991.

86. Fisher B, Costantino JP, Wickerham L et al: Tamoxifen for prevention of breast cancer: report of the National Surgical Adjuvant Breast and Bowel Project P-1 Study, *J Natl Cancer Inst* 90:1371, 1998.

87. Fisher B, Costantino JP, Wickerham L et al: Tamoxifen for the prevention of breast cancer: current status of the National Surgical Adjuvant Breast and Bowel Project P-1 Study, *J Natl Cancer Inst* 97:1652, 2005.

88. Melnikow J, Paterniti D, Azari R et al: Preferences of women evaluating risks of tamoxifen (POWER) study of preferences for tamoxifen for breast cancer risk reduction, *Cancer* 103:103, 2005.

89. Port ER, Montgomery LL, Heerdt AS et al: Patient reluctance toward tamoxifen use for breast cancer primary prevention, *Ann Surg Oncol* 8:580, 2001.

90. Vogel VG: Follow-up of the breast cancer prevention trial and the future of breast cancer prevention efforts, *Clin Cancer Res* 7:4413s, 2001.

91. Cummings SR, Eckert S, Krueger KA et al: The effect of raloxifene on risk of breast cancer in postmenopausal women: results from the MORE randomized trial, *JAMA,* 281:2189, 1999.

92. Baum M, Buzdar A, Cuzick J et al: Anastrozole alone or in combination with tamoxifen versus tamoxifen alone for the adjuvant treatment of post-menopausal women with early stage breast cancer: results of the ATAC (Arimidex, Tamoxifen Alone or in Combination) trial efficacy and safety update analyses, *Cancer* 98:1802, 2003.

93. Cuzick J: Aromatase inhibitors for breast cancer prevention, *J Clin Oncol* 23:1636, 2005.

94. National Cancer Institute: *Clinical trials,* retrieved January 10, 2006, from www.cancer.org.

95. Tsao AS, Kim ES, Hong WK: Chemoprevention of cancer, *CA Cancer J Clin* 54:150, 2004.

96. Steinbach G, Lynch PM, Phillips RKS, et al: The effect of celecoxib, a cyclooxygenase-2 inhibitor, in familial adenomatous polyposis, *New Engl J Medicine* 342:1946, 2000.

97. Lippman SM, Hong WK: Cancer prevention science and practice, *Cancer Res* 62:5119, 2003.

98. Thompson IM, Goodman PJ, Tangen CM et al: The influence of finasteride on the development of prostate cancer, *New Engl J Med* 349:215, 2003.

99. Clark LC, Combs GF Jr, Turnbull BW et al: Effects of selenium supplementation for cancer prevention in patients with carcinoma of the skin. A randomized controlled trial. Nutrition Prevention of Cancer Study Group, *JAMA* 276:1957, 1996.

100. The Alpha-Tocopherol, Beta-Carotene Cancer Prevention Study Group: The effect of vitamin E and beta carotene on the incidence of lung cancer and other cancers in male smokers, *New Engl J Med* 330:1029, 1994.

101. Klein EA, Lippman SM, Thompson IM et al: The selenium and vitamin E cancer prevention trial, *World J Urol* 21:1, 2003.

102. Lippman SM, Goodman PJ, Klein HL et al: Designing the selenium and vitamin E cancer prevention trial (SELECT), *J Natl Cancer Inst* 97:94, 2005.

103. Nagy R, Sweet K, Eng C: Highly penetrant hereditary cancer syndromes, *Oncogene* 23:6445, 2004.

104. Fearon ER: Human cancer syndromes: clues to the origin and nature of cancer, *Science* 278:1043, 1997.

105. National Comprehensive Cancer Network (NCCN): Genetic/familial high-risk assessment: breast and ovarian, version 1.2006, retrieved January 10, 2006, from www.nccn.org.

106. Pharoah PD, Day NE, Duffy S et al: Family history and the risk for breast cancer: a systematic review and meta-analysis, *Int J Cancer* 71:5, 1997

107. American Society of Clinical Oncology: American Society of Clinical Oncology policy statement update: genetic testing for cancer susceptibility, *J Clin Oncol* 21:1, 2003.

108. Carter RF: BRCA1, BRCA2 and breast cancer: a concise clinical review, *Clin Invest Med* 24:147, 2001

109. Kuhl CK, Schrading S, Leutner CC et al: Mammography, breast ultrasound, and magnetic resonance imaging for surveillance of women at high familial risk for breast cancer, *J Clin Oncol* 23:8469, 2005.

110. Lawrence WF, Peshkin B, Liang W et al: Cost of genetic counseling and testing for BRCA 1 and BRCA 2 breast cancer susceptibility mutations, *Cancer Epidemiol Biomarkers Prevent* 10:475, 2001.

111. Phillips J, Belcher A, O'Neil A: Special populations. In Varricchio C, editor: *A cancer source book for nurses,* ed 7, Atlanta, 1997, American Cancer Society.

112. Stromborg MF, Olsen SJ: *Cancer prevention in minority populations: cultural implications for health care professionals,* St Louis, 1993, Mosby.

113. Smith RA, Cokkinides V, Eyre HJ: American Cancer Society Guidelines for the early detection of cancer, 2005, *CA Cancer J Clin* 55:31, 2005.

114. Thomas DB, Gao DL, Ray RM et al: Randomized trial of breast self-examination in Shanghai: final results, *J Natl Cancer Inst* 94:1445, 2002.

115. Humphrey LL, Helfand M, Benjamin KS: Breast cancer screening: a summary of the evidence for the U.S. Preventive Services Task Force, *Ann Intern Med* 137:347, 2002

116. Feig SA: Screening mammography controversies: resolved, partly resolved, and unresolved, *Breast J* 11:S3, 2005.

117. Gates TJ: Screening for cancer: evaluating the evidence, *Am Fam Phys* 63:513, 2001.

118. U.S. Preventive Services Task Force: Screening for colorectal cancer: recommendations and rationale, *Ann Intern Med* 137:129, 2002.

119. Harris R, Lohr KN: Screening for prostate cancer: an update of the evidence for the U.S. Preventive Services Task Force, *Ann Intern Med* 137:917, 2002.

120. Boyd ST, Fremming BA: Rimonabant—a selective CB1 antagonist, *Ann Pharmacother* 39:684, 2005.

121. Cleland JGF, Ghosh J, Freemantle N et al: Clinical trials update and cumulative meta-analyses from the American College of Cardiology: WATCH, SCD-HeFT, DINAMIT, CASINO, INSPIRE, STRATUS-US, RIO-LIPIDS and cardiac resynchronization therapy in heart failure, *Eur J Heart Failure* 6:501, 2004.

122. Fernandez JR, Allison DB: Rimonabant Sanofi-Synthelabo, *Curr Opin Invest Drugs* 5:430, 2004.

123. Henningfield JE, Fant RV, Buchhalter AR, et al: Pharmacotherapy for nicotine dependence, *CA Cancer J Clin* 55:281, 2005.

124. Vocci FJ, Chiang CN: Vaccines against nicotine: how effective are they likely to be in preventing smoking? *CNS Drugs* 15:505, 2001.

125. Hatsukami DK, Rennard S, Jorenby D et al: Safety and immunogencity of a nicotine conjugate vaccine in current smokers, *Clin Pharmacol Ther* 78:456, 2005.

126. Shaw AR: Human papillomavirus vaccines in development: if they're successful in clinical trials, how will they be implemented? *Gynecol Oncol* 99:S246, 2005.

127. Goldie SJ, Kohli M, Grima D et al: Projected clinical benefits and cost-effectiveness of a human papilloma virus 16/18 vaccine, *J Natl Cancer Inst* 96:604, 2004.

128. Arvin AM, Greenberg HB: New viral vaccines, *Virology* 344:240, 2006

129. Christensen ND: Emerging human papillomavirus vaccines, *Summ Expert Opin Emerging Drugs* 10:5, 2005.

130. Washam, C: Two HPV vaccines yielding similar success, *J Natl Cancer Inst* 97:1030, 2005.

131. Koutsky LA, Ault KA, Wheeler CM et al: A controlled trial of a human papillomavirus type 16 vaccine, *New Engl J Med* 347:21, 2002.

132. Emeny RT, Wheeler CM, Jansen KT et al: Priming of human papillomavirus type 11-specific humoral and cellular immune responses in college-aged women with a virus-like particle vaccine, *J Virol* 76:7832, 2002.

133. Harper DM, Fanco EL, Wheeler C et al: Efficacy of a bivalent L1 virus-like particle vaccine in prevention of infection with human papillomavirus types 16 and 18 in young women: a randomized controlled trial, *Lancet* 364:1757, 2004.

134. Truong MT, Munden RF: Lung cancer screening, *Curr Oncol Rep* 5:4, 2003.

135. Swensen SJ, Jett JR, Hartman TE et al: CT screening for lung cancer: five-year prospective experience, *Radiology* 235:1, 2005

136. *What is NLST?* Retrieved January 11, 2006, from http://www.cancer.gov/nlst/what-is-nlst.

137. Recruitment begins for lung cancer screening trial, *J Natl Cancer Inst* 94:21, 2002.

138. Tubiana M: Trends in primary and secondary prevention, *Cancer Detect Prev* 15:1, 1991.

139. Watkins MC: Computerized cancer information sources, *J Med Assoc Ga* 81:143, 1992.

CHAPTER 5

Cancer Diagnosis and Staging

Gail B. Johnson

Early detection and screening are not yet available for all cancers. The diagnosis of cancer may be made during the course of a routine physical examination before a patient has symptoms of disease. It is therefore important that the clinician have a high index of suspicion for abnormal findings, both during the physical exam and in taking the patient's history. Clinicians and the general public should be aware of the American Cancer Society's recommendations for the early detection of cancer in average-risk, asymptomatic people (Table 5-1).[1]

It is commonly known that the risk of developing cancer increases with age.[2] Therefore the elderly are an important target group for screening, early detection, and diagnostic efforts. The presence of comorbities in this group can make it difficult for the elderly to withstand a cancer diagnosis and subsequent treatment. An adequate assessment of functional status and comorbidities is crucial in this group.

The diagnosis of cancer is very complex and provokes high anxiety. It necessitates a team effort that includes the patient, the physician, the nurse, other oncology specialists, pathologists, and technicians. An accurate cancer diagnosis is essential in planning treatment and anticipating treatment outcomes. The current trend is the use of prognostic scoring systems to ascertain the best treatment approaches based on information gained during the diagnostic process. This begins with a careful history and complete physical exam. A high index of suspicion, based on known risk factors, will guide the clinician toward the appropriate testing and procedures required to obtain an accurate diagnosis.

Tumor Markers

Tumor markers may be either a protein product excreted by cancer cells or protein products released in response to the presence of cancer or other conditions. Tumor markers alone are not a sufficient tool to diagnose cancer, since some markers will be elevated in the presence of more than one type of cancer. However, tumor markers in conjunction with a patient's history, physical exam, and other diagnostic tests can aid in the diagnosis of a specific cancer. Tumor markers may also be useful in determining the prognosis of specific cancers, detecting recurrence, and assessing the effectiveness of treatment.

The following tumor markers are used to aid in the diagnosis of cancer, to detect recurrence, or identify regression of a known malignancy.

PROSTATE-SPECIFIC ANTIGEN (PSA)

Prostate-specific antigen (PSA) can be elevated in prostate cancer. However, PSA levels can also be elevated in the presence of benign prostatic hyperplasia, in older men, and in men with larger prostate glands. When screening for prostate cancer, the PSA should be accompanied by a digital rectal exam (DRE) to evaluate the prostate gland for irregularities. The PSA test is also useful in evaluating response to treatment and recurrence in patients treated with surgery or radiation therapy. If the PSA level was elevated at diagnosis, it should fall toward normal levels after definitive treatment. A rising PSA level would suggest recurrence of the disease.

S-100

S-100 is found in melanoma cells. This protein is measured in tissue samples of suspected melanomas. It is usually elevated in patients with metastatic melanoma.

THYROGLOBULIN

Thyroglobulin is a protein made by the thyroid gland. Measured in the blood, it is elevated in many thyroid diseases, including some forms of thyroid cancer. Treatment may include removal of the entire gland, with or without radiation therapy. Afterward, thyroglobulin should fall to undetectable levels. A rise in thyroglobulin levels indicates cancer recurrence.

ESTROGEN AND PROGESTERONE RECEPTORS

To date, there are no tumor markers for the early detection of breast cancer. However, once diagnosed, breast cancer tissue has been tested for the presence of estrogen and progesterone receptors. These markers provide an indication of the aggressiveness of the cancer and how likely the cancer will be to respond to specific types of endocrine therapy.

CA 15-3 AND CA 27-29

Specific for breast cancer, these markers are found in the blood of affected patients and are most useful in evaluating the effectiveness of treatment for individuals with advanced disease. Both tests are commonly used to monitor for recurrence in women who have been treated for breast cancer. The CA 27-29 test may be more sensitive than the CA 15-3.

CARCINOEMBRYONIC ANTIGEN (CEA) AND CA 19-9

These tumor markers are commonly elevated in advanced colorectal cancer. The carcinoembryonic antigen (CEA) has been considered the "gold standard" tumor marker for colorectal cancer for over 20 years. An elevated CEA level before surgical intervention for colorectal cancer may indicate a poorer prognosis. CEA levels are also elevated in other circumstances including breast, lung, thyroid, pancreas, liver, stomach, ovary, and bladder cancers; in noncancer conditions; and in otherwise healthy smokers, as well.

TABLE 5-1 **American Cancer Society Recommendations for the Early Detection of Cancer in Average-Risk, Asymptomatic Persons**

CANCER SITE	POPULATION	TEST OR PROCEDURE	FREQUENCY
Breast	Women, aged ≥ 20 years	Breast self-examination (BSE)	Beginning in their early 20s, women should be told about the benefits and limitations of BSE. The importance of prompt reporting of any new breast symptoms to a health professional should be emphasized. Women who choose to do BSE should receive instruction and have their technique reviewed on the occasion of a periodic health examination. It is acceptable for women to choose not to do BSE or to do BSE irregularly.
		Clinical breast examination (CBE)	For women in their 20s and 30s, it is recommended that CBE be part of a periodic health examination, preferably at least every 3 years. Asymptomatic women aged 40 years and over should continue to receive a clinical breast examination as part of a periodic health examination, preferably annually.
		Mammography	Begin annual mammography at age 40 years.*
Colorectal	Men and women, aged ≥ 50 years	Fecal occult blood test (FOBT),† or fecal immunochemical test (FIT), or	Annual, starting at age 50 years
		Flexible sigmoidoscopy, or	Every 5 years, starting at age 50 years
		Fecal occult blood test (FOBT)† and flexible sigmoidoscopy,‡ or	Annual FOBT (or FIT) and flexible sigmoidoscopy every 5 years, starting at age 50 years
		Double-contrast barium enema (DCBE), or	DCBE every 5 years, starting at age 50 years
		Colonoscopy	Colonoscopy every 10 years, starting at age 50 years.
Prostate	Men, aged ≥ 50 years	Digital rectal examination (DRE) and prostate-specific antigen (PSA) test	The PSA test and the DRE should be offered annually, starting at age 50 years, for men who have a life expectancy of at least 10 more years.§
Cervix	Women, aged ≥ 18 years	Pap test	Cervical cancer screening should begin approximately 3 years after a woman begins having vaginal intercourse, but no later than 21 years of age. Screening should be done every year with conventional Pap tests or every 2 years using liquid-based Pap tests. At or after age 30 years, women who have had three normal test results in a row may get screened every 2 to 3 years with cervical cytology (either conventional or liquid-based Pap test) alone, or every 3 years with a human papillomavirus DNA test plus cervical cytology. Women aged ≥70 years who have had three or more normal Pap tests and no abnormal Pap tests in the last 10 years, and women who have had a total hysterectomy, may choose to stop cervical cancer screening.
Endometrial	Women, at menopause		At the time of menopause, women at average risk should be informed about risks and symptoms of endometrial cancer and strongly encouraged to report any unexpected bleeding or spotting to their physicians.

Continued

TABLE 5-1   American Cancer Society Recommendations for the Early Detection of Cancer in Average-Risk, Asymptomatic Persons—cont'd

CANCER SITE	POPULATION	TEST OR PROCEDURE	FREQUENCY
Cancer-related checkup	Men and women, aged ≥20 years		On the occasion of a periodic health examination, the cancer-related checkup should include examination for cancers of the thyroid, the testicles, the ovaries, the lymph nodes, the oral cavity, and the skin, as well as health counseling about tobacco, sun exposure, diet and nutrition, risk factors, sexual practices, and environmental and occupational exposures.

*Beginning at age 40 years, annual clinical breast examination should be performed before mammography.
†FOBT as it is sometimes done in physicians' offices, with the single-stool sample collected on a fingertip during a DRE, is not an adequate substitute for the recommended at-home procedure of collecting two samples from three consecutive specimens. Toilet-bowl FOBT tests also are not recommended. In comparison with guaiac-based tests for the detection of occult blood, immunochemical tests are more patient-friendly and are likely to be equal or better in sensitivity and specificity. There is no justification for repeating FOBT in response to an initial positive finding.
‡Flexible sigmoidoscopy together with FOBT is preferred to either FOBT or flexible sigmoidoscopy alone.
§Information should be provided to men about the benefits and limitations of testing so that an informed decision about testing can be made with the clinician's assistance.
From Smith RA, Cokkinides V, Eyre HJ: American Cancer Society guidelines for the early detection of cancer, *CA Cancer J Clin* 56:11-25, 2006; retrieved from http://caonline.amcancersoc.org/cgi/content/full/56/1/11.

CA-125

Of women with advanced epithelial ovarian cancer, the most common form of ovarian cancer, 90% will have an elevated CA-125 level. Women with a strong family history of ovarian cancer are often screened with both CA-125 testing and ultrasound. Because of its elevation in other malignancies and conditions, it is not recommended that CA-125 level alone be the determining tool in diagnosing ovarian cancer.

HUMAN CHORIONIC GONADOTROPIN (HCG) AND ALPHA-FETOPROTEIN (AFP)

Female patients with germ cell ovarian tumors and men with nonseminomatous testicular cancer often display elevated levels of human chorionic gonadotropin (HCG) and/or alpha-fetoprotein (AFP). There is no positive correlation between the level of the marker concentration and prognosis. AFP levels are higher than normal in two thirds of patients with cancer. The level increases proportionately to the size of the tumor. AFP levels may also be elevated in chronic hepatitis.

BETA-2-MICROGLOBULIN (B2M)

Beta-2-microglobulin (B2M) is elevated in persons with multiple myeloma, chronic lymphocytic leukemia, and some lymphomas, as well as some types of kidney disease.

HER-2/neu

The HER2/neu marker is overexpressed or elevated in one third of persons diagnosed with breast cancer. It is used to predict response to therapy. Individuals who express this feature respond to a specific type of monoclonal antibody aimed against the HER-2/neu receptor on breast cancer cells.

CHROMOGRANIN A (CgA)

Chromogranin A (CgA) is produced by neuroendocrine tumors including carcinoid, neuroblastoma, and small cell lung cancers. It is the most sensitive tumor marker for carcinoid tumors.

Diagnostic Imaging Methods

The role of imaging is an important one in the diagnosis and staging of cancer. The imaging techniques that have evolved often replace the need for invasive measures to arrive at definitive diagnosis and staging. Imaging techniques can be used to guide the surgeon to the appropriate area for biopsy; they range from the mainstay of the traditional x-ray study to more sophisticated techniques such as positron emission tomography (PET) scans, PET with computed tomography (PET-CT), and magnetic resonance imaging (MRI).

Use of these modalities is guided by information obtained from the patient, by clinical interaction during the history and physical examination, and through collaboration with the radiology specialist.[3]

X-RAY

Radiographic studies allow visualization of internal structures of the body and permit the distinction to be made between normal and abnormal structure and function. X-ray examinations may be site-specific or may view the dynamic function of an organ system.[4]

MAMMOGRAPHY

Mammography is an x-ray study used to screen for malignancies of the breast. Mammography is approximately 80% to 85% sensitive in detecting breast cancers, but is limited in detecting abnormalities in dense breast tissue. Variability in interpretation by radiology professionals can also be a limiting factor in the sensitivity of mammography to detect breast cancers. However, mammography is very useful as a screening tool because of its ability to detect nonpalpable breast masses. To be effective, mammography should be accompanied and correlated with clinical findings.

Full-field digital mammography and computer-aided detection are newer mammography imaging techniques, offering the advantages of detecting and improving visualization of suspicious areas during the actual procedure.

COMPUTED TOMOGRAPHY (CT)

CT uses special x-ray equipment to obtain images from a variety of angles through the body and then employs computer processing to reproduce a detailed cross-sectional image of tissues and organs. CT imaging can be performed with clarity in a wide range of tissue types including lung, bone, soft tissue, and blood vessels. It is usually the preferred method for diagnosis of liver, lung, and pancreatic cancers. The image obtained allows the clinician to confirm the presence and precise location of a tumor. This technique measures tumor size and involvement or spread into adjacent areas. CT is frequently used to plan and properly administer radiation treatment for tumors, guide biopsies, direct surgical intervention, and objectively evaluate response to therapy.

CT examination often requires the use of varied contrast materials to enhance the visibility of certain tissues or blood vessels. The contrast material can be swallowed, injected into the blood stream, or administered via enema. It is important to elicit allergy history, diagnoses of diabetes, heart, or kidney disease. This information determines the patient's potential for both reaction to the contrast material and eliminating the contrast after the exam.

MAGNETIC RESONANCE IMAGING (MRI)

MRI does not use ionizing radiation to provide images. The MRI technology is based on the interaction of atomic nuclei and radio waves placed in a strong magnetic field. The images produced represent intensities of these electromagnetic signals from the hydrogen nuclei in the patient. The technique is based on the premise that abnormal tissue has more free water and will display different characteristics. MRI is the preferred imaging technique for soft tissue structures, neurologic imaging, vascular imaging, and avascular necrosis. Patients are not exposed to radiation with this imaging technique. A number of contrast agents are used, depending upon the target of interest.[3]

ULTRASOUND

Ultrasound uses a set of reflections of high frequency sound waves from internal tissues of the body that have been focused for viewing. It is noninvasive, uses no ionizing radiation and can be used throughout the body. There are a wide variety of high resolution probes and transducers that have been developed over the years that offer improved accuracy and ease of noninvasive diagnosis. Deep vein thrombosis is now easily identified with color-flow Doppler imaging.[3]

NUCLEAR MEDICINE

Nuclear medicine imaging techniques are based on the principle of tagging a physiologic substance in the body and measuring its flow, distribution, or presence in the target organ or system. A radiopharmaceutical agent is injected into the patient, and the radioactive decay events are captured by gamma or PET camera. Most radiopharmaceuticals are gamma emitters. The rate of decay of the radiopharmaceutical agent produces an image of the metabolic process. This technique is excellent for evaluating various metabolic and physiologic changes.

POSITRON EMISSION TOMOGRAPHY (PET)

PET uses radioactive positively charged particles to detect subtle changes in the body's metabolism and chemical activities.[5] The radiopharmaceutical agent (radiotracer) most commonly used

and approved by the U.S. Food and Drug Administration (FDA) is F-fluorodeoxyglucose (F-FDG).[6] Based on the premise that malignant tumors use glucose and grow at a faster rate than healthy tissue, the PET scan locates areas of high F-FDG uptake. False-positive results can occur, because inflammation and infection also increases F-FDG uptake and can mimic a positive malignant tumor finding.[5]

POSITRON EMISSION TOMOGRAPHY WITH COMPUTED TOMOGRAPHY (PET-CT)

PET-CT is the fusion of these two imaging modalities, which results in significantly improved diagnostic accuracy. There is more accurate anatomic localization of PET findings, resulting in fewer false-positive PET interpretations.[6]

LYMPHOSCINTIGRAPHY

Lymphoscintigraphy is a nuclear medicine imaging technique that utilizes radiolabeled monoclonal antibodies to visualize microscopic sites of metastasis or suspected malignancy. A monoclonal antibody against a specific tumor antigen is combined with tracer amounts of radioactive substance and injected either into tissue or intravenously. The activity and locations of the site where the substance migrates can then be imaged with the use of scanner or probe. This provides a guide for the surgeon to the target of interest to more accurately remove any diseased tissue. It is used in the diagnosis and staging of malignant melanoma and breast cancers.

Staging

Staging is the process of describing the extent or spread of a disease from its site of origin. This information is important in determining the choice of therapy, monitoring response to treatment, and assessing prognosis. There are traditionally three types of staging: surgical, clinical, and pathologic. **Surgical staging** utilizes invasive surgical techniques to actually visualize structures and assess the extent of disease. **Clinical staging** is based on professional judgment and measurement of the primary tumor's size, location in the body, and the evidence of disease through physical examination. **Pathologic staging** is the practice of examination of the tissue of interest both grossly and microscopically to evaluate its characteristics and make an assessment as to the aggressiveness of the malignant tumor.

There are a variety of different staging systems utilized today. The most commonly known staging system for solid tumors is the tumor-mode-metastasis (TNM) system, which assesses tumors based on the size or extent of primary tumor (T), absence or presence of regional lymph node involvement (N), and absence or presence of distant metastasis (M). Once ascertained, a stage is designated and typically ranges from stage I through stage IV, with stage I being early-stage disease and IV being advanced disease.[7] This staging system is used for colorectal and breast cancers. Staging systems have evolved and expanded into complex systems as a consequence of the knowledge gained over the past several years. Breast cancer staging is an example of this (see page 104 in Chapter 7).

DIAGNOSIS AND STAGING OF HEMATOLOGIC MALIGNANCIES

The diagnosis and staging of the hematologic malignancies are based, in part, on clinical assessment and history. The leukemias

TABLE 5-2   Leukemia Karyotypes and Associated F-A-B* Classifications/Prognosis

F-A-B	KARYOTYPE	PROGNOSIS
AML M2	t(8;21) (q22;q22)	Favorable
AML M4, M5	t(6;11)(q27;q23)	Poor
	t(10;11)(p12:p23)	Poor
	t(11;19)(q23;p13)	Poor
AML, M5	t (11;17)(q23;q21)	Poor
AML M1, M2, M4, M6	t(3;3)(q23;q26)	Poor
AML, M0, M1, M4, M5,	Inv(3)(q21;q26	Poor
M6, M7	5:5q-7;7q	
ALL, L1	t(1;19)(q23;p13)	Poor
ALL, L3	t(8;14)(q24;q11)	Poor
ALL, L3	t(8;14)(q24;q32)	Moderate
ALL, L1	t(9;22)(q34;q11)	Favorable
ALL, L1	t(4;11)(q21;q23)	Favorable

*French-American-British
From Wujcik D: Molecular biology of leukemia, *Semin Oncol Nurs* 19(2 Suppl): 84, 2003.

have traditionally been characterized by classification systems based on morphology of the cells and clinical information. The most commonly used classification system for the leukemias has been the French-American-British system of classification (see Table 5-2). Our knowledge and ability to further define the behavior of these malignancies more precisely has increased exponentially in recent years. The World Health Organization has proposed a new classification system, incorporating features of the myelodysplastic syndromes with the acute leukemias.

Multiple myeloma is diagnosed and staged using a variety of clinical information: the presence and volume of specific immunoglobulins in urine and/or blood, the hemoglobin level, the presence of plasma cells in the bone marrow, and evidence of bone destruction. Staging has traditionally been based on the Durie-Salmon system and incorporates this information into date regarding renal function. The International Staging System incorporates the use of B2M to assess the stage of multiple myeloma.[8]

The explosion of molecular genetic techniques has made available more accurate information about the nature and biology of hematologic malignancies (see Table 5-2). The roles of cytogenetics and immunophenotyping have become even more important in precisely characterizing the malignancies, particularly hematologic malignancies. This affords the clinician the ability to more effectively prescribe therapies and predict outcomes. For instance, the discovery of the Philadelphia chromosome in the diagnosis of chronic myelogenous leukemia and the subsequent development of an agent specifically targeted against that malignancy have altered the standard of care for that disease.

Cytogenetics. Cytogenetics is the use of molecular biologic testing to observe gene translocations and rearrangements. Myeloid and lymphoid lineage can be determined through cytogenetic testing on bone marrow aspirates. Cytogenetic testing includes chromosome banding, fluorescent in situ hybridization, and polymerase chain reaction. Chromosome banding techniques have been used to screen for chromosome (karyotypic) abnormalities. This technique has been used to identify the Philadelphia chromosome translocation t(9;22).

Fluorescent In Situ Hybridization (FISH). Fluorescent in situ hybridization (FISH) detects structural and numerical abnormalities on chromosomes. FISH is useful because it can be performed on nondividing cells. With this technology, a single gene or entire chromosome can be identified. Polymerase chain reaction (PCR) technique amplifies or copies DNA. With this technology, one abnormal cell in a million can be detected.

Immunophenotyping. Immunophenotyping, which uses antibodies to identify chromosomal aberrations, permits the study of a large number of individual cells in a short period.

Flow Cytometry. Flow cytometry, a technique used to analyze cell surface markers, has been used since the early 1980s. The most common application for flow cytometry is to detect and quantify cellular antigens.[9] In many instances, this has specific and useful application for determining types of therapy. For example, characterization of leukemias using specific information about chromosomal aberrations provides information useful in determining treatment strategies as well as prognostic information.

SURGICAL METHODS USED FOR DIAGNOSIS AND STAGING OF CANCER

Tissue Biopsy. The tissue biopsy is the definitive method for the diagnosis of a malignancy. This is a surgical procedure that involves obtaining a portion of tissue or excising the entire target tissue, which is then examined and subjected to diagnostic testing by the pathologist. In this manner, tissue can be determined to be malignant or benign. Characteristics of the malignant tissue can be examined to delineate tumor grade, aggressiveness, and the presence of other features of malignancy.

Biopsies can be performed within the confines of an outpatient setting or physician's office, or in an operating room environment. There are many different types of biopsies, ranging from the minimally invasive to the most invasive type of procedure. A fine-needle aspiration biopsy is a minimally invasive procedure performed by aspirating the target tissue with a needle. The advantages of this type of biopsy are that it can be done in an outpatient setting and is relatively easy to perform, involving little risk or discomfort to the patient. There may be false-negative findings, especially if the sample yields a low volume of cellular components. A second disadvantage is the inability to distinguish between invasive and in situ disease with this method.

Incisional or Core Biopsy. A core biopsy is one in which a representative sample of the actual target tissue is obtained. This is often accomplished with the aid of imaging techniques to ensure that the area of suspicion is correctly targeted and sampled. With this type of biopsy, further definitive surgery may be indicated if the sampled tissue is positive for malignancy.

Sentinel Lymph Node Biopsy. Sentinel lymph node mapping and biopsy is a new technique that is advancing the staging and treatment of melanoma, breast, and possibly other malignant tumors. In this setting, nuclear medicine imaging studies are performed to help identify the sentinel node. Identification involves injecting a radioactive material, tagged with a cancer antigen–specific monoclonal antibody and blue dye into the area of the tumor. The substance migrates to the sentinel node, allowing detection of the cancer-affected lymph nodes. In this manner, it is possible to remove only the cancerous lymph nodes. In comparison to traditional techniques, the sentinel lymph node removal technique minimizes postoperative complications of pain, numbness, and lymphedema. This method is shown to be an accurate means of determining the stage of breast cancer and still cause fewer complications than the traditional method of lymph node evaluation.[10]

Axillary Lymph Node Biopsy. Axillary lymph node biopsy is a critical step in staging breast cancer. This is a surgical procedure typically carried out under general anesthesia and provides needed information at the time of diagnosis about the cancer and its potential for metastasis.

Conclusion

Diagnosing and staging cancer is a fascinating and ever-changing field. As technology advances, constant updates in testing and tools that aid in the task become available for the clinical use.

Oncology nurses are on the front lines with patients and families who are experiencing a diagnostic work-up for cancer. They are often the first to explain the testing requirements and field questions regarding test results and what those results mean in terms of treatment and prognosis. The human spirit and the family structure can be gravely challenged by a diagnosis of cancer. Therefore, the oncology nurse must not only keep current with diagnostic updates to better care for his or her patients, but also to provide support, resources, and a realistic buffer in this somewhat precarious situation.

REVIEW QUESTIONS

✓ Case Study

Mrs. Conner is a 63-year-old woman referred to the oncology surgeon by the radiologist from the radiology department at St. Vincent's Hospital. The radiologist discovered a suspicious area in Mrs. Conner's right breast during her yearly screening mammogram.

He is recommending further evaluation.

As the clinician working with the oncology surgeon, you are the first person to interact with the patient following her referral. You are responsible for obtaining an initial history from the patient as well as providing information and education and making an initial assessment of the patient.

QUESTIONS

1. What is the most important focus for the initial interaction with this patient?
   a. Assess the findings and the patient's perception of the problem.
   b. Obtain history of any family members with similar illness or any type of cancer.
   c. Ascertain prior personal history of cancer in this patient.
   d. Carefully explain findings of mammography report, and provide an explanation of the appropriate expectations to the patient.
2. During the course of the interview, the patient tells you that she is a new widow and her two adult children live out of state. She is living alone. Anticipating the need for a more thorough evaluation of the mammogram, what is your next course of action?
   a. Arrange for a repeat mammogram to be done at your facility before her leaving today.
   b. Make arrangements for a fine-needle biopsy based on the written report of the first mammogram.
   c. Discuss with the patient her children, her support system, her work, and her usual activities.
   d. Make arrangements for any previous mammogram films to be sent to your facility for comparison.
3. You learn from Mrs. Conner that she has been very faithful in obtaining yearly screening mammogram evaluations, all of which were within normal limits. She is perplexed and in disbelief as to why this happened to her. The correct response(s) to Mrs. Conner include the following (more than one of the following might apply):
   a. You provide positive appraisal of her for following the recommended breast cancer screening guidelines.
   b. You assure her that because she has followed the recommended guidelines, her cancer is probably found in an early, most treatable stage.
   c. You advise that the grief and stress she has experienced from her husband's recent death has precipitated the mammogram change
   d. You state that breast cancer can occur at any time, with or without regularly scheduled mammograms
4. You learn that Mrs. Conner has a sister and a paternal aunt who have had breast cancer in the past. They were in their 50s at diagnosis. Further, her father was diagnosed with prostate cancer at age 54. What significance does this information have for your assessment and planning for Mrs. Conner?
   a. Mrs. Connor is "past" menopause; therefore this family history is not important.
   b. This family history is of no concern because her female siblings had cancer in their 50s, whereas Mrs. Connor is 63.
   c. This family constellation points to a possible genetic link with her developing breast cancer.
   d. All male members of this family should have PSA and DRE done.
5. The surgeon examines Mrs. Conner and determines that there is no focal mass that she can appreciate clinically. She recommends three potential options for Mrs. Conner. Which of the three is the most appropriate?
   a. A lumpectomy to include the area seen on mammogram
   b. An excisional biopsy using an imaging technique to more accurately locate the area of concern
   c. An incisional or core biopsy using an imaging technique to obtain a piece of the tissue to make or rule out a definitive diagnosis of cancer

Continued

REVIEW QUESTIONS—CONT'D

6. Mrs. Conner's biopsy was positive for an infiltrating ductal carcinoma. The surgical options discussed with her are based on which two of the following?
   a. Knowledge of the natural history of this type of cancer
   b. Mrs. Conner's lifestyle and personal preference
   c. The preference of middle-aged and elderly women for more drastic and definitive measures such as total mastectomy
   d. The preference of middle-aged and single women for breast conservation approaches

7. Mrs. Conner then returns and has an excisional biopsy and lumpectomy. What additional testing will likely be ordered to determine distant metastatic spread?
   a. Sentinel lymph node biopsy
   b. CT scans of chest, pelvis, abdomen, and bone
   c. Repeat mammography
   d. CgA and B2M

8. The pathology report for the biopsy Mrs. Conner has undergone reveals an infiltrating ductal carcinoma. What other information about this breast cancer is important to know in planning for treatment options for this patient? Check all that apply.
   a. Her2/neu marker
   b. Lymphoscintigraphy
   c. Full-field digital mammography
   d. Estrogen and progesterone receptors

9. Mrs. Conner's oncologist initially determined the stage of disease based on his expertise and professional judgment, the location of the tumor in the body, the size of the tumor, and evidence of disease through physical examination. How is this staging is defined?
   a. Clinical staging
   b. Pathologic staging
   c. Surgical staging
   d. All of the above

10. Treatment is planned and initiated for Mrs. Conner. What testing will indicate the likeliness and severity of treatment side effects?
    a. CA-125
    b. CA 19-9
    c. CA 15-3
    d. None of the above

ANSWERS

1. **A.** *Rationale:* Initially, further patient assessment should be undertaken from a holistic approach, encompassing the physical, social, practical, informational, psychologic, and spiritual needs of this newly diagnosed elderly patient. In this manner, the clinician may gain an understanding of the patient's level of understanding of the information that she has just received and assess her level of anxiety. Once some of the anxiety has been relieved, the patient can listen more attentively and actively participate in the management of her disease.

2. **C.** *Rationale:* Again, incorporating a more holistic history and assessment you can determine her resources. The patient lives alone. Family cohesiveness can be assessed by learning about her relationship with her children. By discussing her work history, you will glean information about her current social circle, her coping skills, and how she is handling the recent death of her husband.

3. **A & B.** *Rationale:* Studies have indicated that women who use mammography regularly for breast cancer screening are significantly more likely to be diagnosed with an earlier stage of breast cancer and are significantly less likely to die from breast cancer. However, the patient will need to undergo a full diagnostic work-up to determine the extent of disease and accurately stage her breast cancer.

4. **C.** *Rationale:* The information should alert the practitioner that there could be a genetic or familial risk associated with her development of breast cancer. Since the patient has two children, genetic testing or genetic counseling should be offered.

5. **C.** *Rationale:* A decision about which type of surgical intervention Mrs. Conner should have will likely incorporate many factors. She should be provided with thorough information on all three surgical interventions. The options provided should take into consideration the patient's functional abilities, comorbidities, and social situation, and the patient's preference. Comorbidities for this patient may make a surgical intervention under anesthesia an additional risk. A core biopsy carries the risk of sampling error and, if positive, will require further, more definitive surgery if found to be positive for malignancy. However, a core biopsy is usually done in an outpatient setting, using only a local anesthetic. As a person living alone, this may be the preferred option. A lumpectomy or excisional biopsy provides the benefit of being more definitive, but these surgical options require general or systemic anesthesia. There may be increased risk for the patient who has comorbidities or decreased functional capacity.

6. **A & B.** *Rationale:* Further surgical options for Mrs. Conner are based on knowledge of the type of cancer she has and her personal preferences. To further assess and stage her breast cancer, Mrs. Conner will require sentinel lymph node biopsy to assess for the malignant spread of the cancer. Another option for her would be to undergo a mastectomy. The information provided to Mrs. Conner should be based on the natural history of the type of malignancy that has been diagnosed, the size of the tumor, and the extent of the involvement. The benefits and risks of all should be thoroughly discussed. Aging is also a very individual process. Mrs. Connor's decisions should be based on her personal preferences, with an awareness of the benefits and risks of each option.

7. **B.** *Rationale:* Sentinel lymph node biopsy is a technique used to determine lymph node involvement. CgA is a tumor marker in carcinoid tumors. B2Ms are tumor markers that are valuable in tracking multiple myeloma, leukemia, and lymphoma. Repeat mammography would be of no benefit in determining the extent of metastatic spread. CT scan of the chest, the abdomen, and the pelvis, and a bone scan are typically done to ascertain the extent of spread of breast cancers. These areas are evaluated because of the typical spread of breast cancer to the brain, the lung, the liver, and bone.

8. **A. & D.** *Rationale:* The malignant breast tissue is tested by the pathologist for the presence of tumor markers. Estrogen and progesterone receptors indicate the "aggressiveness" of the tumor and how likely it is to respond to specific types of endocrine therapy. The Her2/neu marker will reveal whether or not the cancer will respond to a specific type of

monoclonal antibody. Lymphoscintigraphy is a diagnostic technique that aids in determining microscopic areas of metastasis. Full-field digital mammography is helpful in examining suspicious areas. Both of these are diagnostic in nature. In this instance, the diagnosis has been made; the issue is determining which treatment will be best for the patient.

9. A. *Rationale:* There are traditionally three types of staging: surgical, pathologic and clinical. Surgical staging uses invasive surgical techniques to actually visualize structures and assess the extent of disease. Pathologic staging is based upon the practice of examination of the tissue of interest grossly and microscopically to evaluate the characteristics and aggressiveness of the tumor.

10. D. *Rationale:* CA 15-3 is a marker used to determine the effectiveness of treatment in breast cancer patients. CA 19-9 is commonly elevated in colorectal and pancreatic cancers. CA 125 is elevated in 90% of females with epithelial ovarian cancer. Tumor markers are not used to evaluate one's potential of experiencing side effects.

REFERENCES

1. Smith RA, Cokkinides V, Eyre HJ: American Cancer Society guidelines for the early detection of cancer, *CA Cancer J Clin* 56:11-25, 2006; retrieved from http://caonline.amcancersoc.org/cgi/content/full/56/1/11.
2. von Eschenbach AC: NCI sets goal of eliminating suffering and death due to cancer by 2015, *J Natl Med Assoc* 95(7):637-9, 2003.
3. Galen BA: Diagnostic imaging: an overview. *Prim Care Pract Peer Rev Series* 3(5):461-476, 1999.
4. Groenwald SL, Hansen-Frogge M, Goodman M et al, editors: *Cancer nursing principles and practice*, ed 4, 1997.
5. Lobrano MB, Singha P: Positron emission tomography in oncology, *Clin J Oncol Nurs* 7(4):379-385, 2003.
6. Juweid ME, Cheson BD: Positron emission tomography and assessment of cancer therapy, *N Engl J Med* 354(5): 496-507, 2006.
7. American Cancer Society: *Cancer Facts and Figures, 2003*, Atlanta, 2003, Author, retrieved from http://www.cancer.org/downloads/STT/CAFF2003PWSecured.pdf#search=%22Cancer%20Facts%20and%20Figures%202003%22.
8. Griepp PR, San Miguel J, Durie BG et al: International Staging System for Multiple Myeloma, *J Clin Oncol* 23:3412-3420, 2005.
9. Wujcik D: Molecular biology of leukemia, *Semin Oncol Nurs* 19 (2 Suppl): 2003.
10. Veronesi U, Paganelli G, Galimberti V et al: Sentinel node biopsy to avoid axillary dissection in breast cancer with clinically negative lymph nodes. *Lancet* 349(9069):1864-1867, 1997.

UNIT TWO

Clinical Management of Major Cancers

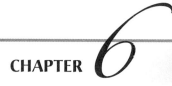

Cancer of the Brain and Central Nervous System

Eileen M. Bohan

Central nervous system (CNS) tumors represent a particular challenge for the oncology practitioner. In many ways, the definitions that apply to cancers in other parts of the body do not apply to these tumors. Some *"benign"* tumors may be located in areas of the brain or spinal cord that cause devastating, even fatal, outcomes. Others may infiltrate the brain or spinal cord parenchyma, making surgical removal impossible and permanent neurologic deficits likely. **Malignant** CNS tumors are aggressive, highly infiltrative and refractory to most of our current treatment modalities.

The neurooncology team is faced with numerous challenges in attempting to treat patients with CNS tumors. Brain and spinal cord tumors have quite different presentations, treatments, and nursing care considerations.

Brain Tumors

Epidemiology

Malignant and nonmalignant brain tumors are reported in 14.8 per 100,000 individuals per year. There are approximately 44,000 new cases of primary brain tumors (originating within the brain) in the United States each year. Of these, 18,500 are high-grade, malignant tumors. Approximately 13,000 deaths from malignant brain tumors were reported in the United States in 2005.[1] Brain tumors account for 1.4% of all cancers. With the exception of meningiomas, incidence of brain tumors is higher in men. There is also a higher incidence among Caucasians and in developed countries.[2]

More than 150,000 metastatic tumors (disseminating to the brain from other organs) are reported in the United States each year.[3,4] Lung and breast cancer make up the most common metastatic lesions to the brain, followed by renal, melanoma, and gastrointestinal cancer.[1,5,6]

Etiology and Risk Factors

There has been a documented recent rise in the incidence of brain tumors. More advanced imaging tools and techniques have contributed to the early detection and treatment of intracranial tumors. It is also postulated that there may be other reasons for this phenomenon. Ionizing radiation has been linked to the development of some central nervous system tumors including meningiomas, gliomas, and nerve sheath tumors. Electromagnetic fields and cellular phones are both topics of extensive study. To date, studies have been unable to link them directly to tumorigenesis. The data do not completely rule out a connection; on the other hand, they do not confirm it either. Further study is needed for more conclusive results.[7]

There are a small number of factors that predispose family members to certain tumor types. Many studies have been undertaken to identify familial influences in the development of brain tumors, and some studies support such a link. A study of twins did not support heredity as a cause. It is also felt that tumors originating in multiple family members may, in fact, have environmental causes.

Dietary habits have been the topic of numerous studies. Researchers have looked at the connection between N-nitroso compounds and brain cancer. There has been a link between increased intake of foods cured with nitrosamines and brain tumors, but other studies show that increased use of some fruits, vegetables, and vitamins may decrease cancer risk.

It is generally believed that gene alterations may be the most likely source of tumor formation. Gain or loss of a number of chromosomes is associated with certain types of brain tumors.[8]

There has been extensive study of risk factors that may cause or predispose one to CNS tumors. It is safe to assume that the development of CNS tumors comes from a number of varied causes and that further study is necessary. The one area that has garnered the most interest is in the field of molecular genetics. Over the next several years, we hope to continue to improve our understanding of the most aggressive and often fatal brain cancers.

Prevention, Screening, and Detection

Because the etiology of brain tumors is still so illusive, it is difficult to initiate prevention and/or screening programs. As with most cancers, early detection is a positive prognostic factor for many CNS tumors. Awareness of the signs and symptoms of brain tumors leads to early diagnosis, fewer neurologic symptoms, and better outcomes. Although there are no known measures available to prevent brain tumors, prevention of irreversible neurologic problems through early diagnosis and treatment increases survival and quality of life.

Classification

The most commonly accepted classification system for CNS tumors is the World Health Organization (WHO) system.[9] Tumors are classified by cell of origin. Some brain tumors are graded (I-IV), based on cell atypia, mitotic activity, microvascular endothelial proliferation, and presence of necrosis. Low-grade tumors are well differentiated and have less mitotic activity. Higher-grade tumors are mitotically active and display increased cell proliferation. The most malignant tumors have evidence of necrosis.

Techniques such as evaluation of Ki-67 (MIB-1) are used to measure cell proliferation and suggest tumor behavior and prognosis. Higher Ki-67 index is predictive of higher grade and aggressiveness.[10,11] Mutations of the *p53* tumor suppression gene are identified in a percentage of astrocytomas and, in combination with other gene alterations, are associated with tumor recurrence.[12] Further delineation is obtained through pathologic chromosomal studies. For example, deletion of the 1p and 19q chromosomes is diagnostic of oligodendroglioma.[13,14]

The four most common primary brain tumors are gliomas, meningiomas, nerve sheath tumors, and pituitary tumors.

Gliomas are most common, accounting for 42% of primary brain tumors and 78% of malignant brain tumors. Glial tumors include astrocytoma, oligodendroglioma, mixed glioma, and ependymoma. The most common sites of origin for gliomas are the cerebral hemispheres—frontal, parietal, temporal, and occipital lobes (65%). Brain stem gliomas account for approximately 4%, cerebellar, 3%, and ventricular, 2%.[1] Gliomas occur in all age groups.

Astrocytomas are divided into four WHO grades:[9]
Grade I: Pilocytic astrocytoma
Grade II: Astrocytoma
Grade III: Anaplastic astrocytoma
Grade IV: Glioblastoma multiforme (GBM) (Fig. 6-1)

Oligodendrogliomas make up approximately 10% of gliomas and are most often low grade, although they can also have malignant features. These tumors are considered slower-growing and more sensitive to treatment than other gliomas.[13] It is not unusual for the neuropathologist to find features of oligodendroglioma and astrocytoma in one tumor specimen (mixed glioma or oligoastrocytoma).

Ependymomas account for approximately 6% of gliomas, they develop from the walls of the ventricles. Therefore, hydrocephalus is of concern in these patients. They are slow-growing, and outcome improves with aggressive surgical resection.

Meningiomas account for 30% of primary tumors and originate from the arachnoid covering of the brain (Fig. 6-2). Less than 10% of these tumors are more aggressive and are classified as atypical, malignant, or anaplastic. They have a higher recurrence rate and require other treatments in addition to surgical resection. Grade I, benign meningiomas comprise over 90% of cases and can be cured with surgery. Recurrence rate is felt to be dependent on tumor location and extent of surgical resection.[1,15,16]

Schwannomas and **pituitary tumors** account for 8% and 7% of primary tumors, respectively. They are usually benign and respond well to treatment, whether surgical, medical, or radiotherapeutic.

Schwannomas develop from the cranial nerve sheath (Fig. 6-3). They are slow-growing and curable with surgery. The most common site of origin is the eighth nerve (acoustic neuroma). These tumors also respond to focused radiation (radiosurgery).[17,18]

Adenomas are the most common pituitary tumor and are also slow-growing. Unlike most other brain tumors, a percentage can be managed with medical treatment, if they secrete certain hormones. Those that are nonsecretory may necessitate surgery at some point. A small number of recurrent adenomas also

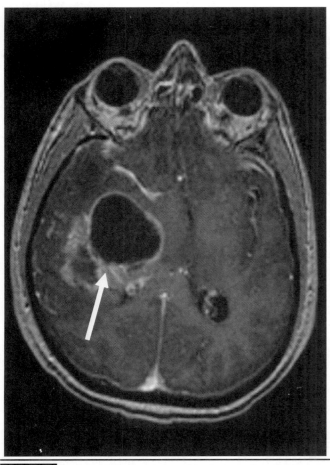

FIG. 6-1   Axial MRI showing enhancing cystic glioblastoma multiforme.

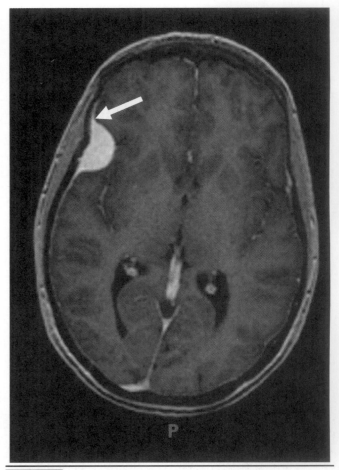

FIG. 6-2   Axial MRI showing meningioma with "dural tail."

necessitate radiation therapy. Like other benign brain tumors, some asymptomatic pituitary tumors are managed with serial imaging studies such as magnetic resonance imaging (MRI) until there is evidence of radiographic or clinical progression.

Unlike primary brain tumors, **metastatic** lesions originate in distant sites and travel to the brain through blood vessels or the lymphatic system. Lung cancer is the most common cause of metastatic brain lesions (35%), followed by breast cancer (20%). Other primary sites of tumors that metastasize to the brain are melanoma (10%), renal cell (10%), and colorectal (5%). Approximately 10% of metastatic lesions to the brain are from an unknown primary tumor. The most common location for these tumors is in the cerebral hemispheres.[1,5,6] Solitary metastases may be surgically resectable. Multiple "mets" often require biopsy for diagnosis followed by adjuvant therapies. Whether one or more lesions are present, radiotherapy is the treatment of choice. Some selected patients may also benefit from chemotherapy (e.g., those with melanoma).[19,20]

For additional information on the seven WHO histologic categories and for further description of the most common tumor types, refer to Table 6-1.[21]

Clinical Features

Patients with brain tumors exhibit a number of clinical features depending on tumor type, biologic characteristics, and location.[22] Symptoms of these tumors are often related to increased intracranial pressure (ICP) caused by blood-brain barrier (BBB) disruption and the development of cerebral edema.[23] Because the brain is enclosed within the rigid cranium, tumor growth can cause displacement of the brain and consequent symptoms. Slow-growing tumors gradually expand and may grow to be quite large before causing symptoms. Rapidly growing tumors are more likely to cause neurologic deficits, because the brain does not accommodate to rapid increases in pressure.

Increasing ICP causes a triad of symptoms including headache, nausea and/or vomiting, and papilledema (swelling of the optic discs). Headaches are a presenting symptom in approximately 50% of patients with brain tumors. Patients complain of headache upon awakening. Those who already suffer from migraines often report headaches with a different characteristic from their "typical" migraine. It is not unusual for patients to have suffered with headaches for weeks or months, thinking that they are related to stress.[24]

Change in mental status is caused by brain shifting associated with increased ICP or with hydrocephalus caused by tumor growth. Many patients complain of mental slowness or inability to concentrate. Aggressive tumors are more likely to cause mental status changes because of rapid growth and pressure exerted on the brain.[25]

Seizures occur as the presenting sign in approximately one third of patients with brain tumors who have supratentorial (cerebral hemispheres) lesions. It is believed that at least 50% of patients have seizure activity at some time during the disease process. Individuals with low-grade or frontal lobe tumors are more likely to experience seizure activity.[26,27]

Headaches, mental status changes, and seizures are considered general symptoms and are not associated with irreversible neurologic damage. Their presence can, in fact, lead to early detection and treatment.[28]

Focal neurologic signs are associated with specific locations and may be reversible if they are related to brain swelling. They are irreversible when they are the result of infiltration and destruction. Table 6-2 outlines specific tumor locations and the associated neurologic symptoms.[29]

Diagnosis

Whether the patient experiences a headache, seizure, or other neurologic symptom, radiologic screening studies are obtained for differential diagnosis. A patient seen in the emergency department (ED) typically undergoes a history and physical exam, blood tests, and computed tomography (CT) to evaluate for hemorrhage, hydrocephalus, or a structural lesion. Once the CT is obtained, MRI with contrast material identifies brain abnormalities and surrounding edema causing increased ICP. Specialized magnetic resonance (MR) images, including diffusion and perfusion weighted sequences, are now able to more accurately differentiate edema from structural lesions, cystic changes, and normal brain tissue, as well as to evaluate stroke.[30]

Magnetic resonance angiography (MRA) utilizes the same technology to specifically identify vascular anatomy, particularly vessels providing blood supply to the tumor (feeding vessels).[31]

A further advance in MR is spectroscopy (MRS), which evaluates the metabolism of the tumor. This is particularly helpful in distinguishing high-grade from low-grade lesions, or for evaluating whether a new area of abnormality in a previously treated tumor may be treatment effect rather than recurrent tumor. Actively growing tumors tend to exhibit increased levels of the metabolites choline and lactate and decreased levels of N-acetylaspartate (NAA). Benign tumors or normal brain should have lower levels of choline and increased NAA. This is a noninvasive study that requires no preparation and can be done at the same time the MRI is being obtained.[32]

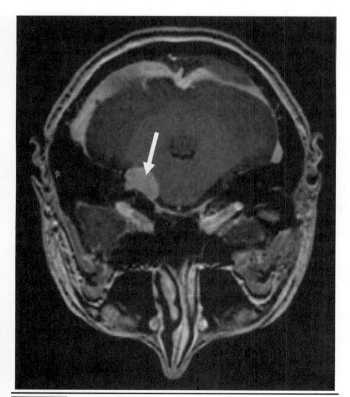

FIG. 6-3   Axial MRI showing cerebello-pontine angle schwannoma.

TABLE 6-1	Classification and Grading of Brain Tumors (Most Common Intracranial Tumors)		
CLASSIFICATION/GRADE	**DESCRIPTION**	**SYMPTOMS**	**TREATMENT/PROGNOSIS**
NEUROEPITHELIAL (approximately 50% of primary tumors)			
Gliomas			
Astrocytic			
WHO Grade I— Pilocytic astrocytoma	Pediatric; 85% cerebellar; slow-growing; well-circumscribed; cystic; benign	Increased intracranial pressure (ICP) Focalneurologic signs	Curable with surgery (craniotomy for tumor removal)
Grade II—Astrocytoma	Infiltrative; slow-growing	Seizures Acute or subtle onset of symptoms	Radiation therapy (RT) for residual tumor; may withhold RT after gross total resection Young age is good prognostic factor
WHO Grade III—Anaplastic astrocytoma	Hypercellular; anaplasia	May have acute onset of symptoms	RT with or without chemotherapy High recurrence rate Age and overall health affect prognosis
WHO Grade IV— Glioblastoma multiforme	Poorly differentiated, with high mitotic rate; highly malignant Most common glioma	Rapid onset of symptoms Increased ICP or focal signs	Infiltrative nature: complete removal of all cells RT with or without chemotherapy not possible Experimental protocols Recurrence in virtually all cases Median survival: 12-18 months
Oligodendroglioma	Well-differentiated; calcified; infiltrative; slow-growing Some tumors are malignant (anaplastic)	Seizures Headaches Subtle onset of symptoms	RT with residual tumor; may withhold after gross total resection RT with or without chemotherapy for anaplastic oligodendroglioma
Mixed glioma (oligoastrocytoma)	May behave more or less aggressively, depending on features	Dependent on location and degree of malignancy	Variable outcome
Ependymoma	Pediatric and young adult patients; originate from lining of the ventricles; frequently in posterior fossa; usually benign	May present with hydrocephalus; symptoms related to location	RT for residual or recurrent disease; craniospinal RT for evidence of spinal disease only Good prognosis
Embryonal (primitive neuroectodermal tumor) medulloblastoma, most common	Pediatric; malignant; occurs mainly in posterior fossa; cerebrospinal fluid (CSF) metastasis in 33% of patients	Symptoms by location Hydrocephalus common	Craniospinal RT Poor prognosis, particularly with CSF dissemination
PERIPHERAL NERVE TUMORS (approximately 8% of primary brain tumors)			
Vestibular schwannoma (acoustic neuroma)	Cerebello-pontine angle; benign; encapsulated Seen in association with neurofibromatosis, type 2	Decreased hearing Tinnitus Balance problems May have other cranial nerve deficits	Curable with surgery Excellent prognosis Cranial nerve deficits may be permanent or temporary; affect quality of life
MENINGEAL TUMORS (approximately 30% of primary brain tumors)			
Meningioma	Composed of arachnoid cells; attached to dura; usually benign; well-circumscribed; may be vascular Common locations: falx; olfactory groove; sphenoid ridge; parasellar region; optic nerve	Headaches may occur from dural stretching Seizures and focal neurologic signs	Degree of resection (and recurrence) associated with location Excellent prognosis with gross total resection Atypical and malignant meningiomas have more aggressive features and less favorable outcomes

TABLE 6-1	Classification and Grading of Brain Tumors (Most Common Intracranial Tumors)—cont'd		
CLASSIFICATION/GRADE	**DESCRIPTION**	**SYMPTOMS**	**TREATMENT/PROGNOSIS**
LYMPHOMAS AND HEMOPOIETIC TUMORS (approximately 3% of primary brain tumors)			
Malignant central nervous system lymphoma	Arise in central nervous system (CNS) without systemic lymphoma; commonly suprasellar; diffuse brain infiltration; may be periventricular and may involve leptomeninges. Solitary or multiple	Neurologic or neuropsychiatric symptoms	Diagnosis commonly via stereotactic biopsy or CSF cytology. Steroids may decrease or temporarily obliterate lesion on computed tomography or magnetic resonance imaging (CT/MRI). RT with or without chemotherapy. High-dose methotrexate used as single agent; some studies defer RT. Increasing incidence in immunocompetent persons; decreasing in AIDS patients. Possible improved survival with newer treatments
GERM CELL TUMORS (approximately 1% of primary brain tumors)			
	Developmental tumors—from gonads and extragonadal sites; germinoma (solid, enhancing on MRI) and teratoma (cystic, with fat and calcification) most common	Symptoms are location dependent. Germinomas are often suprasellar—diabetes insipidus	RT for germinomas; curable. Teratoma has less favorable prognosis; gross total resection means improved survival. Chemotherapy in some cases
SELLAR TUMORS (approximately 7% of primary brain tumors)			
Pituitary adenoma	6.3% of sellar tumors. Benign; originate from adenohypophysis; classification by hormonal content. Microadenoma < 1 cm. Macroadenoma > 1 cm	Hypersecretion prolactin: amenorrhea, galactorrhea. • Growth hormone: acromegaly. • Adrenocorticotropic hormone (ACTH): Cushings. • Thyroid-stimulating hormone (TSH): hyperthyroid (rare). Hyposecretion caused by compression of the pituitary gland. Visual field deficits (bitemporal hemianopia). Headache. Pituitary apoplexy: acute hemorrhage or infarct of gland—emergency treatment indicated	Surgical: transsphenoidal for approximately 95% of surgical cases. Medical: appropriate in some cases of prolactin-secreting and growth hormone-secreting tumors. Radiation for recurrence or for hypersecretory tumors, when medical management has failed
Craniopharyngioma	Benign; calcified, cystic tumors	Endocrine abnormalities. Visual impairment. Cognitive and/or personality changes. May have increased ICP	Gross total resection affects prognosis. RT for residual tumor
METASTATIC TUMORS (approximately 150,000 new cases yearly; occur in 20%-40% of cancer patients)			
	Originate from primary systemic tumors. Discrete, round, ring-enhancing 50% are solitary. Lung and breast are most common primary sites	Symptoms are location dependent	Prognosis dependent on number of tumors, tumor location, systemic disease, and patient age. Improved prognosis with gross total resection and RT

NOTE: For all tumors, biopsy or craniotomy for tumor removal is necessary to establish a definitive diagnosis.
Reprinted and updated from Fitzsimmons B, Bohan E: Common neurosurgical and neurological disorders. In Morton PG, Fontaine DK, Hudak CM et al, editors: *Critical care nursing: a holistic approach*, ed 8, Philadelphia, 2005, Lippincott, Williams & Wilkins.

TABLE 6-2	Neurologic Deficits and Clinical Management in Relationship to Tumor Location		
DEFICITS	**ASSESSMENT***	**INTERVENTIONS**	
Frontal Lobe Contralateral paresis/paralysis; motor aphasia; intellectual impairment; emotional lability; personality changes; urinary frequency, urgency, incontinence; seizures; impaired sense of smell	Motor examination Mental status: observe patient; interview family; assess orientation, general knowledge, spelling ability, and short-term memory	Physical and occupational therapy consultations Neuropsychiatric and/or cognitive therapy Speech therapy Pharmacologic management	
Temporal Lobe Temporal lobe seizures; dysnomia; receptive aphasia; memory problems; perceptual and/or spatial disturbances; vision	Interview of patient regarding seizure history Assessment of ability to follow 1-, 2-, and 3-step commands	Seizure prophylaxis and precautions Teaching regarding items such as seizure diary, driving restrictions Cognitive therapy	
Parietal Lobe Sensory deficits (position, vibration, touch, temperature); calculations; left-right discrimination; visual fields; language; seizures	Test sensation (e.g., to vibration, position awareness)	Occupational therapy for safety, and cognitive retraining	
Occipital Lobe Contralateral homonymous hemianopia (e.g., left lesion leads to loss of vision on right side of each eye); visual hallucinations; seizures	Visual examination to include fields, visual perception, and spatial relationships Interview to include visual hallucinations	Neuroophthalmology evaluation Occupational therapy for visual retraining	
Cerebellum Ipsilateral ataxia; lack of coordination; nystagmus; increased intracranial pressure (ICP)	Coordination testing (finger to nose; rapid alternating movements); evaluation of intention tremor or ataxia	Physical and occupational therapy for balance and coordination Assistive devices Teaching regarding signs of increased ICP	
Brainstem Cranial nerve deficits; sensory and/or motor impairment; vomiting; breathing; heartbeat	Cranial nerve testing	Therapy appropriate to cranial nerve deficit Pharmacologic management	
Intraventricular Increased ICP; hydrocephalus (gait disturbance; cognitive deficits; urinary incontinence); sudden death	Gait testing	Teaching regarding possible shunt Patient and family education regarding obstruction and emergency surgery	

*Each examination is recorded only once, but there are many areas of overlap.
Data from references 68-72, 75.

Positron emission tomography (PET) uses a cyclotron to produce radioactive isotopes, which are injected intravenously. A scanner identifies these isotopes in abnormal areas using computers. Fluorodeoxyglucose-18 (^{18}F) is the most commonly used isotope. The goal is to evaluate metabolically active tumor versus low-grade or treated (quiescent) tumor. It is important for the scanning personnel to be aware of patients with seizure disorders, since this can affect the study results. PET scans are expensive, do not have highly accurate resolution, require special equipment, and are available in only a limited number of centers. However, PET/CT is now being used and may provide added information in the evaluation of tumor metabolism.[33]

Another capability of MR imaging is the functional MRI (fMRI), which is used to assess language, motor, or sensory function in relation to tumor location. Physiologic changes are noted during the performance of certain tasks while the patient is in the MR scanner.[34] This is a noninvasive test and may obviate the need for awake tumor surgery in some cases.

Staging

PROGNOSTIC INDICATORS

Tumor classification, grade, and location are major prognostic indicators. Patient age, overall health, and absence or presence of neurologic deficits also contribute to outcome. Surgical skill determines the amount of tumor removed and the safety of the procedure. Although this is a topic of some controversy, many neurosurgeons believe that survival is directly related to degree of tumor resection. Finally, an accurate histologic diagnosis is crucial to facilitating the appropriate follow-up therapy.

METASTASES WITHIN THE CNS

It is unlikely for primary brain tumors to disseminate systemically because the brain does not have a lymphatic system.[35] They generally recur within 2 cm of the original site. If there is dissemination, it is most likely within the CNS—other areas of the brain or in the spinal cord (drop metastases). As patients live longer and diagnostic tools and techniques improve, leptomeningeal spread to the pia and arachnoid membranes has become more common, with 5% of patients experiencing this devastating outcome. Treatment with radiation or chemotherapy may be attempted, depending on tumor histology, but the outcome is dismal, with a 3- to 6-month median survival reported.[36]

Medical Treatment Modalities and Nursing Care Considerations

SURGERY

Once the patient has come to medical attention, a treatment plan is made, based on clinical and radiographic information. In cases where the patient is asymptomatic and radiographic imaging suggests a benign tumor, a conservative approach with serial CT or MRI may be recommended. Occasionally, the tumor is found incidentally while imaging for another reason (e.g., patient is seen in the ED after a motor vehicle accident) and warrants this conservative approach. Radiographic and clinical indicators, such as edema, mass effect on brain structures, and neurologic deficits warrant exploration for diagnosis and treatment.

Initially, the patient is started on steroid therapy to decrease ICP and relieve symptoms. Dexamethasone, a corticosteroid, is the drug of choice perioperatively. If the patient complains of gastrointestinal symptoms or if a long course of steroid therapy is required, antacids or histamine$_2$ blockers may be used. Anticonvulsants are used for seizure management and are prescribed at the time of seizure onset or preoperatively. Antiepileptic drug (AED) therapy has been vigorously discussed, and several studies have suggested that AED use is not effective or necessary in brain tumor patients who have not had seizures.[37] However, it is still the trend to treat these patients prophylactically with AEDs. A 2005 study by Siomin et al. stated that approximately 70% of neurosurgeons who responded to a survey use AEDs prophylactically for patients with brain tumors.[26] More formal evaluation through clinical trials has been recommended before universal guidelines for AED use in brain tumors can be established.

Once the decision has been made to proceed with surgery, the specific procedure is chosen based on tumor location, surgical goal, and patient performance status. **Stereotactic biopsy** is performed to establish a diagnosis only. It is used for tumors that are deep or in eloquent areas of the brainstem where tumor resection is not feasible. This is also the treatment of choice to differentiate recurrent tumor from treatment effect in previously treated patients.[38] If patients with recurrent tumors opt for an investigational protocol, a biopsy may be required before enrollment in the study.

The goals of **craniotomy** are twofold: to obtain a diagnosis, and to remove tumor and decrease mass effect, if present. In the case of some benign tumors (e.g., meningioma, schwannoma), complete tumor resection may be curative. For infiltrative or malignant tumors, tumor debulking may provide symptom relief

and decrease ICP before initiation of further therapy.[39] It is also an opportunity, in selected cases, to receive additional therapy in the form of biodegradable chemotherapy wafers or implantable devices for radiation.

Although not within the scope of this chapter, it should be noted that there are currently a number of tools used intraoperatively that improve effective tumor removal and minimize patient morbidity. These include frameless stereotaxy, ultrasound, endoscopy, and intraoperative MRI.[40]

Nursing Care Considerations. As with all oncologic problems, the patient receives a great deal of information while simultaneously trying to adjust to a new and potentially life-threatening diagnosis. Often on the first visit to the neurosurgical oncologist, the patient provides a medical history, undergoes a physical exam, discusses the radiographic imaging and potential diagnosis, and reviews consent forms and perioperative routines. It is crucial that the patient and family members have an opportunity to ask questions and to discuss the possibility of obtaining a second opinion.

There are intraoperative therapies (chemotherapy wafers or local radiation treatments) that are discussed and included on the consent form as options if there is pathologic confirmation of malignant tumor. The concepts of adjuvant radiation and/or systemic chemotherapy are often introduced at this time.

Because of the volume and intensity of information, both verbal and written instructions are needed to provide the patient and family with information to discuss and to take home for further study. This includes what should be expected in preparation for surgery, during the hospital stay, and after discharge. Appropriate phone numbers for physician, nurse, and clinical office coordinator are provided.

When available, a social worker meets the patient with a new diagnosis of brain tumor at the initial visit to discuss insurance concerns, possible postoperative rehabilitation needs, home care, and scheduling follow-up. Family members benefit from a discussion of what hospital and community resources may be available if circumstances warrant.

RADIATION THERAPY

Radiation therapy (RT) is an integral part of the treatment of malignant brain tumors. It may be used alone or in combination with chemotherapy or experimental drugs. Once a diagnosis is established via stereotactic biopsy or craniotomy, an RT consultation takes place to assess the most appropriate type/dose of treatment. The radiation oncologist makes a recommendation based on tumor classification, grade, location, and amount of residual tumor. Some benign tumors may also benefit from RT if they are recurrent or if there is significant residual tumor. Many centers withhold RT after gross total resection of low-grade tumors, such as oligodendrogliomas, and continue to evaluate with serial MRI or CT. Once there is evidence of tumor recurrence, a decision is made whether to reoperate and/or to proceed with RT.

Many tumors, such as gliomas, are infiltrative and blend with normal brain tissue. Therefore it is not possible to remove 100% of the tumor. RT is focused to treat the tumor resection cavity and the surrounding brain. It damages DNA as cell division is about to take place. The total dose is divided (fractions) over a 6-week period, with treatment 5 days per week. Rapidly dividing tumor cells are more sensitive to RT than normal brain tissue, and using fractions allows the brain to recover from its effects. However, it is generally accepted that there is a maximum dose from which normal brain cells can recover.

Imaging studies are performed to localize tumor and surrounding tissue to be treated. The patient is in the treatment position, and a mask is made that is used to prevent injury to structures not in the treatment area. This process is referred to as simulation.

The accepted dose for primary brain tumors is 6000 cGy. Studies have shown that this dose is well tolerated and that higher doses do not increase survival.[41] Metastatic lesions receive lower doses and shorter courses (3000 cGy over 10 treatments). The area to be treated depends upon the number and location of metastases. Whole-brain RT, as well as focused radiation, is discussed with the patient. The goal of focused radiation is to provide local control. The option of whole-brain RT may be used at a later date.[42]

A commonly used approach to treatment is 3-dimensional conformal RT (3DCRT), which focuses RT to the entire shape and volume desired. Using special equipment, higher-dose radiation is directed to abnormal areas, sparing normal tissue.[43] Table 6-3 describes the most commonly used treatments, with indications for use.[44-49]

Nursing Care Considerations. If high-grade tumor is suspected, discussion of RT ideally takes place *before* surgery. This helps patient and family plan for not only postoperative recovery, but for an extended treatment of at least 6 weeks. Once the patient has recovered from surgery (RT usually starts after a 2-week recovery period) radiation consultation and simulation take place. Risks and benefits are discussed at that time. These include possible short-term and long-term side effects. RT is often given in conjunction with chemotherapy, especially to treat primary malignant brain tumors. Therefore, medical and radiation oncology consultations are needed. Coordination of appointments is preferred to minimize time, expense, and stress of travel.

The patient will be informed of possible complications and what symptoms should be reported immediately. Although nausea and vomiting are side effects of many oncology therapies, brain tumor patients are instructed to report these symptoms as possible indications of increased ICP, especially when associated with headache. It is not uncommon for the radiation oncologist to add or modify steroid doses during treatment. Symptoms of increased ICP may arise at any time during RT or for several weeks after the end of treatment.[50] It should be noted that local

TABLE 6-3	**Commonly Used Forms of Radiation Therapy**	
TYPE	**DESCRIPTION**	**INDICATION**
Three-dimensional conformal radiation (3-DCRT)	• Beams shaped to match shape of 3-dimensionsal projection of target from each direction • Dose to target and normal tissues calculated throughout the entire relevant 3-dimensional volume	• Used for multiple tumor types and grades
Intensity-modulated RT (IMRT)	• Builds on 3-DCRT • Nonuniform beams in varying patterns and intensities (beam not just shaped as in 3DCRT, but also portions of beam may be increased or decreased in intensity to treat tumor or protect normal tissue)	• Better protects normal brain tissue • Increases dose to tumor
Stereotactic radiosurgery (e.g., gamma knife; linear accelerator; cyber knife; tomotherapy)	• Single large dose to specific, well-defined area that contains minimal normal brain • May also use a small number of fractions • Coordinates obtained under MRI • Very focused beams	• Small (<3 cm) tumors (sometimes used on larger lesions) • Metastatic lesions • Tumor recurrence, when standard RT has already been used
Brachytherapy	• Uses radioactive material • Placed in tumor or tumor resection cavity • May be temporary or permanent • Seeds, balloons, among others	• Local therapy that can be done at the time of surgery • Tumor recurrence, when standard RT has already been used
Radiosensitizers (e.g., efaproxiral)	• Goal is to enhance the effectiveness of RT • Increases delivery of oxygen to tumors, increasing RT effectiveness	• Experimental studies with malignant tumors (e.g., glioblastoma multiforme [GBM])
Boron neutron capture therapy	• Uses atomic energy and nuclear fission to treat tumor • Uses a carrier (i.e., boronated compound) followed by neutron beam RT from a nuclear reactor of RT	• Currently most commonly used for melanoma and GBM • (Very expensive; used in a small number of centers)

Dr. Lawrence Kleinberg, Department of Radiation Oncology, Johns Hopkins University, Baltimore, MD, contributed significant portions of this table.
Data from references 44-49.

radiation in the form of seeds and balloons, among others, is placed at the site of tumor resection during surgery, and can cause increased ICP as it treats dividing tumor cells. Additional side effects associated with RT include fatigue, alopecia, changes in saliva, and taste alterations. Cognitive changes and radiation necrosis (seen on MRI/CT) may be delayed effects of RT.

Verbal *and* written descriptions of treatment, side effects, and hospital resources (with phone numbers) are essential.

CHEMOTHERAPY

As with RT, chemotherapy interferes with cell division and inhibits tumor growth. The role of chemotherapy for both primary and metastatic brain tumors has evolved over the past several years. For primary malignant brain tumors such as grade III and grade IV gliomas, many practitioners have added temozolomide to surgery and radiation therapy, based on recent studies that have shown efficacy.[51] Chemotherapeutic agents including the nitrosoureas (e.g., carmustine, given intravenously, and lomustine, given orally), are also used. In addition, procarbazine and lomustine (+/- vincristine) are used by some practitioners for recurrent malignant gliomas. A biodegradable chemotherapy wafer (Gliadel, MGI Pharma, Minneapolis, MN) that releases carmustine over a period of 2 to 3 weeks can be implanted at the time of craniotomy for tumor debulking (Fig. 6-4). Studies have shown that this approach, used at the time of initial diagnosis or at recurrence, increases survival in patients with malignant gliomas.[52,53] Table 6-4 describes the most commonly used chemotherapeutic agents for primary brain tumors, with uses and side effects.[29]

Chemotherapeutic agents can be used alone or in combination with other treatment modalities. Newer drugs are being explored in clinical trials and/or in combination with currently used therapies.

Metastatic lesions are often treated with surgery (biopsy for multiple lesions; craniotomy for solitary metastasis when appropriate) followed by conventional whole-brain RT or radiosurgery. Some medical oncologists are adding chemotherapy when other approaches have failed or for tumors that are known to be more chemo sensitive.[20]

Nursing Care Considerations. Brain tumor chemotherapy is often well tolerated, having limited toxicities or side effects, although side effects vary with each particular medication.

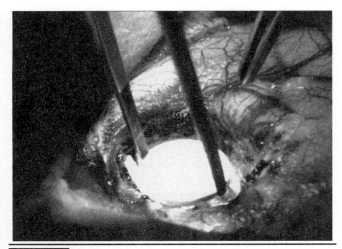

FIG. 6-4   Intraoperative placement of a Gliadel wafer into the tumor resection cavity.

Nausea and vomiting, the most common side effects, are usually experienced at the initiation of therapy, and can be successfully treated with antiemetic drugs. When headache and nausea (with or without vomiting) occur, these are generally related to increased ICP and are treated with steroids. However, unlike RT, systemic chemotherapy does not readily cross the BBB, thus minimizing these problems. Unfortunately, however, the BBB also limits the effectiveness of most chemotherapeutic agents. Local chemotherapy in the form of Gliadel wafers may cause increased ICP, because it is placed in the tumor resection cavity and has a direct effect on residual tumor cells. Use of steroids is recommended for 2 to 3 weeks after wafer placement.[53]

Patients are instructed to report any of the side effects listed, as well as new or worsening symptoms. Written instructions should be given regarding which complaints represent a medical emergency requiring an emergency department visit. Phone numbers for use during business hours, as well as those for after-hours, are included in the patient teaching packet.

OTHER TREATMENT MODALITIES

Medical Treatments. Because the prognosis for patients with malignant brain tumors is so poor, attempts are being made to develop new, innovative ways of treating this challenging disease. New substances are first studied in laboratory animal models and then progress to phase I, II, or III clinical trials to evaluate safety, toxicity, and effectiveness of a new treatment. In addition to surgery, radiation, and chemotherapy, research efforts are directed to other means of disabling tumor growth. Combination therapy approaches are currently in clinical trials, using known treatments either concomitantly or consecutively, with the hope of improving survival statistics. In addition, new systemic and local approaches are under investigation.

Angiogenesis is the ability of a tumor to develop new abnormal vessels and a vascular supply necessary for tumor growth. **Antiangiogenic** substances have been developed to disrupt this process in the hope of retarding blood vessel proliferation.[54]

Gene therapy uses viral vectors (e.g., retrovirus, adenovirus, or human herpes simplex virus) that are unable to replicate. They are injected into dividing tumor cells, making the tumor cells sensitive to antiviral drugs. Antivirals such as ganciclovir are injected into the tumor with the goal of inactivating these "infected" cells. Multiple studies have not yet shown efficacy of this treatment modality.[55,56]

Laboratory studies indicate that certain proteins (cytokines) are overexpressed in some brain tumor cell lines. In clinical trials, **targeted toxins** such as cytokines (e.g., interleukin [IL]–13) in combination with a toxin (e.g., *Pseudomonas aeruginosa*) are injected directly into recurrent malignant gliomas. One such method, convection enhanced delivery (CED), uses catheters placed into the tumor bed for direct delivery by positive pressure diffusion. Phase I and II studies have shown promising results. Phase III studies are currently under way.[57]

Another local approach uses so-called **oncolytic viruses,** developed to replicate in tumor cells but not in normal cells. Once inside the cell, these viruses "infect" tumor cells, releasing proteins that interfere with tumor growth. They replicate and infect surrounding tumor cells. Adenovirus, herpes simplex virus, and others have been followed in clinical trials.[55]

Research efforts continue, both in the laboratory and in clinical trials, using systemic and local therapies. The goal of this work is

TABLE 6-4 **Selected Chemotherapeutic Agents for the Treatment of Malignant Gliomas**

DRUG	DESCRIPTION	DOSE	SIDE EFFECTS	NURSING IMPLICATIONS/ COMMENTS
Carmustine (BCNU)	Nitrosourea Alkylating agent Lipid soluble	150–200 mg/m^2 by intravenous route (IV) every 6–8 weeks	Myelosuppression Gastrointestinal symptoms Pulmonary fibrosis	Teaching regarding need for blood tests and/or office visits Serum blood counts at 3 and 6 weeks Seen after multiple (±6) cycles Pulmonary function tests suggested
Lomustine (CCNU)	Nitrosourea Alkylating agent Lipid soluble Has a short half-life	130 mg/m^2 orally at bedtime every 6 weeks	Same as BCNU Bone marrow toxicity may be more cumulative than BCNU	Teaching regarding need for blood tests and/or office visits Serum blood counts at 3 and 6 weeks
Temozolomide	Methylating agent	150–200 mg/m^2 for 5 days in a 28-day cycle Lower doses used during radiation therapy (RT)	Myelosuppression Gastrointestinal symptoms Fatigue Rash	Blood tests before next dosing Teaching regarding need for blood tests and office visits Studies ongoing regarding adjuvant use in GBM with RT and in recurrent grade III astrocytoma Approximately 10% of patients suffer extended periods of low platelets or other blood count abnormalities, requiring transfusions Once counts recover, lower doses may be used
Procarbazine, CCNU, Vincristine (PCV)	Triple drug therapy	42-day cycle Procarbazine = 60 mg/m^2 from days 8–21 CCNU = 110 mg/m^2 orally on day 1 Vincristine = 1.4 mg/m^2 on days 14 and 29	Myelosuppression Gastrointestinal symptoms Fatigue Pulmonary symptoms Peripheral neuropathy Irreversible myelosuppression possible with multiple nitrosourea regimens	Serum blood counts at 3 and 6 weeks (Some oncologists obtain weekly levels) No survival benefit of PCV over single-agent BCNU Vincristine has been eliminated because of side effects (neuropathy) combined with inability to cross blood–brain barrier (BBB)
Procarbazine	Alkylating agent	56-day cycle 125–150 mg/m^2 for 28 days; no drug for 28 days	Myelosuppression Interactions with some drugs (e.g., monoamine oxidase [MAO] inhibitors)	Serum blood counts This is occasionally used as single agent for recurrence
Gliadel chemotherapy wafers	Carmustine wafers Biodegradable over 2–3 weeks	Implanted at time of tumor surgery Eight 7.7 mg wafers Stored at −20° C	Local brain edema May cause treatment necrosis Studies showed no systemic side effects	Steroids may be required in larger amounts or for longer duration to decrease edema

Data provided by Michel Zeltzman, CRNP, Department of Medical Oncology, Johns Hopkins, Baltimore, MD.

to improve survival while maintaining quality of life for patients with malignant gliomas and other aggressive brain tumors.

Nursing Care Considerations. Patients enroll in investigational protocols for a number of reasons: they would like to be involved in state-of-the-art therapies; they hope to help in the search for more effective treatment modalities for brain tumors; or they have exhausted the more conventional therapies and have limited treatment options. No matter what the reason, patients are aware that these therapies have not yet shown efficacy and may, in fact, have unknown toxicities.

Once the consent form has been discussed with the patient by the principal investigator, the research nurse provides the patient with schedules for treatment and 24-hour contacts for reporting adverse events. It is important to inform the patient and family that withdrawal from the protocol is optional and carries no negative consequences. The patient may then proceed to other conventional treatments or may suspend treatment, if appropriate.

Written instructions are crucial in these cases. The patient and family will receive copies of the consent form, as well as copies of treatment schedules and follow-up appointments. The use of patient teaching sheets with drug description, known side effects, and contact numbers minimizes complications and maximizes patient compliance.

Disease-Related Complications and Treatment

The most common complications of brain tumors, particularly malignant tumors, include the following:

- Increased ICP
- Seizures
- Mental status changes
- Focal neurologic signs
- Deep vein thrombosis (DVT); pulmonary embolus (PE)

The most common complications of brain tumor treatments include all of the above as well as the following:

- Intracranial hemorrhage
- Infection
- Treatment effect: necrosis
- Steroid myopathy
- Immunosuppression
- Cognitive sequelae

Table 6-5 lists the complications of brain tumors and their treatments and identifies nursing care considerations for each complication.[22-25,28,58,59]

Spinal Cord Tumors

Spinal cord tumors make up approximately 4% of CNS tumors[1] (although estimates vary in the literature). Like brain tumors, they may be benign or malignant and may be primary or metastasize from other, primary sites. There are no known risk factors. To date, no prevention or screening measures have been identified. However, patients with severe, consistent back pain (with or without neurologic deficits) should be considered at risk for spinal tumor until proven otherwise.[60] Early detection, before neurologic decline takes place, is key to increased survival and quality of life.

Spinal cord tumors are classified by their location in the spine. Extramedullary tumors are located outside the spinal cord and may be extradural (outside the cord and outside the dura) or intradural (outside the cord but inside the dura). Intramedullary tumors are located within the cord itself.[61]

The most common spinal cord tumors are extradural. Metastases from breast, lung, and prostate cancers, myeloma, and lymphoma are most likely to occur in this location. Ten percent of metastases to the spine are from an unknown primary. These tumors most commonly affect the thoracic or lumbar spine.[62] Pain control is the primary goal of treatment, and 90% of patients with metastatic epidural tumors suffer pain. If tumor is identified early, weakness, numbness, and lack of sphincter control may be avoided. These neurologic symptoms are difficult to reverse.[60] Surgical intervention depends upon tumor location, number of metastatic lesions, extent of primary disease, and the patient's clinical condition. Some metastatic tumors are responsive to RT (e.g., lymphoma, myeloma) and may not require surgery.[63]

Intradural extramedullary tumors are rarely metastatic and are generally benign. Most often seen in this location are meningiomas and schwannomas. Surgery is often the treatment of choice and is performed when complete resection is possible. Recurrence rate is dependent on completeness of resection. Of patients with residual disease, 50% will have tumor recurrence, but recurrence is rare with total tumor removal.[61]

Intramedullary tumors are more likely to be glial—astrocytoma, ependymoma, oligodendroglioma, and others. In adults, ependymoma is most common and is generally well circumscribed. Metastatic tumors occur in the cord in less than 5% of cases. When possible, surgery is recommended for well-circumscribed tumors. Complete resection is difficult with infiltrative tumors such as gliomas. The goal of surgery in the vast majority of these cases is preservation of neurologic function. Close observation with MRI scans is used, and RT may be added for tumor progression.[61]

Table 6-6 describes the most common spinal cord tumors with treatment goals and nursing care considerations.

Considerations for Older Adults

With improvements in nutrition, increased interest in exercise, and better medical screening and care, we are experiencing increased longevity, particularly in developed countries. Older adults are actively involved in maintaining a healthy lifestyle. The media is a source of information on current trends and research initiatives, which aids individuals in keeping up to date with ways to enhance quality of life. As survival increases, so do the needs of the elderly population; with increasing age, they are more likely to develop medical problems. The highest incidence of brain tumors is in the age range between 75 and 84 years.[1]

Insurance and financial concerns make it more difficult for the older patient to get adequate medical care, or they discourage the patient from seeking attention in a timely fashion. Once in the medical system, there are several problems with which the elderly patient may have particular difficulty: medication schedules and dosing; caring for him- or herself at home, whether living alone or with an ailing spouse; returning for follow-up visits; and identifying/reporting new or recurrent symptoms.

Geriatric patients with brain tumors have a unique set of needs and concerns. There may be cognitive issues related to tumor location and/or the side effects of medications and treatments. Visual compromise makes it difficult for the patient to adequately provide his or her own care, even if otherwise capable of doing so. Seizures or other neurologic complaints restrict independence, particularly because of driving limitations. Motor weakness decreases mobility and increases the risk of complications, including DVT, PE, or pneumonia. Sensory or balance difficulties increase the risk of falls and further complications.

It is vital for the neurooncology team to assess patient needs and disabilities and to provide for inpatient and outpatient therapy as necessary. Community resources may be enlisted to provide meals, home health care, financial counseling, explanation of insurance benefits, and hospice care, when appropriate. Involvement of family in decision making and care, which is important for any patient treated for a brain tumor, is even more crucial for the older patient facing surgery and treatment for this disease. Verbal *and* written instructions should include medication doses and schedules, side effects of treatment, emergency situations, appropriate phone numbers, and community resources.

TABLE 6-5   Brain Tumor Complications and Nursing Care Considerations

COMPLICATION	SYMPTOMS	NURSING CARE CONSIDERATIONS
Increased intracranial pressure (ICP)	Headache; nausea/vomiting; papilledema	Patient/family to report symptoms immediately and seek medical care Steroids initiated or increased per physician order when appropriate Instruct patient on steroid side effects
Seizures	May be generalized, complex-partial, or simple-partial	Family to be instructed on safety measures during generalized seizures; when to seek emergency medical attention Provide written instructions on dosage, use, and side effects of each anticonvulsant Instruct patient on driving , restrictions which vary from state to state
Mental status changes	Lethargy, decreased alertness, decreased short-term memory May be related to increased ICP or tumor location	Instruct family on safety measures Notify physician for continued or exacerbated symptoms
Focal neurologic signs	Related to tumor location (see Table 6-2)	See Table 6-2
Deep vein thrombosis and pulmonary embolism (DVT/PE)	DVT: Leg swelling, tenderness; one leg larger than the other PE: Shortness of breath; chest pain or pressure; anxiety	Educate patient regarding • Signs and symptoms • Medical emergency; instruct patient to seek immediate medical treatment Patient should receive computed tomography (CT) of the head before initiating anticoagulation to rule out intracranial hemorrhage Give verbal and written instructions on dosage; side effects; monitoring of blood levels while on anticoagulation; foods that affect efficacy of drugs; contraindicated medications
Intracranial hemorrhage	Severe headache; lethargy; mental status changes; neurologic deficits	This may be a medical emergency Patient may require surgical evacuation of blood Family teaching regarding timely intervention to reverse symptoms and relieve increased ICP
Infection		
• Wound infection	Fevers; wound erythema, tenderness, swelling, drainage	Patient teaching to include that steroid use may mask infection Antibiotic therapy
• Intracranial infection	May cause increased ICP and neurologic symptoms	Hospitalization, reoperation, and antibiotic therapy
• Treatment effect: necrosis	Enhancement on radiographic imaging Increased ICP	Teaching regarding possible side effect of local therapy Magnetic resonance spectroscopy (MRS) or positron emission tomography (PET) may help to differentiate treatment effect from tumor recurrence Possible reoperation to establish a diagnosis
• Immunosuppression	Susceptibility to infection	Patient to report fevers, wound healing problems, malaise Workup includes chest x-ray (*Pneumocistis carinii* pneumonia [PCP], a side effect of steroid therapy); blood tests including CD$_4$ count; urine microscopic exam and culture; CT/magnetic resonance imaging (MRI) to rule out intracranial abscess Examine and/or culture wound if necessary Teaching to include side effects of steroid and chemotherapy use; provide written instructions
Steroid myopathy	Proximal muscle weakness	Patient to report difficulty getting out of chairs, walking up steps, and so on Physical therapy (PT) consultation obtained postoperatively and/or as symptoms develop Encourage ambulation as soon as possible after surgery, and regular exercise as appropriate Discuss with physician steroid dosing and tapering; provide written instructions to patient

TABLE 6-5   Brain Tumor Complications and Nursing Care Considerations—cont'd

COMPLICATION	SYMPTOMS	NURSING CARE CONSIDERATIONS
Cognitive sequelae	Difficulty concentrating; short-term memory problems; emotional lability may be related to medications	Patient and family to report cognitive changes in relation to medication and treatment schedule Importance of differentiating side effects of treatment from symptoms of tumor growth Discuss medication modification with physician when appropriate
Fatigue	Decreased interaction, socialization Difficulty concentrating Increased need for assistance with activities of daily living (ADLs)	May be the effect of tumor growth and ICP, or secondary to treatments/medications Discuss importance of rest and need for naps during treatment Education regarding scheduling activities, work, and treatment to maximize energy levels Reassure patient that fatigue is side effect of therapy and generally improves after treatment Assess drug-related fatigue, particularly with anticonvulsant use

Data from references 22-25, 28, 58, 59.

TABLE 6-6   Classification of Spinal Cord Tumors

LOCATION	CHARACTERISTICS	COMMON TUMOR TYPES	TREATMENT AND TREATMENT GOALS	NURSING CARE CONSIDERATIONS
Extradural Extramedullary	Outside the dura, outside the cord Spine most common site for skeletal metastases 70% in thoracic spine	Metastases most common: lung, breast, prostate, kidney, lymphoma, melanoma, GI	Surgery and/or radiation: depending on tumor type, number, location Pain relief Quality of life Preserve neurologic function Stabilize spine	Pain in 90% of patients Difficult to reverse neurologic symptoms Expedite rehabilitation therapy
Intradural Extramedullary	Inside the dura, outside cord, within Usually slow-growing	Schwannoma Meningioma	Surgery Goal is complete resection Maintain neurologic function	Recurrence rare with complete resection Prevent neurologic complication
Intramedullary	Within the cord Gliomas = 80%-90% Astrocytoma (children) Ependymoma (adults) Hemangioblastoma = 3%-8%	Astrocytoma Ependymoma Hemangioblastoma	Surgery Goal of complete resection is difficult to achieve with infiltrative gliomas	Local recurrence, especially with incomplete resection May require reoperation or radiation therapy (RT)

Data from references 60-63.

Prognosis

A number of brain tumors discussed in this chapter are surgically curable and require no further therapy. The factors affecting outcome include tumor type, age, and location and the patient's overall health. The most common brain tumors are also the most aggressive and have the worst outcomes. Metastatic brain tumors account for greater than 150,000 new brain tumor cases each year. Of the more than 44,000 primary brain tumors diagnosed each year, malignant gliomas comprise approximately 50% and are generally refractory to all treatment we currently have available. Tumor recurrence is common, and 5-year survival for GBM is 4%.[1]

Like brain tumors, many spinal cord tumors are curable with surgery. However the most common spinal cord tumors are metastatic lesions requiring multiple therapies and having poor cure and/or control rates. Quality of life is significantly affected as a result of pain and/or neurologic symptoms.

Younger patients, even those with malignant tumors, tend to respond to treatments for longer periods and with better quality of life. Complications are more common in the older patient population.

Even low-grade, slow-growing tumors can have devastating outcomes, if located in eloquent areas of the brain or spinal cord. Tumors may affect speech, motor strength, or sensation and have an impact on quality of life. A small, slow-growing, histologically "benign" CNS neoplasm can also be rapidly fatal.

Conclusion

In treating patients with all types of CNS tumors, quality of life is as important to consider as survival benefit. Multidisciplinary planning at all stages of the treatment process aids in maximizing quality of life. Choices are based on the patient's neurologic performance status, radiographic tumor progression, risk-benefit ratio of each therapy, and patient preference. Once it is evident that there are no further reasonable alternatives, the neurooncology team recommends comfort measures, and hospice care is discussed with the family and the patient, when appropriate. In recent years, there has been an increase in hospital-based palliative care services, which provide for both inpatient services and home care upon discharge. Home and inpatient hospice care provide the needed medical, nursing, social work, and pastoral services for both patient and family at the terminal stages of this disease. Further improvements in end-of-life care are the responsibility of all members of the multidisciplinary neurooncology team.[64-66]

REVIEW QUESTIONS

✓ Case Study

MG was a 58-year-old, physically active male who was found by a co-worker slumped over his desk, incontinent of urine. The co-worker called 911 and stayed with MG until the ambulance arrived. MG awakened after a few minutes and was somewhat confused. He had no recollection of the event. On the way to the hospital he suffered a generalized seizure with tonic-clonic activity. Once at the ED, he was completely oriented and conversant. Anticonvulsant therapy was administered. After history-taking and physical exam, he was taken for a CT with contrast, which revealed a 3-cm ring-enhancing lesion with significant edema in the left frontal lobe. Steroid therapy was initiated. The patient had no neurologic symptoms or seizures and was discharged to the care of family members. He was subsequently evaluated by his internist and a neurosurgeon.

The following week, he underwent a craniotomy with placement of 8 Gliadel chemotherapy wafers. Final histology was consistent with GBM. He was discharged from the hospital 3 days later with no new neurologic deficits and with instructions for follow-up care. Skin staples were removed and radiation and chemotherapy consults were obtained the following week. RT with low-dose temozolomide was started 18 days postoperatively. After 6 weeks, RT ended and the patient underwent higher-dose temozolomide, monthly, for the next 6 months. He continued to work on a part-time schedule throughout treatment.

Eleven months from initial diagnosis, there was evidence of tumor recurrence on MRI. MG underwent repeat craniotomy followed by an experimental protocol using chemotherapy and an antiangiogenic factor. He gradually began to decline clinically, and the bimonthly MRI scans continued to show evidence of tumor progression. Treatment was discontinued at the request of the patient and his family, and he received home hospice care over a 4-week period. MG died at home in the presence of his family 16 months from original diagnosis.

DISCUSSION

Although the first episode was unwitnessed, the patient most likely suffered a generalized seizure in the office and in the ambulance—a warning sign of an intracerebral abnormality in adults. He went on to receive the appropriate diagnostic workup and treatment in a timely manner. Drug therapy for increased ICP (steroids) and seizures (anticonvulsants) was appropriately initiated. At first, GM received conventional treatment with surgery and implanted chemotherapy wafers, followed by RT and systemic chemotherapy. Quality of life was maintained. Once the tumor recurred, he went on to receive experimental protocols in the hope of treating the recurrence and with the expectation of helping others find information regarding drug toxicity and efficacy. When the tumor progressed after multiple treatments, the patient declined further therapy. The patient, the family, and medical staff made the decision to halt therapy and allow for hospice care, providing the needed support for patient and family in the terminal stage of his disease.

The nurse has a unique opportunity to provide invaluable assistance and information to patients like GM and his family. During the course of the disease process, the nurse will provide teaching regarding diagnostic tests, medications and treatment regimens, surgical interventions, follow-up care, potential complications, and end-of-life care. She or he also provides physical and emotional care to the patient during all phases of the treatment and ensures that team members are communicating with each other as well as with the patient and the family. Accurate, honest answers were appreciated by GM and his family. GM's experience was enhanced by a smooth transition between disciplines during each phase of therapy.

QUESTIONS

1. What is the most common primary brain tumor?
   a. Meningioma
   b. Nerve sheath tumor
   c. Glioma
   d. Lymphoma
2. Which of the following is a risk factor in the development of brain tumors?
   a. Gene alterations
   b. Hypertension (HTN)
   c. Sexually transmitted diseases (STDs)
   d. Lack of exercise
3. Patients receiving local therapies such as Gliadel will need _____ therapy for at least 2 to 3 weeks postoperatively:
   a. Antihypertensive
   b. Speech
   c. Steroid
   d. Physical
4. Which of the following series of goals is appropriate for craniotomy?
   a. Diagnosis
   b. Diagnosis and tumor debulking
   c. Decreasing ICP
   d. Diagnosis, tumor debulking, and decreasing ICP
5. All of the following are commonly used to treat malignant glioma except which one?
   a. Carmustine
   b. Procarbazine
   c. Methotrexate
   d. Temozolomide

6. The nurse is caring for a patient who has undergone left frontal craniotomy for a GBM. On postoperative day 3, she sees that the patient has headache, increased lethargy, and new onset of right-leg weakness. What is the most likely etiology?
   a. Increased ICP
   b. Drug interaction
   c. Pulmonary embolus
   d. Tumor recurrence

7. Steroid therapy is used to reduce which of the following?
   a. Hyperglycemia
   b. Increased ICP
   c. Immunosuppression
   d. Proximal myopathy

8. Mr. W. underwent tumor resection, local chemotherapy implants, radiation, and chemotherapy for a GBM. Follow-up MRI scans show an enlarging ring-enhancing lesion similar to the original lesion. He has no neurologic deficits. Which of the following would be an appropriate initial plan?
   a. Obtain MRI in 6 months
   b. PET scan
   c. Surgery for diagnosis and tumor debulking
   d. Radiation therapy to shrink mass

9. Systemic chemotherapy is effective in only a small percentage of patients with malignant brain tumors; this can be explained as a result of what?
   a. Ineffective drugs
   b. Severe drug side effects
   c. Poor patient compliance
   d. The BBB

10. During the course of their illness, approximately _____% of patients with supratentorial brain tumors experience a seizure
    a. 10%
    b. 25%
    c. 50%
    d. 75%

ANSWERS

1. **C.** *Rationale:* Gliomas make up 42% of primary brain tumors.
2. **A.** *Rationale:* Recent studies suggest a relationship between genetic alterations and many types of brain tumors. To the knowledge of this author, HTN, STDs, and exercise have neither been implicated nor studied.
3. **C.** *Rationale:* Gliadel chemotherapy wafers release carmustine over a 2- to 3-week period. This can cause increased brain swelling and thus increases in ICP. Steroids are used to reduce edema.
4. **D.** *Rationale:* Through craniotomy, tumor is removed and sent to the pathologist for diagnostic purposed. In addition, as much tumor as possible is removed, and this results in decreases in ICP.
5. **C.** *Rationale:* Although methotrexate is used for other brain tumors such as CNS lymphoma, and has even been used in experimental studies with glioma, it is the drug least often used.
6. **A.** *Rationale:* The patient is at the highest risk for increased ICP in the first 72 hours after surgery, and the symptoms described are associated with increased ICP.
7. **B.** *Rationale:* Steroids are used to *treat* ICP. The other three answers are side effects of steroids.
8. **B.** *Rationale:* It is *not* reasonable to wait 6 months to image a patient with a known GBM and possible recurrence. Although surgery is reasonable, a PET scan may give information suggesting treatment effect and obviating the need for surgery at this time. One would not use radiation if there is suspicion of necrosis. Radiation *causes* necrosis.
9. **D.** *Rationale:* Systemic chemotherapeutic agents have difficulty crossing the BBB in significant enough amounts to treat tumor effectively
10. **C.** *Rationale:* Approximately 33% of patients are first seen because of seizures, and approximately 50% have a seizure at some time during the course of their illness

REFERENCES

1. Central Brain Tumor Registry of the United States: Primary brain tumors in the United States, *CBTRUS 1998-2002 Statistical Report*. 2005-2006.
2. Bondy ML, El-Zein R, Wrensch M: Epidemiology of brain cancer. In Schiff D, O'Neill P, editors: *Principles of neuro-oncology,* New York, 2005, McGraw-Hill.
3. Burger PC, Scheithauer BW, Vogel FS: The brain—tumors. In: *Surgical pathology of the nervous system and its coverings* ed 4, New York, 2002, Churchill Livingstone.
4. American College of Surgical Oncology CNS Working Group: The management of brain metastases. In Schiff D, O'Neill P, editors: *Principles of neuro-oncology,* New York, 2005, McGraw-Hill.
5. Brem SS, Panattil JG: An era of rapid advancement: diagnosis and treatment of metastatic brain cancer, *Neurosurgery* 57(5 Suppl): 5-9, 2005.
6. Langer CJ, Mehta MP: Current management of brain metastases, with a focus on systemic options, *J Clin Oncol* 23(25):6207-6219, 2005.
7. Hardell L, Mild KH: Mobile phone use and risk of glioma in adults: results are difficult to interpret because of limitations, *BJM* 332(7548):1035, 2006.
8. Wrensch N, Fisher JL, Schwartbaum JA et al: The molecular epidemiology of gliomas in adults, *Neurosurg Focus* 19(5):E5, 2005.
9. World Health Organization: Classification of tumours. In Kleihues P, Cavenee WK, editors: *Pathology and genetics of tumours of the nervous system,* Lyon, France, 2000, IARC Press.
10. Shaffrey ME, Farace E, Schiff D et al: The Ki-67 labeling index as a prognostic factor in grade II oligoastrocytomas, *J Neurosurg* 102(6):1033-1039, 2005.
11. Neder L, Colli BO, Machado HR et al: MIB-1 labeling index in astrocytic tumors—a clinicopathologic study, *Clin Neuropathol* 23(6):262-270, 2004.
12. Watanabe K, Sato K, Biernat W et al: Incidence and timing of p53 mutations during astrocytoma progression in patients with multiple biopsies, *Clin Cancer Res* 3(4):523-530, 1997.
13. Mason W: Oligodendroglioma. *Curr Treat Options Neurol* 7:305-14, 2005.
14. van den Bent MJ, Looijenga LH, Langenberg K et al: Chromosomal anomalies in oligodendroglial tumors are correlated with clinical features, *Cancer* 97:1276-1284, 2003.
15. Chamberlain MC, Blumenthal DT: Intracranial meningiomas: diagnosis and treatment, *Expert Rev Neurother* 4(4):641-648, 2004.
16. Modha A, Gutin PH: Diagnosis and treatment of atypical and anaplastic meningiomas: a review, *Neurosurg* 57(3):538-50, 2005.
17. Grant GA, Mayberg M: Vestibular schwannomas. In Bernstein M, Berger MS, editors: *Neuro-oncology: the essentials,* New York, 2000, Thieme.

18. Lundsford LD, Niranjan A, Glickinger JC et al: Radiosurgery of vestibular schwannomas: Summary of experience in 829 cases, *J Neurosurg* 102(Suppl):95-99, 2005.

19. Bajaj GK, Kleinberg L, Terezakis S: Current concepts and controversies in the treatment of parenchymal brain metastases: improved outcomes with aggressive management, *Cancer Invest* 23(4):363-376, 2005.

20. Hwu WJ, Lis E, Menell JH, et al: Temozolomide plus thalidomide in patients with brain metastases from melanoma: a phase II study, *Cancer* 103(12):2590-2597, 2005.

21. Fitzsimmons B, Bohan E: Common neurosurgical and neurological disorders. In Morton PG, Fontaine DK, Hudak CM et al, editors: *Critical care nursing: a holistic approach,* ed 8, Philadelphia, 2005, Lippincott, Williams & Wilkins.

22. Wen PY, Teoh SK, Gigas DC et al: Presentation and approach to patient. In Schiff D, O'Neill P, editors: *Principles of neuro-oncology*, New York, 2005, McGraw-Hill.

23. Engelhard HH: Brain tumors and the blood-brain barrier. In Bernstein M, Berger MS, editors: *Neuro-oncology: the essentials*, New York, 2000, Thieme.

24. Wilne SH, Ferris RC, Nathwani A et al: The presenting features of brain tumours: a review of 200 cases, *Arch Dis Child* 91(6):502-506, 2006.

25. Baumgartner K: Neurocognitive changes in cancer patients, *Semin Oncol Nurs Neuro-Oncol* 20(4):284-290, 2004.

26. Siomin V, Angelov L, Li L et al: Results of a survey of neurosurgical practice patterns regarding the prophylactic use of anti-epilepsy drugs in patients with brain tumors, *J Neuro-Oncol* 74:211-215, 2005.

27. Hildebrand J, Lecaille C, Perennes J et al: Epileptic seizures during follow-up of patients treated for primary brain tumors, *Neurology* 65(2):212-215, 2005.

28. Gilbert M, Loghin M: The treatment of malignant gliomas, *Curr Treat Options Neurol* 7:293-303, 2005.

29. Bohan E: Brain tumors. In Barker E, editor: *Neuroscience nursing: a spectrum of care*, ed 3, (in press).

30. Aronen HJ, Perkio J: Dynamic susceptibility contrast MRI of gliomas, *Neuroimaging Clin North Am* 12(4):501-523, 2002.

31. Bullitt E, Zeng D, Gerig G et al: Vessel tortuosity and brain tumor malignancy: a blinded study, *Acad Radiol* 12(10):1232-1240, 2005.

32. Gujar SK, Maheshwari S, Bjorkman-Burtscher I et al: Magnetic resonance spectroscopy, *J Neuroophthalmol* 25(3):217-226, 2005.

33. Spence AM, Mankoff DA, Muzi M: Positron emission tomography of brain tumors, *Neuroimaging Clin North Am* 13:715-739, 2003.

34. Wilkinson ID, Romanowski CA, Jellinek DA et al: Motor functional MRI for preoperative and intraoperative neurosurgical guidance, *Br J Radiol* 76:98-103, 2003.

35. Pignatti F, van den Bent M, Curran D et al: Prognostic factors for survival in adult patients with cerebral low-grade glioma, *J Clin Oncol* 20(8):2076-2084, 2002.

36. Chamberlain M: Neoplastic meningitis, *J Clin Oncol* 23(15):3605-3613, 2005.

37. Forsyth PA, Weaver S, Fulton D et al: Prophylactic anticonvulsants in patients with brain tumor, *Can J Neurol Sci* 30(2):102-112, 2003.

38. Woodworth G, McGirt MJ, Samdani A et al: Accuracy of frameless and frame-based image-guided stereotactic brain biopsy in the diagnosis of glioma: comparison of biopsy and open resection specimen, *Neurol Res* 27(4):358-362, 2005.

39. Weingart J, Brem H: Basic principles of cranial surgery for brain tumors. In Winn HR, editor: *Youmans neurosurgical surgery,* ed 5, Philadelphia, 2003, Saunders.

40. Whittle IR: Surgery for gliomas, *Curr Opin Neurol* 15:663-669, 2002.

41. Scott CB et al: Long-term results of RTOG 90-06. A randomized trial of hyperfractionated radiotherapy to 72Gy and carmustine vs. standard RT and carmustine for malignant glioma patients with emphasis on anaplastic astrocytoma patients, *Proc ASCO* 17:401a, 1998.

42. Martin JJ, Kondiolka D: Indications for resection and radiosurgery for brain metastases, *Curr Opin Oncol* 17(6):584-587, 2005.

43. Khatua S, Jalali R: Recent advances in the treatment of childhood brain tumors, *Pediatr Hematol Oncol* 22(5):361-371, 2005.

44. Fiveash JB, Spencer SA: Role of radiation therapy and radiosurgery in glioblastoma multiforme, *Cancer J* 9(3):222-229, 2003.

45. Pang LJ: Radiation oncology update, *Hawaii Med J* 62(5):109-110, 2003.

46. Yu C, Shepard D: Treatment planning for stereotactic radiosurgery with photon beams, *Technol Cancer Res Treat* 2(2):93-104, 2003.

47. Vitaz TW, Warnke PC, Tabar V et al: Brachytherapy for brain tumors, *J Neuro-Oncol* 73:71-86, 2005.

48. Chan TA, Weingart JD, Parisi M et al.: Treatment of recurrent glioblastoma multiforme with GliaSite brachytherapy, *Int J Radiat Oncol Biol Phys* 62(4):1133-1139, 2005.

49. Kleinberg L, Grossman SA, Carson K et al: Survival of patients with newly diagnosed glioblastoma multiforme treated with RSR13 and radiotherapy: Results of a phase II New Approaches to Brain Tumor Consortium safety and efficacy study, *J Clin Oncol* 20(14):3149-3155, 2002.

50. Rakesh RP, Wolfgang AT, Mehta MP: Radiation therapy for central nervous system tumors. In Rengachary SS, Ellenbogen RG, editors: *Principles of neurosurgery,* ed 2, Philadelphia, 2005, Mosby.

51. Stupp R, Mason WP, van den Bent MJ et al: Radiotherapy plus concomitant and adjuvant temozolomide for glioblastoma, *N Engl J Med* 352:987-996, 2005.

52. Westphal M, Hilt DC, Bortey E, et al: A phase 3 trial of local chemotherapy with biodegradable carmustine (BCNU) wafers (Gliadel wafers) in patients with primary malignant gliomas, *Neurooncol* 5(2):79-88, 2003.

53. Brem H, Piantadosi S, Burgery PC et al: Placebo-controlled trial of safety and efficacy of intraoperative controlled delivery by biodegradable polymers of chemotherapy for recurrent gliomas, *Lancet* 345:1008-1012,1995.

54. Jansen M, de Witt Hamer PC, Witmer AN et al: Current perspectives on antiangiogenesis strategies in the treatment of malignant gliomas, *Brain Res Rev* 45(3):143-163, 2004.

55. Chiocca EA, Broaddus WC, Gillies GT et al: Neurosurgical delivery of chemotherapeutics, targeted toxins, genetic and viral therapies in neuro-oncology, *J Neuro-Oncol* 69:101-117, 2004.

56. Lesniak MS: Gene therapy for malignant glioma, *Expert Rev Neurother* 6(4):479-488, 2006.

57. Shimamura T, Husain SR, Puri RK: The IL-4 and IL-13 *Pseudomonas* exotoxins: New hope for brain tumor therapy, *Neurosurg Focus* 204:E11, 2006.

58. Pruitt AA: Treatment of medical complications in patients with brain tumors, *Curr Treat Options Neurol* 7(4):323-336, 2005.

59. Lovely MP: Symptom management of brain tumor patients, *Semin Oncol Nurs Neuro-Oncol* 20(4):273-283, 2004.

60. Perrin RG, McBroom RJ: Metastatic tumors of the spine. In Rengachary SS, Ellenbogen RG, editors: *Principles of neurosurgery*, Philadelphia, 2005, Mosby.

61. Shedid D, Benzel EC: Neoplastic disease of the spinal cord and the spinal canal. In McLain, RF, editor: *Cancer in the spine: comprehensive care*, New Jersey, 2006, Humana Press.

62. Klimo P Jr, Kestle JRW, Schmidt MH: Treatment of metastatic spinal epidural disease: a review of the literature, *Neurosurg Focus* 15:1-8, 2003.

63. Riley LH 3rd, Frassica DA, Kostuik JP et al: Metastatic disease to the spine: diagnosis and treatment, *Instr Course Lect* 49:471-477, 2000.

64. Fairbrother CA, Paice JA: Life's final journey: the oncology nurse's role, *Clin J Oncol Nurs* 9(5):575-579, 2005.

65. Hanley E: The role of palliative care services, *Care Manag J* 5(3):151-157, 2004.

66. Braunack-Mayer THN, Beilby J: The impact of the hospice environment on patient spiritual expression, *Oncol Nurs Forum* 32(5):1049-1055, 2005.

CHAPTER 7

Breast Cancers

Rebecca Crane-Okada and Molly Loney

Breast cancer is the most common cancer and the leading cause of cancer deaths in women throughout the world; it is a major public health concern.[1] The incidence of breast cancer is increasing throughout the world. Although higher age-specific incidence rates for female breast cancer occur in developed countries, nearly half of the cases of breast cancer diagnosed in the next year will be in developing countries.[1]

In the United States, public awareness of breast cancer has grown considerably in recent years. Women in the public eye have spoken out about their experiences with breast cancer; media coverage includes breast health as well as breast cancer care information; screening mammography is more available under insurance coverage; and women's health care issues are prominent in funded research and foundation projects. It has been less than 40 years since the Halsted radical mastectomy was replaced with more conservative surgery, and since the "one-step" procedure (biopsy with frozen-section diagnosis and immediate surgery) was replaced with a two-step procedure.

Women are expected to be involved in their treatment planning. The knowledge that breast cancer is a systemic disease at the time of diagnosis justifies the use of chemotherapy and hormonal manipulation as adjuncts to surgery that improve survival. Randomized clinical trials continue to assess the value of more dose-intensive and combination therapies in the treatment of women with breast cancer at high risk for recurrence and with advanced disease.

Among questions continually reviewed are these:
1. Which women with negative nodes and smaller tumors benefit most from systemic treatment?
2. What is the optimal timing for initiation of treatment?
3. What is the optimal combination of drugs, the optimal dose size, and the optimal intensity to be used?
4. What is the optimal duration of treatment?

Research has increased our understanding of breast cancer through the recent discovery of two breast cancer susceptibility genes, *BRCA1* and *BRCA2*, and the effects of tumor suppressor genes and oncogenes on breast cancer initiation, on development, and in predicting prognosis. Results of the Breast Cancer Prevention Trial, begun in 1992, led to approval by the U.S. Food and Drug Administration (FDA) in late 1998 of tamoxifen for use as a preventive agent in women at increased risk for breast cancer.[2] A subsequent prevention trial compares the toxicity, the benefits, and the risks of tamoxifen and raloxifene in the prevention of breast cancer in postmenopausal women who are at increased risk for the disease.[3] Other clinical trials, such as the Women's Health Initiative (WHI) and the Women's Intervention Nutrition Study (WINS), have added to our understanding of the effects of dietary fat, obesity, and hormone replacement therapy on breast cancer.[4,5] Each of these lends hope that new and better methods for the prevention and treatment of breast cancer will lead to reductions in mortality.

Early detection remains the key to breast cancer control, with mammography the mainstay for finding breast cancer before it has become clinically detectable. Coupled with regular and thorough examination of the breasts by a professional, and breast self-examination (BSE), breast cancer can be found early, when it is more likely to be cured, often with conservative surgical management.

Socioeconomic and cultural influences on the practice of breast cancer–control activities, stage at diagnosis, and survival establish the need for more attention to these factors in all phases of the breast care continuum. The psychosocial impact of breast cancer screening, diagnosis, and treatment on the individual or family remains a major clinical and research responsibility for nursing, in particular in the arenas of socioeconomic and cultural diversity, the aging female population, and survivorship after breast cancer. Because research results are at times confusing, conflicting, and controversial, women need help in integrating the information they are given, whether regarding risk of developing breast cancer or treatment options after the diagnosis. Nurses have a key role in advocating for women, in both the political arena or at the bedside. Nurses who are knowledgeable about current trends in breast cancer management assist women throughout their treatment process. Nurses are also vital to public education efforts directed at breast cancer screening and early detection.

Epidemiology

The average American woman's lifetime risk for developing invasive breast cancer is 1 in 8. This translates into 211,240 newly diagnosed female cases in the United States during 2005.[6] Men rarely develop breast cancer, by comparison, accounting for only 1690 new cases during the same year. Whereas these numbers reflect cases of invasive breast cancer, carcinoma in situ (CIS) will account for an additional 58,490 new cases of breast cancer in women in 2005, a significant increase since the early 1990s. This can largely be attributed to earlier detection through mammography.[6,7]

Overall, breast cancer incidence rates in women in the United States continued to increase into the 1980s but have leveled off in the 1990s.[7] Mortality rates in the United States have declined since the early 1990s.[7] In some parts of the world, breast cancer mortality rates continue to increase. Since the mid 1980s, more American women have died each year from lung cancer than breast cancer.[7] Breast cancer remains the most common site of cancer in American women.

The highest incidence rates of breast cancer in the world are in developed parts of the world such as North America, Australia, New Zealand, and Europe, with the exception of Japan.[1] In the United States, women who are white have a higher incidence rate than those in other ethnic groups, but African American women have the highest mortality rate.[7] African American women in the United States are more likely to be diagnosed with breast cancer at a later stage, and subsequently have a 5-year relative survival rate that is nearly 15% lower than that for white women.[7]

Etiology and Risk Factors

Research has shown that there is no known single cause of breast cancer. It is a heterogeneous disease, most likely developing as a result of a variety of factors that are different from woman to woman, and most of which are yet unknown. Several characteristics, or **risk factors,** appear to increase the probability of a woman developing breast cancer. A woman diagnosed with breast cancer may or may not have any of the risk factors. In fact, most women do not have any of the known risk factors except gender and age. It is therefore understandable that the concept of risk in breast cancer is often confusing. Many women overestimate their risk of developing breast cancer. This can lead to extremes in response, from avoidance of health care to worry and repeated medical visits. It is important for women and nurses to understand the concept of risk and current risk factors in order to develop individualized care plans for breast health.

UNDERSTANDING BREAST CANCER RISK

Breast cancer risk can be expressed as risk of development of or risk of death from the disease.

Absolute risk is the number of breast cancer cases in a population divided by the number of women in the population, expressed as an **average risk** for every woman in that population. For white women in the United States today, this comes out to be about a 13% chance of developing breast cancer, most commonly expressed as the often-quoted "1 in 8" statistic.[8] This can be deceiving. This percentage is a cumulative lifetime risk based on the sum of risks at different ages (**age-specific risks**) for all women from birth to about 100 years of age.[7,8] This percentage does not take into account an individual woman's situation (her estimated life span, her current age, or the presence of other potentially high-risk factors). Absolute risk is sometimes expressed as age-specific risk for women in different age brackets. For example, American women ages 40 to 59 years have a risk of developing breast cancer during those years that is lower than women ages 60 to 79, because breast cancer occurs more frequently as age increases. However, the cumulative lifetime risk is lower for the 65-year-old woman, because she has fewer years left to be at risk (that is, even if she did live to be 100; because it is still a comparison based on years of life remaining). Because absolute risk can be presented in different ways and does not take individual situations into account, it may be difficult to derive personal meaning from such numbers. Absolute risk may underestimate the risk for some women (e.g., those with a family history of breast cancer) and overestimate the risk for others (e.g., nonwhite women).

Relative risk compares the risk of breast cancer in women with a known or suspected risk factor with women without that risk factor.[8] Summary tables often categorize risk factors by relative risk, based on results of epidemiologic studies of breast cancer.[8] A relative risk greater than 1.0 indicates a greater likelihood of developing breast cancer than individuals without other risk factors.[8] For example, if the relative risk for a woman is 2.0, she is 2 times more likely than the population to develop breast cancer. The relative risk will most likely increase as the number of risk factors increases.

Attributable risk refers to those cancer cases associated with a given risk factor that could potentially be prevented by removing or reducing that risk factor. It is most useful in public health policy and planning for cancer prevention and control. Unlike lung cancer, where there is a clear causal link with smoking, there are no such factors in breast cancer.

RISK FACTORS

The following information covers those risk factors most widely acknowledged or suspected to increase the probability of a woman developing breast cancer.

Gender. Women are more likely than men to develop breast cancer. In the United States, breast cancer accounts for 32% of all invasive cancers in women and less than 1% of the cancers in men.[7]

Age. The incidence of breast cancer increases with age. Most breast cancer cases are diagnosed in women 40 years of age and older, but the majority of cases occur in women over age 50.[8]

Personal History of Cancer. A previous diagnosis of breast cancer increases a woman's lifetime risk for developing a second breast cancer in the opposite (contralateral) breast. Estimates are that the relative risk is 4.0 or greater.[8] A previous history of primary ovarian, endometrial, or colon cancer has been associated with an increased risk of breast cancer (relative risk 1.1 to 2.0).[8]

Family History of Cancer and Genetics. Women with a family history of breast cancer in one first-degree relative (mother, sister, or daughter) have a relative risk of 2.1 to 4.0.[8] Risk is increased if two or more first-degree relatives have had breast cancer (relative risk greater than 4.0), and is increased further if these diagnoses were at a younger age.[8] In some families the clustering of breast cancer may be accounted for only by chance or possibly from interactions among shared environmental and lifestyle factors not yet understood.[8]

Clinical features of possibly hereditary breast cancer include a younger age at diagnosis, bilateral occurrence, multiple family members affected (on maternal *or* paternal side), and the occurrence of cancers in other sites (e.g., ovary). The presence of these features warrants cancer risk counseling and consideration of genetic susceptibility testing. Female carriers of a mutation of the *BRCA1* or *BRCA2* tumor suppressor genes are at great risk of developing breast and/or ovarian cancer. Probably fewer than 10% of breast cancer cases are associated with identifiable genetic mutations.[8] However, in women who are carriers of either mutation, the lifetime risk of breast cancer is significant. (For more information on genetics and cancer, see Chapter 2.)

Hormonal Factors. The exact role of hormones in the etiology of breast cancer has not been precisely determined. **Early onset of menarche** (before age 12), **late menopause** (at 55 or above), and greater total duration of years of regular menses are associated with an increased risk of breast cancer.[8] This increased risk is thought to be due to the total lifetime exposure of the breast to estrogen and progesterone, with fluctuations in cell growth and change in the breast tissues with each ovulatory cycle.

Having no children (**nulliparity**) or the **first full-term pregnancy after age 30** places a woman at increased risk.[8]

The relative risk is higher for the woman who delays childbirth than for the nulliparous woman.[8] Some studies have also shown that as the number of months of breastfeeding increases, an associated reduction occurs in the risk of developing breast cancer.[8]

Numerous studies have evaluated the risk associated with the use of **oral contraceptives (OCs)** or **hormone replacement therapy (HRT)**, suggesting subgroups of women at possibly increased risk based on age at onset of use, duration of use and how recent it was, and dosing regimen. It appears that recent OC use or recent and long-term use of HRT increase a woman's risk of developing breast cancer, especially when HRT includes the addition of a progestin, or when use is prolonged (more than 5 years).[5,9] Nurses can encourage women to learn as much as possible and to discuss and weigh the potential benefits and risks of HRT with their health care provider.

Benign Breast Disease. The term **benign breast disease** encompasses a broad array of histopathologic tissue diagnoses women typically experience clinically at some time in their lives but that are never biopsied. Some question why such a common condition is termed a "disease." Many of these so-called diseases are not associated with any increased risk of breast cancer. "Fibrocystic disease" is a catchall phrase to describe clinical symptoms and findings of local or generalized lumpiness, pain, or cystic changes. **Fibrocystic changes** may be a more appropriate term to describe these often normal breast changes.

Benign breast lesions, when biopsy diagnosis is made, are classified into three groups. **Nonproliferative lesions,** when found alone, are generally not associated with any increased risk of breast cancer. These include cysts, apocrine metaplasia, fibroadenomas, and mild hyperplasia, among others.[10]

Proliferative lesions without atypia, increased growth of epithelial cells in the ductal or lobular tissue of the breast, include ductal epithelial hyperplasias of the usual (common) type, sclerosing adenosis, radial scar, and intraductal papillomas.[10] These are associated with a slightly increased risk (1.5 to 2.0) of breast cancer.[10]

Proliferative lesions with atypia, or **atypical hyperplasia,** is the proliferation of abnormal-looking cells within ducts or lobules. These constitute the third category of benign breast disease and are most associated with increased breast cancer risk.[10] The diagnosis by biopsy of atypical ductal or lobular hyperplasia is associated with a relative risk of developing breast cancer of 2.1 to 4.0. This risk is yet greater with a family history of breast cancer.[8,10]

When the cells within the ductal or lobular tissue are proliferating abnormally yet have characteristics more like cancer cells, these lesions are defined as **carcinoma in situ (CIS),** or cancer confined to the site of origin. The presence of CIS significantly increases a woman's risk of developing an invasive breast cancer. Treatment for CIS is discussed later in this chapter.

Obesity and Dietary Fat. The incidence of breast cancer is increased in industrialized countries with a high socioeconomic status and an increased consumption of **dietary fat,** suggesting a relationship.[1] **Obesity** is associated with an increased risk of breast cancer in postmenopausal women.[8] Most circulating estrogen in postmenopausal women is produced in fat tissue.[8] Dietary fat intake during childhood and adolescence may influence breast cancer risk. Studies of the influence of dietary fat intake have considered fat consumption in total calories from fat, different types of fat intake, and fat intake at specific times in the life cycle, for reducing the risk of both developing breast cancer and of recurrence after treatment for breast cancer.[4,5,11] With 33% of adult women ages 20 to 74 years considered obese in most recent statistics, this is a major public health concern not only for the risk of breast cancer.[11]

Radiation Exposure. A greater than expected incidence of breast cancer has been seen in women exposed to ionizing radiation to the chest, (e.g., for treatment of Hodgkin's disease).[8] Screening mammography in women *over* 40 years of age does not increase risk of breast cancer.

Alcohol Consumption. Several studies have shown an increased risk of breast cancer (relative risk of 1.1 to 2.0) associated with alcohol consumption of 2 or more drinks per day.[8] The age at which drinking begins, amount and type of alcohol consumed, and duration of consumption and how recent it was appear to be important variables in fully understanding the risk that can be attributed to alcohol. Alcohol appears to increase levels of circulating estrogens and androgens.[8] Heavy alcohol consumption may also be associated with poor nutrition or other social and environmental factors that may affect general health, access to care, and stage at diagnosis.

Other Factors. Higher socioeconomic status is associated with a higher risk of developing breast cancer, but lower socioeconomic status is associated with a greater risk of dying from the disease.[7] Ethnicity also is associated with risk, with nonwhite women being at lower risk of developing breast cancer but at greater risk of dying from the disease.[7] No clear associations with increased risk of breast cancer have been found in connection with cigarette smoking, stress, personality type, abortion, antiperspirants, underwire bras, electromagnetic fields, silicone breast implants, caffeine, or hair dyes.[8]

For the woman who appears to have an increased risk based on family history or other factors, a detailed assessment would include assessment of specific risk factors associated with breast cancer, a woman's perceptions of risk, her attitudes toward and beliefs about early detection methods (mammography, clinical breast examination [CBE], BSE) as well as her participation in each and need for information (see also discussion of screening and detection in Chapter 4).

There is no clear preventive intervention. Reduction in alcohol and dietary fat intake, and weight loss if postmenopausal and obese, as well as increasing one's physical activity are some proactive measures nurses can recommend. Prophylactic mastectomy (discussed later in this chapter) may reduce the incidence of breast cancer by as much as 90% and increase life expectancy for women at high risk of breast cancer.[8,12] Current knowledge about risk factors in breast cancer will help the nurse guide the patient in obtaining personally meaningful information.

Prevention, Screening, and Detection

Breast cancer is a **heterogeneous disease;** in other words, it is a disease of many characteristics, varying from woman to woman in its potential for development, growth, and metastasis. The epidemiology of the disease indicates that it is hormonally influenced, with the duration of exposure to elevated levels of circulating estrogens being a primary factor in the promotion of cancer cell development over several years. This period of cell promotion is characterized by reversibility. If this exposure could be reduced or if the adverse effects of the exposure could be prevented, breast cancer might be prevented.

The Breast Cancer Prevention Trial, begun in 1992, evaluated the effectiveness of tamoxifen in preventing the occurrence of invasive breast cancer in a group of women at higher risk for breast cancer development. Over 13,000 women participated in the placebo-controlled trial and were randomized to receive either tamoxifen or a placebo for 5 years. Participants were 60 years of age or older, or 35 to 59 years of age with a 5-year predicted risk for breast cancer of 1.67% or higher, or with a history of lobular carcinoma in situ (LCIS).[2] Besides the risk of breast cancer, the incidence of endometrial cancer, coronary heart disease, and osteoporosis were also closely monitored. This study demonstrated that tamoxifen reduced the risk of invasive and noninvasive breast cancer significantly for women at increased risk for breast cancer, with low toxicity.[2] Thus in 1998, the FDA approved tamoxifen for use in preventing breast cancer in women at high risk for the disease. A subsequent prevention trial, the Study of Tamoxifen and Raloxifene (STAR), compares the effectiveness of tamoxifen and raloxifene in preventing breast cancer in 22,000 postmenopausal women 35 years and older who are at increased risk of the disease.[3] The results of these and other studies evaluating prevention will, in the near future, give us clearer direction in the prevention and treatment of breast cancer.

Early detection is therefore the most important means for control of breast cancer. Survival is directly related to the stage of disease at diagnosis.[6,8] The American Cancer Society (ACS) maintains **screening guidelines** for asymptomatic women that incorporate the following three methods of early detection:[6,8,11]

1. *Mammography* (routine screening mammography) every year beginning at age 40
2. *CBE* by a health professional every 3 years for women ages 20 to 39 and annually beginning at age 40
3. *BSE* monthly by all women beginning at age 20

The nurse can advise women with a known deleterious mutation, or a family history suggestive of the presence of a deleterious mutation, to follow guidelines such as those from the National Comprehensive Cancer Network (NCCN) that suggest initiation of screening at a much younger age and/or more frequently.[13,14] A woman with known risk factors (e.g., family history) or chronic symptomatology needs to consult with her health care provider regarding a personalized schedule for CBEs and mammography. Nurses have a major role in teaching these potentially lifesaving guidelines to all women. For greatest effectiveness, frequency (regular and periodic) and proficiency (skill and thoroughness) are key concepts to consider in each screening method.

MAMMOGRAPHY

Mammography is the only proven means of detecting breast cancer before it can be discovered by CBE or BSE. Screening mammography is used to detect cancer in *asymptomatic* women. Since studies in the early 1960s and 1970s, screening mammography has repeatedly been shown to be effective in reducing the number of deaths associated with breast cancer through the detection of clinically occult lesions. Mammography is also useful in evaluating high-risk women and women with breasts difficult to palpate (e.g., breasts that are large and pendulous or with severe fibrocystic changes). Film-screen mammography has been the gold standard for screening and diagnostic mammography; however, digital mammography, which involves the translation of film-screen images into a computer-generated image, has greater accuracy in younger women and those with radiographically dense breasts.[15]

Ultrasound is helpful in conjunction with mammography to differentiate a fluid-filled cyst from a solid mass. Other methods for imaging the breasts such as thermography, diaphonography (transillumination), and magnetic resonance imaging (MRI) have been evaluated but have not been shown to be effective in routine screening for breast cancer.[13] MRI is useful as an adjunct to mammography for the evaluation of augmented or dense breasts, or in women at high risk for breast cancer. Scintimammography, which involves injection of a radioisotope (technetium Tc-99m-sestamibi) followed by a nuclear medicine scan of the breasts, may be used as an adjunct to mammography in differentiating benign from malignant lesions. Positron emission tomography (PET) is useful in evaluating the breast and the axilla in women with a breast cancer diagnosis.

Screening mammography generally consists of two views of each breast: one from side to side that includes the axilla and the upper outer quadrant of the breast (mediolateral oblique) and one from top to bottom (craniocaudal).[16,17] For each view the breast is compressed to decrease the thickness of the breast and enable better visualization of the structures of the tissue, as well as reduce the amount of radiation. Proper breast compression is one of the most important factors in mammogram quality, and having this information may help women understand the importance of momentary discomfort.[16,17] Premenstrual women should have their screening mammogram after their menses because of the potential for increased breast tenderness just before menses. **Diagnostic mammography** consists of additional views of the breast to help delineate an area of concern found on a screening mammogram or a palpable mass. For example, spot compression allows for greater compression of an isolated area and may be used in conjunction with magnification to enlarge an area of calcifications or asymmetry.

When properly performed, mammography can effectively detect 80% to 90% of breast cancers.[8] It is possible for 10% to 20% of malignant lesions to go undetected. Therefore in women with clinical symptoms, a negative mammogram does not rule out the need for a biopsy. Dense breast tissue, lesions that cannot be seen on mammogram, the skill of the technologist, the experience of the radiologist, and the quality of the equipment may all contribute to false-negative readings. To address the quality of care issues, the Mammography Quality Standards Act (MQSA) was passed by Congress in 1992, took effect October 1, 1994, and was renewed by Congress in 2004.[16] The MQSA sets federal quality standards for equipment, personnel, and record keeping at all mammography facilities. By law a facility must be certified by the FDA as providing quality mammography services, and be inspected annually.[16] The MQSA quality standards require that the following are present:[16]

- Dedicated mammographic equipment with regular quality monitoring
- Radiologic technologists specially trained and experienced in mammography
- Radiologists with demonstrated experience and competence in mammography
- Records of mammography that include comparisons with prior films, findings, recommendations, and communications to health care providers and patients

Despite its value, many women do not get regular mammograms. Fewer than 62% of women 40 years of age and older had completed a mammogram within the past year, according to a 2002 report.[8] The ACS goal is that by 2008, 90% of women ages 40 years and older will have breast screening consistent with ACS guidelines.[11] Reasons women give for not getting a mammogram include fear, pain, embarrassment, a belief that one is not at risk or that other tests (e.g., clinical breast examination) are adequate, exposure to radiation, lack of time, lack of physician referral, and difficult access.[16] Confusion on the part of consumers and health care providers after the debate in the late 1990s about the value of screening mammography in women ages 40 to 49 did not help. The ACS and the American College of Radiology (ACR) have maintained a commitment to the benefits of annual screening mammography in women ages 40 and over, with no upper age limit for the discontinuation of regular mammograms.[8,18] *Healthy People 2010* goals include increasing the proportion of primary care providers who counsel patients about mammograms, from 37% in 1988 to 85% in 2010.[19] Ongoing education for health care providers and the public and health care advocacy efforts remain critical to minimizing each of these known barriers.

BREAST SELF-EXAMINATION

BSE is a free, private, and relatively simple examination. Although recent evidence does not support the value of BSE in reducing mortality from breast cancer, BSE is still a valuable tool by which women learn the appearance and feel of their own breasts and the importance of seeking care for changes from what is normal for them.[6,8] In populations where mammography or professional health care examinations are not consistently available, BSE may have even greater importance in the early detection of breast cancer. For women under 40 years of age, BSE may help identify changes that would not otherwise be noticed. The majority of palpable breast lumps *are* discovered by a woman herself.

Many women in the United States know about BSE, yet few practice BSE regularly or thoroughly. Reasons for not doing BSE may include fear, embarrassment, or lack of knowledge, confidence, motivation, or health care provider recommendation. The best time to perform BSE is 5 to 7 days after the menstrual period (for premenopausal women) when the breasts are less tender. Nonmenstruating or postmenopausal women can select the same day each month to do BSE. Selecting an anniversary or birth date is one suggestion to encourage women to remember this practice. Women who are pregnant or breastfeeding can still examine themselves monthly; when breastfeeding, it is best to do BSE soon after the breasts are emptied. Women who have had breast cancer surgery can continue BSE, with special attention to any surgical scar area and to the chest wall (postmastectomy).

BSE includes inspection and palpation of the breasts in both standing and lying positions. Attention is focused on evaluating for change. It is best done in an atmosphere that is unhurried and most comfortable for the individual woman. A thorough BSE will usually take 20 to 30 minutes. The MammaCare Personal Learning System, for teaching BSE, is perhaps the most comprehensive and researched program, emphasizing proficiency through individualized instruction, the use of specially designed breast palpation models, an instruction manual, and a video program for self-learning.[20] The components of BSE for proficiency in practice include inspection, palpation using the flat **pads of the fingers** at different levels of **pressure** and in a specific **pattern**, most easily done when in a flat or partial side-lying (upper body turned at 45-degree angle) **position** (Fig. 7-1).

Inspection of the breasts is best conducted standing in front of a mirror, with the arms at the sides and both breasts exposed for complete visualization of the skin surface, nipple/areola complex, and breast contour. Turning slightly side to side, the breasts are inspected for any evidence of skin retraction, puckering, dimpling, erythema, vein prominence, presence of other characteristics such as nevi, and position of the nipples. Lifting the breast on either side allows her to inspect the skin on the lower side of the breasts and the chest area. It is normal that one breast may be slightly larger than the other. With hands on the hips pressing in and down, the same observation is repeated. This action is further repeated with the arms over the head and with the arms in front while leaning forward. Palpation is then performed lying down, paying special attention to the upper outer quadrant of the breast, and the central area around the nipple, where most breast cancers occur (see Figure 7-1).

When first performing BSE, a woman is learning her normal breast characteristics so that any future variations or changes can be recognized and evaluated. If she notices a change on one breast, she may want to check the other breast for symmetry. Encourage her to have a plan of action in the event she detects a change that needs evaluation. This plan might be to call her health care provider for an appointment. Encourage her to seek prompt medical attention if any of the clinical features or common symptoms of breast cancer are present.

CLINICAL BREAST EXAMINATION

CBE is an important adjunct to mammography. According to a report for 2002, only 54.1% of women 40 years of age and older had completed both a mammogram and CBE within the past year.[8] *Healthy People 2010* goals are that 80% of U.S. women ages 40 and over will have at least once received a CBE and mammogram, and 70% of women ages 40 and over will have received a mammogram within the prior 2 years.[19] Applying the techniques just described for BSE, the health care provider can conduct a thorough CBE. For CBE to be as effective as possible, the professional performing the examination must be proficient. The MammaCare Learning System for Clinical Breast Examination is a commercially available program, similar to that for BSE but geared to the health care professional who will be performing regular CBEs.[21]

During CBE the health professional can point out a woman's particular normal anatomic variations. Signs and symptoms of breast abnormalities can be discussed and risk factors for breast cancer reviewed, with particular attention to what that means to the individual woman. Further, this is an opportunity to teach BSE technique, explain the rationale for each step, and encourage women to be partners in their care by continuing monthly BSE at home. The establishment of a relationship of trust between the health professional and the patient may lead to improved participation in breast cancer screening activities.

In summary, particular attention must be paid to medically underserved women for all aspects of breast cancer screening.[7,19,22,23] Whether in urban or rural settings, nurses and other health care providers need to find improved ways of reaching these populations with breast cancer screening.

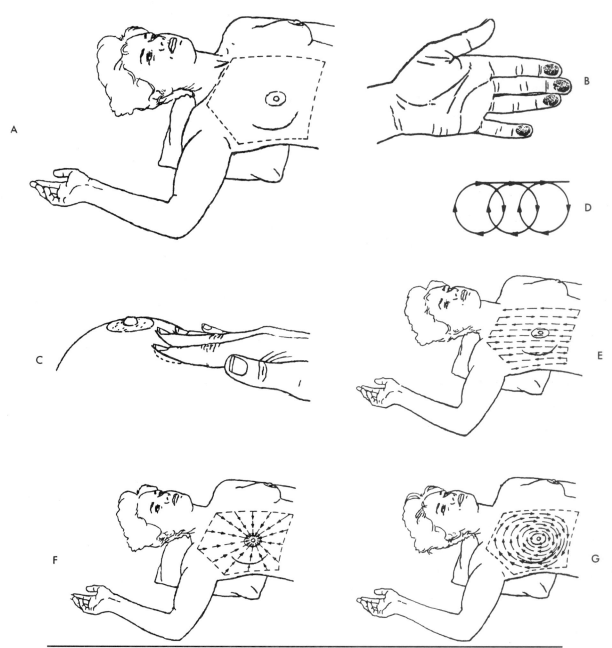

FIG. 7-1 Breast self-examination (BSE). **A,** Perimeter of area to be examined should include all breast tissue. This area is bounded by a line that extends vertically from middle of axilla (armpit) to rib just beneath breast and continues horizontally along underside of breast to midsternum (middle of breastbone). It continues up midsternum to clavicle (collarbone) and along lower border of clavicle to shoulder and back to midaxilla. **B,** Palpation is performed with pads of fingers. **C, D,** Move your fingers (three or four) in small circles about the size of a dime. Varying levels of pressure (light, medium, and firm) should be applied to each spot palpated. Moderate pressure is illustrated. The following patterns can be used for the examination: **E,** vertical strip; **F,** wedge; and **G,** circle. (Courtesy American Cancer Society, California Division.)

Classification

The breast is a gland located on the chest wall (Fig. 7-2). The overlying skin contains hair follicles and sweat and sebaceous glands. The pigmented area surrounding the nipple, known as the **areola**, has sebaceous glands that secrete a lubricant during breastfeeding. Fibrous strands called **Cooper's ligaments** pass through the glandular and fatty tissues from the skin to the underlying muscle, giving the breast support. The glandular tissue is made up of 15 to 20 lobes arranged in a radial pattern, capable of producing milk and connecting with ducts that drain into the nipple. An extensive lymphatic and vascular supply is present. Breast tissue extends to the clavicle, the sternum, the latissimus dorsi muscles, and up into the axilla. The axillary lymph nodes are thought to drain the majority of the lymph fluid from the breast. The axillary nodes are distributed from low in the armpit, at the lateral border of the pectoralis minor muscle

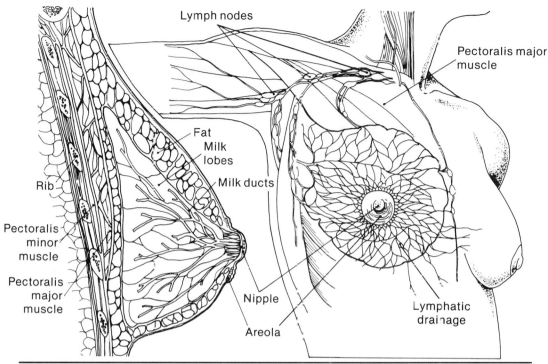

FIG. 7-2   Anatomy of the female breast. (From DiSaia PJ, Creasman WT: *Clinical gynecologic oncology*, ed 5, St. Louis, 1997, Mosby.)

(level I), to midway behind the pectoralis minor muscle (level II), and above at the medial border of the pectoralis minor (level III). Lymph nodes located between the pectoralis major and minor muscles are known as **Rotter's nodes**.

Primary breast cancers are grouped as invasive or noninvasive. A malignancy confined to the ducts or lobules is classified as noninvasive, or CIS. If it arose in the ductal system, it is referred to as **ductal carcinoma in situ (DCIS)**; in the lobule system it is called **lobular carcinoma in situ (LCIS)**. Once the malignant cells penetrate the tissue outside the ducts or lobules, the cancer is described as **infiltrating** or **invasive. Infiltrating ductal carcinoma** accounts for approximately 80% of all breast carcinomas and **infiltrating lobular carcinomas** about 10%. Less common are **inflammatory carcinoma,** characterized by swelling, erythema, and invasion of the dermal lymphatics (giving the classic peau d'orange, or orange peel, appearance), and **medullary, papillary,** and **tubular carcinoma. Paget's disease** of the nipple, one form in which breast cancer presents, occurs infrequently (2% of all cases) and is most often associated with an underlying invasive carcinoma. When noninvasive cancer is found with invasive cancer, the staging and treatment planning are based on the characteristics of the invasive carcinoma.

Clinical Features

In asymptomatic women, mammography can detect microscopic changes indicative of cancer such as a small, irregular mass, indistinct or spiculated margins, microcalcifications, skin thickening, architectural distortion, or asymmetry in the anatomical structures. Palpable breast masses may also have these characteristics, as well as nipple or skin retraction when underlying structures are involved. The Clinical Features box lists additional clinical signs and symptoms of breast cancer at presentation.

Clinical Features of Breast Cancer

Mass (particularly if hard, irregular, nontender) or thickening in breast or axilla
Spontaneous, persistent, unilateral nipple discharge that is serosanguineous, bloody, or watery
Nipple retraction or inversion
Change in size, shape, or texture of breast (asymmetry)
Dimpling or puckering of skin
Scaly skin around nipple
Redness, ulceration, edema, or dilated veins
Peau d'orange skin changes
Enlargement of lymph nodes in axilla

Diagnosis

TISSUE DIAGNOSIS

Breast cancer can be diagnosed with cytologic (cells) or histologic (tissue) evaluation. Examination of tissue will give a definitive diagnosis. **Fine-needle aspiration (FNA) biopsy** for cytology is the preferred technique when dominant masses are palpable. It is a relatively simple procedure involving the aspiration of cellular material from the mass using a syringe and fine-gauge needle. The content of the aspiration is mounted on slides and processed for review. In skilled hands it is highly accurate; false-negative and false-positive results are rare. A negative result in the presence of a suspicious mass warrants further evaluation. Although FNA can lead to the diagnosis of carcinoma, it cannot distinguish whether it is invasive or noninvasive. Advantages of the FNA are the ease with which it can be done in the office setting, use of minimal local anesthesia, and the low incidence of damage to surrounding tissue. When the results show cancer, surgical biopsy will usually not be needed before planning for definitive surgical treatment.

Core needle biopsy provides a core of tissue from a dominant mass. Under local anesthetic, a specially designed 14-, 16- or 18-gauge needle is inserted into the palpable mass. This procedure has been associated with more bleeding and pain than the FNA, especially when deeper lesions are involved. A core needle biopsy may be helpful after a nondiagnostic or suspicious FNA. Because it provides a larger sample of tissue, core needle biopsy can differentiate in situ from invasive cancer. Both the FNA and core biopsy may be done with or without ultrasound guidance. **Stereotactic FNA** or core needle biopsy can be performed on most nonpalpable, suspicious abnormalities found on mammogram, and is available in most breast centers. For this procedure, patients are positioned prone on an examination table, with the affected breast suspended through an opening in the table. The breast is compressed as for mammography, films are taken, the skin anesthetized, and the biopsy needle mechanically and precisely aligned by radiograph and computer to the area of abnormality. Contraindications to the procedure may include lesions close to the chest wall or skin, anticoagulant therapy, obesity, or medical conditions that would make positioning on the exam table difficult. **Incisional biopsy** may be done when the mass is large; it involves removal of only a portion of the mass. Excisional biopsy involves removal of the entire mass and a margin of normal tissue around it. It is used for palpable and nonpalpable lesions.

Nonpalpable abnormalities detected only on mammogram or ultrasound require radiographic guidance before removal. A radiologist localizes the suspicious area using mammogram or ultrasound to direct a small wire, or a needle, into the lesion. The wire (or needle) is then taped to the patient's skin, the patient is transferred to the operating room, and the abnormality at the tip of the wire is removed by the surgeon. The tissue that was removed is then radiographed to verify removal of the suspicious area (or to direct further excision). The tissue is then examined microscopically in permanent sections.

These procedures make it possible to determine a definitive diagnosis of cancer and for a woman to be fully involved in making choices about her surgical treatment plan. Women need to be assured that the interval between diagnosis and definitive treatment, used to obtain recommendations regarding management options, does not adversely affect survival.

Staging

Breast cancer is most frequently staged according to the tumor-nodes-metastasis (TNM) classification system, which evaluates the tumor size (*T*), involvement of regional lymph nodes (*N*), and distant spread of the disease or metastases (*M*) (discussed in detail in Chapter 5). The stages may be simply classified as follows:[24,25]

Stage 0	Carcinoma in situ (Tis-N0-M0)
Stage I	Tumor of under 2 cm with negative nodes (T1-N0-M0) (includes microinvasive T1, less than 0.1 cm)
Stage IIA	Tumor of 0 to 2 cm with positive nodes (including micrometastasis N1, or less than 2 mm), or 2 to 5 cm with negative nodes (T0-N1, T1-N1, T2-N0, all M0)

Stage IIB	Tumor of 2 to 5 cm with positive nodes or greater than 5 cm with negative nodes (T2-N1, T3-N0, all M0)
Stage IIIA	No evidence of primary tumor or tumor of less than 2 cm with involved fixed lymph nodes, or tumor greater than 5 cm with involved movable or nonmovable nodes (T0-N2, T1-N2, T2-N2, T3-N1, T3-N2, all M0)
Stage IIIB	Tumor of any size with direct extension to chest wall or skin, with or without involved lymph nodes, or any size tumor with involved internal mammary lymph nodes (T4-any N, any T-N3, all M0)
Stage IV	Any distant metastasis (includes ipsilateral supraclavicular nodes)

Statistical reports commonly refer to stage as **local** (confined to the breast), **regional** (lymph nodes or surrounding tissue involved), and **distant** (metastasis present). Since 1975 in the United States, the diagnosis of breast cancers that are 2 cm or smaller in diameter has increased. The majority of cases are diagnosed when localized to the breast.[8] However, African American women are still less likely than white women to have their breast cancer diagnosed at a local stage, and to have a poorer 5-year relative survival than white women regardless of stage at diagnosis.[7,8]

Evaluating the extent of disease allows appropriate therapy to be planned, determines the overall prognosis, and permits comparison of research results related to treatment. The clinical staging process routinely begins preoperatively with a thorough history and physical examination, bilateral mammography, complete blood count, and comprehensive chemistry panel, and may include tumor markers. Three tumor markers with some value in breast cancer treatment are **carcinoembryonic antigen (CEA), CA 15-3, and CA 27-29**. CA 15-3 and CA 27-29 may be elevated in benign breast conditions or in inflammatory or malignant conditions of epithelial organs; CEA can also be elevated in smokers. None of these are specific enough to be routinely used for staging and follow-up; however, they are often ordered. If elevated preoperatively, they will be useful markers as treatment progresses.

Evaluation of a patient's bony structure, chest, abdomen, and brain are individualized according to the patient's specific symptoms, laboratory test results, clinical evidence of enlarged axillary nodes, or stage III disease. Testing may include computed tomography (CT) scan of the chest, abdomen, and pelvis, PET or PET/CT, or bone scan. Extensive local surgery might be contraindicated if distant metastases are discovered at the initial diagnosis. Pathologic staging is based on the histologic review of the primary tumor from surgical specimens (type, size, and margins) and, when invasive carcinoma is present, the lymph nodes.

Prognostic Indicators

Tumor size and lymph node status are critical to predicting survival. The staging system provides direction for treatment, but does not provide the means by which to predict which women in a particular stage group will have disease recurrence and which will not. Unfortunately, some women with negative lymph nodes at the time of breast cancer diagnosis will develop a recurrence. Adjuvant therapy would be most appropriately directed to those women if one could identify them more accurately. Several pathologic characteristics have been studied for their ability to determine risk of local recurrence, metastasis, response to therapy, and overall prognosis. Shown in Box 7-1, these are known as **prognostic factors**.

BOX 7-1 Key Prognostic Factors in Breast Cancer

Prognostic Factor	Favorable Range
Tumor size	Noninvasive or <1 cm invasive
Axillary lymph node status	Negative
Estrogen receptors	Positive
Progesterone receptors	Positive
Histologic grade	Well-differentiated
Nuclear grade	Low grade
DNA content	
Ploidy	Diploid (DNA = 1.00%)
S-phase fraction	Low (≤4%)
Oncogenes	
HER2/neu	Low expression
Tumor suppressor genes	
p53	Low expression

TUMOR SIZE

Tumor size is directly related to prognosis. The smaller the tumor size, the less likely there will be axillary lymph node involvement at diagnosis and the less likely the cancer will recur within the breast or axilla. Moreover, with a small tumor there is greater likelihood of eligibility for breast-conserving surgery. The overall 5-year relative survival rate for women with a breast cancer of 2 cm or smaller and negative lymph nodes is 92%.[8]

AXILLARY LYMPH NODE STATUS

The most important predictor of disease recurrence and survival is the presence of axillary lymph node metastasis. The larger the tumor, the greater is the likelihood that lymph nodes will be involved. The more lymph nodes involved, the greater risk that distant disease is present. Survival is directly related to the number of lymph nodes involved. Women with negative lymph nodes have a higher rate of survival than women with involved lymph nodes. U.S. women diagnosed between 1995 and 2001 with localized disease (no lymph node involvement) have 5-year relative survival rates of 98% versus 81% for those with regional disease (any lymph node involvement).[8] Similarly, women with one to three involved lymph nodes do better than women with four or more involved lymph nodes.

BONE MARROW

Bone marrow aspiration and biopsy are not routinely performed in the process of staging of early breast cancer, although some evidence suggests that the presence of metastatic breast cancer cells in bone marrow, when detected with immunohistochemical techniques, may be a better marker than lymph node status in predicting risk of recurrence and survival. This remains under investigation.[26]

ESTROGEN AND PROGESTERONE RECEPTORS

The effects of estrogen and progesterone on human breast cancer cells are mediated by steroid receptors known as estrogen and progesterone receptors (ER/PR). Both normal and cancer cells have these receptors, but they are frequently overexpressed in breast cancer. These receptors are located in the nucleus or on the surface of the cell and bind to circulating steroid hormones. The receptor-hormone complex then works within the cell nucleus to promote cellular growth and division. A biochemical or immunohistochemical analysis routinely done of breast cancer cells removed at the time of tissue diagnosis can quantify the presence of these receptors in noninvasive or invasive breast cancers. Patients are said to be positive or negative for ER and PR based on the level of binding receptors present.

The presence of ER and PR in breast cancer tissue is a predictor of responsiveness to hormonal therapy and chemotherapy, and of survival. The greatest likelihood of response to hormonal therapy is related to high levels of both ER and PR. In addition, receptor status correlates with a variety of clinical and biologic parameters, some of which are also noted as prognostic factors. ER-positive cancers are seen more frequently in postmenopausal women, are associated with other good prognostic factors, and usually have a lower recurrence rate and better overall prognosis.

HISTOPATHOLOGIC GRADE

The **histolopathologic grade** refers to characteristics of the cancer cells (tubule formation, cell appearance, and mitoses). The Scarf-Bloom-Richardson grading system combines these three characteristics into a score (3-9), which is also classified as a grade (1-3).[25] The lower the score or grade, the better the prognosis. Cancers classified as grade 1 tend to have more tubule formation and look more like normal cells, with few mitoses. These cellular characteristics may also be described as well-differentiated. Cancers classified as grade 2 will have less tubule formation, look more varied in their appearance, and have more mitoses. Often referred to as poorly differentiated cancers, grade 3 refers to those that have little tubule formation, the most varied appearance, and many mitoses.

DNA CONTENT

Breast cancer cells are also evaluated for their potential to proliferate, via flow cytometry, which analyzes the cellular DNA content (**ploidy**) of the cells, and according to the percentage of cells in the S phase of cellular division (S-phase fraction, or SPF). Tumors are classified as **diploid** (normal DNA content) or **aneuploid** (abnormal DNA content) and with high or low SPF. In general, a greater risk of recurrence and worse prognosis are associated with aneuploid tumors and cells with a high SPF. This information may be most useful in defining which subsets of node-negative breast cancer patients need systemic adjuvant therapy.

ONCOGENES

Proto-oncogenes are normally involved in regulating cell growth and differentiation. When altered in the cell (**somatic mutation**), these **oncogenes** are responsible for cancer cell growth. Abnormalities of amplification (multiple copies) or overexpression (multiple quantities) of the proto-oncogene HER2/neu (or c-erbB-2) in the DNA of some breast cancers has been associated with tumor growth, more aggressive cancers, local or distant recurrence, and poorer overall survival. The study of oncogenes has greatly enhanced our understanding of the biology of breast cancer and led to the development of new diagnostic techniques as well as treatment options.[27]

OTHER FACTORS

Many other factors are under investigation for their role in predicting cancer cell growth and regulation, response to systemic treatment, or risk of local recurrence and metastasis. Tumor size, axillary lymph node status, ER and PR levels, grade, DNA ploidy, SPF, and HER2/*neu* are the most prominent prognostic factors considered when projecting risk of recurrence and response to systemic therapy. The heterogeneity of breast cancer makes precise determinations of prognosis and response to treatment challenging. Nearly two thirds of all cases of invasive breast cancer diagnosed today will not involve axillary nodes (localized disease).[7] Although a majority of women will be cured without adjuvant chemotherapy, some will face recurrence or metastases. A gene assay was recently validated as an important tool to profile gene expression and indicate risk. The Onco*type* DX test generates a recurrence score from a sample of breast tissue, which can predict which node-negative, ER-positive patients benefit from adjuvant chemotherapy in combination with hormonal therapy. The higher the score, the higher the risk of recurrence in the 10 years after the initial diagnosis: medium risk is a score of 18 to 30, and high risk is a score of 30 or more.[27-29] Further study in genetic profiling is needed to refine measurement techniques and use of prognostic factors as tools to individualize breast cancer treatment.

METASTASIS

Adjuvant systemic therapy has been shown to improve overall survival and prevent or delay the development of metastatic disease. Distant metastases can develop any time after the initial diagnosis. Breast cancer spreads by direct invasion of surrounding tissues, along mammary ducts, or by way of lymphatic or blood vessels. The major site of regional spread is the axillary lymph nodes. The larger the primary cancer, the greater the risk of axillary node involvement. Systemic or distant spread of the disease can occur in a variety of organs and tissues. The most frequent sites are bone, lung, pleura, liver, and adrenals. Symptoms that may be associated with metastasis include bone pain, shortness of breath, loss of weight, or neurologic changes. Elevated serum alkaline phosphatase, calcium, or liver function tests may be indicative of site-specific metastases, when seen in combination with clinical and radiographic findings (see Clinical Features box). Serious complications of metastatic disease, considered oncologic emergencies, can occur (e.g., spinal cord compression, hypercalcemia).

The 5-year relative survival rate for women diagnosed between 1995 and 2001 with metastatic disease is 26%.[8] While metastatic breast cancer is not considered curable, many therapies are available that will control the disease for long periods of time and alleviate symptoms.

Medical Treatment Modalities and Nursing Care Considerations

SURGERY

Historically surgery has been employed for the treatment of breast cancer. The primary goal of surgery has always been to achieve local and regional control of the disease. It has only been within the past century that surgical intervention has shown survival benefits. The use of the Halsted radical mastectomy was based on the theory that breast cancer spreads in an orderly fashion from the breast to the lymph nodes. Thus extensive dissection of lymph nodes and the pectoralis major muscle were included with mastectomy. Newer theories that breast cancer is a systemic disease at diagnosis, and that lymph nodes do not serve as a barrier to metastasis, prompted research into less extensive surgery and the addition of radiation therapy, such that the modified radical mastectomy replaced the radical mastectomy, itself eventually replaced by breast-conserving surgery with radiation therapy for many women with early invasive breast cancer. Removal of regional lymph nodes at levels I and II has been considered the best method for determining nodal status in patients undergoing mastectomy or breast-conserving surgery for invasive breast cancer. Sentinel lymph node biopsy, a new technique to identify the lymph node that receives drainage from the primary site of breast cancer, is allowing preservation of lymph nodes for some women. Box 7-2 describes surgical procedures in the treatment of breast cancer.

Primary Therapy. The type of surgery selected is based on clinical stage of the disease (tumor size, palpable lymph nodes, metastases), mammographic findings (including evidence of cancer cells in other areas of the breast separate from the primary lesion), the tumor location, patient history, available surgical and radiotherapeutic expertise, breast size and shape, and patient preference.

Nearly all patients with operable breast cancer are candidates for **modified radical mastectomy**. For most women with smaller tumors (stages I and II disease), **breast-conserving treatment** is appropriate therapy with proven equivalence to modified radical mastectomy in terms of overall and relapse-free survival rates.[25,30] Breast-conserving surgery without axillary node dissection is also the preferred treatment for most cases of noninvasive breast cancer. Adequate time is needed for full discussion with

---

| BOX 7-2 | **Surgical Procedures in Treatment of Breast Cancer** |

Modified radical mastectomy (also referred to as *total mastectomy with axillary node dissection*). The entire breast is removed along with axillary lymph nodes and the lining over the pectoralis major muscle. The pectoralis major muscle is not removed. The pectoralis minor muscle may or may not be removed.

Total mastectomy (also referred to as *simple mastectomy*). All the breast tissue, including the nipple–areolar complex and the lining over the pectoralis major muscle, is removed. There is no axillary node dissection. Chest wall muscles are not removed.

Lumpectomy/segmental mastectomy (or excision: *tumorectomy*). The cancer is removed with a border of surrounding normal tissue, and the major portion of the breast is left.

Quadrantectomy (also referred to as *partial mastectomy*). The entire quadrant of the breast containing the tumor is removed along with the overlying skin and the lining over the pectoralis major muscle.

NOTE: In each of the breast-conserving surgical procedures (lumpectomy, wide excision, and quadrantectomy), axillary node dissection is usually performed through a separate incision, and surgical intervention is followed by radiation therapy to the remaining breast tissue to treat any undetected cancer and achieve local control.

the patient as to her options, and the advantages and disadvantages of each. Although patients will differ in their desire for and seeking of information, their involvement in the decision-making process is essential.[31-34] Also critical to the success of breast-conserving surgery is appropriate patient selection and a multidisciplinary approach. Patients are selected for breast-conserving treatment based on the factors noted in Box 7-3.[35]

In certain areas of the United States today, breast-conserving treatment is not always administered appropriately. This is due to

---

BOX 7-3   **Considerations in Patient Selection for Breast-Conserving Treatment**

1. *Tumor size.* Local control is best with relatively small tumors. Most published experience in treating patients has been with tumors of a maximum of 4 to 5 cm in diameter. *Contraindications* include stage III or IV disease or the inability to obtain clear margins after repeated attempts at excision of remaining invasive breast cancer.
2. *Tumor location.* The location is not a factor in choosing breast-conserving treatment, although tumors located centrally in the breast, beneath the nipple area, usually require removal of the entire nipple-areolar complex, and cosmesis is then a consideration. *Contraindications* include two or more gross malignancies in other quadrants of the breast or mammographic indications of suspicious calcifications throughout the breast (multicentric disease).
3. *Breast size.* The tumor/breast size ratio influences the cosmetic results. If lumpectomy will result in a large surgical defect, a mastectomy followed by breast reconstruction may be more appropriate. A *contraindication* may be large pendulous breasts because of difficulties encountered with radiation therapy: reproducing the positioning of the patient and availability of equipment to provide dose homogeneity.
4. *Patient preference and attitude, and access to radiation facility.* A woman's desire to save her breast and a willingness to undergo 5 to 6 weeks of daily outpatient radiation therapy are important factors. A short hospital stay may also be required if interstitial implants are used. Some women might consider this extended treatment an unacceptable cost and inconvenience, or they may achieve greater peace of mind with the physical certainty of surgical removal. Living a great distance from a radiation treatment facility may cause additional hardship on some women and their families. Nurses can be supportive of patients in this decision-making process by facilitating communications, providing information, and helping them explore their personal values, relationships, and resources.
5. Other *contraindications* are prior radiation to the chest (e.g., in Hodgkin's lymphoma) that would limit therapeutic dosing to the breast; a history of collagen vascular disorder, which has been associated with poor tolerance of radiation; and pregnancy. Women in the first or the second trimester of pregnancy would be unable to undergo radiation therapy; women in the third trimester could feasibly begin radiation after delivery.

Data from National Comprehensive Cancer Network: *Clinical practice guidelines in oncology. Breast cancer.* Version 2.2006, retrieved December 16, 2005, from http://www.nccn.org/professionals/physician_gls/PDF/breast.pdf.

---

several factors such as distance from radiation facilities, patient age, and surgeon and hospital experience.[36-38] Continued attention must be given to reducing these disparities.

To prevent breast cancer in certain high-risk women, **prophylactic mastectomy** (unilateral or bilateral removal of the normal breast), with or without reconstruction, may be considered after careful discussion of potential risks and benefits. Skin-sparing total mastectomy with the complete excision of breast tissue is the preferred procedure. Women for whom this procedure may be appropriate include those with the following characteristics[39,40]:
1. Strong family history of breast cancer
2. Biopsy-proven DCIS or LCIS or benign breast disease (i.e., atypical hyperplasia) with a family history of breast cancer
3. Personal history of breast cancer in the opposite breast
4. Women with an identified mutation in *BRCA1*, *BRCA2* or other breast cancer susceptibility gene

In women with a moderate to high risk of breast cancer, bilateral prophylactic mastectomies reduce the risk of breast cancer significantly. Nurses can help women who are considering this option by understanding their confidence (or lack of) in breast cancer screening methods and anxieties or worries about cancer risk. **Subcutaneous mastectomy** removes 90% to 95% of the tissue, retaining the skin and nipple-areolar complex. Because of the difficulty removing all the breast tissue and problems with cosmesis, it is not recommended for primary surgical treatment of invasive breast cancer.

DCIS and LCIS, referred to earlier in this chapter, are noninvasive. In the past, these were rarely seen. It is estimated that 15% to 20% of all breast cancers found on mammography are in situ. Incidence rates of DCIS have increased significantly since the early 1980s as a direct result of increased mammography use, because DCIS is primarily discovered on mammography.[8] Lobular CIS accounts for a small percentage of in situ cancers, and has not increased in incidence. It is usually found only coincidentally, when a biopsy is done for other reasons.

DCIS is frequently associated with suspicious clustered microcalcifications seen on mammogram. Calcifications are biopsied via a stereotactic core biopsy or a needle localization excision. It is not known whether all DCIS will progress to an invasive cancer or when. DCIS may also be found incidentally near an invasive cancer. When found outside the area of the primary tumor, DCIS is referred to as **multicentric foci** (sites outside the quadrant of the breast where the primary tumor was found) or **multifocal** (sites within the same quadrant as the primary tumor). Microinvasion, or occult invasion, refers to the presence of a microscopic focus (less than 1 mm) of invasive breast cancer in a specimen containing DCIS. The larger the DCIS, the greater the risk of microinvasion. Mastectomy has been the primary treatment for DCIS, with a cure rate of nearly 100%.[40] Low axillary node dissection is usually included in a mastectomy. For most women with DCIS, breast-conserving surgery (complete removal of DCIS with clear margins of normal tissue) followed by radiation therapy to the remaining breast tissue reduces the risk of local recurrence of DCIS or invasive cancer. Treatment with an antiestrogen may be recommended for the prevention of invasive breast cancer.[25]

LCIS presents different management problems. It is not truly a precancerous lesion but an indicator of the risk of future invasive cancer in either breast, most often invasive DCIS.[12,13,25] It occurs primarily in premenopausal women and may be found diffusely in both breasts. Treatment options for LCIS include no further surgery and close follow-up, tamoxifen, or bilateral total mastectomy with reconstruction.[12,13,25] Neither axillary node dissection nor radiation therapy is indicated for LCIS.[12,13,25] Tamoxifen significantly reduces the risk of invasive breast cancer in these women.[2,12,13,25]

Sentinel lymph node biopsy (SLNB) refers to the removal of the lymph node that is first to receive drainage from the site of a breast cancer. It is based on the hypothesis that cancer cells drain first to the sentinel lymph node before spreading to other lymph nodes. Lymphatic mapping is the procedure by which the sentinel lymph node is located, whether via a nuclear medicine scan (lymphoscintigram) of the breast and axillary areas after injection of the breast with a radioisotope, or with injection of a blue dye, or both. Intraoperatively the blue and/or radioactive sentinel node(s) are located in the axilla after making a small incision in the lower axilla using a handheld probe to detect radioactivity or by visual identification of the blue lymphatic channel and blue-stained lymph node.[41]

The most experienced surgeons have demonstrated that identification of a negative sentinel lymph node is predictive that the remaining lymph nodes are also negative.[41] If the sentinel lymph node is positive for cancer, standard axillary lymph node dissection is indicated, unless the patient is participating in a clinical trial. When no sentinel lymph node can be identified, standard axillary lymph node dissection should be performed. SLNB may be most appropriate for women with invasive breast cancers of 1 cm or less. Contraindications to SLNB include tumors greater than 5 cm in their greatest dimension or in multiple sites in the breast, a large biopsy cavity, presence of a large hematoma or seroma, or the presence of palpable lymph nodes.[25] Surgeons offering SLNB must establish their competency in the technique, in other words that their identification of the sentinel lymph node is truly predictive of the remaining lymph nodes. This is done by first performing standard axillary lymph node dissection along with SLNB on a minimum of 20 to 30 patients.[42,43]

Breast Reconstruction. The disfigurement and loss associated with a mastectomy can be devastating for many women and their sexual partners. A woman's breasts are equated with femininity, sexual attractiveness, and nurturing behavior. The diagnosis and treatment of breast cancer has many psychosexual consequences.[44-47] Consequently, reconstruction has become an important element in a woman's rehabilitation after breast cancer surgery. Improved reconstructive techniques offer women hope for a less altered body image. The goal of breast reconstruction is to replace lost breast tissue and skin, rebuilding the breast mound to symmetry, with or without formation of a nipple and areola. A well-informed patient and a coordinated treatment approach by the surgeon, the medical oncologist, and the plastic surgeon will increase the likelihood of achieving the desired results.

Whether reconstruction should be immediate (at the time of the mastectomy) or delayed to some future date until other treatments have been completed has been the subject of much debate. Concerns about immediate reconstruction delaying the start of adjuvant chemotherapy or impairing the early detection of a local recurrence have generally not been supported by actual experience. Patients undergoing immediate reconstruction have been found to experience less overall trauma with their mastectomy.[48,49] This also eliminates another hospitalization and general anesthesia experience. For most women undergoing mastectomy,

particularly those with stage 0 (in situ) or stage I or IIa breast cancer, there is no scientific justification for delaying reconstruction.

Actual costs for reconstruction vary based on the type of procedure, the surgeon's time, operating room time, and the length of hospitalization. Federal and state laws have provided support to ensure that many insurance providers will include coverage for reconstruction, as well as symmetry procedures on the opposite breast, if they cover mastectomy. Women considering these procedures will need to inquire with their individual insurance plans regarding coverage. Advanced age is not a contraindication for reconstruction as long as the woman is in sufficient health to tolerate the effects of surgery. Obesity, tobacco use, diabetes, or other debilitating diseases are associated with increased postoperative complications and may be contraindications to some types of reconstruction. Treatment of breast cancer is the priority; thus treatment planning within the team will help clarify timing of reconstruction and adjuvant therapies. Ideally, thoughtful discussion of the options for reconstruction is incorporated in the initial treatment planning phase.

Most women with breast cancer preparing to have a mastectomy, particularly those with stage I or II disease, are candidates for reconstruction.[50] The patient's motivation and desire for a restored breast is one of the most important indicators for reconstruction.[50] The reasons women seek breast reconstruction, whether immediate or at a later date, are varied and may include a desire to feel whole again, to maintain a sense of femininity and positive body image, to eliminate an external prosthesis and to have a lasting result, or to reestablish physical symmetry and a sense of balance. Some women will choose mastectomy with reconstruction over breast-conserving surgery (e.g., a desire not to worry about remaining breast tissue or having to undergo radiation therapy). Patients with unrealistic expectations, such as that reconstruction will eliminate the physical and psychologic effects of mastectomy or that it will result in a perfect replication of the lost breast, are more likely to be dissatisfied with the results.

Considerations in the type of reconstructive surgery include the quality and amount of skin, the size and shape of the opposite breast, the initial surgical procedure for cancer, and the patient's goals and general health. There are several breast reconstructive options available.

Silicone gel–filled breast **implants** were first developed in the early 1960s. By 1989, over 1 million implants had been placed in women, with over 80% of these in women for elective breast augmentation and only 20% in women who underwent reconstruction for breast cancer. In response to concerns that silicone gel–filled implants were associated with autoimmune disease, in 1992 the FDA restricted their use to prospective controlled clinical studies with a full discussion of the available options, risks, and benefits for women who have a medically related need for the implant (e.g., breast cancer, rupture of old implant).[51]

Although the concerns have not been substantiated, the restrictions continue. Saline-filled silicone implants, not restricted by the FDA, are available for any woman seeking reconstruction, and currently account for the majority of implants placed today. Implants are placed beneath the muscle. **Tissue expanders** consist of an elastomer or silicone shell liner and a valve or port through which the shell is inflated with saline gradually over several weeks. Also placed beneath the muscle, these are useful in stretching the skin to accommodate a full-size prosthesis.

Some expanders, once fully filled, will remain in the tissue as the permanent prosthesis. Others require a second operation for removal and replacement with a permanent implant.

The most common complication of implants is **capsular contracture,** or hardening of the scar tissue, resulting in firmness of the breast tissue and sometimes distortion of shape. Mechanical problems with inflation or deflation can occur with the tissue expanders but are uncommon. The potential also exists for a missed cancer on mammography, although a knowledgeable and skilled mammography technician will be able to displace the implant and maximize the breast tissue captured in the mammogram.

The **latissimus dorsi myocutaneous flap** from the upper back is useful in women after modified radical mastectomy or breast-conserving surgery. It involves the transfer of fat on the surface of the latissimus dorsi, and overlying skin, to the anterior chest wall mastectomy site. It may be supplemented with an implant for full symmetry. The **transverse rectus abdominis myocutaneous (pedicled or tunneled) flap (TRAM)** from the lower abdomen accomplishes a simultaneous abdominoplasty (similar to a "tummy tuck") and does not require the use of an implant. The rectus abdominis muscle and its blood supply, with overlying fat and skin, is used in the building of the breast mound. Complications with either of these procedures include flap loss from damage to the blood supply, skin necrosis, infection, hematoma, delayed wound healing, and fat necrosis or fibrosis.[50] Hernias at the donor site have occurred with the TRAM flap but are rare. In either procedure an additional scar is left, but the scar from the TRAM procedure is usually hidden within an acceptable "bikini" line. The TRAM flap can also be performed bilaterally. Microsurgical techniques to reconnect blood supplies of

tissue when transferred have enabled other reconstructive procedures using free flaps. These include the **gluteal free flap** (from the buttock area), the **lateral transverse thigh free flap,** and the **TRAM free flap.** For example, in the TRAM free flap transfer, a segment of the rectus abdominis muscle, overlying fat, and skin is taken, and its blood supply microsurgically anastomosed to vessels at the site of implantation (e.g., internal mammary vessels). The added expense of extended operating room time and hospitalization for the TRAM procedures, over other types of reconstruction, may be offset to an extent with defined clinical pathways that facilitate optimum care for patients and high patient satisfaction with these procedures.[52]

Augmentation, mastopexy (breast lift), or **reduction** of the remaining breast is sometimes necessary to achieve **symmetry.** This and any further refinements in the reconstructed breast often are completed before or concurrently with the nipple-areolar complex reconstruction. Saving the nipple-areolar complex at the time of mastectomy for later reconstruction has generally not been recommended, yet new research suggests this may be appropriate for some patients.[53] **Skin transfers** have been the primary means of nipple and areola reconstruction. However, newer and more satisfactory techniques involve the raising of a flap of skin from the reconstructed breast mound and folding back sections of the flap to create the projecting nipple.[50] In all patients, tattooing of the nipple-areolar complex usually follows to achieve color symmetry.[50] Figure 7-3 illustrates reconstructive results.

Nursing Care Considerations. Feelings that arise in the preoperative period of sadness at the anticipated loss (whether part or all of the breast), a sense of readiness for the surgery, and relief (that the cancer will be removed) are often interspersed

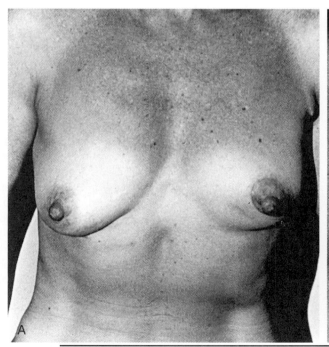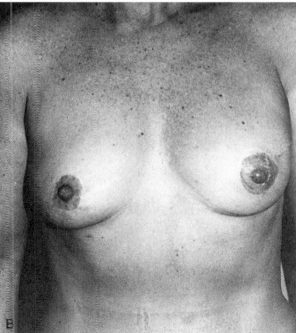

FIG. 7-3   Breast reconstruction results. (From McCraw JB and others: Breast reconstruction following mastectomy. In Bland KI and Copeland EM, editors: *The breast: comprehensive management of benign and malignant diseases,* ed 2, vol 2, Philadelphia, WB Saunders, 1998.)

postoperatively with concern about the final pathology report and the involvement of lymph nodes. Wound care and remobilization of the arm are a focus for the physical recovery during this time. When the best time is to begin mobilization of the arm and shoulder postoperatively has been the subject of many reports in the literature.[54,55] There are concerns about early mobilization (postoperative days 1 to 2), which has been related to the potential for increased drain tube output, delay in drain removal, seroma formation after drain removal, and potential for impaired wound healing and infection. Late mobilization can be a concern in terms of difficulties that may occur with arm and shoulder motion when exercise is not begun sooner. Restricted mobility carries the potential risk of later development of a "frozen shoulder." For women who have undergone an axillary lymph node dissection after lumpectomy or mastectomy, some postoperative exercise to include flexion and extension of the hand, wrist, and elbow and limited movement for simple activities (eating, brushing teeth) seem reasonable immediately after surgery. Exercises, designed to regain full range of motion (ROM) of the shoulder joint, can begin within 3 to 5 days after surgery and gradually be increased. The type of reconstruction after mastectomy may be associated with more limited movement for longer periods. Often exercise programs are designed by a treatment team from nursing, surgery, occupational therapy, and physical therapy.[54] Because surgical admissions are of much shorter duration, much preoperative preparation takes place in the clinic or office setting, as does postoperative education.[56] Nurses have an important role not only in educating but in promoting the expression and exploration of feelings by the patient and her spouse or significant other. It is important to include both individuals in the treatment planning and follow-up (see Treatment-Related Complications box).

Priority interventions for educating, supporting, and assessing women receiving surgical interventions include the following:

1. Inform patient and family about hospital and surgical routines.
2. Describe postoperative activity (positioning and care of the arm on the operative side, drains, pain management, intravenous lines, and ambulation) before surgery so the patient will be prepared to participate appropriately.
3. In the immediate postoperative period, position the arm on the operative side so it is slightly elevated, with a flat pillow or folded towel behind the upper arm until the patient is fully awake and ambulatory. Maintenance of this supported position when reclining may enhance comfort.
4. Reinforce importance of early ambulation, coughing, and deep breathing.
5. All intravenous access sites or venipunctures need to be managed on the nonoperative side.
6. Monitor wound for inflammation, tenderness, swelling, or purulent drainage. Change dressing when ordered, using aseptic technique.
7. Monitor drains and instruct patient simultaneously: they should be intact and secured to the skin or clothing so as not to dangle; check color and amount of fluid output.[57]
8. Assess patient for level of pain or discomfort, and medicate as ordered.
9. Provide information on normal sensations patient will experience postoperatively, such as paresthesias (e.g., numbness, tingling, increased skin sensitivity) of the inner aspect of the upper arm.[58,59] Some women report that rolling up

Treatment-Related Complications

SURGERY	CHEMOTHERAPY
Impaired wound healing/seroma	Marrow suppression
Infection	(bleeding/sepsis)
Nerve injury	Cardiac dysrhythmias,
Lymphedema	congestive heart failure
Shoulder dysfunction	Stomatitis
	Anorexia/nausea/vomiting
	Extravasation/skin necrosis
	Hemorrhagic cystitis
	Excessive tearing
	Peripheral neuropathy
	Hormonal and
	reproductive changes

RADIATION THERAPY	TARGETED THERAPIES
Skin reactions	Flulike symptoms
Lymphedema	Headache
Shoulder dysfunction	Pain at infusion site
Fatigue	Ventricular dysfunction,
Marrow suppression	congestive heart failure

ENDOCRINE THERAPY	
Thrombosis	
Menstrual irregularities	
Hot flashes	
Osteoporosis	
Pulmonary embolism	
Depression	
Fluid retention	
Ovarian and endometrial cancer	

a small towel or washcloth and placing it in the axilla or between the arm and chest helps alleviate some of the discomfort from immediate postoperative paresthesias. "Phantom breast" experiences have also been reported by women after mastectomy.[59,60]

10. Assess readiness to look at incision, and offer support when patient decides to view the incision. Description of the wound appearance may be helpful to some patients before actual viewing. Discuss possible response of patient's spouse/partner toward viewing the incision and patient's readiness for this response.
11. Instruct patient in arm care and postsurgical arm exercises. This intervention will usually require some type of follow-up in the outpatient setting for the first 6 weeks after surgery, although a program of exercise may need to be continued for up to 6 months for full recovery and flexibility. Examples of recommended exercises include squeezing a ball, brushing the hair, shoulder shrugs and circles, and finger climbing up a wall when facing the wall (standing about 6 inches away) and turned perpendicular to the wall. Instruct patient to begin all exercises gently. Gentle stretching of muscles, but not strain, is encouraged. Reach to Recovery volunteers also can demonstrate exercises. Referral to physical therapy may be necessary, if physical therapists were not initially involved in the patient's care or the patient's ROM recovery is not progressing.

MEDICAL TREATMENT: ADJUVANT THERAPY

Radiation Therapy. Radiation therapy has localized effects on breast cancer. It has an important role in combination with other therapies, or sometimes alone, as adjuvant treatment of local and/or regional disease, and for local and/or regional advanced or metastatic disease. In the past, radiotherapy was routinely used after a modified radical mastectomy to decrease the risk of disease recurrence. Now this is primarily reserved for patients who have a high risk for local recurrence of the disease, specifically those women with an advanced primary tumor or with four or more positive nodes.[61] Postmastectomy radiation therapy is given within the first 6 weeks after surgery, targeting both the affected chest wall and regional lymph nodes.[61,52]

Radiation therapy following breast-conserving surgery achieves local control of disease, or reduces the risk of local recurrence, in women with early-stage (I or II) invasive breast cancer. Multiple randomized clinical trials demonstrated lumpectomy followed by radiation to the whole breast resulted in the same overall survival as mastectomy alone.[30,35,63] In stage IIIA disease, preoperative chemotherapy often shrinks the primary tumor enough to allow these women to undergo breast-conserving surgery and radiation. For women with DCIS, radiation has been shown to reduce the risk of subsequent invasive tumor growth.[25,40]

External beam radiotherapy usually begins by 2 to 4 weeks, and no later than 12 weeks, after surgery.[35,40,61] However, some women with invasive breast cancer will be advised to have adjuvant chemotherapy before radiation to minimize cardiac toxicity with anthracycline-based regimens.[61] Treatment planning for radiotherapy is done to ensure homogeneity of dose through consistent, reproducible positioning of the patient and the use of supervoltage equipment.[35] Each field is treated daily, Monday through Friday, to a total whole-breast dose of 4500 to 5000 centigrays (cGy), or rads, at 180 to 200 cGy per fraction, over 4 to 6 weeks.[35,40,61,62] A radiation boost to the original tumor site is given when surgical margins are involved after segmental mastectomy for invasive breast cancer. A boost for women with DCIS remains controversial. The boost dose is usually delivered by electron beam (external boost) and increases the total dose to the primary tumor site to 6000 to 6600 cGy.[35,40,63] Radiation to the axilla is not given after a diagnosis of DCIS, or to women with a diagnosis of invasive breast cancer if a level I and II axillary node dissection or sentinel lymph node biopsy has been done.[35,63] Radiotherapy to the supraclavicular area is recommended after breast-conserving surgery when four or more lymph nodes are involved.[35] Further research is needed to determine if there are subgroups of women who do not need postoperative radiotherapy and/or a boost dose.

New techniques offer more precise imaging to pinpoint the target field and prevent local and regional recurrence after breast-conserving surgery. Three-dimensional (3D) computerized treatment planning helps map out an individualized treatment plan for external beam therapy that conforms to the tumor's dimensions.[27,63] Intensity-modulated radiation therapy (IMRT) delivers low doses of radiation therapy to the tumor bed and surrounding tissue through the use of microleaves. While improving dose homogeneity and expanding the treatment field, IMRT also decreases toxicity to adjacent organs. Long-term effects of IMRT are currently being studied.[63]

Recurrence despite breast-conserving surgery and external beam radiation therapy drove investigation into a new form of brachytherapy, **accelerated partial breast irradiation**. In 2002, the FDA approved the MammoSite, a special device with an intracavitary balloon and catheter that is inserted into the surgical cavity during lumpectomy. MammoSite is indicated for women with small, early-stage tumors that do not lie close to the chest wall. Following surgery, a radioactive source is placed through the catheter into the balloon and withdrawn twice a day for 5 to 7 days. The balloon is then deflated and easily removed by the surgeon. Accelerated treatment that precisely targets the tumor bed offers promising advantages for many women, whose lifestyle can be disrupted by the long duration of external beam radiation therapy.[27,62,63] Research has demonstrated that recurrence control rates are comparable to standard radiation therapy, but long-term evaluation is needed.[25,62,63] For patients with locally advanced disease or those unable to undergo a surgical procedure, radiotherapy may be used alone or in conjunction with chemotherapy and hormone therapy. In metastatic cancer, radiation therapy is palliative for painful bony metastases. It shrinks metastatic brain lesions or tumors compressing the spinal cord, and relieves the symptoms of spinal cord compression or of superior vena cava syndrome.[61]

Nursing Care Considerations. The toxicities associated with radiation therapy are generally mild and reversible. They include local skin changes, generalized fatigue, pain related to temporary inflammation of the nerves or the pectoral muscles in the radiation field, and occasionally sore throat. Extended axillary irradiation can aggravate lymphedema and range of motion difficulties.[61,62] (For a more detailed discussion of the radiation-associated toxicities and specific nursing interventions, see Chapter 20 and the Treatment-Related Complications box.)

Priority interventions for educating, supporting, and assessing women receiving radiation therapy include the following:
1. Briefly explain the rationale behind the planned radiation therapy. Reinforce the goal of preventing recurrence or limiting disease spread.
2. Provide and review educational materials on radiation therapy.
3. Outline the treatment plan and schedule, emphasizing the importance of keeping appointments. Explain how the treatment will be individualized and what to expect with simulation versus actual treatment.
4. Review possible side effects, what symptoms to report, and strategies to prevent or minimize treatment side effects. To minimize breast skin discomfort or breakdown, teach the patient the following strategies:
   a. Use mild, unscented, and nondrying soap.
   b. Pat the radiation field dry instead of rubbing.
   c. Avoid using deodorant on the affected side until after radiation therapy. Some deodorants contain metals that can block the external radiation beam.
   d. Avoid tight tops or underwire bras.
5. Encourage regular skin hygiene for women with large breasts and adjacent skin folds.
6. Encourage talking with another breast cancer survivor who has successfully completed radiation therapy.
7. Monitor for treatment side effects.

SYSTEMIC THERAPY

Breast cancer can spread not only to axillary nodes but also to distant sites through the bloodstream. A percentage of women will therefore have micrometastases at diagnosis.

Chemotherapy, biotherapy, or hormone therapy (or a combination) can prevent, delay, or retard metastatic disease. Chemotherapy and hormone therapy have been in clinical use and studied for the past 30 years, and targeted therapies have recently offered promising results in clinical trials.

Chemotherapy. Chemotherapy offers systemic treatment of breast cancer for women with (1) node-negative disease with high risk of recurrence, (2) axillary node involvement, (3) poor-prognosis, node-negative disease, (4) advanced local and/or regional disease, or (5) distant metastases. Many agents are active against breast cancer. The specific therapy recommended is influenced by the patient's prognostic factors, general medical condition, and treatment preference. Dosages used and the duration of therapy vary, depending on menopausal status, lymph nodes, and ER status. For women with node-negative disease, important factors are histologic or nuclear grade, age, and possibly lymphatic or vascular invasion as well as HER2/*neu* status.[27]

Neoadjuvant chemotherapy is given before surgery to reduce the tumor size and allow for breast-conserving lumpectomy with minimal lymph node removal. Adjuvant chemotherapy is given after the definitive surgical treatment while the tumor burden is small (suspected micrometastases) and the cells are least likely to become drug resistant. Clinical trials have clearly demonstrated that adjuvant chemotherapy delays recurrence and improves disease-free and overall survival in women with early-stage disease up to 70 years of age, as well as those with estrogen-negative tumors, high-risk tumors, and negative lymph nodes.[25,27,28,64]

There is no one optimal drug combination, treatment schedule, or duration of therapy for all patients. Since 1985, the National Institutes of Health (NIH) have gathered panels of experts to evaluate the results of adjuvant clinical trials and to make treatment recommendations.[27,65] For example, clinical trials to date have resulted in a gradual decrease in the total length of time recommended for adjuvant chemotherapy, to the current duration of 4 to 6 months, with chemotherapy administered every 3 to 4 weeks for most patients. The regimens most often used in adjuvant therapy contain a combination of **cyclophosphamide** (C), and an anthracycline such as **doxorubicin** (A), with or without a taxane (**paclitaxel** or **docetaxel**) (T). **Methotrexate** (M) and **5-fluorouracil** (F) or **epirubicin** (E) may also be used, especially

if women have preexisting cardiac disease.[25,66] Table 7-1 summarizes current NCCN practice recommendations for treatment of patients not enrolled in a clinical trial.

No standard treatment recommendations exist for those over 70 years old. Treatment should be individualized and consideration given to comorbid conditions.[25]

In general, women who will most clearly benefit from systemic chemotherapy (with or without hormone therapy) are those at any age with positive lymph nodes, and premenopausal women with large tumors with positive or negative lymph nodes. Women at low risk of relapse, that is, those with tumors of less than 1 cm in diameter and negative lymph nodes, probably do not warrant adjuvant chemotherapy outside of a clinical trial.[25] Further studies in progress will identify the specific subsets of patients who need adjuvant chemotherapy and the most appropriate regimen.

Clinical trials continue to evaluate the benefits of perioperative chemotherapy (begun within hours after surgery), neoadjuvant therapy, short-course intensive chemotherapy, and high-dose chemotherapy with peripheral blood stem cell transplant. Dose-dense chemotherapy is a new scheduling approach that delivers a traditional dose over a shorter period of time. Adjuvant chemotherapy given every 2 weeks has shown sustained drug concentrations and effective cancer cell kill, decreased toxicities, and increased quality of life over chemotherapy given every 3 weeks. The addition of **granulocyte (G-CSF)** and **granulocyte/macrophage colony-stimulating factors (GM-CSF)** to the treatment regimen has enabled more rapid recovery and a reduction of toxicities associated with myelosuppression. New trials are focusing on evaluating the use of oral chemotherapy, such as capecitabine, for metastatic breast cancer, instead of intravenous (IV) chemotherapy every 1 to 3 weeks. Preliminary results have been promising, with sufficient cancer cell kill, lower toxicities from IV chemotherapy, and improved quality of life.[66] Optimum routes of administration for therapy, dose intensity, and scheduling of chemotherapy regimens pose ongoing questions for research.[27,28,67]

Targeted Therapy. In combination with chemotherapy, biotherapy with trastuzumab (Herceptin) is indicated in the treatment of 25% to 30% of women with breast cancer whose tumors overexpress the HER2/*neu* protein (see Table 7-1). Trastuzumab, a monoclonal antibody, blocks HER2/*neu* overexpression and

TABLE 7-1	NCCN Recommendations for Adjuvant Chemotherapy and Biotherapy for ER/PR Negative Invasive Breast Cancer			
TUMOR SIZE	**NODE STATUS**	**HORMONE RECEPTOR STATUS**	**HER2/*NEU* STATUS**	**ADJUVANT CHEMOTHERAPY AND BIOTHERAPY**
≤0.5 cm	Negative	Negative	Positive or Negative	None
	Positive	Negative	Positive or Negative	Consider chemotherapy
0.6–1.0 cm	Negative	Negative	Positive or Negative	Consider chemotherapy
	Positive	Negative	Positive or Negative	Chemotherapy
>1.0 cm	Negative	Negative	Positive	Chemotherapy and trastuzumab
	Negative	Negative	Negative	Chemotherapy
	Positive	Negative	Positive	Chemotherapy and trastuzumab
	Positive	Negative	Negative	Chemotherapy

No standard treatment recommendations exist for those over 70 years old. Treatment should be individualized with consideration of comorbid conditions.
Data from National Comprehensive Cancer Network: *Clinical practice guidelines in oncology. Breast cancer.* Version 1.2007, retrieved February 11, 2007, from http://www.nccn.org/professionals/physician_gls/PDF/breast.pdf.

the resulting proliferation of breast cancer cells. Although first used in women with metastatic disease, trastuzumab has demonstrated significant relapse-free and survival benefits in women with early-stage invasive breast cancer that is HER2/neu-positive.[25,27,28]

OTHER TREATMENT MODALITIES

Endocrine Therapy. **Selective estrogen receptor modulators (SERMs)**, like tamoxifen, make up an important class of drugs that reduce or block the action of estrogen in women with breast cancer. In women with estrogen and progesterone receptor–positive disease, estrogen binds with the estrogen receptors on the surface of breast cancer cells and signals increased cell replication. Tamoxifen competes with estrogen by binding to the cell receptors and blocking estrogen's effects. This therapy is an effective adjunct to surgery and other breast cancer therapies because of its ability to alter the cellular environment that fosters carcinogenesis.[62]

Adjuvant endocrine therapy is recommended for women whose breast cancer expresses hormone receptor protein—regardless of age, menopausal status, tumor size, or involvement of axillary lymph nodes. Tamoxifen has been the gold standard of adjuvant therapy, with a daily dose for up to 5 years' duration.[25,65] For premenopausal women, **ovarian ablation** may be preferred initially or may follow tamoxifen; it serves to reduce the level of circulating estrogen available to stimulate breast cancer cells. This can be achieved with bilateral **oophorectomy** (removal of the ovaries) or with luteinizing hormone–releasing (LHRH) agonists (leuprolide, goserelin).[25]

Tamoxifen not only offers an alternative to ovarian ablation for some premenopausal women, it also decreases the incidence of both ipsilateral and contralateral recurrence and improves survival when combined with chemotherapy in women with invasive hormone receptor–positive breast cancer. When combined with polychemotherapy, tamoxifen further reduces recurrence risk for premenopausal women with early-stage disease. Research is exploring initial evidence that ovarian ablation and hormone therapy enhance the benefits of tamoxifen and may provide an alternative to chemotherapy in premenopausal women with low risk for recurrence.[62,68]

However, recurrence and side effects have restricted tamoxifen's usefulness beyond 5 years' duration. Tamoxifen is generally well tolerated, but side effects may cause a woman to discontinue therapy. Osteoporosis and hot flashes occur frequently along with early menopause, including menstrual irregularities, vaginal dryness, irritation, and impaired sexual functioning. Although rare, depression and thrombosis can be severe. Tamoxifen is also associated with a low risk of uterine or endometrial cancer.[9,65,68]

Recent studies have introduced a promising alternative for first-line and recurrent endocrine therapy in postmenopausal women with estrogen receptor–positive breast cancer. During the Arimidex, Tamoxifen Alone, or in Combination (ATAC) trials, an aromatase inhibitor (AI), anastrazole, was compared with tamoxifen for 5 years in 9366 postmenopausal women with localized disease.[69] Aromatase inhibitors prevent androgens, secreted by the adrenals, from being converted to estrogen. Anastrazole significantly prolonged disease-free survival and decreased the incidence of distant metastases. Anastrazole was noted for fewer side effects, especially menstrual irregularities

and thrombosis, although arthralgias and fractures from loss of bone density were possible side effects. Anastrazole or other aromatase inhibitors (exemestane or letrozole) are now being considered as first-line adjuvant endocrine therapy in place of tamoxifen, to offer a better tolerated and effective therapy at the earliest opportunity.[68-70]

Nursing Care Considerations. The medical decision to recommend adjuvant therapy and the patient's decision to receive it can be complex and challenging. As with decisions about the type of surgical procedure, patients need help understanding the concept of adjuvant therapy and information about its benefits and risks.[34,71,72]

Because the risk for recurrence is highest during the first 2 years after diagnosis, physical examinations may be scheduled every 3 to 6 months during the first 1 to 2 years, every 6 to 12 months during the next 2 to 3 years, and then annually. Some patients will choose to stagger visits to their different specialists so that they see one member of their health care team on a more frequent basis. Mammography may be performed every 6 months for the first 1 to 3 years, then annually thereafter. Blood and imaging tests are performed regularly for individualized follow-up. Any signs or symptoms the patient has at the time of each evaluation will influence what additional tests or imaging studies are ordered, and their frequency.

Difficulties in psychosocial adjustment to breast cancer are not confined to the early phase of the illness but persist over time for both patients and family members. Fear of disease recurrence, role adjustment problems, resource depletion, toxicities of therapy, and changes in body image, self-esteem, and patterns of sexuality are problems the patient and her partner may experience.[45,46,73] Children are also affected and will need support.[74,75,76] Expressions of emotional distress may require referrals to trained counselors or support groups available through the ACS, local hospitals, or community resources. Reintegration into life after treatment may be enhanced through discussion by the nurse, and by structured programs.[54,77-79]

Priority interventions for educating, supporting, and assessing women receiving chemotherapy, targeted therapies, and/or endocrine therapy, and in long-term follow-up include the following:

1. Help explore myths and fears, including those shared by family, friends, or neighbors with breast cancer who have received chemotherapy or biotherapy.
2. Briefly explain the rationale behind treatment (i.e., based on the pathology report). Reinforce the nature of breast cancer as a disease of cells, with the goal of eliminating any residual cancer cells.
3. Provide and review educational materials on chemotherapy and biotherapy.
4. Outline treatment drugs, calendar, and possible side effects, as well as preventive and management strategies. Reinforce what symptoms to watch for and report (see Treatment-Related Complications box).
5. Offer encouragement to take control and prepare for hair loss, which can significantly affect a woman's body image and intimate relationships. Suggest purchasing a wig, scarf, or head covering before starting treatment.
6. Encourage talking about chemotherapy and/or biotherapy with another breast cancer survivor who has undergone similar therapy.

7. Closely monitor for any treatment side effects and reinforce how the symptom(s) can be managed. (See Chapter 21 for side effects.)

8. Reinforce the importance of following the treatment and blood work schedule to gain the most benefit from planned chemotherapy and/or biotherapy.[62,80,81]

9. Encourage partners or significant others to accompany patients at follow-up visits. This allows them to be included in the discussion regarding concerns and problems they are experiencing, whether individually or as a couple.

10. Help patients and significant others to explore quality of life issues individually and as a family.[82]

11. Encourage and facilitate discussion with appropriate medical resources for pregnancy planning.

12. Encourage participation in survivorship activities or group support, if desired.

13. Encourage patient and family to resume participation in activities previously enjoyed.

14. Encourage healthy lifestyle behaviors (e.g., diet, exercise, stress reduction).

Disease-Related Complications and Treatment

Certain patients with features of **locally advanced** disease may be considered inoperable at diagnosis. This includes tumors with direct extension to the chest wall or skin; large, palpable axillary nodes; skin ulceration; and inflammatory changes (stage IIIB, some stage IIIA). Although potentially resectable, the local recurrence rate is high. Some, but not all, of these patients will have distant metastases at the time of diagnosis and need laboratory and radiologic evaluation. Patients with locally advanced disease benefit from preoperative combination chemotherapy. The presence of palpable supraclavicular or infraclavicular lymph nodes or large, nonmovable axillary nodes at the initial diagnosis, as well as the response to chemotherapy will determine whether the subsequent treatment is radiation therapy alone, modified radical mastectomy with radiation therapy, or segmental mastectomy with radiation therapy. The optimum therapy for locally advanced disease has not been determined despite improved responses with this sequential therapy.[25] For women with locally advanced breast cancer (e.g., 10 or more positive lymph nodes), recent studies have evaluated the effectiveness of **autologous bone marrow transplant (ABMT)**, or **peripheral stem cell transplant (PSCT)** (harvesting the

patient's peripheral blood stem cells and reinfusing them after high-dose treatment). There is no evidence of a survival benefit with this treatment, so this is currently recommended only as part of a clinical trial.[83,84]

Lymphedema after breast cancer surgery is the accumulation of lymph fluid in the tissues of the upper extremity, extending from the upper arm and potentially to the hand and fingers. It occurs in 15% to 20% of women who have had an axillary lymph node dissection, although some studies have reported a higher incidence. The risk of developing lymphedema is affected by the extent of lymph node dissection (levels I, II, and III or levels I and II, versus sentinel lymph node biopsy), and radiation therapy to the axilla. It may also be affected by factors such as obesity, poor nutritional status, increased age, and wound infection.[85] Lymphedema may occur any time after surgery, and is caused by the interruption or removal of lymph channels and nodes after axillary node dissection or radiation therapy. These procedures result in less efficient filtration of lymph fluid and a pooling of lymphatic fluid in the tissues. The goals of intervention for lymphedema include the prevention of cosmetic deformity, emotional distress, functional impairment, infection, and discomfort.

Goals of therapy in **metastatic disease** are the control of the disease and palliation of symptoms. Chemotherapy, hormone therapy, targeted therapies, and radiation in combination or alone may achieve temporary regression of the disease in a majority of patients, yet these responses generally last 6 to 12 months. However, some may be alive in 5 years, and a few will become long-term survivors and may be cured. The treatment selection is based on prior adjuvant treatment, prior response, current physical condition, and sites of metastases (e.g., local and/or regional, soft tissue, bone, liver, lung).

CHEMOTHERAPY

In metastatic (or locally advanced) disease, responses to combination drug therapy occur in a majority of patients, and responses generally last from 6 to 12 months. Doxorubicin (Adriamycin) is the most effective single agent in the treatment of metastatic breast cancer. Other active single agents typically used initially in combination regimens may include cyclophosphamide, methotrexate, 5-fluorouracil, mitoxantrone, vinorelbine, or the taxanes (paclitaxel [Taxol], docetaxel [Taxotere]), or the monoclonal antibody, trastuzamab, for women whose tumors overexpress HER2/*neu*. Once initial therapy for distant metastases fails, subsequent treatment regimens may include epirubicin,

$\mathcal{D}$ISEASE-RELATED COMPLICATIONS
Breast Cancers

Local/Regional Advanced Disease or Recurrence	Distant Recurrence
• Ulceration	• Spinal cord compression
• Lymphedema	• Brain/leptomeningeal metastases
• Brachial plexopathy	• Hypercalcemia
• Infection and necrosis	• Pathologic fractures
	• Pleural effusion
	• Lymphangitic spread
	• Pericardial effusion/tamponade
	• Superior vena cava syndrome

mitoxantrone, vinblastine, gemcitabine, mitomycin C, etoposide, and capecitabine. Because there is no "standard" therapy for metastatic disease, new approaches are regularly being tested in phases II and III research. Examples include non–cross-resistant therapy, new phase II agents, standard- versus intensified-dose therapy, intensive chemotherapy and ABMT, chemoendocrine combinations, weekly low-dose chemotherapy, and continuous infusion regimens.

HORMONAL MANIPULATION

Progression or recurrence of disease after tamoxifen or other endocrine therapy or oophorectomy usually necessitates a sequential trial of other endocrine therapies. Metastatic tumors that have responded to one form of hormone therapy are more likely to respond to another type of hormone therapy if there is a recurrence or progression of disease.[25] Women likely to respond to endocrine therapy include those with a combination of the following factors:[25,65,68]

1. Disease-free interval greater than 2 years
2. Disease limited to bone and soft tissue
3. Postmenopausal or late premenopausal
4. Previous response to endocrine therapy

A variety of endocrine therapies are available, but most types require several weeks to be effective. Therefore in women with life-threatening liver, lung, or brain metastases, chemotherapy will likely be preferred. Recent studies have shown that tamoxifen and oophorectomy are equally effective in treating premenopausal women with distant metastases, but tamoxifen is perhaps safer and more tolerable.[25,68]

For the postmenopausal woman who has progression of disease while on tamoxifen, the next treatment choice would be an AI. AIs are drugs that suppress postmenopausal estrogen levels by inhibiting aromatase, an enzyme necessary for estrogen production. This enzyme is more prevalent in breast tissue after menopause and in breast cancer tissue. Nonsteroidal AIs include anastrozole and letrozole. Exemestane and formestane are examples of steroidal AIs. Common side effects include fatigue, nausea and vomiting, and headache.[62,70] Other side effects may include lethargy, dizziness, skin rash, and cushingoid symptoms. AIs alone are contraindicated in premenopausal women with metastatic breast cancer, because the effect of inhibited estrogen production in the ovaries can lead to polycystic ovaries and masculinization from excess androgen production.[70]

Progestins may also be used in postmenopausal women after failure to respond to an AI. The progestins most often used are megestrol acetate (Megace) and medroxy-progesterone acetate (Depo-Provera). Recent studies have shown these drugs to be as effective as other forms of hormone manipulation. The mechanism of action of progestins has not been established. Weight gain is the most frequently experienced side effect, although thrombolytic events have also been reported. **Estrogens** such as diethylstilbestrol (DES) can also result in tumor regressions in postmenopausal women. High doses of estrogen act at the level of the hypothalamus to inhibit the release of luteinizing hormone, which normally stimulates the ovaries to produce estrogen. These drugs are associated with significant side effects (nausea, vomiting, anorexia, vaginal bleeding, breast engorgement, edema) and are contraindicated in patients with a history of cardiac or thrombolytic events.

Androgens, or male hormones, are less effective than estrogens or tamoxifen. Testosterone and fluoxymesterone (Halotestin) have been evaluated. The exact mechanism of action of androgens is unknown. The main side effect of masculinization (facial and body hair, deepening of the voice, alopecia) is often unacceptable.

With any endocrine therapy a "flare reaction" may occur during the first few days to weeks of treatment. The most frequent symptom of a flare reaction is abrupt onset of diffuse musculoskeletal aching, increased pain at sites of known disease, erythema at sites of skin metastases, or hypercalcemia. Hypercalcemia is the most serious manifestation of a flare reaction. This reaction must not be confused with progressive disease and is not an indication of therapeutic response. A transient elevation of tumor markers (e.g., CA15-3 or CA27-29) may also occur in the first month or two in response to endocrine therapy. Women receiving all endocrine therapies must be monitored for this reaction, reassured, and provided treatment for their symptoms.

OTHER THERAPIES

Targeted therapies include trastuzumab for women with breast cancer whose tumors overexpress the HER2/*neu* protein, and two agents under investigation: the monoclonal antibody bevacizumab (Avastin) and gefitinib (Iressa), a molecular inhibitor of epidermal growth factor receptor (EGFR) which is thought to regulate blood vessel formation that supports tumor growth.[62,66]

SUPPORTIVE THERAPIES

Bisphosphanates (e.g., pamidronate, clodronate) may provide symptomatic relief of pain and reduce the risk of pathologic fractures in the patient with bone metastases, but they do not prevent bone metastases or affect overall survival.[86]

NURSING CARE CONSIDERATIONS

Priority interventions for educating, supporting, and assessing women with recurrent or metastatic disease include the following:

1. Provide support when patient is informed of diagnosis and treatment plan.
2. Explain rationale for treatments and anticipated side effects, and their management.
3. Encourage patient and her significant other(s) to discuss their quality of life concerns openly with the health care team.
4. Teach the importance of reporting immediately any signs of swelling or red appearance of the affected arm, or new sensory changes indicative of possible lymphedema. Assessment of patients with a new onset of lymphedema includes collaborative evaluation for possible infection, injury, or obstructive problems (vein thrombosis or tumor recurrence).
5. Interventions for lymphedema include the following:
   a. Gentle range of motion exercises
   b. Not carrying shoulder bags or heavy objects on the affected arm
   c. Prompt attention to unavoidable injuries that break the skin surface (e.g., a scratch, or dry, irritated skin). Meticulous skin care is important.
   d. Elevation of the arm at rest
   e. Referral to a specialist in lymphedema care, which may include complete digestive physiotherapy (which includes a gentle massage known as **manual lymph drainage**,

and bandaging), compression garments, or mechanical decompression with a pneumatic pump

   f. Once a reduction in swelling has been achieved, the patient can be fitted for a compression sleeve and gauntlet that provides gradient pressure to the upper extremity from the hand to the shoulder.

6. With the diagnosis of recurrence, or when conventional treatment fails or is difficult, patients may seek additional help from complementary or alternative therapies. Encourage patients to share this information with the health care team and facilitate patient access to accurate information.

7. Assist patient and family to manage symptoms or complications of disease and/or treatment, such as pain and hypercalcemia.

8. Assess coping and support needs of patient and family. Assist patient and family in the terminal phase to verbalize feelings about the meaning of illness and death.

9. Referrals to supportive resources may be indicated, such as home nursing care and hospice programs, support groups, pastoral care, and professional counselors for therapeutic intervention.

Conclusion

Breast cancer presents nurses with many challenges along a continuum of prevention, early detection, treatment, and survival. The nurse must have many skills and qualities: knowledgeable about breast cancer and its ever-changing management; honest, realistic, and creative when providing support and care; skilled at symptom management; attentive to the patient's concerns within the context of the family or significant others; and ready to be involved in the professional and lay communities to promote breast health for all. Breast health care for elderly women will continue to be a particular concern as the female population ages. (See Considerations for Older Adults box). Early detection outreach to socioeconomically disadvantaged women will also be a focus of breast cancer control efforts, with potential for significant benefit in reducing the number of deaths from breast cancer. Nurses have a pivotal role in all these areas.

CONSIDERATIONS FOR OLDER ADULTS
Breast Cancers

Prevention and Detection

- Incorporate assessments of cognitive function, physical limitations and sensory deficits, and support network into baseline and follow-up assessments.
- Address knowledge, skill, and confidence in breast self-examination (BSE), knowledge and confidence in mammography and clinical breast examination (CBE), and beliefs about benefits of early detection in all patient education.
- Attempt to coordinate care with one or as few providers as possible (e.g., advocate, case manager) to enhance continuity and participation in care.
- Community-based breast cancer screening, going to where the seniors live and socialize, may be beneficial.
- Health care provider education is still needed to encourage regularly scheduled screening of elderly women. Annual screening mammography should begin at age 40 with no upper age limit for discontinuation.*

Diagnosis and Treatment[†]

- Patient involvement in decision making is important at every age.
- Age alone does not determine the type or extent of surgery or subsequent therapy.
- Care throughout the operative phase includes careful preoperative assessment and intraoperative and postoperative physiologic monitoring.
- Early *comprehensive discharge planning* must involve the patient and significant other.
- Side effects with radiation and chemotherapy may be enhanced or prolonged.
- Most trials of systemic therapy have excluded women over 70 years of age.

Rehabilitation[‡]

- Return to or maintenance of precancer level of functioning is a reasonable goal at any age.
- Psychosexual assessment and intervention should be incorporated as appropriate for all ages.
- Physical illness can impair developmental task completion.
- Depression in elderly women may be masked by physical symptoms.

Metastatic Disease

- Differential diagnosis of symptoms must differentiate normal or pathologic changes of aging from signs of metastatic disease.

Data from references 8, 11, 23, 18, and 87.
*References 6, 8, and 11.
†Reference 88.
‡Reference 46.

REVIEW QUESTIONS

✓ Case Study

Cindy is a 38-year-old married mother of three girls (ages 2, 4, and 5) who has just been diagnosed with infiltrating ductal cancer of her left breast following a mammogram and stereotactic core biopsy. She decided to have a mammogram after learning that her maternal aunt and grandmother were diagnosed with breast cancer in the past few months. Her mother was diagnosed with breast cancer 8 years ago at age 50. Her surgeon has asked you to meet with her to offer education and support in making sense of her diagnosis and expected treatment. Her medical history is significant only for starting menstruation early, at age 10, and being chronically 20 to 30 pounds overweight since high school. Her home exercise program includes walking and gardening, and she describes her diet as healthy. She works part-time from home as a science editor, which involves a lot of time on the computer.

QUESTIONS

1. Cindy is asking one question after another, including "Why did this happen to me? What did I do wrong?" Which of the following statements is most appropriate in responding to her questions?
   a. "Following a low-carb diet probably would have helped you lose weight and reduce your risk."
   b. "What did your doctor discuss with you? Did he talk with you about your genetic risk?"
   c. "The average risk for women developing breast cancer is 1 in 8. This isn't your lucky month."
   d. "Breast cancer develops from many factors that are different from one woman to another. We can discuss known risk factors, but they don't imply you did anything wrong."
2. Cindy's history reflects which of the following as a key risk factor for developing breast cancer?
   a. Extended ovulation
   b. Family history of breast cancer
   c. Daily exposure from computer
   d. Being overweight
3. Cindy's breast cancer was detected early—before any clinical symptoms—largely because of what?
   a. Screening mammogram
   b. Diagnostic mammogram
   c. Stereotactic core biopsy
   d. Clinical breast exam
4. Cindy asks about having bilateral mastectomies to prevent breast cancer recurrence even though her surgeon recommends lumpectomy followed by radiation. Which of the following may make bilateral mastectomy preferable?
   a. It is selectively used in strong family history of breast cancer.
   b. It guarantees no cancer recurrence.
   c. No chemotherapy or radiation is needed.
   d. It conserves breast tissue.
5. Cindy may undergo a sentinel lymph node biopsy (SLNB). Which of the following is true regarding SLNB?
   a. If SLNB is negative, an axillary lymph node dissection will be done.
   b. If SLNB is positive, an axillary lymph node dissection will be done.
   c. SNLB will be done in patients with large tumors larger than 5 cm.
   d. SNLB will be performed in patients with multiple tumors in the same breast.
6. What is the current "best" treatment for ductal carcinoma in situ (DCIS)?
   a. Mastectomy followed by systemic chemotherapy
   b. Lumpectomy followed by total body radiation
   c. Lumpectomy followed by aromatase inhibitors
   d. Lumpectomy, radiation, and hormonal therapy
7. Following surgery, Cindy learns that her pathology report has shown the following: Stage IIA, T1 (1.8 cm), N1 (2 of 8 lymph nodes showing cancer), M0 (no metastases), with Grade I, aneuploid, ER/PR-positive, HER2/*neu* positive features. What recommendations for adjuvant treatment would be anticipated for Cindy?
   a. External beam radiation therapy and targeted therapy
   b. MammoSite, chemotherapy, and hormonal therapy
   c. Systemic therapy, hormonal therapy, targeted therapy, and radiation if she chooses breast conservation
   d. No adjuvant therapy is indicated
8. Which of the following is the most important factor determining Cindy's prognosis after treatment?
   a. Family history
   b. ER/PR status
   c. HER2/*neu* status
   d. Lymph node status
9. Once Cindy has completed chemotherapy and targeted therapy, she is started on tamoxifen. She has been taking it for a month and calls the physician's office complaining of aching all over and bone pain. What is the most likely explanation for her symptoms?
   a. Arthritis
   b. Bone metastases
   c. Flu or virus
   d. Flare reaction to tamoxifen
10. During her first-year check-up after successful treatment for breast cancer, Cindy reports some change in sensation in the arm on the affected side of her breast cancer. She has noticed that sleeves to her blouses are tighter than the other side. You concur that indeed that arm is larger than the nonaffected arm. What can you instruct her to do to prevent further swelling?
    a. Vigorous range of motion exercises several times per day
    b. Dependent positioning of the extremity while at rest
    c. Referral to a lymphedema specialist
    d. Ice compresses daily in the morning to reduce swelling

ANSWERS

1. **D.** *Rationale:* Although it is true that a reduction in the patient's weight may have reduced one risk factor for breast cancer, to admonish her for her lack of weight reduction at this time only embarrasses her and jeopardizes the relationship between the two of you. This is a crisis for the patient; she is most likely experiencing high levels of stress and anxiety over this diagnosis. In addition, to quote the

Continued

average breast cancer risk factor of 1:8, and then to add "bad luck" as an issue is insulting. Even if it is an attempt at humor, it is in poor taste at this point. The surgeon has sent the patient to you for supportive counseling and education, and it is likely that he did not broach genetic risk factors with the patient.

2. **B.** *Rationale:* The exact role of a hormonal influence in breast cancer risk is not certain. This patient did start menarche early, at age 10. The case study does not mention whether or not the patient is still menstruating, nor does it mention whether or not she had breastfed her daughters. However, all of her children were born after the patient was 30, which is also felt to have an increased impact on breast cancer risk. Dietary fat does increase the risk of breast cancer, but has more impact in women beyond menopause. There is no clear evidence that exposure to electromagnetic fields (Cindy's computer work) has increased her risk of breast cancer. Clearly, her family history of breast cancer in her own mother (first-degree relative), the patient's own diagnosis at age 38, and multiple family members (two maternal relatives) point to a significant heredity factor for this patient's breast cancer.

3. **A.** *Rationale:* Given current ACS recommendations, and Cindy's being asymptomatic, her request of a mammogram was fortunate. She had no symptoms or abnormalities; therefore a clinical breast exam most likely would not have revealed her breast cancer. Diagnostic mammogram and stereotactic core biopsy are performed when there is a discernable suspicious lesion seen on mammogram or one palpated. In this case, screening mammogram was extremely beneficial in early detection of Cindy's breast cancer.

4. **A.** *Rationale:* No one is granted a "guarantee" of no cancer recurrence. In many areas of the United States, the preferred treatment would be for Cindy to undergo lumpectomy, followed by radiation therapy to reduce local and/or regional recurrence. Bilateral mastectomy may significantly reduce recurrence in the same or the opposite breast; but micrometastasis is a systemic process that may have already occurred, and therefore chemotherapy is often added. In Cindy's case, she is a candidate for bilateral mastectomy on the basis of either her strong family history of breast cancer alone, *or* her biopsy-proven DCIS with strong family history of breast cancer.

5. **B.** *Rationale:* SLNB refers to removal of the lymph node that is first to receive lymphatic drainage from the site of the breast cancer. This procedure is contraindicated in patients with multiple tumors in the same breast, or in patients with tumors larger than 5 cm, or those with palpable lymph nodes. If the patient indeed has a positive sentinel lymph node, or if no sentinel lymph node can be found, an axillary lymph

node dissection should be performed. If negative, it is felt the axillary lymph node dissection is not necessary.

6. **D.** *Rationale:* It is unclear whether most DCIS tumors will progress to an invasive tumor. There is a higher risk of metastasis from DCIS with larger tumors. Mastectomy has long been the treatment for DCIS, which includes a low lymph node dissection. Currently, best treatment is considered to be breast-conserving surgery followed by local radiation to reduce risk of local recurrence, and antiestrogen therapy to reduce risk of invasive disease.

7. **C.** *Rationale:* The lymph node involvement indicates that systemic chemotherapy would be beneficial for Cindy. Her ER/PR-positive status indicates that she should respond to hormonal therapy, possibly tamoxifen. However, the HER2/*neu*-positivity she expresses puts her at risk for proliferation of breast cancer cells. Targeted therapy (trastuzumab) could be of benefit.

8. **D.** *Rationale:* Tumor size and lymph node status are critical to survival. The lymph node status is the most important factor in determining disease recurrence and metastasis. Family history is a predictor of "risk for breast cancer," not prognosis following treatment. ER/PR status is a predictor of how one would respond to hormonal therapy and chemotherapy. HER2/*neu* status is a predictor of tumor growth.

9. **D.** *Rationale:* Overall, most women have tolerated tamoxifen fairly well. There have been reported side effects of osteoporosis and hot flashes occurring, with early menopause symptoms of vaginal dryness and irritation, menstrual irregularities, and decreased sexual functioning. Any hormonal therapy can cause a "flare reaction" within the first few weeks of use, which includes diffuse musculoskeletal pain and aching. Although it is possible that she can have the flu or arthritis, it is more likely due to her use of tamoxifen that she is experiencing a flare. Bone metastases are also seen as a disease progression of breast cancer, but again her achiness began within 1 month of starting tamoxifen, and therefore bone metastases should be considered second to a "tamoxifen flare."

10. **C.** *Rationale:* Lymphedema can occur any time after surgery and is affected by the extent of lymph node dissection and radiation to the axilla. Gentle (not vigorous) range of motion exercises will assist in decreasing the accumulation of fluid. The arm should be elevated as much as possible while she is asleep, rather than in a dependent position. There is no recognized evidence that ice packs will be of any benefit in managing lymphedema. A referral to a specialist who is knowledgeable in the care of lymphedema will optimally lead to access to manual lymph drainage, compression bandaging, mechanical compression, compression garment fitting, and extensive self-care education.

REFERENCES

1. Parkin DM, Bray F, Ferlay J et al: Global cancer statistics 2002, *CA Cancer J Clin* 55(2):74-108, 2005.

2. Fisher B, Costantino JP, Wickerham DL et al: Tamoxifen for the prevention of breast cancer: current status of the National Surgical Adjuvant Breast and Bowel Project P-1 study, *J Natl Cancer Inst* 97(22):1652, 2005.

3. National Cancer Institute: Clinical Trials (PDQ®). Phase III Randomized Study of Tamoxifen and Raloxifene (STAR) for the Prevention of Breast Cancer, retrieved September 25, 2006, from http://www.cancer.gov/clinicaltrials/view_clinicaltrials.aspx?cdrid=67081&version=healthprofessional.

4. National Cancer Institute: Clinical trial results. Low-fat diet may reduce risk of breast cancer relapse. Posted May 16, 2005, retrieved November 4, 2005, from http://www.cancer.gov/clinicaltrials/results/low-fat-diet0505.

5. Rossouw JE, Anderson GL, Prentice RL et al: Risks and benefits of estrogen plus progestin in healthy postmenopausal women: principal results from the Women's Health Initiative randomized controlled trial, *JAMA* 288(3):321-333, 2002.

6. American Cancer Society: *Cancer facts & figures 2005*, Atlanta, 2005, Author.

7. Jemal A, Murray T, Ward E et al: Cancer statistics, 2005, *CA Cancer J Clin* 55(1):10-30, 2005.

8. American Cancer Society: *Breast cancer facts & figures 2005-2006*, Atlanta, 2005, Author.

9. National Heart, Lung, and Blood Institute: Postmenopausal hormone therapy. Facts about menopausal hormone therapy, retrieved November 4, 2005, from http://www.nhlbi.nih.gov/health/women/pht_facts.htm.

10. Santen RJ, Mansel R: Current concepts: benign breast disorders, *N Engl J Med* 353(3):275-285, 2005.

11. American Cancer Society: *Cancer prevention & early detection facts & figures 2005*, Atlanta, 2005, Author.

12. National Comprehensive Cancer Network: Clinical practice guidelines in oncology. Breast cancer risk reduction. Version 1.2007, retrieved February 12, 2007, from http://www.nccn.org/professionals/physician_gls/PDF/breast_risk.pdf.

13. National Comprehensive Cancer Network: Clinical practice guidelines in oncology. Breast cancer screening and diagnosis guidelines. Version 1.2007, retrieved February 12, 2007, from http://www.nccn.org/professionals/physician_gls/PDF/breast-screening.pdf.

14. National Comprehensive Cancer Network: Clinical practice guidelines in oncology. Genetic/familial high-risk assessment: breast and ovarian. Version 1.2006, retrieved November 4, 2005, from http://www.nccn.org/professionals/physician_gls/PDF/genetics_screening.pdf.

15. Pisano ED, Gatsonis C, Hendrick E et al: Diagnostic performance of digital versus film mammography for breast-cancer screening, *N Engl J Med* 353(17):1773-1783, 2005.

16. U.S. Food and Drug Administration, Center for Devices and Radiological Health: Mammography: mammography quality standards act regulations, retrieved November 5, 2005, from www.fda.gov/CDRH/MAMMOGRAPHY/frmamcom2.html.

17. Nass S, Ball J, editors: *Improving breast imaging quality standards,* Washington, DC, 2005, National Academies Press. Also available at www.nap.edu/ or via www.iom.edu.

18. American College of Radiology, Breast Imaging and Intervention: ACR practice guideline for the performance of screening mammography, retrieved November 5, 2005, from www.acr.org/s_acr/bin.asp?CID=549&DID=12281&DOC=FILE.PDF.

19. US Department of Health & Human Services: *Healthy People 2010* (ed 2). *With understanding and improving health and objectives for improving health, 2 vols,* Washington, DC, 2000, U.S. Government Printing Office. Also available at www.healthypeople.gov.

20. Mammatech Corporation: The *MammaCare® personal learning system,* Gainesville, FL, Mammatech, 1995, retrieved November 5, 2005, from www.mammacare.com.

21. Mammatech Corporation: The *MammaCare® learning system for clinical breast examination,* Gainesville, FL, 1993, Mammatech, retrieved November 5, 2005, from www.mammacare.com.

22. Hoehne FM, Taylor E. Trends in breast cancer at a county hospital, *Am Surg* 71(2):159-163, 2005.

23. Mitchell J, Mathews HF, Mayne L: Differences in breast self-examination techniques between Caucasian and African American elderly women, *J Womens Health (Larchmt)* 14(6):476-484, 2005.

24. American Joint Committee on Cancer: *AJCC cancer staging manual,* ed 6, New York, 2002, Springer.

25. National Comprehensive Cancer Network: Clinical practice guidelines in oncology. Breast cancer. Version 1.2007, retrieved Febraury 12, 2007, from http://www.nccn.org/professionals/physician_gls/PDF/breast.pdf.

26. Braun S, Vogl FD, Naume B et al: A pooled analysis of bone marrow micrometastasis in breast cancer, *N Engl J Med* 353(8):793-802, 2005.

27. Boyle S: The evolution and future of breast cancer management, *Oncol Support Care Q* 2(2):14, 2005.

28. Mamounas E: Can we approach zero relapse in breast cancer? *Oncologist* 10(2):9, 2005.

29. Paik S, Shak S, Tang G et al: A multigene assay to predict recurrence of tamoxifen-treated, node-negative breast cancer, *N Engl J Med* 351: 2817-2826, 2004.

30. Fisher B, Anderson S, Bryant J et al: Twenty-year follow-up of a randomized trial comparing total mastectomy, lumpectomy, and lumpectomy plus irradiation for the treatment of invasive breast cancer, *N Engl J Med* 347(16):1233-1241, 2002.

31. Katz SJ, Lantz PM, Janz NK et al: Patient involvement in surgery treatment decisions for breast cancer, *J Clin Oncol* 23(24):5526-5533, 2005.

32. Lantz PM, Janz NK, Fagerlin A et al: Satisfaction with surgery outcomes and the decision process in a population-based sample of women with breast cancer, *Health Serv Res* 40(3):745-767, 2005.

33. Maly RC, Umezawa Y, Leake B et al: Determinants of participation in treatment decision-making by older breast cancer patients, *Breast Cancer Res Treat* 85(3):201-209, 2004.

34. Peele PB, Siminoff LA, Xu Y et al: Decreased use of adjuvant breast cancer therapy in a randomized controlled trial of a decision aid with individualized risk information, *Med Decis Making* 25(3):301-307, 2005.

35. Morrow M, Strom EA, Bassett LW et al: *Standard for breast conservation therapy in the management of invasive breast carcinoma,* Reston, Va, 2002, American College of Radiology.

36. Morrow M, Strom EA, Bassett LW et al: Standards for the management of ductal carcinoma in situ of the breast (DCIS). *CA Cancer J Clin* 52(5):256-276, 2002.

37. Parviz M, Cassel JB, Kaplan BJ et al: Breast conservation therapy rates are no different in medically indigent versus insured patients with early stage breast cancer, *J Surg Oncol* 84(2):57-62, 2003.

38. White J, Morrow M, Moughan J et al: Compliance with breast-conservation standards for patients with early-stage breast carcinoma, *Cancer* 97(4):893-904, 2003.

39. Lostumbo L, Carbine N, Wallace J et al: Prophylactic mastectomy for the prevention of breast cancer, *Cochrane Database Syst Rev,* Oct 18(4):CD002748, 2004.

40. Spear SL, Carter ME, Schwarz K: Prophylactic mastectomy: indications, options, and reconstructive alternatives, *Plast Reconstr Surg* 115(3):891-909, 2005.

41. Giuliano AE, Jones RC, Brennan M et al: Sentinel lymphadenectomy in breast cancer, *J Clin Oncol* 15(6):2345-2350, 1997.

42. Morton D: Intraoperative lymphatic mapping and sentinel lymphadenectomy: community standard care or clinical investigation? *Cancer J Sci Am* 3(6):328-330, 1997.

43. Posther KE, McCall LM, Blumencranz PW et al: Sentinel node skills verification and surgeon performance: data from a multicenter clinical trial for early-stage breast cancer, *Ann Surg* 242(4):593-599, 2005.

44. Cochrane BB, Lewis FM. Partner's adjustment to breast cancer: a critical analysis of intervention studies, *Health Psychol* 24(3):327-332, 2005.

45. Ganz PA, Desmond KA, Leedham B et al: Quality of life in long-term, disease-free survivors of breast cancer: a follow-up study, *J Natl Cancer Inst* 94(1):39-49, 2002.

46. Ganz PA, Guadagnoli E, Landrum MB et al: Breast cancer in older women: quality of life and psychosocial adjustment in the 15 months after diagnosis, *J Clin Oncol* 21(21):4027-4033, 2003.

47. Rowland JH, Desmond KA, Meyerowitz BE et al: Role of breast reconstructive surgery in physical and emotional outcomes among breast cancer survivors, *J Natl Cancer Inst* 92(17):1422-1429, 2000.

48. Al-Ghazal S, Sully L, Fallowfield L et al: The psychological impact of immediate rather than delayed breast reconstruction, *Eur J Surg Oncol* 26(1):17, 2000.

49. Cocquyt VF, Blondeel PN, Depypere HT et al: Better cosmetic results and comparable quality of life after skin-sparing mastectomy and immediate autologous breast reconstruction compared to breast conservative treatment, *Br J Plast Surg* 56(5):462-470, 2003.

50. Hultman CS, Bostwick J 3rd: Breast reconstruction following mastectomy: review of indications, methods, and outcomes, *Breast Dis* 12:113-130, 2001.

51. US Food and Drug Administration, Center for Devices and Radiological Health: Breast implants, retrieved December 14, 2005, from http://www.fda.gov/cdrh/breastimplants/index.html.

52. Hwang TG, Wilkins EG, Lowery JC et al: Implementation and evaluation of a clinical pathway for TRAM breast reconstruction, *Plast Reconstr Surg* 105(2):541-548, 2000.

53. Petit JY, Veronesi U, Luini A et al: When mastectomy becomes inevitable: the nipple-sparing approach, *The Breast* 14:527-531, 2005.

54. Gordon LG, Battistutta D, Scuffham P et al: The impact of rehabilitation support services on health-related quality of life for women with breast cancer, *Breast Cancer Res Treat* 93(3):217-226, 2005.

55. Shamley DR, Barker K, Simonite V et al: Delayed versus immediate exercises following surgery for breast cancer: a systematic review, *Breast Cancer Res Treat* 90(3):263-271, 2005.

56. Burke CC, Zabka CL, McCarver KJ et al: Patient satisfaction with 23-hour "short-stay" observation following breast cancer surgery, *Oncol Nurs Forum* 24(4):645-651, 1997.

57. Dietrick-Gallagher M, Hyzinski M: Teaching patients to care for drains after breast surgery for malignancy, *Oncol Nurs Forum* 16(2):263-265, 1989.

58. Baron RH, Fey JV, Borgen PI et al: Eighteen sensations after breast cancer surgery: a two-year comparison of sentinel lymph node biopsy and axillary lymph node dissection, *Oncol Nurs Forum* 31(4):691-698, 2004.

59. Kwekkeboom K: Postmastectomy pain syndromes, *Cancer Nurs* 19(1):37, 1996.

60. Rothemund Y, Grusser SM, Liebeskind U et al: Phantom phenomena in mastectomized patients and their relation to chronic and acute pre-mastectomy pain, *Pain* 107(1-2):140-146, 2004.

61. Perun J: Radiation therapy. In Hassey Dow K, editor: *Contemporary issues in breast cancer: A nursing perspective,* ed 2, Boston, 2004, Jones & Bartlett.

62. Dell D: Battling breast cancer: help patients make headway in the fight of their lives, *Nursing Made Incredibly Easy* 3(5):4-20, 2005.

63. Arthur DW, Morris MM, Vicini FA: Breast cancer: new radiation treatment options, *Oncology* 18(13):1621-1629, 2004.

64. Geddie P: Adjuvant therapy. In Hassey Dow K, editor: *Contemporary issues in breast cancer: a nursing perspective,* ed 2, Boston, 2004, Jones & Bartlett.

65. National Institutes of Health Consensus Development Program, National Institutes of Health Consensus Development Conference Statement: Adjuvant therapy for breast cancer, November 1-3, 2000, retrieved December 15, 2005, from http://consensus.nih.gov/2000/2000Adjuvant TherapyBreastCancer114html.htm.

66. Gartner E: Novel agents in the treatment of breast cancer, *Breast and colorectal cancer treatment for the 21st* century: what the nurse needs to know, New York, 2005, Medical Communications.

67. Reddy G: Advances in the treatment of early stage breast cancer: integrating chemotherapy as adjuvant therapy, *Clinical Breast Cancer* (February):421, 2005.

68. Gradishar W: Tamoxifen…what next? *Oncologist* 9(4):378-384, 2004.

69. Howell A, Cuzick J, Baum M et al: ATAC Trialists Group: results of the ATAC (Arimidex, Tamoxifen alone, or in combination) trial after completion of 5 years' adjuvant treatment for breast cancer, *Lancet* 365(9453):60-62, 2005.

70. Winer EP, Hudis C, Burstein HJ et al: American Society of Clinical Oncology technology assessment on the use of aromatase inhibitors as adjuvant therapy for postmenopausal women with hormone receptor-positive breast cancer: status report 2004, *J Clin Oncol* 23(3):619-629, 2005.

71. Protiere C, Viens P, Genre D et al: Patient participation in medical decision-making: a French study in adjuvant radiochemotherapy for early breast cancer, *Ann Oncol* 11(1):39-45, 2000.

72. Ravdin PM, Siminoff LA, Davis GJ et al: Computer program to assist in making decisions about adjuvant therapy for women with early breast cancer, *J Clin Oncol* 19(4):980-991, 2001.

73. Northouse L: Helping families of patients with cancer, *Oncol Nurs Forum* 32(4):743-750, 2005.

74. Hilton BA, Gustavson K: Shielding and being shielded: children's perspectives on coping with their mother's cancer and chemotherapy, *Can Oncol Nurs J* 12(4):198-217, 2002.

75. Lewis FM: Shifting perspectives: family-focused oncology nursing research, *Oncol Nurs Forum* 31(2):288-292, 2004.

76. Shands M, Lewis F, Zahlis E: Mother and child interactions about the mother's breast cancer: an interview study, *Oncol Nurs Forum* 27(1):77, 2000.

77. Cimprich B, Janz NK, Northouse L et al: Taking CHARGE: a self management program for women following breast cancer treatment, *Psychooncology* 14(9):704-717, 2005.

78. Manne SL, Ostroff JS, Winkel G et al: Couple-focused group intervention for women with early stage breast cancer, *J Consult Clin Psychol* 73(4):634-646, 2005.

79. Morgan PD, Fogel J, Rose L et al: African American couples merging strengths to successfully cope with breast cancer, *Oncol Nurs Forum* 32(5):979-987, 2005.

80. Geddie P: Acute side effect management. In Hassey Dow K, editor: *Contemporary issues in breast cancer: A nursing perspective,* ed 2, Boston, 2004, Jones & Bartlett.

81. Lenhart C: Relative dose intensity: improving cancer treatment and outcomes, *Oncol Nurs Forum* 32(4):757-764, 2005.

82. Gaston-Johansson F, Lachica EM, Fall-Dickson JM et al: Psychological distress, fatigue, burden of care, and quality of life in primary caregivers of patients with breast cancer undergoing autologous bone marrow transplantation, *Oncol Nurs Forum* 31(6):1161-1169, 2004.

83. Farquhar C, Marjoribanks J, Basser R et al: High dose chemotherapy and autologous bone marrow or stem cell transplantation versus conventional chemotherapy for women with metastatic breast cancer, *Cochrane Database Syst Rev* Jul 20(3):CD003142, 2005.

84. Peters WP, Rosner GL, Vredenburgh JJ et al: Prospective, randomized comparison of high-dose chemotherapy with stem-cell support versus intermediate-dose chemotherapy after surgery and adjuvant chemotherapy in women with high-risk primary breast cancer: a report of CALGB 9082, SWOG 9114, and NCIC MA-13, *J Clin Oncol* 23(10):2191-2200, 2005.

85. McWayne J, Heiney SP: Psychologic and social sequelae of secondary lymphedema: a review, *Cancer* 104(3):457-466, 2005.

86. Hillner BE, Ingle JN, Chlebowski RT et al: American Society of Clinical Oncology 2003 update on the role of bisphosphonates and bone health issues in women with breast cancer, *J Clin Oncol* 21(21):4042-4057, 2003.

87. Wood RY, Duffy ME, Morris SJ et al: The effect of an educational intervention on promoting breast self-examination in older African American and Caucasian women, *Oncol Nurs Forum* 29(7):1081-1090, 2002.

88. Maly RC, Umezawa Y, Leake B et al: Mental health outcomes in older women with breast cancer: impact of perceived family support and adjustment, *Psychooncology* 14(7):535-545, 2005.

CHAPTER 8

Colorectal Cancers

Mary E. Murphy

Colorectal cancer is the third most common malignant tumor in the United States, making up 11% of all cancers and second only to lung cancer in its incidence and mortality. An estimated 145,290 new cases develop each year, with an annual death rate of 56,290 projected in the United States in 2005, accounting for 10% of all cancer deaths. Colorectal cancer, considered separately in both sexes, accounts for the third most common death among men and women.[1-3]

Epidemiology

Colorectal cancer affects both genders, 10% in both male and female, with the incidence increasing significantly in persons over age 50. The incidence rate is 50 times higher in people over the ages of 60 to 79 than those aged 40 years. The disease occurs most frequently in the industrialized countries of North America, Eastern and Western Europe, the Scandinavian countries, New Zealand, and Australia. Individuals from low-incidence countries who move to Western countries develop colorectal cancer at the same rate as the Western population. The incidence varies among race and ethnicity. African Americans, Indians, Hawaiians, and Mexicans have the highest incidence and mortality.[1-5]

Etiology and Risk Factors

The cause of colorectal cancer is unknown, but recent research indicates that diet, age, genetics, environmental, and other predisposing factors such as bowel disorders may play an important role in its development.[1-5]

DIET

The relationship between diet and colorectal cancer remains under investigation, but evidence shows that individuals with diets low in animal fats and high in fiber demonstrate a significantly lower incidence of the disease. Research indicates that fats and meat products may alter the concentration of normal body products such as cholesterol and fecal bile salts and also may change the normal intestinal flora of the bowel. This process may serve as a cancer promoter by damaging the colonic mucosa and increasing the proliferative activity of the colonic epithelium.[6-8]

Reduced dietary fiber may also serve as a promoter of the carcinogenic process by increasing the amount of contact time that the carcinogenic substance has with colonic mucosa, therefore increasing the potential for mutagenic changes in the bowel wall. Increased alcohol and caffeine intake has also been indicated to increase risk of colorectal cancers, but research results have been inconsistent.

Other dietary factors that serve as promoters of the carcinogenic process include genotoxic carcinogens such as charbroiled meats, fish, and fried foods. Dietary deficiencies of vitamins A,

C, and E, selenium, and calcium have also been investigated; dietary recommendations may follow in the future. A recent study demonstrates that dietary calcium and calcium supplements can reduce a women's risk of colorectal cancer. The 2005 U.S. Department of Agriculture (USDA) Food Guide Pyramid and the Dietary Guidelines for Americans provide guidelines. Additional recommendations can be found in Box 8-1.[6-8]

GENETIC FACTORS

Genetic abnormalities and traits represent a new area of scientific technology that may help identify individuals at risk. Progressive genetic changes trigger a multistep process in which chromosomal and oncogenic changes occur and result in colorectal epithelium mutations forming malignant tumors in the colon.

Genetics plays a role in the predisposition to colorectal cancer. The National Cancer Institute (NCI) estimates 5% to 6% of all annual cases of colorectal cancer are related to some type of genetic mutation. Persons with first-degree relatives who have colorectal cancer have a threefold risk of having the disease themselves. Two major genetic syndromes exist, familial adenomatous polyposis (FAP) and hereditary nonpolyposis colorectal cancer (HNPCC), as well as rare genetic syndromes such as Gardner's Syndrome, Turcot's Syndrome, and Peutz-Jeghers. Both FAP and HNPCC are autosomal dominant syndromes and carry specific risk factors related to family history. The Amsterdam

---

BOX 8-1 | **Nutrition Guidelines of the American Cancer Society (Preventing Colorectal Cancer)**

In addition to screening, counsel your patients to do the following:
1. Eat a healthy diet
   - Eat at least 5 servings of fruits and vegetables a day
   - Replace red meat with chicken, fish, nuts, and legumes
   - Take multivitamins containing 0.4 mg of folic acid
   - Limit alcohol intake to 2 drinks/day or less for men and 1 drink/day or less for women
2. Participate in moderate physical activity for at least 30 minutes each day
   - Moderate activity includes brisk walking, dancing, and gardening.
   - Start slowly, and build up to 30 minutes a day.
3. Maintain a healthy weight.
4. Avoid smoking.

Modifying these behaviors will also reduce the risk of other cancers, cardiovascular disease, osteoporosis, and diabetes.

From American Cancer Society: Colorectal prevention, 2003, No. 2431.00.

Criteria-II and the Bethesda Criteria are used to identify risks and set screening recommendations.[4,5]

OTHER PREDISPOSING FACTORS

Other predisposing factors include ulcerative colitis and Crohn's disease. These inflammatory bowel disorders are associated with dysplasia and associated malignant lesions. Potential for the malignant process is correlated to the disease's duration. In addition to inflammatory bowel disease, polyposis adenomas are the most common bowel polyps, accounting for 80% of all types of bowel polyps. These polyps increase their malignant potential as they grow larger and demonstrate cellular changes. This process takes 10 to 15 years from the time of diagnosis. Villous adenomas are another type of polyp that has been associated with increased malignancy and high fatality. These polyps produce excessive mucus and lead to severe fluid and electrolyte disorders. Other relationships have been correlated with a history of breast, endometrial, and ovarian cancer. Aging, itself, is listed as a risk factor, with over 90% of all patients diagnosed after the age of 50.[4,5]

Prevention, Screening, and Detection

The American Cancer Society (ACS) recommends specific protocols for the screening and prevention of colorectal cancers. The ACS recommendations for colon cancer screening for an asymptomatic person includes an annual digital rectal examination and an **annual fecal occult blood test (FOBT)** for persons over age 50. **Proctosigmoidoscopy** should be done every 5 years and **colonoscopy** every 10 years. Table 8-1 shows complete ACS guidelines. Persons at high risk may need screening at an earlier age and more frequently than the general population.

TABLE 8-1   **American Cancer Society Guidelines for Screening and Surveillance for the Early Detection of Colorectal Adenomas and Cancer—Women and Men at Increased Risk or at High Risk**

RISK CATEGORY	AGE TO BEGIN	RECOMMENDATION	COMMENT
Increased Risk			
Persons with a single, small (<1 cm) adenoma	3-6 years after the initial polypectomy	Colonoscopy*	If the exam is normal, the patient can be screened thereafter per average risk guidelines.
Persons with a large (1+ cm) adenoma, multiple adenomas, or adenomas with high-grade dysplasia or villous change	Within 3 years after the initial polypectomy	Colonoscopy*	If normal, repeat examination in 3 years; if normal then, the patient can be screened thereafter per average risk guidelines.
Personal history of curative-intent resection of colorectal cancer	Within 1 year after cancer resection	Colonoscopy*	If normal, repeat examination in 3 years; if that is normal, repeat examination every 5 years thereafter.
Either colorectal cancer or adenomatous polyps in any first-degree relative before age 60, or in two or more first-degree relatives at any age (if not a hereditary syndrome)	Age 40, or 10 years before the youngest case in the immediate family	Colonoscopy*	Every 5-10 years. Colorectal cancer in relatives more distant than first-degree does not increase risk substantially above the average risk group.
High Risk			
Family history of familial adenomatous polyposis (FAP)	Puberty	Early surveillance with endoscopy, and counseling to consider genetic testing	If the genetic test is positive, colectomy is indicated. These patients are best referred to a center with experience in the management of FAP.
Family history of hereditary nonpolyposis colon cancer (HNPCC)	Age 21	Colonoscopy and counseling to consider genetic testing	If the genetic test is positive, or if the patient has not had genetic testing, screen every 1-2 years until age 40, then annually. These patients are best referred to a center with experience in the management of HNPCC.
Inflammatory bowel disease Chronic ulcerative colitis Crohn's disease	Cancer risk begins to be significant 8 years after the onset of pancolitis, or 12-15 years after the onset of left-sided colitis.	Colonoscopy with biopsies for dysplasia.	Every 1-2 years. These patients are best referred to a center with experience in the surveillance and management of inflammatory bowel disease.

*If colonoscopy is unavailable, not feasible, or not desired by the patient, double contrast barium enema alone or the combination of flexible sigmoidoscopy and double contrast barium enema are acceptable alternatives. Adding flexible sigmoidoscopy to DCBE may provide a more comprehensive diagnostic evaluation than DCBE alone in finding significant lesions. A supplementary DCBE may be needed if a colonoscopic exam fails to reach the cecum, and a supplementary colonoscopy may be needed if a DCBE identifies a possible lesion, or does not adequately visualize the entire colorectum.

From Smith RA, Cokkinides V, von Eschenbach AC et al: American Cancer Society Guidelines for the Early Detection of Cancer, *CA Cancer J Clin* 52:8–22: 2002

Because many tumors are found in the lower rectum, abdominal and rectal examinations should be performed at the time of a routine physical examination. **Digital rectal examination (DRE)** should be performed yearly to examine for polyps and cancers of the lower rectum (up to 7 cm) and the anal verge. This should also be done before "scopy" examination or before a barium enema.

The FOBT is an effective and inexpensive screening tool to examine for hidden blood. False-negative and false-positive results may occur for a variety of reasons. The primary cause may be inadequate instruction on sample collection or poor compliance with specific directions, as well as the fact that 50% of most polyps are not actively bleeding at the time of sample collection. Instructions should include various dietary restrictions, medications to avoid during collection, and specific collection procedures.

All individuals should be on a red meat–free, high-residue diet for 3 days before specimen collection. Red meats may contain nonhuman hemoglobin, which yields false-positive tests. Foods with peroxidase activity such as citrus juices, tomatoes, turnips, beets, radishes, cherries, and horseradish should be eliminated, because their consumption will yield a false-positive test. High-residue diets are recommended to encourage bleeding from small colonic lesions.

Medication ingestion may also yield false-negative or false-positive tests. Vitamin C and antacids produce false-negative results even in the presence of active bleeding. Iron, aspirin, cimetidine, cytochromes, halogens, and antiinflammatory medications are known for false-positive results and should be avoided for 7 days before testing. Pathologic gastrointestinal conditions such as diverticulosis and hemorrhoids, among others, have yielded false-positive tests because of an alternate bleeding source.

Sample collection also has a direct impact on test results. Specimens obtained from toilet water may be diluted, resulting in fecal blood loss from the sample, or may be affected by halogens such as chlorine, which may be present in the water. Stool samples either too dry or too wet may also alter results. Testing should be done within 7 days of sample collection, and the sample should not be rehydrated. Newer fecal occult tests with a guaiac base are now available. Hemoccult II, Hemoccult Sensa, and HemeSelect are immunochemical tests that demonstrate improved sensitivity. FOBT collection materials are accessible in physicians' offices, clinics, and even grocery stores. Patients must be reminded that they should call about any positive test reading and that a false-positive result is possible if instructions are not followed completely.[9-11]

A **double-contrast barium enema** should be performed every 5 to 10 years and complement a colonoscopy exam. Barium enemas may yield false readings between 6% and 61% of the time, particularly with smaller lesions; also, they increase costs and offer only evaluation, no possibility of therapeutic intervention if a polyp is identified.

Sigmoidoscopy is also an appropriate method of screening for cancerous lesions of the colon and rectum. Approximately 50% to 65% of all colorectal cancers can be found within the range of this particular instrument (25 cm, or 10 inches). A flexible fiberoptic sigmoidoscope is available that can reach to the splenic flexure (60 cm, or 24 inches). This instrument provides for increased visibility and patient comfort, and the exam should be performed at least every 5 years. Colonoscopy provides complete visualization of the entire colon and is recommended by the ACS as a preventive screening every 10 years. The colonoscopy is considered the most accurate measure but increases cost,

requires increased preparation and time missed from work, and occasionally allows lesions to go undetected if the entire colon cannot visualized. Screening controversies continue to exist because of increased cost per yield of positive cases. Despite these issues, screening remains underutilized among all age and ethnic groups. Emerging technologies to assist with screening include computerized tomographic (CT) colonography (virtual colonoscopy), molecular screening of stool, DNA and RNA protein marker evaluation, and M2A capsule endoscopic exams (ingestible capsules which hold miniature video cameras).[10,12]

Other Preventive Methods

Data are inconsistent regarding use of vitamins, A, C, and E, calcium, and beta carotene. A positive role is hoped to be demonstrated for the use of aspirin and nonsteroidal antiinflammatory drugs (NSAIDs) in the areas of prevention and mortality reduction, but variances in doses and types of NSAIDS require further research. Other areas of consideration include prophylactic surgery methods for high-risk individuals and dietary adjustments related to red meat intake. Fiber and food additives remain under investigation. Other methods require ongoing research for evaluation of their potential impact on prevention.

Table 8-1 summarizes the ACS guidelines for early detection. Patients with family histories or those who have undergone curative surgery will require strict guidelines.[11,12]

Classification

Over 35% of lesions occur in the sigmoid colon. A small percentage may occur as a second primary site (Fig. 8-1).

Most bowel cancers are adenocarcinomas (98%) and are moderately- to well-differentiated cancers. Additional forms of colorectal cancers include epithelioma, squamous cell carcinoma, sarcoma, lymphoma, leiomyosarcoma, and melanoma. Cancer of the anus is rare, but recent research has shown an increase in men with a history of homosexual and bisexual activity, or a

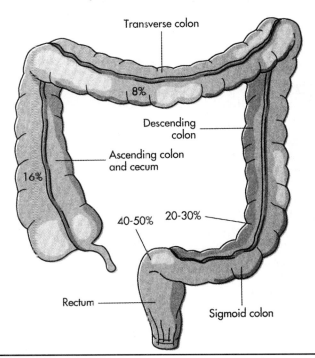

FIG. 8-1   Incidence of cancer in various segments of the colon and rectum. (From Phipps WJ, Sands JK, Marek JF: *Medical surgical nursing: concepts and clinical practice*, St. Louis, 1999, Mosby.)

history of anal condylomata acuminata. Other anal cancers include squamous cell, basal cell, and melanomas.

Clinical Features

General signs and symptoms for all colorectal cancers include a change in bowel habits, blood in the stool, abdominal pain, anorexia, flatulence, and indigestion (Clinical Features of Colorectal Cancer box). Late symptoms include loss of energy, weight loss, and a decline in general health. Symptoms may vary greatly according to size, location, tumor type, and the individual. Often these symptoms are confused with other bowel syndromes. Specific variances are seen between the right and left colon, and the rectum. Patients with right-sided lesions do not display changes in bowel habits because of the liquid nature of the stool. Specific symptoms include a dull, vague abdominal pain radiating from abdomen to back. These tumors present as palpable masses in the right lower quadrant. Dark or mahogany-red blood may be present in the stool. Anemia leads to weakness and malaise, and indigestion and weight loss often occur.

In contrast, patients with left-sided lesions usually display a change in bowel habits, because the area affected is the sigmoid colon and the rectum. Symptoms include cramps, gas pains, a decrease in the caliber of stool, bright red bleeding, constipation, and a feeling of rectal pressure or incomplete evacuation of stool. Obstruction may occur and lead to emergency surgery. Patients with transverse colon tumors have palpable masses, obstruction, a change in bowel habits, and bloody stools. Those with rectal cancers may display similar symptoms, such as changes in bowel habits, bright red bleeding, tenesmus, and a late symptom of severe pain in the groin, the labia, the scrotum, the legs, or the penis. Unfortunately, colorectal cancer may be advanced before symptoms occur. Pain may only be the last symptom to appear, and metastasis may be present before treatment is sought.[13-17]

Diagnosis

Persons at high risk for disease or who have symptoms and are guaiac positive require additional diagnostic testing (Box 8-2). A barium enema provides a clear picture of the large intestine and is useful for detecting smaller tumors. Colonoscopy may be performed at this time, especially if surgery is indicated. This examination provides increased visualization and the ability to biopsy lesions. Potentially metastatic lesions are evaluated using chest x-ray films and liver, bone, and other scans including CT scan, magnetic resonance imaging (MRI), positron emission tomography (PET), and rectal ultrasound. Laboratory work includes a complete blood count (CBC), serum aspartate aminotransferase (AST), serum glutamic-oxaloacetic transaminase (SGOT), lactate dehydrogenase (LDH), alkaline phosphatase (ALP), and blood urea nitrogen (BUN). Other analyses may examine *carcinoembryonic antigen* (CEA), lipid-associated sialic acid (LASA), CA19-9, DNA ploidy, p53, and K-*ras*. This biologic marker is elevated in later stages of colorectal cancer and may have prognostic value at diagnosis or recurrence of disease. Diagnosis is confirmed by tissue biopsy from the suspected site. Additional diagnostic evaluation includes a variety of procedures and varies with the tumor's staging or suspected metastasis.[2,10]

Staging

The most widely used and now replaced method for colorectal surgery is the *Duke's classification* or some modification from its original form, which was developed in 1932. The Duke's system classifies tumors into four major categories based on the degree and depth of tumor involvement and the presence of lymph nodes. Subcategories were developed by Astler and Collier in 1954 in an attempt to delineate the importance of tumor wall penetration.

The variances and minor modifications of various systems of colorectal staging resulted in the promotion of the tumor-node-metastasis system, or **TNM system,** by the Committee of the International Union Against Cancer (UICC). Table 8-2 demonstrates the TNM system.[18] Unlike other tumors, size is not a major factor. The depth of tumor penetration is the best indicator of prognosis. Figure 8-2 shows growth of a colon polyp to invasion stage.

Metastasis

Most colorectal cancers spread by direct extension and penetration into layers of the bowel. Local invasion occurs to surrounding organs. Lymph node involvement and invasion into the vascular bed allow for disseminated disease. Lymphatic disease is present in 37% of all diagnosed cases. Nodal chains follow the

---

Clinical Features *of* Colorectal Cancer

General: Change in bowel habits or shape, color, or size of stool; blood in stool; abdominal pain; anorexia; flatulence; indigestion; alterations in constipation or diarrhea; feeling of incomplete evacuation (tenesmus)

Late symptoms: Weight loss, fatigue, decline in general health, jaundice

Right-sided lesions: Dull, vague abdominal pain radiating to the back, dark red or mahogany-red blood in stool, weakness, anemia, malaise, indigestion, weight loss, liquid stool

Left-sided lesions: Change in bowel habits—cramps, gas pains, decrease in caliber of stool, bright red bleeding, constipation, rectal pressure, incomplete evacuation of stool, abdominal pain

Transverse colon: Palpable masses, obstruction, changes in bowel habits, bloody stools

Rectal: Changes in bowel habits; bright red bleeding; tenesmus; pain in groin, labia, scrotum, legs, or penis; constipation

---

BOX 8-2   Diagnostic Work-Up for Colorectal Cancer

Barium enema
Colonoscopy
Chest x-ray
CT/MRI/PET* scan
Stool for occult blood
Liver scan
Bone scan
CBC, AST (SGOT), LDH, ALP, BUN*
Carcinoembryonic antigen (CEA)
Rectal ultrasound

*See text for abbreviations.

TABLE 8-2   Colon Cancer Staging

STAGE	DESCRIPTION

T = Primary Tumor

TX	Primary tumor cannot be assessed
T0	No evidence of primary tumor
Tis	Carcinoma in situ: intraepithelial or invasion of lamina propria*
T1	Tumor invades submucosa
T2	Tumor invades muscularis propria
T3	Tumor invades through muscularis propria into subserosa or into nonperitonealized pericolic or perirectal tissues
T4	Tumor directly invades other organs or structures, and/or perforates visceral peritoneum**, ***

*Note: Tis includes cancer cells confined within the glandular basement membrane (intraepithelial) or lamina propria (intramucosal) with no extension through the muscularis mucosae into the submocusa.

**Note: Direct invasion in T4 includes invasion of other segments of the colorectum by way of the serosa; for example, invasion of the sigmoid colon by a carcinoma of the cecum.

***Note: Tumor that is adherent to other organs or structures, macroscopically, is classified T4. However, if no tumor is present in the adhesion, microscopically, the classification should be pT3. The V and L subsaging should be used to identify the presence or absence of vascular or lymphatic invasion.

N = Regional Lymph Nodes

NX	Regional lymph nodes cannot be assessed
N0	No regional lymph node metastasis
N1	Metastasis in 1 to 3 regional lymph nodes
N2	Metastasis in 4 or more regional lymph nodes

Note: A tumor module in the pericolorectal adipose tissue of a primary carcinoma without histological evidence of residual lymph node in the nodule is classified in the pN category as a regional lymph node metastasis if the nodule has the form and smooth contour of a lymph node. If the nodule has an irregular contour, it should be classified in the T category and also coded as V1 (microscopic venous invasion) or as V2 (if it was grossly evident), because there is a strong likelihood that it represents venous invasion.

M = Distant Metastasis

MX	Presence of distant metastasis cannot be assessed
M0	No distant metastasis
M1	Distant metastasis

Stage Grouping

0	Tis	N0	M0
I	T1	N0	M0
	T2	N0	M0
II	T3	N0	M0
	T4	N0	M0
III	Any T	N1	M0
	Any T	N2	M0
	Any T	N3	M0
IV	Any T	Any N	M1

*Dukes B is a composite of better (T3 N0 M0) and worse (T4 N0 M0) prognostic groups, as is Dukes C (Any T N1 M0 and Any T N2 M0). MAC is the modified Astler-Coller classification.

G = Histopathologic Grade

GX	Grade cannot be assessed
G1	Well-differentiated
G2	Moderately well-differentiated
G3	Poorly differentiated
G4	Undifferentiated

R = Residual Tumor

R0	Complete resection, margins histologically negative, no residual tumor left after resection
R1	Incomplete resection, margins histologically involved, microscopic tomor remains after resection of gross disease
R2	Incomplete resection, margins involved or gross disease remains after resection

From Greene FL, Page DL, Fleming ID et al, editors: American Joint Committee on Cancer (AJCC) cancer staging handbook, ed 6, New York, 2002, Springer.

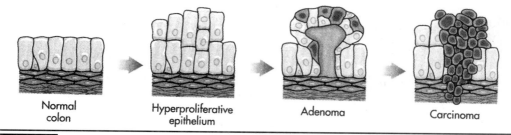

Normal colon   Hyperproliferative epithelium   Adenoma   Carcinoma

FIG. 8-2   The progression to malignancy in bowel cancer. (From Phipps WJ, Sands JK, Marek JF: *Medical surgical nursing: concepts and clinical practice*, St Louis, 1999, Mosby.)

DISEASE-RELATED COMPLICATIONS
Colorectal Cancer

- Bowel perforation
- Obstruction of surrounding genitourinary organs
- Hemorrhage
- Liver failure
- Distant-site metastasis: brain, bone, lung, adrenal glands

pathway of the superior and mesenteric arteries. Colon cancer and cancer of the upper half of the rectum spread by direct extension to the liver. Cancer of the lower half of the rectum spreads to the portal veins and the inferior vena cava. Venous invasion permits distant metastasis, with the liver and the lung as the most common sites. Additional sites include the brain, bone, and the adrenal glands. Anal cancers spread directly into local muscles and to genitourinary organs.

Metastasis involves progressive proliferation and development of vasculature (angiogenesis) and penetration through blood vessels. Metastatic spread at diagnosis significantly alters prognosis and treatment modalities. See Disease-Related Complications box for a summary of complications of colorectal cancer.[19-21]

LIVER METASTASIS

Of all patients diagnosed with colorectal cancer, 25% will have liver metastasis at the time of their diagnosis. As many as 70% will display metastatic disease as the disease progresses. Methods to treat metastatic liver cancer include surgical resection, cryosurgery, regional infusion therapy, radiofrequency ablation (RFA), selective internal radiation therapy, ethanol acid injection, and chemoembolization. Each procedure has specific eligibility criteria based on the extensiveness of the metastatic disease. Risks and benefits vary. To date, no one specific treatment has been documented to successfully manage liver metastasis.[22,23]

Treatment Modalities

SURGERY

Local management can be performed by polyp excision during sigmoidoscopy or colonoscopy. Follow-up and repeated exam are based on the pathology. Other local procedures include laparoscopic colectomy, which is still considered investigational and is part of National Cancer Institute (NCI) clinical trials; this laparoscopic procedure allows for removal of cancerous polyps.[16,22]

Colon resection with disease-free margins remains the surgical goal. Tumor and associated blood vessels are resected en bloc

with the vascular and lymphatic structures to prevent seeding of malignant cells. A biopsy of the liver and regional lymph nodes (sentinel lymph node biopsy) is taken at the time of surgery to evaluate the extent of disease. Extensive procedures may be needed to attain the goal of reanastomosis and return to normal bowel function. Tumor size, tumor location, and additional metastases determine the type and the extent of surgery. Three major surgeries performed for colorectal cancer are *colon resection with reanastomosis, colostomy* (temporary or permanent), and *abdominoperineal resection* (APR) (Fig. 8-3). Table 8-3 outlines site-specific surgeries that may be done for various portions of the colon and rectum.

Localized tumors of the rectum can now be treated with a sphincter-sparing procedure using a reconstructed pouch. Anastomotic stapler devices have allowed greater ease of anostomosis in midrectal tumors and spared patients abdominoperineal resections. Radiolabeled monoclonal antibodies may be given intraoperatively to identify occult disease. Smaller tumors have been removed through colonoscope.

Each case must be evaluated individually to meet specific patient needs. Age, nutritional status, metastases, comorbidities, and complications such as perforation and obstruction may alter the surgical course. Additional surgical modalities may be required for palliation even when cure is not possible.[22,23]

Preoperative Teaching. Patient teaching and preoperative counseling are essential elements of nursing care for the patients preparing for colorectal surgery. Many patients will have already had several diagnostic and laboratory tests in an outpatient setting before they reach the hospital. Often they are aware of their diagnosis but may be in the stage of denial or disbelief. Patients and their families may be anxious or even angry at the diagnosis and will require additional attention and reinforcement of preoperative and postoperative teaching.

Teaching begins with preparation of the colon for surgery. Most regimens include 2 or 3 days of a liquid diet, a combination of laxatives and enemas, and oral antibiotics to sterilize the bowel before surgery. Antibiotics suppress both anaerobic and aerobic colonic organisms and reduce septic complications after surgery. Bowel preparations differ; patients with bowel obstructions do not receive the usual bowel preparation.

The nurse must provide support to an already anxious patient by explaining the rationale for the bowel preparation regimen. Assessment of the patient's tolerance of laxatives and enemas, including the side effects of nausea, vomiting, abdominal discomfort, excessive diarrhea, and the symptoms of electrolyte imbalance, is essential. Elderly and debilitated patients are at the greatest risk for discomfort and complications.

Preoperative Care. Preoperative teaching should include a review of the patient's past experience with surgery. A review of

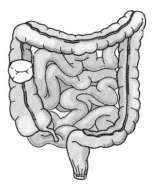

The **ascending colostomy** is done for right-sided tumors.

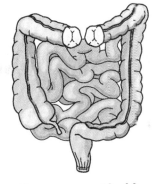

The **transverse (double-barreled) colostomy** is often used in such emergencies as intestinal obstruction or perforation because it can be created quickly. There are two stomas. The proximal one, closest to the small intestine, drains feces. The distal stoma drains mucus. Usually temporary.

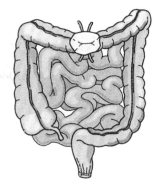

The **transverse loop colostomy** has two openings in the transverse colon, but one stoma. Usually temporary.

Descending colostomy

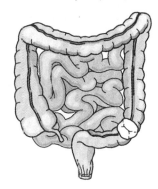

Sigmoid colostomy

FIG. 8-3   Types of colostomies. (From Phipps WJ, Sands JK, Marek JF: *Medical surgical nursing: concepts and clinical practice*, St Louis, 1999, Mosby.)

preoperative routine is included: medications, intravenous lines, recovery room procedures, and placement of a Foley catheter, nasogastric tube, and abdominal dressings. Postoperative exercises, coughing and deep breathing, wound splinting, and leg exercises should be reviewed and practiced. Concerns about pain medication and diet restrictions should be addressed. A basic anatomic review will be helpful in understanding the surgical procedure and possible colostomy placement.

Psychosocial issues and concerns must be addressed and support systems identified. A review of past coping mechanisms allows the individual to evaluate strengths and weaknesses. Ample time to discuss fears and concerns must be permitted to evaluate the dynamics of interpersonal relationships between patients and their support systems. Good preoperative assessment allows for more effective intervention postoperatively.

If a colostomy is performed, a referral to an enterostomal therapist should be made as soon as possible. Preoperative teaching should review the type of surgery, a description of an ostomy, various pouching methods available, and marking of the stoma site. Marking the stoma site is important to eliminate the possibility of future skin problems and difficult pouch applications. Stoma placement should avoid the waistline, folds, scars, and the location of the upcoming abdominal incision. The patient should be able to see and reach the pouch easily. The stoma site will be placed through the rectus abdominis muscle, which runs vertically through the abdomen. Approximately 3 inches (7.5 cm) of skin will be necessary to provide adequate pouch placement. Various positions should be considered before marking the stoma. The stoma should be visualized in sitting, standing, and lying

positions. The site is usually below the umbilicus and at the infraumbilical bulge. The stoma site is then marked with a dye such as methylene blue or gentian violet. Marking the stoma validates the reality of the ostomy. Documentation of the patient's and family's reaction is important to identify future emotional needs.

POSTOPERATIVE CARE

Care during the postoperative period focuses on meeting the patient's physical and metabolic needs. Observing the patient for initial complications includes assessment of vital signs and lung and bowel sounds. The incision is inspected for drainage or bleeding and approximation. The nasogastric tube and Foley catheter are monitored for amount, color, and consistency of drainage, and patency. Accurate record of intake and output is necessary to assure electrolyte balance. The stoma site is observed at each shift for color and size. A postoperative pouch usually covers the stoma, allowing for easy visibility. The stoma should appear pink and moist. If necrosis or ischemia are present, the stoma will appear blue, black, or dusky in appearance, and should be reported at once since it indicates stoma death. Drainage from the stoma should be scant and blood-tinged. A strict postoperative routine of coughing, deep-breathing exercises, early ambulation, and adequate pain control limits potential complications.

Postoperative complications include infection, paralytic ileus, pulmonary complications, anastomotic leak, urinary problems, stoma retraction, and prolapse (Box 8-5). Fevers may indicate infection, respiratory difficulty, urinary infections, or thrombophlebitis. Elderly patients with preexisting medical illness such as diabetes and lung disease are at greatest risk.

TABLE 8-3	Major Surgeries for Colorectal Cancer	
STAGE	DESCRIPTION	TREATMENT OPTIONS
0	Stage 0 colon cancer is the most superficial of all the lesions and is limited to the mucosa within walls of the lamina propia. Because of its superficial nature, the surgical procedure may be limited.	Local excision or simple polypectomy with clear margins Colon resection for larger lesions not amenable to local excision
I	Stage I (old staging: Dukes' A or Modified Astler-Coller A and B1) Because of its localized nature, stage I has a high cure rate.	Wide surgical resection and anastomosis
II	Stage II (old staging: Dukes' B or Modified Astler-Coller B2 and B3)	Wide surgical resection and anastomosis Following surgery, patients should be considered for entry into carefully controlled clinical trials evaluating the use of systemic or regional chemotherapy, radiation therapy, or biologic modifier
III	Stage III (old staging: Dukes' C or Modified Astler-Coller C1-C3) Stage III colon cancer denotes lymph node involvement. Studies have indicated that the number of nodes involved affects prognosis; patients with 1 to 3 involved nodes have a significantly better chance than those with 4 or more involved nodes.	Wide surgical resection and anastomosis For patients who are not candidates for clinical trials, postoperative chemotherapy via 5-FU, leucovorin for 6 months Eligible patients should be considered for entry into carefully controlled clinical trials of various postoperative chemotherapy regimens, including oxaliplatin/irinotecan chemotherapy with or without targeted agents and postoperative radiation
IV	Stage IV (old staging: Modified Astler-Coller D) and recurrent colon cancer Stage IV colon cancer denotes distant metastatic disease. Treatment of recurrent colon cancer sites or recurrent disease demonstrable by physical examination and/or radiographic studies by standard radiographic procedures; radioimmunoscintography may add clinical information affect management.	Surgical resection of locally recurrent cancer. Surgical resection and/or anastomosis or bypass of obstructing or bleeding primary lesions in metastatic cases Resection of liver metastases in selected metastatic patients (5-year cure rate for reoccurrence of solitary or combination metastases exceeds 20%) or ablation in selected patients Resection of isolated pulmonary or ovarian metastases in selected patients Palliative radiation therapy Palliative chemotherapy Surgical resection of isolated metastases (liver, lung, ovaries) Clinical trials evaluating new drugs and biologic therapy Clinical trials comparing various chemotherapy regimens or biologic therapy, or combination
Locally recurrent colon cancer		Locally recurrent colon cancer, such as a suture line recurrence, may be resectable.

Other drug combinations described in this section:
1. AIO regimen (folic acid, 5-FU, irinotecan)
2. Douillard regimen (folic acid, 5-FU, irinotecan)
3. FOLFOX-4 regimen (oxaliplatin, leucovorin, 5-FU)
4. FOLFOX-6 regimen (oxaliplatin, leucovorin, 5-FU)
5. FOLFIRI regimen (folic acid, 5-FU, irinotecan)
6. IFL (or Saltz) regimen (irinotecan, 5-FU, leucovorin)

DISEASE-RELATED COMPLICATIONS
Bowel Surgery

- Infection (wound, urinary, lung)
- Thrombophlebitis
- Paralytic ileus
- Pulmonary embolus
- Hemorrhage
- Anastomotic leaks

Anastomotic leaks are more common in lower resections and often result in fistula formation. Skin care and adequate nutrition are essential components of proper wound healing. Paralytic ileus results from the surgical manipulation of the bowels in surgery and can last up to 14 days or more. Increased abdominal girth, distention, nausea, and vomiting are classic signs of an ileus. Decompression of the bowel with a nasogastric tube, maintenance of the nothing-by-mouth (NPO) status, and increased activity usually result in a return to normal bowel function.

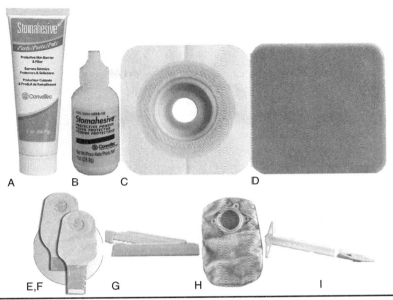

A   B   C   D

E,F   G   H   I

FIG. 8-4 **A**, Stomahesive® Paste; **B**, Stomahesive® Protective Powder; **C**, SUR-FIT Natura® Durahesive® Moldable Convex Skin Barrier with Flange; **D**, Stomahesive® Skin Barrier; **E**, Drainable Pouch with Filter (needs tail clip [G]); **F**, Drainable Pouch with Filter with InvisiClose® Tail Closure System; **G**, Tail clip; **H**, SUR-FIT Natura® Closed-End Pouch; **I**, ConvaTec® Loop Ostomy Rod. All images © E.R. Squibb & Sons, LLC. Reprinted with permission from ConvaTec.

TABLE 8-4	OSTOMY SUPPLIES*
PRODUCT	**USE**
Skin barriers	Paste, wafers, rings, or powders used to protect skin
Skin sealants	Plasticizing agents that produce a thin, protective film around skin
Skin cleaners	Foams, wipes, sprays, or liquids used to clean or remove residue from skin
Skin adhesives	Sprays or liquids used to increase adhesion of ostomy equipment
Pouches	Wafers presized or cut to fit: one-piece or two-piece, disposable or reusable
Belts and binders	Provide support and keep equipment in place
Convex inserts	Provide support and convexity
Pouch covers	Protect skin from moisture and provide concealment
Tail closures	Close end of pouches to prevent leakage
Tapes	Help pouches stay in place; prevent leakage; provide waterproofing
Stoma guide strips	Assist with centering pouches over stoma
Solvents	Assist with removal of residual tape or water residue
Stomocap	Cover for continent ostomy
Irrigation set and insertion cone	Used to irrigate colostomy
Faceplates	Used for retracted stomas

*Patient should be referred to appropriate resources, including the enterostomal therapy nurse, the American Cancer Society, and the United Ostomy Association.

Postoperative wound infection is not a major concern because of the use of prophylactic antibiotics and reduction of wound contamination with postoperative stoma pouching. Patients with abdominoperineal resections are at greater risk for wound complications and infections. Sitz baths, dressing changes, and topical ointments assist in healing, which may be very slow, and meticulous skin care is essential.

Postoperative teaching, support, and addressing the patient's emotional and physical changes may involve referral to outside resources. Postoperative pouch application and stoma care should be a step-by-step process, moving from the simple to the complex components. Ostomy care includes pouch applications, emptying of the pouch, and use of skin care products.

Pouch selection is based on the site of the stoma, the patient's manual dexterity, cost, and patient preference. All pouches should be well fitted, odor-proof, and provide skin protection. Additional special skin barrier products may also be necessary, depending upon the type of effluent discharged. Ileostomy drainage is particularly wet and contains enzymes that cause skin irritation. Sigmoid colostomy effluent is solid; however, it may also cause skin problems. Odor is managed with pouching and ostomy deodorant sprays. The enterostomal therapist is invaluable in selecting appropriate products for the patient.

Colostomy irrigations may be an option for patients with a sigmoid colostomy, whereas other ostomies cannot be regulated by irrigation because the effluent is constant and liquid. Points to emphasize are the advantages of each system, and that irrigation control takes patience. A daily schedule can be established over time. Figure 8-4 and Table 8-4 demonstrate various ostomy supplies.

Dietary needs and restrictions for ostomy patients include adequate fluid intake and the avoidance of certain foods that may cause blockage, odor, or gas. A list of medications that are not absorbed in the intestine and may be expelled through the colostomy should be provided. Foods that contain seeds, nuts, or excessive bulk should be avoided because of blockage potential. Foods that cause gas and odor are frequently the same foods that caused these problems before surgery and usually include beans, cabbage, and brussels sprouts.

By trial and error and with the use of commercial deodorant products, this problem can be eliminated or reduced. Discharge teaching includes specific problems that may be encountered, such as diarrhea or blockage. A dietary consultant can assist the patient in appropriate diet selection. A physician or enterostomal therapist should be notified if these problems arise. Stoma prolapse and stoma retraction can occur if there is undue pressure on the stoma from an appliance, edema, or scar formation. Specific skin problems and use of products are discussed with the patient. Discharge teaching can be overwhelming for a patient who is emotionally and physically drained from the events of surgery. Scheduling short visits that include repetition is the most reliable method of teaching. Readiness to learn has a great impact on ostomy teaching.

Body image and sexuality concerns are discussed preoperatively and postoperatively. Signs of difficulty in dealing with the new ostomy may include failure to look at the stoma, making remarks about the stoma, or not permitting the significant other to assist with care of the appliance. Common concerns are fear of rejection, shame, a sense of disfigurement, and concerns about others' reactions. Continued feelings of low self-esteem can lead to depression, withdrawal, and sexual dysfunction. An ostomy visitor with a similar background may provide the additional support and encouragement needed at this time. Meeting a person who is able to work and continue with outside activities provides the patient with a positive outlook and encouragement.

Sexual counseling begins while the patient is in the hospital. A discussion about sexuality concerns ultimately includes the spouse or significant other. Suggestions to assist couples to deal with sexuality issues should begin with open communication and gradual introduction of sexual activity. Body image concerns may be dealt with by the use of pouch covers, nightgowns and shirts, or other methods to conceal the ostomy until the patient is comfortable with the issue. Altered sexual positions that are more comfortable and less traumatic on the stoma should also be discussed. Patients with abdominoperineal resections require referrals for further counseling, because 30% to 100% of all men with this surgery experience erectile impotence. Damage to the parasympathetic nerve and loss of sensation have a severe impact on sexual performance. Referral to a urologist for a semirigid or inflatable penile implant is necessary if the patient finds he is unable to perform sexually and desires further medical intervention. Research on women with abdominoperineal resections is not conclusive, but reports include changes in sensation that alter the orgasmic process.[22-26]

Rehabilitation. Rehabilitation of the patient with colorectal cancer requires the combined efforts of several professionals. Physical, emotional, and spiritual concerns must be met. The ultimate goal of rehabilitation is to provide patients with the knowledge and support to reach their maximum capabilities within the limits of their condition. The United Ostomy Association and ACS can provide additional support and information for the patient and family. Additional referrals for counseling to deal with emotional and sexual concerns may also be necessary for

long-term support. The availability of an enterostomal therapist and adequate access to ostomy supplies are additional supports for patients who have had ostomy surgery.[20,26,27]

RADIATION THERAPY

The role of radiation therapy in the management of colorectal cancer is based on disease stage and prognostic factors (Table 8-5). Radiation modalities may be used singly or in combination with chemotherapy to reduce tumor border and local recurrence. Radiation therapy serves two roles, one as a new adjuvant reduction of tumor burden to improve resectability; and adjuvant eradication of remaining cancer cells to reduce local recurrences. Adjuvant chemotherapy and radiation protocols are usually part of a clinical trial. Preoperative radiation therapy reduces tumor load and seeding and allows for sphincter preservation. Postoperative radiation has proved effective in rectal cancer for palliation of pain, bleeding, and local control of metastasis. If perforation is present in stage(s) T1, N1, M0, radiation and chemotherapy is necessary. T4, N1-2, M0 protocols include chemotherapy with and without radiation. Additional treatments include endocavity therapy (used in only carefully selected patients instead of surgery) and intraoperative radiation (IOPT), treatment for unresectable tumor, and hyperthermia (still investigational) for rectal cancer.

Patients receiving radiation therapy to the abdominal cavity require emotional and physical support throughout their treatment. Preradiation instruction reviews the frequency and length of treatments, skin markings and their care, and potential side effect management. Ostomy patients who receive radiation therapy may need additional information about skin care of their stomas. Side effects experienced by patients receiving abdominal radiation may include nausea, vomiting, diarrhea, cystitis, sexual dysfunction, bone marrow suppression, local skin reaction, and fatigue (Box 8-6).

TABLE 8-5	Treatment Recommendations for Stages II, III, and IV Colon Cancer
STAGE	**RECOMMENDED TREATMENT**
II	Wide surgical resection and anastomosis
	Patients should be considered for participation in clinical trials of postsurgical adjuvant chemotherapy, radiation therapy, or biologic therapy
III	Wide surgical resection and anastomosis.
	Adjuvant chemotherapy with 5-FU–containing regimens should be considered for patients who are not candidates for clinical trials
	Eligible patients should be considered for entry into clinical trials evaluating postoperative treatments, including chemotherapy, radiation therapy, or biologic therapy, alone or in combination
IV	Surgical resection/anastomosis or bypass of obstructing primary lesions in selected cases
	Surgical resection of isolated metastases
	Chemotherapy
	Clinical trials evaluating new drugs and biologic therapy
	Radiation therapy

Nausea and vomiting are of concern particularly to patients receiving radiation therapy over the abdominal area. This is due to the destruction of the epithelial lining of the bowel wall. The toxic waste production from cellular destruction increases the stimuli to the nausea receptors in the medulla. Prolonged nausea and vomiting may lead to weight loss and dehydration. Appropriate nursing measures include use of antiemetics 1 to 2 hours before radiation therapy and for up to 12 hours after each treatment. Small, frequent meals are encouraged, with high protein and liquid supplements. Weight, dietary intake, and hydration status should be monitored at least weekly. If patients have an ostomy, significant weight loss causes stoma shrinkage, necessitating remeasurement of the stoma and pouch sizes.

Diarrhea is another common symptom, beginning 1 or 2 weeks after the initiation of radiation, and is caused by the rapid proliferation of the epithelial cells in the intestinal wall. Patients experiencing diarrhea should be instructed to eat low-residue, high-protein, high-carbohydrate diets. Fluids high in potassium are encouraged; milk products are discouraged. Antidiarrheal products are effective in controlling diarrhea. Patients should record the number and consistency of bowel movements. Rectal irritation from frequent bowel movements or radiation therapy to the rectum may require assessment by the radiation oncologist and/or enterostomal therapist; sitz baths and use of topical creams may also be needed. Ostomy patients may require more frequent pouch changes, assessment of peristomal skin, and use of a skin barrier to protect their skin. Severe excoriation of the peristomal skin requires a referral to the enterostomal therapist or discontinuation of treatments until symptoms subside.

Abdominal radiation causes inflammation of the bladder, resulting in symptoms of cystitis, burning, back pain, hematuria, and foul-smelling urine. Instructions should be given to increase fluid intake to 2 to 3 quarts of liquids per day and to limit caffeine products. Urine cultures, sensitivity specimens, and monitoring intake and output may be necessary.

Sexual dysfunction occurs for a variety of emotional and physical reasons. Changes in self-concept, decreased libido, impotence, fertility concerns, and changes in the vaginal lining may occur as a result of radiation therapy. Instructions include alternative forms of sexual contact, use of a water-based lubricant, and appropriate referrals for severe sexual concerns and fertility issues.

DISEASE-RELATED COMPLICATIONS
Radiation Therapy

- Skin irritation (erythema, dry or moist desquamation, and hyperpigmentation)
- Proctitis
- Nausea/vomiting
- Diarrhea
- Cystitis
- Bone changes; obstruction, fibrosis, adhesions, fistulas
- Sexual dysfunction
- Myelosuppression
- Fatigue

Bone marrow suppression is the result of the proximity of the radiation dose to the treatment site and the pelvic bones. The depth of suppression depends on the length of treatment cycles, the number of treatments, and the total dose delivered. Patients are monitored for fatigue, infection, bleeding, and fever. Laboratory studies should be monitored weekly. Patient instructions include prudent handwashing to minimize the potential for infection.

Local skin reactions result from the destruction of epithelial tissue. Reactions include itchy, dry skin, darkened areas near the radiation site, and mild excoriation. Patients should avoid excessive heat or cold, and avoid the use of creams or lotions near the treatment site. Only skin products prescribed or applied by the radiation oncologist should be used since other products can increase skin reactions.

Ostomy patients experience increased radiation dermatitis near the peristomal skin site as a result of direct exposure of the mucous membranes to the treatment field. Pouches are often removed before treatment, which causes increased concern for the patient about skin exposure. However this also allows opportunity for assessment of the peristomal skin. Careful skin cleansing and use of skin barriers will provide adequate protection. Severely excoriated areas require the use of additional creams or powders near the stoma site, and a referral to the enterostomal therapist should be made. Treatments are often delayed if symptoms progress.[13,16,17,23,25,27]

CHEMOTHERAPY

Only 37% of all colorectal cancers are diagnosed in early stages. Survival intervention provides a 90% cure rate. For the patient diagnosed in stages III and IV, chemotherapy plays a significant role in the treatment and prognosis.[28-30]

Adjuvant Therapy. 5-FU (Fluorouracil) and leucovorin are currently used for stage II colorectal cancer with a high disease reoccurrence ratio, and for stage III cancer. Infusions may be given via intravenous (IV) bolus daily, once a month (Mayo regimen) or weekly (Roswell Park regimen). Additional combinations of oxaliplatin, 5-FU, and leucovorin (FOLFOX-4) every 2 weeks for 6 months has been added as a improved modality and has been adopted as a standard in adjuvant therapy.[31]

Metastatic Disease. Various protocols are being administered and evaluated as treatment options for metastatic colorectal cancer. Included are the following:

- *IFL—Irinotecan, fluorouracil, leucovorin (Saltz regimen).* Infusions are given weekly for 6 weeks followed by 2-week breaks. Despite improved tumor reduction, the protocol causes increased toxicity related to severe diarrhea.
- *FOLFIRI—*Irinotecan given every other week with infusional 5-FU via a home infusion pump. Caregiver and IV support are necessary.
- *Capiri (Xeliri).* Combined irinotecan and capecitabine (Xeloda). Xeloda is taken twice daily for 2 weeks of a 3-week cycle, and irinotecan is administered on day 1 of the cycle. Diarrhea and palmar-plantar erythrodysthesia (PPE) hand-foot syndrome are the most common side effects.
- *FOLFOX-4—*Oxaliplatin is added to infusional 5-FU and given every other week. Side effects include peripheral neuropathy, immediate response to cold, and cumulative peripheral sensory neuropathy in hands and feet.

- *Other FOLFOX regimens.* Protocols are under investigation that include alteration in doses and infusion methods.
- *Capox (Xelox).* A combination of capecitabine and oxaliplatin. Despite higher response rates, toxicities are also found.[28-30,32-34]

TARGETED THERAPY

Patients expressing EGFR (epidermal growth factor receptor) have demonstrated aggressive tumors, poor prognosis, and shorter survival times. Included in the treatment of colorectal cancer is cetuximab (Erbitux), which has demonstrated improved antitumor effect in colorectal cancer in combination with and without irinotecan. In clinical trials (Bond Trials), adverse affects include acnelike rashes, diarrhea, asthenia, anemia, vomiting, and neutropenia.

Bevacizumab (Avastin) and anti–vascular endothelial growth factor (VEGF) monoclonal antibody (MoAbs) has been approved for metastatic colorectal cancer in combination with 5-FU–based chemotherapy and includes the use of cetuximab, and bevacizumab and cetuximab/bevacizumab/irinotecan protocols.

Additional trials are ongoing to evaluate response to cetuximab and FOLFOX-4 in EGFR-positive metastatic colorectal cancers that demonstrate progression on irinotecan therapy (Explore trial); additional Phase II and III trials are ongoing to evaluate response rates to current protocols.[25,34-36]

OTHER PROTOCOLS

- PTK 787 (Novartis, East Hanover, NJ; and Schering AG, Germany), an oral active VEGF tyrosine kinase inhibitor, is now in phase I, II, and III clinical trials and indicated for use in untreated metastatic colorectal cancers when combined with FOLFOX-4 in varying doses and administration regimens. No additional toxicity has been noted with improved survival rate documented.
- ABX-EGF (panitumumab) now in a phase I clinical trial as monotherapy in patients whose cancer is refractory to 5-FU and irinotecan and/or oxaliplatin.
- Gefitinib (Iressa) and erlotinib (Tarceva) did not demonstrate any clinical affect in recent clinical trials.
- All EGFR inhibitors demonstrated increased side effects including acnelike rash, nausea, vomiting, stomatitis, dyspnea, fever, hypersensitivity reactions, and bone marrow suppression.[34-41]

Interventions. Patients receiving chemotherapy for colorectal cancer may be treated with a single or multidrug protocol as well as a combination of chemotherapy, radiation, and biotherapy. Side effects are usually dose-, drug-, and patient-specific. General side effects include nausea, vomiting, diarrhea, and myelosuppression.

Nursing measures include adequate instructions on potential drug side effects. Diarrhea is of particular concern to the ostomy patient because skin breakdown can easily occur. Use of a protective barrier and additional paste or powder may be necessary. Recording the number and consistency of stools is vital to assess hydration status. Small, frequent, high-protein meals rich in potassium are encouraged. Antidiarrheal agents may be required.

Constipation is treated with fluids, stool softeners, laxatives and, if necessary, irrigations of the stoma. Mucositis is found around the peristomal skin and in the stoma itself. Bowel drainage from infused chemotherapy agents requires the use of protective skin barriers, careful pouch changes, and proper skin cleansing. Fungal infections near the stoma site may also result from prolonged myelosuppression. Antifungal powders near the peristomal skin assist with wound healing. Local trauma from low platelet counts near the stoma can occur. Careful pouch removal is necessary to avoid further trauma.

Nausea and vomiting cause excessive weight loss, which changes stoma size. This often requires a pouch replacement or size change. Consultation should be done to determine the appropriate pouch before any significant changes are made.

Body image and self-esteem disturbances require emotional support, as well as additional changes of hair loss and ostomy formation. Support groups and counseling should be provided for these individuals.

Specialized treatment of metastatic liver cancer may be accomplished with an infusion pump. The Medtronics infusion pump allows patients increased freedom from hospitalization but requires extensive patient teaching concerning the pump's placement and management. A disk-shaped pump is surgically implanted into a subcutaneous pocket, allowing access to the hepatic artery. The pump contains an access port, a chamber for the fluid to be infused, and a chamber filled with fluorocarbon. The vapor pressure of fluorocarbon at normal body temperature results in expansion of the pump and release of the chemotherapeutic drug. Postoperative complications include development of a seroma, an accumulation of sterile fluid in the pump pocket, which may require draining. Infections may also occur within the pocket site and require surgical removal of the pump. Percutaneous access is used to fill the pump on a 2- to 4-week schedule. Each patient's schedule will vary. FUDR (floxuridine, an analogue of 5-FU) and a heparin solution are infused every 2 weeks. Between the doses of FUDR, a solution of normal saline and heparin is used to keep the pump open. Access to the pump for filling is gained using a perfusion scan and injection of radioactive material to assist with proper placement.[6,16,17,27]

Specific teaching concerning the pump includes its use and particular filling schedule. Side effects of FUDR include nausea, vomiting, abdominal pain, diarrhea, fatigue, and chemical hepatitis. Symptoms are treated systemically except for hepatitis, which requires the removal of the drug from the pump. Patients must avoid blunt trauma to the pump site and must limit exposure to extremes of temperature and altitude, which may interfere with drug administration. The effect of intraarterial chemotherapy and its effectiveness in hepatic metastasis are still under evaluation.

Continued patient teaching is needed to support the patient with colorectal cancer through the postoperative course and through various treatment modalities. Patient teaching priorities and implications are summarized in the Patient Teaching Priorities: Colorectal Cancer box.

Considerations for Older Adults

Special considerations should be given to the elderly population, who may demonstrate a lack of awareness of increased risk factors, signs and symptoms, and recommended screening practices for colorectal cancer. Awareness of the ACS guidelines and the availability of community screening programs are imperative to early diagnosis. Once a diagnosis is made and treatment initiated, the elderly patient may experience increased side

*P*atient Teaching Priorities
Colorectal Cancer

Surgery (Preoperative Care)
Turning, coughing, deep breathing
Wound splinting
Ambulation
Pain management
Pouch application
Bowel preparation
Postoperative complications

Chemotherapy
Drug name and regimen
Side effects
Complications
Follow-up schedule

Culture
Relationships
Communication
Values
Sexual concerns
Food habits
Health care beliefs
Teaching and learning process
Religious concerns
Body image
Pain
Beliefs about death and dying

Surgery (Postoperative Care)
Ostomy and skin care
Pouch application
Diet modifications
Complications
Sexuality issues
Rehabilitation
Community support

Radiation
Treatment schedule
Side effects
Skin care
Dietary constraints

Community
Availability of enterostomal therapist services, hospital, clinics,
   ostomy supplier
Support groups
Home care agencies
Housing (privacy/bathroom facilities)
Acceptance of differences
Family resources (financial, emotional, physical
   availability)
Transportation resources
Rehabilitation resources
Community screening programs

---

effects arising from preexisting medical conditions and lack of physical stamina to tolerate aggressive therapy.

Postoperatively, elderly patients are at increased risk for pulmonary, circulatory, and bowel complications. Additional treatment modalities of radiation and chemotherapy impose further complications of fluid and electrolyte imbalance, infection, and skin concerns. Monitoring the immune and nutritional status of this population is essential.

Postoperative teaching of elderly patients may also require added time to allow for any vision and hearing impairment as well as dexterity with pouch applications. Community resources and referrals should be made to assist with physical and financial support.[42-44] The box to the right summarizes considerations for older adults.

Conclusion

Although vast improvements have been made in the public awareness, diagnosis, and treatment of colorectal cancer, it remains a significant health concern of adulthood. Approximately 60% of Americans are expected to develop colorectal cancer in their lifetime, the majority between 60 and 65 years of age, although as a disease, it is 90% preventable and 90% curable when detected early (Table 8-6). Oncology nurses are currently and will continue to be responsible for increasing the public's awareness of current screening guidelines, teaching colorectal cancer prevention strategies, and promoting access to treatment and

*C*ONSIDERATIONS FOR OLDER ADULTS
Colorectal Cancer

Education Needs
- Awareness of screening recommendations
- Knowledge of signs and symptoms
- Understanding of risk factors
- Treatment complications

Surgery
- Pulmonary
- Circulatory
- Bowel

Chemotherapy and Radiation
- Fluid and electrolyte imbalance
- Infection
- Skin impairment

Teaching Concerns
- Vision/hearing impairment
- Dexterity for pouch applications

Community Resources
- Financial
- Home care referral

TABLE 8-6	Prognosis Rates for Colorectal Cancer	
STAGE	**SURVIVAL RATE**
I	90%–95%
II	75%–80%
III	40%–70%
IV	5%
Anal cancer	48%–66%

care including clinical trials, as well as delivering exceptional hands-on nursing care of patients undergoing surgery, radiation, and/or chemotherapy for colorectal cancer. Although the advances discussed here are hope-inspiring, as our population ages, the incidence of colorectal cancer will likely increase—and the oncology nurse will be called upon to care for this targeted population.

REVIEW QUESTIONS

✓ Case Study

John is a 56-year-old male who had a brother succumb to colorectal cancer at age 60, as well as a great-grandfather who had some type of bowel disorder and experienced a sudden death. John is admitted with a 1-year history of abdominal pain, changes in bowel habit, a 10-lb weight loss, indigestion, and a fecal occult blood positive test (FOBT) performed by his family physician. He is currently experiencing nausea and right abdominal, right rib, and hip pain.

His personal health habits include 20-plus years as a smoker; a social drinker, he consumes two to four drinks per day, and despite a 10-lb weight loss, he remains 30 lbs overweight. His diet history is high in red meats.

On admission, labs included CBC, cytidine monophosphate (CMP), BUN and creatinine (CR), and CEA—which was elevated. He underwent colonoscopy and liver and bone scans, as well as a having a normal chest x-ray. Testing revealed a large right mass in the upper colon, abnormal liver scan, and rib cage metastasis.

John has a right hemicolectomy with biliary drains placed for obstructive disease because of his liver metastasis. His postoperative course is uneventful, and he has an oncology consult. John wishes to pursue any possible treatment, stating, "My brother did nothing. I am younger and can fight this." The oncologist recommended FOLFOX-4 therapy based on John's wishes to seek palliative chemotherapy.

QUESTIONS

1. Risk factors for colorectal cancer include the following:
   a. High alcohol intake and abnormal bowel habits
   b. History of constipation and high consumption of red meats
   c. Abnormal bowel habits and tobacco abuse
   d. Combination of factors including diet, genetics, and predisposing factors such as bowel disorders
2. The ACS recommendations for colon cancer screening include which of the following?
   a. FOBT
   b. Persons at high risk to increase screening at an earlier age than the normal population
   c. Proctosigmoidoscopy every year for patients over age 50
   d. Colonoscopy examinations for every rectal bleeding episode

3. Which of the following is a late symptom of colorectal cancer?
   a. Anorexia
   b. Blood in the stool
   c. Change in bowel practices
   d. Weight loss
4. John's diagnostic work-up, based on symptoms, would not include which of the following?
   a. CBC
   b. Bone scan
   c. Liver scan
   d. Sigmoidoscopy
5. Diagnostic tests reveal that John has a staging of T4, N3, M1. What does this diagnosis indicate that John has?
   a. Local disease
   b. Stage II
   c. Stage IV
   d. An inoperable cancer, and he is terminal
6. John's treatment options include the following:
   a. Bone marrow transplant
   b. Liver transplant
   c. 5-FU plus high-dose leucovorin (Roswell Park)
   d. Palliative chemotherapy and radiation, postsurgical debulking
7. Which of the following is not included among appropriate immediate postoperative nursing diagnoses for a patient with colon cancer and a bowel resection?
   a. Sexual dysfunction
   b. Impaired skin integrity
   c. Pain
   d. Risk for infection
8. Immediate postoperative home care teaching excludes discussion of the following:
   a. Dietary modifications
   b. Prevention, screening, and detection guidelines
   c. Potential complications: bleeding, infection
   d. Self-care skin integrity interventions
9. FOLFOX-4 therapy includes the following drugs:
   a. Xeloda, 5-FU
   b. Leucovorin, oxaliplatin, 5-FU
   c. Bevacizumab, oxaliplatin
   d. Cetuximab, 5-FU, leucovorin

10. John's symptoms of confusion, jaundice, and elevated bilirubin are most likely related to which of the following?
    a. Chemotherapy side effects
    b. Bowel obstruction
    c. Liver failure related to liver metastasis
    d. Renal failure

ANSWERS

1. **D.** *Rationale:* No single factor causes colorectal cancer. Known risk factors include a variety of factors with only 5% to 6% of cases due to genetics alone.

2. **B.** *Rationale:* The ACS guidelines for early detection in men and women with average risk over the age of 50 include proctosigmoidoscopy every 5 years, colonoscopy every 10 years, and FOBT every 5 years. High-risk individuals with family history or increased risk based on previous pathology require additional screening based on both risk and pathology.

3. **D.** *Rationale:* Unplanned weight loss with other presenting symptoms is an indicator of advanced disease. The remaining symptoms may be caused by an early-stage malignancy or by other nonmalignant diseases.

4. **D.** *Rationale:* All tests based on symptomatology are appropriate except sigmoidoscopy. The patient displays symptoms of metastatic colorectal cancer. Additional tests would include chest x-ray, CEA, CMP, BUN, CR, colonoscopy, CT scan and MRI.

5. **C.** *Rationale:* Stage IV colorectal cancer denotes distant metastasis, which may be evident as lung, bone, and liver metastasis. Palliative radiation and/or chemotherapy always offers potential treatment options for end-stage disease as well as surgical debulking of tumor mass.

6. **D.** *Rationale:* Bone marrow transplant and liver transplant are not indicated for a patient with metastatic colorectal cancer. The treatment protocol of 5-FU with high-dose leucovorin is for early-stage cancer treatment.

7. **A.** *Rationale:* Sexuality is a significant concern to all patients who have cancer and a bowel obstruction. Only B, C, and D are immediate postoperative concerns.

8. **B.** *Rationale:* Although important, prevention, screening, and detection guidelines do not apply in John's case (stage IV metastatic disease). Based on his family history and John's diagnosis, family teaching when appropriate may be indicated.

9. **B.** *Rationale:* FOLFOX-4 is a protocol used for advanced colorectal cancer and includes leucovorin, 5-FU, and oxaliplatin. Other protocols for advanced colorectal cancer exist. Protocols are based on patient's disease staging, comorbid conditions, ability to tolerate side effects and patient wishes. Treatments including drugs such as irinotecan, 5-FU, and leucovorin, in a variety of protocols, with and without the use of bevacizumab (Avastin) protocols for Stage IV with one site and multiple site metastasis, are under evaluation.

10. **C.** *Rationale:* Based on John's history of liver metastasis and the symptom of jaundice, tea-colored urine, elevated bilirubin, and confusion (all signs of liver disease), John is displaying evidence of liver failure related to increased metastatic progression.

REFERENCES

1. American Cancer Society: *Colorectal facts and figures, special edition,* Atlanta, 2005, Author.
2. Berg A: *Pocket guide to colorectal cancer,* Sudbury, MA, 2003, Jones and Bartlett.
3. Cancer Health Online: Colon cancer risk in U.S. varies by race, ethnicity, retrieved July 24, 2005, from http://Cancer.HealthCentersonline.com.
4. Komaromy M: What is familial colon cancer? Retrieved July 20, 2005, from http://www.GeneticsHealth.com.
5. Jemal A, Murray T, Ward E et al: Cancer Statistics 2005, *CA Cancer J Clin* 55:1, 10-30, 2005.
6. American Cancer Society: *Nutrition for the person with cancer: a guide for patients and families,* Atlanta, 2003, Author.
7. American Cancer Society: Guidelines on nutrition and physical activity for cancer prevention, Atlanta, 2002, Author.
8. Department of Agriculture and U.S. Department of Health and Human Services: *Guidelines for Americans,* 2005. Retrieved December 6, 2006, From http://www.mypyramid.gov.
9. Pullen R: Tips for safe, accurate occult blood testing, *Nursing* 35(3):28, 2005
10. Gangloff J: Screening for colorectal cancer, *Cure* Fall:12-16, 2004.
11. American Cancer Society: *Colorectal cancer prevention guidelines,* Version III, Atlanta, 2003, Author.
12. Smith R, Cokkinides V, Eyre H: American Cancer Society guidelines for early detection of cancer, *CA Cancer J Clin* 56(31):31-44, 2005.
13. Sargent C: Colorectal cancer, *Nursing* 33(2):37-41, 2003.
14. Vogel W, Wilson M, Melvin M: *Advanced practice oncology palliative care guidelines,* New York, 2004, Lippincott, Williams & Wilkins.
15. Metz J, Hampshire M: *OncoLink patient guide to colorectal cancer,* ed 2, New York, 2005, Saunders.
16. Strohl R: Nursing care of the client with cancers of the gastrointestinal tract. In Itano J, Taoka K, editors: *Core curriculum for oncology nursing,* ed. 4, St. Louis, 2005, Saunders.
17. Yarbo CH, Frogge MH, Goodman M et al: *Cancer nursing: principles and practice.* Boston, 2001, Jones & Bartlett.
18. Greene Fl, Page DL, Fleming ID et al, editors: *American Joint Committee on Cancer (AJCC) cancer staging hand book,* ed 6, New York, 2002, Springer.
19. Waldman AR, Crane ME: Surgical aspects of colon cancer. In Burg DT, editor. *Contemporary issues in colorectal cancer: a nursing perspective,* Boston, 2001, Jones and Bartlett.
20. Smith M.: Hepatic colorectal metastases: data remain limited, but treatment approaches appear to offer benefit, *Oncol Times* June:18-23, 2005.
21. Giantonio B: *Update in the medical management of advanced colorectal cancer,* New York, 2004, McMohan.
22. Waldmen AR, Crane ME.: Surgical aspects of colon cancer. In Berg DT, editor: *Contemporary issues in colorectal cancer: a nursing perspective,* Boston, 2001, Jones & Bartlett.
23. Skibber JM, Minsky BD, Hoff PM: Cancer of the colon. In Devita VT, editor: *Cancer principles and practice in oncology,* Philadelphia, 2001, Lippincott, Williams & Wilkins.
24. Hampton BG, Bryant R: *Ostomies and continent diversions,* St. Louis, 1992, Mosby.
25. Vega-Stromberg T: Colon cancer chemotherapy, *Home Health Nurse* 23(3):155-165, 2005.
26. United Ostomy Association: UOAA affiliated support groups, retrieved August 20, 2005, from http://www.UOAA.org/supportgroups.shtml.
27. Bucci MK, Bevan A, Roach M: Advances in radiation conventional 3D, to IMRT, to 4D, and beyond, *CA Cancer J Clin* 55(2):117-134, 2005.
28. Skeel R: *Handbook of chemotherapy,* ed 6, Philadelphia, 2003, Lippincott, Williams & Wilkins.
29. Chu E, Devita V: *Physician's chemotherapy drug manual,* Sudbury, MA, 2005, Jones & Bartlett.
30. Wilkes G, Barton-Burke M: *Oncology nursing drug handbook,* Boston, 2005, Jones & Bartlett.
31. Susman E: NCCN Colon cancer guidelines include adjuvant therapy considerations, *Oncol Times* 28(9):15-17, 2005.

32. Rosenberg L, Burns H: Recent progress in chemotherapy for colon cancer: the X-Act and TREE trials, *Community Oncol* 2(4):4-10, 2005.

33. National Cancer Institute: Colon cancer (PDQ): treatment, retrieved August 20, 2005, from http://www.NCI.NIH.gov/cancertopics/pdq/treatment/colon.

34. Knoop T: Nursing management of patients receiving angiogenesis inhibitors, *Curr Top Colorectal Cancer Targeting VEGF*, March:18-26, 2005, Genetech.

35. Wilkes G: Therapeutic options in the management of colon cancer, *Can J Oncol Nurs* 9(1):31-44, 2005.

36. Ponto J, editor: *Oncology nursing reporter: scientific update from the 30th Annual Congress of the Oncology Nursing Society*, 1-15, 2005.

37. Ponto J, editor: *National peer reviews in colorectal cancer: scientific updates from the 30th Annual Congress of the Oncology Nursing Society*, Orlando, FL, 2-15, 2005.

38. American Society of Clinical Oncology: *Using biologic agents for the treatment of metestatic colorectal cancer*, retrieved August 20, 2005, from http://www.ASCO.org.

39. Franson P, Lapka D: Antivascular endothelial growth factor monoclonal antibody therapy: a promising paradigm in colorectal cancer, *Can J Oncol Nurs* 9(1):55-63, 2005.

40. Wood L, Giantonio B, Gillespie T et al: Novel approaches to patient care targeting colorectal cancer, *Oncology Education Services* 1(2):1-42, 2004.

41. Viale PH, Fuchs C: Colon cancer treatment: progress and prospects, Spotlight on symposia from the ONS 30th Annual Congress in Orlando, FL, 20(8):35-36, 2005.

42. Levitz J, Lichtman S: Adjuvant therapy for colon cancer in the elderly: Treat or don't treat? *Community Oncol* 2(4):331-336, 2005.

43. Overcash J, Balducci L: *The older cancer patient, a guide for nurses and related professionals*, New York, 2005, Springer.

44. Overcash J: Assessing and caring for the older person with cancer: how comprehensive geriatric assessment and multidisciplinary teams can contribute to the caring for older persons with cancer, *Oncol Support Care Q* Oncology Education Services, vol. 2, 2003.

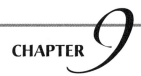

CHAPTER 9

Gastrointestinal Cancers

Ruth Chaplen and Lisa Malburg

Cancers of the digestive system accounted for an estimated 18.4% of the new cases of cancer diagnosed in the United States in 2005 and 23.8% of the cancer deaths in the same period. This represents a total of 253,500 new cases and 136,060 cancer deaths. Unfortunately, these statistics have been relatively stable over the last several years. Gastrointestinal (GI) cancers include esophageal, gastric, hepatocellular, and pancreatic cancers, as well as less common GI cancers: carcinoid, gastrointestinal stromal tumors (GIST), and those occurring in the small intestine, the anal canal, the gallbladder, and the bile ducts.

Cancer of the Esophagus

Epidemiology

Cancer of the esophagus is a fairly uncommon cancer in the United States, accounting for about 1% of the new cancer diagnoses in 2005.[1] This cancer is estimated to have caused 2% of the overall cancer deaths but about 4% of the cancer deaths in men. Esophageal cancer is the eighth leading cause of cancer worldwide and the sixth leading cause of cancer death. In 2002 it was responsible for 462,000 new cases and 386,000 deaths worldwide. In developed countries the survival is poor, with only 16% of those affected in the United States and 10% of those in Europe surviving 5 years. The geographic incidence of this cancer varies widely. A twentyfold difference in incidence is noted between China and Western Africa. The highest areas of risk are China, southern and eastern Africa, south central Asia, and Japan. These differences can be explained in part by geographic variability in environmental carcinogens and genetic predisposition.[2] Worldwide, esophageal cancer is 3 to 4 times more common in men than in women. In the United States, it is about 50% more common among African Americans than Caucasians. Squamous cell cancers are the most common type of esophageal cancer in African Americans and in people outside of the United States. Adenocarcinomas are the most common type of esophageal cancer in Caucasian Americans, and their incidence is rising by as much as 9% per year.[1,3,4]

Etiology and Risk Factors

The exact cause of cancers of the esophagus is unknown. The etiology of esophageal cancer is often associated with environmental factors and conditions that involve chronic irritation of the esophagus. Age is a predominant risk factor, with cases rarely occurring in people under 40. Men are 3 to 4 times more likely to get esophageal cancer than women. Race accounts for a significantly higher incidence of esophageal cancer in African Americans compared to Caucasians in the United States.[3-5] A recent study shows the incidence of esophageal cancer can be lowered by reducing smoking, decreasing obesity, reducing gastroesophageal reflux (GERD), and increasing consumption of fruits and vegetables. Adenocarcinoma has been linked to obesity and smoking.[5] Specific dietary risk factors for esophageal cancer include diets lacking certain fruits, vegetables, and vitamins and minerals; very hot liquids; alcohol; red meats; soft drinks, and foods with nitrosamines. Environmental exposure to chemicals such as dry cleaning agents and lye has also been linked to an increased risk of esophageal caner. Barrett's esophagus, achalasia, tylosis, esophageal webs, and Plummer-Vinson syndrome have been associated with the development of esophageal cancer. Genetics may also affect the development of esophageal cancer through mutations in p53, FHIT, EGFR, and c-erb-2. Mutations of two genes that control alcohol metabolism (ADH2) may explain the high rates of cancer in Japan and populations in the east and southeast of Asia.[2,4,5-8]

Prevention, Screening, and Detection

Avoiding the controllable risk factors discussed in the previous section can reduce risk of esophageal cancer. Risk factors such as age, sex, race, and genetic makeup cannot be altered, whereas avoidance of smoking, limiting alcohol intake, maintaining good nutrition, and decreasing exposure to carcinogens are advantageous. Adenocarcinoma incidence can be decreased by maintaining a healthy weight, treating GERD, and avoiding intake of alcohol and tobacco.[3,9]

Currently there are no routine screening recommendations for esophageal cancer in the United States. In certain areas of the world where esophageal cancer is endemic and it is economically feasible, mass screening can be done, such as in Japan, where the 5-year survival rate is 90%.[3,9] Techniques include balloon cytology and endoscopic mucosal staining. Balloon cytology involves the collection of cells on the outside of a balloon, which is swallowed by the patient and then pulled back through the esophagus.[3] However, this technique is not very effective.[9] Mucosal staining involves the use of special dyes, which are sprayed on the esophageal mucosa during endoscopy in order to identify small lesions that may be missed with the naked eye. This allows identification of early lesions.

In the United States, specific groups are targeted for screening. Although efficacy and cost-effectiveness is not well-established, surveillance endoscopy is routinely performed for persons with Barrett's esophagus every 1 to 4 years depending on the degree of dysplasia present. Persons with lye exposure or tylosis may also benefit from routine surveillance endoscopy.[4,9,10]

Prevention of esophageal cancer focuses primarily on education and public advocacy regarding proper nutrition, alcohol and tobacco cessation, maintaining a healthy weight, and treating GERD. Nutritional recommendations include a diet high in dairy products, fish, vegetables, citrus fruit and juices, dietary fiber, carotenoids, and cereals.[6,11] High-risk individuals should be instructed to report any problems with dysphagia (difficulty in swallowing), odynophagia (pain on swallowing), weight loss, or heartburn. Unfortunately these symptoms often do not occur until the cancer is advanced.[3,4] Recent research has focused on prevention of adenocarcinoma and squamous cell carcinoma of the esophagus using aspirin and nonsteroidal antiinflammatory drugs (NSAIDs). These agents have been found to be effective in high-risk persons.[4,12,13]

Classification

In Europe and the United States, the incidence of esophageal adenocarcinoma has increased from 5% to greater than 50% over the last 30 years. This change in incidence is largely unexplained but may be related to the increase in Barrett's esophagus.[3,4] Squamous cell carcinoma is the second most common subtype in the United States. Worldwide, the majority of esophageal cancers are of the squamous cell type.[2-4] Squamous cell carcinomas arise from the surface epithelium, whereas adenocarcinomas most often occur in the lower portion of the esophagus. Adenocarcinomas frequently arise from the gastroesophageal junction, where metaplasia and eventual dysplasia occur in the epithelium as a result of acid exposure. Adenocarcinomas are rarely found in the upper and middle esophagus. Other, less common, esophageal tumors include mucoepidermoid carcinoma, small cell carcinoma, sarcoma, melanoma, adenoid cystic carcinoma, and lymphoma.[14]

Clinical Features

Dysphagia occurs in 95% of patients and is generally not noted until the esophageal lumen is narrowed to one half or one third normal. Heartburn or GERD symptoms are present in approximately 40% of esophageal cancers and are often associated with adenocarcinoma.[14] Seventy percent of patients present with weight loss, which may be due to the inability to swallow or to metastatic involvement. Pain may be related to swallowing or to extension of the tumor into adjacent structures such as the vertebra, the pleura, or the mediastinum, or to distant bony metastasis. Pain is present in 25% of patients at the time of diagnosis. All of these symptoms generally indicate advanced disease and are associated with a worse prognosis.[3,4,14]

Diagnosis

Most esophageal cancers in the United States are discovered as a result of symptoms. A barium swallow is often the first test to evaluate patients with dysphagia. If a mass is identified, the patient will require a flexible endoscopy to evaluate the lesion, obtain cytology brushings, and obtain biopsy samples. The flexible endoscopy and rigid endoscopy are very accurate in diagnosing malignancy, with an accuracy of 90% to 100% respectively. Endoscopic ultrasonography, computed tomography (CT), and positron emission tomography (PET) are imaging techniques that are used to assist in the staging of a tumor.[3,14-17]

Staging

In 1998, the American Joint Committee on Cancer (AJCC) changed the tumor-node-metastasis (TNM) staging system for esophageal cancer from a clinical to a pathologic format. The TNM staging was modified most recently in 2002 (Table 9-1). Both still

---

TABLE 9-1   TNM Staging System for Esophageal Neoplasms

PRIMARY TUMOR (T)

TX	Primary tumor cannot be assessed
T0	No evidence of primary tumor
Tis	Carcinoma in situ
T1	Tumor invades lamina propria or submucosa
T2	Tumor invades muscularis propria
T3	Tumor invades adventitia
T4	Tumor invades adjacent structures

REGIONAL LYMPH NODES (N)

NX	Regional lymph nodes cannot be assessed
N0	No regional lymph node metastasis
N1	Regional lymph node metastasis

DISTANT METASTASIS (M)

MX	Distant metastasis cannot be assessed
M0	No distant metastasis
M1	Distant metastasis

Tumors of the lower thoracic esophagus:
    M1a Metastasis in celiac lymph nodes
    M1b Other distant metastasis
Tumors of the midthoracic esophagus:
    M1a Not applicable
    M1b Nonregional lymph nodes and/or other
        distant metastasis
Tumors of the upper thoracic esophagus:
    M1a Metastasis in cervical nodes
    M1b Other distant metastasis

STAGE GROUPING

Stage 0	Tis	N0	M0
Stage I	T1	N0	M0
Stage IIA	T2	N0	M0
	T3	N0	M0
Stage IIB	T1	N1	M0
	T2	N1	M0
Stage III	T3	N1	M0
	T4	Any N	M0
Stage IV	Any T	Any N	M1
Stage IVA	Any T	Any N	M1a
Stage IVB	Any T	Any N	M1b

HISTOLOGIC GRADE (G)

GX	Grade cannot be assessed
G1	Well differentiated
G2	Moderately differentiated
G3	Poorly differentiated
G4	Undifferentiated

RESIDUAL TUMOR (R)

RX	Presence of residual tumor cannot be assessed
R0	No residual tumor
R1	Microscopic residual tumor
R2	Macroscopic residual tumor

Regional lymph nodes:
Cervical esophageal tumor: scalene, internal jugular, upper cervical, periesophageal, supraclavicular, cervical not otherwise specified
Intrathoracic esophageal tumor: tracheobronchial, superior mediastinal, peritracheal, carinal, hilar, periesophageal, perigastric, paracardial, mediastinal not otherwise specified

From AJCC *Cancer Staging Handbook*, ed 6, New York, 2002, Springer.

have importance in the staging of esophageal cancer, particularly in patients managed with primary radiotherapy or chemoradiation, where there is no specimen to determine pathologic staging.[14,18] Determining the correct stage is critical to developing the appropriate treatment plan and in formulating a prognosis. A staging evaluation typically includes the endoscopy and barium swallow to assess the stomach in cases where the scope cannot be advanced past a lesion. CT scan of the chest and abdomen determine metastatic disease and aortic or airway involvement by the primary lesion. Endoscopic ultrasound (EUS) and PET scan are new tools that assist in the staging of esophageal cancer. EUS assesses the depth of tumor involvement and evaluates nodal status, particularly when combined with a needle biopsy. PET scans can be used with CT scan to evaluate for metastatic disease and may be more effective in identifying distant metastasis.[14-17]

Two critical prognostic indicators for esophageal cancer are depth of tumor penetration and extent of nodal involvement. The prognosis, according to clinical stage, is demonstrated in Table 9-2. Weight loss is indicative of poor prognosis. Biologic markers are being studied that may aid in estimating prognosis. These include growth factors, oncogenes, tumor suppressor genes, the cell adhesion molecule E-cadherin, carcinoembryonic antigen (CEA), and DNA content. Currently these are not accepted as staging techniques unless performed as part of a research trial.[14,17] In addition, the patient is assessed for risk factors associated with treatment-related morbidity and mortality. This evaluation may include pulmonary function tests (PFTs), electrocardiogram (ECG), echocardiogram, stress test, assessment of nutritional status, and/or liver function studies. Evaluating the patient's performance status is imperative in terms of the aggressiveness of the proposed treatment.[14]

Metastasis

Esophageal cancer can spread to almost any part of the body, and 50% of patients have metastatic or locoregional disease at the time of diagnosis. Distant metastases are found in the liver (35% of newly diagnosed patients), the lungs (20%), the bones (9%), the adrenal gland or the brain (2%), and the spleen, the pancreas, the stomach, the pleura, and the pericardium (1%).[14,16]

Medical Treatment Modalities and Nursing Care Considerations

Standard treatment options that have curative intent for esophageal cancer include surgery, chemotherapy, and radiation therapy or a combination of two or three of these modalities. Surgery is considered the gold standard for cure. Local control is a primary goal of treatment because of the significant impact of dysphagia on quality of life. Selecting the appropriate therapy is often difficult, because a comparison of these options performed in an appropriately controlled fashion is not available in the current research base.[14,19,20] A multimodality approach is generally the most effective.[14,20] The stage at diagnosis and the overall status of the patient determine the best combination of therapy. Surgery alone is used for early-stage lesions for curative intent. Locally advanced disease is often treated with a combination of neoadjuvant chemoradiotherapy if the patient is a good surgical candidate, and chemoradiotherapy alone if the patient is not able to or chooses not to undergo surgery. Newer treatment modalities include photodynamic therapy (PDT) and minimally invasive surgery.[21-23]

SURGERY

Surgery remains the mainstay of treatment for esophageal cancer, both as a single modality in patients with early disease and as part of a multimodality approach in locally advanced disease. The choice of surgical approach for **esophagectomy** remains controversial.[14,18] There are a variety of approaches to resection depending upon the location of the tumor. The main approaches include transthoracic, transhiatal, and minimally invasive.[14] Transthoracic approaches include the Ivor Lewis approach, the McKeown modification of Ivor Lewis, the left thoracectomy with intrathoracic anastamosis, the left thoracotomy with cervical anastamosis, and the thoracoabdominal incision approach. The Ivor Lewis approach involves a laparotomy, right thoracectomy, and high intrathoracic anastomosis. The McKeown modification involves a cervical anastomosis. In most cases, the stomach is used for the reconstruction, with the anastomosis performed in either the chest or the neck. If the patient has had previous surgery involving the stomach, or if the tumor extends so far as to require a total esophagectomy, the esophagus must be reconstructed using a portion of the small or the large intestine. Tumors in the distal esophagus involving the gastroesophageal junction are usually managed with a subtotal esophagectomy. The transhiatal approach (Fig. 9-1) is used for tumors in the cervical region or the upper esophagus. These lesions require a total esophagectomy because of the difficulty in achieving negative margins. Two more extensive operations, the en bloc esophagectomy and the three-field lymphadenectomy, are performed more commonly in Japan than in the United States. These involve extensive resection of lymph nodes and tissue surrounding the esophagus. Studies indicate that these approaches may offer lower incidence of local recurrence; however, they are associated with higher incidence of complications.[18] All of these procedures are associated with significant morbidity. However, postoperative mortality is due to factors beyond just the postoperative complications.[14,24,25]

Due to concerns regarding morbidity and mortality of esophagectomy, minimally invasive procedures have grown in popularity. These approaches include thoracoscopically assisted or laparoscopically assisted esophagectomy or some combination of the two approaches. Decisions regarding minimally invasive procedures should be based on patient preference, history of prior radiation or surgery, and surgical experience. These approaches may decrease postoperative complications and shorten length of stay. One potential complication of these procedures is port-site metastasis.[26]

The nursing care of the patient after esophageal cancer surgery involves preventing further morbidity and mortality, maintaining

TABLE 9-2	Prognosis of Esophageal Carcinoma According to the Clinical Stage	
STAGE (AJCC)	**5-YEAR SURVIVAL (%)**
0 (in situ)	>95
I (T1, N0)	50-80
II (T2-3, N0; T1-2, N1)	10-40
III (T4 or N+)	10-15
IV (M+)	<5

From Hustinx R: PET imaging in assessing gastrointestinal tumors, *Radiol Clin North Am* 42(6):1123-1139, 2004.

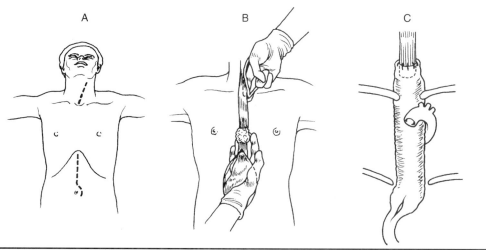

FIG. 9-1   Transhiatal esophagectomy. **A,** The cervical and abdominal incisions. **B,** How manual dissection is used from both above and below. **C,** The stomach anastomosed to the esophagus in the neck. (From Jamieson G, Mathew G: Surgical management of esophageal cancer: the Western experience. In Daly JM, Hennessy TPJ, Reynolds JV et al, editors: *Management of upper gastrointestinal cancer*, Philadelphia, 1999, Saunders.)

nutrition, and enhancing quality of life. Surgical resection of esophageal cancer is associated with high morbidity caused by cardiopulmonary complications, anastomatic stricture, or anastomatic leak. Preventing and/or treating pneumonia is an important factor in decreasing mortality.[24] Immediately after surgery, patients are cared for in the intensive care unit (ICU). Nursing care includes neurologic checks, adequate pain management, pulmonary assessment and care, nutritional support through hyperalimentation or J-tube feedings, and adequate hydration. Five to seven days after surgery, patients undergo fluoroscopic swallowing examination to evaluate for anastomotic leaks before being started on oral fluids or food. Predischarge teaching ensures that the patient can maintain nutrition at home and avoid complications.[27] Psychosocial issues are significant in this population since patients often feel abandoned, lonely, and disappointed if education or support is lacking.[28,29] High intensity of symptoms including reflux, hoarseness, and diarrhea is associated with lower quality of life in esophagectomy patients.[13] Nurses can have a significant impact on the quality of life of these patients by addressing their symptoms and psychosocial concerns early during the postoperative recovery period.[26,30]

RADIATION THERAPY

Because of the low 5-year survival rates of patients treated with surgery as a single modality, a combination approach is often indicated. Radiation therapy (RT) as a primary therapy is rarely used, since studies have shown that chemotherapy plus radiation therapy (chemoradiation) is superior to radiation alone.[14,18] Surgery alone offers a higher survival benefit than preoperative or postoperative radiation alone.

Radiation therapy as a primary treatment is appropriate for patients with obstructing tumors who are not able to receive chemotherapy alone or surgery in combination with chemotherapy. RT for curative intent may be used in patients who have localized disease.[22] Dysphagia is relieved by radiation therapy

alone or used in combination with chemotherapy in 70% to 80% of patients and provides a more durable relief for this symptom than other palliative measures.[18] Intraluminal brachytherapy has been also been explored for palliation in advanced tumors and for patients treated in the curative setting. This allows high doses of radiation to be administered locally to a small volume of tissue. There is no benefit to brachytherapy either alone or in combination with external beam radiation for local disease control. Brachytherapy is effective for palliation of dysphagia and bleeding.[14,18]

Preoperative (neoadjuvant) radiation is done with the hope of improving resectability and decreasing local recurrence. Randomized controlled trials are lacking in this area. Despite the current practices of providing neoadjuvant radiation, the studies to date have not demonstrated a clear improvement of local control or survival.[14,18,31] Induction therapy with radiation does not appear to increase the postoperative complications.[18] Postoperative radiation (adjuvant) has been historically recommended for patients with node-positive disease. To date, the only clear advantage of adjuvant radiation is in patients with positive margins. Radiation alone does not provide a significant benefit in local recurrence or overall survival.[18]

Neoadjuvant-combined chemoradiation has been found to provide improved disease-free survival and a higher frequency of curative resections than either surgery, chemotherapy, or radiation alone. In some cases, the combined modality of chemotherapy and radiation therapy is used when the patient is not a surgical candidate. Although the exact role of neoadjuvant chemoradiation is not yet clear, it appears that survival is improved. The most common chemotherapy agents used are conventional 5-fluorouracil (5-FU), cisplatin, and more recently, paclitaxel. Several trials are currently ongoing in order to better define the role of preoperative chemoradiation[18,32,33]

Nursing care of the patient undergoing radiation involves assessing for complications and educating the patient on how to manage these. Radiation to the esophagus produces both short- and long-term side effects. Most patients experience esophagitis and fatigue. Esophagitis management is critical to completing therapy. Traditional management includes a combination of viscous xylocaine, aluminum hydroxide–magnesium carbonate, and diphenhydramine, or oral liquid narcotics. Medications such as histamine-2 receptor antagonists (H2 blockers) or proton pump inhibitors are also used to reduce injury from gastric acid.[14] New therapies to prevent or improve the severity of esophagitis are under investigation. Among these are amifostine, glutamine, melatonin, omega-3 polyunsaturated fatty acid, transforming growth factors, flavonoid compounds, probucol, and keratinizing growth factor.[34] In a recent metaanalysis, amifostine was found to significantly reduce the severity of mucositis.[35] Long-term effects include esophageal stricture or fistula. Nutritional status is critical, and some patients may require enteral feeding through a J-tube.[18]

CHEMOTHERAPY

Chemotherapy has a role in the management of esophageal cancer patients in the neoadjuvant, adjuvant, metastatic, and combination modality settings. Studies using single-agent chemotherapy have shown some effectiveness. Generally, the response to single-agent chemotherapy is brief and is not associated with any survival benefit.[14] Several agents have been used as single agent therapy in esophageal cancer; these agents include 5-FU, cisplatin, methotrexate, paclitaxel, mitomycin, vindesine, mitoguazone, vinorelbine, doxorubicin, irinotecan, and etoposide.[14] Agents which have demonstrated a 15% to 30% response rate include cisplatin, mitomycin, 5-FU, paclitaxel, and vindesine. However, most of these agents have been tested only in squamous cell cancers. Cisplatin and 5-FU are the most common single agents. Response rates with 5-FU alone have been as high as 85% when given by continuous infusion. The response rate for single-agent cisplatin in newly diagnosed patients may be as high as 73%. The response rate in patients with metastatic or recurrent disease was 21%. Paclitaxel is one of the few new compounds that has been tested in both squamous cell cancers and adenocarcinomas.[18] Most combination chemotherapy regimens contain cisplatin. The most common regimen used is 5-FU and cisplatin. Other recent combinations include paclitaxel combined with cisplatin and/or 5-FU, or irinotecan in combination with cisplatin.[14]

A recent metaanalysis of the benefits of preoperative chemotherapy suggests that neoadjuvant chemotherapy may reduce local recurrence and improve 5-year survival, although this is associated with increased toxicity and mortality associated with the chemotherapy. The most beneficial combination appears to be based on cisplatin and 5-FU.[36] It is suggested that adjuvant chemotherapy improves disease-free survival but shows no significant improvement in overall survival.[14,18]

The nursing care of these patients involves monitoring for side effects and teaching patients side effects management. Patients need to understand when to contact a member of the health care team regarding a side effect or complication. The side effects seen will depend on the chemotherapy drugs used. The common side effects of these agents include nausea, vomiting, myelosuppression, nephrotoxicity, peripheral neuropathy, mucositis, diarrhea, and hand-foot syndrome.

The Diseae-Related Complications: Esophageal Cancer and Treatment box summarizes the potential disease-related and treatment-related complications of esophageal cancer.

DISEASE-RELATED COMPLICATIONS
Esophageal Cancer and Treatment

Disease-Related
Weight loss/anorexia
Hematemesis/melena
Hemoptysis
Dysphonia
Superior vena cava syndrome
Malignant pleural effusion
Malignant ascites
Bone pain
Laryngeal nerve palsy

Treatment-Related
Radiation-Related
Pneumonitis
Stricture
Fistula

Chemotherapy-Related
Nausea and vomiting
Nephrotoxicity
Myelosuppression
Mucositis/diarrhea
Peripheral neuropathy
Skin toxicity (hand-foot-syndrome)

Data from Swisher SG, Ajani JA, Komaki RK et al: Neoplasms of the esophagus. In Kufe DW, Pollock RE, Weichselbaum RR et al editors: *Cancer medicine*, Hamilton (Canada) 2003, BC Decker; Posner M, Forastiere A, Minsky B: Cancer of the esophagus. In Devita VT, Hellman S, Rosenberg SA, editors: *Cancer: principles and practice of oncology*, 2004, Lippincott Williams & Wilkins.

Disease- and Treatment-Related Complications

The most common disease-related complications in patients with esophageal cancer are dysphagia and odynophagia. The treatments discussed above are used to offer palliation for these symptoms. Unfortunately, the treatments may not provide adequate relief of symptoms. In these situations, techniques such as esophageal dilatation, esophageal stenting, laser therapy, and PDT may be used. The morbidity and mortality for these procedures is much less than that for surgical resection, and they often produce a durable palliation of symptoms.[14,18] The quality of life of the patient can be significantly improved by controlling dysphagia and odynophagia. Dysphagia has been found to impact all areas of the patient's life.[37] Management of complications must involve a multidisciplinary team including the physician, the nurse, the speech therapist, the social worker, and the nutritionist.

Prognosis

Although the prognosis for persons with esophageal cancer remains poor, the 5-year survival rate has increased from 4% in Caucasian patients and 1% in African American patients in 1960 to 16% of Caucasian patients and 9% of African American patients in 2005. Even with the improved treatment, 95% of patients diagnosed will die of their disease.[1] Research is ongoing in prevention, screening, diagnosis, treatment, and palliation to improve the survival and quality of life of patients with esophageal cancer.

Cancer of the Stomach

Epidemiology

Adenocarcinoma of the stomach has been the leading cause of cancer-related deaths throughout most of this century. It currently ranks as the second leading cause of death worldwide, second to lung cancer. An estimated 875,000 new cases are diagnosed annually.[1,2,38] The incidence has been gradually declining, mainly because of changes in food preparation and storage. In the United States, the incidence of stomach cancer has declined more dramatically and now ranks seventh as a cause of cancer-related deaths.[18] It accounted for an estimated 21,860 new cancer cases and 11,550 deaths in 2005.[1] The decline in stomach cancers has mainly occurred in cancers of the distal stomach, while cancers of the proximal stomach and esophagogastric (EG) junction have increased markedly in the last 25 years.[38]

The incidence and mortality rates for stomach cancer vary widely in different geographic regions. The highest incidence is in Japan, South America, China, and Eastern Europe, with incidence rates between 30 and 85 cases per 100,000 population. This compares to a rate of less than 8 cases per 100,000 in the United States, Israel, and Kuwait.[38] In the United States, stomach cancer is more common in men than women and is 1.5 to 2.5 times more common in African Americans, Hispanics, and native Americans than Caucasians.[1,38] Two thirds of the patients with newly diagnosed gastric cancer are over 65 years of age. The lifetime risk of developing stomach cancer in a person's lifetime is about 1 in 100.[1]

Etiology and Risk Factors

Several nutritional, environmental, social, genetic, and medical factors have been associated with the development of cancer of the stomach.[38,39] In most patients the development of stomach cancer is multifactorial. Evidence of the environmental and dietary causality of stomach cancer is supported by the study of migrating populations. Several studies have demonstrated that immigrants gradually acquire the incidence rates of the country to which they move.[38,39] Nutritional factors that have been associated with increased incidence of stomach (gastric) cancer include obesity, GERD, poor drinking water, lack of refrigeration, high consumption of foods high in nitrates, smoked or salt-cured food preparation, low dietary fiber, and low dietary intake of vitamins A and C. Smoking and alcohol intake appear to increase the risk of gastric cancer, but the link is stronger for the former than the latter. Smokers have twice the risk of cancers of the proximal stomach than nonsmokers.[5,38,39]

Additional environmental risk factors include occupational and infectious disease–related factors. Metal workers, coal miners, rubber workers, and those exposed to dust from wood and asbestos have all been shown to have a higher than normal incidence. Radiation exposure early in life is also associated with an increased risk of gastric cancer. Gastric cancer has been known to develop as a secondary malignancy following treatment for pediatric Hodgkin's disease.[14,38-40] Stomach cancers involving the body and antrum have a strong association with *Helicobacter pylori* infection. The exact mechanism is not clear, but it is associated with a doubled risk. Epstein-Barr virus has been associated with some stomach cancers, although they tend to be the less aggressive type.[1,38]

Several genetic and medical factors have been linked to the development of gastric cancer. Pernicious anemia, hypertrophic gastropathy (Menetrier's disease), previous gastric resection, adenomatous gastric polyps, chronic atrophic gastritis, intestinal metaplasia, dysplasia, and blood type A seem to be associated with certain types of stomach cancer. Familial occurrence of gastric cancer is rare, accounting for only 8% to 10% of gastric cancers, but a small increase in incidence has been noted in direct relatives. The most notable family with this disease is that of Napoleon Bonaparte. One of the identified genetic mutations associated with hereditary gastric cancer is of *E-cadherin*, which regulates cell adherence. Patients with hereditary nonpolyposis colorectal cancer (HNPCC) or Li-Fraumeni syndrome also have an increased risk of gastric cancer. Familial adenomatous polyposis (FAP) and Peutz-Jeghers syndrome have been linked to an increased risk of gastric cancer in certain populations.[1,38-41]

Prevention, Screening, and Detection

Research on the prevention of gastric cancer has focused primarily on nutritional measures, smoking cessation, use of NSAIDs, and eradication of *H. pylori* infections. Dietary measures include the proper preparation and storage of food and the limitation of foods that are salted, smoked, and pickled. In addition, diets high in fiber, rich in fruits and vegetables, and lower in red meat are advised and will assist in maintaining a healthy weight.[6,42] Specifically, consumption of antioxidants is not recommended.[43] The use of NSAIDs has been studied and is associated with a lower risk of gastric cancer. Because of the significant side effects of these agents, they should only be used in specific situations in high-risk persons as part of a clinical trial.[12,44] Although the identification and treatment of *H. pylori* infection does decrease the risk of development of many gastric cancers, population-based screening and treatment for the purpose of gastric cancer prevention is not recommended at this time. Research continues on the development of a vaccine to treat the *H. pylori* infection.[9,45]

Mass screening and early detection programs have been used and have been successful in Japan and China. In these countries, as many as 50% to 80% of cancers are detected at an early stage. This screening is usually done by **esophagogastroduodenoscopy (EGD)** or upper GI series.[46] The aspiration of gastric secretions to test for pH is useful in some situations.[47] Mass endoscopic screening or radiologic evaluation is not recommended in the United States. High-risk persons with a family history of gastric cancer, a personal history of gastric polyps, FAP, HNPCC, Menetrier's disease, or Li-Fraumeni or Peutz-Jegher's syndrome should undergo surveillance endoscopy every 1 to 2 years.[38,39,46] Diagnosis of gastric cancer is made by examination of histopathology of tissue obtained during endoscopy or by assessment of gastric brushings or washings.[46]

Nurses play a role in the primary and secondary prevention of gastric cancer through education and public advocacy. Nursing interventions include education about identifying and reducing risk factors, identifying appropriate candidates for screening, and identifying signs and symptoms that warrant investigation.[40] The most common symptoms encountered in individuals with stomach cancer are dyspepsia (up to 50% of patients), anorexia, weight loss, epigastric discomfort, nausea, vomiting, early satiety, hematemesis, or melena. The presence of symptoms indicates advanced disease, and in the United States, 80% to 90% of patients present with locally advanced or metastatic tumors. Persons with these symptoms need to be evaluated with physical examination and endoscopy.[38-41,46]

Classification

Adenocarcinomas represent approximately 95% of the malignant tumors of the stomach. Lymphoma, carcinoid, leiomyosarcoma, adenocanthoma, liposarcoma, fibroadenoma, carcinocarcinoma, and squamous cell carcinoma comprise the remaining 5%.[38-40]

Several classification systems are used for stomach cancer. The Borrman classification system divides gastric cancer into five types depending on the macroscopic appearance. Type I are polypoid or fungating tumors. Type II tumors include ulcerating lesions surrounded by elevated borders. Type III lesions are ulcerative lesions that infiltrate the gastric wall. Type IV tumors are diffusely infiltrating, and Type V tumors are unclassifiable. Broder's classification system is based on degree of histologic differentiation. Tumor cells are graded from 1 (well-differentiated) to 4 (anaplastic).[38,40,46]

Siewart and Stein have developed a classification system for adenocarcinoma of the GE junction that recognizes 3 distinctly different cancers arising within 5 cm of the GE junction. Type I is an adenocarcinoma of the distal esophagus, often arising from Barrett's esophagus. Type II is an adenocarcinoma that arises from the cardia. Type III is an adenocarcinoma arising from the subcardial stomach.[38]

The two most commonly used classification systems for gastric cancer are the World Health Organization (WHO) and the Lauren systems. The WHO system grades tumors based on the degree of resemblance to metaplastic intestinal tissue. It consists of 5 subtypes that include adenocarcinoma (diffuse and intestinal), papillary, tubular, mucinous, and signet-ring cell.[46] The most widely accepted system of classification was developed by Lauren in 1965.[38,40,46] This system identifies two main groups of gastric cancers: *intestinal* and *diffuse* gastric cancer. **Intestinal gastric cancers** are characterized by glandular structures with varying degrees of differentiation. These tumors are associated with chronic atrophic gastritis. **Diffuse gastric cancers** are composed of poorly differentiated cells that infiltrate the gastric wall and are not associated with intestinal metaplasia. These are less related to environmental influences, often occur in younger patients, and are associated with familial cases of gastric cancer. This classification system is the most popular, because it correlates well with the differences in pathology, epidemiology, and etiology of gastric cancers.[38,40,46]

Clinical Features

Gastric cancer has no symptoms associated with an early superficial lesion. However, approximately half of the patients with gastric cancer that is, potentially, surgically curable manifest vague GI complaints such as dyspepsia. Unfortunately, because of the lack of symptoms, 80% to 90% of patients are first seen with locally advanced or metastatic tumors. The most common presenting symptoms are weight loss and anorexia. Patients with weight loss have significantly shorter survival. The symptoms experienced often reflect the location of the tumor. Dysphagia is associated with lesions in the cardia and GE junction. Vomiting after meals is seen more often in obstructing tumors of the pyloric region of the stomach. Hematemesis occurs in 10% to 15% of patients. Symptoms of metastatic disease can include ascites, jaundice, palpable mass, hepatomegaly, enlarged supraclavicular lymph node (Virchow's node), left axillary node (Irish's node), or periumbilical lymph node (Sister Mary-Joseph's node).[38,40,46]

Diagnosis and Staging

The most sensitive and specific diagnostic test for gastric cancer is the EGD. This technique allows for direct visualization, evaluation of mucosal involvement, and biopsy for tissue diagnosis. If properly performed, an EGD is 92% to 96% accurate at diagnosing gastric cancer.[38-40,46] EUS, when used in combination with EGD, allows for more accurate assessment of tumor depth and perigastric lymph node involvement. The EUS is extremely useful in preoperative staging and determining resectability.[40,41,46]

Once the initial diagnosis is made, a CT scan of the chest, abdomen, and pelvis is recommended to evaluate tumor extent, nodal involvement, and distant metastasis.[8] CT scans are not useful in determining depth of tumor penetration, but they are very accurate in identifying distant metastasis and somewhat accurate in identifying lymph node involvement. Laparoscopy can be used in combination with CT and EUS for more accurate assessment of serosal infiltration, peritoneal seeding, and hepatic metastasis.[40,46-48] Newer techniques to assist in staging and assessing response to treatment include PET imaging and three-dimensional CT scanning. The added benefit of these techniques to that of the current standard procedures has not yet been established.[17,49] Table 9-3 outlines the AJCC's TNM criteria (sixth edition) for classification and staging of cancer of the stomach. Prognostic factors include stage at diagnosis, histopathologic grade, peritoneal involvement, and weight loss.[39] In addition to staging studies, the patient should have bloodwork including complete blood count (CBC), electrolytes, liver function tests, serum albumin, and tumor markers CEA, CA-125, and CA 19-9.[38,40]

Metastasis

Gastric cancer can spread by direct extension to adjacent structures, through the lymphatics, and by hematogenous dissemination. Direct tumor extension can involve the esophagus, the duodenum, the omentum, the spleen, the adrenal gland, the diaphragm, the liver, the pancreas, or the colon. Peritoneal seeding can also occur. Liver metastasis is the most common distant site of involvement. Other organs that can be involved include the lungs, the bones, and the brain. Skin metastasis have been reported.[38,39,50]

Medical Treatment Modalities and Nursing Care Considerations

Surgery is the mainstay of treatment in local and regional gastric cancers. It is the only curative modality. However, in stages II and III disease, it is not adequate to achieve cure. Surgery can be used alone or in combination with radiation therapy and chemotherapy for the treatment of gastric cancer. Recent research has focused on the combination treatments to produce increased survival with minimal risk of morbidity and mortality.[38,39,46]

SURGERY

Issues to consider in surgical intervention include the extent of both gastric resection and lymph node dissection; the role of splenectomy or pancreatectomy; and the method of reconstruction. Preoperative staging is critical in identification of those who will most benefit from surgical intervention. Surgery is rarely done for palliative purposes alone.[38,39,46]

| TABLE 9-3 | TNM Clinical Classification System for Staging Gastric Carcinoma |

PRIMARY TUMOR (T)

TX	Primary tumor cannot be assessed
T0	No evidence of primary tumor
Tis	Carcinoma in situ: intraepithelial tumor, without invasion of the lamina propria
T1	Tumor invades lamina propria or submucosa
T2	Tumor invades muscularis propria or subserosa
T2a	Tumor invades muscularis propria
T2b	Tumor invades the subserosa
T3	Tumor penetrates serosa (visceral peritoneum) without invasion of adjacent structures
T4	Tumor invades adjacent structures

REGIONAL LYMPH NODES (N)

NX	Regional lymph node(s) cannot be assessed
N0	No regional lymph node metastasis
N1	Metastasis in 1 to 6 regional lymph nodes
N2	Metastasis in 7 to 15 regional lymph nodes
N3	Metastasis in more than 15 regional lymph nodes

DISTANT METASTASIS (M)

MX	Presence of distant metastasis cannot be assessed
M0	No distant metastasis
M1	Distant metastasis

STAGE GROUPING

Stage 0	Tis	N0	M0
Stage IA	T1	N0	M0
Stage IB	T1	N1	M0
	T2a	N0	M0
	T2b	N0	M0
Stage II	T1	N2	M0
	T2a	N1	M0
	T2b	N1	M0
	T3	N0	M0
Stage IIIA	T2a	N2	M0
	T2b	N2	M0
	T3	N1	M0
	T4	N0	M0
Stage IIIB	T3	N2	M0
Stage IV	T4	N1-3	M0
	T1-3	N3	M0
	Any T	Any N	M1

HISTOLOGIC GRADE (G)

GX	Grade cannot be assessed
G1	Well differentiated
G2	Moderately differentiated
G3	Poorly differentiated
G4	Undifferentiated

RESIDUAL TUMOR (R)

RX	Presence of residual tumor cannot be assessed
R0	No residual tumor
R1	Microscopic residual tumor
R2	Macroscopic residual tumor

From *AJCC Cancer Staging Handbook*, ed 6, New York, 2002, Springer.

Options for the surgical management of early gastric cancer (EGC) or T1 lesions include endoscopic mucosal resection (EMR), gastrotomy with local excision, and gastrectomy. These approaches have been observed extensively in the Japanese population, where many gastric cancers are found at an earlier stage. EMR is associated with low complication rates, improved quality of life, and successful complete resection in the majority of cases.[38,51] Recently, surgical local resection has been used as a viable choice for the management of EGC and is a safe and curative option for appropriately selected patients.[52] Laparoscopic surgery has become more popular for the management of EGC. The laparoscopic local resection techniques include laparoscopic wedge resection and intragastric mucosal resection. These procedures are used on patients who are not candidates for EMR. Laparoscopic procedures for more advanced gastric cancers include laparoscopic gastrectomy with minimal or extensive lymph node dissection. There are no current survival data available regarding these procedures, therefore randomized controlled trials are required. Studies show shorter recovery and lower pain levels associated with laparoscopic surgical procedures.[38,51]

The goal of surgery for stages II and III gastric cancer is to perform a macroscopically and microscopically complete resection. The operative procedure depends on the anatomic location of the tumor and the pattern of spread from that particular location. For tumors in the proximal third of the stomach, including the GE junction and the fundus, either a radical subtotal gastrectomy or a total gastrectomy is performed. Currently there appears to be no clear advantage of the total gastrectomy in these patients.[40,46] Tumors in the middle third require a total gastrectomy to obtain tumor-free margins, whereas those located in the distal third are treated with a radical subtotal gastrectomy. A few randomized trials have examined subtotal gastrectomy for distal stomach tumors and found comparable outcomes with fewer long-term sequelae when compared to total gastrectomy.[38,46]

The extent of the lymph node dissection performed with gastric resection remains a controversial issue. Randomized clinical trials comparing limited lymphadenectomy of the perigastric lymph nodes (D1 dissection) to en bloc removal of regional lymph nodes (D2 dissection) have found no difference in survival and a significantly higher rate of complications. However, many of these included splenectomy and pancreatectomy, which increased postoperative complications. Recent prospective studies suggest a survival benefit of D2 resection with pancreas and spleen preservation.[38,46]

Reconstruction procedures after total gastrectomy include a Roux-en-Y, construction of a pouch, or jejunal interposition. Following a subtotal gastrectomy, reconstruction includes a gastroduodenostomy, loop reconstruction, gastrojejunostomy, or Roux-en-Y.[8,18] None of these demonstrates superiority.[39,41] Prophylactic gastrectomy may be performed for *E-cadherin* or *CDH1* mutation carriers because of the potentially high risk of gastric cancer.[53] Gastrectomy or gastrointestinal bypass is considered for palliation of pain, nausea, hemorrhage, dyspepsia, and obstruction. The mortality rate from palliative resection can be as high as 22%.[38]

Postoperative nursing care of the patient with gastric cancer is similar to that of the patient with an esophagectomy and can be reviewed in that section. The major complications include anastomotic leak, hemorrhage, infection, thromboembolism, and pneumonia. A swallow study done 1 week after surgery assesses the anastomosis before oral feedings begin. Enteral feedings are used until oral nutrition is adequate. Patient education regarding long-term sequelae of gastrectomy includes malabsorption of iron, vitamin B_{12}, and calcium, and postprandial symptoms of cramping, sweating, diarrhea, fainting, and dumping syndrome. Techniques such as limiting carbohydrates, eating smaller, more frequent meals, increasing protein intake, and increasing dietary fiber contribute to increased quality of life, which is a significant issue with these patients.[40,54] Postgastrectomy patients experience a struggle to maintain oral nutrition, bodily estrangement, and difficulties with the nutritional treatment regimens.[55]

RADIATION THERAPY

Radiation therapy to control or eliminate recurrent or residual disease may be used either intraoperatively, as an adjuvant, or in the neoadjuvant setting, for the treatment of pain, bleeding or obstruction. Anecdotal experience indicates that radiation may be useful, particularly adjuvant radiation therapy, which seems to improve local control compared to surgery alone.[38] Intraoperative radiation therapy (IORT) has shown both a survival advantage in stages II-IV and improved local control.[39] Radiation therapy is most often combined with chemotherapy such as 5-FU as a radio-sensitizer. This has shown improved overall survival, disease-free survival, and local-regional control.[38,39,56]

Toxicities of radiation therapy include nausea, vomiting, and difficulty in maintaining adequate nutrition. These side effects can be reduced by having patients fast before treatment, and using prophylactic antiemetics and jejunostomy tube feedings. Nurses need to educate patients about side effects management and to monitor nutritional status carefully while receiving radiation therapy.[39]

CHEMOTHERAPY

Chemotherapy is used for gastric cancer as a single agent, in combination, and with or without radiation for neoadjuvant, adjuvant, and palliative therapy. Chemotherapy agents traditionally shown active against gastric cancer include 5-FU, tegafur, doxorubicin, epirubicin, mitomycin C, the nitrosoureas, trimetrexate, methotrexate, and cisplatin. Response rates to single agents are generally less than 20%.[38,39] A widely studied traditional regimen is FAM (5-FU, doxorubicin, mitomycin C). FAM-based regimens have response rates of as high as 42% in patients with advanced gastric cancer. Other studies have used 5-FU, and the nitrosourea methyl-CCNU combined with 5-FU, methyl-CCNU, and doxorubicin, and 5-FU combined with BCNU.[38] The current standard of care is 5-FU in combination with cisplatin for all stages of disease.[40] The taxanes (paclitaxel and docetaxel) and the campthothecin irinotecan are being investigated. These drugs show higher efficacy when used in combination with 5-FU or cisplatin.

In an effort to improve surgical outcomes and long-term survival, preoperative (neoadjuvant) therapy is under investigation. If the patient is responsive, treatment can be continued postoperatively.[53] An example is epirubicin, cisplatin, and continuous infusion 5-FU (ECF), since it appears to have an improved disease-free survival, but it has yet to demonstrate improvement in overall survival. The use of neoadjuvant chemotherapy still requires further controlled research to confirm benefits.[38-40,46]

Several metaanalyses have failed to demonstrate an advantage of postoperative chemotherapy.[38-40,46]

DISEASE-RELATED COMPLICATIONS
Gastric Cancer and Treatment

Disease-Related Complications
- Anorexia/weight loss
- Pain
- Obstruction/vomiting/dysphagia
- Bleeding/hematemesis/melena
- Ascites
- Jaundice
- Bone pain

Treatment-Related Complications
Postoperative Complications

EARLY	LATE
• Infection	• Dumping syndrome
• Hemorrhage	• Reflux esophagitis
• Acute pancreatitis	• Weight loss
• Ileus	• Anemia
• Anastomotic leak	• Hypoproteinemia
• Thromboembolism	• Osteomalacia

Radiation Therapy Complications

DURING TREATMENT	LATE
• Fatigue	• Bleeding
• Nausea	• Ulceration
• Vomiting	• Stricture
• Anorexia/weight loss	

Chemotherapy Complications

• Myelosuppression	• Alopecia
• Oral mucositis/diarrhea	• Fatigue
• Nausea/vomiting	• Nephrotoxicity
• Neuropathy	• Hand-foot syndrome

Data from Pisters W, Kelsen D, Powell S et al: Cancer of the stomach. In Devita VT, Helman S, Rosenberg SA, editors: *Cancer: principles and practice of oncology*, 2004, Lippincott Williams & Wilkins; Mansfield P, Yao J, Crane C: Gastric cancer. In Kufe DW, Pollock RE, Weichselbaum RR et al editors: *Cancer medicine*, Hamilton (Canada), 2003, BC Decker; Waller M: Evaluation and management of gastric adenocarcinoma, *Nurs Clin North Am* 36(3):543-552, 2001; Crookes P: Gastric cancer, *Clin Obstet Gynecol* 45(3):892-903, 2002.

Chemotherapy in advanced gastric cancer has also been investigated. Combination chemotherapy of 5-FU, anthracyclines, and cisplatin produced the highest survival, compared to single-agent 5-FU. The ECF combination has reported response rates of 46%,[39] and is well tolerated, but the impact of treatment-related side effects on the quality of life is unclear.[57] The efficacy of chemotherapy on advanced gastric cancer has been disappointing, with a median survival of less than 1 year.[39]

Current investigational therapies for the treatment of advanced gastric cancer include intraperitoneal chemotherapy with or without hyperthermia, immunotherapy, and the use of the targeted agents Erbitux, Herceptin, Tarceva, Iressa, and Avastin.[38,39,46]

Nursing management of the patient undergoing chemotherapy for gastric cancer is similar to that for esophageal cancer discussed earlier. The box above summarizes the potential disease and treatment-related complications of gastric cancer.

Disease- and Treatment-Related Complications

Common symptoms of advanced gastric carcinoma that can benefit from palliative measures include pain, bleeding, dysphagia, obstruction, and early satiety. Due to the extremely poor prognosis of these patients and the high rate of morbidity and mortality associated with surgery, other measures are used when possible. Long-acting narcotics and celiac plexus blocks can be effective in controlling pain. Chemotherapy may improve quality of life and provide pain control. Radiation therapy is often used to palliate a primary tumor or a metastatic lesion such as a bone metastasis. Topical agents such as lidocaine and sucralfate can provide relief to painful esophageal or gastric mucosa. Bleeding appears to be responsive to chemoradiotherapy. Obstructions can be treated with stenting, radiotherapy, surgical bypass, and laser therapy or PDT. These palliative procedures provide relief for only for a few months.[39] Nursing care can greatly affect symptom management and quality of life.

Prognosis

The prognosis for patients with gastric cancer depends upon the extent of disease and treatment. The 5-year survival rate in the United States is poor, at approximately 23%.[1] Most cases are an advanced stage (III or IV) at diagnosis, and even after surgery, the recurrence rate is 80%.[1]

Cancer of the Liver

Most malignancies identified in the liver are metastatic lesions from other sites. Primary liver cancer is relatively uncommon in the United States, but incidence doubled between 1975 and 1995, and continues to rise.[58,59] Worldwide, it is the fifth most common cancer,[59] with highest incidence found in areas of China and sub-Saharan Africa.[58,60]

Epidemiology

In the United States, liver cancer is reported in combination with intrahepatic bile duct cancer. Therefore, incidence data is not readily available for primary liver cancers only. The estimated number of new cases of liver and intrahepatic bile duct cancers in 2005 was 17,550, resulting in 15,420 deaths.[61] Most primary liver cancers are hepatocellular carcinomas (HCC). Worldwide, HCC results in nearly one million deaths annually.[62] It is twice as common in men as in women in the United States; the male-to-female ratio is much higher in other parts of the world. The mean age at diagnosis is 50 to 60 years, but patients are often diagnosed younger in other geographic areas.[63]

Etiology and Risk Factors

The widespread geographic variance in HCC incidence prompted extensive investigation into causative factors. HCC commonly develops in the presence of chronic liver cell injury, which produces inflammation, leading to hepatocyte regeneration and fibrosis. Repeated cycles of cell death and regeneration ultimately lead to cirrhosis,[58,59] which is found in 60% to 80% of patients with HCC.[58,59,64] Chronic infections with hepatitis B virus (HBV) and hepatitis C virus (HCV) are the most important cause of liver damage worldwide. HBV causes about 80% of HCC in the world, and HCV accounts for 30% to 50% of cases in the United States[63] and is responsible for much of the increased incidence.[59,62] Cirrhosis caused by factors other than viral hepatitis also contributes to the development of HCC. Chronic alcohol use is an important cause of cirrhosis in the United States, and is associated with 15% of HCC cases.[63]

Long-term exposure to toxic chemicals is associated with HCC.[65] Aflatoxins are toxic metabolites produced by several *Aspergillus* species. Aflatoxin B_1 (AFB_1) is produced when foods, especially peanuts and grains, are stored in warm, moist places. AFB_1 has the highest potency among the aflatoxins as a toxin and carcinogen, and is a widespread problem in humid regions of Africa and Asia, where HCC is most common.[58,59,66] Other chemicals that increase the risk of HCC development include androgenic steroids, Thorotrast (a radiology contrast agent used in the past), and oral contraceptives.[63]

Less common risk factors include certain genetic metabolic diseases, such as hereditary hemochromatosis, hereditary tyrosinemia, and antitrypsin deficiency.[62]

Multiple genetic mutations have been identified in HCC, including *p53, p73, Rb, APC, DLC-1, p16, PTEN, BRCA2, c-myc,* and *cyclin D1.* Mutations of *p53* have been detected in approximately 50% of HCCs, and are associated with poorly differentiated tumors and worse prognoses.[59]

Prevention, Screening, and Detection

Efforts to prevent HCC center on the prevention of chronic liver damage and cirrhosis. Universal vaccination of newborns against HBV in endemic areas may dramatically reduce incidence. Interferon-α is an approved treatment to reduce both liver damage and the onset of cirrhosis in chronic HBV, as well as prevent the development of HCC. Refrigerated storage and transportation of food grains should reduce the rate of ingestion of aflatoxins.[63] Continued efforts to reduce chronic alcohol abuse are also important.

Screening high-risk individuals with annual ultrasounds and obtaining an α-fetoprotein (AFP) tumor marker every 4 months has helped to identify HCC at earlier stages.[63,64] High-risk clients include those with HBV and HCV infections, chronic liver disease, and cirrhosis.

Classification

Hepatocellular carcinoma accounts for more than 90% of the adult primary cancers of the liver.[63] These are primarily adenocarcinomas, arising from parenchymal liver cells or hepatocytes.[58] Tumors arising from intrahepatic bile ducts, called cholangiocarcinomas, account for only 10% of liver cancers. Other rare liver tumors include hepatoblastomas and angiosarcomas.[58]

Clinical Features

Early-stage HCC seldom causes symptoms; therefore most patients are first seen with advanced disease. The most common presenting symptoms of HCC are abdominal pain, fatigue, anorexia, weight loss, unexplained fevers, and abdominal swelling (Clinical Features of Hepatocellular Carcinoma box).[63,67] Pain is usually dull or aching and often radiates to the right shoulder.[67] On physical examination, hepatomegaly is found in 50% to 98% of patients.[67] Other signs include ascites, splenomegaly, jaundice, and hepatic arterial bruits.[63,64,67] HCC is also associated with several paraneoplastic syndromes and these may be the presenting signs of the malignancy.[63,67] They include hypoglycemia, hypercalcemia, erythrocytosis, carcinoid syndrome, hypercholesterolemia, osteoporosis, and hyperthyroidism.[63,67]

*C*linical Features *of*

Hepatocellular Carcinoma (HCC)

- Abdominal pain (91%)
- Hepatomegaly (89%)
- Increasing abdominal girth secondary to ascites (43%)
- Anorexia/early satiety/weight loss (35-71%)
- Hepatic arterial bruits (6-25%)
- Jaundice (4-35%)
- Splenomegaly (27-42%)
- Fevers (11-54%)
- Weakness and nonspecific symptoms (25%)
- Paraneoplastic syndromes (hypoglycemia, erythrocytosis, hypercalcemia, hyperthyroidism, hypercholesterolemia, carcinoid syndrome)

Data from Leonard GD, Jarnagin WR, Allegra CJ: Primary cancers of the liver. In Abraham J, Allegra CJ, Gulley J: *Bethesda handbook of clinical oncology*, ed 2, Philadelphia, 2005, Lippincott Williams & Wilkins; Sass DA, Chopra KB: Clinical features and diagnostic evaluation of hepatocellular carcinoma. In Carr BI, editor: *Hepatocellular carcinoma: diagnosis and treatment*, Totowa, NJ, 2005, Humana Press.

Diagnosis

Diagnosis of HCC can be challenging. High-risk patients with elevated AFP levels and patients seen with clinical features of HCC should undergo high-speed helical CT scanning, allowing three-dimensional reconstruction and vascular imaging without invasive angiography.[68] One disadvantage of CT scanning is its inability to distinguish small tumors from macroregenerative nodules in cirrhotic livers.[68] In these situations, magnetic resonance imaging (MRI) is more sensitive.[63,64,68] Ultrasound technology can be beneficial in several ways. Transcutaneous ultrasonography can be used to identify liver lesions, guide percutaneous biopsy, and provide treatment by directing injection or ablation techniques.[68] Intraoperative ultrasound can determine the number and extent of lesions, as well as their association with intrahepatic arteries and veins.[68] Laparoscopic ultrasound probes can exclude the presence of extrahepatic disease on peritoneal surfaces.[68] These techniques reduce the rate of unnecessary exploratory laparotomy, thereby increasing the proportion of patients with successful liver resections.[64,68] PET scanning has not been found useful in the diagnosis of HCC, since many of these tumors do not have significantly higher fluorodeoxyglucose (FDG) uptake than surrounding liver tissue.[64]

The serum tumor marker AFP is also helpful in clinical diagnosis. AFP is elevated in 50% to 90% of HCCs. Both the degree of AFP elevation and the presence of hepatitis are of concern. Patients without hepatitis who have AFP levels above 400 mcg/dl and abnormal liver radiographic findings are likely to have HCC, whereas the AFP level suggestive of HCC in patients positive for hepatitis B surface antigen is over 4,000 mcg/dl.[63]

Preoperative tissue biopsy in resectable HCC is not often recommended because of the potential of tumor seeding and bleeding. Tissue confirmation can be accomplished by CT or ultrasound-guided percutaneous biopsy.[63] Patients with ascites may require palliative paracentesis, and cytology can provide pathologic confirmation of HCC.

Staging

In 2002, the AJCC revised the staging system for primary liver cancers based on the number and size of tumor nodules, extent of vascular invasion, lymph node involvement, and the presence of distant metastasis (TNM).[69] Table 9-4 summarizes this system. Although the TNM system is widely used, it does not reflect the degree of underlying liver disease.[63] Therefore the Child-Pugh scoring system is often added to TNM staging to determine surgical resectability and prognosis of HCC. This system differentiates liver disease into classes A, B, or C, with class C being the most severe. Factors determining class differences are encephalopathy, ascites, serum albumin level, prothrombin time, and serum bilirubin level.[63,64]

TABLE 9-4   TNM Classification and Staging for Primary Liver Cancers, Including Intrahepatic Bile Duct Carcinomas

PRIMARY TUMOR (T)

Tx	Primary tumor cannot be assessed
T0	No evidence of primary tumor
T1	Solitary tumor without vascular invasion
T2	Solitary tumor with vascular invasion or multiple tumors, none more than 5 cm
T3	Multiple tumors more than 5 cm, or tumor involving a major branch of the portal or hepatic vein(s)
T4	Tumor(s) with direct invasion of adjacent organs other than the gallbladder or with perforation of visceral peritoneum

REGIONAL LYMPH NODES (N)

NX	Regional lymph nodes cannot be assessed
N0	No regional lymph node metastasis
N1	Regional lymph node metastasis

DISTANT METASTASIS (M)

MX	Distant metastasis cannot be assessed
M0	No distant metastasis
M1	Distant metastasis

STAGE GROUPING

Stage I	T1	N0	M0
Stage II	T2	N0	M0
Stage IIIA	T3	N0	M0
Stage IIIB	T4	N0	M0
Stage IIIC	Any T	N1	M0
Stage IV	Any T	any N	M1

HISTOLOGIC GRADE (G)

The grading scheme of Edmondson and Steiner is recommended. The system employs four grades.

GX	Grade cannot be assessed
G1	Well differentiated
G2	Moderately differentiated
G3	Poorly differentiated
G4	Undifferentiated

RESIDUAL TUMOR (R)

RX	Presence of residual tumor cannot be assessed
R0	No residual tumor
R1	Microscopic residual tumor
R2	Macroscopic residual tumor

From AJCC *Cancer Staging Handbook*, ed 6, New York, 2002, Springer.

Metastasis

Common sites for distant metastases from HCC, which usually develop late in the disease course, are the lung, bone, and the adrenal glands,.[58,64] Recurrent or progressively enlarging liver lesions are serious conditions, since they greatly affect liver function. Death usually occurs due to liver failure, fatal bleeding from tumor rupture, or esophageal varices.[58]

Medical Treatment Modalities and Nursing Care Considerations

SURGERY

Surgery is the only potentially curative treatment modality for patients with HCC. However, only 30% of patients are first seen with resectable tumors.[60] The size of tumor, the number of tumors, lack of vascular involvement, and absence of extrahepatic disease are factors in determining surgical resectability. Medical comorbidities are equally important. Most patients with HCC have underlying liver dysfunction, which eliminates resection as an option. Cirrhosis can cause easy bleeding and thrombocytopenia, both of which increase the risk of serious hemorrhage. Operative mortality is 10% in cirrhotic patients, compared with 5% in those without cirrhosis.[64] The Child-Pugh scoring system, described previously, is frequently used to evaluate liver function.[60,64]

Partial or total hepatectomy and liver transplantation are surgical options for HCC. The surgery performed depends upon the clinical stage, degree of liver dysfunction, and availability of transplantation.[60,63,64] Partial hepatectomy is performed for early-stage disease in patients with adequate liver function. Small tumors have the best outcome, but recurrence is common in the remaining liver. Repeat partial hepatectomy is possible as long as adequate healthy liver is present.[63,64,68] Patients with significant cirrhosis whose tumors meet criteria regarding tumor size and number are more likely to benefit from transplantation than resection.[64] Indications for liver transplantation include single tumors smaller than 5 cm, three or fewer tumors smaller than 3 cm, and Child-Pugh class B or C. The use of these criteria leads to 5-year survival of 70%.[64] The lack of donor livers and specialty centers performing liver transplantation limits the availability of this procedure.[63,64]

Cryosurgery has become popular in treating unresectable primary and metastatic liver lesions. This procedure involves the ultrasound-guided insertion of probes into the liver. These probes are cooled by liquid nitrogen or argon, which then freezes the complete tumor, plus a 1-cm margin around the tumor(s).[64,68] The benefit is that very little nontumor liver tissue is damaged. It requires general anesthesia and laparotomy, since it cannot be done percutaneously.[64]

Percutaneous ethanol injection can be used to treat small HCCs. This involves the injection of 95% ethanol into the tumor using ultrasound guidance.[64] It has been used for patients with up to as many as three lesions, each less than 5 cm, and for patients with cirrhosis who are ineligible for resection.[63] Tumor necrosis and ischemia result. The technique is usually well-tolerated; however, local recurrences are very common.[63]

Postoperative nursing care of patients with HCC can be very complex; monitoring for bleeding, infections, respiratory complications, and organ failure is essential. Pain management, nutritional support, and patient education are also nursing priorities.

Liver transplantation involves additional concerns regarding organ rejection and immunosuppression.[63,64,68]

CHEMOTHERAPY

Systemic chemotherapy has been ineffective in treating HCC. Studies reporting the use of single-agent chemotherapy reveal response rates less than 25%, and no clear survival advantage.[59] Combination regimes may result in improved response rates, but increased toxicity makes them inappropriate for many patients. The inherent resistance of HCC to chemotherapy and the underlying liver dysfunction makes administration of these agents difficult.[63-65] Since the liver is responsible for metabolism of most chemicals, it a challenge to balance adequate dosage for tumor response with prevention of major side effects. In patients with metastatic HCC, chemotherapy may be the only treatment option available.

Anthracyclines response rates for single-agent treatment have ranged from 10% to 25%. Additional agents that have been evaluated, singly or in combination, include 5-FU, cisplatin, interferon α-2b, gemcitabine, mitoxantrone, and mitomycin C.[64,65] One phase II study evaluating the combination of cisplatin, interferon α-2b, doxorubicin, and 5-FU (PIAF) in 50 patients showed promising results. Although the objective response rate was only 26%, 9 of the 13 responding patients went on to surgical resection, and 4 of those had no viable tumor remaining (complete pathologic response). However, this combination did result in significant toxicity, primarily myelosuppression and mucositis.[70]

A significant number of HCC patients have large, unresectable tumors without extrahepatic spread. Therefore regional chemotherapy has been advocated. This involves infusing agents into the liver via the hepatic artery. Tumor cells derive the majority of their blood supply from the hepatic artery, whereas normal hepatocytes are perfused primarily by the portal circulation.[63,71] Therefore administering chemotherapy through the hepatic artery should result in increased drug delivered to the tumor, while minimizing the effect on normal cells.[64,65,72] Intraarterial chemotherapy is administered through temporary catheters placed into the axillary or femoral arteries it requires bed rest for the duration of the infusion. Complications of this method include hepatic artery thrombosis, catheter displacement, sepsis, and hemorrhage. Drugs can also be administered via an implantable pump, which offers the advantages of allowing the patient to remain ambulatory and reducing catheter-related complications. Insertion of an implantable pump requires a laparotomy, which many patients cannot tolerate.[63,64,72] The agents used most frequently for intraarterial chemotherapy are floxuridine (FUDR), 5FU, mitomycin C, cisplatin, and doxorubicin.[64,71]

Hepatic artery embolization is the selective occlusion of arterial vessels feeding the tumor. Since tumors require blood supply for survival, blocking the blood supply can result in tumor necrosis and ischemia.[71] Embolization is accomplished using gelatin sponges, collagen, alcohol, or microspheres.[63] Chemoembolization involves regional administration of chemotherapy agents, followed by embolization.[63] A randomized clinical trial in HCC patients with Child-Pugh classes A and B liver dysfunction comparing chemoembolization, embolization, and conservative treatment was stopped early because of a significant 2-year survival advantage in the chemoembolization arm (63%, 50%, and 27%, respectively).[73] Drugs used in this application include FUDR, doxorubicin, cisplatin, and mitomycin C.[64,71]

The identification of multiple genetic mutations, combined with the disappointing results of systemic chemotherapy, has prompted intense investigation of molecularly targeted agents in HCC. Targets include growth factors, growth factor receptors, and angiogenesis.[59] Recent data from clinical trials evaluating the epidermal growth factor receptor (EGFR) inhibitor erlotinib, approved for use in non–small cell lung cancer, suggest clinical benefit with acceptable toxicity in patients with HCC.[59,74]

Nursing care of patients receiving systemic treatment for HCC includes monitoring for and managing side effects of chemotherapy and targeted agents, and patient education on measures to prevent or minimize side effects. The primary side effects of chemotherapy are myelosuppression, mucositis, nausea, vomiting, fatigue, and diarrhea. Adverse effects of targeted therapy include infusion-related reactions to monoclonal antibodies, acnelike rash, and diarrhea.[59,70-72,74]

RADIATION THERAPY

Even though HCC is considered a radiosensitive tumor, the use of radiation therapy is restricted by the relative intolerance of the normal liver parenchyma. A cure or long-term remission of HCC requires significantly higher doses of radiation than the liver can tolerate, but lower doses can be used to palliate pain.[63] Radiofrequency ablation (RFA), an alternative to cryosurgery, is performed percutaneously under ultrasound guidance; it causes focal necrosis of tumors via thermal energy.[63,64] RFA does not require laparotomy, but it is more difficult to monitor tumor destruction with this therapy compared with cryosurgery.[64]

Disease- and Treatment-Related Complications

Patients with HCC present many challenges for nurses. Postoperative complications can be life threatening and require intense nursing assessment (see box to right). Since most patients have inoperable disease at diagnosis due to advanced stage or liver dysfunction, palliation of symptoms is important for optimal quality of life. Side effects of systemic and regional chemotherapy present challenges for nurses.

Prognosis

Prognosis of HCC is dependent on the ability to surgically resect the tumor. Survival rates at 5 years for stage I resected tumors are 70% to 75%; this decreases to 60% for stage II tumors and drops to 40% for stage III tumors.[60] Patients with unresectable disease generally survive less than 12 months, with median survival only 3 to 6 months.[60,64]

Cancer of the Pancreas
Epidemiology

Pancreatic cancer is the second most common GI cancer and the fourth leading cause of cancer death in the United States.[61] Cancers of the pancreas fall into two main categories: those arising in the exocrine parenchyma, and those arising in the endocrine cells of the islets of Langerhans.[75] The term *pancreatic cancer* usually refers to cancer of the exocrine pancreas. The estimated new cases of cancer of the pancreas in 2005 was 32,180, resulting in 31,800 deaths. This represents 2% of all cancers diagnosed and 5% of the cancer deaths in the United States.[61]

DISEASE-RELATED COMPLICATIONS
Hepatocellular Carcinoma (HCC)

Disease-Related
- Portal hypertension
- Ascites
- Hemorrhage from tumor or varices
- Abdominal pain
- Coagulopathy
- Jaundice

Treatment-Related
Surgery-Related
- Hemorrhage
- Organ failure (liver and kidney)
- Subphrenic and subhepatic abscesses
- Infection/sepsis
- Portal vein thrombosis
- Pneumonia, pneumothorax

Hepatic Artery Infusion–Related
- Catheter displacement and occlusion
- Arterial thrombosis
- Pump pocket hematoma/seroma
- Localized infection
- Pump malfunction
- Sclerosing cholangitis

Chemotherapy-Related
- Myelosuppression
- Mucositis
- Acnelike rash (EGFR inhibitors)
- Infusion reactions (monoclonal antibodies)
- Fatigue
- Nausea, vomiting, diarrhea

Radiation Therapy-Related
- Nausea
- Vomiting
- Anorexia
- Fatigue

EGFR, Epidermal growth factor receptor.
Data from Weber S, O'Reilly EM, Abou-Alfa GK et al: Liver and bile duct cancer. In Abeloff MD, Armitage JO, Niederhuber JE et al: *Clinical oncology*, ed 3, Philadelphia, 2004, Elsevier; Patt YZ, Hassan MM: Clinical aspects and management of hepatocellular cancer: management options: metastatic hepatocellular carcinoma. In Abbruzzese JL, Evans DB, Willett CG et al, editors: *Gastrointestinal oncology*, New York, 2004, Oxford University Press; Carr BI: Medical therapy of hepatocellular carcinoma. In Carr BI, editor: *Hepatocellular carcinoma: diagnosis and treatment*, Totowa, New Jersey, 2005, Humana Press; Alberts SR, Goldberg RM: Gastrointestinal tract cancers. In Casciato DA, editor: *Manual of clinical oncology*, Philadelphia, 2004, Lippincott Williams & Wilkins.

Pancreatic cancer incidence increased during the twentieth century but has stabilized over the last decade.[76] The incidence increases with age and is diagnosed most often in persons between 65 and 79, rarely in those under 45.[75] Pancreatic cancer is more common in men than women, with a relative risk of 1.5:1, although recent evidence indicates this gap may be narrowing. It is twice as likely to be diagnosed in African Americans as in Caucasians in the United States.[76]

Etiology and Risk Factors

Factors implicated in the development of pancreatic cancer are environmental, disease-related, and genetic (see Box 9-1). The strongest environmental factor is cigarette smoking, and it accounts for 30% of pancreatic cancers, with heavier use for longer periods increasing the risk. Diets high in fat and meat and lower in fruits and vegetables may also play a role, with obesity increasing the risk, whereas physical activity may decrease it.[77]

Risk Factors for Pancreatic Cancer

Cigarette smoking
Diabetes mellitus
Chronic pancreatitis
Dietary factors
Obesity
Familial genetic alterations

Exposure to industrial chemicals, such as those used in metal refining, has also been implicated.[78] Disease-related risk factors include diabetes mellitus and chronic pancreatitis. Although the role of diabetes in the development of pancreatic cancer is unclear, patients diagnosed with pancreatic cancer often appear to have developed diabetes within the previous 2 years, reflecting tumor-associated altered pancreatic function.[76] Longstanding diabetes and chronic pancreatitis also carry increased risk for developing pancreatic cancer, but the causal relationship has not been firmly established, except in hereditary pancreatitis.[79]

Approximately 5% of cancers are found in persons with a family history of pancreatic cancer; the relative risk is about eighteenfold in those with two first-degree relatives, and increases to fiftysevenfold when three or more relatives are involved. This suggests the presence of a familial pancreatic syndrome.[76] Pancreatic cancer is observed in other familial cancer syndromes, including Li Fraumeni, FAP, BRCA2, and familial atypical mole malignant melanoma syndrome. Higher risk is noted in families with hereditary pancreatitis syndrome.[80]

The pathogenesis of pancreatic cancer involves a series of genetic events causing activation of oncogenes and inactivation of tumor-suppressor genes and culminating in a malignant clonal cell population. The most common involve the K-*ras* and HER2/*neu* oncogenes, noted in more than 90% and 50% of pancreatic cancers, respectively. Frequent inactivating mutations involve the tumor-suppressor genes *CDKN2*, *p53* and *DPC4*, which are found in 100%, 70%, and 50% of pancreatic cancers, respectively.[76] Research also demonstrates a stepwise progression of genetic abnormalities ranging from premalignant lesions, defined as **pancreatic intraepithelial neoplasms (PanINs),** to frankly malignant lesions.[79]

Prevention, Screening, and Detection

The lack of proven risk factors for pancreatic cancer makes it difficult to recommend prevention strategies. Avoiding cigarette smoke is clearly indicated. Maintaining a healthy weight by consuming a diet low in fat and high in fruits and vegetables, and engaging in regular physical activity also seem to be prudent.[77]

There is no cost-effective screening test for pancreatic cancer. CA 19-9, a tumor-associated serum antigen elevated in 70% to 90% of pancreatic adenocarcinomas, has a relatively low specificity since it can be elevated in benign conditions such as pancreatitis and biliary inflammation.[81] It is often used in monitoring response to therapy, but it cannot be recommended for screening in asymptomatic individuals.[78]

Classification

Of cancers involving the pancreas, 95% arise from exocrine cells, and ductal adenocarcinoma accounts for 90% of these.[82]

TABLE 9-5 **Presenting Signs and Symptoms of Patients with Pancreatic Cancer**

SIGN OR SYMPTOM	PERCENTAGE OF PATIENTS
Abdominal pain	80
Anorexia	65
Weight loss	60
Early satiety	60
Sleep problems	55
Jaundice	50
Fatigue	45
Weakness, nausea, or constipation	40
Depression	40
Ascites	25

Adapted from Alberts SR, Goldberg RM: Gastrointestinal tract cancers. In Casciato DA, editor: *Manual of clinical oncology,* Philadelphia, 2004, Lippincott Williams & Wilkins.

Less common types of exocrine cancers include acinar cell carcinoma, cystadenocarcinomas, mixed adenosquamous tumors, sarcomas, and lymphomas.[83] Two thirds of these adenocarcinomas occur in the head of the pancreas and the remainder in the body and tail.[82] Less than 5% of pancreatic cancers arise in endocrine islet cells, and they are managed as neuroendocrine tumors.[80]

Clinical Features

The majority of patients have symptoms at the time of diagnosis that may have been present for weeks to months. The presenting symptoms depend on the location of the tumor: lesions in the pancreatic head (especially along the common bile duct and at the ampulla of Vater) may cause jaundice due to biliary obstruction, which may lead to an earlier diagnosis; whereas those in the body and tail tend to produce vague, nonspecific symptoms until the disease is advanced.[76,82,84] The most common presenting symptoms are abdominal and back pain, anorexia and early satiety, weight loss, jaundice, fatigue, and depression.[75] The abdominal pain is described as dull, constant pain radiating to the middle or upper back, often worse while supine. Severe pain is usually indicative of invasion of the celiac and mesenteric plexus, a sign of locally advanced or metastatic disease.[75] Anorexia and weight loss, also common, are caused by multiple factors including tumor obstruction of the duodenum, decreased gastric motility, and increased metabolic activity due to tumor-related cytokines.[76] Table 9-5 summarizes the presenting signs and symptoms of pancreatic cancer.[75]

Diagnosis and Staging

Since complete surgical resection of the tumor with negative margins offers the only chance of long-term survival, it is vital to correctly identify those patients with operable cancers. If the tumor cannot be totally resected, surgery does not offer any survival advantage.[84] Multidetector, multiphase helical CT is the optimal study for clinical staging of pancreas cancer. The objectives of CT are to evaluate for the presence of a primary tumor in the pancreas or periampullary area, identify the presence of peritoneal or liver metastasis, and evaluate the relationship of the tumor to local structures such as the superior mesenteric vein (SMV), the portal vein (PV), the superior mesenteric artery (SMA), the celiac axis, the hepatic artery, and the gastroduodenal artery.

TABLE 9-6   TNM Clinical Classification System for Staging Pancreatic Cancer

PRIMARY TUMOR (T)

TX	Primary tumor cannot be assessed
T0	No evidence of primary tumor
Tis	Carcinoma in situ*
T1	Tumor limited to the pancreas, 2 cm or less in greatest dimension
T2	Tumor limited to the pancreas, more than 2 cm in greatest dimension
T3	Tumor extends beyond the pancreas but without involvement of the celiac axis or the superior mesenteric artery
T4	Tumor involves the celiac axis or the superior mesenteric artery (unresectable primary tumor)

*This includes the "PanInIII" classification.

REGIONAL LYMPH NODES (N)

NX	Regional lymph nodes cannot be assessed
N0	No regional lymph node metastasis
N1	Regional lymph node metastasis

DISTANT METASTASIS (M)

MX	Distant metastasis cannot be assessed
M0	No distant metastasis
M1	Distant metastasis

STAGE GROUPINGS

Stage 0	Tis	N0	M0
Stage IA	T1	N0	M0
Stage IB	T2	N0	M0
Stage IIA	T3	N0	M0
Stage IIB	T1	N1	M0
	T2	N1	M0
	T3	N1	M0
Stage III	T4	Any N	M0
Stage IV	Any T	Any N	M1

HISTOLOGIC GRADE (G)

GX	Grade cannot be assessed
G1	Well differentiated
G2	Moderately differentiated
G3	Poorly differentiated
G4	Undifferentiated

RESIDUAL TUMOR (R)

RX	Presence of residual tumor cannot be assessed
R0	No residual tumor
R1	Microscopic residual tumor
R2	Macroscopic residual tumor

From AJCC Cancer Staging Handbook, ed 6, New York, 2002, Springer.

Studies indicate that up to 80% of tumors deemed resectable by helical CT are actually resectable at the time of surgery.[81] Laparoscopy may be added to the staging work-up in an effort to further define those patients who will benefit from laparotomy. The purpose of laparoscopy is to detect extrapancreatic tumor not seen on CT scans.[85] If a mass is not seen on contrast-enhanced CT, patients undergo EUS and/or endoscopic retrograde cholangiopancreatography (ERCP). If a mass is located, EUS may be used to guide a fine-needle aspiration. However, if tumors are felt to be operable, it is generally unnecessary to obtain tissue confirmation before surgery, unless neoadjuvant therapy is being considered.[85] PET is not routinely used, but studies are ongoing to determine its role.[81,84]

The AJCC has recently updated the staging system for pancreatic cancer based on tumor size and extension, regional lymph node involvement, and presence of distant metastasis using the TNM system.[69] Diagnostic evaluation using this system makes it possible to characterize cancers as operable, locally advanced, or metastatic, in order to make optimal treatment decisions and avoid unnecessary surgical procedures. Table 9-6 depicts the updated TNM classification system.

Metastasis

Fewer than 20% of patients with pancreatic cancer are first seen with potentially resectable disease, and almost half are found to have distant metastasis at the time of diagnosis. Common sites of metastatic spread include the liver, the retroperitoneum, and the lungs.[78,86]

Medical Treatment Modalities and Nursing Care Considerations

Pancreatic cancer continues to be the most difficult of all GI cancers to treat. Surgery, as part of a multimodality approach, is the only potentially curative treatment. Unfortunately, early symptoms are vague and nonspecific and do not become severe until the cancer invades adjacent organs or metastasizes. Fewer than 20% of patients meet the criteria for curative surgery.[78] Both chemotherapy and radiation therapy are being used as neoadjuvant and adjuvant therapy in operable patients and as definitive treatment in locally advanced disease.[87] Patients with metastatic disease are generally offered systemic treatment with chemotherapy, as well as newer, molecularly targeted agents.

SURGERY

Two thirds of pancreatic cancers occur in the head of the pancreas. Patients with operable, localized disease on staging evaluation will undergo curative resection with a pancreaticoduodenectomy (Whipple procedure). This involves removal of the pancreatic head, the gallbladder, the common bile duct, the duodenum, the distal stomach, and regional lymph nodes.[85] A series of three anastomoses are then performed to reestablish gastrointestinal integrity; the first between the pancreatic remnant and the jejunum, a second between the bile duct and the jejunum, and a third between the stomach pouch and the jejunum. Gastrostomy and feeding jejunostomy tubes may be placed to relieve gastric distention and provide nutritional support.[83] Figure 9-2 illustrates reconstruction after the pancreaticoduodenectomy.

A pylorus-preserving pancreaticoduodenectomy may be used for small periampullary lesions; however, this procedure is controversial.[83,85] Although it may result in improved long-term GI function and nutritional status, opponents argue that the nutritional benefit is small and delayed gastric emptying is increased, and that it may compromise complete surgical removal of the tumor with negative margins.[85]

A total pancreatectomy is an extension of the pancreaticoduodenectomy, with removal of the body and tail of the pancreas, the

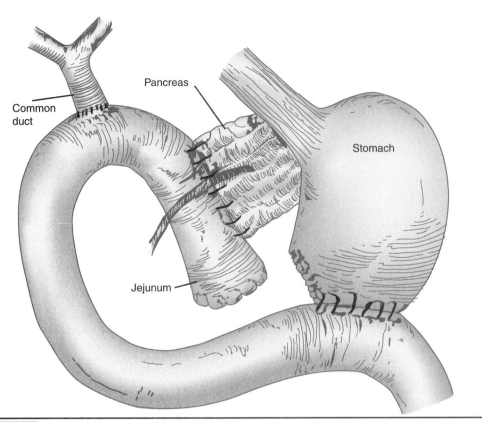

FIG. 9-2   Reconstruction following conventional panreaticoduodenectomy. (From Castillo CF, Warshaw AL: Cancer of the pancreas. In Rustgi AK, editor: *Gastrointestinal cancers: biology, diagnosis, and therapy*, Philadelphia, 1995, Lippincott-Raven.)

spleen, and more extensive regional lymph nodes. This procedure is rarely justified for pancreatic cancer, and results in brittle diabetes and pancreatic exocrine insufficiency.[83]

There are serious postoperative complications following pancreaticoduodenectomy; therefore surgery should only be attempted when there is a reasonable chance of complete tumor resection. Operative mortality and morbidity is inversely associated with surgical volume of this procedure.[80,83,85] Postoperative complications include pancreatic fistulas, intraabdominal abscesses due to leakage of the pancreatic anastomosis, and GI or drain tract bleeding. Long-term complications include delayed gastric emptying, diabetes, and pancreatic insufficiency.[83,85]

In the past, many patients underwent laparotomy with curative intent, but their disease was found to be unresectable. Palliative biliary bypass, by either cholecystojejunostomy or choledochojejunostomy, was performed to relieve obstructive jaundice. With the current availability of percutaneous and endoscopic procedures, palliative surgical bypass is less common. Endoscopic stent placement has a success rate of up to 85%, with a lower rate of complications compared to surgery.[75] Percutaneous biliary drains can be used when endoscopic stent placement is unsuccessful or inappropriate.

Nursing care of surgical patients with pancreatic cancer focuses on monitoring for and managing postoperative complications. Bleeding, infection, anastomotic leaking, blood sugar and electrolyte disturbances, and nutritional deficiencies can all be catastrophic for patients, if not identified and managed early. Pain control, management of GI symptoms, and nutritional support are also priority nursing considerations.[75,76,78,83]

CHEMOTHERAPY

Although pancreatic cancer remains a relatively chemoresistent disease, with single-agent objective response rates below 25%, most patients will receive some form of systemic therapy. Neoadjuvant chemotherapy or chemoradiotherapy may be used in potentially resectable disease; the hope is to shrink the tumor and eliminate micrometastatses.[81,84,85] The standard of care has been 5-FU–based chemotherapy. This therapy is still used, especially when combined with radiation therapy. Capecitabine, an oral 5-FU prodrug, is also combined with radiation. Gemcitabine was found to be active in pancreatic cancer, and was approved based on clinical benefit response (CBR) rather than tumor shrinkage. CBR is a comprehensive assessment of quality of life and considers such factors as pain control, performance status, and weight gain to evaluate treatment benefit in patients with advanced pancreatic cancer. Since its approval in 1996, gemcitabine has been studied extensively in pancreatic cancer and, based on a randomized phase III study showing superiority to 5-FU, is currently considered the standard of care for advanced disease.[88] Gemcitabine is also offered as adjuvant treatment for patients who have undergone surgical resection with negative margins, since recent studies have demonstrated survival benefit when postoperative chemotherapy is given.[81,89,90]

Many chemotherapy agents have been combined with gemcitabine, including cisplatin, oxaliplatin, docetaxel, 5-FU, and irinotecan, with response rates for the cisplatin and oxaliplatin combinations up to 36%, although no definitive survival benefit has been established. Numerous clinical trials are ongoing.[88,91] Patients with better performance status (Eastern

DISEASE-RELATED COMPLICATIONS
Pancreatic Cancer

- Abdominal and back pain
- Obstructive jaundice
- Postoperative complications, including intraabdominal abscesses, fistulas, and bleeding
- Weight loss due to anorexia, malabsorption, and intestinal obstruction
- Side effects from chemotherapy and radiation therapy (myelosuppression, nausea, vomiting, diarrhea, hand-foot syndrome, stomatitis)
- Late complications of surgery and stenting procedures (cholangitis, gastrointestinal ulceration, diabetes mellitus, dumping syndrome)

Data from references 85, 91, and 95-98.

Cooperative Oncolcoy Group [ECOG] 0 or 1) tolerate treatment better and have an increased chance of response. In these situations, combination therapy with two agents is reasonable, since additional agents may increase toxicity with no significant improvement in outcome. When possible, patients should be offered treatment on a clinical trial. The side effects from chemotherapy include myelosuppression, stomatitis, hand-foot syndrome, nausea and vomiting, and diarrhea.[88]

Because pancreatic cancer is relatively chemoresistant, there is interest in the use of molecularly targeted agents, both as single agents, and in combination with chemotherapy. Two EGFR inhibitors, erlotinib and the monoclonal antibody cetuximab, have demonstrated activity when combined with gemcitabine.[91-93] Side effects from EGFR inhibitors are acnelike rash and diarrhea.[74]

Nursing management of patients receiving systemic therapy for pancreatic cancer is similar to that for HCC and can be reviewed in that section. In addition, gemcitabine therapy can cause flulike symptoms. Cisplatin can be renal-toxic and so necessitates adequate hydration and monitoring of kidney function and electrolytes. Also, severe infusion-related reactions are possible with monoclonal antibodies, so nurses must be familiar with protocols for prevention and management of these problems.[75,76,78,88,94]

RADIATION THERAPY

In the United States, radiation therapy is used both preoperatively and adjuvantly in resectable patients, and as definitive therapy in locally advanced disease, with usual doses in the range of 50-60 Gy. It is used in combination with 5-FU–or gemcitabine-based chemotherapy, since improved outcomes have been demonstrated in comparison with radiation therapy alone.[95] Concurrent chemoradiotherapy is the standard of care for locally advanced, unresectable pancreatic cancer. Use in the adjuvant setting is more controversial. Although studies in the United States have supported the use of postoperative radiation therapy, a large European study actually demonstrated poorer survival when radiation was given after surgery.[89] Nausea, vomiting, and fatigue are the primary side effects from radiation therapy for pancreatic cancer.[87,90,95] Nursing care involves monitoring and patient education to help minimize and manage these symptoms.

Disease- and Treatment-Related Complications

Patients with pancreatic cancer present a significant challenge for nurses. For the surgical patient, careful postoperative monitoring for complications, pain control, and nutritional support are essential for optimal recovery. Patients with locally advanced and metastatic disease require extensive supportive care to relieve pain, nausea and vomiting, fatigue, and nutritional deficiencies (see box to left). Patient education about management of side effects from chemotherapy and radiation therapy can help to optimize quality of life.[94] Narcotic analgesics form the cornerstone of pain management, but studies have shown that neurolytic celiac plexis block with alcohol can palliate pancreatic cancer pain for several months.[96,97]

Prognosis

Despite advances in diagnosis and treatment, the overall prognosis for persons with cancer of the pancreas remains poor, with 5-year survival rates for all stages of less than 5%.[76,78,88,98] Thus far, improved surgical techniques and supportive care have not measurably improved overall survival. The 5-year survival rate in patients who have had a pancreatoduodenectomy is 15% to 20%, with a median survival of 11 to 20 months. Patients with locally advanced disease have a median survival of 10 to 12 months, and those with metastatic disease survive only 5 to 7 months.[81,90]

Uncommon Gastrointestinal Cancers

Some uncommon cancers of the gastrointestinal tract include small intestine cancers, carcinoid tumors, cholangiocarcinomas and gallbladder cancer, anal canal cancer, and GIST.

CANCER OF THE SMALL INTESTINES

Neoplasms of the small intestines are rare. They comprise only 2% of GI malignancies. The estimated number of new cases for 2005 was 5420, which resulted in 1070 deaths.[1] More than 40 different histologic types of malignancies have been found in the small intestine. The four most common include adenocarcinoma (22% to 44%), carcinoid (20% to 42%), lymphoma (12% to 27%), and sarcoma or GIST (11%).[99] Risk factors associated with small intestine cancers include FAP, HNPCC, Crohn's disease, celiac disease, Peutz-Jehgers syndrome, Gardner's syndrome, neurofibromatosis, acquired immunodeficiency syndrome (AIDS), and prior history of colorectal, prostate, lung, or breast cancer.[99, 100] Symptoms are vague and nonspecific and include abdominal pain, nausea or vomiting, weight loss, and GI bleeding that occurs when the disease is advanced. Approximately half of the bleeding presents as an acute event, 77% at the time of perforation or obstruction. Endoscopy is used to identify these tumors including wireless capsule endoscopy.[99]

The best curative modality for all tumors found in the small intestine is surgery. The use of other treatment modalities depends on the histologic type of tumor and extent of spread. Lymphoma is often treated with adjuvant chemotherapy or radiation therapy, whereas the role of adjuvant chemotherapy or radiation therapy has not been clearly defined for adenocarcinomas, carcinoid, or GISTs of the small intestine. Chemotherapy for adenocarcinoma of the small intestine consists of 5-FU alone or in combination with other agents. Treatment of lymphoma will depend on the subtype involved. Targeted therapy with is Gleevec is often used in advanced GIST with minimal toxicity. Adjuvant studies with this agent are ongoing. The overall survival for small intestine cancers is approximately 50%.[99]

CARCINOID TUMORS

The GI tract is the most common location (67.5%) for carcinoid tumors, with the small intestine (41.8%), and rectum (27.4%) being the most common GI sites.[99] Little is known about the etiology of these tumors. Growth factors, oncogenes, or tumor suppresser genes may play a role.[101] Symptoms of GI carcinoid tumors include intestinal obstruction and bleeding. Carcinoid syndrome is demonstrated by patients with advanced GI carcinoid tumors and includes facial and neck flushing, diarrhea, and occasionally right-sided heart failure or wheezing.[101] Diagnosis is made by endoscopy. CT and octreotide scan may assist in identifying metastatic disease.[100] Plasma or urine levels of serotonin or its metabolite (5-HIAA) should also be obtained to diagnose carcinoid syndrome. Surgery is the treatment of choice for curative intent. Unfortunately, 45% of patients have metastatic disease when first evaluated, frequently involving the liver. Systemic therapy includes long-acting somatatostatin analogues, hepatic artery embolization, hepatic resection, chemotherapy, and interferon. Additional symptomatic relief of the symptoms associated with carcinoid syndrome may be necessary. Chemotherapy is reserved for aggressive tumors that are unresponsive to somatostatin analogues. The progression of these tumors is slow, and the 5-year survival for patients with distant metastasis is 22%.[101]

BILE DUCT (CHOLANGIOCARCINOMAS) AND GALLBLADDER CANCERS

Cancers of the gallbladder and biliary system are relatively uncommon. In 2005, the estimated incidence was 7480 and deaths, 3340.[61] Gallbladder cancer is more common in women, whereas cholangiocarcinomas occur slightly more frequently in men. Incidence of both increases with age, and most patients are over 60 when diagnosed.[60,64] These cancers arise in the epithelial lining of the gallbladder and bile ducts, and most are adenocarcinomas. Up to 90% are associated with gallstones and chronic inflammation. Risk factors for cholangiocarcinomas include chronic bile duct inflammation from exposure to industrial solvents, liver fluke infestation, primary sclerosing cholangitis, and ulcerative colitis.[60] Diagnostic studies include helical CT, ultrasonography, MRI, and ERCP, and staging follows the TNM staging system.[60,102] Signs and symptoms can be vague and nonspecific and include abdominal pain, weight loss, anorexia, nausea and vomiting, right upper quadrant abdominal mass, and jaundice.

Surgical resection offers the only curative chance for gallbladder and bile duct cancers, and 5-FU–based adjuvant chemoradiation is often given. Locally advanced disease is treated similarly to pancreatic cancer, with 5-FU– or gemcitabine-based chemoradiation therapy. Metastatic disease is treated with single-agent or combination systemic chemotherapy, again primarily gemcitabine- or 5-FU–based.[60,102] Prognosis for early-stage, resectable gallbladder and bile duct cancers includes a 5-year survival rate of 60% to 80%. Unfortunately, most patients are first seen with unresectable disease, and median survival is 12 to 20 months for locally advanced, and 4 to 8 months for metastatic disease.[75,102]

ANAL CANAL CANCERS

Cancer of the anal canal occurs infrequently in the United States, with approximately 4000 cases per year; but risk is increasing, especially among patients positive for human immunodeficiency virus (HIV) and young homosexual males.[103] Risk factors with strong epidemiologic evidence include human papillomavirus (HPV) infection, receptive anal intercourse, history of multiple sexual partners and sexually transmitted disease, history of cervical or vaginal cancer, and immunosuppression. Other evidence implicates long-term use of corticosteroids and cigarette smoking.[75,104] The histologic type of anal canal cancer is dependent on its location, with those occurring distally being primarily squamous cell carcinomas, and those occurring closer to the rectum often cloacogenic (transitional) cell carcinomas.[104] Presenting signs and symptoms include anal bleeding, pain, sensation of a mass, constipation, diarrhea, and pruritus.[104] Diagnosis is made by physical examination and biopsy. Staging is usually by the TNM system, and complete staging generally includes abdominal and pelvic CT, endoscopic ultrasound, chest radiograph, and laboratory studies.[103,104]

Management of small tumors (less than 2 cm) includes simple excision, but larger lesions are usually treated with a multimodality approach of combined chemotherapy and radiation. Anal canal tumors are chemoradiotherapy-sensitive, so cure rate with this treatment is 65% to 75%.[103] The radiation dose given ranges from 40 to 60 Gy, and the chemotherapy consists of 5-FU and mitomycin C. Treatment side effects include perineal skin reactions, at times with moist desquamation, fatigue, nausea, vomiting, diarrhea, dysuria, and rectal and vaginal irritation.[103] Since surgical removal of larger tumors requires a permanent colostomy, it is usually reserved for salvage therapy of recurrent or unresponsive tumors.[75] Prognosis for anal canal cancer depends on tumor size; those smaller than 2 cm have a cure rate of 80%, which drops to 50% for tumors greater than 5 cm.[103]

GASTROINTESTINAL STROMAL TUMORS (GIST)

Historically, gastrointestinal stromal tumors (GISTs) have been uncommon, but recent improvements in pathologic techniques have provided improved identification of these tumors, classified as sarcomas. Approximately 5000 to 6000 cases occur annually in the United States, usually in patients over 50 years of age. Incidence is equal among men and women, and higher in Caucasians.[105] The hallmark of GISTs is the abnormal activation of *KIT* in tumor cells. *KIT* is a receptor expressed on certain cells, involved in various physiologic processes of cell proliferation. Mutations in the *KIT* gene are found in 90% of GISTs, and positive *KIT* staining on tumor cells is diagnostic.[105,106] Presenting signs and symptoms in patients with GISTs include abdominal fullness, discomfort and pain, nausea, vomiting, anorexia, weight loss, and GI tract bleeding.[106] GISTs are most common in the stomach and small intestine. Diagnostic workup includes endoscopic procedures, CT scans, ultrasonograpy, and PET scans, which have been found to be particularly useful in evaluating response to treatment.[105] Although the TNM system is used to stage GISTs, they are generally classified based on their malignant behavior (mitotic rate and proliferation index).[105]

Almost 50% of GISTs are unresectable at presentation; however, complete surgical removal is the only curative treatment. GISTs are generally unresponsive to chemotherapy and radiation therapy, and previously, treatment of inoperable and metastatic disease was difficult. Recently, the molecular biology of GISTs has led to successful treatment targeting abnormal *KIT* activation with

CONSIDERATIONS FOR OLDER ADULTS
Gastrointestinal Cancers

Factors Related to Cancer Prevention and Early Detection

- Encourage low-fat, high-fiber diet within ethnic, social, and economic limitations.
- Encourage smoking cessation and avoidance of exposure to other health hazards (e.g., sun, chemicals, petroleum products).
- Be suspicious of symptoms such as malaise, fatigue, anorexia, weight loss, and altered bowel habits as possible indicators of cancer and not automatically attributable to nonmalignant illnesses associated with aging.

Factors Related to Modalities of Therapy

- Alterations in hepatic and renal function may necessitate adjustment of dosage and schedule of chemotherapy protocols.
- Decreased bone marrow cellularity may place patient at risk for prolonged myelosuppression with chemotherapy as a result of toxic effects on bone marrow.
- Decreased nutritional intake may be exacerbated because of nausea and taste changes associated with many chemotherapeutic agents typically used for GI malignancies.
- Fatigue may be increasing problem after courses of therapy, requiring additional assistance with activities of daily living.
- Comorbid disease (e.g., obesity, poor nutritional status, lung and cardiovascular disease, altered immune function) places the older adult at greater risk for surgical morbidity and mortality.
- Teaching should be tailored to take into account older adult's life experiences and cognitive and physical impairments (e.g., reading comprehension, decreased vision and hearing, altered tactile sense, misconceptions regarding cancer and cancer treatment, past experience with cancer and family members).

Modified from Boyle DM, Engelking C, Blesch KS et al: Oncology nursing society position paper on cancer and aging: the mandate for oncology nursing, *Oncol Nurs Forum* 19(6):913, 1992.

the tyrosine-kinase inhibitor imatinib (Gleevec). Clinical trials demonstrate high objective response rates with imatinib, originally approved for patients with chronic myelogenous leukemia (CML).[105,106] Clinical trials evaluating imatinib for neoadjuvant and adjuvant treatment of GISTs are ongoing. The most common adverse effects associated with imatinib are nausea, vomiting, diarrhea, edema, and skin rash, controlled with antiemetics and diuretics. Rare serious side effects include altered liver function and GI bleeding.[105,106] Survival rates for patients with GISTs vary between 35% and 65%, and median survival has increased from 23 to 50 months with the use of molecularly targeted drug therapy.[106]

Considerations for Older Adults

Older adults are at higher risk for most GI cancers. However, age should not dictate the treatment options for the older patient. Research indicates that age alone does not predict a difference in tolerance to treatment. A multidimensional assessment of older adults should determine the appropriate treatment options and assist in the management of disease and treatment-related complications. This assessment should include an evaluation of functional status, comorbid medical conditions, cognition, psychologic status, social functioning, medication review, and nutritional status. All of these issues should be considered when caring for and educating the older patient. Based on this assessment, the care can be individualized to each patient.[107]

Conclusion

GI tumors continue to challenge the health and quality of life for both patients and family members. Although there have been new advances in the diagnosis and treatment of these disease entities, the morbidity and mortality of the both disease and treatment continue to confound professionals in the field despite recent progress. Nursing's role in the area of GI malignancies continues to grow and necessitate constant vigilance in acquiring current knowledge updates, symptom management, diagnostic improvements, and treatment regimens. Hopefully these efforts will prove to make the arena of gastrointestinal malignancies more manageable, offering some improved patient outcomes and decrease in disease.

REVIEW QUESTIONS

✓ Case Study

BJ is a 57-year-old Caucasian man who comes to see his primary care practitioner with a 6-month history of progressive dysphagia, 2-year history of dyspepsia, and a 20-lb weight loss over the last 6 weeks. BJ has not sought medical care for the last 5 years and has been generally in good health. He has no significant medical or surgical history. He has a 50-pack-year history and consumes 2 to 3 beers a day. He is married and has 3 children, who range in age from 29 to 35 years. He is employed at an auto manufacturing plant, where he works on the assembly line. BJ has no family history of cancer. His review of systems is negative other than the symptoms he first listed. On physical exam he is obese, with a weight of 315 lb; the remainder of his exam is normal.

BJ's primary care doctor sends him for an upper GI study, which reveals an abnormality at the GE junction. He is referred to a gastroenterologist and during EGD is found to have an ulcerative lesion in the lower esophagus near the GE junction, which appears to arise from a Barrett's esophagus. This is biopsied, and the pathology reveals adenocarcinoma. The scope can be passed beyond the lesion. He undergoes a presurgery work-up, which reveals normal CBC and liver function tests. The CT reveals a thickening at the GE junction and borderline lymph nodes in the periesophageal region. A PET scan is done, which does not reveal evidence of liver metastasis. An EUS suggests that the lesion appears to invade the muscularis propria and is suspect for regional lymph node involvement. He appears to have a stage II to III esophageal adenocarcinoma.

The patient is referred for combination neoadjuvant chemotherapy and radiation. He is treated with cisplatin and 5-FU. His treatment is delayed twice because of mucositis and vomiting, but eventually he is able to complete his prescribed therapy. He loses 50 lb during his treatment and requires the placement of a J-tube to prevent further weight loss. A subtotal esophagectomy is performed. The pathology reveals residual adenocarcinoma in the esophagus and in 2 of the 10 lymph nodes in the sample. One week after discharge, he develops right lower extremity edema and is found to have a deep vein thrombosis. He is treated with low-molecular-weight heparin. BJ receives 6 months of adjuvant chemotherapy. He retains his J-tube during
Continued

this time because of difficulty with anorexia. Throughout the course of his treatment and recovery, he is unable to work because of treatment-related toxicity. This causes him significant financial and psychosocial strain. The social worker assists him in identifying community resources. Two months after completing his therapy, he is able to return to work. He undergoes routine blood tests, physical examination, CT and endoscopy 1 year later and is without evidence of disease.

QUESTIONS

1. Which of the following is a known risk factor for esophageal cancer that was present in BJ's case?
   a. Obesity
   b. Young age
   c. Caucasian race
   d. Consumption of well water
2. Which of the following type of esophageal cancer is most common in the United States?
   a. Squamous cell cancer (SCC)
   b. Adenocarcinoma
   c. Lymphoma
   d. Sarcoma
3. Which of the following measures is designed to prevent the development of esophageal cancer?
   a. *H. pylori* eradication
   b. Consuming a high-protein diet
   c. Maintaining a healthy weight
   d. Avoiding pickled foods
4. Which of the following statements is true?
   a. Most of the gastric cancers diagnosed in the United States are found at an early stage.
   b. NSAIDS reduce the risk of esophageal and gastric cancers.
   c. In the United States, routine endoscopy is recommended as screening for esophageal or gastric cancer.
   d. Heartburn is more commonly associated with squamous cell carcinoma than adenocarcinoma.
5. Which of the following are true?
   a. Esophageal stricture is a short-term effect of radiation.
   b. Amifostine has been found to be beneficial in reducing the severity of mucositis related to treatment.
   c. Adjuvant radiation therapy is recommended for node-positive esophageal cancer because it prolongs survival.
   d. Alcohol has been found to be a risk factor for gastric cancer but not esophageal cancer.
6. Which of the following is true concerning cancers of the GI tract?
   a. With the exception of colorectal cancer, pancreatic adenocarcinoma has the highest mortality rate of all GI cancers.
   b. Gallbladder cancers occur more frequently in men than women.
   c. The primary treatment for hepatocellular carcinoma is chemotherapy.
   d. GI stromal tumors (GISTs) respond well to chemotherapy.

7. Which statement regarding pancreatic cancer treatment is true?
   a. Concurrent chemoradiation is the treatment of choice for localized disease.
   b. Chemotherapy is very effective for metastatic disease.
   c. Locally advanced disease is treated with concurrent chemoradiotherapy.
   d. Molecularly targeted agents have proved ineffective in pancreatic cancer.
8. Which of the following statements is *not true* regarding hepatocellular carcinoma?
   a. Surgical resection offers the only opportunity for cure.
   b. Risk factors include HBV and HCV infections.
   c. HCC usually develops in the presence of cirrhosis.
   d. Hepatic artery infusions and chemoembolization are treatments for metastatic disease.
9. Of the following statements about uncommon GI cancers, which is accurate?
   a. Carcinoid tumors occur most commonly in the stomach.
   b. Imatinib is effective in treating GISTs.
   c. Surgery is the treatment of choice for large, nonmetastatic anal canal tumors.
   d. Cancer of the small intestine is treated with concurrent chemoradiation.
10. Which of the following is true concerning care of older adults with GI cancers?
   a. Patients over 65 years of age tolerate chemotherapy poorly.
   b. Studies have shown that using age as the primary factor to determine treatment options is valid.
   c. Older adults always have major organ dysfunction.
   d. Older adults with good functional status can be safely treated with chemotherapy, but should be monitored closely for toxicity.

ANSWERS

1. **A.** *Rationale:* Older age and African American race are risk factors for esophageal cancer, but not applicable in BJ's case. Consumption of well water is a risk factor in stomach cancer. BJ is obese.
2. **B.** *Rationale:* Lymphoma and sarcoma are not common types of esophageal cancer. SCC is the most common type of esophageal cancer world wide.
3. **C.** *Rationale:* H pylori eradication is currently not feasible or cost-effective. Consumption of a high-protein diet increases risk of esophageal cancer. Avoidance of pickled foods is noted as a factor in stomach cancer development, not esophageal cancer.
4. **B.** *Rationale:* In the United States, routine endoscopy is *not* recommended as a screening tool for esophageal or gastric cancer since these cancers are uncommon in the United States compared to China and Japan. Heartburn is more commonly associated with adenocarcinoma of the esophagus, *not* squamous cell carcinoma. Most gastric cancers in the United States are diagnosed at a late stage.

5. **B.** *Rationale:* Esophageal stricture is a late effect of radiation therapy. Adjuvant radiation therapy has not been found to prolong survival. Alcohol is a risk factor for esophageal cancer but has not been shown to be a definite risk factor for gastric cancer.

6. **A.** *Rationale:* Gallbladder cancers are more common in women then in men. Surgical resection is the primary curative treatment for HCC. GIST responds poorly to systemic chemotherapy.

7. **C.** *Rationale:* Localized pancreatic cancer is best treated surgically, whereas chemotherapy is generally ineffective. However, molecularly targeted agents have shown some promise in this disease.

8. **D.** *Rationale:* These statements are true: surgical resection does offer the only opportunity for cure; risk factors do include HBV and HCV; and HCC usually develops in the presence of cirrhosis. Hepatic artery infusions and chemoembolization are treatments not generally used for *metastatic* disease.

9. **B.** *Rationale:* The most common sites for carcinoid tumors are the small intestine and the rectum, not the stomach. Concurrent chemoradiation is the primary treatment in larger tumors. Surgery is the primary treatment modality for cancers of the small intestine. Imatinib *is* effective in treating GIST.

10. **D.** *Rationale:* There is no age limit to treating patients with GI cancers; functional status and comorbidities are most important. Not all older adults have major organ dysfunction. Older adults with good performance status can be treated with chemotherapy, but should be closely monitored for toxicities.

REFERENCES

1. American Cancer Society. *Cancer Facts & Figures, 2005,* Atlanta, 2005, Author.
2. Parkin DM, Bray F, Ferlay J et al: Global cancer statistics, 2002, *CA Cancer J Clin* 55:74-108.
3. Glenn TF: Esophageal cancer facts, figures, and screening, *Gastroenterol Nurs* 24(6):271-275, 2001.
4. Sampliner RE: Epidemiology, pathophysiology, and treatment of Barrett's esophagus: reducing mortality from esophageal adenocarcinoma, *Med Clin North Am* 89:293-312, 2005.
5. Engel LS, Chow WH, Vaughan TL et al: Population attributable risks of esophageal cancers, *J Natl Cancer Inst* 95(18):1404-1413, 2003.
6. Chen H, Ward MH, Graubard BI et al: Dietary patterns and adenocarcinoma of the esophagus and distal stomach, *Am J Clin Nutr* 75:137-144, 2002.
7. Morita M, Saeki H, Mori M et al: Risk factors for esophageal cancer and the multiple occurrence of carcinoma in the upper aerodigestive tract, *Surgery* 131(1):s1-s6, 2002.
8. Lagergren J: Adenocarcinoma of the oesophagus: what exactly is the size of the problem and who is at risk? *Gut* 54(Suppl 1):i1-i5, 2005.
9. Rozen P: Cancer of the gastrointestinal tract: early detection or early prevention? *Eur J Cancer Prev* 13(1):71-75, 2004.
10. Shaheen NJ: Advances in Barrett's esophagus and esophageal adenocarcinoma, *Gastroenterology* 128(6):1554-1566, 2005.
11. Chen H, Tucker KL, Graubard BI et al: Nutrient intakes and adenocarcinomas of the esophagus and distal stomach, *Nutr Cancer* 42(1):33-40, 2002.
12. Wang D, Mann J, Dubois RN: The role of prostaglandins and other eicosanoids in the gastrointestinal tract, *Gastroenterology* 128(5):1445-1461, 2005.
13. Corley DA, Kerlikowske K, Verma R et al: Protective association of aspirin/NSAIDs and esophageal cancer: a systematic review and meta-analysis, *Gastroenterology* 124(1):47-56, 2003.
14. Swisher SG, Ajani JA, Komaki RK et al: Neoplasms of the esophagus. In Kufe DW, Pollock RE, Weichselbaum RR et al editors: *Cancer Medicine,* Hamilton (Canada), 2003, BC Decker.
15. Iyer RB, Silverman PM, Tamm EP et al: Imaging in oncology from the University of Texas M.D. Anderson Cancer Center, diagnosis, staging, and follow-up of esophageal cancer, *AJR, Am J Roentgenol* 181(3):785-793, 2003.
16. Reed CE, Eloubeidi MA: New techniques for staging of esophageal cancer, *Surg Clin N Am* 82:697-710, 2002.
17. Hustinx R: PET imaging in assessing gastrointestinal cancers, *Radiol Clin N Am* 42(6):1123-1139, 2004.
18. Posner M, Forastiere A, Minsky B: Cancer of the esophagus. In Devita VT, Hellman S, Rosenberg SA, editors: *Cancer: principles and practice of oncology,* 2004, Lippincott Williams & Wilkins.
19. Refaely Y, Krasna MJ: Multimodality therapy for esophageal cancer, *Surg Clin N Am* 82(4):729-746, 2002.
20. Lordick F, Stein HJ, Peschel C et al: Neoadjuvant therapy for oesophagogastric cancer, *Br J Surg* 91(5):540-551, 2004.
21. Takahashi I, Emi Y, Hasuda S et al: Clinical application of hyperthermia combined with anticancer drugs for the treatment of solid tumors, *Surgery* 131(1 Suppl):S78-84, 2002.
22. Nozoe T, Saeki H, Ito S et al: Preoperative hyperthermochemoradiotherapy for esophageal carcinoma, *Surgery* 131(1 Suppl):S35-38, 2002.
23. Webber J, Herman M, Kessel D et al: Current concepts in gastrointestinal photodynamic therapy, *Ann Surg* 230(1):12-23, 1999.
24. Atkins BZ, Shah AS, Hutcheson KA et al: Reducing hospital morbidity and mortality following esophagectomy, *Ann Thorac Surg* 78:1170-1176.
25. McCulloch P, Ward J, Tekkis P: Mortality and morbidity in gastro-oesophageal surgery: initial results of the ASCOT multicentre prospective cohort study, *BMJ* 327:1192-1197, 2003.
26. Litle VR, Buenaventura PO, Luketich JD: Minimally invasive resection for esophageal cancer, *Surg Clin N Am* 82:711-728, 2002.
27. Mackenzie DJ, Popplewell PK, Billingsley KG: Care of patients after esophagectomy, *Crit Care Nurse,* 24(1):16-31, 2004.
28. Harris D, Dawson R, Moseley L et al: Patient satisfaction after surgery for GI malignancy, *Gastrointest Nursing* 2(10):25-31, 2004.
29. Olsson U, Bergbom I, Bosaeus I: Patients' experiences of the recovery period 3 months after gastrointestinal surgery, *Eur J Cancer Care* 11:51-60, 2002.
30. Sweed MR, Schiech L, Barsevick A et al: Quality of life after esophagectomy for cancer, *Oncol Nurs Forum* 29(7):1127-1131.
31. Tierney J, Arnott SJ, Duncan W et al: Preoperative radiotherapy for esophageal carcinoma, *Cochrane Database Syst Rev* 19(4):CD001799, 2005.
32. Greer SE, Goodney PP, Sutton JE et al: Neoadjuvant chemoradiotherapy for esophageal carcinoma: a meta-analysis, *Surgery* 137(2):178-179, 2005.
33. Burak WE: Is neoadjuvant therapy the answer to adenocarcinoma of the esophagus? *Amer J Surg* 186:296-300, 2003.
34. Thomas JA: Esophageal cancer and the esophagus: challenges and potential strategies for selective cytoprotection of the tumor-bearing organ during cancer treatment, *Semin Radiat Oncol* 12(1 Suppl 1):62-67, 2002.
35. Sasse AD, Clark LG, Sasse EC et al: Amifostine reduces side effects and improves complete response rate during radiotherapy: Results of a meta-analysis, *Int Radiat Oncol Biol Phys* Sep 27, 2005.
36. Malthaner R, Fenlon D: Preoperative chemotherapy for resectable thoracic esophageal cancer, *Cochrane Database Syst Rev* 1:CD001556, 2001.
37. Bailey K: Management of dysphagia in patients with advanced oesophageal cancer, *Gastrointestinal Nursing* 2(2):18-22, 2004.
38. Pisters W, Kelsen D, Powell S et al: Cancer of the stomach. In Devita VT, Hellman S, Rosenberg SA, editors: *Cancer: principles and practice of oncology,* 2004, Lippincott Williams & Wilkins.
39. Mansfield P, Yao J, Crane C: Gastric cancer. In Kufe DW, Pollock RE, Weichselbaum RR et al editors: *Cancer Medicine,* Hamilton (Canada), 2003, BC Decker.

40. Waller M: Evaluation and Management of gastric adenocarcinoma, *Nurs Clin North Am* 36(3):543-552, 2001.

41. Hohenberger P, Gretschel S: Gastric cancer, *Lancet* 362(9380):305-315, 2003.

42. Terry P, Lagergren J, Ye W et al: Inverse association between intake of cereal fiber and risk of gastric cardia cancer, *Gastroenterology* 120(2): 387-391, 2001.

43. Bjelakovic G, Nikolova D, Simonetti R et al: Antioxidant supplements for the prevention of gastrointestinal cancers: a systematic review and meta-analysis, *Lancet* 364(9441):1219-1228, 2004.

44. Wang W, Huang J, Zheng G et al: Non-steroidal anti-inflammatory drug use and the risk of gastric cancer: a systematic review and meta-analysis, *J Natl Cancer Inst* 95(23):1784-1791, 2003.

45. Roderick P, Davies R, Raftery J et al: Cost-effectiveness of population screening for Helicobacter pylori in preventing gastric cancer and peptic ulcer disease, using simulation, *J Med Screen* 10(3):148-156, 2003.

46. Dicken B, Bigam D, Cass C et al: Gastric adenocarcinoma, review and considerations for future directions, *Ann Surg* 241(1):27-39, 2005.

47. Marshall B, Windsor H: The relation of *Helicobacter pylori* to gastric adenocarcinoma and lymphoma: pathophysiology, epidemiology, screening, clinical presentation, treatment, and prevention, *Med Clin N Am* 89(2):313-344, 2005.

48. D'Ugo D, Pende V, Persiani R et al: Laparoscopic staging of gastric cancer, *J Am Coll Surg* 196(6):965-974, 2003.

49. Bean M, Horton K, Fishman E: Detection and diagnosis of gastric carcinoma with multidetector and 3D computed tomography, *Appl Radiol* 34(3):20-30, 2005.

50. Charalambous C, Zipitiz C, Midwinter M: Gastric adenocarcinoma metastatic to the skin: a report, *Eur J Cancer Care* 11(2):143-144, 2002.

51. Kitano S, Shirashi N: Minimally invasive surgery for gastric tumors, *Surg Clin N Am* 85(1):151-164, 2005.

52. Kobayashi T, Kazui T, 78ura T: Surgical local resection for early gastric cancer, *Surg Laparosc Percutan Tech* 13(5):299-303, 2003.

53. Giarelli E: Prophylactic gastrectomy for CDH1 mutation carriers, *Clin J Oncol Nurs* 6(3):161-162, 2002.

54. Crookes P: Gastric cancer, *Clin Obstet Gynecol* 45(3):892-903, 2002.

55. Olsson U, Bergbom I, Bosaeus I: Patient's experiences of their intake of food and fluid following gastrectomy due to tumor, *Gastroenterol Nurs* 25(4):146-153, 2002.

56. Master S: Gastric carcinoma, *Dis Mon* 50:532-539, 2004.

57. Wagner A, Grothe W, Behl S et al: Chemotherapy for advanced gastric cancer, *Cochrane Database Syst Rev* Apr 18(2):CD004064, 2005.

58. Crawford JM: Liver and biliary tract. In Kumar V, Abbas AK, Fausto N, editors. *Robbins and Cotran Pathologic Basis of Disease*, ed. 7, Philadelphia, 2005, Elsevier.

59. Thomas MB, Abbruzzese JL: Opportunities for targeted therapies in hepatocellular carcinoma, *J Clin Oncol* 23(31):8093-8108, 2005.

60. Choi H, Loyer EM, Charnsangavej C: Neoplasms of the liver and the bile ducts, *Semin Roentgenol* 39(3):412-427, 2004.

61. Jemal A, Murray T, Ward E et al. Cancer Statistics, 2005. *CA Cancer J Clin* 55(1):10-30, 2005.

62. Ahmad J, Rabinovitz M: Etiology and epidemiology of hepatocellular carcinoma. In Carr BI, editor: *Hepatocellular carcinoma: diagnosis and treatment*, Totowa, NJ, 2005, Humana Press.

63. Leonard GD, Jarnagin WR, Allegra CJ: Primary cancers of the liver. In Abraham J, Allegra CJ, Gulley J: *Bethesda handbook of clinical oncology*, ed 2, Philadelphia, 2005, Lippincott Williams & Wilkins.

64. Weber S, O'Reilly EM, Abou-Alfa GK et al: Liver and bile duct cancer. In Abeloff MD, Armitage JO, Niederhuber JE et al: *Clinical oncology*, ed 3, Philadelphia, 2004, Elsevier.

65. Patt YZ, Hassan MM: Clinical aspects and management of hepatocellular cancer: management options: metastatic hepatocellular carcinoma. In Abbruzzese JL, Evans DB, Willett CG et al, editors: *Gastrointestinal oncology*, New York, 2004, Oxford University Press.

66. Hassan MM, Patt YZ: Epidemiology and molecular epidemiology of hepatocellular cancer. In Abbruzzese JL, Evans DB, Willett CG et al, editors: *Gastrointestinal oncology*, New York, 2004, Oxford University Press.

67. Sass DA, Chopra KB: Clinical features and diagnostic evaluation of hepatocellular carcinoma. In Carr BI, editor: *Hepatocellular carcinoma: diagnosis and treatment*, Totowa, NJ, 2005, Humana Press.

68. Curley SA: Treatment of primary liver cancer. In Ajani JA, Curley SA, Janjan NA et al, editors: *MD Anderson cancer care series: gastrointestinal cancer*, New York, 2005, Springer.

69. American Joint Committee on Cancer: *AJCC Cancer staging handbook*, ed 6, New York, 2002, Springer.

70. Leung TWT, Patt YZ, Lau WY et al. Complete pathological remission is possible with systemic combination chemotherapy for inoperable hepatocellular carcinoma, *Clin Cancer Res* 5:1676-1681, 1999.

71. Carr BI: Medical therapy of hepatocellular carcinoma. In Carr BI, editor: *Hepatocellular carcinoma: diagnosis and treatment*, Totowa, New Jersey, 2005, Humana Press.

72. Venook AP: Hepatobiliary cancers. In Furie B, Cassileth PA, Atkins MB et al: *Clinical hematology and oncology*, Philadelphia, 2003, Elsevier.

73. Llovet JM, Real MI, Montana X et al: Arterial embolisation or chemoembolisation versus symptomatic treatment in patients with unresectable hepatocellular carcinoma: a randomized controlled trial, *Lancet* 359:1734-1739, 2002.

74. Philip PA, Mahoney M, Thomas J et al: Phase II open-label study of erlotinib (OSI-774) in patients with hepatocellular or biliary cancer, Presented at 2004 *ASCO Annual Meeting Proceedings*, New Orleans, LA, June 5-8, 2004.

75. Alberts SR, Goldberg RM: Gastrointestinal tract cancers. In Casciato DA, editor: *Manual of clinical oncology*, Philadelphia, 2004, Lippincott Williams & Wilkins.

76. Drebin JA: Carcinoma of the pancreas. In Abeloff MD, Armitage JO, Niederhuber JE et al: *Clinical oncology*, ed 3, Philadelphia, 2004, Elsevier.

77. Michaud DS, Giovannucci E, Willett WC et al: Physical activity, obesity, height, and the risk of pancreatic cancer, *JAMA* 286(8):921-929, 2001.

78. Kim GP, Gulley JL, Takimoto CH: Pancreatic cancer. In Abraham J, Allegra CJ, Gulley J: *Bethesda Handbook of clinical oncology*, ed 2, Philadelphia, 2005, Lippincott Williams & Wilkins.

79. Hruban RH, Wilentz RE: The pancreas. In Kumar V, Abbas AK, Fausto N, editors. *Robbins and Cotran pathologic basis of disease*, ed 7, Philadelphia, 2005, Elsevier.

80. O'Meara AT: Pancreatic cancer: evidence-based diagnosis and treatment, *Clin Obstet Gynecol* 45(3):855-865, 2002.

81. Pisters PW, Wolff RA, Crane CH et al: Combined modality treatment for operable pancreatic adenocarcinoma, *Oncology* 19(3):393-409, 2005.

82. Clark JW: Pancreatic cancer. In Furie B, Cassileth PA, Atkins MB et al: *Clinical hematology and oncology*, Philadelphia, 2003, Elsevier.

83. Stanford P: Surgical Approaches to pancreatic cancer, *Nurs Clin North Am* 36(3):567-577, 2001.

84. Yang GY, Wagner TD, Fuss M et al: Multimodality approaches for pancreatic cancer, *CA Cancer J Clin*, 55:352-367, 2005.

85. Abdalla EK, Pisters PW, Evans DB: Clinical aspects and management of pancreatic adenocarcinoma: management options: potentially resectable pancreatic cancer. In Abbruzzese JL, Evans DB, Willett CG et al, editors: *Gastrointestinal oncology*, New York, 2004, Oxford University Press.

86. McKenna S, Eatock M: The medical management of pancreatic cancer: a review, *Oncologist* 8:149-160, 2003.

87. Willett CG, Czito BG, Bendell JC et al: Locally advanced pancreatic cancer, *J Clin Oncol* 23(20):4538-4544, 2005.

88. El-Rayes BF, Shields AF, Vaitkevicius V et al: Developments in the systemic therapy of pancreatic cancer, *Cancer Invest* 21(1):73-86, 2003.

89. Neoptolemos JP, Stocken DD, Friess H et al: A randomized trial of chemoradiotherapy and chemotherapy after resection of pancreatic cancer, *N Engl J Med* 350:1200-1210, 2004.

90. Wolff RA, Tyler DS, Lu DS: Controversies in the use of adjuvant therapy for patients with pancreatic cancer, In *41st* Annual Meeting of the American Society of Clinical Oncology Educational Book, pgs 308-312, ASCO, 2005.

91. Rothenberg ML, Berlin JD: Clinical aspects and management of metastatic pancreatic cancer. In Abbruzzese JL, Evans DB, Willett CG et al, editors: *Gastrointestinal oncology*, New York, 2004, Oxford University Press.

92. Moore J, Goldstein D, Hamm J et al: Erlotinib plus gemcitabine compared to gemcitabine alone in patients with advanced pancreatic cancer: a phase III trial of the National Cancer Institute of Canada Clinical Trials Group. Paper presented at the *41st* Annual Meeting of the American Society of Clinical Oncology, May 13-17, 2005, Orlando, Fla. Abstract 1.

93. Xiong HQ, Rosenberg A, LoBuglio A et al: Cetuximab, a monoclonal antibody targeting the epidermal growth factor receptor, in combination with gemcitabine for advanced pancreatic cancer: A multicenter Phase II Trial, *J Clin Oncol* 22(13): 2610-2616, 2004.

94. Strohl RA: Nursing care of the client with cancers of the gastrointestinal tract. In Itano JK, Taoka KN, editors: *Core curriculum for oncology nursing*, ed 4, Philadelphia, 2005, *Oncology Nursing Society*.

95. Tempero MA, Termuhlen P, Brand RE et al: Clinical aspects and management of pancreatic adenocarcinoma: management options: locally advanced unresectable pancreatic cancer. In Abbruzzese JL, Evans DB, Willett CG et al, editors: *Gastrointestinal oncology*, New York, 2004, Oxford University Press.

96. Mercadante S, Catala E, Arcuri E et al: Celiac plexus block for pancreatic cancer pain: factors influencing pain, symptoms and quality of life, *J Pain Symptom Manage* 26(6):1140-1147, 2003.

97. Wong GY, Schroeder DR, Carns PE et al: Effect of neurolytic celiac plexus block on pain relief, quality of life, and survival in patients with unresectable pancreatic cancer: a randomized controlled trial, *JAMA* 291(9):1092-1099, 2004.

98. El Kamar FG, Grossbard ML, Kozuch PS: Metastatic pancreatic cancer: emerging strategies in chemotherapy and palliative care, *Oncologist* 8:18-34, 2003.

99. Zeh H: Cancer of the small intestine. In Devita VT, Hellman S, Rosenberg SA, editors: *Cancer: principles and practice of oncology*, 2004, Lippincott Williams & Wilkins.

100. Zawacki K: Hereditary cancer syndromes of the gastrointestinal tract, *AACN Clin Issues*, 13(4):523-539, 2002.

101. Jensen R, Doherty G: Carcinoid tumors and the carcinoid syndrome. In Devita VT, Hellman S, Rosenberg SA, editors: *Cancer: principles and practice of oncology*, 2004, Lippincott Williams & Wilkins.

102. Leonard GD, O'Reilly EM, Allegra CJ: Biliary tract cancer. In Abraham J, Allegra CJ, Gulley J: *Bethesda handbook of clinical oncology*, ed 2, Philadelphia, 2005, Lippincott Williams & Wilkins.

103. Malik U, Mohiuddin M: Cancer of the anal canal. In Abeloff MD, Armitage JO, Niederhuber JE et al: *Clinical oncology*, ed 3, Philadelphia, 2004, Elsevier.

104. Saif MW: Anal cancer. In Abraham J, Allegra CJ, Gulley J: *Bethesda handbook of clinical oncology*, ed 2, Philadelphia, 2005, Lippincott Williams & Wilkins.

105. Steinert DM, Trent J: Gastrointestinal stromal tumors. In Ajani JA, Curley SA, Janjan NA et al, editors: *MD Anderson cancer care series: gastrointestinal cancer*, New York, 2005, Springer.

106. Griffin JM, St. Amand M, Demetri GD: Nursing implications of imatinib as molecularly targeted therapy for gastrointestinal stromal tumors, *Clin J Oncol Nurs* 9(2):161-169, 2005.

107. Hurria A, Muss H, Cohen H: Cancer and aging. In Kufe DW, Pollock RE, Weichselbaum RR, et al editors: *Cancer medicine*, Hamilton (Canada), 2003, BC Decker.

CHAPTER 10

Genitourinary Cancers

Maureen E. O'Rourke

Genitourinary (GU) malignancies include cancers of the urinary and genital organs in men (Fig. 10-1) and urinary organs in women. Taken as a group, the incidence of GU malignancies in the year 2005 is projected to be 343,450, and these GU malignancies are expected to account for 57,600 deaths in the United States alone.[1] Refinements and increased sophistication in both diagnostic approaches and treatment modalities continue to result in improved patient outcomes both in terms of increased survival and enhanced quality of life.

Prostate Cancer

Epidemiology

Prostate cancer is the most frequently diagnosed malignancy and the second leading cause of cancer death in men in the United States, with 232,090 new diagnoses projected in 2005 (American Cancer Society).[1] Incidence rates are expected to rise drastically, and by 2025, as the baby-boom population ages, new cases are estimated to be 38,000 per year.[2] The median age at diagnosis is 71 years, with the incidence rate steadily increasing for each decade after age 50. For African American men the incidence rate is approximately 170 cases per 100,000 men, and the death rate is slightly more than twice that of their Caucasian counterparts. In 1995, 110 cases per 100,000 Caucasian men were diagnosed, and 104 per 100,000 were affected among Hispanic men. Rates for Asian American men were 82 per 100,000.[3] A disturbing trend toward increasing incidence and mortality has been noted among Native Americans. Over the period from 1969 to 1994, prostate cancer developed into the leading cause of male cancer mortality among Native Americans.[4]

The global distribution of prostate cancer reveals predominance in the United States and Canada. Additionally, Scandinavia and parts of the Caribbean have particularly high rates of incidence and mortality, whereas Japan and China have extremely low rates.[3] The highest mortality rates for 2005 are estimated to occur in the Caribbean, South America, and northern and western Europe.[1]

Etiology and Risk Factors

The exact etiology of prostate cancer remains unknown, although it appears to result from interplay between endogenous hormones and environmental influences. Age, ethnicity, and family history are the only well-established risk factors. More than 90% of deaths from prostate cancer and more than 75% of new cases occur in men 65 years of age or older, making age a particularly salient risk factor.[5] Autopsy studies have demonstrated some degree of prostate cancer in at least 30% of men over the age of 50 years.[6]

The differential incidence and mortality among African American males has been suggested to be related to hormonal factors, as higher rates of bioavailable testosterone have been noted among African-American males, along with higher rates of mutations in the prostate susceptibility gene.[7]

Although many links between lifestyle and prostate cancer have been postulated, there remains no conclusive evidence. Increased fat intake, the consumption of red meat, and increased dietary animal fat in general were positively correlated with an increased cancer risk in one prospective cohort study involving 51,529 men.[8] Other factors have been implicated. Although laboratory data identify cadmium as a prostate carcinogen, epidemiologic studies do not convincingly implicate cadmium as a causative factor.[9] Diets high in selenium, vitamins E and D, and lycopene have all been suggested to be protective, yet evidence remains inconclusive at this point.[10] Epidemiologic studies have suggested that vitamin D shows great promise as a chemoprotectant. African American men have greater melanin deposition and have higher prostate cancer rates. Vitamin D synthesis is inhibited by melanin. Men living in higher latitudes with less sun exposure and vitamin D have higher rates of prostate cancer. Older men are often vitamin D deficient, and they also have higher incidence rates of prostate cancer, suggesting a correlation between vitamin D and prostate cancer.[11] Clinical trials have demonstrated that vitamin D can slow the rate of prostate-specific antigen (PSA) rise among men who have experienced biochemical failure after treatment. Hypercalcemia and the formation of renal calculi were limiting factors, however.[12] The effects of dietary lycopene supplementation have been examined in at least one prospective clinical trial. Before undergoing radical prostatectomy, men were fed tomato-based pasta dishes for 3 weeks. Analyses of the prostate glands revealed increased lycopene levels, and increased lycopene levels were also found in the blood, along with reductions in serum PSA levels and oxidative DNA damage.[13]

Occupational exposures have long been suspected to be potentially causative factors in the development of prostate cancer. Farming and pesticide exposure have been correlated with increased prostate cancer incidence, although at this point there are no conclusive data to support any recommendations.[7]

Genetic links are now being examined more extensively. A possible susceptibility locus on chromosome 1 is now thought to be responsible for up to 33% of hereditary cancers; an autosomal dominant pattern of inheritance is suggested.[14] Among men with one affected first-degree relative, the relative risk is 2.5; however, with two affected relatives the risk is fivefold. The relative risk increases to elevenfold if three relatives are affected. Overall, 9% of all malignancies are thought to be hereditary. Chromosomes 1, 8, 10, 16, 17, and 20, as well as the X chromosome, have been associated with prostate cancer, the strongest association being with chromosome 1.[15] Other genetic associations have been implicated in the development of prostate cancer, including *BRCA1* and *BRCA2*.[16]

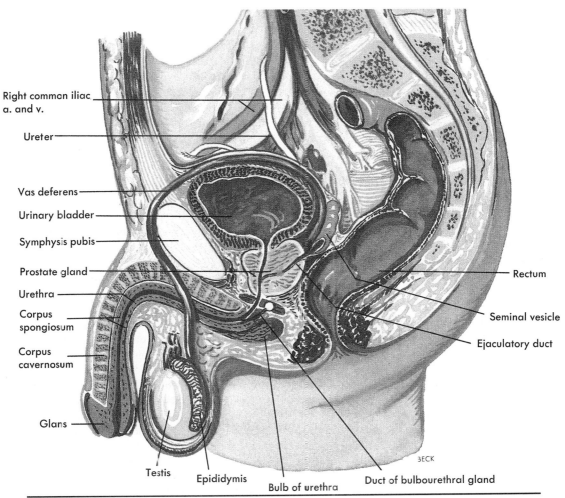

Right common iliac a. and v.
Ureter
Vas deferens
Urinary bladder
Symphysis pubis
Prostate gland
Urethra
Corpus spongiosum
Corpus cavernosum
Glans
Testis
Epididymis
Bulb of urethra
Duct of bulbourethral gland
Ejaculatory duct
Seminal vesicle
Rectum

BECK

FIG. 10-1 Male pelvic organs. (From Thibodeau G, Patton K: Anthony's textbook of anatomy and physiology, ed 16, St Louis, 1999, Mosby.)

The literature is replete with research findings examining the relationship between vasectomy and prostate cancer risk. Although numerous studies have documented a slight increase in relative risk, other studies have failed to demonstrate similar findings. If this risk truly exists, it is small and may be tied in with the fact that men who obtain vasectomies demonstrate health-seeking behaviors and are more likely to be screened for and thus diagnosed with prostate cancer.

Infection has been proposed as a possible risk factor, but research has failed to demonstrate a clear association. This theory appeals to logic, given that numerous cancers are associated with chronic inflammation and prior infection. Despite a century of theorizing, sexual behavior, venereal disease, and fertility fail to demonstrate a clear relationship with the development of prostate cancer.

High-grade prostatic intraepithelial neoplasia (PIN) is a known marker for the later development of prostate cancer. PIN is only detected on biopsy, and does not significantly correlate to elevated PSA. PIN is not detectable by ultrasound. Its presence is highly predictive of the development of prostate cancer within 10 years.[17]

In summary, no single factor has been identified to account for carcinogenesis. Histologic presence of the disease appears to be similar worldwide, whereas clinically significant disease has substantial geographic variation. Current scientific thinking suggests that prostate cancer results from a combination of environmental factors as well as personal risk factors.

Prevention, Screening, and Detection

At this point, no prescriptive recommendations can be made based on clear scientific data. Advising patients regarding a prudent low-fat and high-fiber diet along with consumption of lycopene-rich products may be the best advice that can be offered at this time. Identification of patients at high risk because of family history is another important nursing function. These men should participate in PSA testing regularly and begin at an earlier age.

PSA TESTING

PSA remains the single best test for early diagnosis. PSA is a serine protease produced by malignant cells in the prostate as well as normal and hyperplastic prostate cells. An elevated PSA is not diagnostic of prostate cancer. Any disruption of normal prostate epithelial cell architecture allows PSA to diffuse into the tissue and ultimately into the circulation. Elevated levels are seen following digital rectal examination (DRE) (though this is thought to be clinically insignificant), in men with benign prostatic hyperplasia (BPH) and prostatitis, following transrectal ultrasonography, and in those with urinary retention. A major drawback of PSA testing is its high false-positive rate.

Efforts to enhance the specificity of PSA have included examining PSA density and velocity and the development of age-specific PSA reference ranges. PSA density represents the quotient of serum PSA divided by one half of the prostatic volume. PSA density was thought to be important on the basis of observations that serum PSA values could be normalized by basing them on the volume of the prostate, known to be larger in cases of BPH. Theoretically, data resulting from these calculations could lead to fewer unnecessary prostate biopsies. PSA density testing has lost favor in recent years because of concerns regarding the significant costs associated with subjecting men to transrectal ultrasound (TRUS) with each PSA reading.

PSA velocity refers to the evaluation of serial PSA readings over time. Some researchers have noted that velocity is useful in differentiating men with carcinoma from those without, if three consecutive readings are taken over a 2-year time period. Velocity appeared to be most relevant in men with PSA values greater than 4.0 ng/ml. Others have questioned the value of PSA velocity because it has been found that PSA values vary from day to day; the concern is that normal biologic variations can mask significant PSA changes that may be indicative of carcinoma.[18]

Although a number of researchers have proposed age-specific PSA reference ranges, the predictive value of the 4.0 ng/ml cutoff has withstood the test of time, although 2.5 ng/ml has been suggested as the cutoff for African American men. Research has failed to support the application of age-specific reference ranges.

Substantial controversy surrounds the issues of prostate cancer screening and early detection, and published guidelines by the leading health care authorities reflect a lack of consensus. The central issue is an understanding that screening reveals clinically insignificant tumors that are subsequently treated, perhaps unnecessarily. Such treatment results in significant loss of quality of life (QOL) and increased costs. The most recently updated guidelines published by the American Cancer Society (ACS) recommend that both PSA testing and DRE should be offered annually, beginning at age 50, to men who have at least a 10-year life expectancy and to younger men who are at high risk. High-risk men are identified as those of African American descent and men with a family history of prostate cancer. For these men, the ACS recommends beginning testing at age 45. For men with numerous affected first-degree relatives, the ACS recommends that testing should be initiated at age 40. The ACS further recommends that men should be given specific information regarding the potential risks and benefits of screening. The ACS bases its recommendation on data supporting screening as a means of detecting tumors at a more favorable stage; however, it notes that reductions in mortality from prostate cancer cannot directly be attributed to screening.[19] An abnormal PSA is defined as a value of 4.0 ng/ml or higher.[20] The National Comprehensive Cancer Network (NCCN) recently included in its guidelines for prostate cancer screening that patients with a PSA level of 2.6 ng/ml or higher, even in the presence of a normal a normal DRE, should be considered for a prostate biopsy.[21] The guidelines do not strictly direct physicians to obtain a prostate biopsy for all patients with 2.6 ng/ml or higher but do state that this new level may be considered a cut-off for which to proceed to a biopsy.

Few randomized controlled trials have directly examined the issue of whether screening results in decreased prostate cancer mortality. The Quebec Screening Study randomly assigned men to screening or no screening and then compared mortality over time. Men were screened with PSA and DRE, but only had TRUS if their PSA levels were over 3.0 ng/ml. The trial demonstrated a reduction in mortality of up to 70% among men screened as compared to their unscreened counterparts.[22] However, the trial has been the subject of widespread criticism because of its severe methodologic flaws. Of 46,193 men eligible to participate, only 31,000 were actually invited to participate, and of these only 7100 were actually screened. Both randomization and statistical power were severely compromised. An additional flaw was the lag time of 3 years between "randomization" and screening.

A second Canadian study by Perron and colleagues examined whether the decline in prostate cancer in Quebec could be attributed to PSA screening. Changes in incidence rates between 1989 and 1993 were compared with changes in mortality between 1995 and 1999. Increased screening rates among 15 birth cohorts in 15 regions of Quebec were not significantly correlated with declining prostate cancer mortality rates.[23]

At present, aside from the ACS guidelines, major health care organizations have not formed a clear consensus regarding prostate cancer screening recommendations. The U.S. Preventive Services Task Force found "good" evidence to support PSA screening in detecting early stage prostate cancer, but only "mixed and inconclusive evidence" that early detection improves overall health outcomes.[24] This group does not endorse routine PSA screening. The main factor cited in favor of routine PSA screening is that men who are screened have a higher chance of being diagnosed at an earlier stage that is more conducive to cure. The lack of any clear scientific evidence demonstrating survival benefit from screening-detected prostate cancer is the main factor cited against screening.

Classification

Of all prostate cancers, 95% are adenocarcinomas. The remaining 5% consist of sarcomas and transitional cell tumors.[25] Most neoplasms of the prostate gland develop within the peripheral zone, with malignant growth spreading locally into the seminal vesicles, the peritoneum, and the bladder. Metastases to the lungs, the liver, the kidney, and the bones occur via hematogenous spread. Lymphatic node involvement is common.

Clinical Features

Most men with early-stage disease may be symptom free, because the majority of prostatic neoplasms arise in the peripheral zone. The majority of prostate cancers are detected through routine screening with PSA testing. Although a PSA level of more than 4.0 ng/ml is considered suspicious for malignancies,[26] some men with PSA levels lower than 4.0 ng/ml will still have prostate cancer. Among the 2,950 men in the control group of the Prostate Cancer Prevention Study, 15% were found to have prostate cancer by biopsy at the conclusion of the study, despite having PSA levels lower than 4 ng/ml and no suspicious DRE findings over the 7-year course of the study.[27]

Symptoms may be present in early-stage disease, but generally symptoms such as urinary hesitancy, frequency, and a feeling of incomplete emptying of the bladder occur later in the course and are associated with disease progression. Progression may also cause blood in the semen, decreased ejaculatory volume and, less commonly, impotence. Impotence occurs as the tumor encroaches upon the neurovascular bundles in the periprostatic tissue. Bone pain and pathologic fractures, as well as spinal cord compression, hematuria, and anemia, are late signs and are associated with advanced disease.

Diagnosis

Men may first be seen with an elevated PSA or an abnormal DRE, and yet be symptom free. Alternatively, men may complain of bothersome symptoms. DRE should be performed by a skilled professional health care practitioner. Any change in size, consistency, or contour detected in the gland may represent an inflammatory process, infarction, calculus, or tumor. Only the lateral and posterior areas of the gland can be palpated, precluding estimation of tumor volume and extent, a great disadvantage.

Diagnosis is only established by biopsy. Biopsies are performed transrectally, using TRUS to facilitate visualization of the prostate gland. Biopsies are performed using a spring-loaded biopsy gun, and multiple samples (6 or more) are obtained, sampling all regions of the gland. The sextant biopsy has long been considered the standard, but it is gradually being replaced by a more extended biopsy protocol. Newer protocols include sampling the lateral aspects of the gland, and higher rates of detection have been reported when collating more than 6 samples. An extended 10-core-biopsy protocol was demonstrated to detect 96% of malignancies as opposed to the traditional 6-sextant-biopsy protocol in one major study.[28] The extended protocol was not associated with more pain, but was associated with higher frequency of bloody stools and blood in the semen. King suggests that this extended-biopsy protocol should become the new standard of care, since it has been associated with significantly improved prediction of pathologic Gleason scores.[29]

There is no special prebiopsy patient preparation. The patient is placed in the lithotomy position and local anesthesia is administered. An ultrasound probe is inserted into the rectum to guide needle placement. Patients may experience discomfort as well as a sensation of fullness or pressure. After the procedure, a urine specimen is examined for the presence of hematuria.

Patient education before and after biopsies includes information regarding hematuria, hematochezia, and hematospermia, which may occur for several days to weeks after biopsies. Excessive prolonged bleeding, elevated temperature, fever, chills, or increased urinary difficulties should be reported to the urologist immediately.

Computed tomography (CT) continues to be used for evaluation of nodes, tissue, and organs and to estimate prostatic size. Magnetic resonance imaging (MRI) evaluates extracapsular penetration beyond the gland itself, and evaluates lymph node status and seminal vesicle status. The endorectal coil has been shown to have high positive predictive value, adding important information in the clinical decision making process.[30]

Radionucleotide scanning continues to be a primary modality for detecting or confirming metastatic bone involvement. Bone scans, though highly sensitive, are relatively nonspecific. Findings must be correlated with plain radiographs. Bone scans are recommended for patients with PSA levels of 20 ng/ml or greater to rule out bony metastasis.[21]

Staging and Grading

Prostate cancer is staged using the American Joint Committee on Cancer TNM staging system, wherein *T* refers to the tumor size,

N refers to nodal status, and *M* refers to metastasis. Prostate cancer is graded according to the level of cellular differentiation detected among biopsy specimens. The Gleason score is the most commonly employed grading system. Two scores are assigned. The two most common malignant cellular patterns noted under microscopic examination are rated on a score of 1 to 5. Scores are then summed. Total scores range from 2 to 10. Higher scores indicate more aggressive disease and poorer prognosis.[31]

Treatment Modalities and Nursing Care Considerations

Three basic options are offered for the management of early-stage prostate cancer: radical prostatectomy, radiation therapy (external beam or brachytherapy), or "expectant management," sometimes referred to as "watchful waiting." Cryotherapy has gained popularity as a treatment option as data accumulate and techniques continue to be refined. A substantial body of literature exists examining patient preferences for prostate cancer treatment and the actual decision-making process as experienced by men and their spouses facing a prostate cancer diagnosis.[32] Multiple treatment decision models have been published for physician use, including specific practice guidelines established by the NCCN.[33] The key factors for consideration within each model include the patient's age, projected survival, coexisting medical problems, stage of disease, and tumor factors such as grade and the Gleason score, as well as consideration of potential side effects associated with each treatment modality. The meaning of the cancer experience, the patient's personal or vicarious experiences, and opinions of each treatment option are fundamental issues to be considered (Table 10-1).

SURGERY

In the United States, the radical retropubic prostatectomy (RP) is the mainstay of treatment. This includes complete removal of the prostate gland, with lymph node sampling. RP provides access to regional lymph nodes in the pelvis and affords nerve-sparing potential, improving postoperative potency. Regional lymph node sampling permits assessment of the presence or absence of tumor in adjacent nodes. If the tumor has extended into nodes, radical prostatectomy may be deferred and patients may be treated with palliative as opposed to curative intent.

Immediate postoperative nursing care includes vigilant pain assessment, administration of analgesia, maintaining catheter patency, prevention of thrombophlebitis and pulmonary embolus formation, and prevention of urinary tract infections. Use of an incentive spirometer, compression hose, or sequential compression devices may be indicated. Fluid intake is encouraged to maintain a minimum urine output of 30 cc/hr or more. Rectal manipulation, including rectal temperatures and suppositories, is avoided because of the risk of rectal injury given the close proximity of the prostate to the rectal wall. Teaching includes catheter maintenance following discharge home since it may be in place for several weeks postoperatively; early and progressive ambulation; and avoidance of vigorous activity until cleared by the physician. Nurses should assess patients' knowledge regarding potential incontinence following catheter removal and provide anticipatory teaching in the use of incontinence management aids. Nursing research has demonstrated that patients lack understanding of the potential adverse effects of prostate cancer treatment,

TABLE 10-1	**Prostate Cancer Treatment Options**	
RISK OF RECURRENCE	**LIFE EXPECTANCY**	**TREATMENT**
Clinically localized disease T1–T2a	<10 years	Watchful waiting, XRT or brachytherapy
PSA <10	>10 years	Watchful waiting, XRT or brachytherapy, or RP
Gleason 2–6		
Intermediate disease T2b–T2c	<10 years	Watchful waiting, XRT or brachytherapy, RP
PSA = 10–20	>10 years	XRT or brachytherapy, RP
Gleason 7		
High risk T3	<10 years	Androgen ablation + XRT or brachytherapy, *or* XRT or brachytherapy, *or* RP
PSA >20		
Gleason 8–10	>10 years	same
Locally advanced disease	Any	Androgen ablation of XRT or Brachytherapy
Metastatic disease	Any	Androgen ablation

XRT, External beam radiation therapy; *RT*, radiation therapy, *RP*, radical prostatectomy.
Data from National Comprehensive Cancer Network: Clinical Practice Guidelines, version 2.2005, Prostate cancer, retrieved August 8, 2005, from http://www.nccn.org/professionals/physician_gls/PDF/prostate.pdf.

and that the management of incontinence is a more pressing priority in the immediate postoperative period than management of impotence.[34]

Pelvic floor muscle–strengthening exercises have long been advocated as a means of diminishing incontinence. However, a review of 10 clinical trials conducted among men having RP or transurethral resection of the prostate concluded that 5 studies demonstrated "some value" to the use of pelvic muscle exercises and biofeedback. Evidence was inconclusive regarding the efficacy of the exercises alone, transcutaneous electronic nerve stimulation, and rectal stimulation.[35]

Postoperative complications include incontinence, impotence, urethral stricture, and complications associated with anesthesia and the surgery itself. Morbidity and mortality increase considerably with advanced age. Reports of incontinence following radical prostatectomy vary from 2% to 87% owing to lack of precise definitions of incontinence and inconsistent measurement intervals for assessment.[36] Little additional recovery of continence is expected beyond 12 months after surgery.[37] Research reveals that patients over the age of 70 have considerably higher incidence of incontinence than younger cohorts. Some degree of incontinence immediately following catheter removal is expected in all patients.

Anticholinergic or alpha-adrenergic medications are used for prostatectomy-induced incontinence. Persistent incontinence may require surgical intervention with artificial sphincter placement. Nursing management strategies include scheduled bladder emptying, the use of incontinence pads, sitting to void to facilitate complete emptying, and the use of penile clamps. Restriction of bladder irritants such as alcohol, caffeine, and citrus- and tomato-based products may be beneficial. Stool softeners and increased dietary fiber may reduce bowel pressure on the bladder.

Erectile dysfunction is a significant threat to QOL following radical prostatectomy. Despite nerve-sparing techniques, reports of potency are highly variable in the medical literature. Interpretation of incidence rates is hampered by the lack of standard definitions and the reliance on self-report. Erectile function is affected by surgical procedures, comorbid conditions, and pharmacologic agents such as beta blockers, commonly used by older men.

Nursing responsibilities include patient and partner education and ongoing assessment. Both patients and their partners need reassurance that this condition can be effectively treated and does not signal the end of their sexual relationship. Treatment integrates psychologic, pharmaceutical, and mechanical interventions. The use of sildenafil (Viagra) following RT treatment for prostate cancer has been supported by a single randomized clinical trial,[38] although no randomized clinical trials have tested its efficacy following radical prostatectomy. A single retrospective study suggests four factors are associated with successful use of sildenafil following prostatectomy: the presence of at least one intact neurovascular bundle, preoperative potency, age of 65 years or less, and interval from radical prostatectomy to drug use longer than 6 months.[39] Extended-action medications are now available but have not been tested in the prostate cancer population to date.

Other treatment strategies include the use of vasoconstrictive devices such as vacuum pumps, the use of penile implants, the use of intraurethral prostaglandin suppositories, and intracavernous penile injections to attain erections, although none of these are associated with high levels of patient satisfaction.

RADIATION THERAPY

There are no published randomized clinical trials (RCTs) directly comparing radical prostatectomy with radiation therapy (RT) among men with early-stage prostate cancer. One large-scale RCT that is in progress, the SPIRIT Trial, compares health-related QOL among men treated with RT vs brachytherapy.[40] Nonrandomized retrospective reviews have demonstrated comparable cure rates with external beam RT (XRT) and radical prostatectomy at 5- to 8-year follow-up.[41]

The delivery modes of radiotherapy include external beam RT, three-dimensional conformal radiotherapy (3DCRT), and brachytherapy. External beam radiotherapy can result in long-term remissions paralleling those achieved with radical prostatectomy.

External beam radiation therapy is delivered daily over a 7-week period. The radiation field includes the prostate and the seminal vesicles, with a margin to allow for patient motion. Field sizes depend on patient anatomy. External beam radiation can also be delivered conformally. The goal of this technique is to concentrate high radiation doses to the tumor while sparing critical adjacent structures (bladder and rectum). Three-dimensional conformal radiation therapy uses CT scanning to create a three-dimensional reconstruction of the prostate and surrounding structures. Standard simulation procedures are used in conjunction with three-dimensional reconstructions to facilitate treatment planning. Immobilization casts are used to maintain patient positioning during treatment administration.

The risk of treatment-related side effects is influenced by the dose given to normal tissue and the volume of tissue treated. Radiotherapy-related side effects are categorized as acute and late toxicities. Acute toxicity, occurring within 90 days of treatment, is usually reversible and occurs within rapidly dividing cells. Late reactions occur in more slowly dividing cells and may be permanent. The onset of late effects is variable, occurring anytime after the 90-day period, even months to years after the completion of therapy. (See Chapter 20 for more information regarding general side effects and nursing management of radiation therapy.)

Nursing considerations for men undergoing RT are focused on symptom management. Acute side effects include diarrhea, proctitis, cystitis, fatigue, and local skin reactions. Low-residue diets, antidiarrheal medications, sitz baths, and topical steroid products may provide relief of rectal and anal pain. Adequate nutrition and hydration status are important nursing foci. There are no RCTs to guide nursing care in this area, however. Denton and colleagues summarized the results of six RCTs for the management of chronic proctitis. Although evidence was insufficient for definitive conclusions, the use of rectal sucralfate and the addition of metronidazole to an antiinflammatory regimen did show promise in decreasing rectal bleeding, erythema, and ulceration.[42]

The exact mechanism of radiation-induced fatigue is not known. However, contributing factors may include anemia, cytokine activation, psychologic distress, and medication effects. Nursing management focuses on symptom relief and the identification and correction of potential etiologic factors. Two RCTs provide evidence that moderate aerobic exercise during RT may attenuate fatigue.[43,44]

Erectile function is affected by radiation therapy. Impotence is often multifactorial, and factors such as cardiovascular disease, diabetes, tobacco and alcohol use, and prescription and nonprescription medications must be considered. Patients who are potent prior to external beam therapy tend to remain potent, in contrast to those with poor initial function. Disruptions in potency are caused by radiation damage to the small blood vessels and nerves responsible for erection. The effects of radiation on erectile function may be delayed.

A third method of radiation delivery is through radioactive seed implantation. Brachytherapy may be performed as a solo treatment modality, or before or after external beam radiation therapy. Implants may be permanent or temporary, using palladium-103, iridium-192, and iodine-125 sources. Placement is guided by CT enhancement and TRUS using spinal or general anesthesia. Needles are placed transperineally through a template guide. Radioactive seeds are loaded through the needles directly into the prostate. The needles are withdrawn after all seeds are placed. Following implantation, a cystourethroscopy may be performed to assess for bleeding or to retrieve errant seeds. A Foley catheter may be placed to monitor output for volume and quality. When the urine is free of clots, 200 ml of sterile water is injected into the bladder, and then the catheter is removed. The patient is monitored to determine whether he can spontaneously void. In some cases, patients may be discharged with an indwelling Foley catheter for a period of 24 to 48 hours. Brachytherapy is performed as an outpatient procedure, generally over a period of 1 to 2 hours.

There are no RCTs comparing brachytherapy directly to XRT or radical prostatectomy; however, several retrospective reviews present evidence that brachytherapy is equivalent to XRT and radical prostatectomy for men with low-risk disease. These same studies suggest that brachytherapy is associated with poorer outcomes among men with high-grade disease and higher pretreatment PSA levels.[45]

Nursing care of patients following prostatic brachytherapy includes management of side effects. Mild dysuria, frequency, and mild pain may occur. Patients should report any obstructive symptoms. Patients are encouraged to maintain a high level of fluid intake and to complete the full course of prophylactic antibiotic therapy as prescribed. Rarely, patients may require an indwelling catheter or intermittent self-catheterization if edema causes severe obstructive symptoms. Symptoms generally subside within 3 to 4 months. Hematuria caused by the trauma of needle insertion is common and generally resolves within 72 hours. Patients may resume sexual intercourse within 2 weeks; they are instructed to wear a condom for 2 months to protect their partner from possible seed expulsion. (See Chapter 20 for more detailed information on brachytherapy treatment delivery and radiation safety protocols.) Finally, radiation also plays a role in palliation for prostate cancer. External beam irradiation to selected sites may provide significant pain relief.

HORMONAL THERAPY

Hormonal manipulation is the mainstay of treatment for advanced prostate cancer. Four major types of hormonal manipulation are used, each aimed at the disruption of androgen stimulation bilateral orchiectomy, lutenizing hormone–releasing hormones (LHRH), antiandrogens, and estrogen therapy. An additional approach is total androgen blockade via orchiectomy plus an antiandrogen, or the combination of an LHRH agonist with an antiandrogenic agent.

Although androgen deprivation therapy has traditionally been reserved for metastatic disease, it is increasingly being used in nonmetastatic disease and in the case of biochemical failure (measured by rising PSA levels) following other curative-intent therapies. Neoadjuvant hormonal therapy is used to shrink tumor mass before surgery. Several RCTs have demonstrated reductions in positive surgical margins; however, at 3-year postprostatectomy follow-up, Aus and colleagues noted that the addition of neoadjuvant hormonal therapy did not significantly result in increased progression-free survival.[46]

The central focus of nursing care for men receiving hormonal therapy is patient education, psychosocial support, and the recognition and prompt management of side effects. An excellent review of the side effects with detailed toxicity monitoring and intervention recommendations is presented by Higano.[47] Anemia, loss of bone density, and hot flashes are predominant issues for men receiving hormonal therapy. NCCN Guidelines for Senior Adult Oncology recommend maintaining hemoglobin levels at or above 12 g/dl for older patients.[48] Bone density requires quantitative monitoring and may necessitate bisphosphonate therapy.

The management of hot flashes has not been well researched. Venalfaxine demonstrated promise in one pilot study.[49] Megesterol acetate has been used successfully in the clinical setting, but it has been found to elevate PSA levels even at low doses, raising concern.[50] Black cohosh (*Actaea racemosa*) is a popular remedy for menopausal symptoms, although definitive evidence on safety and efficacy has not been demonstrated, and it is unclear if research findings from menopausal women can be generalized to men with prostate cancer.

EXPECTANT MANAGEMENT OR WATCHFUL WAITING

One option for the management of prostate disease is that of expectant management, surveillance, or watchful waiting (WW). This conservative management strategy involves no local therapy on diagnosis, with initiation of treatment only when the patient becomes symptomatic from either locally advanced disease or metastatic disease. Selection of this option is largely based on patient preference, but it is generally reserved for patients with low-grade disease who are older than 70 years of age, with a life expectancy of less than 10 years. The rationale for expectant management is based on the observation that the incidence rates for prostate cancer far exceed the death rates. More men die "with" the disease than "of" the disease. Proponents of this approach argue that there is significant evidence that aggressive therapy has not improved overall prostate cancer survival but has significantly diminished QOL. Early European and Scandinavian retrospective studies reporting low death rates among men selecting this option are frequently cited in support of this option. In addition, two early RCTs comparing WW with radical prostatectomy found no statistically significant differences in survival between the two groups at 15 and 23 years, respectively.[51,52] More recently, Holmberg and colleagues reported the results of a large RCT comparing WW with radical prostatectomy. At 8-year follow-up, a 50% reduction in cancer-specific mortality and distant metastasis was noted among the radical prostatectomy group as compared with the WW group. Local progression and increased morbidity, including urinary obstruction, was significantly greater in the WW as well. However, overall mortality was similar in both the WW and prostatectomy groups, leaving the question open as to which treatment option is preferable.[53]

Nursing care for men who select WW consists of continuous assessment of both the physiologic and psychosocial dimensions of QOL. In the largest RCT to date comparing WW with radical prostatectomy, Steineck and colleagues examined QOL in both groups. They found overall QOL, anxiety, depression, well-being, and bowel function to be similar between the two groups; however, erectile dysfunction and urinary leakage were significantly more common among the men in the radical prostatectomy group.[54] Galbraith compared QOL and prostate-specific symptoms among men enrolled in several treatment groups: radical prostatectomy, WW, RT, or a combination RT protocol. No significant overall health-related QOL differences were detected,

but post-hoc analyses indicated significantly more gastrointestinal symptoms among RT patients and more sexual dysfunction among men in the radical prostatectomy group.[55] Further research by Wallace noted that QOL among men electing WW was negatively affected by anxiety, uncertainty, and perception of danger.[56]

CRYOTHERAPY

Although initially introduced in the 1960s as a treatment option for prostate cancer, cryotherapy was abandoned because of the high rate of complications experienced. In recent years, there has been a renewed interest in this treatment modality owing to technique refinements. This therapy involves the direct application of ice to the prostate gland via percutaneously inserted cryogenic probes. Probe placement is guided by ultrasound, and continuous temperature monitoring is conducted throughout the procedure. Complications include urethral sloughing, urinary incontinence, bladder neck contracture, and impotence. The advantages of cryotherapy include the fact that it destroys a biologically heterogeneous population of cancer cells and is a relatively noninvasive procedure with minimal blood loss. It can be performed under spinal rather than general anesthesia and thus can be offered to men who are not candidates for surgery because of advanced age, comorbidity, or locally advanced disease. In addition, it can be used to treat men with locally recurrent cancer following prostate radiation therapy, it can be performed more than once and, if necessary, it can be followed by either radiation therapy or radical prostatectomy.[57] The long-term efficacy of cryotherapy as compared to radical prostatectomy or radiotherapy has not yet been established, however.

Nursing care is geared toward education before and after the procedure. Patients and their partners should have a full understanding of the anticipatable side effects. Excessive bleeding, elevated temperature, and symptoms of urinary obstruction should be reported.

LAPAROSCOPIC AND ROBOTIC PROSTATECTOMY

Several reports have documented the feasibility of laparoscopic removal of the prostate gland.[58] To date, however, the laparoscopic approach has achieved inferior results with respect to rates of positive margins, continence, and preservation of potency as compared to open surgical approaches. In addition, no specific advantage has yet been demonstrated for robotic prostatectomy in terms of length of hospital stay, postoperative pain, or blood replacement.[59] This approach is still considered investigational and awaits long-term outcome analysis.

CHEMOTHERAPY

The development of recurrent or progressive disease following curative-intent therapy remains a formidable challenge in the area of prostate cancer management. An additional challenge is the possible development of hormone-refractory disease. Although further treatment options are available, the main focus of care is supportive. Management of distressing symptoms and their impact on QOL poses the greatest nursing challenge. Identified physiologic problems include fatigue, anemia, appetite disturbances, obstruction (both urinary and bowel), spinal cord compression, and pain. Specific side effects related to treatment modalities also require attention. Pain management is a major focus of nursing care.

In the case of advanced disease, selection of further treatment depends on multiple factors, including prior treatment, site of recurrence, comorbid conditions, and individual patient considerations. Although chemotherapy has limited value in the treatment of patients with refractory disease after hormonal therapy, evidence is emerging that chemotherapy may eradicate hormone-resistant cell populations. The benefit of adding chemotherapy to hormone therapy was the subject of a randomized trial conducted by the Radiation Therapy Oncology Group (RTOG) (trial 99-02), in which men with localized high-risk prostate cancer were randomly assigned to androgen deprivation plus radiation therapy alone, or this therapy followed by chemotherapy with paclitaxel, estramustine, and etoposide. Results are pending.[60] Agents that have been used for hormone-resistant prostate cancer include mitoxantrone and related compounds, the taxanes, estramustine, and vinca alkaloids. Additionally, platinum analogues, topoisomerase I inhibitors, and antimetabolites such as cyclophosphamide have demonstrated some clinical activity. As in the case of any chemotherapeutic agent administration, nursing care includes patient education and continuous assessment of QOL. Symptom management with premedication and posttreatment management of nausea and vomiting are critical priorities.

EMERGING THERAPIES

Current efforts are being directed to develop novel strategies for the treatment of prostate cancer. A variety of methods aimed at augmenting immune response are currently under investigation. Phase I and II clinical trials are in progress that investigate the use of cytokine adjuvant therapy, cytokine gene-transduced vaccines, DNA peptide vaccines, and dendritic cell–based vaccines. In addition, gene therapy focused on the introduction of toxic or cell-lytic genes, called "suicide" gene therapy, is under investigation, along with corrective genetic therapies designed to increase or eradicate the expression of specific genes. Therapies targeted at epidermal growth factor and other mechanisms to interfere with metastasis and invasion are also under investigation.

Disease-Related Complications and Treatment

ERECTILE DYSFUNCTION

Erectile dysfunction and impotence are distressing adverse effects that men and their partners encounter following therapy for prostate cancer. Nerve-sparing surgical procedures lessen the incidence of impotence; however, high rates are reported after surgery. Comparison between techniques is hampered by imprecise definitions in the literature and high rates of erectile dysfunction among older men before prostate cancer intervention. For men undergoing brachytherapy, impotence rates range from 6% to 61%.[61]

Options for treatment of erectile dysfunction include pharmacotherapeutic agents such as intracavernous prostaglandin injections, urethral prostaglandin suppositories, and oral agents such as sildenafil or mechanical devices such as penile implants or vacuum pump mechanisms. Assessment of the patient's baseline erection function before treatment, including other potentially contributory factors, can assist the clinician in planning a sexual rehabilitation program. Whenever possible, education and planning should include the partner. Erectile function may return spontaneously up to 2 years after a radical prostatectomy.

INCONTINENCE

Dysfunction in either the storage or emptying of urine can result in urinary incontinence (UI). This problem is significant because of embarrassment and the potential for social isolation, as well as depression and skin breakdown. The incidence of UI following prostate cancer treatment with either surgery or radiation is difficult to determine because of the highly variable rates reported in the literature. In general, younger men report less UI compared with similarly treated men over the age of 65 years.

Medical interventions include the use of anticholinergic and alpha-adrenergic agents combined with pelvic floor strengthening exercises. A metaanalysis of 10 clinical trials failed to support the use of pelvic muscle strengthening exercises as a solo treatment for postprostatectomy incontinence, however.[62] Other management strategies include the use of pads, scheduled bladder emptying, sitting to void to facilitate complete bladder emptying, and the use of penile clamps. Patients may benefit from stool softeners and increased dietary intake of fiber to reduce bowel pressure on the bladder. The restriction of potential bladder irritants such as caffeine, alcohol, citrus, carbonated beverages, and citrus products is often recommended, but is not supported by research.

Acute radiation-induced cystitis may occur within 6 months of treatment and is associated with dysuria, frequency, urgency, nocturia, and hematuria. This acute inflammatory reaction is generally self-limiting, and treatment is symptomatic, including antispasmodics, anticholinergic agents, and urinary analgesics.

Prognosis

Prognosis is influenced by Gleason stage and cellular architectural patterns, tumor size, location, and the presence or absence of metastasis. For Caucasian men with localized disease, the relative 5-year survival is 96.9%; for African Americans it is 85.9%. The 5-year survival for all stages combined is 89.9% for Caucasians and only 65.5% for African Americans, suggesting a need for intense intervention.[1]

Testicular Cancer

Epidemiology

Testicular cancer is the most common malignancy in men aged 15 to 35, although it accounts for only 1% of all solid tumors among men. In 2005, it is estimated that 8010 new cases will be diagnosed in the United States, but only 390 deaths are anticipated.[1] Dramatic increases in survival are a result of a combination of effective diagnostic techniques, improvement in tumor markers, effective multidrug chemotherapeutic regimens, and modification of surgical techniques.

The incidence of testicular cancer has been steadily increasing worldwide since the early 1900s, and this increase has been largely restricted to Caucasian males. Data from the Surveillance Epidemiology and End Results (SEER) database indicate that the overall incidence of testicular germ cell tumors among American men rose 44% (from 3.35 to 4.84 per 100,000 men) between the periods 1973-1978 and 1994-1998, and the incidence of seminoma rose 62%.[63] Testicular cancer is far less common in African Americans, with published ratios between white and African American men ranging from 4:1 to 40:1. Worldwide incidence

CONSIDERATIONS FOR OLDER ADULTS

Prostate Cancer

- Although a variety of genitourinary cancers can affect the elderly, prostate cancer by far has the greatest propensity to occur in older males. More than 70% of all patients with prostate cancer are age 65 or older at the time of diagnosis, thus special attention to the unique concerns of this population is necessary. Developmental demands during this stage of life include a gradual shift in responsibilities, retirement, and reduced income. Relocation and loss of friends and/or spouse may add to these demands.

- Older adults, as a rule, may accommodate symptoms, interpreting them as related to the aging process, which can result in delays in both diagnosis and treatment. Transportation to and from appointments may impede treatment. Decision making regarding treatment in the face of scientific uncertainty may be difficult for older patients more accustomed to a paternalistic, authoritative health care model. Health care providers must be prepared to deal with the significant influence of other family members in the decision-making process.

- Physiologic conditions may influence the available treatment options and contribute to posttreatment complications and side effects. Comorbidities such as diabetes and medications such as beta blockers may contribute to erectile dysfunction. Urinary control may be affected by medications and preexisting conditions, including obesity. In addition, there are many comorbid conditions that can greatly affect therapeutic options. Cardiac and respiratory conditions may preclude surgical intervention. Of older patients, 43% have hypertension, and an estimated 40% have heart conditions.[99] Physiologic changes associated with aging and comorbidities increase the potential for older adults to experience treatment-related complications. Impaired renal function may rule out the use of cisplatin therapy and may be a contraindication for intravenous pyelography. Polypharmacia and age-related hepatic changes may predispose older patients to greater risks of drug reactions.

- Older patients often have sensory impairments that influence teaching and learning. Men often identify their spouse or partner as their most important source of support, thus it is imperative that they be included in all teaching.

- Although progress has been made in the diagnosis and treatment of genitourinary cancers, attention to each patient and his or her individual circumstances—social, physical, emotional and financial—must be considered when guiding and supporting this patient population.

is lowest in Africa and Asia, and highest in the Scandinavian countries, Germany, Switzerland, and New Zealand.[64]

Etiology and Risk Factors

The etiology of testicular cancer is unknown, but certain conditions are associated with an increased incidence of this malignancy. Specifically, testicular tumors are more likely to occur in an atrophic testis or a cryptorchid (undescended) testis. The relative risk of testicular cancer in patients with cryptorchidism

is thought to be 5 times the normal expected risk. Family history of testicular cancer is associated with 3 to 12 times the average risk, history of a prior germ cell testicular tumor is associated with 23 to 27 times the risk, and certain intersex syndromes are associated with greater than 100 times the average risk.[65]

Despite case studies suggesting a link between diethylstilbestrol (DES) use during pregnancy and the development of germ cell tumors (GCTs), no conclusive evidence exists to support this as a risk factor. Case reports have noted that a history of trauma to the testis often precedes diagnosis; however, research findings fail to support a causal association. Epidemiologic studies have also failed to support viral infection as a cause, although increased incidence of testicular GCTs, particularly seminomas, has been described in men who are infected with the human immunodeficiency virus (HIV) compared to HIV-negative men.[66]

Both seminomas and nonseminomatous GCTs are preceded by a premalignant condition termed intratubular germ cell neoplasia of unclassified type (ITGCNU), testicular intraepithelial neoplasia, or carcinoma in situ (CIS). This premalignant condition (ITGCNU) has been found in testicular tissue adjacent to GCTs in approximately 90% of adult cases. Left untreated, the risk of progression to invasive testicular cancer in 5 years is 50%.[67] Other risk factors have been supported by research. A positive family history increases the subsequent risk of development of testicular carcinoma, as does a prior testicular tumor, although specific genetic risk factors have not been defined. Candidate chromosomal regions have been suggested, specifically on chromosome Xq27, and this region is also thought to be related to a predisposition for undescended testicles.[68] Chromosome 12 alterations, specifically increased copies of 12p, in the same chromosome 12 or translocated elsewhere in the genome, have been found in all cases of testicular carcinoma, including CIS, suggesting that this may be the earliest step in carcinogenesis and the main genetic damage of GCT.[69]

Prevention, Screening, and Detection

Prevention of testicular cancer is not a reasonable expectation, because etiologic factors are unknown. The U.S. Preventive Services Task Force and the Canadian Task Force on Periodic Health Examination make no recommendations for the use of routine screening of asymptomatic males for testicular cancer because of the lack of controlled trials in this area. The American Medical Association and the American Academy of Pediatrics do recommend annual clinical testicular examination for teenage males. The ACS recommends annual professional testicular examination and monthly testicular self-examination (TSE). Data suggest that physician teaching of TSE enhances performance, although both teaching and performance rates are low overall, and evidence is currently lacking as to the efficacy of this intervention.[70]

Classification

Cancer of the testes includes a sizeable group of tumors that are diverse in terms of morphology and clinical behavior. General tumor categories include GCTs (seminomas, embryonal cancers, teratomas, choriocarcinomas, and yolk sac tumors), sex cord–stromal or gonadal stromal tumors, mixed germ and stromal cell tumors, adnexal and paratesticular tumors, and other malignancies such as mesothelioma and lymphoma. Additionally, the testes may be the site of metastatic disease. Approximately 95%

of all testicular tumors are GCTs originating in the primordial germ cells essential for spermatogenesis. Testicular cancer is broadly divided into two groups: a pure form or a mixture of cell types. Most clinicians distinguish primarily between seminoma and all others, which as a group are termed nonseminomatous germ cell tumors. α-Fetoprotein (AFP) and human chorionic gonadotropin (HCG) are serum tumor markers of critical importance in the diagnosis and prognosis of testicular cancer. Nonseminomas are associated with elevated HCG or AFP, or both, in 80% to 85% of cases, whereas seminomas are associated with elevated serum HCG alone. Neither of these tumor markers are sensitive enough to be diagnostic.[69]

Diagnosis and Clinical Features

The classic presentation of a testicular tumor is a small, painless mass ranging from several millimeters to centimeters, and confined to one testicle. Patients may first be seen with diffuse pain, swelling, or firmness of the testis. Acute pain is rare and may be caused by epididimitis. Abdominal pain may be related to retroperitoneal node metastasis. Gynecomastia is sometimes present if HCG is increased. A trial of antibiotic therapy is sometimes prescribed on initial presentation if no discrete mass is noted.

A complete history should be taken along with physical examination of the testis. Testicular exam is performed by carefully palpating the organ between the thumb and the first two fingers. The normal testis is homogenous in consistency and freely moveable. Any nodular or fixed mass is an abnormal finding. Attention to possible sites of lymph node metastases, including the abdomen and supraclavicular regions, is imperative. Upon finding a testicular mass, testicular ultrasound should be performed. Other important imaging techniques include chest radiographs and CT scanning of the thorax and abdomen. The utility of MRI and positron emission tomography (PET) scanning have not yet been established. Definitive diagnosis is only established by biopsy. Biopsy is obtained via a radical orchiectomy through an inguinal incision. Scrotal violation at the time of surgery or an attempt to biopsy the testicle should be avoided because of concern for a poorer outcome and high rates of relapse.[71]

Tumor growth proceeds in accordance with the histologic type. Seminomas grow more slowly and have lymphatic involvement, whereas nonseminomas tend to progress more rapidly and have marked hematologic spread. Nonseminomas are often metastatic when first seen. Lymphatic metastasis generally tends to follow the spermatic vessels to primary landing sites in the retroperitoneum. Involvement of the epididymis or spermatic cord may lead to pelvic and inguinal lymph node metastases. Common sites of distant metastases include the lungs, the bone, or the liver and may occur as a direct tumor invasion. Lymphatic metastasis is common to all forms of germinal testicular tumors. Distant metastases occur most frequently to the pulmonary region. Subsequent spread may occur in the liver, the viscera, the brain, or the bone. Bony metastases are encountered late in the course of the disease. Central nervous system metastases may occur.

Staging

Both clinical examination and radical orchiectomy are required for clinical staging. The American Joint Committee on Cancer (AJCC) and International Union Against Cancer (UICC) have established a staging system utilizing the TNM classification adding an "S" category for the serum concentrations of LDH and HCG, because of the independent prognostic significance of these serum markers. The extent of the primary tumor (T) is classified after radical orchiectomy.

Treatment Modalities and Nursing Care Considerations

The International Germ Cell Collaborative Group established a risk stratification system based on tumor type, metastatic status, and marker status (LDH, beta-HCG [bHCG] and AFP). Treatment recommendations are based on risk status.[72]

SEMINOMA THERAPY

Seminomas account for the majority of GCTs, and most present as clinically localized disease confined to the testis. Pure early-stage seminomas exhibit dramatic radiosensitivity. Removal of the affected testicle, or radical inguinal orchiectomy, is the initial treatment for all stages of seminomas. This procedure is performed on an outpatient basis. Following orchiectomy, stage I seminomas (IA,B, or S) are treated with 25 to 30 Gy of radiation (RT) to the infradiaphragmatic area including the para-aortic lymph nodes. Mediastinal prophylaxis is generally not given, since relapse at this site is rare. Surveillance has been studied as an alternative to RT and may be a viable option in selected patients who are committed to vigilant follow-up.[73]

Patients with Stages IIA and IIB seminomas are also treated with postorchiectomy RT, 35 to 40 Gy to the infradiaphragmatic and para-aortic nodes and the ipsilateral iliac nodes. In the case of patients having a horseshoe kidney (a fused kidney, which results from fusion at one pole occurring during embryonic development), RT is not the treatment of choice; rather, these patients are treated with "good-risk" chemotherapy. The recommended regimen consists of four cycles of etoposide plus cisplatin (EP) or 3 cycles of cisplatin, etoposide, and bleomycin (BEP). Approximately 90% of patients with advanced disease will achieve cure with platinum-based chemotherapy regimens.[73]

Nursing considerations are directed at decreasing the treatment-induced symptomatology in the management of seminomas, and fertility-preservation measures and education. One challenge with respect to fertility is that many patients have qualitative and or quantitative deficiencies in spermatogenesis before treatment. Fertility issues must be addressed with regard to both surgery and radiation. Radiotherapy, with its propensity for fatigue, may affect libido but does not affect potency. Azoospermia does result from RT, but recovery is seen up to 80 weeks after therapy. Although retroperitoneal lymph node dissection (RPLND) is still performed in limited cases, modification in techniques to preserve nerve functioning has resulted in preserved anterograde ejaculation. In the event that retrograde ejaculation does occur as a result of RPLND, sperm can be recovered from the urine shortly after ejaculation to be used for assisted reproductive methods.[74] At present, the most effective means to preserve fertility in patients undergoing treatment for testicular cancer is cryopreservation of sperm before the initiation of treatment. All specimens that demonstrate motile or viable sperm should be considered for preservation. Recent technologic advances such as in vitro fertilization (IVF) and sperm micromanipulation have made pregnancy possible even with the poorest quality sperm. The recovery of sperm is independent of the time it has been cryopreserved.

Additional nursing considerations for patients with testicular carcinoma include site-specific side effects related to RT and toxicities associated with chemotherapeutic agents, including synergistic responses. After orchiectomy, measures are taken to promote comfort and to minimize postoperative morbidity. Discussions regarding concerns about body image and sexuality should be encouraged. Reassurance is needed that potency is not permanently impaired. RT to the retroperitoneal area is generally well tolerated. Nausea, vomiting, diarrhea, myelosuppression, and azoospermia may occur as a result of the radiation or chemotherapy. Aggressive treatment with antiemetic therapy is essential. Patients should increase fluid intake and begin a low-residue diet that is high in protein and carbohydrates. Foods or beverages that increase gastrointestinal (GI) motility should be eliminated. Measures should be taken to prevent infection and bleeding from chemotherapy-induced myelosuppression.

NONSEMINOMA THERAPY

The majority of nonseminomas have more than one cell type. Tumors with mixed cell types are treated as nonseminomas. Two treatment options exist for Stage IA nonseminoma: nerve-sparing RPLND or observation. The cure rate for either approach is approximately 95%, but is predicated on vigilant follow-up and chemotherapy for those 30% of patients who relapse. Follow-up for patients selecting observation includes pelvic and abdominal CT scans every 2 to 3 months for the first year and every 3 to 4 months during the second year, along with serum marker studies and chest x-rays monthly for year 1, and every 2 months for the year 2. For those patients with stage 1B tumors, treatment options include nerve-sparing RPLND, observation, or chemotherapy, with RPNLD being the preferred option. Chemotherapy generally consists of two cycles of BEP. Patients with stage 1S disease and no radiographic evidence of disease are treated with chemotherapy: four cycles of EP or three cycles of BEP. These patients tend to have disseminated disease, and thus chemotherapy is preferable to RPLND.[73]

Stage II nonseminoma treatment is largely influenced by serum tumor marker status, with elevated levels indicating a need for aggressive chemotherapy with either BEP or EP regimens. Chemotherapy for more advanced disease such as extragonadal primary sites is based on the risk stratification system of the International Germ Cell Cancer Collaborative Group, and may include chemotherapy and RT. Poor prognostic indicators include nonpulmonary metastases and high serum tumor marker concentrations, or mediastinal primary site.[73] These patients may choose to investigate clinical trials.

The psychologic and physical experiences of the diagnosis and treatment of testicular cancer are severe. Yet, given the remarkable success associated with aggressive treatment, the promotion of compliance with prescribed therapeutic regimens is of paramount importance. A multidisciplinary approach is necessary. Promoting an atmosphere of trust and openness is a nursing priority. Diligent attention to symptom management and QOL issues will promote compliance with treatment.

Penile Cancer

Epidemiology

Penile carcinoma is a rare disease in industrialized countries. The estimated number of new cases of penile cancer, combined with other male genital organ malignancies (excluding testes and prostate) is 1470 for the year 2005, with an expected 390 deaths.[1] However, incidence rates are higher in less developed countries, accounting for 10% to 20% of all malignancies in parts of Africa, Asia, and South America, most notably in Paraguay.[75] In the United States, SEER data from the National Cancer Institute suggest that African American men are first seen at a later stage of disease and have significantly worse survival than their white counterparts.[76]

Etiology and Risk Factors

Penile cancer is generally associated with older age, with most cases being diagnosed in men in the sixth or seventh decade of life. Cases have been reported in younger men and in children. The etiology is unknown, although several risk factors have been identified. Poor hygiene and the accumulation of smegma and other irritants are postulated to be contributing factors. Dillner and colleagues presented a detailed evidence-based analysis of etiologic factors.[77] Strong risk factors include phimosis and chronic inflammatory conditions including balanoposthitis and lichen sclerosus et atrophicus, as well as psoriasis treatment with psoralen and ultraviolet A photochemotherapy (PUVA). Consistent associations were noted between penile cancer and smoking, and these were dose dependent. A threefold to fivefold increase in penile cancer risk was associated with sexual history and history of condyloma. Although cervical cancer in female partners has been suggested as a risk factor, a consistent association was not detected. Neonatal circumcision was associated with a threefold decreased risk, although evidence does not support a benefit from circumcision later in life. Human papillomavirus (HPV) DNA has been identified in penile neoplastic tissue in large numbers of cases.[77,78]

Prevention, Screening, and Detection

The evidence regarding risk factors for penile cancer suggests that preventive measures include circumcision and the prevention of phimosis, treatment of chronic inflammatory conditions, limiting PUVA treatment, smoking cessation and education, and education regarding prevention of HPV infection. Because of the low incidence of penile cancer, no screening methods are in place other than screening through periodic physical examination by a health professional.

Classification

Histologic differentiation ranges from well-differentiated to poorly differentiated grades. High-grade tumors and the basaloid and sarcomatoid subtypes are associated with nodal metastases and poor survival, whereas verrucous cancers rarely metastasize.[78] The TNM staging system is most widely used clinically; and the Jackson system, which does not discuss depth of penetration, is no longer considered clinically useful.

Clinical Features

Clinical presentation of penile cancer is variable and can range from a small papule or pustule to an extensive fungating wound. Patients generally arrive to be seen for evaluation of nonhealing ulceration, and may experience burning or itching under the foreskin. If neglected, lesions will progress and foul-smelling discharge may be seen exuding from beneath a phimotic, nonretractive prepuce. Eventually, disease extension along the penile shaft is seen, and ultimately the corpora cavernosa becomes involved. Rarely, patients are first seen with inguinal adenopathy, bleeding, urinary fistulas, and urinary retention. The distribution of penile cancers anatomically is estimated as follows: glans (48%), prepuce (21%), glans and prepuce (9%), prepuce, glans, and shaft (14%), coronal sulcus (6%), and shaft (less than 2%).[79] Although metastasis is rare in the absence of lymphatic involvement, metastatic sites include the liver, the lungs, the bone, and the brain. Lesions must be differentiated from those of sexually transmitted infectious diseases.

Diagnosis

Diagnosis is established by incisional biopsy, which must be of sufficient size and depth to assess involvement of the surrounding tissues. Evaluation includes urethroscopy and cavernosography with contrast media. Ultrasound examination and MRI are also used to view adjacent structures. Lymph nodes are assessed by direct palpation, with fine-needle aspiration performed on suspicious nodes. Although sentinel node biopsy techniques were originally developed for use with penile cancer, false-negative rates as high as 22% have been reported,[80] thus sentinel node biopsy is not yet an evidence-based standard of care.

Treatment Modalities and Nursing Care Considerations

SURGERY

Penile carcinoma is basically a local and/or regional disease with a low incidence of distant metastasis. The aim of treatment is complete removal of the tumor while maintaining a reasonable QOL. Partial or total penile amputation is the gold standard of therapy. In the absence of lymphatic involvement, partial penectomy may allow preservation of enough penile stump to allow for upright micturition and sexual function. Wide excisions or partial penectomies are generally the treatment of choice for small, localized tumors. A 2-cm margin of clearance has been considered standard surgical technique, but has become controversial. Wedge resections are associated with high rates of recurrence.

Conservative treatment with Mohs micrographic surgery (MMS) is also used; it involves the systematic excision of cancerous tissue under complete microscopic control. In one series of 35 men treated with MMS, the 5-year cure rate was 74%, and local control of the primary tumor was achieved in 94%.[81] Laser surgery with CO_2, Nd:YAG, argon, and potassium titanyl phosphate represents another form of less invasive management and is routinely performed for superficial lesions, precancerous lesions, and CIS. In addition, laser surgery has been used for the treatment of T1 and T2 tumors and for local recurrence following partial or total penectomy. Because of the relative infrequency of penile cancer, case series are small and tend to be from single institutions, providing insufficient evidence as to the long-term efficacy of these conservative management strategies.

Nursing management is aimed at the prevention and treatment of surgical complications. Additionally, the psychosocial implications of surgery cannot be overemphasized. Assisting patients and their partners to adjust to major body image alterations may require referral for counseling. The relative rarity of penile cancer and the intimate nature of the diagnosis and treatment make this particularly difficult to deal with.

RADIOTHERAPY

RT offers a conservative approach for small T1N1 tumors less than 4 cm in diameter. Both external beam and brachytherapy are used. Circumcision is performed before brachytherapy. Brachytherapy entails the use of an iridium-192–containing silicone mold and interstitial therapy with implanted iridium-192 wires. This device is generally worn for 8 to 10 hours daily and is removed for micturition and nursing care. Because squamous cell carcinomas are relatively radio-resistant, high doses are required and result in frequent, significant complications including edema, secondary infection, and urethral mucositis. Nursing management of these anticipatable side effects is crucial and mainly focused on pain management and education regarding hygiene and the necessity to take antibiotic therapy as directed. Common later complications include necrosis, fistula formation, urethral stricture, and stenosis of the meatus.[82] Treatment of urethral meatus stenosis involves dilation or surgical repair.

CHEMOTHERAPY

Squamous cell penile tumors do respond to chemotherapy, although RCTs are generally lacking in this area. Several agents such as cisplatin, methotrexate, bleomycin, and 5-fluorouracil (5-FU) have been shown to produce responses either alone or in combination in the palliative setting. Toxicities remain problematic, and the tradeoff must be weighed when palliation is the goal. Nursing care aimed at the minimization of distressing side effects, including nausea and vomiting, is essential. Chemotherapy is also used as adjuvant and as neoadjuvant therapy. Long-term survival of patients with penile cancer is directly related to nodal status.

When diagnosed early (stages I and II), penile cancer is highly curable, although cure rates decrease sharply for stages III and IV. Clinical trials specifically for penile cancer are infrequent, owing to the low incidence of this malignancy in the United States. A search through the National Cancer Institute (NCI) website (*www.cancer.gov*) revealed only one active trial involving docetaxel for advanced disease. Patients with stages III and IV cancer may be candidates for phase I and II clinical trials testing new drugs, biologic agents, or surgical techniques to improve local control and distant metastases. Nurses can be instrumental in educating patients and their families about these possibilities.

Bladder Cancer

Epidemiology

Bladder carcinoma is the most common malignant tumor of the urinary tract, with approximately 63,210 new cases and 13,180 deaths anticipated in the United States in the year 2005.[1] Incidence rates are high in African counties, most especially in Egypt, where schistosomiasis is endemic.[83] There is a marked male predominance. Men in the United States are 4 times more likely than women to be diagnosed with bladder cancer, and whites are 2 times more likely than African Americans. African Americans continue to lag behind in the area of survival, with 62% 5-year relative cancer survival as compared to 82% among whites.[1] Bladder cancers are rarely diagnosed before the age of 40, the median age of diagnosis being 65 years.[84]

Etiology and Risk Factors

The first reports linking chemical carcinogenic exposure to bladder cancer date back to the 1890s when bladder cancer was observed among workers in a German dye factory. Since then, numerous investigations have demonstrated a relationship between bladder cancer and exposure to aromatic amines. Specific compounds that have been identified include 2-naphthylamine, 4-aminobiophenyl, benzidine, chlornaphazine, and 4-chloro-o-toludine. These chemicals are used in textile, rubber and cable, paint, and printing industries.[85] Cigarette smoking is considered the most significant risk factor, contributing to some 50% to 66% of all cases in men and 25% in women.[86] The mechanism by which damage occurs is thought to be related to changes in the uroepithelium, and cellular changes are dose and duration sensitive. Some occupations are associated with higher than average risk, including aluminum workers, motor vehicle operators, drycleaners, chemical workers, pesticide applicators, miners, chimney sweeps, and cooks. Recently, several other occupations have become suspect. A modest increase in bladder cancer incidence has been noted among truck and bus drivers, and this has been attributed to diesel fuel exhaust exposure, but the level of evidence is unclear.[87] There is conflicting evidence regarding the increased risk of bladder cancer that has been noted among hairdresser and barbers. One large population-based study found a fivefold risk, which is postulated to be related to long-term exposure to hair dyes.[88] No significant association has been found with personal use of hair dye.

A high consumption of fried meats and fats has been associated with increased risk, whereas a combination of vitamins A, B_6, and E and zinc has been suggested to be highly protective.[89] A review of 13 case-controlled studies failed to convincingly demonstrate an increased risk of bladder cancer in people exposed to saccharin or cyclamates.[90] Likewise, although caffeine exposure has been investigated by multiple researchers, evidence at this point is inconsistent and weak. Exposure to certain drugs such as phenacetin and cyclophosphamide is associated with increased risk.[91,92] Phenacetin was subsequently labeled as a human carcinogen and removed from analgesic medications in 1987.

An increased risk for developing secondary bladder cancer has been associated with pelvic radiation, with a relative increase of 1.5 to 4 times the risk. The risk is dose related, and the latency period to development is typically short. These secondary malignancies tend to be high-grade and invasive at diagnosis. Radiation-related bladder cancer has a relatively short latency period (5 to 10 years), and is characteristically high-grade and muscle-invasive at diagnosis.[93] Parasitic infection with *Shistosoma haemotobium* has a long-established, strong association with increased risk of bladder cancer development. Recurrent urinary tract infections have been associated with increased risk of squamous cell carcinoma, especially among paraplegics with indwelling Foley catheters and recurrent bladder calculi.[94]

Prevention, Screening, and Detection

Smoking cessation is a key factor in risk reduction. Identification of persons at high risk because of environmental and work exposures is also a priority. Urine cytology may be of screening value in industrial settings and can be used to detect lesions at an early stage. Education regarding the signs and symptoms of bladder cancer is critical for patients who have undergone pelvic irradiation or who have received cytotoxic therapy with cyclophospahamide. Such patients should have urinalyses performed with microscopic evaluation at follow-up visits. Screening is not currently recommended by any major preventive group in the United States.

Classification

The TNM system developed by the AJCC is the most commonly employed staging tool. Clinical staging is determined by the depth of the tumor's invasion of the bladder wall. This determination requires a cystoscopic examination under anesthesia that includes a biopsy. Urothelial carcinoma (formerly called transitional cell carcinoma) is the most common carcinoma of the bladder in the United States, accounting for 90% of cases. The remainder of bladder cancers are squamous cell carcinoma (5%) and adenocarcinoma (less than 1%). The most significant prognostic indicators include the depth of invasion at presentation, multifocality, history of prior urothelial lesions, tumor size, and tumor grade.[95] Bladder tumors are now classified as either low- or high-grade; this replaces the previous classification system, which included an intermediate grade. The histologic grade is based upon the degree of resemblance to the normal tissue architecture, including cellular atypia, nuclear abnormalities, and number of mitotic features.

Metastasis occurs via direct extension into adjacent organs including the colon, the rectum, the prostate, the uterus or the vagina. Tumors may also obstruct ureters or the bladder neck. Metastasis also occurs by lymphatic and hematogeneous routes to the lymph nodes, the liver, the lung, and the bones.

Clinical Features

The most common presenting sign of bladder cancer is gross hematuria. This hematuria is often described as "painless," with or without bladder irritability (urgency, dysuria, or frequency). Intermittent bleeding is characteristic and may lead to delayed diagnosis since either the patient or the physician may postpone further investigation if the urine clears. Because urinary tract infections (UTIs) are often seen, patients with cancer of the bladder are treated with antibiotics for what is thought to be hemorrhagic cystitis, a common phenomenon in women. The presence of unexplained gross or microscopic hematuria should always be evaluated. Obstructive symptoms are associated with large tumor burden or metastases. Tumor pushing on the urethral orifice may cause urinary hesitancy or decrease in stream force. Patients may experience flank pain caused by hydronephrosis if ureteral obstruction occurs. Back pain, rectal pain, or suprapubic pain may suggest metastatic disease.

Diagnosis

Physical examination generally reveals no suggestive signs of bladder cancer, although rarely a mass may be detected on rectal examination. The diagnostic steps indicated in a patient with hematuria include microscopic urinalysis, cystourethroscopy, urinary cytology, and an evaluation of the upper tracts, since urothelial malignancy can be multifocal, with lesions at any site between the renal pelvis and the proximal urethra. Evaluation of the upper tract includes a CT scan of the pelvis and abdomen with intravenous pyelography.

Cystoscopy is used to verify the presence of a bladder tumor and to characterize its gross appearance, and as a means of obtaining a biopsy specimen. Areas of erythema may represent CIS. Cystoscopy with multiple random bladder biopsies is performed with the patient under local anesthesia, using an intraurethral topical anesthetic with or without intravenous sedation. Associated procedures, such as transurethral resection, bimanual examination, or retrograde studies of the upper tracts, are more readily performed with the patient sedated. A bimanual pelvic examination helps to determine the presence of a palpable or fixed mass. In addition to tissue biopsies, cells may be captured from bladder mucosa through bladder washings or voided urine.

Flow cytometry, a technique that allows examination of the DNA content of cells within the urine, is useful for providing information for staging and grading purposes. Flow cytometry can be performed on bladder-wash specimens, urine specimens, and biopsy specimens. High grade and aneuploidy (large amounts of DNA per cell) are associated with poor prognosis. The limitations of cytology and the invasiveness of cystoscopy has generated the development of noninvasive diagnostic tools, including urine immunocytochemistry (ImmunoCyt test) and proteomics assays for the tumor marker nuclear matrix protein NMP22 (NMP22 Bladder Check test). These tools are expected to improve early diagnosis.[96] Chest x-ray, abdominal CT or MRI, and bone scans may be necessary to rule out metastatic disease.

Treatment Modalities and Nursing Care Considerations

The management of bladder cancer is based on multiple factors. Recurrence and progression depend on the initial anatomic and histologic classification, the depth of invasion at presentation, multifocality, history of prior urothelial lesions, tumor size, and tumor grade. The patient's age and general stage of health, functional status, self-care abilities, and personal preferences, and presence of associated GU problems (e.g., infection, obstruction, and compromised renal function) factor into the treatment decision. Treatment planning is based on the depth and degree to which the cancer has penetrated into the bladder wall. Before treatment, it is essential to determine if the tumor has seeded downward from the renal pelvis or has originated as a ureteral primary tumor. Metastasis occurs by lymphatic and hematogeneous routes and usually spreads to the lymph nodes, the liver, the lung, and the bones. The bladder is also a common site for contiguous spread from malignant lesions of neighboring organs such as the uterus, the colon, and the rectum.

NONINVASIVE TUMORS

The goals of therapy are to eradicate existing disease, prevent disease progression and invasion, avoid loss of the bladder, and prevent the development of recurrent disease. Historically, most patients with noninvasive stage I bladder cancer have been managed with transurethral resection (TUR) and fulguration using electrical current or laser, with or without intravesical therapy.[84] Following resection, an indwelling catheter may be left in place. The catheter may be connected to gravity drainage or a continuous irrigation system. The catheter is left in place for 2 to 3 days or until the urine is clear. Patients must be monitored for any signs of clot retention and urinary outlet obstruction. They should be informed that they may experience some bleeding on urination as the postoperative site heals.

Intravesicular therapy has been found to be more effective than TUR alone in preventing tumor recurrence.[97] Tumors confined to the mucosa have a 10% to 70% recurrence rate within 5 years, with a similar risk of developing a new urothelial tumor.[85] Chemotherapeutic or immunotherapeutic agents may be instilled directly into the bladder postoperatively. Intravesicular chemotherapy offers an advantage over systemic chemotherapy because it allows active agents to come into direct contact with the uroepithelium. In addition, this mode of delivery reduces the occurrence of systemic toxicity, although this varies depending on the agents selected. Intravesicular therapy usually begins within 10 to 14 days after resection. Patient preparation involves restricting fluids in an attempt to limit urine output and to facilitate retention of chemotherapy or immunotherapy for the requisite 2 hours. A urinalysis is performed before the procedure; infection is a contraindication. A Foley catheter is inserted. Topical lidocaine may be applied to the urethra to minimize discomfort. The prescribed agents are slowly instilled into the catheter by gravity. The catheter is clamped to retain the therapeutic agents, and patients are repositioned every 30 minutes to allow maximal bladder tissue exposure. Following catheter removal, patients may be discharged and instructed to increase fluid intake to flush residual medication from the bladder and minimize irritation. Patients receiving Bacille Calmette-Guerin (BCG), a live attenuated form of *Mycobacterium bovis*, remain at the treatment center until they have voided to ensure proper disposal of contaminated urine. Patients are instructed that burning, frequency, and urgency are expected side effects. These may be managed with topical anesthetics, antispasmotic agents, and nonsteroidal antiinflammatory agents (NSAIDs). Blood in the urine or any signs of infection should be reported to the health care provider immediately. BCG is the most commonly used agent for intravesicular therapy. Bladder instillation is usually performed weekly for 6 weeks. BCG is contraindicated in patients with immune system compromise due to HIV, steroid use, active urinary tract infection, or past reaction to tuberculosis strains,[97] thus a thorough nursing history is critical before the instillation procedure.

If recurrent or persistent disease is detected at the first 3-month follow-up, a second course of BCG is indicated. Detection of disease at the next 3-month follow-up is an indication for mitomycin or, less commonly valrubicin or α-interferon as an alternative to cystectomy.[84] Patients must be monitored for allergic reactions and the potential for the development of myelosupression. Myelosuppression is less common with the aforementioned agents as compared to the low-molecular-weight thiotepa, which was formerly used and had a high propensity for systemic absorption.

INVASIVE TUMORS

The standard treatment for tumors invading the muscle is surgical removal of the bladder by radical cystectomy. If distant disease is detected on MRI, CT, or bone scan, systemic treatment is required. In the absence of distant disease, an exploratory laparotomy with pelvic node dissection is performed. For men, the procedure involves a cystoprostatectomy. Women generally undergo both cystectomy and hysterectomy.[84] Pretreatment chemotherapy using methotrexate, vinblastine, doxorubicin, and cisplatin (MVAC) has been demonstrated to double survival rates for patients with advanced bladder cancer as compared to surgery alone[98] and is recommended by the NCCN. Urinary diversions are created in the form of ileal conduits or by directing urine flow into an internal urinary reservoir with drainage to the abdominal wall or to the urethra.

The ileal conduit is constructed from a small piece of bowel. A portion of the ileum is isolated and the proximal end closed, and then the end is brought out through an opening in the abdominal wall. This is sutured to the skin, creating a stoma. An external collection device is used. Continent ileal reservoirs provide an intraabdominal pouch for urine storage. Typically these have a nipple valve stoma to prevent urine reflux. The stoma is generally placed below the undergarment line to avoid irritation. No external collection device is needed since urine remains in the internal reservoir until the patient self-catheterizes through the stoma approximately every 6 hours.

Preoperative consultation and education with an enterostomal therapist (ET) are essential to treatment and rehabilitation. Preoperative determination of the optimal ileal stoma site should be done jointly with the surgeon and the ET while the patient is in the supine, sitting, and standing positions. Optimal stoma placement is crucial for postoperative management. The standard of care for urinary diversion focuses on patient adjustment to body image and QOL.

Postoperative nursing management includes assessment of patients for complications including signs of peritonitis related to an anastomotic leak. This should be suspected if there is a sudden decrease in urinary output or the presence of malodorous urine, elevated temperature, leukocytosis, or abdominal distention and/or tenderness. The surgical site should be monitored for infection, and pain management is a priority. Urinary output is monitored hourly and maintained at a minimum of 30 cc/hr. Decreased urinary output may be a sign of obstruction, anastomotic failure, or early renal failure.

Teaching priorities include early identification of signs and symptoms of infection and the necessity for increased fluid intake. Instruction regarding the normal appearance of the stoma includes information that edema will decrease within 1 to 2 weeks. A normal stoma can be compared to the mucosal lining of the oral cavity. A dusky appearance ranging from purple to black indicates impaired circulation and should be reported immediately. Patients and/or caretakers should be able to demonstrate the ability to change the drainage pouch to straight drainage for nighttime use. In addition, the ability to demonstrate proper selection and sizing of pouches and cleansing of the stoma are important teaching outcomes. Consultation with an ET is recommended for selection of collection devices and appropriate skin barrier selection. For patients with continent reservoirs, demonstration of the ability to self-catheterize is essential. Significant others should be included in teaching.

BLADDER PRESERVATION THERAPIES

Bladder preservation–therapy strategies include external beam RT and multimodality therapy combining TUR, RT, and systemic chemotherapy. Concurrent RT and chemotherapy with cisplatin is the most studied regimen. Four weeks of radiation to the whole bladder for a total dose of 40 Gy is recommended, with cisplatin given in weeks 1 and 4. Following therapy completion, a cystocopy is performed. If residual disease is detected, cystectomy is recommended. If no disease is detected, a boost of 25 Gy is administered with one additional dose of cisplatin.[83]

Early reactions to radiation usually occur during the first 3 to 4 weeks of therapy. Urinary frequency, urgency, and dysuria may occur as bladder capacity is reduced. Hematuria may result from mucosal inflammation. Patients may require a respite from

CONSIDERATIONS FOR OLDER ADULTS
Bladder Cancer

- Older patients often have sensory impairments that influence teaching and learning. In addition, they often have comorbid conditions that influence therapeutic options. Cardiac and respiratory conditions may preclude surgical intervention. Of older patients, 43% have hypertension, and an estimated 40% have heart conditions.[99] Physiologic changes associated with aging and comorbidities increase the potential for older adults to experience treatment-related complications. Impaired renal function may rule out the use of cisplatin therapy and may be a contraindication for intravenous pyelography. Polypharmacia and age-related hepatic changes may predispose older patients to greater risks of drug reactions.

treatment as symptoms intensify or as skin integrity becomes compromised. Pharmacologic treatments provide relief and are used to prevent infection. Antispasmodics or parasympathetic blockers provide relief of symptoms and promote analgesia. Patients are instructed to empty the bladder frequently and increase intake of fluids, such as water and cranberry juice. Caffeine, alcohol, tobacco, and spices may irritate the bladder mucosa and should be avoided. Reactions may be exacerbated as a result of the synergistic effects of combined modality therapy.

Late effects of radiation can occur 1 year or more after treatment. Internal fibrosis, telangiectasia, chronic urinary frequency, and permanent diminished bladder capacity may occur. Combined modalities of surgery and RT may lead to fistula formation, although the occurrence is rare. Development of a fistula after treatment may indicate tumor recurrence.

Renal Cell Cancer

Epidemiology

Kidney cancer is relatively rare in the United States. In 2005, 38,500 new cases were expected, and renal cancer was expected to cause 12,000 deaths during the same period, with more than 8000 of these being among men.[1] Incidence rates have been rising since 1973,[100] although this may be related to high-resolution imaging. Approximately two thirds of renal carcinomas are discovered incidentally during pelvic or abdominal scanning.[101]

Etiology and Risk Factors

The etiology of renal cancer is unknown. A wide variety of environmental, genetic, cellular, and hormonal factors have been examined including obesity, dietary fat intake, tobacco use, phenacetin use, and occupational exposures to asbestos and petroleum. Numerous epidemiologic studies suggest that tobacco plays a significant role. An increase in renal cell carcinoma has been observed among persons with autosomal dominant polycystic kidney disease and tuberous sclerosis, and among persons with von Hippel-Lindau syndrome, associated with autosomal dominant genetic changes on chromosome 3p.[102] The highest incidence occurs in the sixth decade of life.[101] There is marked male predominance, with 1.5 cases in men for every 1 case in women.[101]

Prevention, Screening, and Detection

With the identification of certain etiologic factors, lifestyle or environmental modification to decrease the risk of developing kidney cancer is a reasonable goal. Specifically, encouraging cessation of tobacco use, avoidance of developing a tobacco habit in youth, and stressing dietary modification to decrease or limit high fat content are positive steps in decreasing cancer risk. Minimizing occupational or lifestyle exposure to petrochemicals is also suggested. Owing to the extremely low incidence rates, there are currently no screening recommendations. Persons with multiple affected relatives should be referred for genetic counseling.

Classification and Staging

The AJCC TNM staging system is the primary system for staging renal carcinoma. Revision in 2002 included the creation of a subdivision of T1 lesions into T1a—tumors of 4 cm or less, and T1b—tumors of greater than 4 cm but less than 7 cm. A T stage is assigned preoperatively, and a pathologic (P) stage is established postoperatively. Of renal cancers, 90% are renal cell carcinomas; and of these, 85% are of the clear cell variety. These occur in hereditary and sporadic forms and are thought to arise from the proximal renal tubule. Other, less common cell types include papillary, chromophobe, and collecting duct or Bellini's duct carcinomas. An "unclassified" category has been maintained for those tumors that do not fit other categories. Sarcomatoid is no longer considered a distinct category.[103]

Clinical Features

Renal cell carcinomas generally remain clinically occult until signs of metastasis prompt diagnostic evaluation. The classic triad of pain, hematuria, and flank mass is noted in less than 10% of patients and signals advanced disease.[100] Renal cell carcinomas locally invade the capsule, are highly angio-invasive, often spread to the renal vein and the vena cava, and result in widespread hematogeneous and lymphatic metastases. The most common sites for nonlymphatic metastases are lung, bone, liver, adrenals, and brain. Renal cell carcinoma can metastasize to unusual sites, such as the testes and skin. Renal cell carcinomas have been reported to regress spontaneously. Renal cell carcinomas are known to secrete hormones, including parathyroid hormone and erythropoietin, resulting in hypercalcemia and erythrocytosis. Hypertension is often encountered and may be mediated by tumor secretion of renin. Unfortunately, approximately one third of patients have metastases at diagnosis. A number of paraneoplastic syndromes are associated with renal carcinoma. They are detailed in Box 10-1.

Diagnosis

Early-stage renal cell cancer is usually "silent" and is coincidentally detected when the patient is undergoing work-up for a non–cancer-related procedure such as cardiac angiography or gallbladder ultrasound. There appears to be high variability in symptom presentation. The differential diagnosis includes a variety of conditions including benign inflammatory processes such as abscess and pyelonephritis; in addition, hematomas, cystic masses, and hydronephrosis must be considered. Kidney, ureters, and bladder radiography is performed before and after intravenous pyelography. Renal ultrasounds and pelvic and abdominal CTs are also employed. Renal angiography is less commonly

BOX 10-1   Syndromes Associated with Renal Carcinomas

Syndromes and Serologic Factors
Hypercalcemia
Nonmetastatic hepatopathy
Hypertension
Erythrocytosis
Pyrexia
Galactorrhea
Cushing's syndrome
Gynecomastia
Serum glucose abnormalities
Prostaglandins
Alkaline phosphatase
Neuromyopathy
Amyloidosis
Coagulation factors
Iron metabolism
α-Fetoprotein
Vasculitis
Fibroblast growth factor

Adapted from Sufrin et al: Paraneoplastic and serologic syndromes of renal adenocarcinoma, *Semin Urol* 7(3):159, 1989

performed, but may be indicated if the renal mass is large and renal artery embolization is planned. MRI is particularly important if vena caval involvement is suspected. CT-guided fine-needle biopsy is the current diagnostic standard. There is no known tumor or molecular marker to confirm diagnosis, progression, or relapse at this point.

Treatment Modalities and Nursing Care Considerations

Since 1960, radical nephrectomy has proved to be an efficient treatment modality for localized renal carcinomas. Radical nephrectomy includes the excision of the kidney, the surrounding lymph nodes, fat, and the fascia, as well as the adrenal gland on the affected side.[101] Nephron-sparing surgery is now more commonly practiced and may be equally effective as radical nephrectomy in selected patients.[104] Laparoscopic partial nephrectomy is now becoming widely accepted for patients with solitary tumors of 4 cm or less.[105]

Nephrectomy remains the standard of care for patients with stage II renal disease. The focus of care for patients with stage IV disease is palliation. Renal cell carcinomas are unresponsive to radiotherapy; however, RT is indicated for the palliative management of skeletal tumors. Adjuvant chemotherapy has not improved survival, although current clinical trials are investigating the use of gemcitabine with and without 5-FU, bevacizumab, and antivascular endothelial growth factors.[106] Clinical trials continue to investigate the use of cytokine therapy consisting of α-interferon and interleukin 2 (IL-2). Gene therapy is also under investigation and may provide new options in the future.

Nursing management focuses on preoperative and postoperative teaching to minimize complications. Pain management is a top priority since pain, related to extensive tissue trauma, may be severe. Postoperative bleeding is a significant risk because of the highly vascular nature of the kidney. Profuse drainage and distention at the suture line is a sign of massive hemorrhage. The nephrectomy dressing should be closely observed for signs of bleeding. Urine output must be maintained at a minimum of 30 cc/hr. Nephrectomy patients are at risk for paralytic ileus as a result of bowel manipulation during surgery and the extensive need for narcotic analgesia. Auscultation of bowel sounds and repositioning to promote peristalsis are appropriate interventions. A bowel regimen should be initiated to accompany narcotic use.

Postoperative teaching focuses on protecting the function of the remaining kidney. Patients should avoid any potentially nephrotoxic drugs, including NSAIDs. Although resumption of normal activities is the goal, care must be taken to avoid trauma to the remaining kidney. Early recognition of urinary tract infection is essential for prompt initiation of antibiotic therapy. Patients should consult their physician before the initiation of any over-the-counter medications, dietary supplements, or complementary therapies. Follow-up examinations should include periodic CT scans, chest x-rays, and bone scans to rule out metastatic disease. Blood pressure monitoring is essential.

Prognosis

Unfortunately, the prognosis for any patient with treated renal cancer who has relapsing, recurring, or progressing disease, regardless of stage or cell type, is poor. Survival is equated with early diagnosis of incident carcinoma. Five-year survival for all stages is 64%. Five-year survival for organ-contained local disease is 91%, although this decreases to 59% and 9% for regional and distant disease, respectively.[1]

Conclusion

Genitourinary malignancies represent a broad array of carcinomas. Despite the variability in incidence and prognosis, each of the GU malignancies represents a significant threat to life and quality of life. The uniqueness of this group of malignancies lies in their intense threat to body image and sexuality. Although it is encouraging to note the major treatment advances over the past decade, it is more encouraging still to note the increased emphasis on quality of life. Nurses are challenged to retain and refine their focus on quality of life, especially in the face of increasingly aggressive multimodality therapy.

REVIEW QUESTIONS

 Case Study

The patient was a 52-year-old male. He reported having numerous bouts of prostatitis over a 10-year period, which became increasingly severe. PSA levels rose from an initial 3.0 to 5.5 ng/ml. At that point, biopsies revealed malignancy in both lobes, at clinical stage II. The couple was presented with treatment options by the urologist: radiation, radical prostatectomy, or "doing nothing." The urologist discussed the potential treatment-related side effects in great detail with the patient and his wife of 27 years, who was a former registered nurse. They ultimately chose surgery, which they described as a "couple decision." They related that although the subsequent risk of incontinence and impotence were high, they chose the treatment that they felt had the best odds of cure.

The patient recovered from surgery without complications, although he did report problems with incontinence and impotence. Both he and his wife were disappointed to learn that final pathology indicated seminal vesicle involvement. Initially the patient was depressed and stated that he wanted no further treatment, although his wife was not ready to "give up." When the bone scan was negative, he reconsidered further treatment, opting for external beam RT. He received 30 treatments over the course of 6 weeks.

Because of difficulties managing urinary leakage and bowel urgency, he retired at age 54, much earlier than he had originally anticipated. They down-sized to a smaller, more manageable home.

They attempted several methods of dealing with the erectile dysfunction, including a vacuum device, urethral prostaglandin suppositories, and sildenafil, without success. They state that "we can live with it," referring to the changes in their sexual relationship. The couple states that they are closer now than ever before. Four years after the completion of treatment, the patient's PSA remains at 0.1 ng/ml; however, he is plagued with worry that the disease will return.

DISCUSSION

The psychologic sequelae of learning that the disease was not confined to the prostate gland included depression and an inability to fully consider further treatment. Waiting for the results of the bone scan proved to be a period of increased stress related to uncertainty. During this time the couple needed additional psychologic support in the form of telephone calls from the office nurse. Once bone metastasis was ruled out, the patient, with the help of his spouse, was able to reconsider additional therapy with a more hopeful outlook for the future.

The timing of intervention regarding impotence is critical. Immediate concerns tend to focus on cure, followed by dealing with incontinence. Sexual activity is difficult if a patient continues to have urinary control issues. Although this couple tried several methods of dealing with erectile dysfunction, none were successful. They did manage to come to terms with this as they considered the totality of their marital relationship.

The continued uncertainty 4 years following completion of treatment, in spite of encouraging PSA levels, may suggest the need for a counseling referral.

QUESTIONS

1. Which of the following is a risk factor for the development of prostate cancer?
   a. Affected brother
   b. History of tobacco use
   c. Affected uncle
   d. History of venereal disease

2. Which of the following can be said of high-grade prostatic intraepithelial prostate neoplasia?
   a. It is suspected if the PSA is elevated above 4.0 ng/ml.
   b. It is detectable by ultrasound.
   c. It is detectable by biopsy.
   d. It is detectable by MRI.
3. Which of the following statements is accurate regarding the practice of pelvic floor strengthening exercises following radical prostatectomy?
   a. There is strong evidence to support their use in the prevention of incontinence.
   b. There is no evidence to support their use in the prevention of incontinence.
   c. There is inconclusive evidence to support their use in the prevention of incontinence.
   d. There is a lack of clinical trials to evaluate their use in the prevention of incontinence.
4. Watchful waiting (WW) as a treatment option is usually considered in patients with which of the following characteristics?
   a. Are asymptomatic and under the age of 60
   b. Have extension of tumor beyond the capsule of the prostate
   c. Have an additional cancer diagnosis other than prostate
   d. Are older than 70 and have life expectancy less than 10 years and low-grade disease
5. Which if the following would be considered *the most important immediate postoperative nursing interventions* for this patient?
   a. Signs and symptoms of infection and urinary obstruction
   b. Pain management and adequate urinary output
   c. Foley catheter management
   d. Anticipated treatment related side effects
6. Erectile dysfunction is multifactorial. In prostate cancer patients treated with radiation, the following most likely contribute to erectile dysfunction:
   a. Pain and urethral stricture
   b. Depression, decreased quality of life
   c. Prescription and nonprescription medications
   d. Radiation to small blood vessels and nerves
7. Successful use of sildenafil (Viagra) for erectile dysfunction following surgery for prostate cancer depends the following factors, among others:
   a. Size of tumor, tumor penetration, and nerve involvement
   b. Postoperative infection, inflammation, and presurgical potency
   c. Age, postoperative Foley catheter use, and current voiding pattern
   d. Age less than 65, 6-month postoperative period before sildenafil use, preoperative potency
8. For men undergoing radiation therapy for prostate cancer, treatment side effects are affected most by which of the following?
   a. Age and previous cancer therapies
   b. Dose given to normal tissue and the volume of tissue treated
   c. Time interval between diagnosis and start of treatment
   d. Presence of bone metastases

9. The timing of supportive and emotional intervention for this couple is critical. Which psychologic/emotional issue *arouses the greatest concern* and requires long-term assessment and intervention?
   a. Depression, anxiety
   b. Incontinence issues, pain management
   c. Metastatic spread, further treatment
   d. Sexual intimacy, erectile dysfunction
10. Which of the following describes "high-risk" men who should be considered for early PSA testing? Check all that apply.
   a. All men over the age of 50
   b. African American males with family history of prostate cancer
   c. Men with a history of sexually transmitted disease and who exhibit symptoms of urinary obstruction
   d. Men who have had urinary incontinence who are maintained by catheterization for greater than 6-week period

ANSWERS

1. **A.** *Rationale:* The exact cause of prostate cancer is unclear. There are several issues that seem to play a contributing role, primarily a combination of environmental and endogenous factors. Smoking does not seem to play a role in prostate cancer, nor does a history of sexually transmitted disease. There has been interest in a genetic link in the development of prostate cancer, and a man's risk increases as the number of first-degree relatives with prostate cancer increases.
2. **C.** *Rationale:* Most men with early-stage disease may be symptom free, because the vast majority of prostatic neoplasms arise in the periphery. Although most patients are initially detected with PSA testing, over 4.0 ng/ml, there are false-negative results (prostate cancer found in a patient with a reading *less than 4.0 ng/ml*). A transurethral ultrasound can aid in visualization of the prostate, but it is not diagnostic. MRI evaluates extracapsular extension beyond the prostate gland, into the lymph nodes and seminal vesicles. True, definitive diagnosis is obtained by biopsy of the prostate.
3. **C.** *Rationale:* Although there has been long-term interest and some advocacy in the use of pelvic floor strengthening exercises to diminish incontinence, evidence is inconclusive as to their efficacy for that purpose.
4. **D.** *Rationale:* Watchful waiting, (also called expectant management or surveillance) is conservative management which involves no local therapy on diagnosis. Treatment is initiated if the patient becomes symptomatic from either local or metastatic disease. Factors likely to lead one to consider an aggressive therapy are having disease which extends beyond the capsule of the prostate; a diagnosis of an additional malignancy; being asymptomatic and under the age of 60 years.
5. **B.** *Rationale:* Nursing interventions for this couple are numerous. Although education regarding surgical procedure, recovery path, and anticipated side effects are important, these topics should be approached initially preoperatively, with review and recap postoperatively. The maintenance of the Foley catheter, as well as signs and symptoms of infection, are important to cover before discharge since the couple will be dealing with these issues at home. Immediately after surgery, it is essential to maintain adequate urinary output and provide pain management.

Continued

REVIEW QUESTIONS—CONT'D

6. D. *Rationale:* Erectile dysfunction is a distressing outcome that may result from prostate cancer or its treatment. Although A, B, and C represent contributing factors, radiation damage to small vessels and nerves is the main cause of erectile dysfunction.

7. D. *Rationale:* Although numerous factors could contribute to erectile dysfunction, the text discusses a retrospective study in which four factors are associated with successful use of sildenafil for postprostatectomy erectile function. These include the following: age less than 65 years, a 6-month lag between surgery and initiating sildenafil, a minimum of one intact neurovascular bundle, and preoperative potency.

8. B. *Rationale:* Side effects of radiation therapy are most dependent upon the amount of normal tissue in treatment margins affected during treatment and the dose and/or volume of radiation administered.

9. A. *Rationale:* The diagnosis of prostate cancer has caused the couple a fair amount of loss, such as the downsizing into a smaller home and the patient's early retirement. In addition, the time lag in awaiting bone scan results caused levels of high anxiety. Currently, even though his PSA markers have been within normal limits for 4 years, the patient continues to obsess about the possibility of recurrence. A referral for counseling and management of depression and anxiety would be of benefit.

10. A. *Rationale:* Although there is much controversy regarding PSA velocity testing, the findings of false-negative, and the initiation of age-specific references, current recommendations regarding "who is at high risk" and in need of PSA includes African American males and men with a family history of prostate cancer. This group should begin PSA at age 45 years. For patients with numerous first-degree relatives with prostate cancer, screening should begin at 40 due to increased risk. All men over age 50 are not considered high risk.

REFERENCES

1. American Cancer Society: *Cancer facts and figures 2005*, Atlanta, GA, 2005, Author.
2. Scardino P: The prevention of prostate cancer—The dilemma continues, *N Engl J Med* 349:297-299, 2003.
3. Routh JC, Leibovich BC: Adenocarcinoma of the prostate: epidemiological trends, screening, diagnosis, and surgical management of localized disease, *Mayo Clin Proc* 80:899-907, 2005.
4. Gilliland FD, Key CR: Prostate cancer in American Indians, New Mexico, 1969–1994, *J Urol* 159:893-897, 1998.
5. Stanford JL, Stephenson RA, Coyle LM et al: *Prostate cancer trends 1973-1975*. SEER Program, National Cancer Institute: NIH Publication No.99-4543, retrieved August 1, 2004, from http: //seer.cancer.gov/publications/prostate/
6. Scott R, Mutchnik DL, Laskowski TZ et al: (1969). Carcinoma of the prostate in elderly men: incidence, growth characteristics and clinical significance, *J Urol* 101:602-607, 1969.
7. Brawley OW, Barnes S: The epidemiology of prostate cancer in the United States, *Semin Oncol Nurs* 17:72-77, 2001.
8. Giovanucci E, Rimm EB, Colditz GA et al: A prospective study of dietary fat and risk of prostate cancer, *J Natl Cancer Inst* 85:1571-1579, 1993.
9. Sahmoun AE, Jackson SA, Schwartz GG: Cadmium and prostate cancer: a critical epidemiologic analysis, *Cancer Invest* 23:256-263, 2005.
10. Gann PH, Ma J, Giovanucci E et al: Prostate risk in men with elevated plasma lycopene levels: results of a prospective analysis, *Cancer Res* 59:1225-1230, 1999.
11. Polek TC, Weigel NL: Vitamin D and prostate cancer, *J Androl* 23:9-17, 2002.
12. Gross C, Stamey T, Hancock S et al: Treatment of early recurrent prostate cancer with 1,25 dihydroxyvitamin D3 (clacitrol), *J Urol* 159:2035-2039, 1998.
13. Chen L, Stacewicz-Sapuntzakis M, Duncan C et al: Oxidative DNA damage in prostate cancer patients consuming tomato sauce-based entrees as a whole food intervention, *J Natl Cancer Inst* 93(24):1872-1879, 2001.
14. Cooney KA, McCarthy JD, Lange E el al: Prostate cancer susceptibility locus on chromosome 1q: a confirmatory study, *JNCI* 89:955-959, 1997.
15. Johns LE, Houllston RS: A systematic review and meta-analysis of familial prostate cancer risk, *Br J Urol* 91:789-794, 2003.
16. Ekman P: Genetic and environmental factors in prostate cancer genesis: identifying high-risk cohorts, *Eur Oncol* 35:362-369, 1999.
17. Bostwick DG:. Prostatic intraepithelial neoplasia, *Curr Urol Rep* 1:65-70, 2000.
18. Brawer MK: Prostate-specific antigen, *Semin Surg Oncol* 18:3-9, 2000.
19. Smith RA, Conkkindes V, Eyre HJ: American Cancer Society guidelines for early detection of cancer, 2003, *CA Cancer J Clin* 53:27-43, 2003.
20. von Eschenbach A, Ho R, Murphy GP et al: American Cancer Society Guidelines for the early detection of prostate cancer, *Cancer* 80:180, 1997.
21. National Comprehensive Cancer Network: Clinical Practice Guidelines, version 1. 2005, Prostate cancer early detection, retrieved August 8, 2005, from http://www.nccn.org/professionals/physician_gls/PDF/prostate_detection.pdf.
22. Labrie F, Candas B, Supont A et al: Screening decreased prostate cancer death: first analysis of the 1988 Quebec prospective randomized controlled trial, *Prostate* 38:83-91, 1999.
23. Perron L, Moore L, Bairati I et al: PSA screening and prostate cancer mortality, *CMAJ* 166:586-591, 2002.
24. United States Preventive Services Task Force: Screening for prostate cancer: recommendation and rationale, *Ann Int Med* 137:915-916, 2002.
25. Frank I, Granham S, Neighbors W: Urologic and male genital cancers. In Holleb A, Fink D, Murphy G, editors: *American Cancer Society textbook of clinical oncology,* Atlanta, 1991, American Cancer Society.
26. Mettlin C, Littrup PJ, Kane RA et al: Relative sensitivity and specificity of serum prostate specific antigen (PSA) level compared with age-referenced PSA, PSA density, and PSA change. Data from the American Cancer Society National Prostate Cancer Detection Project, *Cancer* 74:1615-1620, 1994.
27. Thompson IM, Pauler DK, Goodman PJ et al: Prevalence of prostate cancer among men with a prostate-specific antigen level ≤4 ng/milliliter, *N Engl J Med* 350:2239-2246, 2004.
28. Presti JC Jr, Chang JJ, Bhargava V et al: The optimal systematic prostate biopsy scheme should include 8 rather than 6 biopsies: results of a prospective trial, *J Urol* 163:163-166, 2000.
29. King CR, McNeal J, Gil IL et al: Extended prostate cancer biopsy scheme improves reliability of Gleason grading: implications for radiotherapy patients, *Int J Radiat Oncol Biol Phys* 59:386-391, 2004.
30. Brassel SA, Krueger WR, Choi JH et al: Correlation of endorectal coil magnetic resonance imagine of the prostate with pathologic stage, *World J Urol* 22:289-292.
31. Gleason D, Mellinger G: Prediction of prognosis for prostatic adenocarcinoma by combined histological grading and clinical staging, *J Urol* 11:58-61, 1974.
32. O'Rourke ME: Narrowing the options: the process of deciding on prostate cancer treatment, *Cancer Invest* 17:349-359, 1999.

33. National Comprehensive Cancer Network: Clinical Practice Guidelines, version 2.2005, Prostate cancer, retrieved August 8, 2005, from http://www.nccn.org/professionals/physician_gls/PDF/prostate.pdf.

34. O'Rourke ME: Urinary incontinence as a factor in prostate cancer treatment selection, *J WOCN* 27:146, 2000.

35. Hunter KF, Moore KN, Helgessen F et al: Conservative management of post prostatectomy incontinence, *Cochrane Database Systematic Reviews* 2:CD001843, 2004.

36. Palmer MH: Postprostatectomy incontinence: the magnitude of the problem, *J WOCN* 27:129-137, 2000.

37. Cespedes RD, Leng WW, McGuire WJ: Collagen injection for post-prostatectomy incontinence, *Urology* 54:597-602, 1999.

38. Incrocci L, Hopp WC, Slob AK: Efficacy of sildenafil in an open-label study as a continuation of a double-blind study in the treatment of erectile dysfunction after radiotherapy for prostate cancer, *Urology* 62:116-120, 2003.

39. Raina R, Lakin MM, Agarwal A et al: Efficacy and factors associated with successful outcome of sildenafil citrate use for erectile dysfunction after radical prostatectomy, *Urology* 63:960-966, 2004.

40. American College of Surgeons Oncology Group (ASCOSOG): Health-related quality of life in patients with low risk, localized prostate cancer randomized to radical prostatectomy or brachytherapy, Study synopsis, retrieved August 10, 2005, from https://www.acosog.org/studies/synopses/Z0071_Synopsis.pdf.

41. Kuban DA, Thames HD, Levy LB et al: Long-term multi-institutional analysis of stage T1-T2 prostate cancer treated with radiotherapy in the PSA era, *Int J Radiat Oncol Biol Phys* 57:915-928, 2003.

42. Denton A, Forbes A, Andreyev J et al: Non surgical interventions for late radiation proctitis in patients who have received radiotherapy to the pelvis, *Cochrane Database Systematic Reviews* 1:CD003455, 2002.

43. Mock V, Dow KH, Grimm PM et al: Effects of exercise on fatigue, physical functioning, and emotional distress during radiotherapy for breast cancer, *Oncol Nurs Forum* 24:991-1000, 1997.

44. Windsor PM, Nicol KF, Potter J: A randomized controlled trial of aerobic exercise for treatment-related fatigue in men receiving external beam radiotherapy for localized prostate carcinoma, *Cancer* 101:550-557, 2004.

45. D'Amico AV, Whittington R, Malkowicz SB et al: Biochemical outcome after radical prostatectomy, external beam radiation therapy, or interstitial radiation therapy for clinically localized prostate cancer, *JAMA* 280:969-974, 1998.

46. Aus G, Abrahamsson PA, Ahlgren G et al: Hormonal therapy before radical prostatectomy: a 3-year followup, *J Urol* 159:2013-2016, 1998.

47. Higano CS: Side effects of androgen deprivation therapy: monitoring and minimizing toxicity, *Urology* 61(2 suppl 1):32-38, 2003

48. National Comprehensive Cancer Network: Practice guidelines: senior adult oncology: v1.2005, retrieved August 10, 2005, from http://www.nccn.org/professionals/physician_gls/PDF/senior.pdf.

49. Quella SK, Loprinzi CL, Sloan J et al: Pilot evaluation of venlafaxine for the treatment of hot flashes in men undergoing androgen ablation therapy for prostate cancer, *J Urol* 162:98-102, 1999.

50. Sartor O, Eastham JA: Progressive prostate cancer associated with the use of megestrol acetate administered for control of hot flashes, *South Med J* 92:415-416, 1999.

51. Graversen PH, Nielsen KT, Corle DK et al: Radical prostatectomy versus expectant treatment in stages I and II prostate cancer. A fifteen-year follow-up, *Urology* 36:493-498, 1990.

52. Iversen P, Madsen PO, Corle DK: Radical prostatectomy versus expectant treatment for early carcinoma of the prostate. Twenty-three year follow-up of a prospective randomized study, *Scand J Urol Nephrol Suppl* 172:65-72, 1995.

53. Homberg L, Bill-Alexson A, Helgessen F et al: A randomized trial comparing radical prostatectomy with watchful waiting in early prostate cancer, *N Engl J Med* 347:781-786, 2002.

54. Steineck G, Helgessen F, Adolfsson J et al: Quality of life after watchful waiting, *N Engl J Med* 347:790-796, 2002.

55. Galbraith ME, Ramirez JM, Pedro LW: Quality of life, health outcomes, and identify for patients with prostate cancer in five different groups, *Oncol Nurs Forum* 28:55-60, 2001.

56. Wallace M: Uncertainty and quality of life of older men who undergo watchful waiting for prostate cancer, *Oncol Nurs Forum* 30:303-309, 2003.

57. Perrotte P, Litwin MS, McGuire EJ et al: Quality of life after salvage cryotherapy: the impact of treatment parameters, *J Urol* 162:398-402, 1999.

58. Guillonneau B, Vallancien G: Laparoscopic radical prostatectomy: the Montsouris experience, *J Urol* 163:418-422, 2000.

59. Smith JA: Robotically assisted laparoscopic prostatectomy: an assessment of its contemporary role in the surgical management of localized prostate cancer, *Am J Surg* 188(4A Suppl):63S-67S, 2004.

60. Radiation Therapy Oncology Treatment Group: A phase III protocol of androgen suppression (AS) and RT v. AS and RT followed by paclitaxel, estramustine and etoposide for localized high-risk prostate cancer, retrieved September 20, 2005, from http://www.rtog.org/members/protocols/99-02/99-02.pdf.

61. Abel L, Dafoe-Lambie J, Butler WM et al: Treatment outcomes and quality of life issues for patients treated with brachytherapy, *Clin J Oncol Nurs* 7:48-54, 2003.

62. Hunter KF, Moore KN, Cody DJ et al: Conservative management of post prostatectomy incontinence, *Cochrane Database Systematic Reviews* 2:CD001843, 2004.

63. McGlynn KA, Devesa SS, Sigurdson AJ et al: Trends in the incidence of testicular germ cell tumors in the United State, *Cancer* 97:63-70, 2003.

64. Nichols CR: Testicular cancer, *Curr Probl Cancer* 22:187-274, 1998.

65. Ulbright TM: Testis risk and prognostic factors: the pathologist's perspective, *Urol Clin North Am* 26:611-626, 1999.

66. Powles T, Bower M, Daugaard G et al: Multicenter study of human immunodeficiency virus-related germ cell tumor, *J Clin Oncol* 21:1922-1927, 2003.

67. Dieckmann KP, Skakkebaek NE: Carcinoma in situ of the testis: review of biological and clinical features, *Int J Cancer* 83:815-822, 1999.

68. Rapley EA, Crockford GP, Teare D et al. Localization to Xq27 of a susceptibility gene for testicular germ-cell tumours. *Nat Genet* 24:197-200, 2000.

69. Gori S, Porozzi S, Roila F et al: Germ cell tumors of the testis, *Critical reviews in oncology/hematology* 53:141-164, 2005.

70. Adelman WP, Joffe A: Controversies in male adolescent health: varicocele, circumcision, and testicular self-examination, *Curr Opin Pediatr* 16:363-367, 2004.

71. Clark PE, Ransil BJ, Loughlin KR: A review of scrotal violation in testicular cancer: is adjuvant local therapy necessary?. *J Urol* 153:981-985, 1995.

72. International Germ Cell Cooperative Group: International Germ Cell Consensus Classification: a prognostic factor- based staging system for metastatic germ cell cancers, *J Clin Oncol* 15:594-603, 1997.

73. National Comprehensive Cancer Network (NCCN): Testicular cancer practice guidelines-v.1.2005 retrieved September 10, 2005 from http://www.nccn.org/professionals/physician_gls/PDF/testicular.pdf.

74. Simon B, Lee SJ, Partridge AH et al: Preserving fertility after cancer, *CA Cancer J Clin* 55:211-228, 2005.

75. Parkin DM, Muir CS: Cancer incidence in five continents. Comparability and quality of data, *IARC Sci Publ* 120:45-173, 1992.

76. Rippentropp JM, Josyln SA, Konety BR: Squamous cell carcinoma of the penis: evaluation of data from the surveillance, epidemiology, and end results program, *Cancer* 101:1357-63, 2004.

77. Dillner J, von Krogh G, Horenblas S et al: Etiology of squamous cell carcinoma of the penis. *Scand J Urol Nephrol Suppl* 205:189-193, 2000.

78. Cubilla AL, Reuter V, Velazquez E et al. Histologic classification of penile carcinoma and its relation to outcome in 61 patients with primary resection, *Int J Surg Pathol* 9:111-120, 2001.

79. Misra S, Chaturvedi A, Misra N: Penile cancer: a challenge for the developing world, *Lancet Oncol* 5: 240-247, 2004.

80. Tanis PJ, Lont AP, Meinhardt W et al: Dynamic sentinel node biopsy for penile cancer: reliability of a staging technique, *J Urol* 168:76-80, 2002.

81. Mohs FE, Snow SN, Larson PO: Mohs micrographic surgery for penile tumors, *Urol Clin North Am* 19:291-304, 1992.

82. Pizzocaro G, Piva L, Bandieramonte G et al: Up-to-date management of carcinoma of the penis, *Eur Urol* 32:5-15, 1997.

83. el-Mawala NG, el-Bolkainy MN, Khaled HM: Bladder cancer in Africa: Update, *Semin Oncol* 28:174-178, 2001.

84. National Comprehensive Cancer Network: Clinical practice guidelines: Bladder cancer including upper tract tumors and uroepithelial carcinoma of the prostate, v1.2005, retrieved September 20, 2005, from http://www.nccn.org/professionals/physician_gls/PDF/bladder.pdf.

85. Pashos CL, Botteman MF, Laskin BL et al: Bladder cancer: epidemiology, diagnosis, and management, *Cancer Pract* 10:311-322, 2002.

86. Marcus PM, Hayes RB, Vineis P et al: Cigarette smoking, N-acetyltransferase w acetylation status, and bladder cancer risk: a case series meta-analysis of a gene-environment interaction, *Cancer Epidemiol Biomarkers Prev* 9:461-7, 2000.

87. Bofetta P, Silverman DT: A meta-analysis of bladder cancer and diesel exhaust exposure, *Epidemiology* 12:125-130, 2001.

88. Gago-Dominguez M, Castelao JE, Yuan JM et al: Use of permanent hair dyes and bladder–cancer risk, *Int J Cancer* 91:575-579, 2001.

89. Kammat AM, Lamm DL: Chemoprevention of urological cancer, *J Urol* 161:1748-1760, 1999.

90. Armstrong BK: Saccharin/cyclamates: epidemiological evidence, *IARC Sci Publ* 65:129-143, 1985

91. Piper JM, Tonascia J, Matanoski GM: Heavy phenacetin use and bladder cancer in women aged 20 to 49 years, *N Engl J Med* 313:292-295, 1985.

92. Travis LB, Curtis RE, Glimelius B et al: Bladder and kidney cancer following cyclophosphamide therapy for non-Hodgkin's lymphoma, *J Natl Cancer Inst* 87:524-530, 1995.

93. Sella A, Dexeus FH, Chong C et al: Radiation therapy-associated invasive bladder tumors, *Urology* 33:185-188, 1989.

94. Groah SL, Weitzenkamp DA, Lammertse DP et al: Excess risk of bladder cancer in spinal cord injury: evidence for an association between indwelling catheter use and bladder cancer, *Arch Phys Med Rehabil* 83:346-51, 2002.

95. Reuter VE: Bladder cancer: risk and prognostic factors—a pathologist's perspective, *Urol Clin North Am* 26:481-492 1999.

96. Grossman HB, Messing E, Soloway M et al: Detection of bladder cancer using a point-of-care proteomic assay, *JAMA* 293:810-816, 2005.

97. Duque JL, Loughlin KR: An overview of the treatment of superficial bladder cancer: intravesicular chemotherapy, *Urol Clin North Am* 27:125-135, 2000.

98. Grossman HB, Natale RB, Tangen CM, Speights VO, Vogelzang NJ et al: Neoadjuvant chemotherapy plus cystectomy compared with cystectomy alone for locally advanced bladder cancer, *N Engl J Med* 349:859-866, 2003.

99. Yanick R: Cancer burden in the aged: an epidemiologic and demographic overview, *Cancer* 80:1273-1283, 1997.

100. Vogelzang NJ, Stadler WM: Kidney cancer, *Lancet* 352: 1691-1696, 1998.

101. Zweizig SL: Cancer of the kidney, *Clin Obstet Gynecol* 45:884-891, 2002.

102. Choyke PL: Hereditary renal cancers, *Radiology* 226:33-46, 2003.

103. Pantuck AJ, Zisman A, Belldegrun A: Biology of renal cell carcinoma: changing concepts in identification and staging, *Semin Urol Oncol* 19:72-79.

104. Novick AC, Streem S, Montie JE et al: Conservative surgery for renal cell carcinoma: a single-center experience with 100 patients, *J Urol* 167:878-883, 2002.

105. Albqami N, Janetschek G: Laparoscopic partial nephrectomy, *Curr Opin Urol* 15:306-311, 2005.

106. National Comprehensive Cancer Network: Clinical practice guidelines in oncology: kidney cancer, v2.2005, retrieved September 23, 2005, from http://www.nccn.org/professionals/physician_gls/PDF/kidney.pdf.

CHAPTER 11

Gynecologic Cancers

Rebecca Allan

The American Cancer Society (ACS) estimates that 79,480 women were diagnosed with a malignancy of the genital system in 2005. Although dramatic improvements have occurred during the past decade in the prevention, diagnosis, and treatment of women with gynecologic cancers, an estimated 28,910 women were expected to die from gynecologic malignancies in 2005.[1] The term *gynecologic cancers* encompasses cervical, endometrial, ovarian, vulvar, vaginal, fallopian tube disease, and gestational trophoblastic neoplasia.

Cervical Cancer

Epidemiology

Cervical cancer is the second most common cancer in women worldwide, with 10,370 women expected to be diagnosed with invasive cervical cancer in 2005.[1,2] Although incidence rates of cervical cancer have steadily declined over the past several decades in both Caucasian and African American women, it is one of the leading causes of morbidity and mortality in women.[1,3] This decline can be attributed to successful screening with the use of the Papanicolaou (Pap) smear, with an increase in the diagnosis of preinvasive cancer.[3] Cervical cancer varies by age and socioeconomic status. It is typically seen in patients who fall into two main age groups, 30 to 39 years and 60 to 69 years, with the mean age of 51.4 years, and is rarely seen in women younger than 25 years of age.[4,5] In the United States, large racial and ethnic variance in incidence rates is observed. The highest age-adjusted rates are reported among Vietnamese, Hispanic, Native Alaskan, Korean, and African American women, and the lowest rates are reported among the Japanese and non-Hispanic whites.[6] Approximately 80% of all cervical cancer will occur in less developed regions of the world, with the highest incidence in Central and South America, southern and eastern Africa, and the Caribbean.[5,7]

The cervix is the lower part of the uterus and is divided into two major, contiguous parts: the endocervix and the exocervix. Squamous epithelial cells line the outside surface of the cervix, and columnar epithelial cells line the rest of the cervix and the uterus. The area where the columnar epithelium of the endocervix joins the squamous epithelium of the exocervix is called the squamocolumnar junction, often referred to as the transformation zone.[5] Most cases of cervical carcinoma originate at this junction.[2,4] Cervical cancer begins with a neoplastic alteration of the squamocolumnar junction. Abnormal cells can progress to involve the full thickness of the epithelium and invade the stromal tissue of the cervix.[5]

Cervical cancer develops over a period of 2 to 3 decades.[8] Lesions are usually low-grade in nature during adolescence. The majority of these will spontaneously regress back to normal. Those that do not regress undergo cellular changes ranging from cervical intraepithelial neoplasia (CIN) (premalignant changes) to CIS (carcinoma in situ), and eventually invasive disease (Fig. 11-1).[3] With Pap smear screening for early detection of preinvasive and invasive disease becoming more common over the last 50 years, incidence and mortality rates for cervical cancer have declined in most developed countries. However, even with widespread use of the Pap smear, some 3710 women were expected to die of cervical cancer in 2005.[1]

Etiology and Risk Factors

The exact etiology of cervical cancer is unknown. Epidemiologic evidence has long suggested a strong association between sexual history and practices and an increased risk for cervical cancer. Sexual practices associated with an increased risk include multiple sexual partners and early age at first coitus. Tobacco use, hormonal and diet factors such as a diet low in folate, carotene, and vitamin C, immunosuppression, unavailability or lack of screening, ethnicity, and diethylstilbestrol (DES) exposure in utero are associated with the development of the disease.[5] A history of sexually transmitted viruses has been linked to the development of cervical cancer, such as herpes simplex virus type 2 (HSV-2) and the human papillomavirus (HPV), specifically, subtypes 16, 18, 33, 35, and 45. HPV has been implicated in more than 99% of cervical cancer cases.[6,9] Most HPV infections disappear within several months to 2 years. Persistent infection by the virus is a hallmark for the development of invasive cervical cancer.[9] However, although HPV is the most common sexually transmitted disease (STD), only a small portion of those infected will go on to develop cancer.[7] Women infected with the human immunodeficiency virus (HIV), are also at risk for cervical cancer. According to Jhingran et al, "HIV-positive women have been reported to have higher rates of cervical abnormalities, larger lesions, higher-grade lesions, and higher recurrence rates than HIV-negative women."[6]

From the 1940s through 1971, DES, a nonsteroidal estrogen, was used to prevent pregnancy loss in women who had a threatened abortion or previous spontaneous abortions. In 1971, a study showed links between DES exposure and clear cell carcinoma of the cervix and vagina, as well as other gynecologic and obstetric complications.[10] At that time DES was banned from use by the U.S. Food and Drug Administration (FDA).

Prevention, Screening, and Detection
PREVENTION

Prevention is the key strategy for the eradication of cervical cancer. Counseling adolescents and women of all ages regarding STD screening, use of barrier types of contraceptives, and limiting the number of sexual partners is recommended to reduce the risk of cervical cancer.[3] In addition, strategies to prevent or to

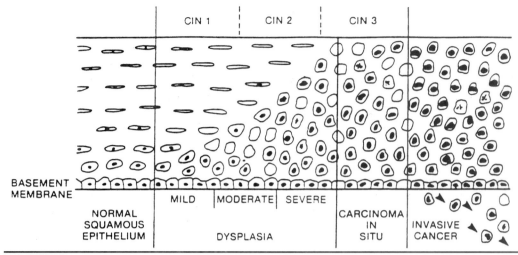

FIG. 11-1 Progression of cervical intraepithelial neoplasia (CIN). (From Jones HW, Wentz AC, Burnett LS: *Novak's textbook of gynecology,* ed 11, Baltimore, 1988, Williams & Wilkins.)

discourage tobacco use should be recommended. Adolescents are targeted primarily because it is known that sexually active adolescents are frequently infected with HPV.[11] Studies are currently under way focusing on vaccines to prevent HPV infections.[5,12]

SCREENING

The primary screening test for cervical cancer is the Pap smear. The Pap smear is a relatively accurate, effective, and economical screening technique to detect cervical changes. Traditionally, an Ayre's spatula and endocervical brush are used to collect squamous and endocervical cells. This sample is then smeared on a glass slide, with the spatula first and then with the endocervical brush. A fixative is then sprayed on the sample.[5] Recently, a new, liquid-based cytology method has been introduced. When using this technique, the cellular collection is not smeared onto a slide but is transferred to a vial containing a liquid medium. This type of testing is more expensive than standard Pap tests, but offers the advantages of greater accuracy and the added possibility of HPV testing[4,5]

In 2005, the ACS recommended that screening for asymptomatic women should begin approximately 3 years after a woman begins having vaginal intercourse, but no later than 21 years of age. Annual Pap smears are necessary, or every 2 years using liquid-based tests. Women 30 years of age or older who have had three normal test results in a row may get screened every 2 to 3 years. Cervical cancer screening with HPV DNA testing and conventional or liquid-based cytology could be an alternative performed every 3 years. Doctors may suggest that those women with certain risk factors be tested more frequently. Those women 70 years and older who have had three or more consecutive normal Pap smears in the last 10 years may choose to stop cervical cancer screening. Screening after a total hysterectomy is not necessary, unless the surgery was done as a treatment for cervical cancer or dysplasia.[1]

DETECTION

A thorough history and bimanual physical examination is used to detect cervical cancer in asymptomatic women.[3,4] At this time,

gross extension of the tumor to adjacent structures such as the bladder, the rectum, the vagina, and paracervical tissues can also be evaluated.[5] A clinical examination is performed to visualize the cervix, obtain a Pap smear, conduct a colposcopic examination, and palpate the cervix, the liver, and the lymph nodes to exclude metastatic disease, as well as adjacent tissues. A rectal exam is also necessary to best determine the size of the cervix, as well as extension of the disease into the parametrium.[4]

A colposcopic examination may be performed in women with an abnormal Pap smear or those who are at high risk for developing cervical cancer. A colposcopy uses a binocular microscope that magnifies and illuminates the cervical tissues. After application of a 3% to 5% acetic acid solution to the cervix, the clinician then evaluates the epithelium of the cervix and the lower genital tract for abnormalities in color and contour of tissues and vascular patterns (Fig. 11-2). The clinician obtains a cervical biopsy for definitive diagnosis if abnormal areas are seen on colposcopy.[4]

Classification

Cervical cancers are classified histologically by their tissue of origin. There two main types of cervical carcinoma: squamous carcinoma and adenocarcinoma. Squamous carcinoma is most common and is identified in 80% to 90% of cervical cancer. Squamous carcinoma originates in the squamocolumnar junction and often is associated with CIS, microinvasive disease, and invasive carcinoma. Grades 1 through 4 are assigned: G1 is well-differentiated, G2 is moderately differentiated, G3 poorly differentiated, and G4 is undifferentiated. Adenocarcinomas comprise 10% to 20% of cervical cancer and carry a poorer prognosis. They carry a greater risk owing to the tumor's arising within the endocervical mucous-producing gland cells. Tumors produced here can become quite bulky, which makes the tumor harder to treat. This type of cancer has a high rate of local recurrence and is more difficult to detect. Oral contraceptives have been associated with higher rates of adenocarcinoma in women. This may be especially true if oral contraceptives were used during adolescence, when the cervix is not fully mature.[5,6]

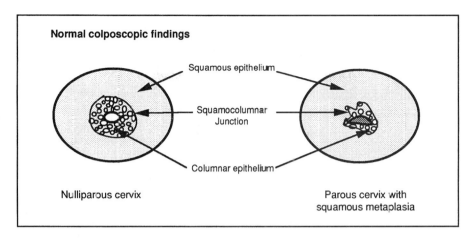

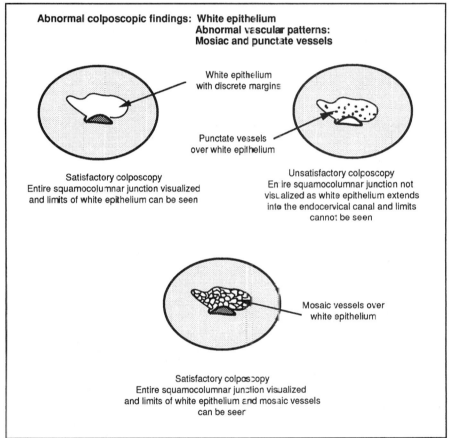

FIG. 11-2   Graphic representation of cervical findings using the colposcope.

Currently, the Bethesda system is used to help clinicians in the reporting of abnormal Pap tests. In addition to this system, cervical biopsies are reported using the CIN classification.[3,11]

Clinical Features

Women usually remain asymptomatic during preinvasive and early stages of cervical cancer, until the disease is advanced. The most common presenting symptom is abnormal vaginal bleeding. Women may experience postcoital, intermenstrual, or post-menopausal bleeding or an increase in length and amount of menstrual flow. A common complaint is a thin, watery, serosanguineous, or yellow, and sometimes malodorous, vaginal discharge.

Late symptoms include dysuria, urinary retention, urinary frequency, hematuria, and hydronephrosis, as well as bowel symptoms such as rectal bleeding, bowel obstruction, and constipation, which suggest tumor invasion of the bladder or the rectum. Lymphatic obstruction may result in edema to the lower extremities, whereas pelvic or sciatic pain suggests nerve involvement.[3,4,7]

Diagnosis and Staging

Diagnosis and staging form the basis of treatment for cervical carcinomas. It is critical that the extent of the lesion be determined as accurately as possible before the start of treatment.[5]

To determine the extent and severity of the lesions, a Pap smear, colposcopy, and colposcopically-directed biopsies are used. Typically, colposcopy-directed biopsies and the products of endocervical curettage provide a firm diagnosis in most patients.[2] If the Pap smear reveals preinvasive lesions, the woman has several options, all based on the extent of the disease, the woman's wishes to preserve reproductive function, and the ability to comply with follow-up.[5]

Clinical staging for cervical cancer occurs concurrently with planned surgical intervention.[6] The most commonly used staging system is the International Federation of Gynecology and Obstetrics (FIGO) system. (See Table 11-1 for Cervix Uteri Definition of TNM.) Data are obtained from diagnostic testing (i.e., chest and skeletal radiographs, intravenous pyelograms [IVP], barium enemas, blood chemistry studies, cystoscopy, and rectosigmoidoscopy), and are used to assist in the staging process.[3,5] Computed tomography (CT) and magnetic resonance imaging (MRI) can be helpful in identifying enlarged lymph nodes, and CT scanning also enables evaluation of the liver, the urinary tract, and bony structures.[5] However, CT is unable to distinguish between cancer and normal soft tissue of the cervix and uterus. MRI provides improved evaluation of tumor size and stromal invasion. Data from the physical exam, including bimanual pelvic and rectovaginal exam, are also included.[4] Positron emission tomography (PET) scans can also be helpful since, in combination with CT or MRI, they have the potential to more accurately delineate the extent of the disease.[5]

METASTASIS

Cervical carcinomas are slow-growing tumors that directly invade adjacent tissues. Metastasis includes extension into the uterus, the vagina, the parametrium, the abdomen, the pelvis, the rectum, and the bladder. Both regional and distant lymphatic

---

TABLE 11-1   **American Joint Committee on Cancer Definitions and Stage Grouping**

CERVICAL CANCER: DEFINITION OF TNM

Primary Tumor (T)

TNM Categories	FIGO Stages	Description
TX		Primary tumor cannot be assessed
T0		No evidence of primary tumor
Tis	0	Carcinoma *in situ*
T1	I	Cervical carcinoma confined to uterus (extension to corpus should be disregarded
*T1a	IA	Invasive carcinoma diagnosed only by microscopy. Stromal invasion with a maximum depth of 5.0 mm measured from the base of the epithelium and a horizontal spread of 7.0 mm or less. Vascular space involvement, venous or lymphatic, does not affect classification
T1a1	IA1	Measured stromal invasion 3.0 mm or less in depth and 7.0 mm or less in horizontal spread
T1a2	IA2	Measured stromal invasion more than 3.0 mm and not more than 5.0 mm with a horizontal spread 7.0 mm or less
T1b	IB	Clinically visible lesion confined to the cervix or microscopic lesion greater than T1a/IA2
T1b1	IB1	Clinically visible lesion 4.0 cm or less in greatest dimension
T1b2	IB2	Clinically visible lesion more than 4.0 cm in greatest dimension
T2	II	Cervical carcinoma invades beyond uterus but not to pelvic wall or to lower third of vagina
T2a	IIA	Tumor without parametrial invasion
T2b	IIB	Tumor with parametrial invasion
T3	III	Tumor extends to pelvic wall and/or involves lower third of vagina, and/or causes hydronephrosis or non-functioning kidney
T3a	IIIA	Tumor involves lower third of vagina, no extension to pelvic wall
T3b	IIIB	Tumor extends to pelvic wall and/or causes hydronephrosis or non-functioning kidney
T4	IVA	Tumor invades mucosa of bladder or rectum, and/or extends beyond true pelvis (bullous edema is not sufficient to classify a tumor as T4)

*All macroscopially visible lesions—even with superficial invasion—are T1b/IB.

Regional Lymph Nodes (N)

NX	Regional lymph nodes cannot be assessed
N0	No regional lymph nodes metastasis
N1	Regional lymph node metastasis

Distant Metastasis (M)

MX		Distant metastasis cannot be assessed
M0		No distant metastasis
M1	IVB	Distant metastasis

TABLE 11-1	American Joint Committee on Cancer Definitions and Stage Grouping—cont'd

STAGE GROUPING (AJCC/UICC/FIGO)

Stage	TNM	Regional Lymph Nodes	Distant Metastasis
Stage 0	Tis	N0	M0
Stage I	T1	N0	M0
Stage IA	T1a	N0	M0
Stage IA1	T1a1	N0	M0
Stage IA2	T1a2	N0	M0
Stage IB	T1b	N0	M0
Stage IB1	T1b1	N0	M0
Stage IB2	T1b2	N0	M0
Stage II	T2	N0	M0
Stage IIA	T2a	N0	M0
Stage IIB	T2b	N0	M0
Stage III	T3	N0	M0
Stage IIIA	T3a	N0	M0
Stage IIIB	T1	N1	M0
	T2	N1	M0
	T3a	N1	M0
	T3b	Any N	M0
Stage IVA	T4	Any N	M0
Stage IVB	Any T	Any N	M1

HISTOLOGIC GRADE (G)

GX	Grade cannot be assessed
G1	Well differentiated
G2	Moderately differentiated
G3	Poorly differentiated
G4	Undifferentiated

RESIDUAL TUMOR (R)

RX	Presence of residual tumor cannot be assessed
R0	No residual tumor
R1	Microscopic residual tumor
R2	Macroscopic residual tumor

From American Joint Committee on Cancer: *AJCC Cancer Staging Manual*, ed 6, Chicago, 2002, AJCC.

invasion occurs via lymphatic channels. Cervical cancer may also spread by hematogeneous routes; the most common organs involved are the lungs, the liver and bone, although more widespread metastasis has also been reported.[3,4]

Treatment Modalities

SURGERY

Surgical treatment is based upon the extent of disease, involving appropriate management for the primary lesion and potential sites of metastatic disease.[4] Treatment decisions depend on the size and location of the lesion, desire for childbearing, and physician skills and preference (Fig. 11-3).[3] Women who have preinvasive disease may be treated with cryotherapy and laser therapy as a conservative approach. Cryotherapy is effective and consists of using liquid nitrogen to freeze the cervix. Laser therapy uses laser beams, which are directed under colposcopic control. Thermal damage of the specimen obtained may occur, making it difficult to rule out invasive carcinoma.[5] A loop electrosurgical excisional procedure (LEEP) is an option, if the woman has obvious tumor growth or ulceration; an advantage of this procedure is that larger wedges of tissue may be obtained.[3,5] A conization involves the removal of a cone-shaped piece of tissue from the exocervix and the endocervix using a scalpel. This procedure is used if there is no gross lesion found but a tumor is still suspected, if colposcopy is inadequate, or if biopsy results reveal invasive disease (Fig. 11-4). A LEEP and a cold-knife conization procedure may be used for the same purpose.

Localized cervical carcinoma is divided into two stages, IA1 and IA2. IA1 may be treated with surgery alone. Surgical procedures include a total abdominal hysterectomy (TAH) or a total vaginal hysterectomy (TVH) if the patient does not desire childbearing in the future. Conization provides a definitive diagnosis when microinvasion is present, and can be used in poor surgical candidates and for those who wish to preserve their fertility. The 5-year survival rate in patients with properly staged cervical cancer is nearly 100%.[4,5]

For stage IA2 disease, a modified radical hysterectomy with pelvic lymphadenectomy is performed. In women for whom childbearing is still a concern, a radical trachelectomy with

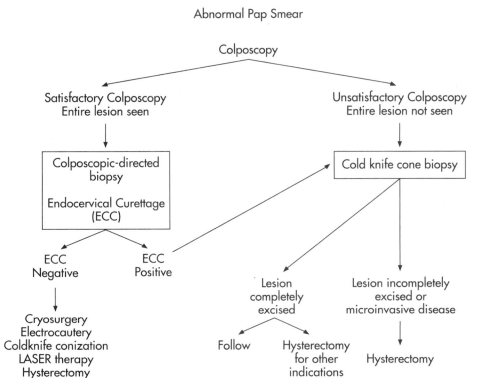

Abnormal Pap Smear

FIG. 11-3 Decision tree for management of cervical intraepithelial neoplasia (CIN). (From Flannery M: Reproductive cancers. In Clark JC, McGee RF, editors: *Core curriculum for oncology nursing,* Philadelphia, 1992, Saunders.)

laparoscopic pelvic lymphadenectomy preserves uterine morphology and reproductive function.[2,4] Cervical incompetence is almost inevitable. Therefore these patients must be managed by a high-risk pregnancy obstetric team.[7,13]

Stages IB and IIA may be treated with radical abdominal hysterectomy and pelvic lymphadenectomy, although equal cure rates have been obtained with primary radiation therapy.[4] Surgery may be preferred to radiation so that ovarian function may be preserved.[5] Radical hysterectomy includes removal of the uterus, the upper third of the vagina, the entire uterosacral and uterovesical ligaments, all of the parametrium, and pelvic node lymphadenectomy (Box 11-1). Women who prefer radiation therapy can avoid postoperative complications and receive their radiation treatment in an outpatient setting.[5] According to Duenas-Gonzalez and colleagues, cisplatin-based chemoradiation is now the standard of care in patients with locally advanced disease. The cure rate for stage IB disease using radiation or surgery is approximately 80% to 90%.[5,14]

Advanced cervical carcinoma, stages IIB through IV, are treated primarily with radiation therapy alone, although the role of chemotherapy is currently receiving more attention. Randomized clinical trials have shown that patient outcomes significantly improve with combined chemotherapy and radiation, as compared to radiation alone. However, there was an increase in early toxicity compared to radiation therapy as a single modality. Hyperbaric oxygen and the use of hyperthermia are also being studied.[15] Five-year survival rates for patients with stage IIB disease are 60% to 79%; for those with stage III, 25% to 50%; and with stage IVA, 18% to 34%.[5]

Of women with invasive cervical cancer, 35% will have recurrent or persistent disease. One-year survival rates after recurrence

are 10% to 15%. Diagnosis of recurrence is difficult because of distortion of the cells from radiation therapy. Signs and symptoms include unintentional weight loss, unilateral leg edema, serosanguineous vaginal discharge, pain in the buttocks, the pelvis, and the thighs, cough, chest pain, hemoptysis, and supraclavicular lymph node enlargement (usually on the left side).

The goal of treatment is palliation, since disease control or cure is rare. For women with central pelvic recurrence, a pelvic exenteration may be appropriate. This surgical procedure cannot be performed for disease contained outside the pelvis, with positive lymph nodes present, and disease that has spread to the pelvic wall. Inoperable disease is found in 60% of candidates for this procedure; therefore it is done in a select group of patients.[5] If a patient meets criteria for a pelvic exenteration, the bladder, the uterus, the vagina, the anus, the rectum, and the sigmoid colon are removed, while creating a permanent colostomy and urinary stoma. Variations of this procedure, including anterior and posterior exenteration, are determined by the extent of disease (Fig. 11-5).[4] Anterior exenterations preserve the rectum, whereas posterior exenterations preserve the bladder.[4] Nursing interventions include teaching the patient urostomy and/or colostomy care and referring her to a wound care specialist, as well as to social workers for support in regard to coping, body image disturbances, and functional or psychologic changes she may be having (Box 11-2).[2]

RADIATION

Radiation therapy is an option for patients with recurrent cervical disease. External and intracavitary implants may afford excellent palliation or cure for women previously treated with surgery, and can provide local control to relieve symptoms (Box 11-3).[3,5]

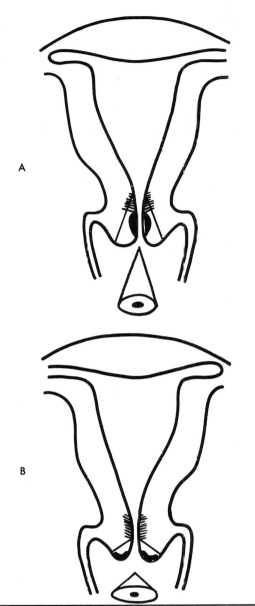

FIG. 11-4 Cone biopsy for endocervical and exocervical disease. **A,** Endocervical disease: increased depth of cone biopsy to remove all abnormal areas. **B,** Exocervical disease: increased width of cone biopsy to remove all abnormal areas. (From DiSaia PJ, Creasman WT: *Clinical gynecologic oncology,* ed 4, St. Louis, 1997, Mosby.)

CHEMOTHERAPY

Use of antineoplastic agents in recurrent or metastatic disease is merely palliative, used to relieve symptoms and prolong life (Box 11-4).[21,22] Single-agent cisplatin (Platinol) is the single most active agent in metastatic or recurrent disease. Additional agents are cyclophosphamide (Cytoxan), ifosfamide (Ifex), paclitaxol (Taxol), vinorelbine (Navelbine), topotecan (Hycamptin), irinotecan (Camptosar), carboplatin (Paraplatin), 5-fluorouracil (5-FU), methotrexte (Mexate), chlorambucil (Leukeran), melphalan (Alkeran), doxorubicin (Adriamycin) vincristine (Oncovin), and altretamine (Hexamethylmelamine). In phase 2 clinical trials, gemcitabine (Gemzar) exhibited antitumor activity.[3,5]

BOX 11-1   **Surgical Complications of a Radical Hysterectomy with Nursing Interventions**

Bowel and bladder dysfunction—Teach bladder training before discharge, and assess for fistula formation.

Pelvic infection—Assess for fever, and drainage, odor, and redness at surgical site.

Pulmonary embolus—Teach patient about use of compression stockings and heparin or Lovenox injections if ordered.

Lymphedema of the lower extremities—Teach specific exercises to improve drainage, and assess and protect skin integrity.

Bowel obstruction—Teach patient the importance of bowel decompression and bowel rest. Patient may or may not have a nasogastric tube.

Hemorrhage—Assess blood counts; assess surgical site for increased and/or uncontrolled bleeding.

Data from Hacker NF: Cervical cancer. In Berek JS, Hacker NF: *Practical gynecologic oncology,* ed 4, Philadelphia, 2005, Lippincott, Williams & Wilkins; Vogt Temple S: Cervical cancer: In Henke Yarbro C, Hansen Frogge M, Goodman M: *Cancer nursing: principles and practice,* ed 6, Sudbury, Mass, 2005, Jones & Bartlett.

Treatment during Pregnancy

Increasing incidence of preinvasive and invasive cervical cancer in younger women raises the issue of treatment during pregnancy. Overall, there is an incident rate of 0.24 to 0.45 of genital tract malignancies per every 1000 pregnancies. Treatment decisions require careful discussion among the woman, her partner, the gynecologic oncologist, and the obstetrician.[23] Vaginal bleeding, vaginal discharge, pelvic pain, and postcoital bleeding are common symptoms. Bleeding that can be attributed to the pregnancy itself instead of to malignancy may delay diagnosis.[4] Twenty percent of women are asymptomatic, and over 90% of early invasive lesions are detected on routine screening.[4,23] A colposcopic evaluation is necessary, and because of physiologic alteration during pregnancy, interpretation of the findings can be difficult. A definitive diagnosis is made with a biopsy of the gross cervical lesion.[4] For patients with stage IA disease and clear margins after cervical conization, it is reasonable to follow the pregnancy to term and to anticipate a vaginal delivery. For women with stage IB and early IIA disease, radical hysterectomy and pelvic lymphadenectomy is the preferred method of surgery, performed with the fetus in utero before 20 weeks of gestation. Women between 20 and 32 weeks of pregnancy will experience treatment delays to ensure survival of the fetus. Once the fetus has reached sufficient maturity, a Caesarean section is usually performed, followed by a radical hysterectomy and pelvic lymphadenectomy. Vaginal delivery would increase the risk of complications such as hemorrhage, cervical laceration, dissemination of malignant cells into the lymphatic or vascular channels, sepsis, and tumor implantation at the episiotomy site.[23]

With stages IIB, III, and IV disease, radiation is the treatment of choice. Early in pregnancy, external beam irradiation is given, which ultimately results in an abortion. Brachytherapy completes treatment once the fetus is evacuated. Radiation therapy complications appear similar to those in nonpregnant women. Patients in

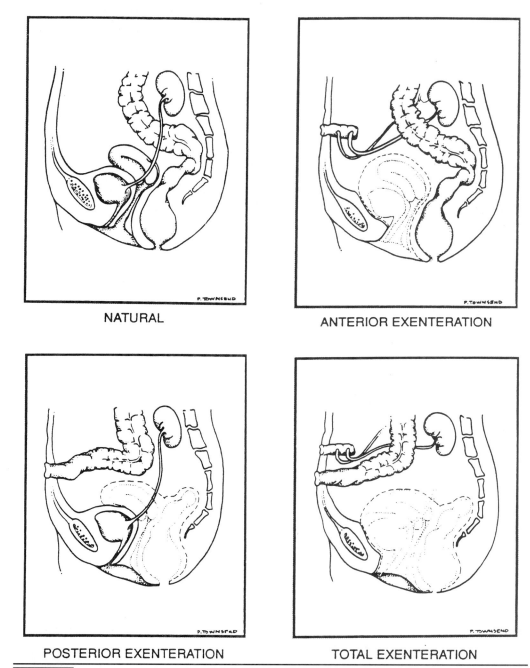

NATURAL

ANTERIOR EXENTERATION

POSTERIOR EXENTERATION

TOTAL EXENTERATION

FIG. 11-5   Pelvic exenteration for treatment of cervical cancer. (From DeStefano MS, Bertin-Matson K: Gynecologic cancers. In McCorkle R et al, editors: *Cancer nursing: A comprehensive textbook*, ed 2, Philadelphia, 1997, Saunders.)

the second and third trimesters will have treatment delayed to achieve fetal viability, then Caesarean section followed by radiation therapy.

Chemotherapy is avoided during the first trimester, when fetal organs are being developed. After 13 weeks of gestation, organogenesis is completed and the risk of fetal anomalies is low, although intrauterine growth restriction is predicted. Because of potential risks for the fetus, chemotherapy should be avoided during pregnancy.[23]

Follow-Up after Cervical Cancer Treatment

Patients are usually seen in follow-up every 3 months for 2 years, every 6 months until 5 years have passed, and annually thereafter.

Recurrences are often detected as a result of patient symptomatology, and any symptoms should be asked about at each visit. The physical exam should include a Pap smear, and abdominal and rectovaginal examination including supraclavicular and inguinal node assessment; it is worth noting that 72% of vaginal recurrences are asymptomatic.[4]

Prognosis

The most significant prognostic factor in patients with invasive carcinoma of the cervix is the clinical stage of the disease. Other determinants of survival include age, race, socioeconomic status, general health, tumor size and location, and lymph node involvement. Patients without lymph node involvement show a higher 5-year survival compared to those with para-aortic or pelvic lymph

BOX 11-2 | **Nursing Management of the Patient Who Has Had Pelvic/Abdominal Surgery**

Assess vital signs and respiratory status.

Assess surgical site for bleeding, drainage, and signs and symptoms of infection.

Assess for acute pain, and review nonpharmocologic methods of relief (i.e., massage, music, guided imagery, diversional techniques). Administer analgesics as ordered

Review blood counts.

Teach coughing and deep breathing exercises.

Teach importance of ambulation early after surgery.

Assess intake and output.

Assess nutritional status to support wound healing (i.e., is the patient nauseated or vomiting?).

Discuss with the patient her fears and concerns regarding surgery (i.e., body image and sexual dysfunction), and assess coping strategies. Refer to support services if necessary.

Vaginal reconstruction may be an option for patients who have had an exenteration.

Include patient in self-care activities (i.e., wound dressings, care of colostomy or urostomy). Teach patient how to care for drains and tubes.

Teach patient what signs and symptoms to report.

Discuss plan for further treatment and follow-up.

Data from Vogt Temple S, Umstead CH: Nursing care of the client with reproductive disorders. In Itano JK, Taoka KN: *Core curriculum for oncology nursing*, ed 4, St Louis, 2005, Saunders; Szopa TJ: Nursing implications of surgical treatment. In Itano JK, Taoka KN: *Core curriculum for oncology nursing*, ed 4, St Louis, 2005, Saunders; Barclay, MM: Cancer surgery. In Nevidjon BM, Sowers KW: *A nurse's guide to cancer care*, Philadelphia, 2000, Lippincott.; Thompson SD: Gynecologic cancers. In Shelton BK, Ziegfeld CR, Olsen: *Manual of cancer nursing*, ed 2, Philadelphia, 2003, Lippincott, Williams & Wilkins.

BOX 11-3 | **Nursing Management of the Patient Who Has Pelvic/Abdominal Radiation**

Assess vital signs and respiratory status.

Note any special radiation precautions for the patient or nursing staff, if applicable.

Assess skin integrity and site of radiation therapy. The site of treatment determines what side effects will occur (i.e., diarrhea with pelvic radiation). Teach patient to use warm water and mild soap when cleansing. Pat—do not rub—the skin dry.

Assess nutritional status to support wound healing.

Assess intake and output.

Teach patient about the specific radiation regimen.

Teach patient side effects management, especially proper skin care to increase comfort, as well as when to report side effects.

Teach importance of water-soluble lubrication and use of vaginal dilator if patient is not sexually active to minimize the effects of the radiation therapy.

Include patient in self-care activities.

Discuss with the patient her fears and concerns (i.e., body image and sexual dysfunction), and assess coping strategies. Refer to support services if necessary.

Discuss plan for further treatment and follow-up.

Skin reaction, fatigue, pain, nausea, vomiting and bone marrow suppression may also occur.

Data from Vogt Temple S, Umstead CH: Nursing care of the client with reproductive disorders. In Itano JK, Taoka KN: *Core curriculum for oncology nursing*, ed 4, St Louis 2005, Saunders; Vogt Temple S: Cervical cancer: In Henke Yarbro C, Hansen Frogge M, Goodman M: *Cancer nursing: principles and practice*, ed 6, Sudbury Mass, 2005, Jones & Bartlett; Witt, ME: Nursing implications of radiation therapy. In Itano JK, Taoka KN: *Core curriculum for oncology nursing*, ed 4, St Louis, 2005, Saunders; Almadrones, L: Endometrial cancer. In Henke Yarbro C, Hansen Frogge M, Goodman M: *Cancer nursing: principles and practice*, ed 6, Sudbury, Mass, 2005, Jones & Bartlett.

node metastasis. Metastatic lymph node involvement and a tumor with deep stromal invasion is a predictor of less than 2 years' survival and a greater incidence of recurrence compared to patients with small tumors. For women with preinvasive lesions, the survival rate is nearly 100%. Survival rates 1 year after diagnosis are approximately 90%, and the 5-year survival rate is 73%. Treatment of invasive cervical cancer is highly successful when detected at an early stage.[1,2]

Endometrial Cancer

Epidemiology

Endometrial cancer is the most common gynecologic malignancy and the fourth most common cancer in women in the United States.[3] It primarily affects postmenopausal woman aged 55 to 70 years.[18] Approximately 5% of women will be diagnosed before the age of 40, with 20% to 25% being premenopausal.[20] Incidence rates for endometrial cancer are higher in Caucasian women compared to African American women.[24] Incidence rates in developing countries and Japan are 4 to 5 times lower than in Western industrialized nations, with the lowest rates seen in India and South Asia.[25] The ACS estimated that 40,880 women would be diagnosed in 2005.[1]

The uterus is located in the pelvis between the bladder and the rectum. It is divided into two structural parts: the body (corpus) and the cervix. The uterus is composed of three inner layers: the endometrium, the myometrium, and the parietal peritoneum. The endometrium is a highly vascular mucous membrane lining that provides a nutrient supply for a fetus. It also responds to variations in estrogen and progesterone levels in a cyclic fashion.[3]

Etiology and Risk Factors

Although the etiology of endometrial cancer is unknown, it is believed to be complex, involving both endogenous and exogenous factors. Some cases of endometrial cancer clearly have a hereditary basis, but most cases are thought to be sporadic in nature.[26] The major risk factor for this disease is a high cumulative exposure to estrogen.[1] Estrogen replacement therapy and obesity are two factors that dramatically increase estrogen exposure. Women who are more than 50 pounds overweight have a tenfold risk of developing endometrial cancer. Other risk factors include estrogen replacement without progesterone, never having children, late menopause, irregular menstrual history, failure to ovulate, and history of infertility. Diabetes and hypertension play a role but are no longer considered independent risk factors for endometrial cancer.[20] Women who have a history of tamoxifen

---

BOX 11-4   Nursing Management of the Patient Receiving Chemotherapy

Assess vital signs and respiratory status.

Assess patient's knowledge about chemotherapy, and teach patient about any special precautions to take.

Review common chemotherapy side effects and which ones to report to the physician.. Chemotherapy side effects are determined by the specific drug being given. Chemotherapy agents work best on rapidly dividing cells. Examples of these include the skin, the hair, the mucous membranes, and the bone marrow. The following are examples of such side effects:

- Nausea and vomiting
- Bone marrow suppression
- Alopecia
- Fatigue

Follow special safety precautions when administering or monitoring chemotherapy.

Assess nutritional status.

Assess intake and output.

Teach patient about care of central lines, if applicable, and include patient in self care activities.

Discuss with the patient her fears and concerns regarding treatment (i.e., hair loss, N/V) and refer to support services if necessary.

Discuss plan for further treatment and follow-up.

Data from Thompson SD: Gynecologic cancers. In Shelton BK, Ziegfeld CR, Olsen MM: *Manual of cancer nursing*, ed 2, Philadelphia, 2003, Lippincott, Williams & Wilkins; Poniatowski BC, Vogt Temple S: Nursing implications of antineoplastic therapy. In Itano JK, Taoka KN: *Core curriculum for oncology nursing*, ed 4, St. Louis, 2005, Saunders.

---

use and of hereditary nonpolyposis colon cancer (HNPCC) are also at increased risk for endometrial cancer.[1]

Prevention, Screening, and Detection

PREVENTION

As knowledge of the etiology of endometrial cancer evolves, the primary focus of prevention is on high-risk women. Of all endometrial cancer, 95% occurs in women 40 years of age and older. Prompt recognition of precursor lesions such as endometrial hyperplasia can prevent disease progression.[26] In addition, it is also known that oral contraceptive use has a protective effect against the development of endometrial cancer. Other behaviors that are recommended in preventing endometrial cancer include controlling for obesity, diabetes, and hypertension, as well as adding progesterone to estrogen replacement. Avoiding tamoxifen use and a high-fat diet are also recommended.[20]

SCREENING AND DETECTION

Currently, there are no screening tests for endometrial cancer recommended for asymptomatic women.[20] Only occasionally will endometrial cancer be detected by Pap smear. Endometrial biopsy is 90% effective in detecting cancer, but is not recommended at this time for screening purposes. In addition, a physical exam is important in order to inspect and palpate the vulva, the vagina, and the cervix to exclude metastatic disease.

Rectovaginal exam should also be performed to asses the fallopian tubes and ovaries.[25] According to ACS guidelines, all women at the time of menopause should be informed about the risks and symptoms of this disease, and are strongly encouraged to report any unexpected bleeding or spotting to their physician. Candidates for annual endometrial biopsies are women age 35 years and older who have or are at risk for HNPCC.[1]

Classification

The majority of endometrial cancers are adenocarcinomas; these account for more than 80% of the endometrial cancers that are seen. Less frequently seen endometrial cancers include clear cell, papillary serous, mucinous, and squamous cell.[20,27] Uterine papillary serous and clear cell carcinomas have a high relapse rate and poor survival.[27] In addition to being extremely rare, uterine sarcomas are the most malignant amongst all of uterine tumors.[28] Histologic grading is used to differentiate the various endometrial carcinomas. Grade 1 tumors are well-differentiated, grade 2 are moderately differentiated, and grade 3 are poorly differentiated and frequently have a poor prognosis.[25,26]

Clinical Features

The most common presenting symptom is abnormal vaginal bleeding, either postmenopausal or heavy, irregular menstrual flow, in a premenopausal patient.[18] Additional symptoms include serosanguineous vaginal discharge and pain in the lumbosacral, hypogastric, or pelvic regions. Women with advanced disease may be seen with bowel obstruction, ascites, jaundice, hemorrhage, or respiratory distress.[3,18]

Diagnosis and Staging

The diagnostic evaluation encompasses a physical exam, tissue sampling, radiography, and laboratory studies to determine the histologic type, degree of differentiation, and extent of disease. A complete pelvic work-up with rectovaginal bimanual examination, and assessment of the lymph nodes, the abdomen, and the lungs for metastatic disease should be performed. Additional diagnostic studies include endometrial biopsy to sample the endometrial tissue, which is considered a reliable diagnostic technique. Further testing is needed if symptoms persist and the biopsy is negative. A fractional dilatation and curettage is done to obtain a differential diagnosis. Laboratory studies include blood chemistries, liver and renal function tests, and a CA-125 level. MRI, CT, hysterography, ultrasonography, and lymphangiography may be used to evaluate the size of the tumor and to determine nodal involvement.[20] Contrast MRIs are valuable in assessing the degree of myometrial invasion, but may not be appropriate for all patients. Because of its high sensitivity, transvaginal ultrasonography is used to determine endometrial thickness. Endometrial disease is more prevalent in women with a thick endometrium.[29] A full pelvic and para-aortic lymphadenectomy is used as a staging tool in patients who are suspected of having lymph node involvement.[30] Cystoscopy, IVP, proctoscopy, and barium enema may be necessary in patients in whom urologic involvement is suspected.[18,20]

Depth of endometrial invasion, lymph node metastases, histologic type and grade, extent of cervical involvement, and metastatic disease are considered in surgical staging.[26] This involves, at minimum, an abdominal and pelvic exploration with biopsy, a TAH and bilateral salpingo-oophorectomy (BSO), samples of peritoneal fluid for cytologic evaluation, and pelvic and para-aortic lymph node sampling.[20] The FIGO staging system is used.[25] See Table 11-2 for the AJCC definitions and staging system for endometrial cancer.

METASTASIS

The majority of endometrial cancers originate in the fundus of the uterus and spread by direct extension to the entire endometrium, the myometrium, the endocervix, and the cervix, as well as through the lymphatic system, usually to the pelvic and the para-aortic lymph nodes. The disease may spread outside the uterus into the abdominal cavity, the vagina, the fallopian tubes, the ovaries and the omentum if peritoneal seeding occurs. Endometrial cancer metastasizes through hematogenous spread to sites including lung, liver, brain, and bone.[20]

Treatment Modalities

Treatment is based upon the stage and grade of the disease, depth of myometrial invasion, and presence or absence of prognostic factors, as well the woman's general health.[3]

SURGERY

The primary treatment for early-stage disease is a TAH-BSO. Many women with early-stage disease will not need additional therapy beyond this initial surgery. Laparoscopically-assisted vaginal hysterectomy has also been a successful technique, although not an option for high-risk surgical patients or morbidly obese patients.[20] The TAH–BSO, accompanied by a pelvic and para-aortic lymphadenectomy and possible omental biopsy, is the treatment of choice in women with grades 2 and 3 lesions.[3]

TABLE 11-2   Endometrium (Corpus Uteri): American Joint Committee on Cancer Definitions and Stage Grouping

DEFINITIONS (CLINICAL)

Primary Tumor (T)

FIGO recommends surgical/pathologic staging. Clinical staging is done with 1971 FIGO as follows:

TNM	FIGO	Definitions
(c)Tis	0	Carcinoma *in situ*. Histological findings suspicious of malignancy
(c)T1	I	Carcinoma is confined to the corpus including the isthmus
(c)T1a	IA	Length of the uterine cavity is more than 8 cm

Stage I cases should be subgrouped with regard to the histological type of the adenocarcinoma as follows:

G1		Highly differentiated adenomatous carcinoma
G2		Moderately differentiated adenomatous carcinoma with partly solid areas
G3		Predominantly solid or entirely undifferentiated carcinoma
(c)T2	II	Carcinoma has involved the corpus and the cervix, but has not extended outside the uterus
(c)T3	III	Carcinoma has extended outside the uterus, but not outside the true pelvis
(c)T4	IV	Carcinoma has extended outside the true pelvis or has obviously involved the mucosa of the bladder or rectum (Bullous edema as such does not permit a case to be allotted to stage IV)
(c)T4a	IVA	Spread of the growth to adjacent organs as urinary bladder, rectum, sigmoid colon, or small bowel

Stage 0 cases should not be included in any therapeutic statistics

DEFINITIONS (PATHOLOGIC)

Primary Tumor (T)

TNM	FIGO	Definitions
TX		Primary tumor cannot be assessed
T0		No evidence of primary tumor
Tis	0	Carcinoma *in situ*
T1	I	Tumor confined to corpus uteri
T1a	IA	Tumor limited to endometrium
T1b	IB	Tumor invades less than one-half of the myometrium
T1c	IC	Tumor invades one-half of the myometrium
T2	II	Tumor invades cervix but does not extend beyond uterus
T2a	IIA	Tumor limited to the glandular epithelium of the endocervix. There is no evidence of connective tissue stromal invasion
T2b	IIB	Invasion of the stromal connective tissue of the cervix
T3	III	Local and/or regional spread as defined below
T3a	IIIA	Tumor involves serosa and/or adnexa (direct extension or metastasis) and/or cancer cells in ascites or peritoneal washings
T3b	IIIB	Vaginal involvement (direct extension or metastasis)
T4	IVA	Tumor invades bladder mucosa and/or bowel mucosa (bullous edema is not sufficient evidence to classify a tumor as T4)

Continued

| TABLE 11-2 | Endometrium (Corpus Uteri): American Joint Committee on Cancer Definitions and Stage Grouping—cont'd |

Regional Lymph Nodes (N)

NX   Regional lymph nodes cannot be assessed
N0   No regional lymph node metastasis
N1   Regional lymph node metastasis to pelvic and/or para-aortic lymph nodes

Distant Metastasis

MX   Distant metastasis cannot be assessed
M0   No distant metastasis
M1   Distant metastasis includes metastasis to intraabdominal lymph nodes other than paraaortic, and/or inguinal lymph nodes; excludes metastasis to vagina, pelvic serosa, or adnexa

GROUPING (AJCC/UICC/FIGO)

Stage	TNM	Regional Lymph Nodes	Distant Metastasis
0	Tis	N0	M0
I	T1	N0	M0
IA	T1a	N0	M0
IB	T1b	N0	M0
IC	T1c	N0	M0
II	T2	N0	M0
IIA	T2a	N0	M0
IIB	T2b	N0	M0
III	T3	N0	M0
IIIA	T3a	N0	M0
IIIB	T3b	N0	M0
IIIC	T1	N1	M0
	T3	N1	M0
	T3	N1	M0
IVA	T4	Any N	M0
IVB	Any T	Any N	M1

HISTOLOGIC GRADE (G)

GX   Grade cannot be assessed
G1   Well differentiated
G2   Moderately differentiated
G3–G4   Poorly differentiated or undifferentiated

HISTOPATHOLOGY—DEGREE OF DIFFERENTIATION

Cases of carcinoma of the corpus should be grouped with regard to the degree of differentiation of the adenocarcinoma as follows:

G1   5% or less fo a nonsquamous or nonmorular solid growth pattern
G2   6% to 50% of a nonsquamous or nonmorular solid growth pattern
G3   More than 50% of a nonsquamous or nonmorular solid growth pattern

RESIDUAL TUMOR

RX   Presence of residual tumor cannot be assessed
R0   No residual tumor
R1   Microscopic residual tumor
R2   Macroscopic residual tumor

From American Joint Committee on Cancer: *AJCC Cancer Staging Manual*, ed 6, Chicago, 2002, AJCC.

RADIATION THERAPY

Radiation is the primary treatment in patients with all stages of disease who are not surgical candidates.[3] Most patients undergo surgery initially, based upon features obtained from the pathology report.[26] In patients with stage I disease, high-dose brachytherapy alone has proven highly effective; with very low morbidity rates, it is considered a safe alternative to external beam radiation therapy.[31] Radiation therapy can be used preoperatively in both patients with extensive lesions involving the cervix and those with high-grade lesions. It is also used postoperatively in women with recurrent disease.[3]

HORMONAL THERAPY

Hormone therapy is used for both recurrent disease and for adjuvant treatment. In women with advanced or recurrent endometrial cancer, progesterone therapy has been successful, with response rates from 10% to 30%. Unfortunately, two thirds of these patients will not respond.[24] Patients with well-differentiated tumors have better response rates. Common progestational agents currently used include megestrol (Megace), medroxyprogesterone (Depo Provera), and tamoxifen (Nolvadex).[3]

CHEMOTHERAPY

Antineoplastic agents have a limited role in the treatment of endometrial cancer. Chemotherapy has not been shown to be effective as adjuvant therapy, but may be used for disease recurrence. Chemotherapy agents that have shown activity in women include doxorubicin, cisplatin, hexamethylmelamine, cyclophosphamide, and 5-FU, with combination therapy of cisplatin and doxorubicin producing response rates of 66% but not improving median survival. Doxorubicin is the single most active agent in stage IV disease.[25]

Prognosis

The most significant prognostic variable for women with endometrial cancer is the stage of the disease, followed by histologic grade. Studies have shown that patients with stage II, grade 1 tumors have a better prognosis than patients with stage I, grade II lesions.[25] The 5-year relative survival rate for endometrial cancer is 96% for localized disease, 67% for regional disease, and 26% for distant disease.[1]

Ovarian Cancer

Epidemiology

Ovarian cancer is the fifth most common cancer in women in the United States and ranks as the fourth leading cause of death from malignancy in women. Two thirds of cases or more are seen at diagnosis with advanced disease, which may be attributable to the nonspecific symptoms of ovarian cancer. An estimated 22,220 new cases of ovarian cancer were expected to be diagnosed in 2005.[1] Peak incidence is in women between 60 to 64 years of age, but it can also be seen in women between 40 and 65 years old.[3] A strong hereditary component contributes to 10% of cases identified. The overall lifetime risk of developing ovarian cancer is approximately 1 in 70.

The incidence of ovarian cancer varies throughout the world. In Japan, epithelial ovarian tumors are considered rare compared to Western countries, including the United States and the United Kingdom, where the incidence rate of ovarian cancer is 3 to 7 times greater.[32] Caucasian women develop ovarian cancer 1.5 times more frequently than African Americans.[33]

Etiology and Risk Factors

The etiology of ovarian cancer remains unknown. However, prior reproductive history and the number of ovulatory cycles appear to have the greatest impact on the development of the disease, with low parity, early menarche, and late menopause increasing risk.[32] Environmental and genetic factors also have roles in the development of ovarian cancer.[33]

Risk factors for ovarian cancer include nulliparity, a history of pelvic inflammatory disease, low serum gonadotropin, prior use of talc, family history of breast or ovarian cancer, living in industrialized countries, and being of Jewish descent. Family history, specifically the number of family members with ovarian cancer, defines an individual's degree of risk. Hereditary ovarian cancer and family history of ovarian cancer are separate risk categories. Hereditary breast-ovarian cancer and HNPCC put a woman at increased risk for ovarian cancer.[33] Further research is necessary to determine whether fertility-enhancing drugs increase the risk of ovarian cancer.[32] Women who use oral contraceptives decrease their risk of ovarian cancer by 30% to 60%, depending on the length of use. Lactating during pregnancy and breastfeeding appears to have a protective effect.[33]

Prevention, Screening, and Detection
PREVENTION AND SCREENING

Because the etiology of ovarian cancer remains unclear, no recommendations exist for prevention of the disease. Women who have experienced the birth of at least one child have a risk reduction of 0.3 or 0.4%. Prophylactic oophorectomy will reduce but not eliminate the risk for development of ovarian cancer.[32] Current screening methods include pelvic examinations, measuring the levels of tumor markers (CA-125), and pelvic ultrasonography in high-risk women.[34] CA-125 is a tumor antigen that is commonly present in increased levels in women with ovarian cancer. These serial levels monitor and confirm disease relapse.[33] Although 80% of women with advanced stages of disease will have alterations in their CA-125 level, only 50% to 60% with early disease will have plasma elevations. CA-125 levels can also be elevated in pregnancy, pelvic inflammatory disease, endometriosis, and inflammatory colon cancer. Therefore, CA-125 is not helpful in the screening process in the general population.

Transvaginal ultrasound, where a probe is placed into the vagina, is used to evaluate the ovaries. Proteomics, the study of human proteins under different conditions, is currently being researched as a method of detecting early-stage ovarian cancer.

DETECTION

Women with early-stage ovarian cancer are often asymptomatic, making early detection difficult. A Pap smear is not a screening method in ovarian cancer, and the success rate in bimanual palpation depends upon the size of the mass.[28] Palpation of a pelvic mass, or a palpable ovary in postmenopausal women, should be cause for further investigation. Chest x-rays and CT scans are used to evaluate metastatic disease.[33]

Classification

Ovarian carcinomas are classified according to the structures of the ovary from which they are derived, such as epithelial, sex cord–stromal, or germ cell tumors. Epithelial tumors account for approximately 90% of the ovarian carcinomas, while the remaining 10% are nonepithelial tumors. Epithelial tumors are then further classified as either serous or mucinous. Patients who are 40 years of age or older tend to have epithelial tumors, whereas women under the age of 30 exhibit germ cell tumors, which account for 3% of ovarian malignancies. The most common malignant germ cell tumor is the dysgerminoma.[32,33,35] Sex cord–stromal tumors account for only 7% of malignant ovarian neoplasms, are of low malignant potential, and are associated with a favorable long-term prognosis. Usually these tumors are diagnosed in patients before they reach the age of 40.[36]

Clinical Features

Early symptoms of ovarian cancer are vague and diffuse. These include gastrointestinal (GI) distress, dyspepsia, abdominal discomfort, back pain, loss of appetite, changes in bowel habits, bloating, eructation, increase in pelvic pressure, and vaginal bleeding. In addition, women may experience genitourinary symptoms such as burning, urgency, and frequency. The most common symptom seen in women is abdominal bloating and/or discomfort.[18] Late symptoms include a palpable abdominal mass, ascites, increased abdominal girth, pleural effusion, shortness of breath, weight loss, nausea and vomiting, intestinal obstruction, and vaginal bleeding. Ascites occurs when lymphatic channels are blocked or when the tumor produces excessive fluid. Comfort can be provided by positioning the patient on the left side to decrease weight on the organs and having her eat frequent, smaller, high-protein meals. Parenteral nutrition may be indicated on a temporary or permanent basis. One third of patients are seen at diagnosis with ascites; therefore abdominal girth should be obtained. Ovarian cancer patients who have undergone surgery with lymph node removal may experience lymphedema in their lower extremities. Patients who present with pleural effusion may experience shortness of breath. Thoracentesis or pleurodesis may be necessary. Although these are all signs of late disease, often they are the first symptoms experienced.[18,33]

Diagnosis and Staging

Exploratory laparotomy provides a thorough evaluation of all areas at risk. Specimens for cytology and biopsies are obtained. Methodical and meticulous staging is imperative, since postoperative treatment is based upon the stage of the disease.[36] The goal of surgery is to leave no tumor greater than 1 cm. For patients with advanced-stage disease, cytoreductive surgery, or debulking, is performed during the exploratory laparotomy to remove the primary tumor and all the associated disease; it provides the basis of treatment decisions.[33] Removing all accessible tumor alleviates ascites, nausea, and early satiety and in addition may restore adequate intestinal functioning if intestinal metastases are found. Debulking is helpful in eliminating areas that are resistant to treatment (i.e., chemotherapy agents). Reducing tumor burden can also decrease the production of immunologically suppressive substances that large tumors may have. The FIGO staging system is used (see Table 11-3).[35]

Before surgical exploration, a series of tests is performed: CT, ultrasound, and MRI help the evaluation of the size and location of the pelvic mass. Barium enema, colonoscopy, proctoscopy, sigmoidoscopy, chest x-rays, measurement of CA-125 levels, and IVP may also be performed.[18]

METASTASIS

Ovarian cancer spreads by direct extension to adjacent organs, such as the opposite ovary, the uterus, the fallopian tubes, the omentum, the bladder, and the rectum. Peritoneal seeding can occur when ovarian cancer penetrates through the surface of the

TABLE 11-3	Ovary: American Joint Committee on Cancer Definitions and Stage Grouping

DEFINITIONS

Primary Tumor (T)

TNM Classifications	FIGO Stages	Definitions
TX		Primary tumor cannot be assessed
T0		No evidence of primary tumor
T1	I	Tumor limited to ovaries (one or both)
T1a	IA	Tumor limited to one ovary; capsule intact, no tumor on ovarian surface. No malignant cells in ascites or peritoneal washings*
T1b	IB	Tumor limited to both ovaries; capsule intact, no tumor on ovarian surface. No malignant cells in ascites or peritoneal washings*
T1c	IC	Tumor limited to one or both ovaries with any of the following: capsule ruptured, tumor on ovarian surface, malignant cells in ascites or peritoneal washings
T2	II	Tumor involves one or both ovaries with pelvic extension
T2a	IIA	Extension and/or implants on uterus and/or tube(s). No malignant cells in ascites or peritoneal washings
T2b	IIB	Extension to and/or implants on other pelvic tissues. No malignant cells in ascites or peritoneal washings
T2c	IIC	Pelvic extension and/or implants (T2a or T2b) with malignant cells in ascites or peritoneal washings
T3	III	Tumor involves one or both ovaries with microscopically confirmed peritoneal metastasis outside the pelvis**
T3a	IIIA	Microscopic peritoneal metastasis beyond pelvis (no macroscopic tumor)**
T3b	IIIB	Macroscopic peritoneal metastasis beyond pelvis 2 cm or less in greatest dimension**
T3c	IIIC	Peritoneal metastasis beyond pelvis more than 2 cm in greatest dimension and/or regional lymph node metastasis

TABLE 11-3   Ovary: American Joint Committee on Cancer Definitions and Stage Grouping—cont'd

Regional Lymph Nodes (N)

NX		Regional lymph nodes cannot be assessed
N0		No regional lymph node metastasis
N1	IIIC	Regional lymph node metastasis

Distant Metastasis

MX		Distant metastasis cannot be assessed
M0		No distant metastasis
M1	IV	Distant metastasis (excludes peritoneal metastasis)**

STAGE GROUPING (AJCC/UICC/FIGO)

Stage	TNM	Regional Lymph Nodes	Distant Metastasis
I	T1	N0	M0
IA	T1a	N0	M0
IB	T1b	N0	M0
IC	T1c	N0	M0
II	T2	N0	M0
IIA	T2a	N0	M0
IIB	T2b	N0	M0
IIC	T2c	N0	M0
III	T3	N0	M0
IIIA	T3a	N0	M0
IIIB	T3b	N0	M0
IIIC	T3c	N0	M0
	Any T	N1	M0
IV	Any T	Any N	M1

HISTOLOGIC GRADE (G)

GX	Grade cannot be assessed
GB	Borderline malignancy
G1	Well differentiated
G2	Moderately differentiated
G3–G4	Poorly differentiated or undifferentiated

RESIDUAL TUMOR

RX	Presence of residual tumor cannot be assessed
R0	No residual tumor
R1	Microscopic residual tumor
R2	Macroscopic residual tumor

*The presence of non-malignant ascites is not classified. The presence of ascites does not affect staging unless malignant cells are present
**Liver capsule metastasis T3/III, liver parenchymal metastasis M1/Stage IV. Pleural effusion must have positive cytology for M1/Stage IV.
From American Joint Committee on Cancer: *AJCC Cancer Staging Manual*, ed 6, Chicago, 2002, AJCC.

ovarian capsule, which allows malignant cells into the peritoneal cavity. Once in the peritoneal cavity, malignant cells follow the continuous circulation of peritoneal fluid and implant themselves on the diaphragm. Peritoneal seeding can also occur through lymph and vascular channels. This allows for metastasis to the lungs and the liver through hematogenous spread in about 2% to 3% of patients.[33,35] Spread via the lymphatic system is common, particularly in advanced disease (Fig. 11-6).[35]

Treatment Modalities

SURGERY

Surgery and chemotherapy are current treatment modalities, used alone or in combination. The primary treatment for early-stage epithelial ovarian cancer is a TAH-BSO with surgical staging. Surgery plays a major role in diagnosis, primary treatment, evaluation of treatment response, and palliative care. In addition, surgery is also the primary treatment for women with borderline tumors of the ovary. Conservative treatment (a unilateral oophorectomy) is appropriate for young patients who have borderline tumors and wish to preserve their fertility. Beyond a TAH-BSO, surgical resection of the bulk of remaining tumor is attempted. The goal of cytoreductive therapy is to remove all primary cancer and metastatic disease. The extent to which this goal can be met and influence survival is limited by the extent of metastasis. The use of "second-look" surgery is not a standard procedure but may be performed on a patient who has no clinical evidence of disease.[35] The intent is to thoroughly reexplore the

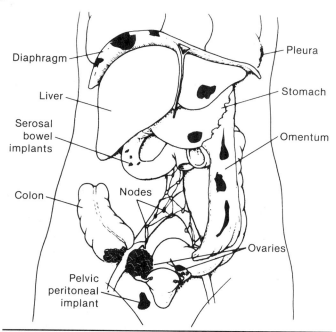

Diaphragm

Pleura

Liver

Stomach

Serosal
bowel
implants

Omentum

Colon

Nodes

Ovaries

Pelvic
peritoneal
implant

FIG. 11-6 Patterns of metastasis for ovarian cancer. (From DiSaia PJ, Creasman WT: *Clinical gynecologic oncology*, ed 4, St. Louis, 1997, Mosby).

peritoneal cavity and selected retroperitoneal structures to detect residual disease, debulk the remaining tumor, and determine further treatment.[3,36,37] There is no current evidence that surgery after initial chemotherapy prolongs survival.[38] Second-look surgery has been used as a means of providing palliative care in patients with advanced disease, for example, to relieve recurrent bowel obstructions.[3]

RADIATION THERAPY

Radiation therapy in ovarian cancer is controversial. Specific criteria have been established to select patients for abdominal pelvic radiation who have primary ovarian cancer and are in need of adjunctive treatment. These criteria include patients who have residual disease or a tumor of less than or equal to 2 cm, early-stage disease, cell type and grade, and whether the tumor site is located within the radiation field. In addition, the patient's physical status must be able to tolerate the radiation. Complications of radiation therapy in ovarian cancer include lung fibrosis, bone necrosis, and secondary malignancies such as leukemia, melanoma, and breast cancer.[39]

CHEMOTHERAPY

For women with high-risk early-stage epithelial ovarian cancer, single-agent or multiagent chemotherapy has been used.[36] The chemotherapy agent used depends upon the patient's overall health status. Carboplatin and paclitaxel are the most commonly preferred agents, and this combination is equally effective, less toxic, and easy to administer in an outpatient setting.[33,35] Researchers have explored the use of antineoplastic agents intraperitoneally to treat metastatic disease within the peritoneal cavity. Cisplatin is most frequently used.[33]

Autologous bone marrow transplantation using high-dose chemotherapy and peripheral stem cell support is being researched in patients with advanced ovarian cancer. Patient selection for this type of treatment is under discussion.[40]

Prognosis

Prognostic factors for ovarian cancer include age and response to treatment. Patients over 69 years of age have poorer survival rates compared to those under the age of 50. In addition, histologic type, grade, and tumor stage are significant. The volume of the disease remaining after surgery is also an important determining factor; the greater the tumor burden remaining, the poorer the prognosis. Overall 5-year survival for ovarian cancer is 53%.[3]

Vulvar Cancer
Epidemiology

Vulvar carcinoma is an uncommon disease; there were approximately 3870 cases in the United States during 2005, comprising 3% to 5% of all gynecologic cancers.[1,41] Preinvasive disease, or vulvar intraepithelial neoplasia (VIN), has increased significantly over the past 20 years. VIN is used to denote vulvar epithelial abnormalities.[41] VIN occurs most often in women who are in their forties and fifties but may also affect women in their thirties. Although VIN is considered preinvasive disease, 3% to 5% of women will develop invasive vulvar carcinoma.[42]

Etiology and Risk Factors

Although the etiology of vulvar carcinoma is unknown, several factors have been associated with an increased incidence of the disease. Concurrent illnesses and conditions such as hypertension, diabetes, obesity, HPV type 16, venereal warts, herpes simplex type 2, syphilis, multiple sexual partners, chronic vulvar disease, a history of smoking and of immunosuppression, age greater than 60 years, and previous malignancy of the genital tract are currently considered to be risk factors.[41,43]

Prevention, Screening, and Detection
PREVENTION AND SCREENING

There are no screening measures specific to vulvar cancer. Screening includes a Pap smear with careful examination of the vulva, the mons pubis, the labia majora, the labia minora, the clitoris, the vagina, and the Bartholin glands, particularly in women with the high-risk factors previously mentioned. Of patients with early-stage lesions, 50% are asymptomatic; therefore careful screening is critical.[41,44]

DETECTION

Women may fail to report symptoms because of denial or embarrassment attributed to the disease. A complete history and careful physical exam is imperative in detecting vulvar carcinoma. Early squamous cell carcinoma lesions are not detectable by palpation, and a gross examination with colposcopy should be performed.[44] The physical exam should include evaluation of the entire vulva, the perineum, the perianal area, the vagina, and the cervix. Lymph nodes in the groin should be palpated and biopsied if they are suspicious.[41]

Classification

Ninety percent of vulvar carcinomas are of the squamous cell type. Other, less frequent types include melanomas, sarcomas, basal cell, adenocarcinoma, and tumors arising in the Bartholin glands.[3,45]

VIN is classified into three categories: VIN I comprises mild dysplasia, VIN II is moderate dysplasia, and VIN III, also known as CIS, is classified as severe dysplasia.[41]

Clinical Features

The most common presenting symptoms of vulvar carcinoma include vulvar pruritus, irritation, and a mass in the vulvar area. Late signs and symptoms are vulvar bleeding, discharge, and dysuria.[3] Clinical features of squamous cell vulvar carcinomas include a raised lesion, which may be fleshy, ulcerated, or warty in appearance.[41]

Diagnosis and Staging

Forty percent of patients are not diagnosed until their cancer has reached advanced stage.[44] The diagnosis is made by a wedge biopsy including the surrounding skin, the underlying dermis, and connective tissue. The procedure can be done in an outpatient setting under local anesthesia. Careful examination is critical to detect abnormalities. Patients may also have additional testing such as chest x-rays, CT, MRI, cystoscopy, IVP, barium enema, and proctosigmoidoscopy. Vulvar carcinoma is staged using the FIGO staging system (see Table 11-4).[18,41]

Metastasis

Vulvar cancer usually remains localized, but may metastasize to adjacent structures such as the vagina, the urethra, and the anus, and can progress into the mucosa of the rectum and the bladder. [41,44,45] Lymphatic embolization to regional lymph nodes can occur early in this disease. Hematogenous spread is uncommon in patients with vulvar cancer, but metastases may occur in the lungs, the liver, and bone.[44,45]

Treatment Modalities

SURGERY

Surgical intervention is the most common treatment for vulvar cancer, with emphasis on the most conservative approach that is also consistent with the cure of disease.[45] The age of the patient with VIN will help to determine surgical approach, along with the clinician's consideration of function and cosmesis.

Surgical approach can vary from a wide local excision to a skinning vulvectomy (excision of the vulvar skin while conserving fat, muscle, and glands below the skin) for women with multicentric disease, to local treatment with use of cautery,

---

TABLE 11-4	Vulva: American Joint Committee on Cancer Definitions and Stage Grouping

DEFINITIONS

Primary Tumor (T)

TNM Classifications	FIGO Stages	Definitions
TX		Primary tumor cannot be assessed
T0		No evidence of primary tumor
Tis	0	Carcinoma *in situ* (preinvasive carcinoma)
T1	I	Tumor confined to the vulva or vulva and perineum, 2 cm or less in greatest dimension
T1a	IA	Tumor confined to the vulva or vulva and perineum, 2 cm or less in greatest dimension, and with stromal invasion no greater than 1 mm*
T1b	IB	Tumor confined to the vulva or vulva and perineum, 2 cm or less in greatest dimension, and with stromal invasion greater than 1 mm*
T2	II	Tumor confined to the vulva or vulva and perineum, more than 2 cm in greatest dimension
T3	III	Tumor of any size with contiguous spread to the lower urethra and/or vagina or anus
T4	IVA	Tumor invades any of the following: upper urethra, bladder mucosa, rectal mucosa, or is fixed to the pubic bone

Regional Lymph Nodes (N)

NX		Regional lymph nodes cannot be assessed
N0		No regional lymph node metastasis
N1	III	Unilateral regional lymph node metastasis
N2	IVA	Bilateral regional lymph node metastasis

Distant Metastasis

MX		Distant metastasis cannot be assessed
M0		No distant metastasis
M1	IVB	Distant metastasis (including pelvic lymph node metastasis)

STAGE GROUPING (AJCC/UICC/FIGO)

Stage	TNM	Regional Lymph Nodes	Distant Metastasis
0	Tis	N0	M0
I	T1	N0	M0
IA	T1a	N0	M0
IB	T1b	N0	M0

Continued

| TABLE 11-4 | Vulva: American Joint Committee on Cancer Definitions and Stage Grouping—cont'd |

STAGE GROUPING (AJCC/UICC/FIGO)

Stage	TNM	Regional Lymph Nodes	Distant Metastasis
II	T2	N0	M0
III	T1	N1	M0
	T2	N1	M0
	T3	N0	M0
	T3	N1	M0
IVA	T1	N2	M0
	T2	N2	M0
	T3	N2	M0
	T4	Any N	M0
IVB	Any T	Any N	M1

HISTOLOGIC GRADE (G)

GX	Grade cannot be assessed
G1	Well differentiated
G2	Moderately differentiated
G3	Poorly differentiated
G4	Undifferentiated

RESIDUAL TUMOR

RX	Presence of residual tumor cannot be assessed
R0	No residual tumor
R1	Microscopic residual tumor
R2	Macroscopic residual tumor

*The depth of invasion is defined as the measurement of the tumor from the epithelial–stromal junction of the adjacent most superficial dermal papilla to the deepest point of invasion.

From American Joint Committee on Cancer: *AJCC Cancer Staging Manual*, ed 6, Chicago, 2002, AJCC.

cryosurgery, laser ablation, topical creams, and photodynamic therapy. The wide local excisional approach is approximately 83% to 91% effective in eradicating VIN.

Management of regional lymph nodes is the single most important factor in decreasing mortality from early-stage disease. Women with less than 1 mm of stromal invasion on the wedge biopsy will not require a groin dissection. However, the incidence of women with less than 1 mm is small.

In stage III disease, with tumor spreading to the urethra, the vagina, the anus, and the lymph nodes, a radical vulvectomy is indicated. This procedure often removes a portion of the distal urethra or the vagina, and excision of a portion of the anus is possible.[41] Metastasis to the upper urethra, the bladder, the rectal mucosa, or the pelvic bone, with regional or distant lymph node involvement or distant metastases is characteristic of stage IV vulvar cancer. Surgical treatment depends upon the extent of the metastasis. A radical vulvectomy or a total pelvic exenteration, or both, may be indicated.[18]

RADIATION THERAPY

Radiation therapy for vulvar carcinoma continues to evolve. Indications include preoperative radiation therapy to reduce the extent of the tumor and thus the necessary surgery, or postoperatively to treat the pelvic and inguinal lymph nodes in patients with metastasis. It is also used for women who are at high risk for surgery.[41] Combination therapy protocols for radiation and surgery may be used to help maintain urinary or fecal continence. Complications of radiation therapy are wet desquamation of the skin and mucosa, edema of the labia, ulceration of the vulva, and

stenosis of the vagina or the urethra.[39] Aims of nursing care are maintaining skin integrity and pain management. Topical ointments, frequent sitz baths, and exposure to air can help to minimize skin reactions.[41] Studies have shown that radiation used concurrently with chemotherapy has resulted in greater response rates than radiation alone.[41]

CHEMOTHERAPY

Chemotherapy alone has not been shown to be effective as adjuvant therapy for vulvar cancer, although it has been used for palliation for women with stage IV disease.[18] The most common agents used include 5-FU, cisplatin, mitomycin C, bleomycin, and methotrexate.[18,41] Studies showing concurrent use of radiation and chemotherapy are promising.[41]

Prognosis

Survival rates for vulvar carcinoma depend upon the extent of lymph node involvement. In addition, tumor stage, grade, and size affect patient outcomes. Women who have invasive disease without lymph node involvement show survival rates are as high as 90%. As the number of positive nodes increases, the survival rate decreases.

Vaginal Cancer

Epidemiology

Carcinoma of the vagina is rare, representing less than 2% of all gynecologic malignancies.[41,46] The upper third of the vagina is most commonly involved. The majority of vaginal carcinomas represent metastases from some other gynecologic malignancy site.[46,47] Vaginal cancer occurs most often in women between the ages of 50 and 70 years, but it is on the rise in younger women.[47] It is rare in women under 40 years of age.[41]

Etiology and Risk Factors

The exact etiology of vaginal cancer is unknown; however, there is an association with HPV in more than 50% of cases. Prior radiation therapy, abdominal hysterectomy, DES exposure in utero, and age place a woman at higher risk for the disease.[41] A previous history of CIS or invasive cervical cancer treatment in the last 5 years places a woman at an approximate risk of 30% of developing primary vaginal carcinoma.[48]

Prevention, Screening, and Detection

PREVENTION AND SCREENING

There are no current recommendations for the prevention and screening of vaginal cancer. Inspection, palpation, and annual Pap smears are encouraged.[41]

DETECTION

Most women with vaginal carcinoma are asymptomatic.[41] Detection of preinvasive disease and invasive lesions requires a thorough examination of the vagina. Small lesions, particularly in the lower two thirds of the vagina, are often missed on Pap exam in spots where they may be covered by the blades of the speculum.[48] An inspection of the vagina should be performed at the time the Pap smear is completed.[41]

Classification

Of vaginal cancers, 85% are of squamous cell origin. Other types seen, although rarely, include melanoma, clear cell, adenocarcinoma, and sarcomas. Vaginal intraepithelial neoplasia (VAIN), is considered precancerous and can precede invasive vaginal cancer. VAIN is classified into three categories. Mild dysplasia is referred to as VAIN I, and VAIN II refers to moderate dysplasia.[41] VAIN III indicates premalignant lesions and severe dysplasia.

Clinical Features

The most common presenting symptom is abnormal vaginal bleeding; it is usually postmenopausal but may occur after sexual intercourse. Other symptoms include vaginal discharge, dysuria, palpable mass, and pain in the perineum. Patients may also display symptoms related to the tumor location, such as urinary retention with spasms, and hematuria. Tumors compressing the posterior vaginal wall often cause blood in the stool and constipation.[41]

Diagnosis and Staging

The diagnosis of primary, metastatic, or recurrent vaginal carcinoma is made with a thorough physical examination, including digital palpation of the vagina, colposcopy with biopsy, and cytologic evaluation. Biopsies of the cervix will rule out primary cervical cancer. A biopsy under anesthesia may be necessary for a thorough evaluation of the vagina.

Chest x-rays, barium enemas, IVP, cystoscopy, proctoscopy, complete blood count (CBC), and biochemical profiles may be used to determine the extent of the disease. Lymph nodes are assessed using MRI or CT.[41,47] Vaginal cancer is staged according to the FIGO staging system (see Table 11-5).

METASTASIS

Squamous cell carcinoma of the vagina spreads by direct extension to adjacent organs of the bladder and the rectum, pelvic soft tissue, and pelvic bones. The disease may disseminate via

---

TABLE 11-5   **Vagina: American Joint Committee on Cancer Definitions and Stage Grouping**

DEFINITIONS

Primary Tumor (T)

TNM Classifications	FIGO Stages	Definitions
TX		Primary tumor cannot be assessed
T0		No evidence of primary tumor
Tis	0	Carcinoma *in situ*
T1	I	Tumor confined to vagina
T2	II	Tumor invades paravaginal tissues but not to pelvic wall*
T3	III	Tumor extends to pelvic wall
T4	IVA	Tumor invades mucosa of the bladder or rectum and/or extends beyond the true pelvis (bullous edema is not sufficient evidence to classify a tumor as T4)

Regional Lymph Nodes (N)

NX	Regional lymph nodes cannot be assessed
N0	No regional lymph node metastasis
N1	Pelvic or inguinal lymph node metastasis

Distant Metastasis

MX		Distant metastasis cannot be assessed
M0		No distant metastasis
M1	IVB	Distant metastasis

Continued

TABLE 11-5	Vagina: American Joint Committee on Cancer Definitions and Stage Grouping—cont'd

STAGE GROUPING (AJCC/UICC/FIGO)

Stage	TNM	Regional Lymph Nodes	Distant Metastasis
0	Tis	N0	M0
I	T1	N0	M0
II	T2	N0	M0
III	T1-T3	N1	M0
	T3	N0	M0
IVA	T4	Any N	M0
IVB	Any T	Any N	M1

HISTOLOGIC GRADE (G)

GX	Grade cannot be assessed
G1	Well differentiated
G2	Moderately differentiated
G3	Poorly differentiated
G4	Undifferentiated

RESIDUAL TUMOR

RX	Presence of residual tumor cannot be assessed
R0	No residual tumor
R1	Microscopic residual tumor
R2	Macroscopic residual tumor

*Pelvic wall is defined as the muscle, fascia associated neurovascular structures, or skeletal portions of the bony pelvix.
From American Joint Committee on Cancer: *AJCC Cancer Staging Manual,* ed 6, Chicago, 2002, AJCC.

the pelvic and para-aortic lymph nodes. Hematogenous dissemination occurs in late disease and spreads to distant sites such as the lungs, the liver and the bones.[48]

Treatment Modalities

Because of the low incidence of vaginal cancers, treatment is individualized according to the stage of the disease and site of vaginal involvement.[47]

SURGERY

Surgery has a limited role but may be an option for a select group of women. A radical vaginectomy or radical hysterectomy with pelvic lymphadenectomy may be used for lesions that are superficial. Pelvic exenteration is often warranted for larger tumors without pelvic sidewall involvement.[41]

RADIATION THERAPY

Radiation therapy is the most widely used treatment of choice for all stages of vaginal cancer.[41,48] For women with stages I and II lesions, brachytherapy alone is sufficient, with treatment encompassing intracavitary and interstitial therapy. External beam radiation is used for larger tumors with lymph node involvement and is followed by brachytherapy.[48] Complications of radiation therapy include vaginal dryness, fibrosis, strictures, loss of blood supply, loss of elasticity, and chronic proctitis.[41]

CHEMOTHERAPY

Chemotherapy may be an option, but very few studies have been reported. The most common chemotherapeutic agents used

are 5-FU and cisplatin. Further studies are needed to determine the therapeutic effects of concurrent chemotherapy and radiation therapy.[47]

Prognosis

Because of treatment difficulties and the commonly advanced stage at time of diagnosis, the overall 5-year survival rate is approximately 44%. Surprisingly, patients with stage I disease also have a 5-year survival rate of approximately 70%, which is less when compared to carcinoma of the cervix or vulva. This is likely due to advanced stage at diagnosis and the close proximity of other organs. One study has shown the 5-year survival rate of stage IVB to be 0%.[48]

Fallopian Tube Cancer

Epidemiology

Cancer of the fallopian tubes accounts for 1% of all gynecologic malignancies.[49] The annual incidence rate is 3.6 million women per year in the United States. The incidence is lower in African Americans compared to Caucasian and Hispanic women. The mean age is 55 years of age, but it can occur in women as young as 18 years and as old as 88 years of age. Most patients diagnosed with this disease are postmenopausal.[50]

Etiology and Risk Factors

The etiology of cancer of the fallopian tube is unknown. Researchers have hypothesized that chronic tubal inflammation, infertility, salpingitis, and tubal endometriosis may contribute to the development of the disease.[49] Evidence of mutations in either the *BRCA1* or the *BRCA2* gene have emerged as causal factors in the last 5 years.[51] Cytogenic studies show an association with an overexpression of *p53*, HER2/*neu* and c-*myc*.[49]

Prevention, Screening, and Detection
PREVENTION AND SCREENING

Currently, there are no recommendations for the prevention and screening of women for fallopian tube cancer. Some researchers have advocated for the use of the Pap smear as a preoperative screening tool in patients with nonspecific symptoms.

DETECTION

The rarity of primary malignancies of the fallopian tubes makes difficult a diagnosis that is already complicated by presenting signs resembling salpingitis, ectopic pregnancy, and pelvic inflammatory disease.[51] Physical examination is important in these patients because a pelvic mass is present in 60% of women.[35]

Classification

Papillary serous adenocarcinoma is the most common histologic type seen and accounts for 90% of all fallopian tube cancers. Other histologic types include clear cell and endometiral carcinoma, whereas sarcomas, germ cell tumors, and lymphomas are rare histologic types. The grading system for serous tumors is based on the extent of differentiation and solid components.

Clinical Features

Women with fallopian tube cancers are frequently seen with vaginal bleeding, unexplained serosanguineous vaginal discharge, and pelvic pain.[49,50] Dull or colicky pain is significant because of the fact that cervical, endometrial, and ovarian cancer symptoms do not cause pain until obvious disease is present.[50] Approximately 15% of patients are first seen with Latzko's triad of symptoms: pelvic pain, pelvic mass, and intermittent, profuse serosanguineous vaginal discharge.[49,50] The vaginal discharge is termed *hydrops tubae profluens*, denoting a sudden emptying of the accumulation of fluid in the distended fallopian tubes. Pelvic mass is the most common physical finding.[49]

Diagnosis and Staging

The signs and symptoms of fallopian tube cancer resemble those of other conditions, and it can be difficult to diagnose. Diagnostic techniques under investigation include nuclear medicine imaging technology with radioactive nucleotides, CT, MRI, ultrasound, and measurement of tumor markers. CA-125 is a tumor marker used in the diagnosis of ovarian cancer, but more than 80% of patients with fallopian tube cancer have elevated pretreatment serum CA-125 levels. The FIGO staging system is used (see Table 11-6).[49]

Metastasis

Carcinoma of the fallopian tube metastasizes in a similar manner to epithelial ovarian malignancies. Metastasis to the peritoneum and distant spread are most common. Metastasis to the lymph nodes, and para-aortic and pelvic lymph nodes is

---

TABLE 11-6   Fallopian Tube: American Joint Committee on Cancer Definitions and Stage Grouping

DEFINITIONS

Primary Tumor (T)

TNM Classifications	FIGO Stages	Definitions
TX		Primary tumor cannot be assessed
T0		No evidence of primary tumor
Tis	0	Carcinoma *in situ* (limited to tubal mucosa)
T1	I	Tumor limited to the fallopian tube(s)
T1a	IA	Tumor limited to one tube, without penetrating the serosal suface; no ascites
T1b	IB	Tumor limited to both tubes, without penetrating the serosal surface; no ascites
T1c	IC	Tumor limited to one or both tubes with extension onto or through the tubal serosa, or with malignant cells in ascites or peritoneal washings
T2	II	Tumor involves one or both fallopian tubes with pelvic extension
T2a	IIA	Extension and/or metastasis to the uterus and/or ovaries
T2b	IIB	Extension to other pelvic structures
T2c	IIC	Pelvic extension with malignant cells in ascites or peritoneal washings
T3	III	Tumor involves one or both fallopian tubes, with peritoneal implants outside the pelvis
T3a	IIIA	Microscopic peritoneal metastasis outside the pelvis
T3b	IIIB	Macroscopic peritoneal metastasis outside the pelvis 2 cm or less in greatest dimension
T3c	IIIC	Peritoneal metastasis more than 2 cm in diameter

Regional Lymph Nodes (N)

NX		Regional lymph nodes cannot be assessed
N0		No regional lymph node metastasis
N1	IIIC	Regional lymph node metastasis

Continued

TABLE 11-6	Fallopian Tube: American Joint Committee on Cancer Definitions and Stage Grouping—cont'd

Distant Metastasis

MX		Distant metastasis cannot be assessed
M0		No distant metastasis
M1	IV	Distant metastasis (excludes metastasis within the peritoneal cavity)

STAGE GROUPING (AJCC/UICC/FIGO)

Stage	TNM	Regional Lymph Nodes	Distant Metastasis
0	Tis	N0	M0
I	T1	N0	M0
IA	T1a	N0	M0
IB	T1b	N0	M0
IC	T1c	N0	M0
II	T2	N0	M0
IIA	T2a	N0	M0
IIB	T2b	N0	M0
IIC	T2c	N0	M0
III	T3	N0	M0
IIIA	T3a	N0	M0
IIIB	T3b	N0	M0
IIIC	T3c	N0	M0
	Any T	N1	M0
IV	Any T	Any N	M1

HISTOLOGIC GRADE (G)

GX	Grade cannot be assessed
G1	Well differentiated
G2	Moderately differentiated
G3	Poorly differentiated
G4	Undifferentiated

RESIDUAL TUMOR

RX	Presence of residual tumor cannot be assessed
R0	No residual tumor
R1	Microscopic residual tumor
R2	Macroscopic residual tumor

From American Joint Committee on Cancer: *AJCC Cancer Staging Manual*, ed 6, Chicago, 2002, AJCC.

common, because the fallopian tubes are richly permeated with lymphatic channels.[35]

Treatment Modalities

SURGERY

Surgery is the definitive treatment for fallopian tube cancer. Typically, a TAH-BSO is performed followed by a node dissection (specifically, retroperitoneal), and peritoneal cytologic studies and biopsies should be performed along with an omentecomy.[49,51]

RADIATION THERAPY

It has been shown that for postoperative treatment for fallopian tube carcinoma, whole abdominopelvic irradiation produces a better survival compared with pelvic radiation alone. Current research is studying the use of chemotherapy and radiation for women with advanced disease. One study suggests that this method is superior to whole abdominopelvic irradiation alone.

More research is needed to determine the role that radiation plays in fallopian tube carcinoma.[50]

CHEMOTHERAPY

The most active agents are the platinum and the taxane compounds. Research has shown that cisplatin in combination with paclitaxel is able to provide a complete response.[35] Other studies have shown that paclitaxel-containing regimens, in addition to the standard chemotherapy combination of cyclophosphamide, adriamycin, and platinum, are effective.[49]

Prognosis

The prognosis for patients with fallopian tube cancer is related to the stage of the disease at diagnosis. The overall 5-year survival rate is 56%, and it is as high as 84% with stage I disease. Patients with fallopian tube cancer have a higher 5-year survival when compared to ovarian cancer patients because of early disease stage at diagnosis.[36]

Gestational Trophoblastic Disease

Epidemiology

Gestational trophoblastic disease (GTD) consists of a spectrum of interrelated diseases including hydatidiform mole, invasive mole, placental site trophoblastic tumor (PSTT), and choriocarcinoma.[52] This group of diseases is characterized by an abnormal proliferation of trophoblastic tissue, with persistently elevated serum human chorionic gonadotropin (HCG) levels.[53] The incidence of GTD varies dramatically around the world, with 1 in 1500 live births in the United States, whereas the frequency of molar pregnancies in Asian countries is about 7 to 10 times greater than in North America and Europe. The variation in incidence may be due to differences in reporting.[51] Today, this group of diseases is considered the most curable gynecologic cancer.[53]

Etiology and Risk Factors

The etiology of GTD is unknown; however, several risk factors have been associated with an increased incidence. Specific risk factors include socioeconomic and nutritional factors (decreased intake of carotene), advanced maternal age (women over 40 years of age), history of spontaneous abortions and infertility, and hormonal factors.[3,54] The greatest risk factor appears to be a previous molar pregnancy.[3]

Prevention, Screening, and Detection

PREVENTION AND SCREENING

No recommendations for prevention and screening of asymptomatic women for GTD are available.

DETECTION

The HCG test is essential in the detection of GTD. This test has a high diagnostic sensitivity, approaching 100%.[53] In addition to the HCG test, physical exam and review of the patient's reproductive history are also important in the detection of the disease.

Classification

Hydatidiform moles are studied as two distinct diseases, complete and partial moles. Both have the ability to become an invasive mole, which is another classification of GTD. Partial moles have a lower frequency of progressing to choriocarcinoma. Choriocarcinoma is a malignant tumor of the trophoblast. The term *gestational trophoblastic neoplasia* was added in in 2000. It was used for patients whose serum HCG level failed to regress in the absence of a normal pregnancy and who had a history of either a normal or abnormal antecedent pregnancy.[53]

Clinical Features

The most common presenting symptom of GTD is vaginal bleeding in women with a complete molar pregnancy.[55] Marked increases in HCG are present in complete moles but are less common with partial moles.[54] Hyperemesis, toxemia, and hyperthyroidism may be clinically evident.[55] Excessive uterine size relative to gestational age may also be noted. Patients with partial moles are generally not seen with the same symptoms as those with complete moles. These patients are usually seen with the signs and symptoms of an incomplete or missed abortion.[54]

Diagnosis and Staging

A thorough assessment of the extent of the disease is required before treatment is initiated. This includes a complete history, physical examination, measurement of the serum HCG value, hepatic, thyroid, and renal function tests, and blood counts. Ultrasonography is a reliable technique for detecting complete and partial moles. The marked swelling of the chorionic villi with complete moles produces a characteristic pattern visible by ultrasound.[52,54] A metastatic work-up should be included consisting of chest x-ray, and CT of the abdomen and pelvis and the brain. For patients with choriocarcinoma and/or metastatic disease, HCG levels should be measured in the cerebral spinal fluid to exclude cerebral involvement if the CT scan of the brain is negative.[55]

The following staging system has been adopted by FIGO: stage I, lesions confined to uterus; stage II, metastasis to vagina and pelvis; stage III, metastasis to lung; and stage IV, distant metastasis to brain and liver (see Table 11-7).[52,55]

Metastasis

Metastatic GTN can invade locally, or it can metastasize to distant sites. After evacuation of a complete mole, 15% of

---

TABLE 11-7 Gestational Trophoblastic Tumors: American Joint Committee on Cancer Definitions and Stage Grouping

DEFINITIONS

Primary Tumor (T)* TNM** Classifications	FIGO Stages	Definitions
TX		Primary tumor cannot be assessed
T0		No evidence of primary tumor
T1	I	Disease limited to uterus
T2	II	Disease outside of uterus but limited to genital structures (ovary, tube, vagina, broad ligaments)
Distant Metastasis		
MX		Metastasis cannot be assessed
M0		No distant metastasis
M1		Distant metastasis
M1a	III	Lung metastasis
M1b	IV	All other distant metastasis

Continued

TABLE 11-7	Gestational Trophoblastic Tumors: American Joint Committee on Cancer Definitions and Stage Grouping—cont'd

STAGE GROUPING* (AJCC/UICC/FIGO)

Stage	Primary Tumor	Distant Metastasis	Risk Factors
I	T1	M0	Unknown
IA	T1	M0	Low risk
IB	T2	M0	High risk
II	T2	M0	Unknown
IIA	T2	M0	Low risk
IIB	T2	M0	High risk
III	Any T	M1a	Unknown
IIIA	Any T	M1a	Low risk
IIIB	Any T	M1a	High risk
IV	Any T	M1b	Unknown
IVA	Any T	M1b	Low risk
IVB	Any T	M1b	High risk

RESIDUAL TUMOR

RX	Presence of residual tumor cannot be assessed
R0	No residual tumor
R1	Microscopic residual tumor
R2	Macroscopic residual tumor

PROGNOSTIC INDICATORS SCORING INDEX

Prognostic Factor	Risk Score 0	1	2	4
Age	<40	≤40		
Antecedent pregnancy	Hydatidiform mole	Abortion	Term pregnancy	
Interval months from index pregnancy	<4	4-<7	7-12	>12
Pretreatment hCG (IU/ml)	$<10^3$	$=10^3-<10^4$	$10^4-<10^5$	$\geq10^5$
Largest tumor size, including uterus	<3 cm	3-<5 cm	≥5 cm	
Site of metastases	Lung	Spleen, kidney	Gastrointestinal tract	Brain, liver
Number of metastases identified		1-4	5-8	>8
Previous failed chemotherapy			Single drug	Two or more drugs
Total score				

Low risk is a score of 7 or less. High risk is a score of 8 or greater.
*See prognostic indicator section for substage definitions.
**There is no regional nodal staging for this tumor.
From American Joint Committee on Cancer: *AJCC Cancer Staging Manual*, ed 6, Chicago, 2002, AJCC.

patients experience local invasion and 4% of patients experience metastatic disease.[55] Choriocarcinoma is usually associated with disease metastases and has the propensity for early vascular invasion and dissemination. The lungs are the most common site for metastasis, followed by vaginal metastasis in 30% of patients, and hepatic and cerebral metastases in approximately 10%.[52]

Treatment Modalities

SURGERY AND CHEMOTHERAPY

Treatment decisions are based on whether or not the patient wishes to preserve fertility. A hysterectomy may be performed for patients with stage I disease who no longer desire to preserve fertility. A hysterectomy does eliminate risk of local invasion, but does not prevent metastasis. In these women, the hysterectomy may be followed by adjuvant chemotherapy.[54,55] Single-agent chemotherapy, such as actinomycin-D or methotrexate, has achieved excellent remission rates in both nonmetastatic and low-risk GTN.[55] Etoposide has been reported to induce a complete remission with nonmetastatic and low-risk metastatic GTN; however, it has been reported that etoposide increases the risk of later secondary tumors.[54,55] Hysterectomies are also recommended in those patients who have nonmetastatic PSTT because of their poor response to chemotherapy. For patients who wish to have children, evacuation—specifically, suction curettage—is performed to remove the uterine contents. This eliminates the mole while preserving fertility.[54] Patients with stage IV disease should be treated with primary intensive combination chemotherapy and the selected use of radiation and surgery. Primary combination chemotherapy is used to manage patients with metastases.[55]

RADIATION THERAPY

Radiation does not have a significant role in the treatment plan for GTD. If the disease metastasizes to the liver or the brain, external beam radiation may be used.[39]

Prognosis

Women who develop hydatidiform mole can anticipate a normal reproductive future. Weekly HCG levels are followed for 3 weeks, and then monthly until normal for all patients with stages III and IV disease. Patients with stage IV disease are followed for at least 24 months rather than on a monthly basis until normal. This is due to the increased risk of recurrence of the disease.[54]

Conclusion

Many patients with preinvasive disease or invasive cancer face many psychosocial issues when diagnosed with a gynecologic neoplasm. Depending on the specific disease or treatment, organs may have been removed, skin may have been disfigured, or the patient may have to deal with the chance of cancer returning for the duration of her life. Nurses caring for these patients must remain sensitive to these issues. Interventions must be supportive and may require referrals to other members of the health care team, such as social workers to help patients deal with sexual dysfunction, body image, and coping issues, as well as grief.[56]

CONSIDERATIONS FOR OLDER ADULTS

- Older clients may be treated with less invasive treatment methods
- Common comorbities in older adults that may add complications to a cancer diagnosis and treatment include hypertension, cardiovascular disease, diabetes, obesity, visual and/or hearing impairment, and dementia and depression.
- Teach patients the need for annual health examinations and preventive health behaviors.
- Encourage patients to report new symptoms or any abnormalities to their health care provider immediately.
- Assess the need for emotional support, social services, and discharge planning. Issues that they may experience might be related to coping, grief, body image disturbances, or sexual dysfunction issues. Make referrals to support services as needed.
- Assess nutritional status. Socioeconomic factors may play a role for older adults who live alone. These older adults may have a poor nutritional status, which may cause delayed wound healing in the surgical patient.
- When teaching older adults: Present the most important information first, provide large, easy to read instructions or materials, speak slowly and enunciate, be specific, clarify with examples, and offer encouragement and praise.

Holland BE, McCurren C: Health promotion in older adults. In Black JM, Hokanson Hawks J: *Medical surgical nursing: clinical management for positive outcomes,* ed 7, St. Louis, 2005, Saunders; DeGaetano C, Lichtman SM: Care of elderly women with ovarian cancer, *Geriatr Nurs* 25(6):331, 2004.

REVIEW QUESTIONS

✔ Case Study

Lucille, a 40-year-old Caucasian woman, came in to be seen and complained of abnormal vaginal bleeding for the past 4 months, occurring after coitus and between menstrual periods. She was married and had a 9-year-old child. She had been diagnosed with the human papilloma virus 5 years earlier. Lucille enjoyed good health, and her family history was unremarkable.

Previous Pap smear, 2 years earlier, showed mild cervical dysplasia. At that time a colposcopy with biopsy were done, and she was instructed to return for a repeat Pap smear in 6 months; however, she did not return until today's appointment.

At this visit, the nurse discussed the importance of yearly Pap smears and pelvic examinations on all women unless they are both over the age and 30 and have had three consecutive normal Pap smears. Because of the results of her previous Pap smear and current symptoms, the Pap smear and colposcopy were repeated today. On physical exam, genitalia appeared normal and the cervix was firm. The results of the colposcopy revealed a 3.5-cm cervical lesion positive for invasive cervical cancer, stage IB1. Lucille was surprised at the diagnosis but wanted to do whatever was necessary to prevent the disease from getting any worse.

The best option was to have radical hysterectomy with pelvic lymphadenectomy. Radiation is also an option but is typically reserved for patients who are poor surgical candidates. Surgery would also avoid potential radiation damage to

adjacent organs, namely, the bowel and the bladder. Lucille discussed these options with her husband, particularly in light of the fact that she would not be able to have additional children.

Surgery was performed 1 month later and, overall, Lucille recovered very well postoperatively. One day before discharge, her catheter was removed and she had difficulty voiding. Nursing staff instructed Lucille on the technique of home self-catheterization, which they anticipated would be necessary for approximately 2 weeks. This was distressing, since no one had told Lucille that an expected complication of a radical hysterectomy was voiding difficulties. The nurse discussed Lucille's fears and concerns, affirming that her feelings were normal. The nurses explained that her difficulty voiding was due to the nerves being affected during surgery and that in most cases this resolves itself. Intermittent self-catheterization retrains the bladder to work normally. The nurse gave Lucille written directions and equipment such as a mirror, straight catheters, and cleansing materials; also provided were instructions for care of the catheters and a chart to record voiding volume. A list of adverse signs and symptoms and possible complications was provided and reviewed; it included specific instructions regarding when to call the physician. Her technique was observed several times, and with encouragement and feedback, Lucille gained confidence. The nurse discussed the importance of following up after surgery to monitor for recurrence.

Continued

REVIEW QUESTIONS—CONT'D

QUESTIONS

1. Cervical cancer can be best prevented by teaching patients about what?
   a. Quitting smoking
   b. Eating a high-fat diet
   c. Having an annual Pap smear
   d. Having only one child

2. What sexually transmitted disease is associated with a high number of cervical cancer cases?
   a. Syphilis
   b. Gonorrhea
   c. Herpes simplex 2
   d. Human papillomavirus

3. Why was it suggested that Lucille have a radical hysterectomy instead of radiation therapy, if both options provide equal cure rates?
   a. Treatment for radiation therapy would be longer
   b. Less damage to adjacent organs (bowel, bladder, and vagina)
   c. Lucille wanted to preserve her fertility
   d. Lucille had a history of radiation therapy and could not have any more treatments

4. If Lucille's bleeding became chronic and she delayed seeking a medical opinion, what problem was she likely to experience?
   a. Electrolyte imbalance
   b. Lymphedema
   c. Bowel obstruction
   d. Anemia

5. What is a late sign of cervical cancer?
   a. Foul-smelling, serosanguineous, yellow discharge
   b. Hair loss
   c. Hematuria
   d. Numbness/tingling of the legs

6. Which of the below is true regarding cervical cancer prevention?
   a. Screening should begin 5 years after a woman begins having sexual intercourse.
   b. Screening should start no later than 16 years of age.
   c. Pap tests are necessary only if you experience symptoms.
   d. A woman who has had a total hysterectomy does not need Pap smears, unless the surgery was done for cervical cancer.

7. The most important prognostic indicator in patients with invasive cervical cancer is the clinical stage of the disease at diagnosis. Which patient scenario below depicts the poorest prognosis?
   a. Patient who is 65 years old with metastatic lymph node involvement and deep stromal tumor
   b. Patient who is 40 years old with stage IIB cervical cancer who had previously been treated for breast cancer
   c. Patient who is 24 years old and a mother of 2, who is currently pregnant and diagnosed with cervical cancer, stage IA
   d. Patient who is 50 years old nulliparous, smokes, has had three lifetime sexual partners, and has a preinvasive cervical lesion

8. In the case study described, what is the physiologic reason that Lucille is taught bladder training after her radical hysterectomy surgery?
   a. It is important to know exactly how much she is voiding at home.
   b. The cervical cancer must be prevented from metastasizing to the bladder.
   c. There is a loss of sense to void and inability to empty the bladder.
   d. It is important to prevent formation of a rectovaginal fistula.

9. What procedure assists in staging the extent of cervical disease in patients who undergo radical hysterectomy?
   a. Pelvic lymphadenectomy
   b. CT scan
   c. CBC
   d. CA-125

10. Postoperative nursing assessment after radical hysterectomy includes detecting which of the following potential complications?
    a. Proctitis
    b. Ascites
    c. Ulceration of the vulva and labial edema
    d. Infection and hemorrhage

ANSWERS

1. **C.** *Rationale:* Although it is important to discourage patients from smoking, and although high-fat diets may contribute to cancer, at this time neither are considered risk factors for cervical cancer. There is no information that supports the idea that having only one child prevents cervical cancer. However, having an annual Pap smear can help to detect cervical changes early, before invasive cancer is found.

2. **D.** *Rationale:* The human papillomavirus (HPV), specifically, subtypes 16, 18, 33, 35, and 45, have been implicated in more than 99% of cervical cancer cases.

3. **B.** *Rationale:* Radiation can cause damage to the organs listed, which leads to a difficult situation to manage; it is also an ongoing form of treatment, longer that a surgical procedure. Surgery allows for more accurate staging and therefore allows treatment to be targeted to the individual. Radiation is ideal for patients who are not candidates for surgery. A radical hysterectomy would not preserve her fertility, and she did not have a history of radiation therapy.

4. **D.** *Rationale:* An electrolyte imbalance can be the result of numerous physiologic conditions such as nausea, vomiting, or renal failure, to name a few, but it is not usually associated with blood loss. Lymphedema occurs from blocked lymph channels, and bowel obstructions can be caused by a tumor pressing on or entwining itself around the bowel. Both of these complications would more likely be seen in a patient with a large ovarian tumor. Anemia, the result of blood loss, is accompanied by decreases in hemoglobin and hematocrit, indicating that oxygen and iron are not circulating proficiently. Patients who are anemic may experience fatigue, pallor, weakness, and shortness of breath. Lucille's condition may not have progressed this severely, but her complete blood count would be affected.

5. C. *Rationale:* An early symptom would include foul-smelling, serosanguineous, yellow discharge. Hair loss is not a side effect of the the disease itself but rather of the treatment. Usually a late sign would be edematous lower extremities, not numbness and tingling. Hematuria is the correct answer; it is the late sign that cervical cancer has affected the urinary system.

6. D. *Rationale:* Cervical cancer screening with Pap smears should begin by the age of 21 and/or 3 years after a woman begins having sexual intercourse (whichever is earlier), not at 16 years of age. Cervical cancer is usually asymptomatic until late in the disease, which is why screening is imperative. A woman who has had a total hysterectomy does not need Pap smears, unless the surgery was done for cervical cancer,

7. A. *Rationale:* Three of these patients have issues of concern that raise questions regarding prognosis: a previous diagnosis of breast cancer, diagnosis of cervical cancer while pregnant, and risk factors of null parity, smoking, and multiple partners. However, the fact that patient A has a deep stromal tumor with metastatic lymph node involvement points to a poor prognosis.

8. C. *Rationale:* The amount the patient voids is important but not the reason for teaching her bladder training.

Although a rectovaginal fistula is a possible complication of a radical hysterectomy, bladder training will not prevent that from occurring, nor will it prevent disease metastasis. Bladder training helps empty the bladder in patients who have lost the sensation of bladder fullness and the ability to start micturition.

9. A. *Rationale:* CT scan is not able to distinguish between cancer and normal soft tissue of the cervix and uterus. CBC can provide information regarding reported blood loss and potential anemia but is not diagnostic for cervical cancer. Tumor marker CA-125 is commonly increased in patients with ovarian cancer, not cervical cancer. Pelvic lymphadenectomy, usually done at the time of surgical intervention, is valuable both in determining the extent of regional disease and estimating the potential for distant metastases.

10. D. *Rationale:* Proctitis is a side effect of radiation therapy to the abdominal cavity. Ascites is more common in patients with late-stage ovarian carcinoma. Vulvar ulceration and labial edema are potential complications of radiation therapy for vulvar cancer. Patients undergoing radical hysterectomy may have postoperative infection and hemorrhage.

REFERENCES

1. American Cancer Society: *Cancer Facts and Figures 2005*, Atlanta, 2005, Author.
2. Randall ME, Michael H, Ver Morken et al: Uterine cervix. In Hoskins WJ, Perez CA, Young RC et al: *Principles and practice of gynecologic oncology*, ed 4, Philadelphia, 2005, Lippincott, Williams & Wilkins.
3. Vogt Temple S, Umstead CH: Nursing care of the client with reproductive disorders. In Itano JK, Taoka KN: *Core curriculum for oncology nursing*, ed 4, St Louis, 2005, Saunders.
4. Hacker NF: Cervical cancer. In Berek JS, Hacker NF: *Practical gynecologic oncology*, ed 4, Philadelphia, 2005, Lippincott, Williams & Wilkins.
5. Vogt Temple S: Cervical cancer: In Henke Yarbro C, Hansen Frogge M, Goodman M: *Cancer nursing: principles and practice*, ed 6, Sudbury, Mass, 2005, Jones & Bartlett.
6. Jhingran A, Eifel PJ, Taylor Wharton J et al: Neoplasms of the cervix. In Holland JF, Frei E: *Cancer medicine 6*, vol 2, Hamilton, Ontario, 2003, BC Decker.
7. Todd RW, Shafi M: Invasive cervical cancer, *Curr Obstet Gynecol* 14(3): 200-206, 2004.
8. Cronje HS: Screening for cervical cancer in developing countries, *Int J Gynaecol Obstet* 84(2):103, 2004.
9. Cuschieri KS, Cubie HA: The role of human papillomavirus testing in cervical screening, *J Clin Virol* 32(1):36, 2005.
10. Tedeschi CA, Rubin M, Krumholz BA: Six cases of women with diethylstilbestrol in utero demonstrating long-term manifestation and current evaluation guidelines, *J Genital Tract Dis* 9(1) 12, 2005.
11. Guido R: Guidelines for screening and treatment of cervical disease in the adolescent, *J Pediatr Adolesc Gynecol* 17(5):310, 2004.
12. Herzog TJ: New approaches for the management of cervical cancer, *Gynecol Oncol* 90(3):27-28, 2003.
13. Plante M, Claude Renaud M, Hoskins IA et al: Vaginal radical trachelectomy: a valuable fertility-preserving option in the management of early-stage cervical cancer. A series of 50 pregnancies and review of the literature, *Gynecol Oncol* 98(1):3-10, 2005.
14. Duenas-Gonzalez AM, Lopez-Graniel C, Gonzalez A et al: Induction chemotherapy with gemcitabine and oxaliplatin for locally advanced cervical carcinoma, *Am J Obstet Gynecol* 26(1):22-23, 2003.
15. Serkies K, Jassem J: Chemotherapy in the primary treatment of cervical carcinoma, *Crit Rev Oncol Hematol* 54(3):197-198, 2005.
16. Szopa TJ: Nursing implications of surgical treatment. In Itano JK, Taoka KN: *Core curriculum for oncology nursing*, ed 4, St Louis, 2005, Saunders.
17. Barclay, MM: Cancer surgery. In Nevidjon BM, Sowers KW: *A nurse's guide to cancer care*, Philadelphia, 2000, Lippincott.
18. Thompson SD: Gynecologic cancers. In Shelton BK, Ziegfeld CR, Olsen MM: *Manual of cancer nursing*, ed 2, Philadelphia, 2003, Lippincott, Williams & Wilkins.
19. Witt, ME: Nursing implications of radiation therapy. In Itano JK, Taoka KN: *Core curriculum for oncology nursing*, ed 4, St Louis, 2005, Saunders.
20. Almadrones, L: Endometrial cancer. In Henke Yarbro C, Hansen Frogge M, Goodman M: *Cancer nursing: principles and practice*, ed 6, Sudbury, Mass, 2005, Jones & Bartlett.
21. Painter J: Chemotherapy administration. In Nevidjon BM, Sowers KW: *A nurse's guide to cancer care*, Philadelphia, 2000, Lippincott.
22. Poniatowski BC, Vogt Temple S: Nursing implications of antineoplastic therapy. In Itano JK, Taoka KN: *Core curriculum for oncology nursing*, ed 4, St. Louis, 2005, Saunders.
23. Sivanesaratnam V: Gynaecological malignancies in pregnancy, *Rev Gynecol Pract* 4(3):162-168, 2004.
24. Rahaman J, Cohen CJ: Endometrial cancer. In Holland JF, Frei E: *Cancer medicine 6*, vol 2, Hamilton, Ontario, 2003, BC Decker.
25. Hacker NF: Uterine cancer. In Berek JS, Hacker NF: *Practical gynecologic oncology*, ed 4, Philadelphia, 2005, Lippincott, Williams & Wilkins.
26. Trope CG, Alektiar KM, Sabbatini PJ et al: Corpus: epithelial tumors. In Hoskins WJ, Perez CA, Young RC et al: *Principles and practice of gynecologic oncology*, ed 4, Philadelphia, 2005, Lippincott, Williams & Wilkins.
27. Homesley HD, Manetta A: Cancer of the uterine corpus. In Manetta A: *Cancer prevention and early diagnosis in women*, Philadelphia, 2004, Mosby.
28. Chamarro T: The gynecologic cancers. In Nevidjon BM, Sowers KW: *A nurse's guide to cancer care*, Philadelphia, 2000, Lippincott.
29. Timmerman D, Van den Bosch T: Diagnostic strategies in endometrial cancer, *Int Congres Ser* 1279:141-148, 2005.
30. Mourits MJ, Aalders JG: Surgical staging in endometrial cancer, *Int Congres Ser* 1279:158-161, 2005.
31. Solhjem MC: Vaginal brachytherapy alone is sufficient adjuvant treatment of surgical stage I endometrial cancer, *Int J Radiat Oncol Biol Phys* 62(5):1384. 2005.
32. Berek JS, Bast RC: Ovarian cancer. In Holland JF, Frei E: *Cancer medicine*, ed 6, Vol 2, Hamilton, Ontario, 2003, BC Decker.
33. Martin VR: Ovarian cancer. In Henke Yarbro C, Hansen Frogge M, Goodman M: *Cancer Nursing: principles and practice*, ed 6, Sudbury, Mass, 2005, Jones & Bartlett.

34. Breedlove G, Busenhart C: Screening and detection of ovarian cancer, *J Midwifery Womens Health* 50(1):51, 2005.

35. Berek JS, Hacker NF: Nonepithelial ovarian and fallopian tube cancers. In Berek JS, Hacker NF: *Practical gynecologic oncology*, ed 4, Philadelphia, 2005, Lippincott, Williams & Wilkins.

36. Ozols RF, Rubin SC, Thomas, GM: Epithelial ovarian cancer. In Hoskins WJ, Perez CA, Young RC et al: *Principles and practice of gynecologic oncology*, ed 4, Philadelphia, 2005, Lippincott, Williams & Wilkins.

37. Berek JS: Epithelial ovarian cancer. In Berek JS, Hacker NF: *Practical gynecologic oncology,* ed 4, Philadelphia, 2005, Lippincott, Williams & Wilkins.

38. Martin VR: Straight talk about ovarian cancer, *Nurs 2005* 35(4): 36-41, 2005.

39. Brown D, Lewis LC, Axiak A: Use of radiation in gynecologic and breast malignancies. In Moore-Higgs GJ, Almadrones LA, Colvin-Huff B et al: *Women and cancer: a gynecologic oncology nursing perspective*, ed 2, Sudbury, Mass, 2003, Jones & Bartlett.

40. Stiff PJ, Veum-Stone J, Lazarus HM et al: High-dose chemotherapy and autologous stem-cell transplantation for ovarian cancer: an autologous blood and marrow transplant registry report, *Ann Int Med* 133(7): 504, 2000.

41. Guarnieri C: Vulvar and vaginal cancer. In Henke Yarbro C, Hansen Frogge M, Goodman M: *Cancer nursing: principles and practice*, ed 6, Sudbury, Mass, 2005, Jones & Bartlett.

42. McFadden K, Cruickshank M: New developments in the management of VIN, *Rev Gynecol Pract* 5(2):103, 2005

43. Moore DH, Koh, WJ, McGuire WP et al: Vulva. In Hoskins WJ, Perez CA, Young RC et al: *Principles and practice of gynecologic oncology*, ed 4, Philadelphia, 2005, Lippincott, Williams & Wilkins.

44. Tyring SK: Vulvar squamous cell carcinoma: guidelines for early diagnosis and treatment, *AM J Obstet Gynecol* 189(3):18-19, 2003.

45. Hacker NF: Vulvar cancer. In Berek JS, Hacker NF: *Practical gynecologic oncology,* ed 4, Philadelphia, 2005, Lippincott, Williams & Wilkins.

46. Rotmensch J, Yamada SD: Neoplasms of the vulva and vagina. In Holland JF, Frei E: *Cancer medicine,* ed 6, vol 2, Hamilton, 2003, BC Decker.

47. Cardenes HR, Roth LM, McGuire WP et al: Vagina. In Hoskins WJ, Perez CA, Young RC et al: *Principles and practice of gynecologic oncology,* ed 4, Philadelphia, 2005, Lippincott, Williams & Wilkins.

48. Hacker NF: Vaginal Cancer. In Berek JS, Hacker NF: *Practical gynecologic oncology,* ed 4, Philadelphia, 2005, Lippincott, Williams & Wilkins.

49. Ajithkumar TV, Minimole AL, John MM: Primary fallopian tube carcinoma, *Obstet Gynecol Surv* 60(4):247-252, 2005.

50. Cohen CJ, Rahaman J: Neoplasms of the fallopian tube. In Holland JF, Frei, E: *Cancer medicine,* ed 6, vol 2, Hamilton, 2003, BC Decker.

51. Markman M, Zaino RJ, Fleming PA et al: Carcinoma of the fallopian tube. In Hoskins WJ, Perez CA, Young RC et al: *Principles and practice of gynecologic oncology,* ed 4, Philadelphia, 2005, Lippincott, Williams & Wilkins.

52. Berkowitz RS, Goldstein DP: Gestational trophoblastic disease. In Holland JF, Frei E: *Cancer medicine,* ed 6, vol 2, Hamilton, Ontario, 2003, BC Decker.

53. Seki K, Matsui H, Sekiya S: Advances in the clinical laboratory detection of gestatational trophoblastic disease, *Clin Chim Acta* 349(1-2):1-3, 2004.

54. Berkowitz RS, Goldstein DP: Gestational trophoblastic disease. In Hoskins WJ, Perez CA, Young RC et al: *Principles and practice of gynecologic oncology,* ed 4, Philadelphia, 2005, Lippincott, Williams & Wilkins.

55. Berkowitz RS, Goldstein DR: Gestational trophoblastic neoplasia. In Berek JS, Hacker NF: *Practical gynecologic oncology,* ed 4, Philadelphia, 2005, Lippincott, Williams & Wilkins.

56. Wenzel LB, Cella D: Quality of life issues in gynecologic cancer. In Hoskins WJ, Perex CA, Young RC et al: *Principles and practice of gynecologic oncology,* ed 4, Philadelphia. 2005, Lippincott, Williams & Wilkins.

CHAPTER 12

Head and Neck Cancers

Virginia Braden Bowman

Epidemiology

Head and neck cancer is the fifth leading cause of cancer death worldwide[1] and will account for approximately 3% of new cancers in the United States in 2005. The most common location for head and neck cancers is the oral cavity (48%),[2] with approximately 30,000 new cases and 7300 deaths expected in the United States in 2005.[3] Cancer of the oral cavity occurs more frequently in males and in African Americans.[2] The larynx is the second most common location (25%)[2]; cancer occurs there in an expected 10,000 new cases yearly,[3] again more commonly in males. Of new head and neck cancers in 2005, 10% will occur in the oropharynx.[2]

Head and neck cancer most often affects Americans over the age of 60 years, although incidence in younger adults is increasing.[1] The 5-year survival rate is greater than 80% when only local disease is found at diagnosis[2]; however, the overall 5-year survival rate for head and neck cancers is only 59%, the result of most cases being diagnosed at later stages.[1]

Other head and neck cancers occur in the nasopharynx (2%), hypopharynx (rare), and salivary glands (3% to 5%).[1,2] Cancers of the nasopharynx are often seen in peoples of Asian or North African descent. Nasopharyngeal cancer (NPC) represents 18% of all cancers in southern China.[2]

Etiology and Risk Factors

The number-one risk factor for head and neck cancer is tobacco. Smokers are 6 times more likely to have cancer of the head and neck than nonsmokers.[1,2,4] This includes users of cigarettes, cigars, and pipes and is associated with cancers of the oral cavity, oropharynx, and larynx, as well as cancers of the paranasal sinuses and nasal cavity. Tobacco has such a strong carcinogenic effect in the head and neck region that 15% of patients are seen with a second cancer in the same anatomic area, and 10% to 40% will develop a second primary site in another region of the head and neck.[5]

The use of oral or "smokeless" tobacco is strongly linked with cancers of the oral cavity. The risk may be as much as 50 times higher in those individuals who use these products than for those who do not, and the risk increases with the amount of tobacco and the length of time it is used.[5,6]

Alcohol is an important promoter of carcinogenesis and is believed to contribute to the development of 75% of head and neck cancers, particularly in those who drink alcohol heavily in combination with tobacco use.[1,5] People who drink alcohol but do not use tobacco are still at higher risk if their drinking is excessive, though it is the synergistic effect of alcohol and tobacco combined that is of greater concern.[1]

Additional controllable risk factors for head and neck cancers are specific to the site of the cancer. See Table 12-1 for site-specific risk factors. Poor oral hygiene and mechanical irritation are considered risk factors for cancers of the oral cavity. Certain occupational exposures, such as wood, nickel, and leather dusts, are risk factors for nasopharyngeal (NPC) and paranasal sinus cancers. Ingestion of certain preservatives and salty foods increases the risk for NPC, as does the presence of the Epstein-Barr virus. The human papilloma virus (HPV) is considered a risk factor for cancer of the larynx and the oropharynx, as is gastroesophageal reflux disease, or GERD. Sun is considered a significant risk factor for cancer of the lip, and asbestos exposure increases a person's risk of laryngeal cancer. The only proven risk factor for the development of cancers of the salivary gland is radiation exposure.[4-7]

It is not possible to control all risk factors. NPC is more common in the Asian population,[7] and African Americans have 50% more cancers of the head and neck than do Caucasians.[8] Overall, males are 3 times more likely to develop a cancer of the head and neck.[1] Although cancer of the hypopharynx is rare, individuals with Plummer-Vinson syndrome are at increased risk.[5-7]

Prevention

The primary prevention techniques directed toward head and neck cancers are related to education about the dangers of tobacco use. The American Cancer Society (ACS) and other organizations have recognized this and offer educational programs addressing tobacco use. The American Academy of Otolaryngology-Head and Neck Surgery strongly emphasizes the dangers of smokeless tobacco, and the Society of Otorhinolaryngology and Head-Neck Nurses has committed time and resources to a nationwide effort to educate our nation's young people about this issue and to provide information to assist nurses in addressing the issue, as well.[9] Although tobacco cessation is extremely challenging, studies have shown that patients with head and neck cancer who continue to smoke during diagnosis and treatment have a higher risk of recurrence and/or treatment failure.[10]

Combating excessive alcohol consumption is of prime importance in any program focusing on the prevention of head and neck cancer. Again, education is focused toward youth and regards outcomes and risk factors of tobacco and heavy alcohol consumption; this education should begin at an early age.[11]

The primary nursing roles in the prevention of head and neck cancer are assessment and education. Nurses must ask pertinent questions during health assessments and address the findings. Emphasis on the importance of routine medical exams, with age-appropriate screening, and knowledge of the signs and symptoms to report are essential. Patients who report tobacco use should be offered information about tobacco cessation; and nurses should be aware of the programs available in their areas. An accurate assessment of alcohol consumption and the educational resources available for reduction or cessation of alcohol use are important.

Screening and Detection

There has been a great deal of controversy regarding cancer screening recommendations for head and neck cancer, since there is insufficient evidence to support a screening program for asymptomatic persons.[12] Despite this, the ACS recommends making an oral exam part of any cancer-related exam.[11] It is unlikely that screening for laryngeal cancer will become a standard part of an exam, since this requires an invasive procedure. Emphasis should be placed on teaching health care professionals and the public about the early signs and symptoms of head and neck cancer and the importance of regular dental examinations.

Screening for head and neck cancer includes a thorough physical exam, with an intraoral exam involving both visualization and palpation of the structures within the oral cavity, including the tongue.[1] Flexible fiberoptic laryngoscopy, a more invasive exam, enables visualization of the pharynx, the larynx, and the subglottis. The patient is awake, and the exam requires only topical anesthetic.[13] Though extremely helpful in patients with suspected lesions in this area, this exam is generally done by a specialist and is unlikely to be performed for routine screening in asymptomatic subjects unless multiple risk factors are present.

Clinical manifestations of head and neck cancer are related to changes in function caused by injury to the involved tissues.[2] Patients may report that symptoms have been present for some time. Therefore, many head and neck cancers are not diagnosed until they are in an advanced stage.[1,2,4]

Symptoms are related to the location of the tumor. Symptoms considered to be "red flags" for any cancer which should be investigated immediately include an unexpected/unexplained weight loss and a persistent lump or mass.[1,2] Symptoms specific to the head and neck are persistent earache, blood-tinged sputum, difficulty swallowing, hoarseness, and a unilateral lump in the neck.[1,2,5] See Table 12-2 for site-specific signs and symptoms.

Classification

Carcinomas arising in the head and neck region are classified according to *anatomic regions* rather than cell type. The regions

TABLE 12-1   Risk Factors for Head and Neck Cancer by Site

Oral cavity	Tobacco, alcohol, HPV, gender, betel nuts
Lip	Sun exposure
Oropharynx	Poor oral hygiene, mechanical irritation, HPV, betel nuts
Larynx	Tobacco, alcohol, asbestos, GERD, HPV
Nasopharynx/ nasal cavity	Ethnicity (Asian), occupational exposure (leather, wood, nickel), preservatives, EBV
Salivary gland	Radiation exposure
Hypopharynx	Plummer-Vinson syndrome

EBV, Epstein-Barr virus; *GERD,* gastroesophageal reflux disease; *HPV,* human papilloma virus.
Data from National Cancer Institute: Head and neck cancer: questions and answers, retrieved December 5, 2005, from http://www.cancer.gov/cancertopics/factsheet/Sites-Types/head-and-neck; Carr, E. Nursing care of the client with head and neck cancer. In Itano, JK and Taoka, KN editors: *Core curriculum for oncology nursing,* ed 4, St. Louis, 2005, Saunders.

TABLE 12-2   Major Subdivisions of Aerodigestive Tract

SITE	FUNCTION	ANATOMIC RELATIONSHIP	CLINICAL FEATURES OF CANCERS
Oral cavity	Maintain oral competency for swallowing, articulation	Sensory motor innervation of tongue is bilateral; central chamber of salivary system; sensory innervation mediated by lingual nerve (V); motor innervation to muscles by hypoglossal nerve (XII) Lymphatic drainage to submaxillary and upper cervical lymph nodes and retropharyngeal lymph nodes	*Early symptoms:* painless "white spot," persistent ulcerations, difficulty with denture fit, difficulty swallowing, blood-tinged sputum
Oropharynx	Mouth and pharynx perform together in alimentary functions of swallowing and emesis, and respiratory functions of crying, speaking, coughing, and yawning	Boundaries include soft palate, tonsils, tonsillar fossa, and base of tongue; glossopharyngeal nerve (IX) mediates motor and sensory innervation to pharynx and posterior one third of tongue; soft palate and pharynx innervated by vagus nerve (X) Lymphatic drainage to jugulodigastric (tonsillar) node and retropharyngeal lymph nodes	Irregular ulcerations of mucosal surfaces, painless growth, dysphagia, pain on swallowing, otalgia, persistent sore throat *Late symptoms:* speech difficulties, palatal incompetence with resultant nasal regurgitation, dysphagia with or without aspiration, trismus
Nasal cavity	Conditions affecting inspired air before entrance: olfaction humidification, temperature control, cleansing, and antibacterial and antiviral protection	First cranial nerve (olfactory) innervates mucous membranes to mediate sense of smell Drainage into submandibular nodes	Similar to chronic sinusitis

TABLE 12-2	Major Subdivisions of Aerodigestive Tract—cont'd		
SITE	**FUNCTION**	**ANATOMIC RELATIONSHIP**	**CLINICAL FEATURES OF CANCERS**
Nasopharynx	Anatomic boundary that lies behind nasal cavities and above soft palate	Open space situated just below base of skull behind nasal cavity; inferior wall bordered by soft palate, pharyngeal orifice of eustachian tube, abducens nerve (VI), oculomotor nerve (III), trochlear nerve (IV), and optic nerve (II) Behind eustachian tube lies internal carotid artery; internal jugular vein; and glossopharyngeal (IX), vagus (X), spinal accessory (X), and hypoglossal (XII) nerves Lymph node chain that drains these areas: posterior cervical triangles, supraclavicular nodes, and jugular chain	Persistent, poorly localized frontal headaches; temporal, parietal, and orificial pain; decreased hearing, tinnitus; multiple nerve palsies, sensory losses Blood in postnasal drip very significant Profuse epistaxis an infrequent presenting symptom
Paranasal sinuses	Air-filled cavities within bones of skull lined by mucous membranes that drain into nasal cavities	Four pairs of maxillary, ethmoid, and frontal sphenoid tumors drain into submaxillary, retropharyngeal, and jugular lymph nodes	Chronic sinusitis, bump on hard palate, swelling, numbness and/or pain of cheek, swelling gums, toothache, increased lacrimation Visual changes: diplopia and exophthalmos Persistent unilateral rhinorrhea: epistaxis
Hypopharynx	Anatomic boundary extending from tip of epiglottis to lower border of cricoid cartilage Structures important for swallowing and airway protection	Lower subdivision of oropharynx, also called laryngopharynx, divided into pyriform sinuses and posterior cricoid area; posterior and lateral pharyngeal walls Pharyngeal constrictions innervated by glossopharyngeal (IX) and vagus (X) nerves Lymphatic drainage: primary along internal jugular vein and retropharyngeal and paratracheal nodes	Painless, enlarged cervical lymph nodes; odynophagia accompanied with progressive dysphagia and rapid weight loss Otalgia on same side of tumor Hoarseness, dysphagia
Larynx	Serves for speech production, maintenance of airway, and airway protection	Located directly below hypopharynx; sensory innervation supplied from internal laryngeal branch of superior laryngeal nerve of vagus and recurrent laryngeal nerve Divided into three anatomic sites: (1) supraglottic, (2) glottic, and (3) subglottic Lymph drainage to anterior jugular nodes	Persistent hoarseness, change in quality and pitch of voice, pain, hemoptysis, dysphagia, cough, aspiration
Salivary glands	Production of saliva	Divided into major glands: paired parotid, submandibular, sublingual, and minor salivary glands Lymphatic drainage usually to deep jugular or intraglandular or paraglandular lymph nodes; innervation of this area includes mandibular branch of seventh cranial, lingual, and hypoglossal (XII) nerves	Painless, rapidly growing mass with or without associated nerve paralysis
Thyroid gland	Endocrine gland	Highly vascular gland located in anterior and lower part of neck; composed of small central part, isthmus, and two lobes; isthmus covers second, third, and fourth tracheal rings; thyroid related medially to esophagus and recurrent laryngeal nerve and laterally to carotid sheath, containing carotid artery; internal jugular vein and vagus nerve Lymphatic drainage of thyroid gland mainly through lymphatic vessels that accompany arterial blood supply	Neck pain, tightness or fullness in neck, hoarseness, dysphagia, dyspnea

include (1) oral cavity, (2) oropharynx, (3) nasal cavity, (4) naso-pharynx, (5) paranasal sinuses, (6) hypopharynx, (7) larynx, and (8) salivary glands. These regions are subdivided into specific sites (Fig.12-1 and Table 12-2). The tumor characteristics, therapeutic management, and prognosis may differ depending on the disease's natural history, the sites of metastases, and the biologic behavior of the disease.[14]

Clinical Features

More than 90% of head and neck cancers are squamous cell in origin,[1,5] and although grading of the tumor cells is part of a routine pathology review, this system has not proven helpful in determining prognosis in head and neck cancers. Multiple cell types can be seen in salivary gland tumors. In fact, salivary gland tumors represent the most heterogenous group of tumors of any tissue in the body. Four types of cancer cells are most commonly seen in the salivary gland: mucoepidermoid carcinoma, adenoid cystic carcinoma, acinic cell carcinoma, and adenocarcinoma.[5] In addition, a multitude of rare cell types are seen in benign salivary gland tumors.

Diagnosis

Optimal treatment and patient survival require accurate identification of the primary tumor, local and regional spread and invasiveness, distant metastasis, and synchronous second primaries. After a complete review of systems and medical and surgical histories, patients should undergo a thorough head and neck examination using a mirror for indirect laryngoscopy, a fiberoptic nasopharyngolaryngoscope, as well as a thorough visual exam and bimanual palpation. Endoscopic evaluation should include the nasopharynx, the oropharynx, the hypopharynx, the larynx, and the upper esophagus, and should also be followed by a chest x-ray and barium swallow.[1] In patients who first complain of a suspicious mass or lump in the neck, a thorough exam often reveals the primary lesion.[1] Radiologic examinations may also include computed tomography (CT), magnetic resonance imaging (MRI), and positron emission tomography (PET).[1] Ideally, all radiographic studies should be completed before obtaining biopsies. The biopsy process can alter the mucosa and bone detail and may cause misinterpretation of films. Direct laryngoscopy with multiple biopsies performed under general anesthesia is the definitive diagnostic and staging procedure.[1] Fine-needle aspiration (FNA) of any suspicious node is performed if no obvious primary is identified. Because open biopsy may jeopardize curative therapy, it is a last resort, used if radiologic studies and FNA fail to identify a primary site or histopathology.[14] An essential element in head and neck staging is the physician's documentation, including a precise diagram and written description of the extent of disease, to provide all consulting disciplines with accurate data.

Staging

Head and neck cancer is staged based on anatomic location and uses the criteria established by the American Joint Committee on Cancer (AJCC).[15] This system contains staging guidelines for lip and oral cavity, pharynx, larynx, nasal cavity and paranasal sinuses, and major salivary gland cancers (Box 12-1).[1,2,15] This staging system has three components: tumor size (T), lymph node involvement (N), and metastatic spread (M). See Table 12-3 for criteria related to staging for laryngeal cancer. The latest updates to the AJCC staging system (2002) include distinctions among larger tumors (stage IV), those considered resectable, and nonresectable.[15] This information can be important when evaluating a patient's response to treatment, especially in a research environment.[1]

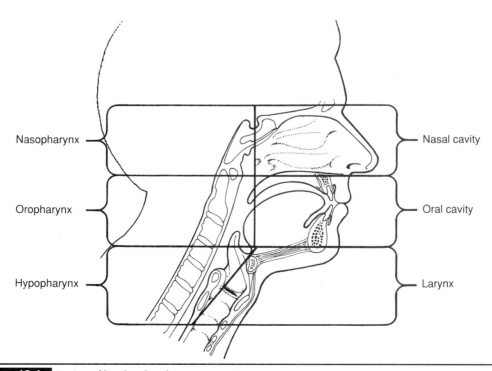

Nasopharynx

Oropharynx

Hypopharynx

Nasal cavity

Oral cavity

Larynx

FIG. 12-1 Region of head and neck.

Information Needed for Staging Head and Neck Tumors

Facts about Tumor
Exact location
Histologic type
Estimated degree of local invasion
Cytologic grade
Involvement of other structures

Local Lymph Node Involvement
Location of all suspicious nodes (unilateral and/or bilateral)
Size
Firmness
Presence of extracapsular spread

Distant Metastasis
Organ system involved
Degree of tumor replacement

Presence or Absence of Second Cancer

TABLE 12-3   ### Staging for Laryngeal Cancer

Stage 0	Tis	N0	M0
Stage I	T1	N0	M0
Stage II	T2	N0	M0
Stage III	T3	N0	M0
	T1	N1	M0
	T2	N1	M0
	T3	N1	M0
Stage IVA	T4a	N0	M0
	T4a	N1	M0
	T1	N2	M0
	T2	N2	M0
	T3	N2	M0
	T4a	N2	M0
Stage IVB	T4b	Any N	M0
	Any T	N3	M0
Stage IVB	Any T	Any N	M1

Data from AJCC: *Cancer Staging Handbook*, ed 6, New York, 2002 Springer.

PROGNOSTIC INDICATORS

Accurate documentation of *disease stage at time of diagnosis* is of primary importance when discussing the prognosis of head and neck cancers. Prognosis is based on tumor site, location, regional lymph node involvement, vascularity, perineural invasion, and distant metastatic disease.[1,2] Prognosis can vary by anatomic site.

In **cancer of the lip and oral cavity,** the presence of a positive margin during surgical resection or a tumor depth greater than 5 mm significantly increases the risk of local recurrence. However, if the cancers are first seen in the early stages (I or II), the cure rate is 90% to 100%.[16] **Oropharyngeal cancer,** which encompasses the base of the tongue, the tonsillar region, the soft palate, or the pharyngeal walls, often is first seen at later stages.

Again, lymph node involvement and large tumor size suggests a potentially poorer outcome.[17]

The most important prognostic factor for **laryngeal cancer** is also tumor size and nodal involvement; patients with smaller, earlier-stage cancers (no lymph node involvement) have more than a 75% cure rate, depending upon site, tumor burden, and degree of infiltration.[18] Patients with large, locally advanced disease and clinically involved lymph nodes have a much poorer prognosis and a greater risk of distant metastasis, even when local disease is controlled.[18]

Major prognostic factors for **nasopharyngeal cancer** include large tumor burden and the presence of involved lymph nodes in the neck. With treatment, patients with small lesions of the nasopharynx have shown survival rates of 80% to 90%. However, survival rate drops to less than 50% for patients with advanced lesions, especially those with clinically positive cervical lymph nodes.[19] These cancers are often associated with a poorer prognosis related to early perineural and skull base invasion.[2]

RECURRENCE AND METASTASIS

Cancers of the head and neck have a high rate of local recurrence and the development of second primary tumors in the head and neck, the esophagus, and/or the lung.[1,5] There is a high incidence of regional spread to lymph nodes at diagnosis, and nodal involvement in the neck can be predicted according to the anatomic location of the tumor (see Fig 12-2).[2] The frequency of distant metastasis varies in the literature, ranging from 4% to 26% in the clinical setting, and 37% to 57% in autopsy findings.[20] **Distant metastasis** is diagnosed when a head and neck cancer is found to have spread below the clavicle and is found in the lymph nodes, such as mediastinal nodes, or in distant organs. The most common sites for **distant organ metastases** are the lungs, the liver, and bone.[20]

Complications of local disease and/or disease recurrence are related to tumor location in the head and neck. As a general rule, lymph node involvement in the upper neck is less ominous than involvement of nodes in the lower neck.[2] Over 25% of patients with **laryngeal cancer** have lymph node involvement when they are first seen for treatment, and these patients are at highest risk for recurrence in the first 2 to 3 years following treatment.[18] In patients with cancer of the hypopharynx, 50% are first seen with cervical lymph node involvement, and 25% have a second primary.[21] **Cancers of the hypopharynx** have a higher rate of distant metastases at diagnosis (17% to 24%) than for all other head and neck cancers (11%).[22] Patients with **tumors of the nasal cavity and paranasal sinuses** often arrive for treatment at advanced stages, and these may recur rapidly after treatment. The tumors can spread directly into the skull, leading to a 5-year survival rate of less than 50%.[23]

When patients are seen with recurrent or metastatic disease, the focus of care shifts from cure to comfort. Health care providers use different prognostic indicators to determine this (Box 12-2). Recurrent and/or metastatic disease is not necessarily an indication to stop treatment, but providers consider the patient's overall status when discussing further treatment options. Factors for review include tumor burden, length of disease-free interval, major organ function, and response to previous treatment.[14] Each of these are examined in the context of the patient's performance status, as well as the quality of life (QOL) desired by the patient. The presence of bony metastases and cutaneous metastases, and

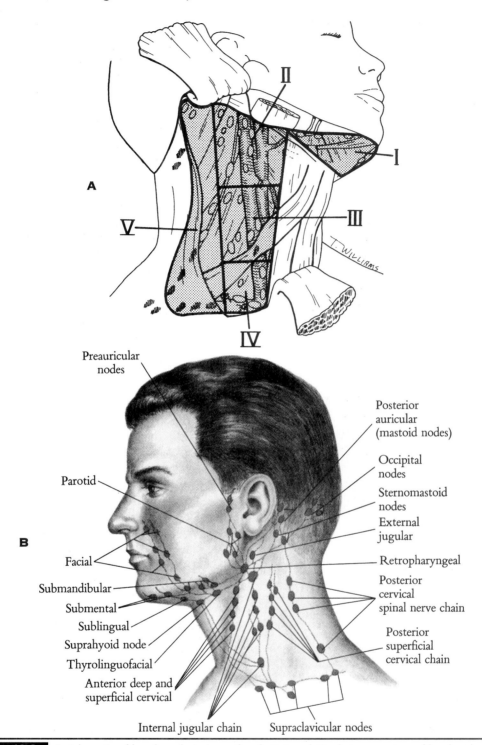

FIG. 12-2   **A,** Schematic of lymph node regions of neck. **B,** Lymphatic drainage system of head and neck. (**A** from Cummings CW et al, editors: *Otolaryngology–Head and neck surgery,* ed 3, St. Louis, 1999, Mosby; **B** from Seidel HM et al: *Mosby's guide to physical examination,* ed 3, St. Louis, 1995, Mosby.)

the failure of radiotherapy and/or adjuvant chemotherapy are poor prognostic factors.[24]

Treatment Modalities

SURGERY

Surgery and radiation remain the primary treatments for head and neck cancer.[7] See Table 12-4 for comparison of treatment options.

For early disease (stages I and II), surgery is often the primary therapy of choice. Depending upon tumor location and the potential for functional impairment, primary radiation therapy may be used. The treatment of advanced disease (stages III and IV) usually requires multimodality therapy.

The choice of surgical treatment for squamous cell carcinomas (SCC) of the head and neck is dictated by the anticipated functional and cosmetic results, as well as the availability of a skilled

BOX 12-2 **Prognostic Factors in Recurrent and Systemic Head and Neck Cancer**

Good Prognostic Factors

Good performance status
Minimal disease
Local recurrence only
No bony erosion
Good response to induction (adjuvant) chemotherapy
Good response to previous chemotherapy
Long disease-free interval
First-line chemotherapy
Good organ function
Complete response to chemotherapy

Poor Prognostic Factors

Poor performance status
Bulky disease
Systemic and/or visceral disease
Bone metastasis and/or hypercalcemia (and local bone invasion)
Lymphangitic spread (skin)
Failure of radiotherapy (persistent disease)
Failure of induction (adjuvant) chemotherapy
Patients receiving first-line chemotherapy for recurrent and/or systemic cancer
Organ impairment
Less than complete response to chemotherapy

Modified from Al-Sarraf M: Head and neck cancer: chemotherapy concepts, *Semin Oncol* 15(1):70, 1988.

surgical oncologist and/or reconstructive surgeon.[5] Surgical considerations include adequate removal of the disease, preservation of cosmesis, and functionality related to speech, chewing, and swallowing.[1,9]

Mohs Surgery. Mohs surgery, also known as Mohs micrographic surgery (MMS), is an advanced treatment procedure for skin cancer used primarily to treat basal and squamous cell carcinoma.[25-27] It is used in areas where function or cosmesis is important, such as the nose, the ears, the lips and the eyelids. MMS is also a surgical option for treatment of small skin cancers in the head and neck region. MMS is performed by highly specialized surgeons trained in dermatology, pathology, and the reconstructive techniques commonly used after the Mohs procedure.[26]

MMS is performed using local anesthesia and involves taking small slices of tissue that are immediately reviewed microscopically. The surgeon continues to remove slices until cancer cells are no longer visible during microscopic examination. This procedure reduces the amount of normal tissue removed, allowing a more favorable cosmetic result.[6] After all tumor cells are removed, the surgeon will individualize the plan for wound closure. with sutures, a skin graft, or a flap.[26]

Nursing management for these patients begins with a complete preoperative assessment including clotting parameters, and medications, particularly aspirin, nonsteroidal medications, or warfarin, which are often discontinued for several days before the procedure. A complete history and assessment including whether the patient has a pacemaker, prosthetic valves or joints, heart murmurs, or mitral valve prolapse would necessitate discussion with the surgeon and possible prophylactic antibiotic treatment. Inquiry regarding drug allergies should include information regarding topical antibiotic use, which could affect what is prescribed as postoperative wound care.[26] For patients with certain medical conditions such as severe hypertension, heart failure, or dysrhythmias avoid the use of lidocaine with epinephrine, when possible.[25] The nurse should also be aware that only hand-held electrocautery is recommended in patients with pace makers and/or implanted defibrillators.[25]

TABLE 12-4 **Advantages and Disadvantages of Treatments for Head and Neck Cancers**

MODALITY	ADVANTAGES	DISADVANTAGES
Surgery	Ability to remove central-resistant hypoxic tumor cells Immediate reconstruction Provides most accurate estimate of disease extent No carcinogenic effect No biologic resistance by tumor	Potential for structural, functional, or cosmetic loss Only provides local and regional treatment May leave behind viable malignant tissue Must sacrifice some healthy tissue to excise malignancy effectively
Radiation therapy	Curative if disease is small and localized Acute side effects generally disappear after treatment Limited residual deformity or functional loss (in most patients) Focused delivery of tumoricidal dose	Time consuming Not effective as single treatment for large tumors Potential long-term sequelae: soft tissue damage May have carcinogenic effects Some tumors radioresistant
Chemotherapy and/or biologic therapy	Potential chemopreventive systemic treatment for killing lymphatic and hematogenous metastasis Minimal residual deformity or loss of function	Limiting factors: normal tissue tolerance and tumor responsiveness

The postoperative care is physician-specific. Most surgeons recommend a pressure dressing for 24 to 48 hours, daily cleansing of the wound with saline, and application of a topical antibiotic ointment or cream.[25] Patients need to be instructed to immediately report bleeding, elevated temperature, erythema, or purulent discharge from the wound.

Neck Dissection Neck dissection refers to the removal of cervical lymph nodes of various levels in the neck (Fig. 12-2), and was first performed in 1906 in an effort to manage metastatic head and neck cancer.[27] The original surgical procedure has been modified many times, leading to the development of a classification system for neck dissections by the American Head and Neck Society and the Committee for Head and Neck Surgery and Oncology of the American Academy of Otolaryngology.

This classification system was initiated in 1991 and revised in 2002.[27] Table 12-5 details various neck dissection procedures.

A **radical neck dissection (RND)** involves the removal of all ipsilateral (same-side) cervical lymph nodes, levels I-V, the spinal accessory nerve (SAN), the internal jugular vein, the submandibular gland, and the sternocleidomastoid muscle (SCM). Indications for this procedure include (1) multiple lymph node metastases in an untreated patient; (2) a patient who has been previously treated with surgery, radiation, and/or chemotherapy; and (3) one or more clinically positive lymph nodes with extracapsular spread involving the SAN and the internal jugular vein.[4]

The radical neck procedure results in significant functional and cosmetic deformity, primarily because of the removal of the SCM and the SAN.[28] The SCM normally provides contour to the neck on

TABLE 12-5 Neck Dissection Procedures

PROCEDURE	STRUCTURES REMOVED	ADVANTAGES	DISADVANTAGES
Radical neck dissection	En bloc removal of nodal regions I to VI and all lymph node-bearing tissues on one side of neck, superficial and deep fascia, sternocleidomastoid muscle, omohyoid muscle, submandibular gland, tail of parotid gland, internal and external jugular veins, connective tissue of carotid sheath, transverse cervical vessels, spinal accessory nerve, greater auricular nerve, cutaneous branches of the cervical plexus; excision may also include external carotid artery, portion of digastric muscle, branches of vagus nerve, and hypoglossal nerve	Low probability of leaving nodal disease behind	Trapezius muscle dysfunction with shoulder drop, resulting in pain and limitation in motion Mild to moderate neck deformity If bilateral procedure is performed, cerebral edema may persist Painful neuromas may occur Loss of carotid artery
Modified radical neck dissection	Unilateral removal of nodal regions I to V with preservation of spinal accessory nerve and internal jugular and/or sternocleidomastoid muscle	Low incidence of shoulder drop and shoulder disability Carotid artery not sacrificed Cosmetic deformity not as severe as with comprehensive neck dissection If cervical plexus preserved, decreased incidence of sensory deficit and painful neuromas	Possible omission of occult positive nodes Increased risk of hematoma under sternocleidomastoid muscle Increased risk of surgeon cutting into positive nodes and seeding neck Increased difficulty in performing secondary procedure and if disease recurs
Type I	Spinal accessory nerve preserved		
Type II	Spinal accessory nerve and internal jugular preserved		
Type III (functional or Bocca) neck dissection	Spinal accessory nerve, internal jugular, and sternocleidomastoid preserved		
Selective neck dissection	Spinal accessory, internal jugular, and sternocleidomastoid muscles preserved	Same as for modified neck dissection, plus improved lymphatic drainage because selected lymph node groups retained	Increased possibility of cutting into or omitting occult positive nodes

TABLE 12-5	Neck Dissection Procedures—cont'd		
PROCEDURE	**STRUCTURES REMOVED**	**ADVANTAGES**	**DISADVANTAGES**
Lateral neck dissection	En bloc removal of nodal regions II, III, and IV		
Anterolateral neck dissection	Supraomohyoid neck dissection: en bloc removal of nodal regions II, III, and IV Expanded supraomohyoid neck dissection: en bloc removal of nodal regions I, II, III, and IV		
Posterolateral neck dissection	Removal of suboccipital and retroauricular lymph node groups and nodal regions II, III, IV, and V		
Extended neck dissection	Any neck dissection extended to include lymph node groups not usually removed or structures not routinely removed (e.g., carotid artery, levator scapular muscle)	Lower probability of leaving occult disease behind	Increased risk of cerebrovascular accident (stroke) if carotid is resected Increased risk of shoulder dysfunction if levator scapular muscle excised

Data from Robbins KT: Neck dissection. In Cummings CW and others, editors: *Otolaryngology–Head and neck surgery*, ed 3, St. Louis, 1999, Mosby.

the affected side, whereas the absence of the SAN results in limited mobility, specifically range of motion to the shoulder. Patients undergoing this procedure often face chronic pain, decreased shoulder function, and shoulder droop on the affected side. [6,27,28]

Nursing intervention for these patients includes education regarding incision care and the need to care for a wound drainage system (Jackson Pratt) at home, care of the patient while hospitalized, and home care instructions, which will vary according to institutional standards and physician preferences. Patients with neck dissection require physical therapy education regarding exercises to strengthen and maintain shoulder function on the affected side, and range of motion exercises for the neck (Fig. 12-3). Patients who have had radical neck procedures experience changes in self-image as a result of the affected side of the neck appearing concave and noticeably different from the unaffected side. Most patients will have a permanent shoulder droop and chronic pain. Nurses must emphasize the importance of following the exercise and/or physical therapy plan and the timely reporting of any changes to the health care provider. [29]

Modified neck dissection differs from a radical neck dissection in the amount of tissue removed, which depends upon the size and extent of disease found in the neck. [6] This procedure is designed to preserve the SCM, the great auricular nerve, and the SAN. All five levels of lymph nodes are removed, though great care is taken to prevent the loss of the jugular vein and other structures affected by a radical neck dissection. [29]

A **selective neck dissection** refers to the dissection of "select" groups of lymph nodes based on the spread of disease to the neck and the location of the primary tumor. Removal of levels 1, 2, and 3 constitute a supraomohyoid neck dissection; levels 2, 3, and 4 an anterior neck dissection; and levels 2 through 5 an anterolateral neck dissection. [28,29] These procedures have proven to be as effective as an RND for patients with early disease without known involvement in the neck. However, the finding of even one positive node in the neck greatly increases the likelihood of another, unexpected node. [29] This requires careful consideration

by the surgeon and the rest of the oncology team in determining the appropriate procedure for each patient and what, if any, follow-up treatment (radiation, chemotherapy) is needed.

Total Laryngectomy. A **total laryngectomy** includes the removal of the entire larynx, as well as the hyoid bone, the true vocal cords (or vocal folds), the false vocal cords (or vestibular folds), the epiglottis, the cricoid cartilage, and two to three tracheal rings. [30] This surgery is most often performed for advanced laryngeal cancers, often in conjunction with radiation therapy. [28] It is also indicated for extensive glottic carcinomas, subglottic tumors, and extensive tumors of the base of the tongue that invade the larynx. [28] Table 12-6 details the structures affected or removed during laryngectomy surgeries.

A total laryngectomy results in the loss of voice (aphonia) and a permanent tracheostomy, where the trachea is sutured to the anterior wall of the neck, creating a permanent opening for breathing. [28,30] The upper aerodigestive tract (nose and mouth) can no longer take in air, resulting in the loss of ability to warm, filter, and humidify air. The patient loses the ability to sneeze and blow the nose; also the sense of smell is lost, which causes a decrease in the sense of taste. [28,31]

This also permanently separates the patient's airway from the digestive tract, and patients are able to swallow without risk of aspiration. Initially, however, patients may receive nutrition through a feeding tube (a nasogastric tube or a gastrostomy tube), until the surgical incisions heal sufficiently to prevent any leakage of saliva or food; this is used in particular with patients who have been previously treated with radiation to the surgical field. The risk for fistula formation, wound infection, and/or wound breakdown is much greater in patients who have received previous radiation therapy to the surgical field. [31]

Nursing care for patients undergoing a total laryngectomy begins before surgery with comprehensive patient education about the procedure itself and postoperative expectations. Education should include family and significant others. Postoperatively, maintaining a patent airway is a priority. The head of the bed

The following exercises have been developed to increase the movement and strength in your neck, arms, and shoulders.

Neck Range of Motion

1. Bring chin to chest in a relaxed way and then let it fall gently backwards so a stretch on the neck muscles is felt.
2. Slowly turn head as far as possible to one side as if attempting to look over that shoulder. Do the same to the other side.
3. Bend the head toward the shoulder on the unaffected side. A stretching will be felt on the operated side.

Shoulder Mobility

1. Standing with shoulders relaxed and head facing forward, let arm on the affected side hang freely. Make circles with the shoulder by moving it:
   a) forward
   b) upward
   c) backward
   d) downward
2. With a wand or cane in front of body and shoulders and arms relaxed, raise wand as high as possible keeping elbows extended. After you are able to raise it directly overhead, slowly lower it behind the neck. Raise wand overhead and return it to starting position.
3. Stand facing a wall with your feet a few inches from it. Slide the hand on your affected side up the wall as far as possible, using the wall for support. Perform the same exercise with your affected side facing the wall. Repeat the motion of sliding your hand up the wall but do not turn your body when doing this exercise.

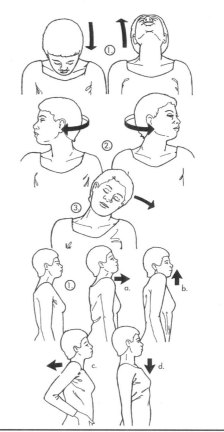

FIG. 12-3 Exercises after neck dissection. (From Sigler BA, Schuring LT: *Ear, nose, and throat disorders,* St. Louis, 1993, Mosby.)

remains elevated, and patients are observed closely for any signs of respiratory distress such as restlessness and agitation or diminished air exchange from the laryngectomy tube. Patients are also assessed for signs of wound infection. Education about stoma and wound care should begin early in the postoperative period so the patient and family are performing these activities independently before discharge. After laryngectomy, patients are instructed to cover their stoma when coughing, rather than their nose, and about the use of humidification to help maintain some moisture in the airway.[14]

Following laryngectomy, patients cannot generate the pressure to perform a Valsalva maneuver. This change, combined with the use of narcotic analgesics and postoperative changes in oral intake, can result in constipation. All laryngectomy patients need a bowel management program to prevent ongoing problems.[31]

The laryngectomy patient may need enteral nutrition support for several days to weeks postoperatively, as well as education regarding the use of the tube, flushing techniques and schedules, medication administration, and insertion site care. Working with a dietician ensures that patients will receive the appropriate caloric and nutritional formula for their needs and to promote wound healing. Patients and families should receive written instructions indicating situations that require immediate intervention.

Special instructions for bathing and the need to keep water from splashing into the stoma are essential; as well as the avoidance of any water sports (e.g., swimming and boating), since they no longer have the ability to seal their airway to keep water out.

Voice rehabilitation is a major consideration for any patient undergoing a total laryngectomy, and there are several options available to these patients. These include the use of an electrolarynx,

development of esophageal speech, or using a tracheoesophageal voice puncture (TEP).[28] All laryngectomy patients will need access to writing materials for immediate postoperative communication. Dry erase boards and picture boards are excellent tools for patients during this period. Working closely with a speech pathologist, most patients learn to use an electrolarynx in the immediate postoperative period and may transition to esophageal speech or the use of a TEP.

A surgically created tracheoesophageal fistula is the initial step for TEP (Fig. 12-4).[28] This can be done during the original surgery or as a separate procedure at a later date. During the immediate postoperative period, a red rubber catheter is placed in the new opening. Once the fistula has begun to mature (7 to 10 days), the catheter is replaced with a prosthesis that includes a one-way valve that diverts pulmonary air, causing vibration of the pharyngeal-esophageal wall and resulting in voice production.[28] Most patients consider the sound produced with TEP to be superior to the electrolarynx or esophageal speech.

The psychosocial impact of a laryngectomy is significant. Patients and families need support in the adjustment to this new way of life. Organizations that provide information and support for patients and families include the ACS, the International Association of Laryngectomees (IAL), Support for People with Oral and Head and Neck Cancer (SPOHN), and the Head and Neck Cancer Community, among others.[2]

There are also a variety of surgical procedures referred to as partial laryngectomies. These include cordectomy, vertical partial laryngectomy, supracricoid laryngectomy, and other types of hemilaryngectomies.[28] These were developed in an effort to preserve laryngeal function and voice production in selected

TABLE 12-6   Functional Loss Associated with Laryngectomy

PROCEDURE	STRUCTURES REMOVED	STRUCTURES REMAINING	FUNCTIONS
Total Laryngectomy Loss of laryngeal sphincter mechanism may lead to aspiration. Swallowing mechanism must be intact so that when food lands on vocal cords, patient coughs to remove it and swallows instantly.	Hyoid bone Entire larynx Epiglottis, false and true cords Cricoid cartilage Two to three rings of trachea	Tongue Pharyngeal walls Lower trachea	Loss of voice (resulting from tracheal laryngectomy) Normal swallowing
Partial Supraglottic/Horizontal Laryngectomy During supraglottic laryngectomy, muscles that elevate larynx are transected, thereby limiting elevation of larynx. This, along with loss of supraglottic structures, further downgrades swallowing. Because cough is necessary to clear larynx, patient's pulmonary functions must be adequate.	Hyoid bone Epiglottis False cords	True cords Cricoid cartilage Trachea	Normal voice Increased risk for aspiration Normal airway
Hemivertical Laryngectomy Interferes very little with swallowing. Removal of arytenoid cartilage may cause aspiration in a small percentage of patients. Free or pedicled muscle or submucosal cartilage grafts may prevent aspiration. If surgical resection extends to base of tongue, swallowing may be affected related to inability to move bolus. Aspiration may occur.	One true cord, one false cord Arytenoid cartilage One half of thyroid cartilage	Epiglottis One true cord, one false cord Cricoid	Hoarse but serviceable voice Normal airway Normal swallowing
Partila Laryngectomy/Laryngofissure Procedure may affect predominantly deglutition and phonation.	One vocal cord	All other structures	Hoarse but serviceable voice Normal airway Normal swallowing

patients. The operation selected depends upon the structures, the location, and the extent of disease.

A tracheotomy is performed during the surgery to ensure an adequate airway, since edema of the larynx and the surrounding tissues during the immediate postoperative period is anticipated.[28] The patient may be discharged with a tracheostomy tube still in place, to be removed at a follow-up visit. One problem that can occur following partial laryngectomy is swallowing. The removal of structures such as the epiglottis changes the normal swallowing function and can result in impaired swallowing. Referral to a speech pathologist familiar with head and neck procedures will help ensure a positive outcome. Patients experiencing aspiration can use techniques that will help guide food and liquids into the esophagus, bypassing the airway. These patients are closely monitored for signs of dehydration, poor wound healing, and infection.

Maxillectomy. Squamous cell carcinoma of the maxillary sinus is the most common type of cancer found in the paranasal sinuses.[32] The procedure of choice for patients with antral maxillary sinus tumors is a limited or subtotal maxillectomy, whereas more extensive lesions invading the orbit will necessitate a total maxillectomy and orbital exenteration.[33] The procedure is classified based on the number of maxillary sinus walls resected. A limited maxillectomy indicates that a single antrum wall is removed.

Subtotal maxillectomy refers to a procedure in which at least two walls are removed, and a total maxillectomy includes the removal of the entire maxilla.[34] In addition, a medial maxillectomy involves the en bloc resection of the lateral nasal wall, the ethmoid labyrinth, and the medial portion of the maxilla. This preserves the orbital rim, the eye, and the palate, among other structures.[34]

Patients need preoperative dental consultation to assess the need for an obturator, a prosthetic device resembling an upper denture, to fill any surgical defect and allow the patient to speak and swallow after surgery.[28,33] Dental obturators are removed daily and cleaned, similar to the care required for dentures; the surgical cavity is also cleaned daily. Because of the potential for speech and swallowing difficulties, a speech pathology consultation before surgery and postoperatively is imperative.

Free Flaps. Many head and neck procedures result in significant surgical defects. Removing a malignancy while maintaining or restoring function and appearance is a challenge for the surgical team.[28] In recent years, great advances have been made in the use of microvascular free flaps to reconstruct surgical defects in head and neck surgery patients. The free flap donor site is selected on the defect to be filled, considering both cosmesis and function (Figs. 12-5 and 12-6). A multidisciplinary team including both a head and neck surgeon and a reconstructive surgeon is needed.

An opening (fistula) has been created between the tracheostoma (windpipe) and esophagus (food passage) in order to place a speech valve (prosthesis). Temporarily, a red rubber catheter will stent the fistula open. Once healing has taken place, a speech prosthesis will replace the catheter.

If the Prosthesis Comes Out

1. Insert a red rubber catheter (10, 12, 14 Fr) into fistula approximately 6-8 inches.
2. Tie a knot in the external end of the catheter to prevent passage of stomach contents.
3. Tape external end of catheter to skin of chest.
4. If catheter cannot be inserted, contact your physician or speech therapist immediately. This may indicate closure of the fistula.

Replacing the Prosthesis

1. Remove prosthesis.
2. Cleanse neck and stoma.

3. Using inserter that is supplied with prosthesis, reinsert clean prosthesis into fistula.
4. Tape in place.
5. Clean prosthesis with hydrogen peroxide and water. Rinse well.
6. The voice prosthesis will last from 2 weeks to several months between changes. The length of time a prosthesis remains in place is dependent upon you. If food or fluid leaks around the prosthesis, it should be changed. If leakage continues, contact your speech therapist for a new size or length of prosthesis.

To Use the Prosthesis

1. Cover your stoma with your thumb. This will allow air from your lungs to pass through the opening of the prosthesis into the esophagus. The walls of your throat and the structures in your mouth will form the words for speech.

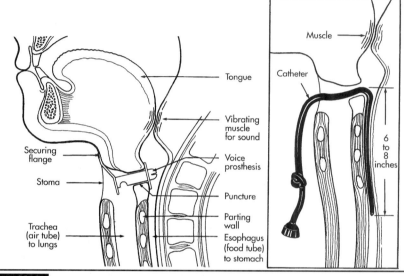

FIG. 12-4 Tongue flap used for reconstruction of lateral oropharynx. (From Genden EM, Thawley SE, O'Leary MJ: Malignant neoplasms of the oropharynx. In Cummings CW et al, editors: *Otolaryngology—Head and neck surgery,* ed 3, St. Louis, 1999, Mosby.)

Careful evaluation of the patient's medical and surgical history, extent of disease, and potential postoperative needs will be conducted before determining appropriate disease management and reconstruction. Common free flap donor sites used in head and neck surgery are the radial forearm, the fibula, and the anteriolateral thigh. Choice is based primarily on the function of the tissue being reconstructed and the size of the defect to be filled (Table 12-7).[28]

Nursing care of the patient with a free flap includes monitoring both the flap surgical site and the donor site. In the immediate postoperative period, the flap is monitored hourly for arterial and venous blood flow, color, temperature, and capillary refill. Slow capillary refill, fullness, and/or changes in color or temperature can indicate problems with the flap and may constitute a surgical emergency.[14]

Patients with reconstructive surgery of the head and neck face issues related to self-image and feelings of loss. Patients are given the opportunity to express their feelings of fear or anxiety; nurses use the multidisciplinary team members to assist patients with these sensitive issues. Patients and family members are referred to support groups, as well.

RADIATION THERAPY

In addition to surgery, radiation therapy remains one of the primary treatments of head and neck cancer. It can be used as a primary treatment for early-stage disease or in conjunction with surgery or chemotherapy. Radiation also has a role in palliative treatment for tumors that are unresectable or for patients with recurrent disease. Treatment planning is based on the location, size, and stage of disease, as well as the patient's general health and comorbid conditions. A multidisciplinary approach is used when planning radiation treatment for patients with head and neck cancer. The patient is seen and evaluated by a surgeon and medical oncologist, as well as the radiation oncologist, to determine the treatment options and the best approach for each individual situation. Once radiation is selected as the treatment of choice, the patient undergoes a pretreatment work-up, including a physical and a dental exam. Any dental caries or other dental problems are best managed before the initiation of radiation therapy. After a patient has received radiation to the head and neck region, any dental work must be done by a practitioner familiar with the long-term effects that radiation has on the teeth, gums, mucosa, and mandible.

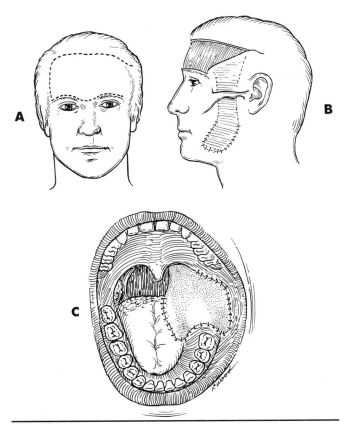

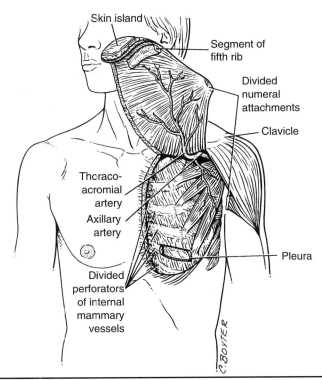

FIG. 12-6 Diagrammatic representation of myocutaneous flap procedure. (From Mathes S, Nahal F: *Clinical applications for muscle and musculocutaneous flaps*, St. Louis, 1982, Mosby.)

FIG. 12-5 **A,** Forehead flap based on superficial temporal artery and portions of occipital artery. **B,** Rotation of forehead flap medial to zygomatic arch for reconstruction of oropharynx. Flap is pulled interiorly to fill resected area. **C,** Completion of forehead flap reconstruction. (From Genden EM, Thawley SE, O'Leary MJ: Malignant neoplasms of the oropharynx. In Cummings CW et al, editors: *Otolaryngology–Head and neck surgery*, ed 3, St. Louis, 1999, Mosby.)

TABLE 12-7	Factors That Affect Surgeon's Choice of Flaps
TISSUE CONSIDERATIONS	**PHYSICIAN CONSIDERATIONS**
Size of arc	Will the flap cover the defect?
Vascular supply	Will the flap survive?
Accessibility	How close to the defect is the new tissue?
Donor site	Functional loss and contour of donor site
Sensation	Maintain nerve supply

There are several methods of radiation therapy used in the treatment of head and neck cancer. The most common are conformal radiotherapy, intensity-modulated radiotherapy (IMRT), and brachytherapy. Conformal therapy and IMRT both involve external beam radiation, also known as teletherapy. In conformal therapy, the patient is treated using a linear accelerator; a beam, or beams, of radiation are directed at the identified site, with shields (called blocks) used to block the radiation from surrounding tissue to some degree. The downside to this type of therapy is a wide range of toxicities to normal tissues such as mucositis, xerostomia, pain, dental complications, and dysphagia.[35] IMRT, on the other hand, is a much more specific form of conformal therapy that allows the physician to design a treatment field around normal structures while still providing an optimal dose of radiation to the tumor and other at-risk areas.[36] Treatment is planned using three-dimensional CT images and computerized dose calculations. The linear accelerator is then programmed to modulate the intensity of the radiation beam to focus the higher dose of radiation on the tumor while greatly minimizing exposure to vital structures such as salivary glands. Most IMRT treatment involves a combination of fields and beam directions to produce a customized treatment for each individual patient.[35]

Brachytherapy involves the placement of a radioactive source into the site. In head and neck cancers, this is usually done intraoperatively by placing catheters close to the tumor itself and then loading in the radioactive material at a later time, usually in 3 to 5 days. There are also radioactive "seeds" that can be implanted into the tissue surrounding the tumor. Whichever method is used, the radiation is released over a period of time based on the half-life of the isotope that is used. Low-dose-rate (LDR) brachytherapy has been used effectively in the treatment of head and neck cancers and has the advantage of delivering more radiation to the tumor while sparing surrounding tissue and critical structures.[36] In recent years, there has been increased interest in the use of high-dose-rate (HDR) brachytherapy for the treatment of head and neck cancers. In 2001, the American Brachytherapy Society (ABS) convened a panel of experts to perform a literature review on HDR for the purpose of making recommendations related to its use in tumors of the head and neck. This panel offered treatment recommendations for the use of HDR and identified areas for further investigation.[36]

Nursing care of the patient undergoing head and neck radiation focuses on symptom management, specifically xerostomia, dysphagia, and pain; related to these are oral hygiene, nutrition, and skin care. Oral hygiene is a key factor for this patient population. Many radiation fields for the treatment of head and neck cancers include at least one major salivary gland, if not more. These glands are adversely affected by the radiation, which changes the production and consistency of the patient's saliva, leading to xerostomia or excessive dryness of the mouth due to the decrease in saliva production. This condition makes it difficult for patients to speak and swallow; over time, this can also lead to dental caries, since saliva regulates the pH of the oral cavity, controlling bacterial flora. The patient's oral cavity is examined at each visit during and after radiation, and the patient is instructed on the use of daily fluoride treatments to help preserve dentition. Patients are also encouraged to carry a bottle of water or some other noncaffeinated liquid with them to help lessen the effects of the xerostomia on speech and swallowing.

In recent years, studies have been conducted testing several agents thought to be radioprotectants. The agent found to be an effective cytoprotectant in head and neck radiation is amifostine. Administration of this drug before radiation has been shown to decrease the radiation-induced toxicity to normal cells in the head and neck region, thus reducing the occurrence of xerostomia. In an open-label phase III randomized trial, it was concluded that daily pretreatment with amifostine reduced the incidence of acute and chronic xerostomia during radiotherapy of the head and neck, while preserving the antitumor effect of the radiation.[37] This study used intravenous (IV) administration of the drug; further studies are being done to compare the efficacy of IV administration to that of subcutaneous administration.

Patients are instructed about the side effects common with amifostine. These include hypotension, nausea and vomiting, and rash. Patients are encouraged to take in several glasses of water or sports drink, either by mouth or gastrostomy tube, on the morning of the injection. They are also encouraged to take extra fluids throughout the day, avoiding caffeine and alcohol. They are monitored during infusion of the drug and afterward for any signs of dehydration or hypotension, as well as any anaphylactic reactions. Prophylactic antiemetics are given before the amifostine, and patients are given a prescription for antiemetics that can be taken at home on an as-needed basis. Nurses administering amifostine assess the patient daily for any adverse reactions. Amifostine should be permanently discontinued for any severe cutaneous reaction, or any cutaneous reaction associated with fever.[38]

Pain is a serious side effect of radiation to the head and neck region. The site of the pain depends upon the area being treated; however, pain is assessed at each visit, and the efficacy of their pain management regimen is also reviewed. Mucositis and skin reactions cause pain in these patients. Pain management includes nonsteroidal antiinflammatory drugs (NSAIDs) and/or, in many cases, narcotics.[39]

Infection is a risk factor in patients receiving oral cavity radiation, which is related to the disruption of the normal balance of bacterial flora present in the mouth. Patients are taught to rinse the mouth frequently with an alkaline solution and to keep mucous membranes moist by adequate hydration. Dental evaluation and repair before treatment are essential.[39]

Laryngeal edema is another potential side effect of radiation therapy to the head and neck.[40] This occurs as the dose of radiation accumulates. Patients who complain of increasing hoarseness are examined for any increasing inflammation. Though voice changes are anticipated with treatment to the larynx, careful assessment is needed to ensure that the patient is not in immediate danger of losing the airway. Steroids can be given to help reduce acute inflammation. Stridor and/or dyspnea may require a tracheostomy. Depending upon the size and location of the mass before treatment, a tracheostomy can also be planned before beginning treatment to prevent an emergent situation.[40]

Nutrition is a key factor in QOL during treatment for head and neck cancer. Weight loss affects as many as 50% of patients with head and neck cancer.[41] Decreased saliva, oral pain, mucositis, and difficulty swallowing all combine to potentially decrease food intake during and after radiation treatment.[42] In recent studies, 50% of patients undergoing radiotherapy for locally advanced head and neck cancer lost more than 10% of body weight, and 6% lost more than 20%.[42] It has also been shown that these patients are often in need of enteral nutritional support, either with a nasogastric tube or a gastrostomy tube. The type of tube selected is based on patient assessment, preference, and length of expected treatment, as well as any preexisting medical factors that may influence the decision. The enteral route is preferred since it allows the patient to maintain the normal function of the gut, as well as having fewer risks and lower costs than parenteral nutrition.[42] Some institutions require gastrostomy tube placement for any patient undergoing concurrent chemotherapy and radiation therapy.[42]

Nutritional assessment before beginning therapy includes height, weight, recent weight loss or gain, and normal eating patterns, as well as any known food allergies or intolerance. The consulting dietician determines the patient's caloric needs during and after treatment, as well as follows the patient's progress through treatment and recommends changes based on the patient's response.

Nurses play a vital role in patient assessment for those receiving radiation for head and neck cancer. Assessment includes pain, skin condition, respiratory status, and nutritional status, as well as signs and symptoms of infection and fatigue. Skin changes in the treatment field are anticipated. The skin will darken to a deep red, and some patients experience desquamation. The desquamation can be moist or dry, moist being more severe and painful. See Table 12-8 for some of the common terminology criteria (CTC) used by the Radiation Therapy Oncology Group (RTOG) when scoring skin reactions during radiotherapy.

Skin care during treatment varies by institution, since there is a lack of empiric evidence regarding choice of topical agents to use for skin reactions.[43] However, there is agreement on basic guidelines for patients to follow. These include using only lukewarm water and a mild soap for cleansing; avoidance of any tight clothing over the area; avoidance of extreme heat or cold to the area, such as hot or cold packs; and not rubbing or scratching the skin in the treatment area.[39] Patients are asked not to apply any moisturizers to the treated skin for 2 hours before their radiation treatment; however, most institutions will recommend the use of a specific lotion or petroleum-based cream for application after treatment each day. Any topical agents containing metal, such as zinc, should be strictly avoided since these can increase the amount of radiation absorbed at the skin level.[43]

Careful dental follow-up is essential for patients undergoing radiation therapy. For those whose oral cavity is included in the treatment field, daily fluoride treatment is prescribed to protect any teeth remaining. Fluoride trays are made for the patient before the initiation of treatment, and instructions are given for use. It is recommended that this treatment be continued for the

TABLE 12-8	**RTOG Scoring for Skin Reactions**					
DERMATOLOGY/SKIN		**GRADE**				
ADVERSE EVENT	***SHORT NAME***	***1***	***2***	***3***	***4***	***5***
Atrophy, subcutaneous fat Also consider: Induration/fibrosis	Same	Detectable	Marked	-	-	-
Bruising (in absence of Grade 3 or 4 thrombocytopenia	Same	Localized in a dependent area	Generalized	-	-	-
Burn Refers to all burns, including radiation and chemical	Same	Minimal symptoms; intervention not indicated	Medical intervention; minimal debridement indicated	Moderate to major debridement or reconstruction indicated	Life-threatening consequences	Death
Hair loss/alopecia	Alopecia	Thinning or patchy	Complete	-	-	-
Hyperpigmentation	Same	Slight or localized	Marked or generalized	-	-	-
Induration/fibrosis (skin and subcutaneous tissue)	Induration	Increased density on palpation	Moderate impairment of function not interfering with ADLs; marked increase in density and firmness on palpation with or without minimal retraction	Dysfunction interfering with ADLs; very marked density, retraction, or fixation	-	-
Rash: dermatitis associated with radiation Select: Chemoradiation Radiation	Dermatitis	Faint erythema or dry desquamation	Moderate to brisk erythema; patchy moist desquamation, mostly confined to skin folds and creases; moderate edema	Moist desquamation other than skin folds and creases; bleeding induced by minor trauma or abrasion	Skin necrosis or ulceration of full-thickness dermis; spontaneous bleeding from involved site	Death

ADLs, Activities of daily living; *RTOG*, Radiation Therapy Oncology Group.
Selected data from the Common Terminology Criteria for Adverse Events (CTCAE v3.0); Used with permission from the National Cancer Institute; retrieved May 14, 2006 from *http://www.cancer.gov.*

patient's lifetime to reduce the incidence of caries and the risk of osteoradionecrosis.

The nurse needs to inform the patient that the majority of acute side effects resolve over time, after the completion of treatment. Education regarding the management of potentially long-term effects, such as xerostomia, trismus, and fibrosis is central to the nurse's role; the nurse should also emphasize continued follow-up with the radiation oncologist or surgeon for management of both short- and long-term side effects and prevention or detection of recurrent disease or a second primary.

CHEMOTHERAPY

The use of chemotherapy in the treatment of head and neck cancer is still evolving. Until recently, chemotherapy was primarily used only in patients with advanced and/or recurrent disease and did not show significant long-term benefit.[44] However, the relatively low 5-year survival rates for patients with locally advanced disease have driven continued research in this area.

Chemotherapy has traditionally been given in one of three ways in the treatment of head and neck cancers: (1) adjuvant postoperative or postradiotherapy; (2) in metastatic disease; or (3) preoperative induction. Various agents and regimens have been used, but the primary agents have been platinum-based. In the 1990s, trials began looking at concurrent chemotherapy and radiotherapy regimens for the patient with head and neck cancer. Now, **postoperative concurrent chemoradiation** with a platinum-based agent is considered standard treatment for locally advanced head and neck cancers.[44] **Adjuvant chemotherapy** for patients with low risk of recurrence is not the standard of care, though it is being evaluated in clinical trials.[2]

Chemoradiation is being studied in the preoperative setting in patients with locally advanced disease, with the goal of tumor regression and, ultimately, organ preservation. Conversely, the increase in acute side effects often experienced with chemoradiation may offset the benefits for some patients.[45] A large number of patients undergoing chemoradiation experience severe mucositis, which may require a break in radiation treatments.[45] In all studies, xerostomia and dysphagia were the most commonly reported side effects; only 50% of patients were able to resume their normal dietary habits after treatment was completed.[45] However, even with the increased incidence of acute side effects, QOL studies have shown that patients treated with chemoradiation that leads to organ preservation have a better QOL than those treated with induction chemotherapy, followed by surgery and radiotherapy alone.[45]

The most commonly used chemotherapy agents for head and neck tumors are platinum-based, such as cisplatin and carboplatin. Historically, the most common regimen has been cisplatin with 5- fluorouracil (5-FU) for three cycles before surgery, with further cycles given after surgery and/or radiation. Cisplatin or carboplatin alone are generally the agents given with radiotherapy in concurrent treatment regimens.[24] Newer agents, such as docetaxel and paclitaxel, are now in clinical trials in combination with the platinum-based drugs.[46] Patients generally exhibit significant toxicities, noted especially in the skin and oral cavity with moist desquamation and mucositis.

Patients undergoing chemotherapy alone or chemoradiation for head and neck cancer need comprehensive education on the side effects of treatment and management of these side effects. A comprehensive physical exam, as well as a dental exam, is done before the beginning of treatment. Patients with comorbid conditions such as diabetes, hypertension, renal disease, or cardiac disease are medically evaluated before treatment to assess their ability to tolerate the proposed regimen. Any dental needs are addressed before the initiation of treatment to decrease the threat of oral infections during treatment.

Supportive care for the patient undergoing chemotherapy is imperative. This includes comprehensive patient education about the agents being used, their side effects, and any potential adverse effects. (Additional information can be obtained in Chapter 21.)

Mucositis can be very troubling in the head and neck patients undergoing concurrent chemoradiation, especially when the oropharynx is within the treatment field. Mucositis is characterized by oral erythema, ulceration, and pain[47] and is a common side effect of both chemotherapy and radiation therapy. In a recent review, it was noted that whereas chemotherapy normally affects specific tissues in the oral cavity, and radiation affects only the tissue in the field, in combined treatment for head and neck patients, no tissue is spared.[47]

Patients often complain of such pain from mucositis that oral intake is significantly affected. This can result in the need for narcotic pain medications, as well as consideration for enteral feeding either via nasogastric or gastrostomy tube. Patients undergoing chemotherapy or radiation therapy alone, as well as those undergoing concurrent treatment, need an oral exam at every visit in which mucositis can be graded and the efficacy of any management strategies assessed.

Management of treatment-induced mucositis remains essentially palliative.[47] Overall, recommendations include good oral hygiene, avoidance of oral irritants, and topical anesthetic use, along with oral pain medication. Patients can be given a list of acceptable mouthwashes, as well as instructions on gentle brushing after each meal. Assessment of the oral cavity is a key nursing component each time the patient is seen. (Mucositis is further addressed in the Symptom Management section in Chapter 29).

Patients undergoing chemotherapy are also instructed about the potential adverse effects of treatment, such as thrombocytopenia, neutropenia, and anemia. Comprehensive patient education should include a discussion of signs and symptoms of infection, bleeding, and when to call and report changes.

NEW THERAPIES

There are a number of new therapies and treatment approaches in development for head and neck cancers. These include immunotherapy, in the form of vaccines and cytokine immunostimulation,[48] as well as monoclonal antibodies targeting epidermal growth factor receptor (EGFR) and vascular endothelial growth factor (VEGF).[49] Also, cancer gene therapy (CGT) is under investigation; this entails the delivery of specific genetic sequences to the tumor itself by introducing genes that mediate a cytotoxic effect within the tumor. Additional research is being done with genetic sequencing designed to introduce genetic material in to normal tissues to direct the immune system to attack the cancer cells.[50]

Considerations for Older Adults

Because of the rising number of elderly Americans, the medical and nursing communities are faced with treating more and more patients over the age of 70. Since the prevalence of cancer increases with age, nurses caring for patients with head and neck cancer will see an increase in that population. It is suggested that nearly half of the new cases of head and neck cancer seen annually occur in patients over the age of 65.[51] Historically, standard treatment is less likely to be used in the elderly, despite retrospective studies showing that radical surgery can be performed safely in this population.[52] It appears that the lack of randomized clinical trials specific to the elderly has led to a lack of consistency in regard to the treatment of this population.[53] Genden and colleagues emphasize that treatment should be based on the patient's medical condition and patient preference, *not age*. There have been several studies published on head and neck cancer in the elderly; however, the focus has primarily been on therapeutic consequences. Little has been done in the area of research related to psychosocial factors that can influence the choices made by elderly patients and or their physicians.[53]

Nutrition is a major concern in the treatment of elderly patients with head and neck cancer, since the adverse effects of any treatment are made even worse when the patient becomes nutritionally depleted. Healing of surgical wounds and/or radiation skin reactions can be significantly affected by poor nutrition, and it has been shown that elderly patients are more likely to refuse the placement of a gastrostomy tube for nutritional support.[53]

When a cisplatin-based chemotherapy regimen is used for the elderly, studies have reported an increase in nephrotoxicity, diarrhea, and thrombocytopenia.[51] Pretreatment evaluations must include renal and cardiac function, and these are monitored closely during treatment as well. Education about adequate hydration is emphasized and reinforced throughout the course of therapy.

Studies have shown that older patients respond to external beam radiation and tolerate it as well as younger patients.[53] However, the definition of "elderly" is not always clear when looking at both efficacy and side effects of treatment regimens.[53] The older population needs thorough pretreatment assessment and careful monitoring throughout the course of treatment so that any side effects are addressed quickly to avoid possible adverse outcomes.

Conclusion

As with many types of cancer, the prognosis for patients diagnosed with head and neck cancer depends on a number of factors: location of the tumor, extent of disease at diagnosis, age, and comorbid conditions. Although treatment options, regimens, and surgical techniques are evolving, the 5-year survival rate for patients diagnosed with advanced or recurrent disease remains low, approximately 56%.[4]

One way nurses can have an impact is to advocate strongly for smoking abstinence and cessation from use of all forms of tobacco. Smokers are at an increased risk of developing a second primary head and neck cancer, and this risk is even greater for those who continue to smoke or use other forms of tobacco.[4] Cancer of the head and neck is a devastating disease for all involved, and elimination of causal factors is therefore imperative.

REVIEW QUESTIONS

✓ Case Study

Mr. Jones is a 45-year-old African American male with a 3- to 4-month history of a sore throat that has been treated with antibiotics twice during the past 6 weeks. There has been no alleviation of the symptoms. He says that his reason for coming to be seen at the clinic today is a sore throat, left ear pain, and nasal congestion. You notice that he appears short of breath after walking down the hall, and he is favoring his right leg. When asked, he denies any distress or shortness of breath. Mr. Jones does not drink alcohol or use recreational drugs, but does have a history of smoking two packs of cigarettes daily since the age of 15. Past medical and surgical history is unremarkable, with the exception of moderate hypertension that is currently being treated with oral hydrochlorothiazide. Vital signs are the following: T 36.9° C, BP 142/78, HR 88, and R 24; his height is 5' 10" and his weight 250 lb. Mr. Jones is married and has two children, ages 19 and 22. He lives with his wife, and the children attend college out of town. Today, he is accompanied by his wife, who expresses concern that "something is wrong—he is so tired all the time."

After examining Mr. Jones, the physician recommends a direct laryngoscopy under anesthesia and biopsy of his larynx and a left neck lymph node. He also informs Mr. Jones that tracheostomy may be necessary if his shortness of breath worsens. All of this, including possible risks and complications, is explained to the patient. Mr. Jones gives consent for the procedure.

QUESTIONS

1. Mr. Jones has which of the following risk factors for a cancer in the head and neck region?
   a. Gender, race, smoking, and obesity
   b. Race, smoking, and age
   c. Gender, smoking, and race
   d. Smoking, hypertension, and age
2. Which of the following of Mr. Jones's symptoms are suspicious for laryngeal cancer?
   a. Throat and ear pain
   b. Hypertension
   c. Pain in the right leg
   d. Nasal congestion
3. Which of the following cell types is most likely to be found on the biopsy?
   a. Melanoma
   b. Merkel cell carcinoma
   c. Squamous cell carcinoma
   d. Basal cell carcinoma

4. Mr. Jones required a tracheostomy during this procedure. What is the most probable reason?
   a. Convenience for future intubation
   b. Asthma attack
   c. Hypertensive episode
   d. Size of mass involving the larynx, laryngeal edema
5. Mr. Jones and his wife ask you if he can still talk. What is your best response?
   a. "No, the tracheostomy prevents airflow through the vocal cords."
   b. "Yes. We will work with the speech therapist to teach you how to speak with the tracheostomy tube in place."
   c. "I don't know. I'll have to look at the operative report."
   d. "No. The tracheostomy procedure removed your larynx."
6. Mr. Jones was discharged after learning to care for his new tracheostomy. He returns for follow-up to discuss treatment options. Which of the following are possible options for his treatment?
   a. Concurrent chemoradiation
   b. Total laryngectomy and neck dissection
   c. Partial laryngectomy followed by radiation therapy
   d. All of the above
7. Mr. Jones has chosen to undergo concurrent chemoradiation with cisplatin. Which of the following side effects are an important part of his patient education?
   a. Risk for infection related to decreased white cell counts
   b. Mucositis
   c. Cystitis
   d. Constipation
8. After 3 weeks of treatment, Mr. Jones is complaining of dysphagia and has lost 20 lb since beginning treatment. What option would you consider best to ensure adequate nutrition for Mr. Jones?
   a. Nasogastric tube for purpose of enteral feeding
   b. Pureed and liquid diet, especially protein shakes
   c. Total parenteral nutrition
   d. Gastrostomy tube placement for enteral feeding
9. Two months after completing treatment, Mr. Jones has had resolution of his laryngeal mass and neck mass. He asks the physician about removing his tracheostomy and his feeding tube. The physician agrees to decanulation and gives the following response regarding the feeding tube:
   a. "It can be removed today."
   b. "The feeding tube can be removed when you can maintain your current weight for 1 month with oral intake only."

Continued

REVIEW QUESTIONS—CONT'D

c. "You will be dependent on the feeding tube for the rest of your life."

d. "We will consider taking it our when you are cancer free for 1 year."

10. Mr. Jones has a recurrence in his neck after 18 months. The surgeon recommends a modified neck dissection to remove any involved nodes. What is one of the potential complications?

a. Poor tissue healing related to previous radiation therapy

b. Hoarseness from damage to laryngeal nerve

c. Difficulty swallowing

d. Loss of function of left arm

ANSWERS

1. **C.** *Rationale:* Smoking is the greatest risk factor for cancer of the head and neck. African Americans and males also have a greater incidence of head and neck cancer (HNC). Age is a risk factor for HNC for those over 60. Hypertension and obesity have not been identified as factors for HNC.

2. **A.** *Rationale:* Sore throat and ear pain are common symptoms of a laryngeal mass. While nasal congestion can be seen in other types of head and neck cancer, it is not indicative of a laryngeal mass. There is no evidence that the leg pain or hypertension is related to his diagnosis.

3. **C.** *Rationale:* Over 90% of HNC is squamous cell in origin. Melanoma and basal cell carcinoma are more commonly seen in the skin of the head and neck region. Merkel cell is a cell type seen in salivary gland cancer.

4. **D.** *Rationale:* Size of mass and/or laryngeal edema could have prevented intubation, thus requiring a tracheostomy. Although an acute asthma attack could necessitate an emergency tracheostomy, there is no history of asthma with Mr. Jones. Hypertension in the operative setting would be controlled with medication; convenience for potential future intubation would not be considered appropriate medical care.

5. **B.** *Rationale:* The speech therapist will demonstrate the technique for occluding the end of the "trach tube" to force air up through the vocal cords, thereby enabling Mr. Jones to speak. This can be achieved with the patient's finger or with the use of a special one-way valve placed on the end of the tube. The other options show a lack of understanding of the procedure that was performed on Mr. Jones.

6. **D.** *Rationale:* All of these are potential treatment options for Mr. Jones. The decision is based on stage of disease and patient condition, as well as patient choice after discussion regarding the pros and cons of each option.

7. **A, B.** *Rationale:* Decreased white cell count and mucositis are common side effects of treatment with platinum-based chemotherapy. Mucositis is also common with radiation for head and neck cancer. Cystitis and constipation are not considered likely side effects from cisplatin.

8. **D.** *Rationale:* A gastrostomy tube feeding is the best choice for Mr. Jones. A nasogastric tube would not only be less comfortable, it would also add trauma to the area being treated. It is always preferable to use enteral feeding when possible; total parenteral nutrition would be a last resort in this situation.

9. **B.** *Rationale:* It is best to be confident that the patient will be able to maintain his weight on oral intake for a specific time before removing the tube. If the tube is removed prematurely, it will require an invasive procedure to replace it. If Mr. Jones can maintain his weight with oral intake, there is no need to wait an entire year.

10. **A.** *Rationale:* Tissue healing in a previously radiated area is a major concern. The changes to the tissue created by radiation make healing slower, and the risk of incision breakdown is greater. The laryngeal nerve should not be affected in a neck dissection, nor is there concern about swallowing. Although a radical neck procedure can cause shoulder droop and decreased mobility, that risk is greatly reduced with the modified procedure.

REFERENCES

1. Diaz EM, Sturges EM, Laramore GE et al: Head and neck. In Holland, Frei, editors: *Cancer medicine*, ed 6, London, 2003, BC Decker.

2. Carr E: Head and neck malignancies. In Yarbro CH, Frogg MH, Goodman M, editors: *Cancer nursing, principles and practices*, ed 6, Sudbury, Mass, 2005, Jones & Bartlett.

3. American Cancer Society: *Cancer facts and figures 2005*, Atlanta, 2005, Author.

4. Kadkade P, Hale K: Cancer of the mouth and throat, 2003, retrieved September 12, 2005, from http://www.emedicinehealth.com/fulltest/25733.htm.

5. National Cancer Institute: Fact sheet: head and neck cancer: Questions and answers, retrieved October 27, 2005, from http://www.cancer.gov/cancertopics/factsheet/sites-types/head-and-neck.

6. American Cancer Society: Oral cavity and oropharyngeal cancer, retrieved October 11, 2005, from http://www.cancer.org.

7. Carr E: Nursing care of the client with head and neck cancer. In Itano JK, Taoka KN, editors: *Core curriculum for oncology nursing*, ed 4, St. Louis, 2005, Elsevier.

8. Dropkin MJ, Clarke LK: Introduction. In Dropkin MJ, Clarke LK, editors: *Head and neck cancer*, Pittsburgh, 2005, Oncology Nursing Society.

9. Krioukov LF: Principles for professional nursing practice. In Harris LL, Huntoon MB, editors: *Core curriculum for otorhinolaryngology and head-neck nursing*, New Smyrna Beach, Fl, 1998, Society of Otorhinolaryngology and Head-Neck Nurses.

10. Sharp LS, Tishelman C: Smoking cessation for patients with head and neck cancer, *Cancer Nurs* 28(3): 226-235, 2005.

11. American Cancer Society: *Cancer prevention and early detection facts & figures 2005*, Atlanta, 2005, Author.

12. Colwill ML, Lazio-Stegall H: Prevention and early detection. In Dropkin MJ, Clarke LK, editors: *Head and neck cancer*, Pittsburgh, 2005, Oncology Nursing Society.

13. Andresen HG, Baker KH, Caplan S et al: Diagnostic exams and procedures. In Harris LL, Huntoon MB, editors: *Core curriculum for otorhinolaryngology and head-neck nursing*, New Smyrna Beach, Fl, 1998, Society of Otorhinolaryngology and Head-Neck Nurses.

14. Haggood, AS: Head and neck cancers. In Otto SE: *Oncology nursing*, ed 4, St. Louis, 2001, Mosby.

15. Greene FL, Page DL, Fleming ID et al, editors: *AJCC cancer staging manual*, ed 6, New York, 2002, Springer.

16. National Cancer Institute: Lip and oral cavity cancer (pdq): treatment, health professional version, 2005, retrieved August 18, 2005, from http://www.cancer.gov/cancertopics/pdq/treatment/lip-and-oral-cavity/healthprofessional.

17. National Cancer Institute: Oropharyngeal cancer (pdq): Treatment, health professional version, 2005, retrieved August 18, 2005, from http://www.cancer.gov/cancertopics/pdq/treatment/oropharyngeal/healthprofessional.

18. National Cancer Institute: Laryngeal cancer (pdq): treatment, health professional version, 2005, retrieved August 18, 2005, from http://www.cancer.gov/cancertopics/pdq/treatment/laryngeal/healthprofessional.

19. National Cancer Institute: Nasopharyngeal cancer (pdq): treatment, health professional version, 2005, retrieved December 1, 2005, from http://www.cancer.gov/cancertopics/pdq/treatment/nasopharyngeal/healthprofessional.

20. Leon X, Quer M, Orus C et al: Distant metastases in head and neck cancer patients who achieved loco-regional control, *Head Neck* 22(7): 680-686, 2000.

21. American Cancer Society: Laryngeal and hypopharyngeal cancer, retrieved November 9, 2005, from http://cancer.org.

22. Helliwell TR: Best practice No 169: evidence based pathology: squamous carcinoma of the hypopharynx, *J Clin Pathol*, 56(2): 81-85, 2003

23. National Cancer Institute: Paranasal sinus and nasal cavity cancer (pdq): Treatment, health professional version, 2005, retrieved October 19, 2005, from http://www.cancer.gov/cancertopics/pdq/treatment/paranasalsinus/healthprofessional.

24. Al-Sarraf M: Treatment of locally advanced had and neck cancer: historical and critical review, *Cancer Control* 9:5, 2002.

25. Jiang SB: Mohs surgery, 2005, retrieved December 7, 2005, from http://www.emedicine.com/ent/topic29.htm.

26. American College of Mohs Micrographic Surgery and Cutaneous Oncology: about Mohs micrographic surgery, 2005, retrieved December 7, 2005 from http://www.mohscollege.org/aboumms.html.

27. Robbins KT, Clayman G, Levine PA et al: Neck dissection classification update: revisions proposed by the American Head and Neck Society and American Academy of Otolaryngology-Head and Neck Surgery, *Arch Otolaryngol Head Neck Surg* 128:751-758, 2002.

28. Scarpa R, Zevallos J: Surgical management of head and neck malignancies. In Dropkin MJ, Clarke LK, editors: *Head and neck cancer,* Pittsburgh, 2005, Oncology Nursing Society.

29. Joseph E: Head and neck cancer: squamous cell carcinoma, retrieved October 20, 2005, from http://www.emedicine.com/plastic/topic376.htm.

30. Cyr MH, Higgins TS, McGuire MA: Laryngeal, hypopharyngeal conditions and care. In Harris LL, Huntoon MB, editors: *Core curriculum for otorhinolaryngology and head-neck nursing,* New Smyrna Beach, Fl, 1998, Society of Otorhinolaryngology and Head-Neck Nurses.

31. Sievers AEF: Postoperative management of the head and neck surgical patient. In Dropkin MJ, Clarke LK, editors: *Head and neck cancer,* Pittsburgh, 2005, Oncology Nursing Society.

32. American Cancer Society: Nasal cavity and paranasal sinuses cancer, retrieved October 11, 2005, from http://cancer.org.

33. Higgins TS, Kun SS, LeGrand MS et al: Nasal cavity, paranasal sinuses, nasopharynx conditions and care. In Harris LL, Huntoon MB, editors: *Core curriculum for otorhinolaryngology and head- neck nursing,* New Smyrna Beach, Fl, 1998, Society of Otorhinolaryngology and Head-Neck Nurses.

34. Spiro RH, Elliot WS, Shah JP: Maxillectomy and its classification, 1996. Cited in Nazar G, Rodrigo JP, Lorente JL et al: Prognostic factors of maxillary sinus malignancies, *Am J Rhinol* 18:4, 2004.

35. Hong TS, Wolfgang AT, Haran, PM: Intensity-modulated radiation therapy in the management of head and neck cancer, *Curr Opin Oncol* 17:231-235, 2005.

36. Nag S, Cano ER, Demanes DJ et al: The American Brachytherapy Society recommendations for high-dose-rate brachytherapy for head-and-neck carcinoma, *Int J Radiat Oncol Biol Phys* 50(5):1190-1198, 2001.

37. Brizel M, Wasserman TH, Henke M et al: Phase III randomized trial of amifostine as a radioprotector in head and neck cancer, *J Clin Oncol* 18(19):3339-3345, 2000.

38. Subcutaneous administration of amifostine for radioprotection: frequently asked questions, *Oncol Nurse Pract Consult* 1:1, 2004.

39. MD Anderson Cancer Center: Head and neck radiation: about your treatment, Houston, TX, 2004, MD Anderson Cancer Center.

40. Blevins LL: Radiation treatment and symptom management. In Dropkin MJ, Clarke LK, editors: *Head and neck cancer,* Pittsburgh, 2005, Oncology Nursing Society.

41. Petruson KM, Silander EM, Hammerlid EB: Quality of life as predictor of weight loss in patients with head and neck cancer, *Head Neck* 27(4): 302-310, 2005.

42. Colasanto JM, Prasad P, Nash MA et al: Nutritional support of patients undergoing radiation therapy for head and neck cancer, *Oncology* 19(3): 371-379, 2005.

43. Porock D, Kristjanson L: Skin reactions during radiotherapy for breast cancer: the use and impact of topical agents and dressings, *Eur J Cancer Care* 8:143-153, 1999.

44. Bernier J, Cooper JS: Chemoradiation after surgery for high-risk head and neck cancer patients: how strong is the evidence? *Oncologist* 10: 215-224, 2005.

45. Nguyen NP, Sallah S, Karlsson U et al: Combined chemotherapy and radiation therapy for head and neck malignancies, *Cancer* 94:4, 2002.

46. Monnerat C, Faivre S, Temam S et al: End points for new agents in induction chemotherapy for locally advanced head and neck cancers, *Ann Oncol* 13:995-1006, 2002.

47. Scully C, Epstein J, Sonis S: Oral mucositis: a challenging complication of radiotherapy, chemotherapy, and radiochemotherapy. Part 2: Diagnosis and management of mucositis, *Head Neck* 26(1): 77-84, 2004.

48. Ferris RL: Progress in head and neck cancer immunotherapy: can tolerance and immune suppression be reversed? *ORL* 66:332-340, 2004.

49. Caponigro F, Formato R, Caraglia M et al: Monoclonal antibodies targeting epidermal growth factor receptor and vascular endothelial growth factor with a focus on head and neck tumors, *Curr Opin Oncol* 17: 212-217, 2005.

50. Harrington KJ, Nutting NM, Pandha HS: Gene therapy for head and neck cancer, *Cancer Metast Rev* 24:147-164, 2005.

51. Argiris A, Li Y, Murphy BA et al: Outcome of elderly patients with recurrent metastatic head and neck cancer treated with cisplatin-based chemotherapy, *J Clin Oncol* 22:5, 2004.

52. Derks W, de Leeuw JRJ, Hordijk GJ et al: Reasons for non-standard treatment in elderly patients with advanced head and neck cancer, *Eur Arch Otorhinolaryngol* 262:21-26, 2005.

53. Genden EM, Rinaldo A, Shaha AR et al: Treatment consideration for head and neck cancer in the elderly, *J Laryngol Otol* 119:169-174, 2005.

CHAPTER 13

Leukemia

Rosanne Elbe Ososki and Kim O'Riley

The leukemias are a complex collection of heterogenous diseases with distinct biologic and clinical characteristics. The two major classifications of leukemia are **acute** and **chronic.** These two types of leukemia are similar in that they are the result of a dysfunctional bone marrow, but they differ dramatically in disease presentation, treatment, and prognosis. The cell line of origin is characterized as **myeloid** or **lymphoid.** Much of the scientific knowledge of adult leukemia is derived from studies done on pediatric leukemia.

Pathophysiology

Leukemia is a malignant hematologic disorder characterized by a proliferation of abnormal white blood cells (WBCs) that infiltrate the bone marrow, peripheral blood, and other organs. Circulating blood cells are formed in the bone marrow through a process called **hematopoiesis.** Bone marrow in the vertebrae, the clavicle, the scapula, the sternum, the ribs, the skull, the proximal ends of long bones, and the pelvis produces blood cells. In adults, most of the blood cells are produced in the pelvis, the sternum, and the vertebrae. All circulating blood cells arise from a small pool of **hematopoietic stem cells (HSCs),** also known as **pluripotent stem cells.** These cells have the ability to self-renew and maintain their numbers. HSCs have the capacity to proliferate and differentiate into all cell lines (Pool 1 in Fig. 13-1). Whether they proliferate or differentiate is determined by the body's current needs.

With every stem cell division, one daughter cell remains in the stem cell pool. An injury to the stem cell pool, such as a lethal dose of radiation, prevents the production of blood cells and results in marrow aplasia. The stem cell pool cannot be assessed by a routine bone marrow examination. Studies of the stem cell population are called **colony-forming assays** and are performed by **in vitro** culturing. Proliferation of stem cells is mediated by specific **colony stimulating factors (CSFs)** acting on HSC to give rise to a pool of committed progenitor cells (Pool II in Fig. 13-1).[1]

Committed progenitor cells mature in the bone marrow within a framework of supporting cells and blood vessels that supply nutrition and growth factors. This second pool of cells is the precursor to all mature blood cells. A stem cell becomes committed to a certain blood cell line when it leaves the stem cell pool. In the second pool the cells differentiate and mature. Figure 13-1 illustrates the steps of cell differentiation and maturation. In the second pool, cells at the blast phase of development cannot function as mature blood cells, but they can undergo mitosis. At this stage of development the **blast cells** (the least differentiated cells with commitment to their bloodline) are responsive to specific CSFs. Each cell divides multiple times at early stages, as shown. As the cells divide, they differentiate, enabling them to carry out only specific functions, losing their proliferative response to CSFs. The exact process by which stem cells undergo self-renewal or commitment to differentiate is unknown.[2]

When the precursor cells of the second pool are mature, they are released into the **peripheral circulation,** which is the third pool. Each kind of mature blood cell performs a specific function (red blood cells [RBCs]—oxygen transport; granulocytes—phagocytosis; platelets—clotting). Mature circulating cells cannot undergo mitosis and must be replaced at the end of their life span (RBCs—120 days; granulocytes—6 to 8 hours; platelets—8 to 10 days). Mature blood cells are released from the bone marrow in response to the body's needs.[2]

In patients with leukemia, the control factors regulating the orderly differentiation and maturation of the blood cells are absent. This lack of regulatory control results in the arrest of the maturation process of a specific cell line. The involved cell form proliferates and accumulates in the bone marrow, resulting in crowding of the normal marrow cells. This marrow crowding impairs the production and function of normal cell lines; eventually, leukemic cells, which are released into the circulating blood, replace the marrow. The leukemic cells may also invade body organs.

The specific type of leukemia depends on which stem cell line is affected (myeloid or lymphoid) and the point of maturation at which growth is arrested. Acute leukemias result from arrest of immature blood cells; chronic leukemias involve more mature blood cells.

Epidemiology

An estimated 35,000 new cases of leukemia were expected to be diagnosed in the United States in 2006. Acute leukemias account for nearly 45% of cases, with chronic leukemias accounting for 41%. Most cases occur in older adults; more than half of all cases occur after age 67 years. Leukemia was expected to affect 9 times as many adults as children in 2006. (About 31,000 adults compared with 3500 children, ages 0-19 years). About 30% of cancers in children ages 0-14 years are leukemia. The most common form of leukemia among children under 19 years of age is acute lymphocytic leukemia (ALL).

The most common types of leukemia in adults are acute myelogenous leukemia (AML), with an estimated 11,930 new cases in 2006, and chronic lymphocytic leukemia (CLL), with about 10,020 new cases in 2006. Chronic myelogenous leukemia (CML) is estimated to affect about 4500 persons, and ALL will account for about 3930 cases. Other, unclassified forms of leukemia account for the 4690 remaining cases[3] (Table 13-1).

An estimated 13,000 new cases (3.5 to 12.6 per 100,000) of myelodysplastic syndromes (MDS) will be diagnosed yearly in the United States. The incidence increases with age, with the median age of diagnosis being over age 70.[4] MDS can be primary (arising de novo), as occurs in 70% to 80% of cases, or secondary, as in 20% to 30% of cases. The incidence is higher in males than females.

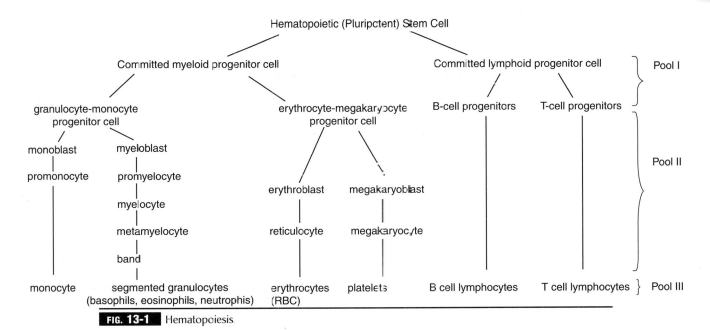

FIG. 13-1 Hematopoiesis

TABLE 13-1 Estimated New Leukemia Cases in the United States in 2006			
TYPE	INDIVIDUALS	MALE	FEMALE
Acute lymphoblastic leukemia (ALL)	3,930	2,150	1,780
Chronic lymphoblastic leukemia (CLL)	10,020	6,280	3,740
Acute myelogenous leukemia (AML)	11,930	6,350	5,580
Chronic myelogenous leukemia (CML)	4,500	2,550	1,950
Other, unclassified forms of leukemia	4,690	2,670	2,020
Total	35,070	20,000	15,070

Data from American Cancer Society, *Facts and Figures*, Atlanta, 2006, Author.

Etiology and Risk Factors

Acute leukemias are recognized as a genetic disease resulting from a series of acquired or inherited mutations in the structure of certain genes. These mutations are passed from the original transformed progenitor cell to its clonal offspring. Most of these genetic changes cause leukemia by destroying normal cell cycle controls, inhibiting differentiation of cells, or resisting therapeutic apoptosis (cell self-destruction) in leukemic blasts.[5]

Prevention, Screening, and Detection

Currently, there is no way to prevent leukemia, and screening is not done. Because symptoms often resemble other, less serious conditions, it may be difficult to diagnosis leukemia early.

Acute Leukemias

Acute leukemia is a severe and aggressive disease characterized by rapid onset and a rapid terminal course if untreated. There are two types of acute leukemia: **lymphocytic** or **lymphoblastic (ALL)** and **myeloid** or **myelogenous (AML).**

In acute leukemia, the leukemic or blast cells function abnormally and accumulate in the peripheral blood, the bone marrow, the reticuloendothelial system (RES), and sometimes the central nervous system (CNS). The overproduction of leukemic cells in the bone marrow impairs normal hematopoiesis, resulting in anemia, granulocytopenia, and thrombocytopenia.

ACUTE LYMPHOCYTIC (LYMPHOBLASTIC) LEUKEMIA
Etiology and Risk Factors

The exact etiology of ALL is unknown. High-dose radiation, chemicals, drugs, viruses, and genetic abnormalities have been implicated in the etiology of this disease.[3] There is a strong association between Epstein-Barr virus (EBV) and human immunodeficiency virus (HIV) in patients with mature B-cell ALL.[6]

Acute lymphocytic leukemia has a bimodal age distribution. The initial peak in children occurs between ages 2 and 4 years and decreases during childhood. The second peak occurs after age 50.[6]

Classification

ALL is a hematopoietic malignancy that originates in the bone marrow precursor lymphoid cell. The World Health Organization (WHO) classification defines leukemias using morphology, immunophenotype, genetic features, and clinical features. WHO's classification of ALL divides it into precursor B lymphoblastic leukemia/lymphoma (B-cell ALL) (75% of patients) or precursor T lymphoblastic leukemia/lymphoma (T-cell ALL) (25% of patients). Marrow involvement of 20% lymphoblasts or more, with or without a mass lesion, classifies the disease into leukemia. The disease is termed lymphoma when most of the tumor bulk is in the mediastinum or other nodal structures and there are fewer than 20% blasts in the bone marrow.[7,8]

Previously, the French-American-British (FAB) classification, based on cell morphology, was used to classify ALL. The WHO classification has replaced this. Lymphoblast morphology does not distinguish between B- and T-cell lineage. Assessing the reactivity of antigens on the cell surface to antibodies using flow cytometry, a process called immunophenotyping (also called cell surface marker studies), establishes their cell lineage. Different antigens are expressed as the cell matures, which aids in identification.[9]

Cytogenetic characteristics are one of the most important prognostic factors for B-cell ALL. Genetic changes are not prognostic in T-cell ALL. Abnormalities can be related to the number of chromosomes or structural characteristics. In children, **ploidy** (increased number of chromosomes) is the most important prognostic factor; those with more than 50 chromosomes have the best prognosis. Structural cytogenetic abnormalities are thought to either generate a novel gene (an oncogene) whose protein product acts on the host cell to induce malignancy; or it may cause a loss or inactivation of genes whose proteins normally suppress cancer (a tumor suppressor gene). These structural abnormalities take the form of chromosomal translocation, inversions, or deletions.[10]

See Table 13-2 for the most common cytogenetic abnormalities for B-cell ALL.

Clinical Features

The most common presenting complaints are the result of anemia, neutropenia, and thrombocytopenia caused by a rapidly expanding leukemic cell population. Symptoms are malaise, fatigue, bony pain, bleeding, bruising, fever, night sweats, and infections. Pain, especially in children, results from increased blasts in the bone marrow. CNS involvement is present in 50% of patients with Burkitt's leukemia, but is rare in other ALLs.[11,12] Most CNS manifestations involve cranial nerves VI, III, IV, and VII and lead to double vision, abnormal ocular movements, facial dysesthesia, and facial droop. Chin numbness is often overlooked.[6] Parenchymal involvement of the brain is rare in leukemia, as is testicular involvement at diagnosis. Enlargement of the testes is usually asymmetrical and painless.[11] Hepatosplenomegaly and lymphadenopathy are found in 20% of cases, mostly with T-cell and Burkitt's leukemia. Evidence of tumor lysis and disseminated intravascular coagulopathies (DIC)

are present in 10% to 20% of patients. Mediastinal disease is common in T-cell ALL.[12]

Diagnosis

The diagnosis of acute leukemia is often obvious from the peripheral blood smear; however, a bone marrow evaluation is essential to finalize the diagnosis and provide specimens for further histochemical staining, immunophenotyping, and cytogenetic testing.

The WBC count is greater than 10,000/mm³ in 50% to 60% of patients at diagnosis and greater than 100,000/mm³ in 10%. Leukemic cells may be seen in the blood. Despite high WBC counts, absolute neutrophil counts are low. Anemia is almost universal: two thirds of patients are first seen with a platelet count less than 50,000/mm³.[13] Bone marrow aspirate is used to obtain the **differential** count, which reveals the percentage of each hematologic component in the marrow. Lymphoblasts comprise at least 20% of the marrow cells in ALL.

Smears of the bone marrow aspirate are stained to reveal the cell morphology. A portion of the bone marrow aspirate is heparinized for cytogenetic analysis and flow cytometry. Recurrent cytogenetic abnormalities occur in 80% of children and in 60% to 70% of adults. Distinct subtypes of ALL can be identified; these have implications for prognosis and choice of treatment.[6] A core biopsy of the bone is obtained during the bone marrow procedure. This specimen is used to determine the marrow cellularity. **Cellularity** refers to the ratio of hematopoietic tissue to adipose tissue in the marrow. The amount of blood-forming, or **red,** marrow decreases with the aging process and is replaced by fat, or **yellow,** marrow. Normocellular marrow cellularity for an adult is 30% to 40%. Young adults and children have bone marrow that is much more cellular. Older adults have more fat in their marrow. These age-related changes are reflected in marrow cellularity definitions: **normocellular** marrow has normal proportions of the hematopoietic cells and adipose cells; **hypocellular** marrow has a reduced number of hematopoietic cells and an increase in adipose elements; and **hypercellular** marrow has an increased number of hematopoietic cells and a decreased amount of adipose tissue.[2] The bone marrow from a newly diagnosed ALL patient is usually hypercellular with increased lymphoblasts (e.g., cellularity = 90%; lymphoblasts = 80%).

Infiltration of the cerebrospinal fluid (CSF) by leukemic cells is seen in 3% to 5% of adults.[11] The CSF specimen is centrifuged

TABLE 13-2   B-Cell ALL Cytogenetics

IMMUNOPHENOTYPE LINEAGE	CYTOGENETIC ABNORMALITY (KARYOTYPE)	FUSION GENE	INCIDENCE	PROGNOSIS	TREATMENT CHOICE
cALL	t(9;22)	BCR/ABL	30%–35%	Poor	SCT in 1st CR; possibly imatinib
Pre- B-cell ALL	t(1;19)	E2A-PBX1	3%–4%	Poor	Intensive treatment
Pro- B-cell ALL	t(4;11)	MLL-AF4	3%–4%	Poor	SCT in 1st CR
Pro- B-cell ALL	11q23 aberrations	Aberrant MLL	<5%	Poor	SCT in 1st CR
Pre- B-cell ALL	t(12;21)	ETV6-AML1	1%–3%	Undetermined	Standard-dose chemo
Mature B-cell (Burkitt's)	t(8;14) or t(8;2) or t(8;22)	MYC-IGH	5%	Favorable	High-dose chemo; no maintenance

ALL, Acute lymphoblastic leukemia.
Data from Ludwig W, Haferlach T, Schoch C: Classification of acute leukemias. In Pui, C, editor: Treatment of acute leukemias, new directions for clinical research, Totowa, NJ, 2003, Humana Press; and Hoelzer D, Gökbuget N, Ottmann O et al: Acute lymphoblastic leukemia, *Hematology 2002* (Am Soc Hematol Educ Prog):10-34, 2002.

TABLE 13-3	Physical Findings and Laboratory Results in ALL and AML Patients	
	ACUTE LYMPHOCYTIC LEUKEMIA	**ACUTE MYELOGENOUS LEUKEMIA**
Physical Examination		
Fever	Often present	May be present
Infection	Frequently present	30% have serious infections
Bleeding	Mild in 30%	30% have significant bleeding or petechiae
		75% have intracutaneous bleeding
Adenopathy	Present in 80%	Rare
Splenomegaly with or without hepatomegaly	Frequently present	Occurs in 25%
Gingival hypertrophy	Rare	Present with monocytic element
Neurologic findings	Headaches, visual disturbances	Rare
Laboratory Values		
White blood cell count (WBC)	50%–60% WBC >10,000/mm^3	30% decreased
	30%–40% WBC <100,000/mm^3	30% normal
	10% WBC >100,000/mm^3	30% increased
	Often neutropenic	WBC >50,000/mm^3 in 25%
	Most have blasts	10% have no blasts
Platelets	<50,000/mm^3 in 60%	<20,000/mm^3 common
Uric acid	Increased	Increased in 50%
Lactate dehydrogenase (LDH)	Increased	Typically increased
Bone Marrow		
Cellularity	Hypercellular	Hypercellular
Blasts	20% or greater	20% or greater
Erythroid elements	Decreased	Increased
Morphology	Normal	Bizarre granulation of mature granulocytes
Cerebrospinal Fluid		
Cytology: infiltration with leukemic cells at presentation	Children: 5% Adult: <10%	<5% occurrence: greater risk in M$_4$ and M$_5$ greater risk with WBC >100,000/mm^3

ALL, Acute lymphoblastic leukemia; *AML*, acute myelogenous leukemia.

and stained to determine the presence of leukemic cells. A low glucose level or a high protein level may indicate either leukemic infiltration or an infectious process. Patients with high numbers of circulating blast cells may have their CSF specimens contaminated with circulating blast cells. This may lead to an inaccurate diagnosis of CNS involvement.

Table 13-3 presents the physical findings, laboratory values, bone marrow, and CSF results in ALL and AML.

Staging/Prognostic Indicators

There is no staging system for acute leukemias. Treatment is based on classification of the disease as described above. Age and cytogenetic features are the most important predictors of prognosis in adult ALL. Adults have a poorer prognosis than children, with those older than 60 years having the poorest. Adverse prognostic factors are listed in Table 13-4.

Medical Treatment Modalities and Nursing Care Considerations

The treatment goal in ALL is to achieve a cure and is divided into phases. Induction chemotherapy is the initial treatment designed to clear the bone marrow of overt disease. A complete remission (CR) bone marrow biopsy will show a return of normal hematopoiesis and lymphoblasts below 5%, neutrophils above 1500/mm^3, and platelet count above 150,000/mm^3. Consolidation therapy further reduces the residual leukemic burden in patients

TABLE 13-4	Adverse Prognostic Factors in ALL
Clinical characteristics	Higher age: >50 yrs
	High WBC: >30,000/mm^3 in B-cell ALL
	High WBC: >100,000/mm^3 in T-cell ALL
Immunophenotype	Pro B
	Early T
	Mature T
Cytogenetic features and molecular genetics	t(9;22)/BCR/ABL or 11q23 abnormalities
Treatment response	Late achievement of CR: >4 weeks
	multiple drug resistance (MDR) positivity
	Presence of blasts in BM at day 14

ALL, Acute lymphoblastic leukemia.
From Faderi S, Jehna S, Kantarjian HM: The biology and therapy of adult acute lymphoblastic leukemia, *Cancer* 98(7):1340, 2003.

who are in morphologic remission. The intensity of consolidation varies, depending on the risk of relapse based on cytogenetic features and patient age. Lower-dose maintenance chemotherapy continues for 18 to 24 months. CNS prophylaxis is an important part of all therapies.[11] (See Table 13-5 for sample treatment.)

INDUCTION CHEMOTHERAPY

The primary chemotherapeutic agents used to induce remission are (1) vincristine, (2) a corticosteroid, and (3) anthracycline. Remission rates range from 72% to 92%, with a low mortality rate resulting from induction. Some induction regimens use additional drugs (L-asparaginase, cyclophosphamide, methotrexate, 6-mercaptopurine (6-MP), cytarabine (Ara-C), which do not appear to increase response rates.[6] Exceptions appear in the use of higher doses of cytarabine in T-cell ALL and in the use of high-dose cyclophosphamide, alternating with high doses of methotrexate and cytarabine in mature B-cell ALL.[6] The use of growth factors such as granulocyte CSF (G-CSF) has decreased the otherwise profound myelosuppression and its complications. This allows for timely administration of dose-intensive regimens.[14]

CENTRAL NERVOUS SYSTEM TREATMENT

The CNS may serve as a "sanctuary" site for leukemia cells. Leukemic involvement in the CNS at the time of diagnosis is seen in 3% to 5% of adults.[11] If the CNS is not treated, as many as 30% to 50% of adults will develop CNS involvement. This number is reduced to less than 10% with CNS prophlaxis.[15] Cranial irradiation plus intrathecal (IT) chemotherapy with methotrexate or

cytarabine was the standard for children with ALL. This resulted in neuropsychologic deficits and endocrine dysfunction in some children. Newer treatments include IT cytarabine or methotrexate (or both) without cranial irradiation and high-dose systemic chemotherapy with CNS penetration (e.g., high-dose methotrexate or cytarabine). In adults at high risk for CNS disease, the combination of high-dose chemotherapy with IT chemotherapy given early during induction prevented CNS recurrence in 98% of patients.[16]

Patients who have CNS leukemia should be treated more aggressively. This includes cranial irradiation and intraventricular chemotherapy via an Ommaya reservoir. The advantages of drug administration through an Ommaya include ease of access to CSF, and higher, more predictable levels of the drug in ventricular CSF than when administered by lumbar puncture.[12]

POSTREMISSION THERAPY

Without some form of postremission therapy, ALL will almost certainly recur. The goal is to eliminate minimal residual disease (MRD). The optimal form of this therapy remains controversial, but the two most widely used types of therapy are consolidation/intensification and maintenance.

Consolidation/Intensification Therapy. The role of consolidation/intensification in children has improved prognosis in those with high-risk features. The role in adults is less clear. Consolidation or intensification is early treatment with chemotherapy after obtaining CR with a combination of drugs of comparable intensity given in repeated courses over several months. Intensification uses higher doses than given in consolidation and

---

TABLE 13-5   CALGB Protocol for ALL

INDUCTION AND EARLY INTENSIFICATION	CNS PROPHYLAXIS AND INTERIM MAINTENANCE	LATE INTENSIFICATION	PROLONGED MAINTENANCE
COURSE I: INDUCTION (4 WK)	*COURSE III: CNS PROPHYLAXIS AND INTERIM MAINTENANCE (12 WK)*	*COURSE IV: LATE INTENSIFICATION (8 WK)*	*COURSE V: PRONLONGED MAINTENANCE*
CTX 1,200 mg/m² IV on day 1 DNR 45 mg/m² IV on days 1-3 VCR 2 mg IV on days 1, 8, 15, 2 PSE 60 mg/m²/d PO/IV on days 1-21 L-Asp 6,000 international units/m² subQ on days 5, 8, 11, 15, 18, 22	Cranial RT 2,400 cGy on days 1-12 MTX 15 mg IT on days 1, 8, 15, 22, 29 6-MP 60 mg/m² PO on days 1-70 MTX 20 mg/m² PO on days 36, 43, 50, 57, 64	Dox 30 mg/m² IV on days 1, 8, 15 VCR 2 mg IV on days 1, 8, 15 Dex 10 mg/m²/d PO on days 1-14 CTX 1,000 mg/m² IV on day 29 6-TG 60 mg/m²/d PO on days 29-42 Ara-C 75 mg/m²/d subQ on days 29, 32, 36-39	VCR 2 mg IV on day 1 of q4wk PSE 60 mg/m²/d on days 1-5 of q4wk MTX 20 mg/m² PO on days 1, 8, 15, 22 6-MP 80 mg/m²/d PO on days 1-28
COURSE II: EARLY INTENSIFICATION 4 WK; REPEAT ONCE			
MTX 15 mg IT on day 1 CTX 1,000 mg/m² IV on day 1 6-MP 60 mg/m²/d PO on days 1-14 Ara-C 75 mg/m²/d subQ on days 1-4, 8-11 VCR 2 mg IV on days 15, 22 L-Asp 6,000 international units/m² subQ on days 15, 18, 22, 25			

ALL, Acute lymphoblastic leukemia; *IT,* intrathecal; *IV,* intravenous route; *PO,* by mouth; *subQ,* subcutaneously; *CALGB,* Cancer and Leukemia Group B; *CTX,* cyclophophamide; *DNR,* daunorubicin; *VCR,* vincristine; *L-Asp,* L-asparaginase; *MTX,* methotrexate; *DOX,* doxorubicin; *Dex,* dexamethasone; *PSE,* prednisone; *6-MP,* 6-mercaptopurine; *Ara-C,* cytarabine; *6-TG,* thioguanine.

may include stem cell transplant. Current treatment protocols address the subtype and genetic abnormalities and try to match treatment to the risk.[6]

Maintenance Therapy. Maintenance therapy is lower-dose treatment given continuously for 2 to 3 years, usually consisting of daily 6-MP and weekly oral methotrexate, and monthly pulses of vincristine and prednisone. The optimal drugs and dosage remain unknown. In T-cell ALL, the benefit of maintenance chemotherapy has been questioned. No maintenance therapy is given to patients with Burkitt's leukemia.[6]

STEM CELL TRANSPLANTATION (SCT)

SCT can be used as a form of intensification in high-risk patients. Trying to compare the outcomes of adults receiving allogeneic SCT versus chemotherapy in first CR is difficult, because 70% either do not have a matched sibling or have comorbidities or infections that prevent randomization to SCT.[17] The International Bone Marrow Transplant Registry compared patients receiving intensive postremission chemotherapy with SCT. Disease-free survival (DFS) rates at 9 years were 32% for chemotherapy and 34% for SCT. Disease recurrence was the cause of death in the chemotherapy arm, whereas treatment-related mortality was the reason in the SCT group.[18] A large French study compared SCT with a control group. Overall survival rate at 10 years was 49% with SCT versus 39% for chemotherapy in the standard risk group. In the high-risk group, survival rates at 10 years were 44% with SCT and 11% with chemotherapy alone.[19] Another trial has a 5-year event-free survival (EFS) rate of 54% in SCT as compared to 34% in the chemotherapy group. Better EFS was found for both high-risk and standard-risk groups with SCT.[20] Currently SCT is offered only to high-risk ALL in first CR or in second CR after relapse for standard risk. If the data from this study are confirmed, allogeneic SCT may be offered sooner in the treatment protocol for standard-risk patients. Autologous SCT has not shown to have an advantage to chemotherapy alone.[6]

PHILADELPHIA-POSITIVE DISEASE

Patients with t (9:22) or Philadelphia (Ph+) chromosome have a dismal prognosis, and most relapse within 6 to 11 months.[21] The incidence of Ph+ increases with age and seems to stabilize at 30% of patients over age 60.[22] Patients with Ph+ ALL have similar CR rates, but shorter median duration of remission and survival. Long-term survival is less than 10%.[10] SCT is recommended for all patients with Ph+ ALL who achieve a CR and have a matched donor.

The Ph+ chromosome results in the production of BCR-ABL oncoproteins, resulting in uncontrolled tyrosine kinase activity. Imatinib, a tyrosine kinase inhibitor, has been used extensively in CML with elimination of BCR-ABL. Treatment of polymerase chain reaction (PCR)–positive BCR-ABL (see later section on minimal residual disease) after SCT in ALL patients has resulted in 52% of patients testing negative for PCR after starting on imatinib with 91% and 54% remaining PCR negative at 12 and 24 months. Patients who continued to test positive for BCR-ABL had survival rates of 8%.[23] Another trial used imatinib after induction and consolidation and before SCT. This provided a good-quality CR and survival advantage.[21] These results are encouraging, and clinical trials are under way incorporating imatinib into different stages of therapy.

THERAPY FOR RECURRENT AND REFRACTORY DISEASE

Up to 25% of adult ALL patients have primary resistant disease. These patients do not obtain remission, and the majority of those

achieving CR will relapse. Salvage regimens are based on promising induction regimens and adding high-dose cytarabine. SCT is used, if a donor can be identified and the patient achieves a second CR.[24] Clofarabine (Clolar), a new-generation nucleoside analogue, was granted U.S. Food and Drug Administration (FDA) approval in 2004 for pediatric relapsed or refractory ALL. CR was obtained in 12% of patients refractory to at least two prior regimens.[25] Clofarabine is currently in clinical trials for elderly adults with AML.[26] Nelarabine (Arranon), given as a daily 1-hour infusion consecutively for 5 days in refractory pediatric ALL patients, had an overall response rate of 31%, and patients with T-cell malignancies achieved 54% response. The dose-limiting side effect is neurotoxicity, mostly peripheral neuropathy.[27] Both drugs will undergo clinical trials for adults in the future.

Most ALL relapses occur within the first 2 years of remission. Patients who relapse after completing maintenance therapy have a better chance of attaining second remission than those who relapse while receiving therapy. The outcome of salvage therapy in adult ALL is poor, and response rates are low (20% to 40%).[12] Salvage therapies are patterned according to promising therapies used in induction and consolidation. High-dose cytarabine may be added with other therapies. Patients who have a matched donor may proceed to SCT.[6]

MINIMAL RESIDUAL DISEASE

Minimal residual disease (MRD) is a term used to describe subclinical levels of disease that can lead to relapse. Standard definition of CR in acute leukemia is a bone marrow with less than 5% blasts. The sensitivity for detecting residual disease is limited to 5% when only 20 to 40 metaphase cells are examined. A patient in clinical remission can harbor 10^{10} leukemic cells. This is equal to finding one leukemic cell for every 20 to 100 normal cells. Using PCR techniques to assess for MRD may detect 1 to 5 blast cells per 100,000 normal cells.[28] Relying on routine microscopic and cytogenetic determination of CR may allow for a residual blast count up to 300 times greater than the number needed for a relapse.[28]

Different methods are available to evaluate MRD including immunophenotyping, PCR, fluorescent in situ hybridization analysis (FISH), and southern blotting. PCR-based methods look for the known molecular rearrangements such as the fusion genes noted in Table 13-2. If a patient does not have a known rearrangement at diagnosis, PCR will not be useful. PCR is most useful in Ph+ ALL. Current experience with MRD is not yet sufficient to make treatment decisions. Presence of the original clonal marker does not always predict relapse. Ongoing clinical trials are designed to answer these questions.

MULTIDRUG RESISTANCE

Drug resistance may be an important factor in treatment failure in adult ALL. The best-known mechanism of multiple drug resistance (MDR) is regulated by P-glycoprotein (Pgp). Pgp acts as an efflux pump and results in decreased chemotherapy levels in the malignant cells. Attempts to inhibit the Pgp function with verapamil and cyclosporine have not been successful.[29] MDR gene overexpression increases from 10% at diagnosis to 50% at relapse.[12] Additional mechanisms of drug resistance in ALL are being studied. We currently do not know the best way to overcome MDR.

Disease-Related Complications and Treatment

Disease-related complications for ALL, AML, and MDS will be discussed in the AML section.

Prognosis

In adult ALL, complete CR rates of 80% to 85% and cure rates of 30% to 40% can be achieved. Specific subgroups such as T-cell ALL or mature B-cell ALL can have cure rates greater than 50%, whereas patients with Ph+ ALL have cure rates less than 10%.[30] Intensified consolidation with high-dose methotrexate or cytarabine have improved outcomes in some subtypes. New treatment modalities targeting molecular changes such as tyrosine kinase inhibitors in BCR/ABL show promise for the future.

The most important prognostic factors in adult ALL are age, WBC count, immunophenotype, cytogenetic features, and molecular genetic features at diagnosis. Time to achieve CR is also important. Table 13-4 lists the adverse prognostic factors in ALL.

ACUTE MYELOID LEUKEMIA
Etiology and Risk Factors

Some specific predisposing factors have been identified in AML. People with certain genetic disorders such as Down syndrome (trisomy 21), as well as other genetic disorders, are at increased risk to develop AML.[3] Cigarette smoking and exposure to certain chemicals such as benzene, a chemical in gasoline and cigarette smoke, are risk factors. Farmers exposed to pesticides also have a higher rate of myeloid leukemias. Leukemia has been associated with exposure to ionizing radiation.[3] Electromagnetic field (EMF) exposure has been implicated, but a review of all the literature to date reveals a doubtful link between EMF exposure and leukemia.[31]

Improvements in multimodality therapy over the past decade have resulted in increased survival and a potential cure for patients with a variety of cancers. Long-term survival now allows evaluation of late effects of cancer therapy. The incidence of secondary malignancies related to cytotoxic therapy, particularly therapy-related acute myeloid leukemias (T-AMLs) has increased dramatically over the past decade. Two types of chemotherapy-related leukemias have been identified: (1) alkylating drug–induced, usually preceded by myelodysplastic syndrome and occurring about 5 years after treatment; and (2) epipodophyllotoxin topisomerase–induced, where the incubation is about 2 years.[31]

Classification

The pathophysiology of AML can be explained by genetic changes in bone marrow stem cells. Either a complete block or partial block in maturation occurs. The genetic changes in chromosomes lead to formation of growth-promoting oncogenes, inactivation of tumor suppressor genes, or changes in transcription factors.[31] The natural history of AML arising de novo in young adults is believed to be a disease of committed stem cells, which is different from the disease arising from a primitive stem cell typical of secondary AML and the AML seen in the elderly.[32]

AML is currently classified by the use of immunologic markers (usually by flow cytometry), histochemical stains, genetic alterations, and morphology. WHO has taken the FAB classification

and further refined it to allow for better identification of subtypes. Table 13-6 lists the various subtypes and prognoses. Marrow involvement of 20% or more myeloblasts is diagnostic of AML. Although AML is due to a genetic change in the bone marrow stem cell, not all AMLs exhibit cytogenetic abnormalities. The most common cytogenetic abnormalities are listed in Table 13-7 and grouped according to probability of long-term remission.

Clinical Features

As with ALL, AML symptoms are related to the rapidly expanding leukemic cell population. AML patients usually are first seen with symptoms of anemia, as well as an infection not responsive to oral antibiotics. Easy bruising, epistaxis, or gingival bleeding reflect thrombocytopenia. Unlike ALL patients, virtually all AML patients are symptomatic when they enter the health care system.

Abnormal findings on physical examination are related to leukemic infiltration of an organ, granulocytopenia, or thrombocytopenia. A thorough and systematic physical examination confirms many of the patient's complaints and is an integral part of the diagnosis. Table 13-3 lists possible physical manifestations of both ALL and AML. Gingival infiltrates and skin nodules are frequently seen in acute myelomonocytic and monocytic leukemias and may precede other manifestations by 2 to 4 weeks.

Diagnosis

A diagnosis of AML is strongly indicated when the examination of peripheral blood smears shows an increased number of immature blast cells associated with anemia and thrombocytopenia. The presence of Auer rods suggests a diagnosis of AML before other diagnostic results are available. The total WBC count in AML may be normal, decreased, or increased. A small percentage of AML patients may first be seen without peripheral blast cells. Platelet counts of less than 20,000/mm³ are common in AML. Abnormalities in one or more organ systems may result from leukemic cell infiltration or metabolic complications related to leukemia. Rarely, a solid mass of leukemic cells will develop called a **granulocytic sarcoma** or **leukemic infiltrate.**

As with ALL, the marrow aspirate is used to obtain the differential count, and biopsy is used to establish an assessment of cellularity and evaluate fibrosis. Myeloblasts comprise at least 20% of the nucleated cells in AML, and the marrow is hypercellular. A "packed" bone marrow with cellularity of 90% to 100% may be seen in AML patients. Immunophenotyping and cytogenetic analysis is routine at time of diagnosis. This is needed to determine appropriate therapy.

Prognostic Indicators

The two major prognostic factors are age and chromosome status.[33] Adults over 60 years are considered older in terms of treatment for leukemia.[32] In younger adults, 30% to 40% of newly diagnosed patients can be cured. In adults over 60 years, overall survival is 10% to 15%.[34] Elderly patients with the same "favorable" cytogenetic features as younger patients still do more poorly. AML seems to be intrinsically more resistant to treatment in the elderly.[35,36] Table 13-7 identifies the most common chromosomal abnormalities and their impact on prognosis. It is important to note that most prognostic factors have focused on patients less than 60 years of age whereas most patients with AML are over 60.[35,36]

Most patients belong to the standard-risk group. This group is highly heterogenous, and new molecular markers have been

TABLE 13-6   **AML Classification***

WHO CLASSIFICATION	FAB	PROGNOSIS
AMLs with Recurrent Cytogenetic Translocations		
AML with t(8;21)(q22;q22)		Good
APL (AML with t(15;17)(q22;q11-12) and variants	M3	Good
AML with abnormal bone marrow eosinophils (inv 16)(p13q22)		Good
AML with 11q23 (MLL) abnormalities		Poor
AML with Multilineage Dysplasia		
With prior MDS		Poor
Without prior MDS		Poor
AML and Myelodysplastic Syndrome, Therapy-Related		
Alkylating agent–related		Poor
Epipodonphyllotoxin-related (some may be lymphoid)		Poor
AML not Otherwise Characterized		
AML minimally differentiated	M0	Treatment resistant
AML without maturation	M1	
AML with maturation	M2	
Acute myelomonocytic leukemia	M4	
Acute monocytic leukemia	M5a, M5b	
Acute erythroid leukemia	M6	
Acute megakaryocytic leukemia	M7	
Acute basophilic leukemia		Very rare, may be result of CML in blast crisis
Acute panmyelosis with myelofibrosis		All three myeloid cell lines affected with significant fibrosis
Acute biphenotypic leukemia		Myeloid and either B or T lymphocyte; rare

*Not all WHO classifications have a corresponding FAB classification.
AML, Acute myelogenous leukemia; AMML, acute myelomonocytic leukemia; FAB, French-American-British; CML, chronic myelogenous leukemia; MDS, myelodysplastic syndrome; WHO, World Health Organization.
Information from Harris NL, Jaffe ES, Diebold J et al: World Health Organization Classification of neoplastic diseases of the hematopoietic and lymphoid tissues: report of the Clinical Advisory Committee Meeting-Airlie House, Virginia. November 1997, J Clin Oncol 17:3835–49, 1999 and Todd WM: Acute myeloid leukemia and related conditions. Hematol Oncol Clin North Am,16(2):301-19, 2002.

TABLE 13-7   **AML Cytogenetics**

CYTOGENETIC ABNORMALITY	FUSION GENE	FREQUENCY IN ADULTS	RISK OF RELAPSE
Favorable			30%
t(8;21)	AML 1/ETO	5%-8%	
Inv 18	CBFβ/MYH11	10%	
t(15;17)	PML-RAR α	15%	
Intermediate			57%
+8		10%	
normal		15%-20%	
Unfavorable			75%
Any 11q23 abnormality	MLL	5%-7%	
t(6;9)	DEK/CAN	<1%	
t(3;3)		1%-2%	
-5/del(5q)		<10%	
-7/del(7q)		<10%	

AML, Acute myelogenous leukemia.
Adapted from Giles FJ, Keating A, Goldstone AH, et al: Acute myeloid leukemia, Hematology 2002 (Am Soc Hematol Educ Prog) 2002:73–110, 2002.

developed to further define this group. Fms-like tyrosine kinase 3, known as FLT3, plays an important role in survival and self-renewal of early hematopoietic stem cells, monocyte precursors, and in early lymphoid development. Mutations in FLT3 are found in 30% of AML patients, including patients with favorable cytogenetic features, but are not detectable in normal hematopoiesis. The presence of FLT3 mutations may explain the variability in prognosis among patients who have the same karyotypes. Testing for FLT3 is currently done only under research protocols.[37] Patients who develop AML related to prior treatment do poorly, often having multiple cytogenetic abnormalities.

Medical Treatment Modalities and Nursing Care Considerations

The treatment goal of AML, as in ALL, is cure. Treatment is divided into two phases: induction and postremission therapy. Currently, maintenance therapy is not recommended in the treatment of AML.

A complete remission in AML is defined as less than 5% marrow blasts in a normocellular marrow. Peripheral blood counts must return to normal, and preexisting adenopathy or organomegaly must be absent.

INDUCTION CHEMOTHERAPY

Successful treatment of AML requires the control of bone marrow and systemic disease, and specific treatment of CNS disease, if present. Cytarabine, 100 to 200 mg/m² per day by continuous intravenous (IV) infusion for 7 days, plus daunorubicin, 45 to 60 mg/m² per day by IV bolus for 3 days, is the standard treatment. This 7 + 3 regimen results in a CR rate of approximately 65%.[31] Idarubicin has been substituted for daunorubicin, with reports of higher CR, but no difference in DFS. High-dose cytarabine (HIDAC) has been studied in various schedules, with no clear benefits over the 7 + 3 regimen.[31]

A bone marrow examination is repeated on day 14 from the first day of chemotherapy to assess for antileukemic response. A positive response is indicated by a hypocellular, aplastic marrow. Peripheral blood studies reflect marrow aplasia, with profound neutropenia and thrombocytopenia at the 14-day nadir. If the day 14 bone marrow shows persistent leukemia, a second induction is started despite severe pancytopenia. Once blood counts have recovered, generally 3 to 4 weeks after the start of induction, a bone marrow aspirate and biopsy is done to assess for response. If evidence of leukemia persists, further therapy is needed with the choice of drugs dependent on the degree of response to the initial induction.

POSTREMISSION THERAPY

If further chemotherapy is not administered to patients in CR, patients will relapse within 6 to 8 months.[38] Postremission therapy options include consolidation therapy with standard-dose chemotherapy, intensification using higher-dose chemotherapy, or ablative therapy. Treatment decisions are based on the patient age, comorbidities, and risk stratification.

Patients aged 18 to 60 are discussed here. "Good-risk" patients with cytogenetic abnormalities t(8,21) or inv(16) benefit from intensification chemotherapy. HIDAC at 2 to 3 g/m^2 for 6 to 12 doses is used. Three or four cycles of HIDAC can produce a cure rate of 60% to 70%.[31,33] There is no benefit to using transplants in these patients in first CR. Patients who relapse are then evaluated for transplant.

Therapy with HIDAC increases the risk for ocular problems and neurotoxicity. Corticosteroid eye drops prevent these ocular problems. Increased neurotoxicity, especially cerebellar toxicity, is more common in the elderly. Pretreatment assessment of the patient's neurologic status, gait, speech, eye movements, and ability to perform alternating movement rapidly should be assessed before administering each dose of HIDAC.[39] Refer to Chapter 21 for specifics on each type of chemotherapy. It is important to remember that chemotherapeutic doses given to treat acute leukemias will always result in bone marrow suppression. Mucositis secondary to chemotherapy is also evident.

Patients who have high-risk cytogenetic features, therapy-related AML, or AML resulting from MDS, and who also have a matched sibling donor (less than one third of patients) should receive allogeneic transplant in first CR.[31] Patients lacking a donor should have an unrelated donor search started as soon as possible after diagnosis. Patients who have either sibling or unrelated transplants have DFS rates of 40% to 45% for those younger than 45 years.[33] The graft-versus-leukemia (GVL) effect is important in helping prevent relapse.

The treatment choice for patients with standard-risk cytogenetic features is not as clear. Choices include intensification with HIDAC, autologous transplant, or allogeneic transplant for those without significant comorbidities.[33] Autologous (auto) stem cell transplant allows higher doses of chemotherapy than intensification, but lacks the GVL effect of allogeneic (allo) stem cell transplant. It also has the potential complication of reinfusion of leukemic cells. Allotransplant has the GVL effect but higher treatment-related mortality than the other two strategies.

Patients unable to tolerate HIDAC or SCT will be given standard consolidation with cytarabine, 100 to 200 mg/m^2 per day

by continuous infusion for 5 days, and 1 to 2 doses of an anthracyline for 2 to 4 courses.[31]

RECURRENT DISEASE

Most patients who achieve CR later relapse with AML and die. Achieving remission after relapse is difficult, and patients who do achieve a second remission rarely survive more than a year. The likelihood of achieving a second CR depends on the length of the first CR. Those patients refractory to initial therapy or with a 6- to 12-month first remission do poorly. For patients eligible for allogeneic transplant, this is the first treatment of choice. Those not eligible for SCT should consider investigational treatment if the first CR is less than 1 year or should repeat the original induction if longer than 1 year.[31]

MULTIDRUG RESISTANCE

MDR to chemotherapy has been attributed to overexpression of the *MDR1* gene and its protein product, P-glycoprotein (Pgp). Pgp functions as a pump, transporting anthracyclines and etoposide out of malignant cells. This results in decreased chemotherapy levels in the malignant cells and affects response rate.[40]

Pgp expression has been shown to be a predictor of chemoresistant disease, especially in the elderly. Cyclosporine's analogue PSC833 is being used as part of induction therapy in some clinical trials. In addition to its role as an efflux pump, a possible role for Pgp as an inhibitor of apoptosis in AML cell survival has been proposed.[40]

Disease-Related Complications and Treatment

Disease-related complications and treatment of lymphoid, myeloid, and myelodysplastic syndromes are similar. The presenting symptoms and severity may differ depending on whether the disease is chronic or acute. The complications and treatment will be discussed in this section. Patient education is an important component of all aspects of care. The Patient Teaching Priorities box below summarizes key teaching priorities for the leukemic patient.

NEUTROPENIA AND INFECTION

Neutropenia and infection are the presenting symptoms in acute leukemia and/or result from treatment. The absolute neutrophil

*P*atient Teaching Priorities
Leukemia

Normal hematopoiesis; purpose of red blood cells, white blood cells, and platelets

Pathophysiology of leukemia

Goals of planned treatment

Treatment schedule and method of administration

Expected side effects and related interventions

Plan for symptom management

Neutropenia and bleeding precautions

Plan for patient and family participation in treatment and shared decision making

Explanation of any procedures, e.g., bone marrow biopsy, catheter insertion

Exploration of patient coping methods and assistance as needed count (ANC) is the total WBCs multiplied by the combined percentage of segmented (mature) neutrophils and band cells. Infection risk increases when the ANC falls below 500 cells/mm³ for longer than 1 week. Sepsis is lethal in 47% of infected patients with neutrophil counts less than 0.1×10^9/L, compared to 14% when counts are more than 1×10^9/L.[41] The duration of neutropenia is significant since there is almost 100% risk of infection if the ANC is below 100/mm for 3 weeks. Most infections are due to bacteria, with most fatal infections caused by fungus.[42]

The patient's own microbial floras pose the greatest risk of infection that results from the severe neutropenia. The nurse's role focuses on reducing this risk by reducing hospital exposure (when appropriate), antimicrobial therapy, colony-stimulating factors, HEPA filtration, private rooms, personal hygiene and skin decontamination, aseptic management of central venous catheters, and clean food and water.[43] A review of the evidence-based literature showed that many hospitals use low microbial diets, but no recent studies link dietary restrictions to decreased infections.[43] Oncology Nursing Society (ONS) guidelines do not recommend protective isolation or food restrictions for care of neutropenic patients.[44] There are contradictory studies confirming a decrease in infection when neutropenic patients use antiseptic bathing.[43] Much of the routine care that is used for neutropenic patients is not evidence-based practice. Patients with CLL have infections that result from a defect in humoral immunity. Even if not neutropenic, they may be infected with *Streptococcus pneumoniae* or *Haemophilus influenzae*.[42]

There is an increased risk of infection when mucositis is present and allowing movement of endogenous flora into the bloodstream. A break in the skin can also allow entry into the blood stream. Long-term venous catheters (LTVC) may have infection rates as high as 60% when patients are severely neutropenic for more than 1 week. Corticosteroids may suppress the immune system and mask signs of infection.[42]

An elevated temperature is often the only sign of infection. Redness, swelling, and pus formation are absent or delayed because of a lack of WBCs. Pain and tenderness may be the presenting signs. Older adults may not demonstrate an elevated temperature, but instead come to attention because of a new onset of delirium.[45] High-risk areas for infection include the perirectal area, the oral mucosa, the sinuses, the lung, and the skin. Blood cultures should be drawn before instituting IV antibiotic therapy. The Infectious Disease Society of America recommends using two sites for blood cultures if a LTVC is present, whereas the National Comprehensive Cancer Network (NCCN) guidelines focus on adequate volume. There is no consensus on culturing techniques, and further studies are needed. Patients at home need to understand the importance of an elevated temperature and not to mask the symptoms by taking an antipyretic. Febrile neutropenia is treated with empiric, broad-spectrum antibiotics.[42]

Hospitalized patients have vital signs assessed every 4 hours and full physical assessment at least daily. Visitors should be screened for infections. Good personal hygiene with an emphasis on oral care is emphasized for all patients. Ambulation is encouraged to promote lung expansion. Good handwashing is stressed for caregivers.[42] Growth factors have been studied in the elderly.

THROMBOCYTOPENIA AND BLEEDING

Thrombocytopenia and bleeding can also occur either at presentation or secondary to chemotherapy in acute leukemias.

Wandt and colleagues studied 105 leukemic patients and found an 18% incidence of bleeding complications in leukemia patients undergoing active treatment when a threshold for platelet transfusion of 10,000/mm³ was used and 17% when 20,000/mm³ was used. The incidence of fatal hemorrhages was less than 1%, and the fatal bleeding actually occurred in patients with counts of 36,000/mm³ and 50,000/mm³.[46] These data support the importance of making platelet transfusion decisions based on the patient's condition as well as the platelet count.

American Society of Clinical Oncology (ASCO) guidelines for platelet transfusion recommend a threshold of 10,000/mm³ for prophylactic platelet transfusion. Multiple randomized trials demonstrate that this approach is equivalent to the use of the 20,000/mm³ threshold. Higher levels may be necessary in patients with signs of hemorrhage, high fever, hyperleukocytosis, rapid fall of platelet count, or coagulation abnormalities (e.g., acute promyelocytic leukemia- APL).[47] The threshold for bone marrow aspirate/biopsy is 20,000/mm³, although many centers use lower numbers. Surgical or invasive procedures require 40,000 to 50,000/mm³.[47]

Platelet counts should be checked 15 minutes to 1 hour after transfusion to assess the increment of platelet increase. This also enables evaluation of possible alloimmunization and the need for a different platelet product. Alloimmunization occurs because the antigens on the transfused platelets react with the patient's antibodies, and the platelets are destroyed. Using platelets that have been leukoreduced and/or irradiated can decrease the risk. If a poor response still occurs, single-donor or HLA-matched platelets may be used. When patients develop fever, chills, or hives during transfusions, they may be premedicated with diphenhydramine and/or hydrocortisone.[47]

Avoiding injury is important in thrombocytopenia. Venipunctures are kept to a minimum and subcutaneous or intramuscular injections are avoided if at all possible. Direct pressure must be applied for longer than the usual period to stop bleeding. The use of electric razors, soft toothbrushes, and stool softeners to decrease straining, and avoidance of rectal manipulation (no enemas no suppositories or rectal exams) is advised. Aspirin and aspirinlike medications, including herbal medications, should be avoided.

HYPERLEUKOCYTOSIS

AML patients with WBC counts greater than 100,000/mm³ are more likely to experience leukostasis. Blast cells are stickier than normal cells and clot more easily. Clinical symptoms are usually related to CNS and pulmonary involvement. This medical emergency necessitates immediate reduction of circulating WBCs. Starting chemotherapy and giving high doses of hydrea can bring the counts down. Allopurinol must also be given to decrease uric acid. If patients are not able to begin chemotherapy, leukopheresis may be used to lower the WBC count. Chronic leukemia patients may have WBC counts greater than 100,000/mm³ without an increased chance of leukostasis.[12]

DISSEMINATED INTRAVASCULAR COAGULATION

DIC is most common in acute promyelocytic leukemia (APL), but the use of all-trans retinoic acid (ATRA), has decreased the incidence with treatment. However, patients with DIC may still be seen at the time of diagnosis with APL and, less commonly, with AML and ALL.

TUMOR LYSIS SYNDROME

Tumor lysis syndrome is the result of massive cell death. It is more frequent in ALL than AML. It is treated with hydration, diuresis, urine alkalinization, electrolyte correction, oral phospate binders, and hemodialysis if needed.

Future Directions

Molecules capable of blocking *FLT3* tyrosine kinase activity are thought to kill transformed cell lines. PKC-412 has been identified as an inhibitor of *FLT3* mutations. Clinical trials incorporating the addition of PKC-412 into induction therapy with daunorubicin and cytarabine are currently in process.[37] Mutations in the *ras* gene are thought to allow autonomous cell growth. These mutations have been described in 10% to 50% of AML patients. Farnesyl transferase inhibitors (FTIs) are agents that inhibit the *ras*-mutated cell lines. R115777 (tipifarnib) and BMS-214662 are examples of drugs in this class currently under investigation.[33]

Prognosis

Median CR duration is 12 to 18 months with only 20% to 25% of complete responders remaining as long-term disease-free survivors.[31] The CR rate for older patients is 45%, compared to 75% for those younger than 60. Long-term DFS is 10% to 15% for older patients[35] and 35% for adults under 40.

ACUTE PROMYELOCYTIC LEUKEMIA

APL is a form of AML with distinct clinical characteristics. It was cytogenetic features and morphology distinct from other types of AML.

Etiology and Risk Factors

The etiology of APL is unknown, but Latinos have the highest incidence. Obesity is thought to increase risk. Secondary APL is seen in patients treated with topoisomerase II inhibitors such as etoposide and doxorubicin. Patients with APL are commonly 30 to 40 years of age.[48]

Classification

Under the old FAB classification, APL is known as M3. In the WHO classification of myeloid malignancies, it is classified as acute promyelocytic leukemia with t(15;17).[7]

Clinical Features

APL is discovered either on routine complete blood count (CBC) or when patients arrive for care with heavy bleeding or in frank DIC (40% of cases). The bone marrow is filled with blasts resembling heavily granulated progranulyocytes. It is typical for patients to first be seen with low blood counts; however, at first visit a few patients manifest a WBC count above10,000/mm³.[48] Presenting symptoms may be infection, fever, bleeding, fatigue, or anemia.

Diagnosis

The diagnosis of APL is confirmed with a bone marrow aspiration and biopsy. The aspirate is sent for analysis of flow cytometry, cytogenetic features, and molecular genetics (PCR) for the presence of PML/RARα. The t(15,17) forms the *PML/RARα* fusion gene that produces the PML/RARα-fusion protein that blocks the differentiation of hematopoietic precursor cells.[48]

Prognostic Indicators

WBC count at presentation less than 10,000/mm³ and age less than 30 are favorable prognostic indicators. Patients who present with platelet counts over 40,000/mm³ at diagnosis have an increased rate of relapse at 3 years.[49]

Medical Treatment Modalities and Nursing Care Considerations

Before the introduction of ATRA (Vesanoid; also called tretinoin), mortality and long-term prognosis of this subtype of AML was poor, with high rates of mortality from DIC and bleeding complications. ATRA, which promotes cell differentiation, has changed the course and outcome of this disease, which now has the best long-term prognosis and cure of the acute myeloid leukemias.

As soon as the diagnosis of APL is confirmed, the patient is started on induction chemotherapy. If DIC is present, the coagulopathies should be aggressively managed. ATRA can be given for a few days before chemotherapy, which effectively stops the coagulopathies associated with APL. ATRA is given orally at a dose of 45mg/m² until CR is obtained, generally in 30 to 45 days. Remissions are not sustained with ATRA alone. Trials have shown improved long-term responses that include the use of ATRA with an anthracycline, either daunorubicin or idarubicin, with or without cytarabine. Once remission is attained, consolidation therapy is given for an additional two cycles with an anthracycline plus ATRA. Maintenance therapy with ATRA is given for at least a year following completion of consolidation. There are data that suggest that the addition of 6-MP and methotrexate as part of maintenance can improve long-term survival. Bone marrow testing including use of PCR for MRD should be done after consolidation to assess response.[49]

Complications

APL DIFFERENTIATION SYNDROME

APL differentiation syndrome or retinoic acid syndrome (RAS) occurs with both ATRA and arsenic. The exact mechanism of action is not fully known or understood. It is a cardiorespiratory distress syndrome occurring in about 25% of patients receiving ATRA. Early recognition of signs and symptoms can prevent the severe respiratory complications, including mortality, associated with it (Box 13-1). RAS is treated with dexamethasone 10 mg every 12 hours given IV or orally for 3 to 5 days or until symptoms resolve. ATRA should be held for moderate to severe cases and restarted once RAS has resolved. Diuretics may also be given for fluid retention.[48]

HYPERLEUKOCYTOSIS

A rapid rise in WBC count may occur with use of ATRA alone. Chemotherapy given with or a few days after initiation of ATRA has decreased symptoms. Leukopheresis is generally not indicated.[50]

RELAPSED DISEASE

Most patients will convert to testing negative by PCR for PML/RARα after consolidation chemotherapy. This is not predictive of cure; however, becoming PCR positive for PML/RARα is predictive of overt relapse generally within months.[49]

Twenty to thirty percent of patients will develop relapsed disease. Patients who relapse can be divided into two groups: those who relapse after maintenance is completed and those who relapse while on ATRA. Patients in the first group should be reinduced with ATRA plus chemotherapy. Patients in the second group are considered ATRA refractory.

Arsenic as a single agent has been shown to produce remission in about 80% of patients who have relapsed or refractory disease. Table 13-8 provides an overview of side effects. Electrocardiograms (ECGs) must be obtained since arsenic can prolong the QT interval and cause torsades de pointes. Potassium and magnesium levels, along with ECGs for prolongation of the QT interval, must be checked throughout administration of arsenic.[51] Table 13-9 describes recommended testing while on arsenic therapy. A bone marrow assessment should be done at day 30 to assess response. If the patient is not in remission, an additional 30-day induction is given. Once CR is obtained, consolidation with arsenic is started 3 to 6 weeks after induction is given. Up to four cycles of consolidation can be given.[52]

BONE MARROW TRANSPLANT

Autologous transplant is an option in patients in second CR who test PCR negative for PML/RARα. Allogeneic transplant should be considered for patients who continue to test PCR positive for PML/RARα if a donor is available.[49]

| BOX 13-1 | Retinoic Acid Syndrome (RAS) |

Early Signs and Symptoms
Fever
Edema
Weight gain
Arthralgias
Musculoskeletal pain
May or may not have leukocytosis

Late Symptoms
Respiratory distress
Interstitial pulmonary infiltrates
Pleural effusions
Pericardial effusion
Chest pain
Acute renal failure
Acute respiratory distress syndrome (ARDS)

| TABLE 13-8 | Side Effects of Arsenic Therapy |

Vasomotor effects	Flushing, headache, tachycardia, dizziness
Cardiac dysrhythmia	QT interval prolongation can progress to ventricular tachycardia and torsades de pointes
Retinoic acid syndrome	Cardiac-respiratory distress syndrome
Gastrointestinal (GI) disturbances	Nausea may occur Diarrhea occurs in 50% of patients
Fatigue	Monitor for anemia
Peripheral neuropathy	Wide range of symptoms Degree is dose related
Skin rash	Macropapular pruritic type on trunk

Future Therapies

Clinical trials are in progress to determine the benefit of adding arsenic to ATRA and anthracyclines in induction or consolidation. There are also trials to determine if the addition of oral chemotherapy agents along with ATRA improves long-term response rates or cure.[49] There are data indicating that gemtuzumab ozogamicin (Mylotarg) as a single agent may be utilized for salvage therapy.[53]

Prognosis

The prognosis for APL has changed to being one of the most fatal to one with a cure rate of 70% to 80%.[49]

MYELODYSPLASTIC SYNDROMES
Etiology and Risk Factors

The exact etiology of de novo MDS is not known. Therapy-related MDS occurs 3 to 8 years after treatment with alkylating agents for lymphoma, multiple myeloma, or breast or ovarian cancer. After therapy with DNA topoisomerase II inhibitors, secondary MDS or AML occurs 2 to 3 years later. Radiation exposure and chemical injury are also risk factors.[54] In about 35% to 40% of patients, the disease transforms to AML.[55]

Classification

The pathophysiology of MDS is thought to begin with involvement of the primitive bone marrow stem cell. Additional abnormalities with the granulocyte-monocyte progenitor cell have been identified. Other studies reported decreased or absent growth of the erythrocyte-megakaryocyte progenitor cell. Abnormalities in the bone marrow environment may also be present.[56] Cytogenetic abnormalities have been found in as many as 70% of patients studied. During the course of the disease, 20% to 30% of patients have developed additional abnormalities.[57]

As with AML, the FAB classification was the initial method of classifying this heterogenous group; it relied on morphology. WHO revised this in 1997 to further refine the categories. Refractory anemia with excess blasts in transformation (RAEB-t) has been reclassified in the WHO system to AML with multilineage dysplasia following MDS. Chronic myelomonocytic leukemia (CMML) is considered a myeloid stem cell disorder with both proliferative and myelodysplastic features. Both systems rely on correctly identifying cell morphology (see Table 13-10).[7]

| TABLE 13-9 | Monitoring While on Arsenic Therapy |

	BEFORE STARTING	TWICE WEEKLY	WEEKLY	OTHER
Electrocardiogram (ECG)	X		X	And prn
Chemistry panel	X		X	And prn
Electrolytes		X		And prn
Magnesium		X		And prn
Complete blood count (CBC)	X		X	And prn

TABLE 13-10 Myelodysplastic Syndromes

FAB CLASSIFICATION	WHO CLASSIFICATION	PERIPHERAL BLOOD	BONE MARROW
RA	RA	Anemia No blasts	Blasts <5% Ringed sid <15%
RARS	RARS	Anemia No blasts	Blasts <5% Ringed sid > 15%
	RCMD	Mono <1000/mm³ Cytopenias (bi- or pan) No or rare blasts	Ringed sid<15% Dysplasia ≥10 % of cells in 2 or more cell lines Blasts <5%
	RCMD-RS	Mono<1000/mm³ Cytopenias (bi-or pan) No or rare blasts	Ringed sid ≥15% Dysplasia ≥10% of cells in 2 or more cell lines Blasts <5%
RAEB	RAEB-1	Cytopenias Blasts <5% Mono <1000/mm³	Uni- or multilineage dysplasia Blasts 5%-9%
	RAEB-2	Cytopenias Blasts ≤5%-19% Mono <1000/mm³ Auer rods + or –	Uni- or multilineage dysplasia Blasts10%-19% Auer rods + or –
	MDS-U	Cytopenias Blasts <1%	Unilineage dysplasia Blasts <5%
	MDS, del(5q) Isolated	Anemia Blasts <5% Plt normal or increased	Blasts <5% Isolated del(5q) Normal or increased mega
	Reclassified from MDS to:		
RAEB-t	AML, with multilineage dysplasia following MDS	Multilineage dysplasia Blasts >20% Cytopenias	Multilineage dysplasia Blasts >20% Cytopenias

Chronic myelomonocytic
    leukemia
	Myelodysplastic/
	    Myeloproliferative
	    Diseases		

FAB, French-American-British; *MDS-U*, myelodysplastic syndrome unclassified; *mega*, megakaryocytes; *mono*, monocytes; *RA*, refractory anemia; *RAEB*, RA with excess blasts; *RARS*, refractory anemia with ringed sideroblasts; *RCMD*, refractory anemia with multilineage dysplasia; *RCMD-RS*, RCMD with ringed sideroblasts; *sid*, sideroblasts; *WHO*, World Health Organization; *Plt*, platelets.

Clinical Features

Presenting symptoms depend on the subtype of MDS. Those with early disease will have minimal symptoms, whereas those with advanced subtypes can have symptoms indistinguishable from AML. The disease may be identified coincidently with routine blood work. Patients may first arrive to be seen with anemia, neutropenia, or thrombocytopenia. A peripheral smear will demonstrate morphologic abnormalities. Easy bruising, bleeding, or bacterial infections may precede the diagnosis. Physical findings reflect the underlying hematologic disturbance. Patients with CMML often have massive splenomegaly (25%), hepatomegaly, lymphadenopathy, and nodular cutaneous leukemic infiltrates, which is rare in other types of MDS.

Diagnosis

Careful review of the clinical presentation, in addition to bone marrow and peripheral blood examination, is important. Medications and viral infections may cause morphologic changes similar to MDS. Bone marrow cellularity must be assessed.

Cytogenetic assessments should be performed on all patients with suspected MDS. Defining characteristics of MDS include clones of immature cells with chromosomal abnormalities, and a high rate of apoptosis in the bone marrow, causing cytopenias.

Prognostic Indicators

The International Prognostic Scoring System (IPPS) (Table 13-11) was developed to stratify the risk of MDS by the International MDS Risk Analysis Workshop.[55] The patient's IPPS risk category is used in planning therapeutic options. Median survival of 184 patients without transplant when stratified by IPPS score were 141.1, 62.9, 22.5, and 4.9 months for the low, INT-1, INT-2, and high-risk groups, respectively.[4]

Medical Treatment Modalities and Nursing Care Considerations

Historically the treatment for MDS for most patients has been supportive care. Supportive care includes treatment with antibiotics for infections, transfusions as needed for anemia and

TABLE 13-11   International Prognostic Scoring System (IPPS) for MDS

PROGNOSTIC VARIABLE	SCORE VALUE				
	0	0.5	1.0	1.5	2.0
BM blasts (%)	<5	5-10	—	11-20	21-30
Karyotype*	Good	Intermediate	Poor		
Cytopenias	0/1	2/3			

*Karyotypes:
Good: normal, -Y, del(5q), del(20q)
Poor: complex (> or = 3 abnormalities) or chromosome 7 anomalies
Intermediate: other abnormalities
Scores for risk groups are as follows: low, 0; intermediate-1, 0.5-1.0; intermediate-2, 1.5-2.0; and high, ≥2.5.

thrombocytopenia, and psychosocial support. A group of clinicians comprising the MDS Panel for Practice Guidelines of the NCCN suggested that therapeutic decisions should be based on age, performance status, and IPPS score. Treatments were categorized as supportive or high or low intensity. High intensity requires hospitalization with significant risk for treatment-related mortality. It may include SCT or intensive combination chemotherapy. Low intensity is defined as outpatient treatment and may include hematopoietic growth factors, differentiation-inducing agents, biologic response modifiers, and low-intensity chemotherapy.[58] High-intensity therapy is generally reserved for patients under age 60 with an IPPS score of INT-2, or high risk. Low-intensity or supportive therapy would be the choice for most other patients. Supportive care is also a part of low- or high-intensity treatment choices.

LOW INTENSITY

Azacitidine (Vidaza) is the first drug approved for the treatment of MDS by the FDA. It is an antimetabolite that acts as a hypomethylating agent and inhibits DNA methyltransferases, resulting in gradual suppression of the abnormal clone. The suppressive effect is thought to lead to an increase in the expression of genes necessary for differentiation, resulting in a gradual improvement of anemia and granulocytopenia following a rise in the platelet counts.[59] A randomized phase III study comparing azacitidine to supportive care showed a complete or partial response in 23% of patients and hematologic improvement in 35% of patients. Hematologic improvement occurred in all three cell lines in 37% of patients, two cell lines in 30% of patients and one cell line in 35% of patients. Median duration of CR has not been reported, but experience suggests that ongoing maintenance is required.[60] Between 40% and 60% of patients experienced grade 3 or 4 hematologic toxicities with neutropenia and thrombocytopenia. Monitoring of hepatic and renal function is required since the drug is excreted through the kidneys, and its use is contraindicated with advanced hepatic tumors or hepatic failure. Subcutaneous injection administration causes ecchymosis, rash, and erythema, necessitating site rotation. Premedication for nausea should be given. The drug is generally given at a dose of 75 mg/m² per day subcutaneously for 7 days monthly for 4 to 6 months. Responses may not be seen for 3 to 4 months.[60]

Decitabine (Dacogen), another drug that inhibits DNA methylation and is capable of inducing cell differentiation, is

currently in clinical trials. Cytogenetic responses were noted in 31% of patients with toxicities of fever (27%), infection (20%), sepsis (11%), neutropenia (12%), anemia (11%), and thrombocytopenia (5%).[57]

Patients with low levels of circulating erythropoietin (EPO) may benefit from either EPO or EPO plus G-CSF, administered subcutaneously. Responses have been higher in patients with low or INT-1 IPPS scores. Arsenic is being studied in clinical trials.[54]

Lenalidomide (Revlimid), a thalidomide derivative, is an oral immunomodulatory agent that does not have the neurologic toxicities or teratogenic effects of thalidomide. It increases both the immune response and erythropoietin-receptor signaling. Dose-dependent myelosuppression is the most common dose-limiting toxicity, with diarrhea, pruritus, and urticaria being the most common adverse events. *Forty-nine percent of patients had a 2 gm increase in hemoglobin or became transfusion independent.* An increase in platelet count (10%) and neutrophils (17%) was also noted. Some normalization of karyotypes occurred in 50% of patients.[57]

Allogeneic SCT is the only known cure for MDS. The older age of many patients with MDS and the lack of available donors limit this option. Approximately 25% of patients with MDS are younger than age 60, and SCT may be considered. A recent analysis was performed using individual patient risk-assessment data from transplantation and nontransplantation registries for all four IPFS risk groups, including adjustments for quality of life to examine the optimal timing of SCT. For low-risk and INT-1 patients, delayed SCT was associated with maximal life expectancy. For INT-2 and high-risk patients, immediate transplantation was associated with maximal life expectancy.[4]

Chronic Leukemias
CHRONIC MYELOGENOUS LEUKEMIA

CML is a myeloproliferative disorder that arises in the hematopoietic stem cell and is characterized by proliferation in the granulocyte cell series. Chronic leukemias differ from acute leukemias in that the malignant WBCs appear mature and are well-differentiated. A second difference is the progression of CML through three distinct phases: chronic, accelerated, and blast crisis.

Etiology and Risk Factors

The incidence of CML increases with exposure to high-dose radiation but is not clearly associated with any other factors.[61]

Classification and Clinical Features

PHILADELPHIA CHROMOSOME

The hallmark of CML is the presence of the Ph+ chromosome, an abnormality that occurs when a portion of chromosome 22 is translocated to the long arm of chromosome 9. This chromosomal translocation creates the hybrid *BCR/ABL* oncogene. The *BCR/ABL* fusion gene activates multiple signal transduction pathways with increased tyrosine kinase activity, resulting in the malignant CML cell undergoing more divisions than a normal cell.[62] This process leads to the large number of granulocytes. The Ph+ chromosome can be detected by cytogenetic analysis of bone marrow aspirate or peripheral blood with increased WBC count, by FISH on peripheral blood or marrow aspirate, or by molecular analysis of *BCR/ABL* by reverse transcriptase polymerase chain reaction (RT-PCR) analysis.[62]

CHRONIC PHASE

The presenting symptoms of chronic-phase CML are related to the expansion of the granulocytic mass. Symptoms may include fatigue, night sweats, pallor, dyspnea, anemia, anorexia, weight loss, and sternal tenderness. The most common finding at diagnosis is splenomegaly. The spleen may be minimally enlarged on palpation to severely enlarged, filling most of the abdominal cavity. The splenomegaly is caused by infiltration of WBCs and can cause symptoms of left upper quadrant pain, early satiety, and abdominal fullness. Many patients are diagnosed on routine blood work and are asymptomatic. Eighty-five percent of patients are diagnosed in chronic phase, which has a median duration of 5 to 6 years. The chronic phase is the initial indolent form of CML (Table 13-12).

A very high WBC count in CML neither leads to complications nor requires emergency leukopheresis. Thrombocytosis is present in about one third of patients, with platelet counts being greater than 1 million/mm^3. WBC and platelet counts may fluctuate in 30- to 60-day cycles without any therapy.[61]

ACCELERATED PHASE

Accelerated phase refers to patients who have been under treatment and show signs of disease progression but do not meet the criteria for blast crisis. The cells acquire more chromosomal abnormalities, with loss of differentiation and increasing numbers of more immature cells. The time to progression is variable and greatly affects length of survival. The leukocyte doubling time shortens to 20 days or less during this stage. Evidence of progression to accelerated phase includes cytogenetic clonal evolution and platelet counts of less than 100,000/mm^3 unrelated to therapy, and for clinical trials, peripheral blasts between 15% to 30% of WBC. WHO criteria define accelerated phase as 10% to 19% of blasts.[63]

Physical exam reveals increased fatigue, increasing anemia, recurrence of splenomegaly, and thrombocytopenia (or thrombocytosis). Occasionally fever of unknown origin, lymphadenopathy, hepatomegaly, and basophilia are present. The patient may exhibit signs of hypermetabolism, including night sweats, decreased appetite, and weight loss. Periosteal infiltrates and lytic lesions may cause bone pain. The survival for patients in accelerated phase can be estimated at about 6 to 9 months.[61]

BLAST PHASE/BLAST CRISIS

Patients with CML inevitably enter blast phase or blast crisis, defined as an aggressive, rapidly terminal phase of the disease that is refractory to treatment. Two thirds of patients have cells with predominantly myeloblastic characteristics; one third exhibit lymphoblastic features. The blast phase resembles either AML or ALL, but neither myeloid nor lymphoid blast crisis responds well to conventional chemotherapy. Median survival of blast crisis is less than 6 months. The defining criterion of blast crisis is when 20% or more of white cells are blasts. Clinical trial definitions still use the 30% or higher number of blasts. Many patients die from complications of infection or bleeding during blast crisis.[61]

Diagnosis

The diagnosis of CML is established by hematologic evaluation. Table 13-12 describes blood and bone marrow findings. A bone marrow aspiration and biopsy with cytogenetic assessment is necessary to evaluate for the presence of the Ph+ chromosome (BCR-ABL) and is required to confirm the diagnosis of CML. The 5% to 10% of patients, previously described as CML with Ph− chromosome, are now considered to have a diagnosis of myeloproliferative syndrome, unclassifiable.[63]

Medical Treatment Modalities and Nursing Care Considerations

Once the diagnosis of CML is confirmed by the presence of the Ph+ chromosome or FISH positivity for BCR-ABL, treatment for CML is initiated. Traditional therapies have included use of busulfan or hydroxyurea (Hydrea), or interferon with or without cytarabine. Chemotherapeutic agents such as busulfan and hydroxyurea only control blood counts and thus produce hematologic responses, but do not eliminate the presence of BCR-ABL.[64] Interferon alone or with the addition of cytarabine produces a 5% to 20% cytogenetic response rate.[64] There has been a significant change in the treatment of CML in the last few years with the introduction of imatinib mesylate (Gleevec), an oral tyrosine kinase inhibitor. Despite the introduction of imatinib, bone marrow transplant continues to be the only curative option available for CML. All patients 65 or younger should be evaluated for a bone marrow transplant to assess the availability of a matched sibling or unrelated donor.[65]

IMATINIB MESYLATE

Imatinib was developed as a molecular targeted therapy with the goal of eliminating production of the malignant clone. Imatinib acts as a selective competitor at the binding site of the tyrosine kinase protein of the *BCR-ABL* oncogene (Fig. 13-2). Imatinib binds at the site instead of the BCR portion of chromosome 22, stopping the cycle of continuous tyrosine kinase production. The binding effect is to shut off production of BCR-ABL and production of the Ph+ chromosome by interfering with the pathways that signal growth of the abnormal cell or signal transduction inhibitors.[66] Imatinib was approved for use in the United States in May 2001, when phase I and II trial data demonstrated complete cytogenetic responses in patients previously treated with interferon.[64] Original phase II trials were completed for chronic phase,

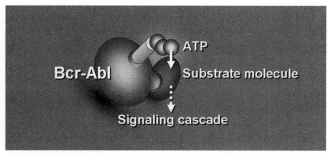

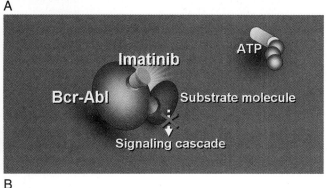

A

B

FIG. 13-2 Imatinib mesylate. Courtesy Jeffrey Zonder, MD.

accelerated phase, and blast crisis. For patients in chronic phase, the results revealed a 95% complete hematologic response (normalization of blood counts), a 60% major cytogenetic response (1% to 30% positivity of BCR-ABL), and a 41% complete cytogenetic response (absence of BCR-ABL). Patients in accelerated phase had a 53% complete hematologic response, 24% had a major cytogenetic response, and 17% had a complete cytogenetic response. Patients in blast crisis attained a 7% complete cytogenetic response. Results in accelerated and blast crisis were not sustained. In the phase 2 study for patients in chronic phase, the median survival has not been reached as of the 5-year mark.[67] Because of these data, a trial with newly diagnosed patients in chronic phase was started comparing imatinib with interferon plus low-dose cytarabine. Results of the IRIS (International Randomized Study of Interferon and STI-571) trial with newly diagnosed CML patients showed an 81% cytogenetic response for the imatinib arm compared to 34.7% for interferon in combination with the low-dose cytarabine arm.[68] The IRIS trial compared both imatinib and interferon alpha (IFN-α) for both response and quality of life.[69] The results showed imatinib was superior in both respects, leading to the early data release from the trial.

TABLE 13-12   Chronic Myelogenous Leukemia

	CHRONIC	ACELERATED	BLAST
Peripheral Blood	WBC often >100,000/mm³ → Blasts < 5%	Basophils to >20%	
	Mature and immature granulocytes, segmented neutrophils predominate ↑ Basophils	Blasts >15% Blast + promyelocytes >30%	Blasts >30% Plus all the same as accelerated phase
		Thrombocytopenia <100,000/mm³ unrelated to toxicity	
	↑ Eosinophils ↑ Megakaryocytes	Hgb <7.0 WBC difficult to control after being stable	
	Mild anemia Normal or ↑ platelets		
Bone Marrow	Hypercellular Blasts <5% ↑ Basophils ↑ Eosinophils	Blasts >10% Basophils or eosinophils >10% Cytogenetic—additional changes Fibrosis beginning	Blasts in clumps Blasts >30% Fibrosis Leukemic infiltrates lymph nodes palpable
	↑ Megakaryocytes in clusters		
Fever	Resolves once WBC controlled	Symptoms recur after being previously controlled	Symptoms recur after being previously controlled
Night Sweats	Resolves once WBC controlled	Symptoms recur after being previously controlled	Symptoms recur after being previously controlled
Weight Loss	Resolves once WBC controlled	Symptoms recur after being previously controlled	Symptoms recur after being previously controlled
Splenomegaly	Resolves once WBC controlled	Symptoms recur after being previously controlled	Symptoms recur after being previously controlled
Bone Pain	Resolves once WBC controlled	Symptoms recur after being previously controlled	Symptoms recur after being previously controlled
Survival	5–6 years	6 mo to 1 year	3–6 mo

Hgb, Hemoglobin; *WBC*, white blood cells.

TABLE 13-13	Side Effects of Imatinib		
		INCIDENCE	MANAGEMENT
Hematologic			
Neutropenia		35%	Monitor blood counts weekly when starting drug
Thrombocytopenia		20%	Stop for ANC less than 1.0, platelets less than 50,000/mm³
Anemia		7%	Restart drug when counts return
GI			
Nausea		57%	Take drug with a meal and full glass of water
Vomiting		24%	Antiemetic as needed
Diarrhea		30%	Antidiarrheal as needed
GI upset		19%	Proton pump inhibitors or H_2 blockers
Muscle cramps		50%	Calcium, magnesium, or potassium
Myalgia		20%	Supplements may help
Anthralgia		20%	Do not take Tylenol or Tylenol-containing OTC meds
Muscle pain		20%	
Edema		61%	Diuretics as needed
Rash		35%	Benadryl if pruritus occurs
Weight gain		30%	Diuretics as needed
Fatigue		18%	Epogen if anemic

ANC, Absolute neutrophil count; *GI,* gastrointestinal; *OTC,* over-the-counter.

Newly diagnosed patients in chronic phase are started on a dose of a 400 mg daily. Patients in accelerated phase should be started at a dose of 600 mg daily. Doses less than 300 mg a day are considered subtherapeutic. The most common side effects are listed in Table 13-13.

Blood counts should be obtained weekly when starting imatinib, since blood counts rapidly decrease. The drug should be held for an ANC less than 1.0 or platelets less than 50,000/mm³. When blood counts normalize, the drug should be restarted at the original daily dose. Blood chemistry studies are monitored since the drug can increase liver enzymes. The drug is metabolized through the P450 pathway. Drugs that interfere with metabolism when used in combination with imatinib are noted in Box 13-2.

Women should not become pregnant while taking imatinib. Adequate birth control measures should be used in females of childbearing potential. Women who become pregnant while on imatinib have the option to discontinue imatinib. They must assess the risk of discontinuing the drug, causing the loss of the cytogenetic response. There are no controlled data on whether discontinuation of imatinib followed by restarting of the drug will allow for another cytogenetic response. There are limited data in men whose partners have become pregnant while the men were on imatinib and women who became pregnant while on imatinib, but not enough for any recommendation except to avoid pregnancy. There are also data that suggest that imatinib can decrease sperm count, decrease testosterone levels, and cause gynecomastia in men.[66,70]

It is essential to evaluate cytogenetic response. This is done most easily by FISH testing for BCR-ABL every 3 months on peripheral blood. Any change in the FISH (from no presence of BCR-ABL to any positive result) requires bone marrow aspiration and biopsy with full cytogenetic testing to assess for resistance. Patients who do not attain a complete hematologic or cytogenetic response are considered refractory. Patients who lose a complete hematologic or cytogenetic response are considered

BOX 13-2	Drugs that Interfere with Metabolism When Used with Imatinib (Gleevec)

Drugs that may Increase Plasma Levels of Imatinib
Clarithromycin
Erythromycin
Itraconazole
Ketoconazole

Drugs that may Decrease Plasma Levels of Imatinib
Carbamazepine
Dexamethasone
Phenobarbital
Phenytoin
Rifampin
St. John's wort

Drugs Whose Plasma Levels may be Increased by Imatinib
Acetaminophen
Cyclosporin
Ca⁺⁺ channel blockers
Statin drugs, e.g., simvastatin
Pimozide
Triazolo-benzodiazepines
Warfarin

Other Substances that Interfere with Imatinib Effectiveness
Grapefruit juice

to be resistant. The dose of imatinib may be increased to 400 mg by mouth twice daily for patients who lose their response. Patients either resistant or refractory to imatinib should be evaluated for either a clinical trial or stem cell marrow transplant.[65]

STEM CELL TRANSPLANTATION

Allogeneic bone marrow transplantation remains the only curative therapy for CML despite the advent of imatinib. Best results occur when the transplant is performed early in the chronic phase. All patients should be evaluated at diagnosis for the presence of a matched sibling or unrelated donor. The quandary for younger patients in chronic phase continues to be the mortality associated with transplant versus the excellent response the majority of patients attain with imatinib. The current recommendation is to proceed to transplant if there is any change in a previous cytogenetic response, or if the patient is refractory to imatinib, or intolerable of side effects of imatinib.[66]

FUTURE TREATMENTS

There are also data on giving increased doses of imatinib to increase initial complete cytogenetic responses. The increase in dose does increase the incidence of side effects.[67] There also are multiple ongoing clinical trials available for patients resistant or refractory to imatinib, including 600-mg daily doses with the addition of other drugs. Trials include approved agents such as cytarabine or interferon, or experimental drugs such as 17-AAG, a protein shock inhibitor; RAD-001, an oral agent that is an mTOR inhibitor; or tipifarnib (Zarnestra), an oral agent that is a farnesyl transferase inhibitor. Dasatinib (Sprycel) was approved in June 2006 for patients refractory or intolerant to imatinib with CML or for Ph+ ALL. New oral agent AMN-107 is in phase I/II trials, and results are not available at present. AMN-107 is given instead of imatinib, with action taking place at a different site on the tyrosine kinase pathway. These drugs were developed specifically to act at a different point in the cell-signalling pathway, adjusting for changes at the binding site where mechanisms are located that cause resistance to imatinib.[66]

NURSING CONSIDERATIONS

Nurses can assist patients using oral therapies by assessing medication use, compliance, side effects, and side effect management. Patients may be unsure if symptoms they are experiencing are side effects of the drug and therefore hesitate to discuss what they are feeling. Many CML patients are very knowledgeable about their disease and become anxious about the cytogenetic results. Even though the side effects of imatinib are significantly less than those of interferon, it is still an emotional challenge for newly diagnosed patients. They have been told they have a malignant disorder that is chronic and not curable without stem cell transplant. Significant psychosocial issues arise in the context of a chronic diagnosis including noncompliance, depression, or increased anxiety over lab test results. The nurse is key in determining support systems and facilitating access to resources such as the Leukemia Lymphoma Society, support groups, or individual counselling, which can help patients cope and live with the diagnosis of a chronic malignant disease.

CHRONIC LYMPHOCYTIC LEUKEMIA

CLL is a malignant chronic lymphoproliferative disorder characterized by proliferation and accumulation of functionally incompetent lymphocytes. The vast majority of cases (95%) are B-cell. The remaining 5% are T-cell in origin.[71] The following discussion focuses on B-cell CLL.

Etiology and Risk Factors

The development of CLL is a result more of genetic predisposition than environmental influences. It is not associated with radiation or drug exposure. A familial tendency has been suggested, but no pattern of inheritance has been reported.[72] CLL has a variable clinical picture, with many patients living a normal life span without treatment whereas others will die within months of diagnosis.[71]

Classification

There are several methods of classifying and distinguishing CLL from other lymphoid malignancies. The two most common staging systems are based on physical findings and lab abnormalities. They are the Rai (used in the United States) and the Binet (used in Europe) systems, summarized in Table 13-14.[73,74] The Rai system has been modified into risk groups rather than the original five stages.[75] Both systems fail to identify subsets of early patients, that is, lymphocytosis alone in Binet stage A and splenomegaly alone in Rai O. They also do not identify subsets that will progress quickly.[71]

TABLE 13-14	**The Rai and Binet Staging Systems**			
STAGING SYSTEM	**STAGE**	**MODIFIED THREE-STAGE SYSTEM**	**CLINICAL FEATURES**	**MEDIAN SURVIVAL (Y)**
Rai	0	Low risk	Lymphocytes in blood and marrow only	>10
	I	Intermediate risk	Lymphocytosis + lymphadenopathy + splenomegaly ± hepatomegaly	7
	II			
	III	High risk	Lymphocytosis + anemia and/or thrombocytopenia	1.5
	IV			
Binet	A		<3 Node-bearing areas	>10
	B		≥3 Node-bearing areas	5
	C		Anemia and/or thrombocytopenia	2

From Zwiebel JA, Cheson BD: Chronic lymphocytic leukemia: staging and prognostic factors, *Semin Oncol* 25(1):43, 1998.

Clinical Features

Chronic lymphocytic leukemia is discovered on routine physical examination or routine laboratory work in the 25% of patients who are asymptomatic. Because CLL is a disease of immunoglobulin-secreting cells, recurrent skin and respiratory infections may be elicited from the patient's history. Nearly 50% of the bone marrow is infiltrated before peripheral blood counts are compromised. Progressive accumulation of the abnormal lymphocytes into nodal structures and advancing marrow involvement yields symptoms of malaise, anorexia, fatigue, and lymphadenopathy, particularly in patients with advanced disease. Gastrointestinal and genitourinary complaints are related to enlarging abdominal lymph nodes. Splenomegaly may cause abdominal discomfort and/or early satiety.

Physical findings may or may not illicit splenomegaly in patients with early-stage disease.

Advanced patients with anemia and thrombocytopenia display bruising or petechiae, as well as shortness of breath (SOB), fatigue, pallor, and weakness. Hepatosplenomegaly may be seen, in addition to splenomegaly, if portal obstruction is related to abdominal adenopathy. Infections are common as the disease progresses and are generally the cause of death in CLL.[76]

Diagnosis

The National Cancer Institute (NCI)–sponsored working group (NCI-WG) has developed guidelines for diagnosis of CLL:[77]

1. Peripheral blood lymphocytosis: an absolute lymphocyte count greater than 5000/mm^3, with cells that appear morphologically mature.
2. Immunophenotype of blood lymphocytes that coexpress B-cell antigens CD19, CD20, and CD23, as well as T-cell antigen CD5; monoclonal expression of either kappa or lambda light chain; and low-density surface immunoglobulin secretion.
3. Bone marrow examination is not a requirement when both of the above criteria are met, but it is useful for prognostic information. Lymphoid cells must constitute more than 30% of cells.
4. The peripheral blood is sent for flow cytometry to assess the immunophenotype of the cells.

Lymph node biopsy of enlarged nodes demonstrates histology indistinguishable from that of small lymphocytic lymphoma.[7]

It must be remembered that CLL is a **heterogeneous disease** even when patients are at the same stage of disease. There are subsets of patients who will have variable courses, some never requiring therapy for many years ranging to those needing treatment within months of diagnosis and resulting in a poorer outcome. Ongoing research efforts are aimed at predicting which of these factors are most predictive of clinical outcomes. Treatment decisions are currently not based on prognostic factors except in clinical trials.

Prognostic Indicators

Clinical stage at time of diagnosis remains the strongest predictor of survival in patients with CLL.

AGE AND SEX

Increased age demonstrates a poorer prognosis in CLL. When compared by stage, some of the differences may be attributed to comorbid conditions of the elderly. Females survive longer than males.

LYMPHOCYTE DOUBLING TIME (LDT)

LDT, the rate at which the lymphocyte count increases, correlates with survival. Those with a LDT longer than 12 months have a better outcome.

β_2-MICROGLOBULINS

Low or high serum β_2-microglobulin (β2M) levels are associated with good and poor survival times, respectively, in the intermediate- and high-risk groups. The increased serum β2M levels correlate with bulky disease.

VH GENES/ZAP-70/CD38 EXPRESSION

There are multiple reports that mutations of the immumoglobulin heavy-chain variable region, commonly referred to as Vh genes, constitute a good prognostic indicator and unmutated Vh genes a negative prognostic indicator. Genotyping is not commercially available. The focus of ongoing research has been to develop a surrogate marker for the presence of Vh genes. Initial reports that testing for CD38+/− and ZAP-70, both done on blood or bone marrow by flow cytometry, could potentially be substituted in place of assessing Vh gene expression; however, data analysis in larger study groups has demonstrated that each of these tests is an individual prognostic indicator. The presence of CD-38+ on the cell surface and expression of the ZAP-70 protein generally correlates with disease that is more aggressive. Increased availability and improved reliability of these tests will increase their use outside of clinical trials.[78-80]

CYTOGENETICS

The most unfavorable abnormality is deletion of part of chromosome 17 (deletion 17p) and is associated with disease refractory to fludarabine (Fludara). An intermediate risk is deletion of 11q22-23. More favorable abnormalities include 13q14 deletion and trisomy 12.[79,81]

Medical Treatment Modalities and Nursing Care Considerations

INDICATIONS FOR TREATMENT

One of the most difficult decisions in CLL is when to initiate treatment. At present, no cure exists for CLL. There are a wide variety of treatment options available, ranging from no treatment or watchful waiting to unrelated allogeneic transplants for subsets of younger patients.

Treatment is aimed at alleviating symptoms. The absolute WBC count is not an indication for treatment. Patients with low-risk prognostic factors should not be treated. There is no survival advantage, and early treatment has had detrimental effects in some studies. The NCI-WG recommends starting treatment when disease-related symptoms are present. These include the following symptoms: weight loss greater than 10% in 6 months, profound fatigue, fever without infection, night sweats, increase in anemia or thrombocytopenia, autoimmune anemia or thrombocytopenia, massively increased lymph nodes or spleen, repeated infections or a rapid increase in WBCs, or high-risk Rai stage.[80,82]

Research is ongoing to develop specific tests and prognostic indicators to determine which groups of patients will benefit from treatment at an early stage. Treatment of patients according to risk stratification remains controversial since no outcome data are yet available.

SINGLE-AGENT CHEMOTHERAPY

Chlorambucil (Leukeran), an alkylating agent, is the earliest agent used in CLL patients. It is given orally in 6- to 14-mg doses every 2 to 4 weeks until maximum response is achieved, generally for 4 to 6 months. Response rates range from 40% to 70%. Combinations with prednisone have shown increased clinical response but not an overall survival advantage.[76]

Cyclophosphamide (Cytoxan) is as effective as chlorambucil, and its non–cross-resistance makes it useful in treating patients unresponsive to chlorambucil. There are minimal data in giving cyclophosphamide as a single agent.[76] Prednisone has been used to control leukocytosis but should be limited because of the increased risk of infection. The use of steroids should be limited to its treatment of autoimmune hemolytic anemia or immune thrombocytopenia.

NUCLEOSIDE ANALOGUES

Fludarabine is the nucleoside analogue used most often in the treatment of CLL. A comparison of fludarabine, chlorambucil, and fludarabine plus chlorambucil showed increased response rates and longer duration of remission and progression-free survival with fludarabine, but no increase in overall survival. The fludarabine plus chlorambucil arm showed significantly increased toxicity and increased incidences of both MDS and acute leukemia, and was stopped early. [83] It is often used as front-line treatment, especially in younger patients.

Cladribine (Leustatin; 2-chlorodeoxyadenosine, 2-CdA) and pentostatin (Nipent) also have shown activity in CLL, but there are fewer studies supporting their use.[82] Clofarabine (Clolar) has recently been approved for pediatric leukemia, and clinical trials are ongoing in CLL.[80] The major toxicity of purine analogues is myelosuppression, requiring close monitoring for infections.

COMBINATION CHEMOTHERAPY

Current combinations include fludarabine with cyclophosphamide (FC),[84,85] fludarabine and rituximab (Rituxan) (FR),[86,87] and clinical trials using all three drugs in combination (FCR).[88] Response rates range from 30% to 80%, but long-term data demonstrating improved survival over previous treatments are not available. The major side effect associated with administration of combination regimens is infections. Fludarabine plus cytoxan caused grade 3 to grade 4 neutropenia, with sepsis occurring in 48% of patients. Fludarabine plus rituxan has an overall response rate of 87%[89] with the major side effects of infection and infusion-related side effects of the rituxan. Grade 3 to grade 4 hematologic toxicity occurred in about 25% of patients. Most combination studies use growth factors and prophylaxis with an antiviral agent for herpes, and trimethoprim-sulfamethoxazole (Bactrim) for bacterial infections and *Pneumocystis carinii* pneumonia (PCP) prophylaxis.

MONOCLONAL ANTIBODIES

Rituxan and alemtuzumab (Campath) are the two approved monoclonal antibodies used in CLL. Rituxan, a CD20 chimeric monoclonal antibody most commonly used in non-Hodgkin's lymphoma has been used alone and in combination with other drugs, usually with fludarabine, to treat CLL.[86] Considerations must be given when rituxan is used in a patient with a WBC count over 30,000/mm³ since frequent, severe, and life-threatening infusion reactions have been reported. When rituxan is administered as a single agent, the dose is divided into three weekly administrations. Premedication is essential to decrease the incidence of reactions.[89] Patients must take allopurinol until their WBC count decreases, and they are monitored for tumor lysis syndrome.

Alemtuzumab is a CD52+ humanized monoclonal antibody indicated for the treatment of CLL resistant to fludarabine. Single-agent response rates range from 33% to 89%, with bulky lymphadenopathy having a poorer response. Alemtuzumab can be given either IV or subcutaneously 3 times weekly with an infusion time of 2 hours.[90] The first dose is given at 3 mg followed by dose escalation daily (3 mg, 10 mg, 30 mg) until the maintenance dose of 30 mg is reached. Once a patient tolerates a dose of 30 mg, the dose is given 3 times a week (e.g., Monday, Wednesday, and Friday) for up to 12 weeks. Premedications include diphenhydramine and acetaminophen with or without hydrocortisone (depending upon institutional protocol). Because of a significant decrease in both B and T cells (CD4 and CD8 cell counts), patients must receive prophylaxis with agents to prevent viral, fungal, and bacterial infections. Lynn, Williams, and Sickler have provided specific drug administration guidelines.[91]

SPLENECTOMY/RADIATION THERAPY

Neither splenectomy nor the use of radiation therapy has demonstrated influence on survival in CLL patients, but they may be beneficial for palliation of symptoms in selected cases.[82]

STEM CELL TRANSPLANTATION

Both autologous and allogeneic SCTs have been utilized in younger patients with high-risk disease as a potentially curative measure in CLL. Autologous transplant has a lower mortality rate and a better response rate when there is minimal disease at time of transplant. There is a statistically significant longer overall survival benefit for autologous transplant in patients with unmutated Vh gene status.[92] The United Kingdom Medical Research Council pilot study had a very low mortality rate in their auto transplant group of 1.5% with a 5-year overall and disease-free survival of 77.5% and 51.5%, respectively.[93] However, clinical and molecular relapses are observed in all series of autologous SCT, which provides evidence against the curative potential of autologous SCT in CLL.[94] Allogeneic transplantation is the only curative mechanism for CLL and has been performed in patients with unmutated Vh gene status, where MRD becomes undetectable with the graft-versus-leukemia effect. This study was on a small sample size.[95] The European BMT Registry reported OS at 10 years was 41% in a series of 54 patients.. The role of reduced intensity conditioning (RIC) in allogeneic SCT is also being explored, and early data demonstrate promise, with many centers using RIC over full myeloablative transplants. The final comparisons will depend on the outcome of large multicenter randomized clinical trials. Any type of transplant for CLL should be performed in a clinical trial setting to collect long-term data and determine the best treatment option.[94]

NURSING CONSIDERATIONS

Nursing considerations for patients with CLL include patient education. Education regarding prevention of infection is essential, as is education about signs and symptoms of infection (bacterial, viral, and fungal). In addition, patients must be aware of medication side effects and what to report to the health care team. The nurse administering chemotherapy or immunotherapy must be alert to infusion-related side effects when giving these drugs and what actions to take if they occur. Assessment of psychosocial needs and the provision of emotional support and resources should be addressed. (See previous sections for additional details.)

Prognosis

Table 13-14 lists prognosis according to stage. As mentioned previously, this varies greatly based on other risks such as Vh gene status and cytogenetics.

HAIRY-CELL LEUKEMIA
Etiology and Risk Factors

Hairy-cell leukemia (HCL) is a rare chronic lymphoproliferative disorder of unknown etiology. There does not seem to be an association with ionizing radiation or other environmental factors. The disease is usually diagnosed in middle-aged patients and is quite rare, representing less than 2% of adult leukemias with a 4:1 increased incidence in males.[96]

Classification

No accepted staging system is useful for both prognosis and therapy. For the purpose of treatment decisions, it is best to consider this disease in two broad categories: untreated and progressive.

Clinical Features

Clinical manifestations of HCL are related to excessive infiltration of the bone marrow or the spleen, or both, with "hairy cells." This results in underproduction or excessive peripheral sequestration of circulating cells manifested as granulocytopenia, anemia, or thrombocytopenia.[96] Half of the patients are first seen with constitutional symptoms (weakness, lethargy, or fatigue) or bruising, bleeding, or infection. Another 25% of patients are diagnosed incidentally when a routine CBC reveals abnormalities. Physical findings are limited to splenomegaly, which is seen in as many as 90% of patients. The spleen may be massively enlarged and measure over 8 cm. Patients are more susceptible to infections, usually by gram-negative bacteria.

Diagnosis

The hallmark of HCL is the presence of the peculiar hairy cell in the blood, the bone marrow, and the reticuloendothelial organs. This cell is characterized morphologically by its hairlike projections. Cytochemical stains demonstrate the presence of tartrate-resistant acid phosphatase (TRAP). Flow cytometry has replaced the use of TRAP in most centers. Flow cytometry reveals strong expression of the B-cell markers including CD19, CD20, CD22, and CD25. CD5 is usually not expressed. The presence of CD103 positivity and/or CD11c, with the coexpression of other pan–B cell markers, is very suggestive of HCL. Patients are diagnosed based on the presence of cytopenias, hairy cells in the peripheral blood, splenomegaly, and bone marrow aspiration and biopsy. The bone marrow is frequently fibrotic and usually not aspirable. Splenomegaly is seen without peripheral lymphadenopathy.[96]

Medical Treatment Modalities and Nursing Care Considerations

Hairy-cell leukemia is a highly treatable and often a curable disease. Patients who are asymptomatic with acceptable blood counts can be observed until the disease progresses and requires treatment. Treatment is required when cytopenias become symptomatic, splenomegaly increases, or infectious complications exist.

Deoxycoformycin (dCF) (pentostatin), is a purine analogue first reported to have activity in HCL in 1984. This drug is given as a short infusion every other week for 3 to 6 months. Overall response to pentostatin was 96%, with a CR of 81% and a median DFS of 15 years.[97]

Cladribine (2-CdA), another purine analogue, has similar activity to dCF. The drug is given intravenously daily for 1 week and has shown an overall response rate of 100%, with CR of 95% with overall survival of 97% at 9 years.[98] Recovery of blood counts has ranged from 11 to 268 days.[99]

Relapse rates at 5 years were 24% with pentostatin and 33% with cladribine; at 10 years they were 42% with pentostatin and 48% with cladribine. The drugs were shown to have equivalent efficacies in HCL, with DFS showing no plateau.[97] The majority of patients who relapse can be successfully retreated with cladribine.[98]

NURSING CONSIDERATIONS

Even though the treatment is short when administering cladribine, blood counts can remain low indefinitely, which requires vigilant observation for signs and symptoms of infection. Blood counts are monitored, and transfusions are given as supportive care until blood counts recover.

Considerations for Older Adults

Care considerations for older adults vary depending upon the hematologic diagnosis and are delineated in the following material.

ACUTE LYMPHOCYTIC LEUKEMIA

Approximately 15% to 30% of adults with ALL are over 60 years of age. The biology of ALL in older patients seems to be significantly different than in younger patients, with the incidence of the Ph+ chromosome being much higher and T-cell ALL being less common. The median overall survival in older patients treated curatively is 3 to 14 months, and 1 to 14 months for those treated palliatively.[100]

Patients over age 60 have the worst prognosis of all adults, and those over 70 years of age have the highest incidence of induction mortality. Cumulative toxicity of chemotherapy is one of the main factors influencing results. Comorbid conditions also play a role, particularly impaired cardiac function, which can limit the use of anthracyclines.[22]

ACUTE MYELOCYTIC LEUKEMIA

Treatment of AML in older patients is complicated not only by comorbidities, but also the prevalence of AML subtypes that are more resistant to treatment. There appears to be an intrinsic difference in the biology of the leukemia itself in adults over 60, displaying several biologic overlaps with secondary AMLs including multilineage involvement, unfavorable cytogenetic features, and elevated activity of multidrug-resistant genes.[101,102] The AML in these patients is more likely to originate from a proximal bone marrow stem cell with abnormalities in more than one cell line. This patient group is also more likely to have had previous chemotherapy, radiation, another malignancy, or previous MDS.[32]

Treatment-related mortality may be as high as 25% in this age group; as a result, decisions must be made whether aggressive induction therapy or supportive care with blood product support and antibiotic therapy is the best choice for each patient, based on comorbidities and performance status. In addition to the standard 7 + 3 regimen, clinical trials have substituted mitoxantrone or idarubicin for daunorubicin, with no statistical differences. The DFS was 14 months for elderly patients treated with standard 7 + 3. Nonmyeloablative allogeneic stem cell transplants are being studied.[32] HIDAC is generally not used in older adults for consolidation because of an increased incidence of cerebellar dysfunction and no increase in survival compared to standard 7 + 3 therapy.[32]

Gemtuzumab ozogamicin is a humanized monoclonal antibody that targets the CD33 antigen, expressed in 90% of patients with AML.[103] It is conjugated to the chemotherapy agent calicheamycin. Gemtuzumab is approved as single-agent therapy for first recurrence in older patients. It has CR rates ranging from 5% to 20%. Current trials are evaluating the use of gemtuzumab in combination with cytarabine, anthracyclines, and fludarabine for patients younger than 60.[103]

Reduced-intensity transplants have been used in patients over age 50. Two-year DFS in first CR was reported at 50%; those transplanted in relapse had survivals of 15%.[33]

The goal of research is to develop chemotherapy regimens that are more tolerable for older adults and reduce drug resistance. The use of growth factors has not led to a reduction in treatment-related morbidity and mortality.

Table 13-15 summarizes the body system changes that occur in varying degrees in older adults. The amount of change can range from minimal to extreme. More than 80% of people older than 65 years of age have at least one comorbid condition. Polypharmacy increases the chance of adverse drug reactions.

The use of medications other than chemotherapy that use the cytochrome P450 system in the liver may interfere with excretion of the chemotherapy medications.[45] Mental status, available support systems, and stage of disease are all important. The patient's overall fitness level is more important than actual age. Pretreatment nutritional status should be evaluated; older persons often have decreased albumin levels.

ACUTE PROMYLEOCYTIC LEUKEMIA

Age is not a prognostic factor in APL, but many studies have identified that the CR rate and survival during induction is less in older adults than in younger adults.

MYELODYSPLASTIC SYNDROME

Older adults with MDS need to be evaluated for other comorbid conditions. Patients in poor clinical condition should receive supportive care. Patients who are able should be offered either demethylating drugs or enrollment in clinical trials.

CHRONIC MYELOGENOUS LEUKEMIA

Of patients diagnosed with CML, 30% are over age 60. Many patients over 65 are not candidates for SCT. Imatinib can be given to older adults with no significant change in the side effect profile.[104] For older adults who do not respond or who become resistant to imatinib, clinical trials should be considered.

CHRONIC LYMPHOCYTIC LEUKEMIA

Older adults may benefit from administration of single-agent regimens such as chlorambucil alone. Each patient needs to be assessed on an individual basis for comorbidities and functional status.[82] Many older adults may never require treatment for their CLL. Supportive care measures, including transfusions as needed and prevention of and treatment of infections, may be the best treatment choice for some patients. Chlorambucil and cyclophosphamide orally as single agents are well tolerated with few side effects. Their use may decrease lymphocyte burden and improve blood counts.

TABLE 13-15 Age-Related Changes in Older Adults

ORGAN	NORMAL PHYSIOLOGIC CHANGES	EFFECT ON MEDICATIONS
Gastrointestinal	Decreased GI motility, saliva, gastric secretions Prolonged gastric emptying Decreased liver function	Increased drug absorption = increased toxicities Decreased drug absorption = decreased drug effectiveness Decreased metabolism of antineoplastic agents
Renal	Decreased glomerular filtration rate and urinary concentrating ability and limited ability to excrete some electrolytes	Decreased ability to excrete toxins = increased toxicities
Body composition change	Increased body fat Decreased plasma volume Decreased total body water Decreased plasma albumin Decreased ratio of lean body weight to fat	Increased concentration of lipid soluble drugs Decreased volume of distribution and increased plasma concentration of hydrophilic drugs
Hematopoiesis	Decreased stem cell (SC) mass Decreased ability to mobilize SC from marrow	Decreased hematopoietic recovery after chemo
Cardiac	Decreased cardiac reserves	Increased CHF
Neurologic	Decreased brain mass Minor declines in memory and cognitive and motor functions	Cerebellar dysfunction Peripheral neuropathy

Conclusion

Great progress has been made in the knowledge of the biologic nature and treatment of leukemia during the past decade. Advances in supportive care of the immunosuppressed patient have dramatically improved survival in leukemia patients. Much research is still required to define more effective therapies to increase DFS and decrease relapse rates.

The challenges and opportunities for nurses are numerous in the field of leukemia. The acuity level of patient care for those with leukemia depends on the disease variables and the practice setting. Hospital-based nurses provide care for the leukemic patient who is acutely ill. The intensity and complexity of the nursing care required for many of these patients rival those of intensive care units. Other patients with leukemia, such as those in chronic phase CML, early CLL, AML, or ALL in remission, or those receiving milder continuation therapy, are seen in the clinic or outpatient setting.

The NCI's Cooperative Group Outreach Program (CGOP) and the Community Clinical Oncology Program (CCOP) provide the opportunity to enroll leukemia patients in cooperative group clinical trials. All patients diagnosed with leukemia should be enrolled in a clinical trial if there is one available. The intensity and complexity of caring for leukemic patients are both rewarding and frustrating. Providing direct care to an acutely ill patient in a life-threatening situation fosters very close relationships with both the patient and the members of his or her support system. These relationships can be intensely rewarding. At the same time the intensity of care can lead to frustration and exhaustion when the patient does not respond to therapy or dies. Sudden and unexpected medical crisis and death do occur in this population of patients. Nurses caring for patients with leukemia must be cognizant of their own feelings and needs. The most valuable support system oncology nurses have is the support and understanding of their peers. These are the people who experience the same joys, fears, pain, and frustrations of caring for the acutely ill patient. The most important self-care aspect of the nurse caring for the patient with leukemia is recognizing the level of investment and acknowledging the emotional peaks and valleys that accompany this investment.

REVIEW QUESTIONS

✓ Case Study

Mrs. M. is a 54-year-old Caucasian female with AML, M2 with cytogenetic abnormality t(6:9). She received induction chemotherapy with standard-dose cytarabine and idarubicin (7 + 3). Complications during induction included becoming refractory to platelet transfusions with development of platelet antibodies and blood cultures positive for *Staphylococcus* from both LTVC and peripheral cultures. She experienced no problems with bleeding complications during treatment. Her blood counts returned to normal after 45 days. The bone marrow biopsy showed a remission marrow after induction therapy.

Her sibling was not a match for SCT. A search for an unrelated donor for SCT was initiated after induction therapy. She received HIDAC for consolidation therapy for three cycles. She was discharged after HIDAC while still neutropenic. She was seen in the outpatient clinic 3 times weekly for follow-up and transfusions as needed. Her platelet counts averaged 30,000/mm³, and she continued to be platelet refractory, requiring transfusions with HLA-matched platelets. She had minimal petechiae and occasional nosebleeds, but no other bleeding. During her first consolidation she was admitted with neutropenic fever with the LTVC infected with *Streptococcus viridans* resistant to cefepime, but sensitive to vancomycin. During her next two consolidations she received prophylactic oral clindamycin. She did not require admission with neutropenic fever during those cycles. Her follow-up bone marrow after cycle 3 continued to show a remission.

An unrelated donor was identified 1 month after completion of treatment. The patient relapsed 1 month after completion of treatment. She was retreated with another induction treatment using HIDAC but did not achieve remission. Mrs. M. was taken to SCT in relapse. She tolerated SCT with minimal complications, engrafted, and was discharged home after 30 days. Her bone marrow showed a remission marrow with normal cytogenetics. She was readmitted with an infection and died of complications.

QUESTIONS

1. Why was Mrs. M. considered high risk at the time of diagnosis?
   a. The type of leukemia
   b. The cytogenetic abnormality
   c. Her age
   d. Because of being platelet refractory
2. What precautions may have been instituted for a platelet count of 3000 mm³?
   a. No suppositories or rectal exam, minimal venipunctures
   b. Platelet transfusions for platelet count less than 50,000 mm³
   c. Bed rest
   d. Neupogen administration
3. Identify the side effects unique to treatment with HIDAC.
   a. Bone marrow suppression
   b. Mucositis
   c. Neurotoxicity and ocular problems
   d. Nausea and vomiting
4. What discharge instructions would the patient receive before leaving the hospital after receiving HIDAC chemotherapy?
   a. Take acetaminophen for any temperature greater than 100° F.
   b. Feel encouraged to resume all normal activities.
   c. Call and report immediately any increased temperature of 100.5° F or higher.
   d. Eat five servings of fresh fruits and vegetables a day.
5. What is the most important means of avoiding infection in neutropenic patients?
   a. Wearing a mask when caring for the patient
   b. Prophylactic antibiotics for all patients
   c. Proper hand washing by patient and caregivers
   d. Use of HEPA filters
6. With a neutropenic patient and an initial temperature of 101° F, what is the best order for what interventions?
   a. Start IV antibiotics ASAP; then draw blood cultures.
   b. Draw blood cultures; then start IV antibiotics.

   c. Increase IV fluids, give Tylenol, and start IV antibiotics.

   d. Give Tylenol, obtain urine for culture and sensitivity testing, and give oral antibiotics.

7. Even though Mrs. M.'s bone marrow showed remission, why did she relapse?

   a. The bone marrow assessment was done incorrectly.

   b. Her cytogenetics revealed a poor prognosis.

   c. She did not receive enough chemotherapy.

   d. She did not take her prophylactic antibiotics.

8. Why did the patient not go into remission after receiving chemotherapy for her relapsed leukemia?

   a. Her leukemia became resistant to HIDAC.

   b. She had an infection.

   c. It was too soon after her last chemotherapy.

   d. She was platelet refractory.

9. What method will decrease the risk of alloimmunization to platelet products?

   a. Give platelet products that are leukopoor.

   b. Premedicate with Benadryl.

   c. Give Demerol for chills.

   d. Give all patients HLA-matched platelets.

10. Patient education for the neutropenic patient with leukemia should stress which of the following?

   a. Importance of handwashing, monitoring temperature, and calling health care provider if febrile

   b. Discussion of fertility and sexuality issues

   c. Informed consent for treatment decision making

   d. Baseline assessment of chemotherapy knowledge

ANSWERS

1. **B.** *Rationale:* t(6:9) is a rare cytogenetic abnormality with a poor prognosis. The best outcomes are seen when transplant is done during first remission.

2. **A.** *Rationale:* Bed rest and Neupogen administration will not particularly affect thrombocytopenia. Parameters for platelet transfusions vary depending upon institutional guidelines and the individual patient. Certainly a platelet count of 50,000/mm³ is not uncommon in a leukemia patient. Avoiding injury is extremely important since it may be difficult to stop the bleeding.

3. **C.** *Rationale:* Although most chemotherapy regimens have the potential to produce side effects of bone marrow suppression, mucositis, and nausea and vomiting, the HIDAC protocol, in particular, commonly causes neurotoxicities and ocular problems.

4. **C.** *Rationale:* Fever is the primary symptom of infection. In neutropenic patients, acetaminophen will mask fever, and therefore initial signs of infection may be missed. Therefore acetaminophen should not be used. Patients should notify their physician immediately of any temperature elevation. Fresh fruits and vegetables are usually avoided to reduce any opportunity for infection from uncooked foods.

5. **C.** *Rationale:* Prophylactic antibiotics are not routinely prescribed, to avoid setting the patient up for antibiotic-resistant strains such as methicillin-resistant *Staphylococcus aureus* (MRSA). HEPA filters and face masks will reduce the amount of airborne organisms. However, the strongest defense against infections is diligent, frequent, and thorough handwashing by staff, visitors, and the patient.

6. **B.** *Rationale:* Blood cultures should be drawn immediately once a fever is suspected. Then initiation of antibiotic therapy can begin. In this manner, the offending organism can be identified and appropriately treated.

7. **B.** *Rationale:* Poor-risk cytogenetic abnormalities predict the possibility of relapse. A remission bone marrow often remains with fewer than 5% blasts. A patient may harbor 10⁻⁰ residual leukemic cells. The cytogenetic abnormality may still be present in some cells and not be seen on routine cytogenetics.

8. **A.** *Rationale:* Leukemic cells can develop multidrug resistance after exposure to chemotherapy. There is no known way to prevent or overcome multidrug resistance.

9. **A.** *Rationale:* Giving leukocyte-poor platelets can decrease exposure to antigens found on donor leukocytes that may be present in platelet transfusions. Repeated exposure to antigens results in having antibodies in the patient that can react against antigens on donor platelets.

10. **A.** *Rationale:* The most important factor in a leukemia patient's education is the prevention of, identification of, and notification regarding infection. All remaining responses are also valuable but not unique to leukemia patients.

REFERENCES

1. Sieff, CA: Overview of hematopoiesis and stem cell function, *Up ToDate*, v14.2, 2006, retrieved October 4, 2006, from www.uptodate.com.

2. Bondurant MC, Koury MJ: Origin and development of blood cells. In Greer JP, Foerster J, Lukens J et al, editors: *Wintrobe's clinical hematology*, Philadelphia, 2004, Lippincott, Williams & Wilkins.

3. American Cancer Society: *Cancer facts and figures—2006*, Atlanta, 2006, Author.

4. Cutler CS, Lee SJ, Greenberg H et al: A decision analysis of allogeneic bone marrow transplantation for the myelodysplastic syndromes: delayed transplantation for low-risk myelodysplasia is associated with improved outcome, *Blood* 104(2):579-585, 2004.

5. Ludwig W, Haferlach T, Schoch C: Classification of acute leukemias. In Pui C, editor: *Treatment of acute leukemias, new directions for clinical research*, Totowa, NJ, 2003, Humana Press.

6. Faderi S, Jeha S, Kantarjian HM: The biology and therapy of adult acute lymphoblastic leukemia, *Cancer* 98(7):1340, 2003.

7. Harris NL, Jaffe ES, Diebold J et al: World Health Organization Classification of neoplastic diseases of the hematopoietic and lymphoid tissues: report of the Clinical Advisory Committee Meeting-Airlie House, Virginia, November 1997, *J Clin Oncol* 17:3835-49, 1999.

8. Freedman AS, Harris NL: Clinical and pathologic features of precursor T and precursor B lymphoblastic leukemia/lymphoma, *Up ToDate*, v14.2, 2006, retrieved October 4, 2006 from www.uptodate.com.

9. Paraskevas F: Clinical flow cytometry. In Greer JP, Foerster J, LukensJ et al, editors: *Wintrobe's clinical hematology*, Philadelphia, 2004, Lippincott, Williams & Wilkins.

10. LeBeau MM, Larson RA: Cytogenetics in acute lymphoblastic leukemia, *Up ToDate*, v14.2, 2006 retrieved October 4, 2006, from www.uptodate.com.

11. O'Donnell MR: Acute leukemias. In Pazdur R, Coia LR, Hoskins WJ et al, editors: *Cancer management: a multidisciplinary approach to medical, surgical, & radiation oncology*, Lawrence, Ks, 2005, CMP Media.

12. Garcia-Manero G, Kantarjian HM, Schiffer CA: Adult acute lymphocytic leukemia. In Kufe DW, Pollack RE, Weichselbaum RR et al, editors: *Holland-Frei Cancer Medicine*, ed 6, Hamilton, ON, 2003, BC Decker.

13. Cortes JE, Kantarjian H: Acute lymphoblastic leukemia. In Pazdur R, editor: *Medical oncology: a comprehensive review*, ed 2, New York, 1996, Huntington.

14. Larson, RA, Dodge RK, Linker CA et al: A randomized controlled trial of filgrastim during remission induction and consolidation chemotherapy for adults with acute lymphoblastic leukemia, CALGB study 9111, *Blood* 92(5):1556-1564, 1998.

15. Surapaneni UR, Cortes JE, Thomas D et al: Central nervous system relapse in adults with acute lymphoblastic leukemia, *Cancer* 94(4): 773-779, 2002.

16. Cortes, J, O'Brien SM, Pierce S et al: The value of high-dose systemic chemotherapy and intrathecal therapy for central nervous system prophylaxis in different risk groups of adult acute lymphoblastic leukemia, *Blood* 86(6):2091-2097, 1995.

17. Martin TG, Gajewski JL: Allogeneic stem cell transplantation for acute lymphocytic leukemia in adults, *Hematol Oncol Clin North Am* 15(1):97-120, 2001.

18. Zhang M, Hoelzer D, Horowitz M et al: Long-term follow-up of adults with acute lymphoblastic leukemia in first remission treated with chemotherapy or bone marrow transplantation, *Ann Intern Med* 123(6):428-431, 1995.

19. Thiebault A, Vernant JP, Degos L et al: Adult acute lymphocytic leukemia study testing chemotherapy and autologous and allogeneic transplantation. A follow-up report of the French protocol LALA 87, *Hematol Oncol Clin North Am* 14(6):1353-1366, 2000.

20. Rowe JM, Richards S, Burnett AK et al: Favorable results of allogeneic bone marrow transplantation (BMT) for adults with Philadelphia (PH)-chromosome-negative acute lymphoblastic leukemia (ALL) in first complete remission (CR): results from the International ALL Trial (MRC UKALL XII/ECOG E2993), *Blood* 98:481a, 2001 (abstract).

21. Lee S, Kim YJ, Min CK et al: The effect of first-line imatinib interim therapy on the outcome of allogeneic stem cell transplantation in adults with newly diagnosed Philadelphia chromosome-positive acute lymphoblastic leukemia, *Blood* 105(9):3449-3457, 2005.

22. Pagano L, Mele L, Trape G, et al: The treatment of acute lymphoblastic leukemia in the elderly, *Leuk Lymphoma* 45(1):117-123, 2004.

23. Wassmann B, Pfeifer H, Stadler M et al: Early molecular response to posttransplantation imatinib determines outcome in MRD+ Philadelphia-positive acute lymphoblastic leukemia, *Blood* 106(2):458-63, 2005.

24. Larson RA: Treatment of acute lymphoblastic leukemia in adults, *Up ToDate*, v14.2, 2006, retrieved October 4, 2006, from www.uptodate.com.

25. Pui CH, Jeha S: Clofarabine, *Nat Rev Drug Discov* May Suppl:S12-3, 2005.

26. Faderl S, Gandhi V, Keating MJ et al: The role of clofarabine in hematologic and solid malignancies-development of a next generation nucleoside analog, *Cancer* 103(10):1985-1995, 2005.

27. Kurtzberg J, Ernst TJ, Keating MJ et al: Phase I study of 506U78 administration of a consecutive 5-day schedule in children and adults with refractory hematologic malignancies, *J Clin Oncol* 23(15):3396-3403, 2005.

28. Stock W, Estrov Z: Detection of minimal residual disease in acute lymphoblastic leukemia, *Up ToDate*, v14.2, 2006, retrieved October 4, 2006, from www.uptodate.com.

29. Henze G, von Stackelberg: Treatment of relapsed acute lymphoblastic leukemia. In Pui C, editor: *Treatment of acute leukemias*, Totowa, NJ, 2003, Humana Press.

30. Hoelzer D, Gökbuget N, Ottmann O et al: Acute lymphoblastic leukemia, *Hematology 2002* (Am Soc Hematol Educ Prog) 2002:10-34, 2002.

31. Schiffer CA, Stone RM: Acute myeloid leukemia in adults. In Kufe DW, Pollack RE, Weichselbaum RR et al, editors in *Holland-Frei Cancer Medicine*, ed 6, Hamilton, ON, 2003, BC Decker.

32. Sekeres MA, Stone RM: The challenge of acute myeloid leukemia in older patients, *Curr Opin Oncol* 14(1):24-30, 2002.

33. Stone RM, O'Donnel MR, Sekers MA: Acute myelogenous leukemia, *Hematology 2004* (Am Soc Hematol Educ Prog) 2004:98-117, 2004.

34. Giles FJ, Keating A, Goldstone AH et al: Acute myeloid leukemia, *Hematology 2002* (Am Soc Hematol Educ Prog) 2002:73-110, 2002.

35. Lichtman MA, Rowe JM: The relationship of patient age to the pathobiology of the clonal myeloid diseases. *Semin Oncol* 31(2):185-197, 2004.

36. Avivi I, Rowe JM: Prognostic factors in acute myeloid leukemia, *Curr Opin Hematol* 12(1):62-67, 2004.

37. Weisberg E, Boulton C, Kelly LM, et al: Inhibition of mutant FLT3 receptors in leukemia cells by the small molecule tyrosine kinase inhibitor PKC412, *Cancer Cell* June (1): 433-443, 2002.

38. Buchner T, Urbanitz D, Hiddemann W: Intensified induction and consolidation with or without maintenance chemotherapy for AML: two multicenter studies of the German AML Cooperative Group, *J Clin Oncol* 3(12):1583-1589, 1985.

39. Waldman AR: High-dose post remission therapy. Wujik D, editor: *Nursing care issues of adult acute leukemia*, New York, 1995, Huntington.

40. Pallis M, Turzanski J, Higashi Y et al: P-glycoprotein in acute myeloid leukaemia: therapeutic implications of its association with both a multidrug-resistant and an apoptosis-resistant phenotype, *Leuk Lymphoma* 43(6):1221-1228, 2002.

41. Giamarellou H, Antoniadou A: Infectious complications of febrile leucopenia, *Infect Dis Clin North Am* 15(2):457-482, 2001.

42. Wujcik D: Infection. In Yarbro CH, Frogge MH, Goodman M, editors: *Cancer symptom management*, ed 3, Boston, 2004, Jones & Bartlett.

43. Larson E, Nirenberg A: Evidence-based nursing practice to prevent infection in hospitalized neutropenic patients with cancer, *Oncol Nurs Forum* 31(4):717-723, 2004.

44. Brown K, Esper P, Kelleher L et al: *Chemotherapy and biotherapy: guidelines and recommendations for practice*, Pittsburgh, PA, 2001, Oncology Nursing Society.

45. Green JM, Hacker ED: Chemotherapy in the geriatric population, *J Clin Oncol* 8(6):591-597, 2004.

46. Wandt H, Frank M, Ehninger G et al: Safety and cost effectiveness of a 10×10 9/L trigger for prophylactic platelet transfusions compared with the traditional 20×10 9/L trigger: a prospective comparative trial in 105 patients with acute myeloid leukemia, *Blood* 91(10):3601-3606, 1998.

47. Schiffer CA, Anderson KC, Bennett CL et al: Platelet transfusion for patients with cancer: clinical practice guidelines of the American Society of Clinical Oncology, *J Clin Oncol* 19(5):1519-1538, 2001.

48. Larson R: Clinical features and treatment of acute promyelocytic leukemia in adults, *Up toDate*, v14.2, 2006, retrieved October 4, 2006, from www.uptodate.com.

49. Tallman MS, Nabhan C, Feusner JH et al: Acute promyelocytic leukemia: evolving therapeutic strategies, *Blood* 99(3):759-767, 2002.

50. Schiffer C: Clinical features, diagnosis, and prognosis of acute myeloid leukemia, *Up toDate*, v.14.2, 2006, retrieved October 4, 2006, from www.uptodate.com.

51. Unnikrishnan D, Dutcher JP, Varsneya N et al: Torsades de pointes in 3 patients with leukemia treated with arsenic trioxide, *Blood* 97(5): 1514-1516, 2001.

52. Soignet SL, Frankel SR, Douer D et al: United States Multicenter Study of arsenic trioxide in relapsed acute promyelocytic leukemia, *J Clin Oncol* 19(18):3852-3860, 2001.

53. Lo-Cocco F, Cimino G, Breccia M et al: Gemtuzumab ozogamicin (Mylotarg) as a single agent for molecularly relapsed acute promyelocytic leukemia, *Blood* 104(7):1995-1999, 2004.

54. Hoffman WK, Koeffler HP: Myelodysplastic syndrome, *Annu Rev Med* 56:1-16, 2005.

55. Greenberg P, Cox C, LeBeau MM et al: International scoring system for evaluating prognosis in myelodysplastic syndromes, *Blood* 89(6): 2079-2088, 1997.

56. Silverman LR: The myelodysplastic syndrome. In Kufe DW, Pollack RE, Weichselbaum RR et al, editors in *Holland-Frei Cancer Medicine*, ed 6, Hamilton, ON, 2003, BC Decker.

57. Estey EH, Schrier SL: Treatment and prognosis of the myelodysplastic syndromes, *Up toDate*, v14.2, 2006, retrieved October 4, 2006, from www.uptodate.com.

58. NCCN practice guidelines for the myelodysplastic syndromes, *J of Natl Comp Can Network* 1:456, 2003, retrieved July 1, 2005, from http://www.nccn.org/professionals/physician_gls/PDF/mds.pdf.

59. Silverman LR, Demakos EP, Peterson BL et al: Randomized controlled trial of azacytidine in patients with the myelodysplastic syndrome: a study of the Cancer and Leukemia Group B, *J Clin Oncol* 20(10):2429-2440, 2002.

60. Kornblith AB, Herndon JE, Silverman LR et al: Impact of azacytidine on the quality of life of patients with myelodysplastic syndrome treated in a randomized phase III trial: a Cancer and Leukemia Group B study, *J Clin Oncol* 20:2441-2452, 2002.

61. Van Etten RA: Clinical manifestations of CML, *Up toDate*, v 14.2, 2006, retrieved October 4, 2006, from www.uptodate.com.

62. Goldman JM, Melo JV: Chronic myelogenous leukemia-Advances in biology and new approaches to treatment, *N Eng J Med* 349(15):1451-1464, 2003.

63. Vardiman J, Harris NL, Brunning RD: The World Health Organization (WHO) classification of the myeloid neoplasms, *Blood* 100(7):2292-2302, 2002.

64. Kantarjian H, Sawyers C, Hochhaus A et al: Hematologic and cytogenetic responses to imatinib mesylate in chronic myelogenous leukemia, *New Engl J Med* 346(9):645-652, 2002.

65. NCCN practice guidelines for the chronic myelogenous leukemia, v1.2006, retrieved September 22, 2005, from http://www.nccn.org/professionals/physician_gls/PDF/mds.pdf.

66. Denninger M., Buchdunger E, Druker B: The development of imatinib as a therapeutic agent for chronic myeloid leukemia, *Blood* 105(7):2640-2653. 2005.

67. Kantarjian H, Talpaz M, O'Brien S et al: High-dose imatinib mesylate therapy in newly diagnosed Philadelphia chromosome-positive chronic phase chronic myeloid leukemia, *Blood* 103(8):2873-2878, 2004.

68. O'Brien S, Guilhot F, Larson R et al: Imatinib compared with interferon and low-dose cytarabine for newly diagnosed chronic-phase chronic myeloid leukemia, *New Engl J Med* 348(11):994-1004, 2003.

69. Hahn E, Glendenning A, Sorensen M et al: Quality of life in patients with newly diagnosed chronic phase chronic myeloid leukemia on imatinib versus interferon alfa plus low-dose cytarabine: results from the IRIS Study, *J Clin Oncol* 21(11):2138-2146, 2003.

70. Hensley ML, Ford JM: Imitinib treatment: specific issues related to safety, fertility, and pregnancy, *Semin Hematol* 40(2 Suppl 2):21-25, 2003.

71. Shanafelt TD, Feyer SM, Kay NE: Prognosis at diagnosis: integrating molecular biologic insights into clinical practice for patients with CLL, *Blood* 103(4):1202-1210, 2004.

72. Goldin, LR, Pfeiffer RM, Li X et al: Familial risk of lymphoproliferative tumors in families of patients with chronic lymphocytic leukemia: results from the Swedish Family-Cancer Database *Blood* 104(6):1850-1854, 2004.

73. Rai KR, Sawitsky A, Cronkite EP et al: Clinical staging of chronic lymphocytic leukemia, *Blood* 46(2):219-234, 1975.

74. Binet JL, Auquier A, Dighiero G et al: A new prognostic classification of chronic lymphocytic leukemia derived from a multivariate survival analysis, *Cancer* 48(1):198-206, 1981.

75. Rai K: A critical analysis of staging in CLL. In Gale RP, Rai, K, editors: Chronic lymphocytic leukemias: recent progress, future directions. New York, 1987, Alan R Liss.

76. Rai K, Keating MJ: Clinical manifestations and diagnosis of chronic lymphocytic leukemia, *Up toDate*, v14.2, 2004, retrieved October 4, 2006, from www.uptodate.com.

77. Cheson BD, Bennet JM, Grever M et al: National Cancer Institute sponsored Working Group guidelines for diagnosis and treatment, *Blood* 87(12):4990-4997, 1996.

78. Rassenti LZ, Huynh L, Toy TL et al: ZAP-70 Compared with immunoglobulin heavy-chain gene mutation status as a predictor of disease progression in chronic lymphocytic leukemia, *N Engl J Med* 351(9):893-901, 2004.

79. Chiorazzi N, Rai KR, Ferrarini M: Chronic lymphocytic leukemia, *N Engl J Med* 352(8):804-815, 2005.

80. Abott BL: Advances in the diagnosis and treatment of chronic lymphocytic leukemia, *Hematol Oncol* 23(1):34-40, 2005.

81. Rai K, Keating MJ: Pathophysiology and cytogenetics of chronic lymphocytic leukemia. *Up toDate*, v14.2, 2006, retrieved October 4, 2006, from www.uptodate.com.

82. Rai K, Keating MJ: Treatment of chronic lymphocytic leukemia, *Up toDate*, v14.2, 2006, retrieved October 4, 2006, from www.uptodate.com.

83. Rai K, Peterson BL, Appelbaum FR et al: Fludarabine compared with chlorambucil as primary therapy for chronic lymphocytic leukemia, *N Engl J Med* 343(24):1750-1757, 2000.

84. Flinn IW, Byrd JC, Morrison C et al: Fludarabine and cyclophosphamide with filgrastim support in patients with previously untreated indolent lymphoid malignancies, *Blood* 96(1):71-75, 2000.

85. O'Brien SM, Kantarjian H, Cortes J et al: Results of the fludarabine and cyclophosphamide combination regimen in chronic lymphocytic leukemia, *J Clin Oncol* 19(5):1414-1420, 2001.

86. Byrd JC, Rai K, Peterson BL et al: Addition of rituximab to fludarabine may prolong progression-free survival and overall survival in patients with previously untreated chronic lymphocytic leukemia: an updated retrospective comparative analysis of CALBG 9712 and CALBG 9011, *Blood* 105(1):49-53, 2005.

87. Schulz H, Klein SK, Rehwald U et al: Phase 2 study of a combined immunochemotherapy using rituximab and fludarabine in patients with chronic lymphocytic leukemia, *Blood* 100(9):3115-3120, 2002.

88. Keating MJ, O'Brien S, Albitar M et al: Early results of a chemoimmunotherapy regimen of fludarabine, cyclophosphamide, and rituximab as initial therapy for chronic lymphocytic leukemia, *J Clin Oncol* 23(18):4079-4088, 2005.

89. Byrd JC, Murphy T, Howard RS et al: Rituximab using a thrice weekly dosing schedule in B-cell chronic lymphocytic leukemia and small lymphocytic lymphoma demonstrates clinical activity and acceptable toxicity, *J Clin Oncol* 19(8):2153-2164, 2001.

90. Mavromatis B, Cheson BD: Monoclonal antibody therapy of chronic lymphocytic leukemia, *J Clin Oncol* 21(9):1874-1881, 2003.

91. Lynn A, Williams ML, Sickler J: Treatment of chronic lymphocytic leukemia with alemtuzumab: a review for nurses, *Oncol Nurs Forum* 30(4):689-694, 2003.

92. Dreger P, Stilgenbauer S, Benner A et al: The prognostic impact of autologous stem cell transplantation in patients with chronic lymphocytic leukemia: a risk-matched analysis based on the Vh gene mutational status, *Blood* 103(7):2850-2858, 2004.

93. Millligan DW, Fernandes S, Dasgupta R et al: Results of the MRC pilot study show autografting for younger patients with chronic lymphocytic leukemia is safe and achieves a high percentage of molecular responses, *Blood* 105(1):397-404, 2005.

94. Byrd JC, Stilgenbauer S, Flinn IW: Chronic lymphocytic leukemia, *Hematology 2004* (Am Soc Hematol Educ Prog) 2004:163-183, 2004.

95. Ritgen M, Stilgenbauer S, von Neuhoff N, et al Graft-versus leukemia activity may overcome therapeutic resistance of chronic lymphocytic leukemia with unmutated immunoglobulin variable heavy-chain gene status: implications of minimal residual disease measurement with quantitative PCR, *Blood* 104(8):2600-2602, 2004.

96. Tallman M: Clinical features and diagnosis of hairy cell leukemia, *Up toDate*, v13.4, 2006, retrieved October 4, 2006, from www.uptodate.com.

97. Else M, Ruchlemer R, Osuji N et al: Long remissions in hairy cell leukemia with purine analogs, *Cancer* 104(11):2442-2448, 2005.

98. Goodman GR, Burian C, Koziol JA: Extended follow-up of patients with hairy cell leukemia after treatment with cladribine. *J Clin Oncol* 21(5):891-896, 2003.

99. Dearden CE, Matutes D, Hilditch E: Long-term follow up of patients with hairy cell leukaemia after treatment with pentostatin or cladribine, *Br J Haematol* 106(2):515-519, 1999.

100. Robak T: Acute lymphoblastic leukemia in elderly patients: biological characteristics and therapeutic approaches, *Drugs Aging* 21(12):779-791, 2004.

101. Pinto A, Zagonel V, Ferrara F: Acute myeloid leukemia in the elderly: biology and therapeutic strategies, *Crit Rev Oncol Hematol* 39(3):275-287, 2001.

102. Godwin JE, Smith SE: Acute myeloid leukemia in the older patient, *Crit Rev Oncol Hematol* 48 (Suppl):S17-26, 2003.

103. Giles F, Estey E, O'Brien: Gemtuzumab ozogamicin in the treatment of acute myeloid leukemia, *Cancer* 98(10):2095-104, 2003.

104. Cortes J, Talpaz M, O'Brien S et al: Effect of age on prognosis with imatinib mesylate therapy for patients with Philadelphia positive chronic myelogenous leukemia, *Cancer* 98(6):1105-1113, 2003.

14

Lung Cancer

Amy J. Hoffman and Audrey G. Gift

In our efforts to understand and meet the challenges of cancer, there are moments in time that remind us of the seriousness of the problem. On August 7, 2005, the news announced the death of the renowned anchorman, Peter Jennings. He had died at his home from lung cancer. Sadly, the next day, Emmy-winning "Dallas" star Barbara Bel Geddes also lost her life to lung cancer. A few days later, the courageous wife of America's "Superman" and later a heroine in advocacy for spinal cord research, Dana Reeve, a lifelong nonsmoker, revealed to the public that she, too, had lung cancer. In March 2006, less than a year after she announced she had lung cancer, Dana Reeve died. These popular people bring an urgent awareness to the unknown faces that will be directly affected by this common aggressive cancer. Even the grandfather of one of the chapter authors (Hoffman), William D. Lawton, who was a surgical technician overseas in World War II, died shortly after diagnosis while trying to combat the disease.

Lung cancer is the second most common cancer irrespective of gender in the United States,[1] and the most common cancer throughout the world.[2] In addition, lung cancer is one of the most lethal of all cancers, accounting for approximately 29% of all cancer deaths that were to occur in 2006.[1] However, despite the prevalence of lung cancer, national media attention and research initiatives pale in comparison to other, less common fatal forms of cancer.[3,4] Moreover, from 2002 to 2004, less was spent on research per lung cancer death than was spent on breast, prostate, and colorectal cancer combined.[5] The Global Lung Cancer Coalition states that the negative perception and stigmas surrounding lung cancer have a direct impact on government funding committed to fighting this disease.[4] Besides a lack of funding, there are no famous spokespersons, no races for a cure, and no movies of the week about persons living with lung cancer. Therefore, the priority becomes education about risk factors, in an effort to prevent the disease. Moreover, promoting research efforts are imperative to optimize care for those who are suffering from the disease and the effects of its treatment.

Epidemiology

Lung cancer was considered a rare disease in the nineteenth and early twentieth centuries.[6] In fact, in 1912, Adler found it difficult to identify 374 persons with lung cancer worldwide to describe the manifestations of this disease.[7] In contrast, by the close of the twentieth century, lung cancer had become the most lethal cause of cancer mortality. The abrupt increase in deaths related to lung cancer started around 1935 (4300 deaths), and it was expected that 174,470 persons would be diagnosed with lung cancer in 2006. Each year, lung cancer kills more people than prostate, breast, and colorectal cancer combined, and it has been the leading cause of cancer deaths among men since the 1950s.[1] Since 1987, death rates related to lung cancer among women continue to exceed those of breast cancer, and lung cancer

remains the leading cause of cancer mortality in women.[1] Peak incidence for both men and women is between 60 and 79 years of age, when the disease affects 1 in 17 men and 1 in 26 women.[8] The American Cancer Society (ACS) reports that the average incidence of lung cancer among African American men during 1997-2001 was 47% higher than among Caucasian men, whereas the incidence rate is comparable among African American and Caucasian women.[8]

Within the United States, approximately 80% of all lung cancer diagnoses are non–small cell lung cancer (NSCLC), and the other 20% are from small cell lung cancer (SCLC). The 5-year survival rate for all stages of lung cancer is a dismal 15%, and this improves to 50% if the disease is detected early while it is still localized.[1] Life-extending and palliative polychemotherapy regimens for persons with NSCLC cancer have a 1-year survival rate of 30% to 40%.[9] A recent, important study indicates greater length of survival for those with resected early-stage NSCLC with adjuvant vinorelbine plus cisplatin.[10] However, greater survival time comes at a cost to the patient's quality of life, given the many unpleasant symptoms, such as fatigue, that occur.[10]

Etiology and Risk Factors

Lung cancer is one of the few cancers that are known to result from specific carcinogens. Evidence exists that lung cancer is the end stage of an interplay of multiple factors resulting in genetic damage as a result of ongoing exposure to carcinogens (e.g., persons exposed to tobacco smoke).[11]

ACTIVE SMOKING: THE PRIMARY RISK FACTOR

The increase in lung cancer incidence occurred after the introduction of cigarettes manufactured with addictive properties in the beginning of the twentieth century.[12] Increased tobacco use during the twentieth century was also propelled by the marketing of cigarettes, which glamorized and instilled a culture of smoking acceptance for men in the 1930s and for women in the 1960s. A prospective study by Hammond in 1954 first demonstrated the relationship between smoking and the risk of developing lung cancer. In subsequent years the association of smoking with the development of lung cancer is one of the strongest and most extensively documented causal relationships in biomedical research.[12] Tobacco has been noted as a complete carcinogen, since approximately 3500 different chemical substances containing at least 20 proven pulmonary carcinogens exist in tobacco.[12]

Smoking accounts for 87% of lung cancer deaths.[1] Increased incidence rates in lung cancer have been associated with increased smoking rates with a lag time that can range from less than 2 years up to 20 years between the start of smoking and development of lung cancer.[12] Likewise, mortality from lung cancer is 23 times higher for current male smokers and 13 times higher for current female smokers, compared with lifelong nonsmokers.[1]

The risk of developing lung cancer increases for smokers who started at an early age, smoked for a number of years, and smoked a greater number of cigarettes per day. Women smoking the same amount as men have a twice the risk of developing lung cancer than men.[13] Cigar and pipe smoking have independently been associated in studies as an increased risk for the development of lung cancer.[14,15] Patients with chronic obstructive pulmonary disease (COPD) have a 4 to 6 times the risk of developing lung cancer, independent of their smoking history.[16]

NONSMOKERS

Cigarette smoking is by far the greatest risk factor for lung cancer in the United States, causing an estimated 80% of lung cancer cases in women and 90% in men. However, approximately 15% of lung cancers are caused by something other than cigarette smoking.[17] Nevertheless, the announcement of Dana Reeve's diagnosis with lung cancer and her never-smoking status strongly illuminates the fact that lung cancer does occur in people who have never smoked. Nonsmokers make up 10% of men with lung cancer, but they comprise 20% of women with the disease.[17] Also, like Dana Reeve, lung cancer occurs in 3% of people under the age of 45 years.[17]

There is a growing body of literature on differences in tumor biology between smokers and nonsmokers. Genetic analyses have shown that widespread chromosomal abnormalities are frequent in lung adenocarcinoma in smokers but are infrequent in never-smokers.[18,19] For example, smokers are exposed to direct and repeated tobacco-related carcinogens that are known to induce genetic damage. Such a genetic environment would alter oncogenes and tumor suppressor genes and lead to tumor progression and resistance. Knowing about risks can help clinicians and patients make decisions about health care behaviors, such as offering and taking opportunities for lung cancer screening. Using a prediction tool such as the Memorial Sloan-Kettering Cancer Center Lung Cancer Risk Assessment, available online at *http://www.mskcc.org/mskcc/html/12463.cfm*, can facilitate informed patient care.

PASSIVE SMOKING

Passive smokers inhale a complex mixture of smoke that is termed environmental tobacco smoke (ETS). Accumulating evidence from epidemiologic studies spurred a report by the Surgeon General that judged ETS to be a cause of lung cancer. This inference was validated in 1992 by the United States Environmental Protection Agency (EPA), and ETS was classified as a known human (class A) carcinogen. Exposure to ETS accounts for approximately 3000 deaths annually in the United States.[12]

RADON

This colorless, odorless, radioactive gas is produced as a result of the decay of uranium and radium. The EPA, the World Health Organization (WHO), and the U. S. Department of Health and Human Services (DHHS) classified radon as a human carcinogen in 2000. Exposure to indoor radon gas presents a significant risk of lung cancer, causing an estimated 7,000 to 30,000 deaths in the United States each year.[20] Radon exposure can occur in places such as homes where there is reduced air turnover and ventilation, and in underground mines. Radon emits tiny airborne radioactive elements that situate themselves in the lungs and emit ionizing radiation to the surrounding epithelial tissue, which increases the risk for lung cancer development.[20]

ASBESTOS

Epidemiologic studies have documented the association between asbestos and lung cancer. Many Americans believe that the use of asbestos in products was banned years ago. However, asbestos is still being imported and sold in the United States and is used in many products such as gaskets and in roofing and friction products.[21] Asbestos exposure may occur not only during the mining and manufacture of asbestos materials but from contact with such materials in the home, in school, or in the workplace. Furthermore, not only is asbestos a carcinogen itself, but exposure to asbestos acts synergistically with cigarette smoking in the development of lung cancer.[21]

OCCUPATIONAL HAZARDS AND AIR POLLUTION

Occupational exposures to carcinogens account for 9% to 15% of reported lung cancer cases.[12] Examples of hazards in the work place can include coal gasification, coke production, exposure to tar and soot, and a number of metals.[12] Outdoor air pollutants have been incriminated in the etiology of lung cancer. Nevertheless, although high rates of lung cancer occur in areas of greater urbanization, no definite association to lung cancer incidence has been found.[12] Indoor air pollution includes the quality of the air indoors and out, as well as the indoors pollutants such as ETS, building materials, radon, household products, and combustion from heating and cooking. The two most important indoor air pollutants that influence the development of lung cancer in developed countries are radon and ETS.[12]

GENETIC SUSCEPTIBILITY

Smoking has been associated with great risk for development of lung cancer. However, relative to never-smokers, the absolute lifetime risk of a smoker developing lung cancer is estimated at 10% to 20%, which leads to the inference that susceptibility is determined by inheritance.[22] The genes that contribute most to the development of lung cancer have been found to be *CYP1A1*, *CYP2D6*, and *GSTM1*.[22] In addition, having a family history of lung cancer has been associated with increased risk. Family members of Caucasian lung cancer patients have 1.48 times the risk of that borne by relatives of healthy Caucasians. In contrast, family members of African Americans with lung cancer have a risk of developing lung cancer that is 2.3 times greater than the relatives of the African American control group members.[23]

DIETARY FACTORS

Diet has been of interest as a potential determinant of the risk of lung cancer, specifically in smokers and pertaining to beta-carotene and vitamin A. Data from three studies indicate that smokers (current and ex-smokers analyzed together) who received high-dose retinoid (B-carotene) supplementation had an increased risk for lung cancer.[23] In the only published randomized control trial studying Vitamin E (alpha-tocopherol) supplementation, it was found to have no effect on lung cancer incidence.[24] A class of nutrients, isothiocyanates, found only in cruciferous vegetables such as broccoli, cauliflower, cabbage, watercress, and bok choy, were found to be protective against lung cancer in a study of a sample of 18,244 males ages 45 to 69 years in Shanghai, China. The study also showed a gene-diet interaction. Subjects genetically deficient in an enzyme (GSTM1) that quickly eliminates isothiocyanates from the body got the most benefit from cruciferous vegetables, presumably because isothiocyanates stayed around longer to confer their protective effect.[25]

ADVANCING AGE

Lung cancer is a disease that is relatively age-dependent, with nearly 9% of patients affected in their 50s, 23% in their 60s, 36% in their 70s, and 30% in their 80s and beyond.[26] Since lung cancer most commonly occurs with advancing age, persons with lung cancer generally have some degree of comorbidities. In addition, aging determines physiologic changes in organ functions and pharmacokinetics. Although anticancer treatment modalities potentially have positive benefits, they have the ability to cause considerable morbidity and even mortality. Thus a comprehensive approach to assessing elderly people with lung cancer should include a geriatric assessment to best gauge the optimal health-related quality of life (HQL) for treatment considerations.[27] However, less is known about effective treatment regimens for elderly populations with lung cancer. The role of clinical trials is to enlighten clinical practice to the best therapeutic options, but the elderly are largely underrepresented in cancer trials.[28] The true effect of treatments in relation to HQL may be confused by pre-existing comorbidities.[29]

RACE

Disparity in the incidence and the mortality rates of cancer among African Americans as compared to white Americans has been on the rise since the 1950s. The incidence of lung cancer had its most dramatic increase for African Americans during the years from 1988 to 1992, when it increased 170% for men and 464% for women.[30] Moreover, one study found that being African American with lung cancer carried a reduced chance of being referred to a specialist and of receiving chemotherapy.[31]

Prevention

The overall *Healthy People 2010* objective for cancer is to "reduce the overall cancer death rate as well as illness, disability, and death by cancer."[32] Since the majority (at least 87%) of lung cancer deaths are smoking related, it is imperative to focus primary prevention efforts within this risk factor category. Of the 564,830 estimated cancer deaths in 2006, about 162,460 (29% of all cancer deaths) will be caused by lung cancer, that is, about 456 persons each day.[1] It is important to note that people who quit smoking, regardless of age, live longer than people who continue to smoke.[1] Furthermore, people who quit smoking before age 50 cut their risk of dying in the next 15 years in half compared to those who continue to smoke.[1] With the cessation of smoking, the risk of lung cancer decreases over time. Approximately 10 years after quitting, an ex-smoker's risk of dying from lung cancer is 30% to 50% less than the risk for those who continue to smoke.[33] Clinicians should encourage all smokers to quit smoking. Guidelines to support clinicians in this effort can be ordered on the Agency for Healthcare Research and Quality National Guideline Clearinghouse website, *www.guidelines.gov*. Additional resources to support smoking cessation can be found on the *Healthy People 2010* website, *www.healthypeople.gov/healthfinder/*. In July 2003, the American Society of Clinical Oncology (ASCO) published an updated policy statement on tobacco control whose goal is to reduce cancer incidence and save lives. This can be found on the Internet at *www.jco.org/cgi/reprint/21/14/2777*.

Prevention targeted towards reducing other risk factors is also important in meeting the *Healthy People 2010* objective for cancer. Clinicians should assess patients for their risk of being exposed to environmental carcinogens such as ETS, radon, and asbestos. Equally important is educating patients about the synergistic effects of concurrent tobacco smoking and exposure to environmental carcinogens in increasing the risk of developing lung cancer. Since lung cancer risk may be inherited and is greater in those with a history of lung disease, a comprehensive patient history is essential. Implementation of prevention practices is imperative, since lung cancer is difficult to detect early and symptoms do not appear until the disease is advanced.

Chemoprevention is the use of chemical or synthetic substances to reduce the risk of developing cancer, or reduce the risk that cancer will reoccur.[34] To date, chemoprevention studies in lung cancer have failed to reduce lung cancer mortality.[24] However, continued progress in the understanding of the molecular and biologic basis of lung carcinogenesis may raise new possibilities for the chemoprevention of lung cancer.

Primary chemoprevention is prevention in persons who are healthy, high-risk smokers. Evidence suggests that high intake of fruit and vegetables is associated with a decreased risk of lung cancer.[35] Consequently, it has been hypothesized that the nutrients in the diet may act to inhibit cancer. However, as previously discussed, phase III trials with retinoids and alpha-tocopherol (vitamin E) have not demonstrated risk reduction. Alpha-tocopherol was found to be more protective in younger men with fewer years of smoking, which suggests that if high levels of serum alpha-tocopherol are present during the early stages of carcinogenesis, this may inhibit the development of lung cancer.[36] In addition, in the Women's Health Study including 39,876 women, researchers found that there was a trend in reduction of the risk for lung cancer for those who regularly took low-dose aspirin.[37] The researchers conclude that a protective effect on lung cancer or a benefit of higher doses cannot be ruled out. At present, researchers are investigating the use of nonsteroidal antiinflammatory drugs (NSAIDs) to reduce the risk of developing lung cancer. A recent metaanalysis to examine this phenomenon support an inverse relationship between NSAIDs use and risk of lung cancer, but do not suggest a causal relationship.[38,39]

Secondary chemoprevention seeks to prevent the development of cancer in people with precancerous lesions. Carcinogenesis of lung cancer is a multistep process evolving into preinvasive and invasive disease. There are targets along the carcinogenic pathway for preventing this progression. Four phase IIb trials evaluated the capability of alpha-tocopherol, beta-carotene, retinol, and retinyl palmitate or isotretinoin to reverse changes in smokers with metaplasia or sputum atypia. Only smoking cessation was correlated with significant reduction in metaplasia and cell proliferation, and isotretinoin administration plus smoking cessation further decreased metaplasia.[24] In a randomized phase IIb study, 112 former or current smokers were randomly assigned to receive a placebo or anethole dithiolethione (ADT), an organosulfur compound found in many vegetables.[16] Results showed no difference between the two groups, but the progression rate in the ADT group was statistically lower than the placebo group. Thus ADT may possibly be effective in chemoprevention for lung cancer. Secondary chemoprevention research is focusing on the identification of biologic markers to reverse premalignancy in lung cancer.[24]

Tertiary chemoprevention focuses on persons who have a previous diagnosis of lung cancer. The goal is to prevent recurrence. Persons with early-stage lung cancer are at high risk for developing secondary tumors. Ongoing research is in progress to identify chemopreventive agents to avert such an event. Selenium, a mineral that has been found in animal studies to prevent the growth of tumors, is now being investigated in the prevention of recurrence of secondary tumor growth in NSCLC.

Screening and Detection

Symptoms of lung cancer do not often appear until the disease has spread, making early detection difficult. Many lung cancers are diagnosed during work-up for other medical conditions. If detected early at a localized stage, lung cancer treatment is more successful, thus enhancing survival. The 5-year survival rate for localized lung cancer that has not metastasized is 50%.[1] However, there are no current standard recommendations for screening to detect lung cancer.

To date, studies involving screening with chest x-ray (CXR) and/or CXR in combination with sputum cytology studies have not demonstrated increased survival benefits for persons with lung cancer. CXR for screening lacks sensitivity in detecting lung cancer since it is not sensitive to lesions smaller than 2 cm.[16] Barriers to detection include size and location of the lesion, image quality, and the skill of the person interpreting the results.

Sputum cytology studies have shown no improvement in reducing lung cancer mortality over CXR. They are particularly helpful in patients with centrally located tumors who have hemoptysis. It is the least invasive means of screening, but testing depends upon the rigor of specimen sampling (at least three samples are most effective) and preservation techniques, as well as the location and size of the tumor. An average overall sputum cytology sensitivity of 0.66 and specificity of 0.99 has been reported.[40]

Currently, low-dose spiral (or helical) chest computed tomography (CT) is the method most likely to offer superiority over CXR for detecting early lung cancer. Chest x-ray examination has been shown to fail to detect up to 77% of CT-detected cancers.[41] These CT scanners noninvasively obtain images by scanning the entire chest in 5 to 10 seconds, during a single breath-hold. The Early Lung Cancer Action Project (ECLAP) demonstrated that false-positive rate results can be kept low (15% for baseline cycles and 6% for subsequent cycles) and that CT screening can be managed with no excess in percutaneous or surgical biopsies when following a well-defined protocol. Furthermore, the relative frequency of finding presurgical stage I lesions is over 80%, most of which are genuine cancers that would lead to death if undetected and untreated.[42]

Bronchoscopy is commonly used for acquiring tissue for diagnosis of cancer, but is limited in detecting clinically occult preinvasive lesions. Autofluorescence bronchoscopy is able to detect preinvasive lesions. However, autofluorescence bronchoscopy has difficulty distinguishing between preinvasive lesions and other, benign epithelial changes.[43] Thus, two newer bronchoscopic techniques have been introduced that demonstrate promising diagnostic sensitivity with varying specificity for each type of change: light-induced fluorescence endoscopy (96.7%, 36.6%) and autofluorescence imaging bronchovideoscope (80%, 83.3%).[44]

Key Components to the Initial Clinical Evaluation

Persons with lung cancer come to the attention of health caregivers with serious, multiple symptoms.[45,46] Among oncology patients aged 65 years and older, those with lung cancer have reported a greater number of symptoms than patients diagnosed with other solid tumors.[47] Greater number of symptoms adds to the overall level of distress and interferes with the person's ability to function physically, psychologically, and socially. Salient patient information important in the initial component of the history includes an assessment of the person's presenting symptoms.

Lung cancer disease and treatment has a negative effect on one's fitness level and hinders participation in physical activities.[47,48] Among the highly prevalent symptoms reported by persons with lung cancer, fatigue heightens the overall symptom burden and interferes with functional status.[49-51] A decreased capacity to perform activities interferes with their independence, leading to a reduction in their health-related quality of life (HQL). It is important to assess the person's ability to participate in typical daily physical activities. This will help the clinician, in collaboration with the patient, develop a plan of care that allows the person to carry out his or her daily activities. It is important to ask whether patients have had any difficulty with work or other activities as a result of their symptoms.[52]

Persons with lung cancer were found to have cognitive deficits before treatment, particularly in verbal memory and frontal lobe executive functions.[53] Various responses have been documented to treatment regimens as they relate to cognitive function. The severity of these deficits and the responses to treatment can vary, both before and after chemotherapy, and after prophylactic whole brain irradiation treatment.[54] Persons with lung cancer can also experience profound levels of emotional distress, particularly depression, which affects those who are also physically compromised.[55] Research has shown that a person's functional status is directly related to symptoms. Questions pertaining to the extent to which their physical and/or psychological symptoms interfere with patients' normal social activities are important (see Chapter 32).[56-60]

Symptoms the person first reports of and exhibits on an ongoing basis should be fully assessed in terms of location, severity, duration, quality, and aggravating and/or alleviating factors, as well as the person's ability and resources to manage the symptoms.[61] Specific respiratory symptoms, such as cough, dyspnea, sputum production, hemoptysis, wheezing, and chest pain, should be assessed in detail. Persons with lung cancer may also experience symptoms such as pain, fatigue, dyspnea, disturbed sleep, nausea, memory loss, anorexia, dry mouth, vomiting, numbness, tingling, diarrhea, fever, cough, constipation, weakness, alopecia, and hot flashes or nightsweats.[51,62] Using a reliable symptom assessment tool, such as the MD Anderson Symptom Inventory (MDASI), the report of the severity of the patient's symptoms and the impact of these symptoms on daily functioning within the past 24 hours can be assessed. The MDASI can be located on the University of Texas MD Anderson Cancer Center's website, at *http://www.mdanderson.org/departments/prg/display.cfm?id=0ee78c60-6646-11d5-812400508b603a14&pn=0ee78204-6646-11d5-12400508b603a14&method=displayfull.*

The patient's past medical history and exposure to risk factors should be assessed. It is imperative to determine any previous treatment for respiratory illnesses (e.g., bronchitis, COPD, asthma, pneumonia, and frequent respiratory infections), as well as ascertain any tobacco and smoke type (e.g., cigarettes, cigars, pipes, smokeless tobacco, and recreational drugs such as marijuana), age at initiation, average use per day, number of years of use, and number of years since quitting. While collecting information on the tobacco history, opportunities may arise to provide tobacco cessation information and counseling as well as information pertaining to other amendable risk factors.

The physical exam includes all body systems, with emphasis on the pulmonary and lymphatic systems. Special note should be taken of the following, which are all signs of respiratory compromise: altered mental status; cough; nasal flaring; cyanosis of the skin, mucous membranes, and nailbeds; use of accessory muscles; asymmetrical chest movement; and asymmetry of the trachea. The presence of prominent vascular markings on the chest wall may indicate a possible superior vena cava syndrome or thrombosis. Palpation, percussion, and auscultation help evaluate potential signs of complications related to lung cancer such as pleural effusion, pericardial effusion, pneumothorax, COPD, asthma, and/or bronchitis, and pneumonia. The lymphatic system is assessed via palpation of the lymph nodes and the abdomen for signs of abnormal spleen or liver enlargement. Any areas where symptom(s) are reported should be examined; for example, after a report of back discomfort, subsequent palpation of the spine may reveal metastatic disease.

DIAGNOSTIC STUDIES

Noninvasive Testing. For persons with suspected lung cancer, noninvasive diagnostics will validate the type of tumor and the clinical stage of disease, and will help provide an evidenced-based, tailored plan of care.[63,64]

Laboratory tests include complete blood count (CBC), chemistry profile, and liver enzymes. Results will show the status of concurrent comorbidities, possible metastatic disease, or the presence of paraneoplastic syndromes; alternatively, normal results may occur even in the presence of lung cancer. If indicated, pulmonary function tests and an electrocardiogram (ECG) with cardiac assessment should be completed, particularly if any chest radiotherapy (RT) will be performed.

Chest x-ray examination is used to assess the primary tumor as well as the presence of any other pulmonary abnormalities such as pleural or pericardial effusions, pneumonia, or congestive heart failure (CHF). Chest CT (including upper abdomen) facilitates assessment of the suspected primary tumor, the status of the mediastinal lymph nodes, bony involvement, and possible tumor invasion of other structures, such as liver and adrenals.[63] CT scan of the chest is effective because lung cancer tumors are highly vascularized and can be distinguished by the intravenous contrast material.

Magnetic resonance imaging (MRI) is used selectively and may provide information about invasion of the pericardium, superior sulcus tumors invading the brachial plexus, vertebral invasion into the spinal cord, or central nervous system (CNS) metastases.[65,66]

Bone imaging is most sensitive for detection of bone metastases. Problems can arise with false-positive scans due to trauma or degenerative disease that may exist.[66] A plain x-ray film can rule out traumatic or degenerative lesions that are detected on a bone imaging test. Bone imaging tests have 50% sensitivity and 92% specificity.[65]

Positron emission tomography (PET) scanning is an imaging technique based on the biologic activity of neoplastic cells compared to normal cells. Lung cancer cells use glucose at a higher rate of glycolysis. Using radiolabeled glucose F-fluoro-deoxy-D-glucose (FDG), areas of high FDG uptake seen by PET indicate tumor growth. PET results should be interpreted in conjunction with CT to correlate the anatomic information. When used to diagnose and stage lung cancer, whole-body PET has resulted in changing the patient management plan 41% of the time, either because lesions that had gone undetected with standard diagnostic imaging were revealed, or because lesions that had appeared suspect on standard diagnostic imaging proved negative on PET.[65] Consequently, PET has an increasingly important role in the evaluation of lung cancer, particularly in distinguishing resectable stage IIIA from nonresectable stage IV NSCLC.[63] Further information about noninvasive testing can be found at the National Cancer Institute (NCI) website at *http://imaging.cancer.gov/imaginginformation/cancerimaging/page1.*

Invasive Diagnostic Testing. Tissue sampling is necessary to diagnose the type of lung cancer, determine the presence of metastatic disease, and ascertain whether mediastinal lymph nodes as identified on radiography are benign or malignant.

The Primary Tumor. The level of invasiveness required depends upon the tumor location and size. In a person with lung cancer, the distinction between NSCLC and SCLC is vital because the treatment prescribed is radically different. A positive pathologic or cytologic diagnosis of NSCLC is reliable, given the following diagnostic testing procedures.[40] However, a possibility of erroneous diagnosis of SCLC on a cytology specimen must be kept in mind if the clinical presentation or clinical course is not consistent with SCLC. In such cases, further testing should be done to determine cell type.[40]

The least invasive approach in obtaining cells is through sputum cytology. This is useful in diagnosing centrally located tumors in persons who have hemoptysis. To ascertain an accurate diagnosis, it is important that health care organizations have an established policy for sputum collection and processing.[40]

Bronchoscopy is commonly used in collecting tissue. Bronchoscopy may be performed on an outpatient basis with sedation and is generally tolerated well. If the findings from a bronchoscopy are normal despite an abnormal CT or PET test, then further attempts should be made to confirm tissue identification.[40]

In conjunction with CT guidance to help localize the lesion at the time of aspiration, transthoracic needle aspiration (TTNA) offers greater sensitivity for tumors of increased size (larger than 2 cm).[40] TTNA can provide a diagnosis in persons with peripheral lesions that cannot be reached by bronchoscopy. Like bronchoscopy, the procedure is generally tolerated well, and a nonconfirmatory result requires further investigation. TTNA complications include bleeding and/or pneumothorax.[40]

In the absence of evidence for metastatic disease, a thoracoscopy or thoracotomy may be the first procedure performed in a person who has a small, inaccessible tumor or a single pulmonary nodule that is found to be suspect via CT or PET scan.[40]

The Mediastinum. Accurate evaluation of the mediastinal lymph nodes greatly affects a person's prognosis and plan of care, since the presence of mediastinal lymph node involvement may indicate stage IIIA (operable) or IIIB (inoperable) NSCLC.[67] Noninvasive diagnostic techniques depend on lymph node size (e.g., CT, endoscopic ultrasound) or metabolism (e.g., PET), but they do not provide definitive tissue diagnosis and are not sufficient for determining nonsurgical treatment.[67] ASCO guidelines recommend biopsy for any mediastinal lymph nodes larger than 1 cm found on CT or positive on FDG-PET scanning.[68]

Mediastinoscopy is the gold standard for evaluation of lymph nodes. It is necessary to consider comorbidities, the degree of suspicion for metastatic disease, the location of the suspicious nodes, and the availability of the procedure with experienced physicians to perform and interpret the results.[67] Mediastinoscopy is performed under general anesthesia on an outpatient basis. The procedure necessitates a small incision at the suprasternal notch to sample most mediastinal lymph nodes.

Endobronchial ultrasound is a newer technique in evaluating the mediastinum and represents an alternative to mediastinoscopy. A biopsy needle catheter is passed through the working channel of an endoscope through the esophageal wall and guided ultrasonographically toward mediastinal nodes of interest. Advantages include imaging, sampling of smaller nodes, and a qualitative assessment of these nodes. A major disadvantage is its inability to sample all nodal stations.[67]

Metastatic Disease. The ASCO 2003 guidelines recommend an FDG-PET scan for the staging of distant metastatic disease when there is no evidence of distant metastatic disease on CT scan of the chest. Suspected metastatic disease in the adrenal glands or liver should be confirmed by biopsy in patients who would be considered as operative candidates.[68]

Overview of Small Cell and Non–Small Cell Lung Cancer

The WHO has identified numerous categories of lung cancer, which include four major histologic types: (1) small cell carcinoma, (2) squamous cell carcinoma, (3) adenocarcinoma, and (4) large cell carcinoma. These classes are further subdivided, and there are also other, less common lung tumors such as carcinoid. For clinical purposes, lung cancer is discussed in two major categories: NSCLC, which comprises 80% of all lung cancer diagnoses in the United States, and SCLC, which accounts for the remaining 20%. Accurate typing and staging are critical to prognosis and selecting treatment options, including entry into clinical trials.

SMALL CELL LUNG CANCER
Cell Type

Biologically and clinically, SCLC behaves differently from all other cell types, which are referred to as NSCLCs. Distinctive to SCLC is its rapid cell growth, its relentless spread with a tendency to be widely disseminated at the time of diagnosis, and its great sensitivity to chemotherapy and RT. Consequently, 60% of patients have metastatic disease on diagnosis. Because of its large growth fraction and aggressive nature, if left untreated the median survival from diagnosis is 2 to 4 months.[69] With the incorporation of chemotherapy regimens into the treatment program, survival is prolonged with at least a four- to fivefold improvement in median survival compared to those who receive no treatment.[69] However, overall survival at 5 years is 5% to 10%.[69] A strong relationship between SCLC and cigarette smoking exists.[70] SCLC is believed to arise from a type of neuroendocrine cell in the basal cell lining of the bronchial mucosa that secretes peptide hormones, called Kulchitsky's cell.[70] The current pathologic classification of SCLC recognizes three classes: (1) small cell carcinoma (most common, comprising more than 90% of all SCLCs); (2) mixed-cell and large cell variant; and (3) combined small and non–small cell carcinoma.

Clinical Presentation

SCLC most often arises in a central endobronchial location (Fig. 14-1). Common signs and symptoms include the following, among others: (1) cough, dyspnea, wheezing, and hemoptysis; (2) postobstructive pneumonia and atelectasis; (3) hilar adenopathy; (4) superior vena cava syndrome (fewer than 10% of patients); and, (5) compression of other mediastinal structures such as the laryngeal nerve (hoarseness) and the esophagus (dysphagia).[70] Frequent sites of distant metastases with corresponding signs and symptoms may include the following: (1) CNS (headache, seizures, visual disturbances); (2) liver (jaundice, asymptomatic elevations in liver enzymes); and (3) bone marrow (anemia, leukopenia, or thrombocytopenia). Weight loss, anorexia, and fatigue are often found in SCLC. Paraneoplastic syndromes occur as a result of secreted polypeptide hormones in SCLC patients and include (1) Eaton-Lambert syndrome (proximal muscle weakness); (2) hyponatremia from syndrome of inappropriate antidiuretic hormone (SIADH, secretion of excess atrial natriuretic peptide); (3) Cushing syndrome (from ectopic adrenocorticotropic hormone [ACTH]); and, (4) various neurologic syndromes.

Staging

The tumor, node, metastasis (TNM) staging classification is rarely used for SCLC because most patients have locally advanced or systemic metastases at the time of diagnosis. Pathologic nodal evaluation is not required since surgery is not a primary treatment in SCLC management. The TNM staging classification may be helpful for the uncommon circumstance when the disease is not extensive (stage I) and the patient may benefit from surgical resection. SCLC is most frequently staged via the Veterans Administration Lung Cancer Study Group, which is a two-staged

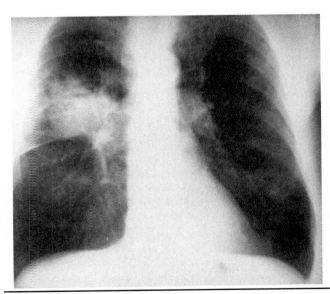

FIG. 14-1 Patient with small-cell cancer in which large tumor mass is centrally located and adjacent pleura is thickened. There is fluid in fissure and possible postobstructive signs of atelectasis. (Courtesy of Dr. Norman Martin, Diagnostic Radiology, University of Kansas Medical Center.)

system: limited- and extensive-stage disease. Thirty percent of patients with small cell carcinoma are diagnosed with limited-stage disease (LD). LD is defined as a tumor confined to one hemithorax of origin, the mediastinum, and the supraclavicular nodes, which can be encompassed within a tolerable radiation therapy port.[69] There is no uncontroversial, universally accepted definition of LD, and patients with pleural effusion, massive pulmonary tumor, and contralateral supraclavicular nodes have been both included within and excluded from LD by various groups. Patients who attain a 2-year disease-free survivorship are generally classified with LD. A small number of these patients may benefit from surgery with or without chemotherapy and thus experience this improved prognosis.[69] Extensive-stage disease (ED) is any stage of disease beyond the LD classification. Patients with distant metastases are always considered to have ED.

Prognostic Factors

In a prospective multicenter study the pretreatment clinical and laboratory values of 436 persons with SCLC were examined.[71] For persons having LD, hemoglobin level, performance status, neuron-specific enolase (a biomarker), and total white blood cell count were significant prognostic indicators for survival, whereas performance status, weight loss, normal lactate dehydrogenase, number of metastases, liver metastasis, and brain metastasis were identified as independent prognostic factors in ED. In a second study consisting of 516 persons with SCLC, similar prognostic factors were found.[57] Complete response (CR) to treatment was achieved in 26.8% of patients and partial response in 40.1%. In addition, the median survival was 10.5 months, and the 2-year survival rate was 12%. The stage of the disease and performance status were major prognostic factors for survival, duration of response, and CR. Female gender was a favorable predictor for CR, whereas superior vena cava syndrome carried a poor prognostic factor for survival and duration of response. Weight loss and age (60 years or above) were predictors of poor response. The sites of metastases affected survival, duration of response, and degree of response. Normal alkaline phosphatase was a favorable prognostic factor for survival, duration of response, and degree of response. Normal lactate dehydrogenase and thoracic irradiation were favorable prognostic factors for survival and duration of response.

Treatment
SURGERY

SCLC is termed a systemic disease because of its propensity for early hematogenous dissemination, and as a result it is rarely treated surgically. However, although controversial, a very small subset are classified as stage I LD patients who are first seen with isolated lesions and no node involvement and who may benefit from surgical resection.[72] Adjuvant combination chemotherapy is advised for surgically treated patients. Phase III trials have demonstrated benefits of preoperative or postoperative chemotherapy with surgical resection. Depending on the extent of the primary tumor and nodal involvement, 5-year survival rates range from 10% to 50%.[72] A recent study of 69 patients who underwent complete resection of SCLC of various stages reported that those who received adjuvant chemotherapy survived longer than those who did not.[73] Pathologic nodal status and chemotherapy were reported as predictors of survival.

CHEMOTHERAPY, RADIATION THERAPY, AND COMBINED THERAPY

SCLC is generally highly chemosensitive and radiosensitive. Chemotherapy has been the cornerstone of treatment for both LD and ED. Chemotherapy in combination with RT has shown to be highly effective with LD SCLC. RT aims to prevent local recurrence of disease by eliminating deposits of tumor cells at the primary site and to palliate symptoms from local and metastatic disease. However, SCLC usually manifests with immense mediastinal lymphadenopathy in combination with tumor mass and atelectasis in the lung parenchyma. This necessitates a large area of thoracic tissue being irradiated, which presents challenges in minimizing undesirable toxicities and side effects such as esophagitis, pneumonitis, and radiation myelopathy. For both the lungs and the esophagus, the risk of toxicity depends not only on the dose, but the volume of tissue irradiated. A goal of RT is to deliver the minimal appropriate target volume and dose.

Intracranial metastasis is identified in 39% of patients with SCLC. Most chemotherapeutic agents do not readily cross the blood-brain barrier. Thus the underlying premise for prophylactic cranial irradiation (PCI) is that moderate doses of radiation administered to patients without detectable CNS involvement might eliminate actual metastases, improve CNS control, and prolong survival. Both randomized and nonrandomized studies demonstrate that PCI is effective in preventing cerebral metastasis. Individual studies do not have sufficient power to show survival benefit. A metaanalysis of seven trials with 987 patients with SCLC in CR compared cranial PCI to no PCI.[74] The study reported a 5.4% increase in the rate of survival at 3 years for those undergoing PCI (15.3% in the control group as opposed to 20.7% in the treatment group). Moreover, higher doses of RT (i.e., 30 to 36 Gy) tended to have better results than lower doses (i.e., 20 Gy). However, this was not a randomized comparison, and survival was not dose dependent. Furthermore, it has been reported that acute and late neurologic toxicity rates are high when PCI is administered in high doses (greater than 40 Gy)[69] and concurrently with chemotherapy.[54] However, data from a prospective trial found cognitive impairment in more than 97% of patients (n = 30) with LD SCLC before undergoing PCI.[75] Baseline cognitive impairment did not seem to deteriorate further in any patients on completion of therapy or at 2-year follow-up. Therefore, PCI is strongly recommended for patients with LD with CR and should be considered for those with ED in CR.[64] PCI is not recommended for persons with multiple comorbidities, poor performance status, or impaired mental function. Furthermore, PCI should not be administered concurrently with systemic chemotherapy because of the risk of increased toxicity. See the National Comprehensive Cancer Network (NCCN) Practice Guidelines in Oncology for specifics on the most current recommended treatment agents and regimens, found online at *http://www.nccn.org/professionals/physician_gls/PDF/sclc.pdf.*

LIMITED-STAGE DISEASE

Several chemotherapeutic agents exist, and a variety of combination treatment regimens are currently used. Current chemotherapy programs deliver overall objective response rates of 65% to 90% and CR rates of 45% to 75%.[69] The combined treatment of chemotherapy and RT has been demonstrated to improve survival over chemotherapy alone.[76,77] The benefit of combined therapy in overall survival at 3 years was 5.4%. The combined therapy was noted to also have increased survival advantages for younger patients, in other words, those younger than 55 years of age as opposed to those older than 70 years of age. Thus chemoradiation is the standard of care throughout the world for persons with LD SCLC, but optimal dosing and sequencing remains controversial. Concurrent combined therapy has demonstrated a survival advantage compared with the sequential plan.[69] The combination of etoposide and cisplatin chemotherapy with concurrent chest RT has now been used in multiple single institutional studies and in cooperative group studies. These studies have consistently achieved median survivals of 18 to 24 months, and 40% to 50% 2-year survival with less than 3% treatment-related mortality.[69]

EXTENSIVE-STAGE DISEASE

Like LD SCLC, combinations of chemotherapeutic agents are required to produce the best result in persons who have ED SCLC. Current chemotherapy doses and schedules provide overall response rates of 70% to 85% and CR rates of 20% to 30% in persons with ED.[69] Platinum-based chemotherapy is most commonly used for ED SCLC. Use of non–platinum-containing cyclophosphamide-based regimens, such as cyclophosphamide, doxorubicin, and vincristine (CAV), has not improved survival over combined etoposide and platinum.[78] There have been no large randomized studies comparing cisplatin to carboplatin in ED patients, but carboplatin appears to be as active as cisplatin.[78] In clinical practice, carboplatin is often substituted in combination with etoposide, has significantly less treatment toxicities, and provides improved tolerability.[78,79] Intensifying the dose of chemotherapy has not increased survival time but leads to increased toxicities and side effects.[69] No obvious improvement in survival occurs when the duration of chemotherapy exceeds 6 months, and no clear evidence is available that maintenance chemotherapy will improve survival duration.[69] Unlike LD SCLC, the addition of thoracic RT to chemotherapy treatment in those with ED has shown no improvement in prognosis compared to chemotherapy alone.[69] However, RT is important in palliation of the symptoms caused by the primary tumor and areas of tumor metastases.

Recurrent Disease

While most persons with SCLC respond to first-line treatment, the majority will relapse. Regardless of the stage, the prognosis for those that relapse is dismal with an expected median survival of 2 to 3 months.[69] Patients who relapse less than 3 months after completing treatment are considered chemoresistant or refractory and should be considered for palliative care or clinical trials.[69] Second-line therapy for early relapsers may be considered, depending on the person's performance status, comorbidities, and sites of progression. Those who initially responded and relapsed more than 3 months after completing treatment are considered chemosensitive and are more likely to respond to additional chemotherapy.[80] Consequently, 20% to 50% of chemosensitive patients respond to second-line chemotherapy, with a median survival time of 6 months.[64] For patients with localized sites of metastasis (e.g., bone, CNS), RT can provide excellent palliation of symptoms.

NON–SMALL CELL LUNG CANCER
Cell Type

Squamous cell carcinoma represents 30% of all lung cancers.[81] These tumors predominantly originate as central tumors arising in the proximal bronchi (Figs. 14-2 and 14-3). They progress

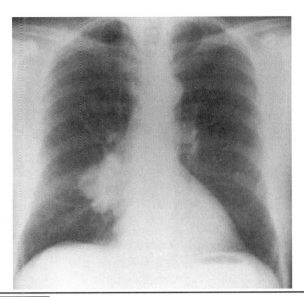

FIG. 14-2   Patient with squamous cell carcinoma that developed centrally (right middle lobe) with left hilar prominence showing regional lymph node spread. (Courtesy of Dr. Norman Martin, Diagnostic Radiology, University of Kansas Medical Center.)

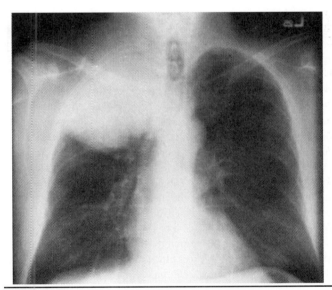

FIG. 14-3   Classic Pancoast tumor in patient with squamous cell carcinoma of lung. Large right upper apex mass with nearly complete right first rib bony destruction and right supraclavicular fullness. (Courtesy of Dr. Norman Martin, Diagnostic Radiology, University of Kansas Medical Center.)

from noninvasive metaplasia and dysplasia to carcinoma in situ. Once a carcinoma in situ penetrates the basement membrane, involving the lamina propria, it becomes invasive and has the ability to metastasize.[82] Histologically, squamous cell carcinoma appears as sheets of epithelial cells that range from well to poorly differentiated. Three features are key to the diagnosis: keratin formation, keratin pearl formation, and intercellular bridges. Most frequently, hypercalcemia is associated with squamous cell carcinoma. It tends to be slow growing and progresses from in situ to a clinically apparent tumor in 3 to 4 years.[82]

Adenocarcinoma is the most common type of lung cancer and the most commonly occurring cell type in nonsmokers.[64]

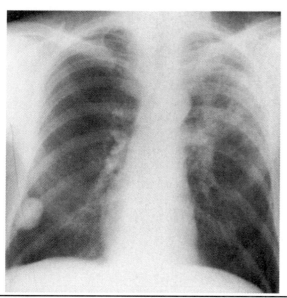

FIG. 14-4   Adenocarcinomas can present as clearly defined peripheral lesions. Patient with right lower lobe lesion. (Courtesy of Dr. Norman Martin, Diagnostic Radiology, University of Kansas Medical Center.)

Adenocarcinoma arises from the alveolar surface of the epithelium or bronchial mucosal glands where it produces mucin.[70] Adenocarcinoma usually manifests itself in the periphery of the lung (Fig. 14-4), and is usually associated with fewer pulmonary symptoms than the other, more centrally located cancers. It has been hypothesized that filtered cigarettes cause smokers to inhale more deeply, exposing the deeper, more peripheral airways to the carcinogens[82] and resulting in greater incidence of adenocarcinoma rather than squamous cell carcinoma. Adenocarcinoma may originate as a single pulmonary lesion or as multifocal disease. Adenocarcinomas grow more slowly than small cell carcinomas; however, they invade lymphatic and blood vessels early, and for this reason they have a worse stage-for-stage prognosis compared to small cell carcinomas. Of the many adenocarcinoma subtypes, bronchioloalveolar carcinoma (BAC), although more uncommon, is of particular interest because of its increase in incidence. This type typically is seen in younger patients and women who are nonsmokers. BAC has a lesser tendency for extrathoracic metastases, with a better survival rate than NSCLC at a similar stage.[83]

Large cell carcinoma represents approximately 15% of all lung cancers. These tumors are less well differentiated than adenocarcinoma tumors and do not exhibit glandular or squamous characteristics on light microscopy.[82] Large cell carcinomas tend to be found at the periphery of the lung, invading subsegmental bronchi or larger airways. Central necrosis is common, but cavitation of the airways is rare. These cells typically contain neuroendocrine features associated with a poorer prognosis.[82] Giant cell carcinoma is a subtype of large cell carcinoma and has a poorer prognosis as compared to large cell carcinoma.[82]

Clinical Presentation

NSCLC presents as a central or peripheral tumor and can grow within the lung parenchyma or the bronchial wall.[84] Spread of NSCLC by direct extension to the chest wall, diaphragm, or lymphatic invasion may occlude the airway and compress the pulmonary areas of the vasculature, the nerves, and the alveolar structures. The pulmonary lymphatics and vasculature provides a

mechanism for metastases to local (intrapulmonary and hilar), regional (hilar and mediastinal), and distant (supraclavicular) nodal sites. Metastatic disease commonly involves the bone, the liver, the adrenal glands, the pericardium, and the brain (Figs. 14-5 to 14-7). Thus the clinical presentation of NSCLC is variable and depends upon the manifestations of the local tumor growth, the regional spread, the distant metastases, and the presence of any paraneoplastic syndromes. However, the overwhelming majority of persons with lung cancer are symptomatic at the time of diagnosis,[45,47] and many persons are seen at diagnosis with signs and symptoms of oncologic urgencies and emergencies (e.g., superior vena cava syndrome, pericardial effusion, cardiac tamponade, pleural effusion, and malignant spinal cord compression).[85]

Staging

The staging system applied to NSCLC is the TNM system, revised in 1996. The American Joint Committee on Cancer (AJCC) and the Union Internationale Contre le Cancer adopted the revisions, which were published in 1997.[86] The purpose of the revisions was to refine the placement of persons with lung cancer into strategies with similar survival rates and therapeutic options. Accurate staging is imperative to make decisions about curative or palliative treatment. The 5-year survival rate for patients with surgical stage IA is 67%, which drops to 57% at stage IB. However, the 5-year survival rate diminishes in patients with more advanced stages: 55% for stage IIA and 38% to 39% for stage IIB; 23 to 25% for stage IIIA and 3% to 7% for stage IIIB; and 1% for stage IV disease.[64] Further information about the staging system can be found in the NCCN Practice Guidelines in Oncology online at *http://www.nccn.org/professionals/physician_gls/f_guidelines. asp#site.*

Prognostic Factors

Prognostic factors predictive of survival in persons with NSCLC include the patient's performance status, which is key in predicting not only the patient's ability to receive therapy, but also survivability.[87,88] Other favorable prognostic factors include early stage of disease at time of diagnosis, no significant weight loss (not more than 5%),[64] fewer comorbidities,[87] and being female.[64] Histology affects prognosis. Persons with large cell carcinoma are reported to have a poorer prognosis (followed by those with adenocarcinoma) than those with squamous cell or bronchioloalveolar carcinoma of the lung.[70] The presence of symptoms that reflect advancing disease also affects survivability.[46] New biologic markers such as p53, activation of k-*ras* oncogenes, and lack of H-*ras* p21 expression are associated with a poor outcome.[64] Other factors reported that demonstrate a poorer prognosis are hemoglobin (Hgb) levels of 10 g/dl or lower compared to Hgb above 10 g/dl[89]; tumor size greater than 5 cm as compared to those measuring 3.1 to 5 cm[90]; and concurrent COPD with the presence of a worsening pulmonary function (last forced expiratory volume 1 [FEV1] percentile versus first FEV1 percentile).[91]

Treatment

Treatment for NSCLC is determined by the stage of disease in consideration with other patient characteristics (e.g., performance status, comorbidities, symptoms). Surgery, RT, and chemotherapy represent common modalities to treat NSCLC. Depending on the status of the disease, the approach may be used singly or in combination.

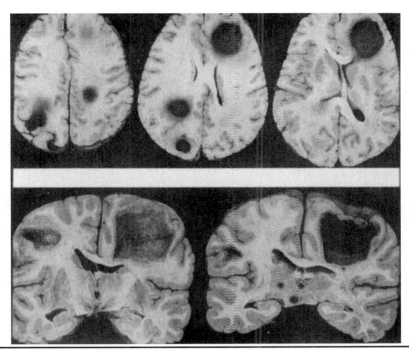

FIG. 14-5   Brain metastases. *Top,* Gross specimens show metastatic deposits of an undifferentiated large cell lung carcinoma. The metastases form essentially necrotic masses with peripheral enhancement and peritumoral edema. *Bottom,* Occasionally, extensive necrosis transforms metastases into cysts lined by only a thin rim of viable tumor.

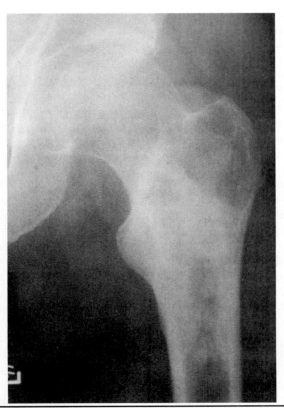

FIG. 14-6   Osteoblastic metastatic lesion to hip from adenocarcinoma of lung.

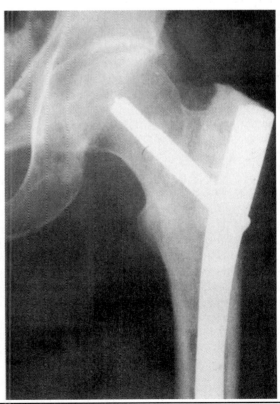

FIG. 14-7   Example of a prophylactic Zickel hip nailing from metastatic adenocarcinoma of lung.

SURGERY

Surgery is the treatment of choice and the primary hope for cure for stages I and II NSCLC. Some selected stage IIIA patients may benefit from surgical resection in terms of improved survival. Nearly none of stage IIIB patients are surgical candidates. The type of surgical procedure chosen depends on the tumor location, the patient's comorbidities, and the cardiopulmonary reserve of the patient. For those who are able to withstand surgical intervention, the recommended procedure is lobectomy or pneumonectomy. A lobectomy involves removal of the lobe as well as the lymph nodes draining that lobe and is ideal for a tumor confined to a single lobe. A pneumonectomy involves removal of a whole lung and is used for more centralized tumors. Studies are under way to determine whether mediastinal lymph node sampling as opposed to complete lymph node dissection provides the most benefit.[64] For those who are unable to withstand more extensive procedures, lesser surgical interventions such as a wedge resection are recommended. A wedge resection removes a triangle-shaped slice of tissue targeting the area of the tumor. Patients with early-stage NSCLC have the best long-term survival rates following surgical resection. However, systemic recurrences remain a problem in the majority of these patients. Thus the rationale for treating patients with early-stage NSCLC with combined-modality therapy (chemotherapy and surgery) is compelling, and several randomized trials are currently in progress.[92]

Nursing Management

Nursing management of persons undergoing pulmonary surgical interventions is complex. High mortality and morbidity associated with pulmonary resection necessitates sound preoperative and postoperative nursing management. A majority of these patients are current or former smokers and may also have tobacco-related comorbidities. Thus the patient's cardiopulmonary status is important. Implementation of a smoking cessation program before surgery may reduce the incidence of morbidity and mortality due to thoracic surgery.[93] In a study of 180 patients undergoing various thoracic surgical interventions, 27% of the patients developed a total of 80 postoperative complications, and 2% died from those complications.[94] Postoperatively, nursing care is multidimensional, but three areas of major focus should include pulmonary, cardiac, and pain and symptom management. Pain management is essential to facilitate participation in early mobility and recovery. See Chapter 39 for pain-relief techniques.

A common postoperative symptom is dyspnea.[95] This can be attributed to the thoracotomy incision and diminished lung capacity related to removal of the involved portion of the lung. Over time, with increased mobility and pain control, dyspnea may become more controlled. Patients having pulmonary resection are at risk for atrial dysrhythmias because of the irritation of the vagus nerve.

Emotional support for the patient and family also affects the course of recovery. Practice guidelines have been established about the perioperative evaluation and management of patients having thoracic surgery. The American College of Cardiology and the American Heart Association have published such guidelines, which are found online at *http://circ.ahajournals.org/cgi/content/full/105/10/1257.*[96]

CHEMOTHERAPY

Chemotherapy is administered for NSCLC using various approaches such as adjuvant and neoadjuvant treatment,

multimodality treatment, treatment for patients with unresectable stage III disease, and treatment for patients with stage IV disease. Most trials evaluating chemotherapy have enrolled patients at different disease stages (usually stages II and III). Currently, trials use platinum-based regimens since these agents are most active against NSCLC.[97]

Resectable NSCLC (Stages I-IIIA). In patients with NSCLC who undergo resectable surgery but are at risk for recurrence, adjuvant chemotherapy may provide an increased chance for a cure. The International Adjuvant Lung Cancer Trial randomized 1867 patients to either 3 or 4 cycles of cisplatin-based adjuvant chemotherapy or to observation.[98] The results showed a survival improvement of 4.1% in the adjuvant therapy group as compared to observation only. This is consistent with a metaanalysis of cisplatin-based adjuvant chemotherapy that could produce an absolute overall survival advantage of 5% at 5 years.[99] This survival benefit is consistent with that found with adjuvant therapy for other cancers, such as breast, colon, ovarian, and bladder cancers.[100] However, prior trials employing adjuvant chemotherapy in persons with resectable NSCLC were unable to demonstrate any survival benefit. Another metaanalysis consisting of 19 studies further supported the efficacy of adjuvant chemotherapy in resectable stages I and II NSCLC.[101] Thus the results of this trial have the potential to change the current standard treatment for resected NSCLC from observation to adjuvant chemotherapy.

Neoadjuvant chemotherapy is theoretically administered to downstage the disease before surgery and decrease perioperative tumor seeding to facilitate a curative outcome. Two randomized control trials evaluated neoadjuvant chemotherapy (cisplatin-based) before surgery versus surgery alone.[102,103] Although both studies had small sample sizes (n = 60), an increased survival advantage was reported. A third randomized control trial with a larger group of patients (n = 356) undergoing surgery for early-stage NSCLC evaluated the use of neoadjuvant chemotherapy.[104] Although results did not indicate a significant survival advantage, the study did show a lower risk of distant recurrence in the chemotherapy group, revealing the possibility that chemotherapy eradicated microscopic metastases. Consequently, the larger study and the two smaller studies are in conflict with each other. The Bimodality Lung Oncology Team reported on their study, where neoadjuvant carboplatin and paclitaxel followed by surgery and adjuvant chemotherapy were used in persons with stages I and II disease. While 45% of the patients were unable to finish adjuvant chemotherapy after surgery, an overall survival rate of 85% was attained at 1 year and 56% at 2 years.[105] A second trial administering gemcitabine and cisplatin found comparable results.[106] Based upon the results cited, ongoing research is being conducted to validate the usefulness of neoadjuvant chemotherapy in persons with early-stage NSCLC.

Advanced-Disease NSCLC. At present, patients with advanced disease, stage IIIB or IV, will not be cured. Chemotherapy is the standard course of treatment for unresectable stages III and IV, but the response rates are low, and survival time is poor. In advanced NSCLC, gains in survival occur when chemotherapy is used as compared with the best supportive care. Increased survival of 2 to 4 months and increases in the 1-year survival rate from 10% to 20% have been reported.[97] However, the goal of treatment becomes not only survival but also optimization of QOL. ASCO treatment guidelines recommend that treatment should start right after diagnosis, without delay, to prevent deterioration in performance status or the development of weight loss, which will have a deleterious effect on survival advantage. The ASCO guidelines recommend a two-drug combination that may or may not include platinum agents. The ASCO 2003 treatment guidelines can be located online at *http://www.jco.org/cgi/content/full/22/2/330*.[68] The ASCO guidelines recommend docetaxel as second-line therapy, since most first-line therapy incorporates a platinum-based agent. Patients who develop a single site of metastasis with a solitary lesion may benefit from resection of the lesion. Patients who undergo resection of a solitary brain metastasis followed by whole-brain radiation therapy can gain a 10% to 20% 5-year survival rate.[97]

RADIATION THERAPY

The goal of RT is the same in NSCLC as it is in SCLC. RT is important in management of all stages of NSCLC. RT is an integral treatment for medically inoperable early-stage NSCLC; for patients with early-stage unresectable disease; as prophylactic treatment (e.g., for impending superior vena cava syndrome, malignant spinal cord compression); or to palliate symptoms caused by metastases.

Adjuvant RT is recommended for patients who are otherwise healthy and found to have N2 disease (i.e., metastasis to ipsilateral mediastinal and/or subcarinal lymph nodes) at resection and/or positive surgical margins. This recommendation is derived from a study that found a decrease in recurrence but no improvement in overall survival with the use of adjuvant RT.[97] In addition, a more recent metaanalysis reported that postoperative RT was detrimental, which includes an increased risk of death.[107] It is important to note that this study was completed before the institution of newer approaches to RT techniques.[97] Studies using neoadjuvant RT in combination with chemotherapy for resectable and nonresectable NSCLC have mixed reports, with both positive and negative results.[97] In advanced NSCLC, palliative RT improves symptom status as well as survival.

Symptom Management

Symptoms are the "perceived red flags of threats to health."[108] Symptoms are the experience of the person, the consequence of the disease and its treatment that affects the person's HQL. Treatment may relieve some of the disease-related symptoms, but other symptoms may ensue owing to the side effects of the treatment itself. Persons with lung cancer experience multiple serious symptoms that influence their ability to perform their daily activities. A recent study of 220 newly diagnosed persons with lung cancer reported having 1 to 27 symptoms with a mean of 11 symptoms.[45] In this study, fatigue (79%), pain (60%), dyspnea (58%), and nausea (34%) were frequently reported symptoms with appreciable levels of severity. This study illustrates the imperative role of nursing in the management of symptoms for persons with lung cancer. Symptom management protects the patient from harm during treatment; improves daily HQL; and enhances survival time. However, despite the worldwide advances in symptom research resulting in clear practice guidelines for symptoms, too many patients continue to suffer from unrelieved symptoms like fatigue, pain, dyspnea, and nausea.[109-112] Thus a priority becomes management of symptoms, to optimize HQL from diagnosis of the disease and throughout the living trajectory.

Over a decade ago, researchers identified salient principles of symptom management relevant and applicable to the challenges of today.[113] Knowing from the empirical literature that fatigue, pain, dyspnea, and nausea are frequently reported as severe symptoms by persons with lung cancer, and knowing that they may occur simultaneously around the time of initial diagnosis, should prompt clinicians to act with anticipatory watchfulness. Consequently, a symptom management plan should be established to pre-empt the symptoms by allocating the resources required to prevent the onset of symptoms. Preventing the development of symptoms is imperative in promoting wellness at the end-of-life.

Secondly, symptom management is an ongoing process of assessment, intervention, and evaluation. Persons with lung cancer already face an aggressively lethal chronic health condition, and the addition of any other unremitting conditions should be circumvented at all costs. Thus, a culture of active symptom management to promote comfort and well-being in people with lung cancer is possible by integrating an anticipatory and ongoing approach to symptom assessment, intervention, and evaluation.

Considerations for Older Adults

The incidence of lung cancer increases with age. Therefore, with the "graying of America," nurses will be caring for and treating an increasing number of persons with lung cancer. With the elderly come co-morbidities such as hypertension, diabetes, cardiovascular disease, obesity, sensory impairments, and dementia or depression, all of which may add complications to a cancer diagnosis. In addition, emotional losses and a decrease in social support structure, resources, independence, and physical stamina may have their impact on the patient, their disease, and the choice and tolerability of treatment options. The fact that most clinical trials are not created for or offered to the elderly makes it difficult, at best, to gauge beneficial options against potential risks and side effects, and the potential for decreasing QOL.

It is important, therefore, that nurses act as advocates and educators with elderly patients and their families, giving a realistic view of what the treatment, side effects, and ongoing care requirements will entail. Oncology care in the lung cancer patient can be a significant undertaking, but choices for the elderly should be based on potential treatment options and their efficacy, managing side effects, and maintaining what the patient defines as his or her QOL. Each patient should be viewed as an individual. The option to treat should not be withheld because of age.

Conclusion

In August 2005, the NCI announced a three-pronged, integrated plan to eliminate the suffering and death due to lung cancer by 2015. The primary cause of lung cancer is tobacco use. Consequently, the plan starts with stepping up efforts to drive down the initiation and continued use of tobacco as well as exposure to secondhand smoke. However, tobacco use is not the only cause of lung cancer. Reducing the burden of lung cancer means targeting efforts against the other environmental factors as well. Improving and discovering new techniques to maximize early detection of lung cancer will increase the likelihood for chances of a cure from the disease. Thus, continued research into use of CT scanning and the development of proteomic (proteins expressed by a genome) and other expression technologies on tissue samples is needed. Third, research efforts are required to develop novel targeted therapies to combat the disease. Nevertheless, until the disease is eradicated and a cure is found, clinicians must launch a tailored, evidence-based plan of care for each patient to alleviate the suffering associated with the devastating symptoms from lung cancer and the treatment itself.

REVIEW QUESTIONS

☑ Case Study

Ms. Teresa Brown, 42 years old, has been experiencing increasing neck and shoulder pain for 2 weeks. She does full-time factory work and thought the discomfort was due to an injury. The pain became intolerable, and she came in to be seen at the emergency room since she had no health benefits. She has been a smoker since the age of 16, averaging 1½ packs per day. Her concerns included increased fatigue, and increased shortness of breath (SOB) over the past 6 weeks, with no change in her smoker's cough or sputum production. She attributed the fatigue and dyspnea to a lingering upper respiratory infection, even though she had recently completed two courses of antibiotic therapy. The MRI showed a tumor in the cervical area of her neck, and further tests revealed stage IV NSCLC, with a maximum survival prognosis of 2 to 4 months. She selected a course of palliative medical treatment in preparing for end-of-life care.

Ms. Brown was widowed and had two children, ages 9 and 11. She lived with her children in an apartment in the same small town as her 73-year-old mother, her primary support system. Ms. Brown was admitted to the hospital under a hospitalist physician with an oncologist for consultation when needed. A hospital discharge planning nurse assisted Ms. Brown in applying for Medicaid health insurance benefits. However, without discussing plans with Ms. Brown, the nurse arranged for Ms. Brown's discharge to a nursing home with hospice services 50 miles from her home. The nurse practitioner working in collaboration with the oncologist was unaware of the discharge arrangements made by the hospital discharge planning nurse. She was fully informed of Ms. Brown's health care benefit status and began to discuss discharge placement options with her. One of the options included a hospice that was not a nursing home but was located in her home town. While Ms. Brown and the nurse practitioner were discussing options for discharge, the hospital discharge nurse entered the room and, upon hearing their conversation, announced to the patient, the patient's mother, and the nurse practitioner that Ms. Brown would be discharged to a nursing home the following morning. The patient, in her bewildered state, started to cry and said, "I'm too young to go in a nursing home. I won't be able to see my children. We live an hour away from there. No, I'm not going." The discharge planning nurse informed the patient that the discharge arrangements had already been made and they would not be changed; after all, a hospice was a hospice. Then she abruptly left Ms. Brown's room.

QUESTIONS

1. What reason do you believe prompted the discharge nurse to act so abruptly with Ms. Brown when announcing her discharge plans?
   a. The discharge planning nurse felt that hospice was the appropriate option for Ms. Brown, and she did not want to miss the opportunity for placement.
   b. The discharge policy at the hospital determines the hour and date of discharge for all patients.

   c. Her own bias and the assumption that the lung cancer diagnosis is Ms. Brown's fault led to her behavior.
   d. For patients on federal or state assistance, the discharge nurse is not required to discuss plans with the patient.
2. What is included among patient teaching priorities for prevention and detection of lung cancer?
   a. Avoid tobacco use; know environmental carcinogens that increase risk, and personal and family history
   b. Limit tobacco use; know environmental carcinogens that increase risk, and personal and family history
   c. Limit tobacco use; know work-related carcinogens that increase risk, and personal and family history
   d. Avoid tobacco use; know work-related and environmental carcinogens that increase risk, and personal and family history
3. Currently, the best method of screening for lung cancer includes which of the following?
   a. Sputum cytology and CXR
   b. CXR alone
   c. Sputum cytology alone
   d. Low-dose spiral (or helical) chest CT
4. What does research indicate is seen in persons with lung cancer at diagnosis?
   a. Fewer number of symptoms compared with persons with other solid tumor composition
   b. Greater number of symptoms compared with persons with other solid tumor composition with appreciable levels of symptom severity
   c. Fewer number of symptoms and lower levels of symptom severity compared with persons with other solid tumor composition
   d. No symptoms at diagnosis
5. SCLC usually arises in a central endobronchial location. What would common symptoms include?
   a. Fatigue, weight loss, and anemia
   b. Wheeze, cough, and hemoptysis
   c. Fever, night sweats, and hilar lymphadenopathy
   d. Headache, dizziness, and visual disturbances
6. In collecting data regarding possible metastases, the following statement is accurate:
   a. Plain film will detect previous trauma, but not degenerative disease.
   b. PET will detect bone metastasis.
   c. Biopsy will detect metastatic lesions in the adrenals or liver.
   d. Mediastinoscopy is used to determine distant metastasis.
7. Ms. Brown states to the nurse that the diagnosis of NSCLC is a tremendous shock to her. What makes this likely?
   a. There is always early symptomatology in most lung cancers.
   b. The patient had been a long-term smoker, but "did not contemplate" that someone her age could get lung cancer.

c. Being treated for a lingering respiratory infection should never raise a "red flag" of a serious illness of lung cancer for Ms. Brown.

d. Because of the physical nature of her work, there were no plausible reasons why her shoulder and neck could ache.

8. Favorable prognostic criteria for patients with early-stage NSCLC include which of the following?

a. Squamous cell or bronchoalveolar carcinoma of the lung

b. Large cell carcinoma or adenocarcinoma

c. Tumor size between 5 and 7 cm

d. Male gender

9. Which of the following characteristics applies to SCLC?

a. Early hematogenous spread; highly chemo- and radiosenstive; frequent metastases to CNS, the liver, and the bone marrow

b. Chemosensitive but radio-resistant; sites of distant metastases are brain, bone, and pericardium; responds well to first-line therapy but relapses to NSCLC

c. Spreads commonly via lymphatics; surgical intervention efficacious; resistant to chemotherapy and radiation therapy

d. Secondary malignancies as lymphoma in approximately 25% of patients; patient therefore does not relapse with lung cancer

10. What are included among characteristics associated with NSCLC?

a. All NSCLCs are associated with smoking; they tend to grow in the central bronchus of the lung, with numerous pulmonary symptoms.

b. Giant cell carcinoma is associated with hypercalcemia and neuroendocrine features.

c. Squamous cell carcinoma invades the blood stream and lymphatics quickly and shows a worse stage-for-stage prognosis.

d. Adenocarcinoma is associated with nonsmokers and is seen in the periphery of the lung with fewer pulmonary symptoms.

ANSWERS

1. **C.** *Rationale:* A lung cancer diagnosis carries a stigma in which others assume the patient has "brought this illness on him- or herself by smoking," and therefore deserves no sympathy or consideration of needs or desires.

2. **D.** *Rationale:* The most broad-reaching personal effort to prevent lung cancer would include no smoking (direct, smokeless, or passive), and awareness of work and environmental carcinogens and personal and family history.

3. **D.** *Rationale:* Currently, sputum cytology studies have not improved lung cancer mortality since they are efficacious in centrally located tumors, and dependent upon the rigor of the specimen. Chest x-ray results are dependent upon the image quality and the skills of the practitioner interpreting the film. CT helical scanning has been shown superior and has detected up to 77% more of lung cancer lesions compared to chest x-ray.[41]

4. **B.** *Rationale:* Persons with lung cancer are seen with serious multiple occurring symptoms. In particular, patients over 65 years of age usually have more symptoms than patients diagnosed with solid tumors.

5. **B.** *Rationale:* Owing to the local central bronchial location of SCLC, the most likely symptoms include hemoptysis, wheeze, and cough.

6. **C.** *Rationale:* Plain x-ray films will show both previous trauma and degenerative disease. PET acts to measure the biologic activity of neoplastic cells compared to normal lung cells. Mediastinoscopy is the gold standard for evaluation of lymph nodes in the mediastinal area. Biopsy would be used to detect distant metastasis in the liver or the adrenal glands.

7. **B.** *Rationale:* The diagnosis of lung cancer is often made coincidentally while investigating other illnesses. Symptoms of early disease are often vague, making diagnosis difficult. The lingering respiratory infection not responsive to usual antibiotic therapy is a common finding in those diagnosed with lung cancer. Ms. Brown's factory work may have exposed her to long-term toxic carcinogens. Lung cancer is not age discriminatory; although it is more commonly diagnosed in the age range of 50 to 75 years, young people do get lung cancer.

8. **A.** *Rationale:* NSCLC is a devastating disease, but there are a few patient characteristics which demonstrate a more favorable prognosis. These include being female, having a tumor less than 5 cm with histologic features of either squamous cell carcinoma or bronchoalveolar carcinoma.

9. **A.** *Rationale:* SCLC disseminates early and rapidly via hematogenous route. There is a good responsiveness to both chemotherapy and radiation therapy; however, most will relapse. Common metastatic sites are CNS, liver, and bone marrow.

10. **D.** *Rationale:* NSCLC encompasses the following types: squamous cell, adenocarcinoma, large cell carcinoma, and giant cell carcinoma. Squamous cell carcinoma originates as a central tumor in the proximal bronchi; adenocarcinoma arises in the alveolar surface of the epithelium or the bronchial mucosal glands, usually in the periphery; large cell carcinomas present in the periphery and invade subsegmental bronchi or large airways, and tend to have neuroendocrine features.

Spread and invasion occurs as follows: adenocarcinomas invade the lymphatics and the bloodstream early during the course of the disease, whereas squamous cell carcinoma invades the lamina propria and erodes the basement membrane. Once there is it likely to metastasize.

Adenocarcinomas tend to be diagnosed in nonsmokers, and younger patients who are female.

REFERENCES

1. American Cancer Society: *Cancer facts and figures 2006*, Atlanta, 2005, Author.
2. Parkin D, Bray F, Ferlay J et al: Global cancer statistics 2002, *CA Cancer J Clin* 55:74-108, 2005.
3. Blum D, Kennedy VN, Boerckel W et al: Lung cancer under reported in the media. Paper presented at: *American Society of Clinical Oncology*, May 15, 2001.
4. The Global Lung Cancer Coalition: No one in the world deserves lung cancer: call to action to lessen stigma of the disease and pressure governments to increase funding, 2003, retrieved August 1, 2005, from http://www.lungcancercoalition.org/pressc12.html.
5. National Cancer Institute: Cancer research funding, U.S. Department of Health and Human Services, 2003, retrieved May 28, 2004, from http://cis.nci.nih.gov/fact/1.htm.
6. Cooley ME, Kaiser L, Abraham J et al: The silent epidemic: tobacco and the evolution of lung cancer and its treatment. *Cancer Invest* 9(7):739-751, 2001.
7. Adler I: *Primary malignant growths of the lungs and bronchi*, New York, 1912, Longmans, Green.
8. American Cancer Society: Cancer facts and figures for African Americans 2005-2006, retrieved August 1, 2005, from http://www.cancer.org/downloads/STT/CAFF2005AACorrPWSecured.pdf.
9. Ramalingam S, Belani CP: Meaningful survival in lung cancer patients, *Semin Oncol* 29(1 Suppl 4):125-131, 2002.
10. Winton T, Livingston R, Johnson D et al: Vinorelbine plus cisplatin vs. observation in resected non-small cell lung cancer, *New Eng J Med* 352(25):2589-2597, 2005.
11. National Cancer Institute: Lung Cancer Prevention, retrieved August 1, 2005, from http://www.nci.nih.gov/cancertopics/pdq/prevention/lung/HealthProfessional/page3.
12. Alberg A, Samet J: Epidemiology of lung cancer, *Chest* 123:21S-49S, 2003.
13. Siegfried J: Women and lung cancer: does oestrogen play a role? *Lancet Oncol* 2(8):506-513, 2001.
14. Shapiro J, Jacobs EJ, Thun MJ: Cigar smoking in men and risk of death from tobacco-related cancers, *J Natl Cancer Inst* 92(4):333-337, 2000.
15. Boffetta P, Pershagen G, Jockel K et al: Cigar and pipe smoking and lung cancer risk: a multicenter study from Europe, *J Natl Cancer Inst* 91(8):697-701, 1999.
16. Soria J, Kim E, Fayett J et al: Chemoprevention of lung cancer, *Lancet Oncol* 4(11):659-669, 2003.
17. Lung Cancer Alliance. Lung cancer risks retrieved August 1, 2005, from http://www.lungcanceralliance.org/facing/about.html.
18. Wong M, Fung L, Wang E et al: Chromosomal aberrations of primary lung adenocarcinomas in nonsmokers, *Cancer* 97(5):1263-1270, 2003.
19. Sanchez-Cespedes M, Ahrendt S, Piantadosi S et al: Chromosomal alterations in lung adenocarcinoma from smokers and nonsmokers, *Cancer Res* 61(4):1309-1313, 2001.
20. U.S. Environmental Protection Agency: A citizen's guide to radon: the guide to protecting yourself and your family from radon, retrieved August 1, 2005, from http://www.epa.gov/iaq/radon/pubs/citguide.html.
21. National Cancer Institute: Asbestos exposure: Questions and answers, retrieved August 1, 2005, from http://cis.nci.nih.gov/fact/3_21.htm.
22. Alberg A, Malcolm B, Samet J: Epidemiology of lung cancer: looking to the future, *J Clin Oncol* 23(14):3175-3185, 2005.
23. Cote M, Kardia S, Wenzlaff A et al: Risk of lung cancer among white and black relatives of individuals with early-onset lung cancer, *JAMA* 293(24):3036-3042, 2005.
24. Winterhalder R, Hirsch F, Kotantoulas G et al: Chemoprevention of lung cancer—from biology to clinical reality, *Ann Oncol* 15(2):185-196, 2004.
25. National Institutes of Health: Nutrient in cruciferous vegetables protects against lung cancer in study of 18,244, retrieved August 1, 2005, from http://www.nih.gov/news/pr/sep2000/niehs-18.htm.
26. National Cancer Institute: Surveillance, epidemiology, and end results cancer statistics review 1973-1999 for lung and bronchus, retrieved August 1, 2005, from http//:seer.cancer.gov/csr/1973-1999/lung.pdf.
27. Hey JC: Lung cancer in elderly patients, *Clin Geriatr Med* 19(1):139-155, 2003.
28. Lewis JH, Kilgore ML, Goldman DP et al: Participation of patients 65 years of age or older in cancer clinical trials, *J Clin Oncol* 21(7):1383-1389, 2003.
29. Repetto L, Venturino A, Fratino L et al: Geriatric oncology: a clinical approach to the older patient with cancer, *Eur J Cancer* 39(7):870-880, 2003.
30. Cooley ME, Jennings-Dozier K: Lung cancer in African Americans. A call for action, *Cancer Pract* 6(2):99-106, 1998.
31. Earle CC, Neumann PJ, Gelber RD et al: Impact of referral patterns on the use of chemotherapy for lung cancer, *J Clin Oncol* 20(7):1786-1792, 2002.
32. Healthy People 2010: *Healthy People 2010* vol I: Objectives for improving health, retrieved August 1, 2005, from http://www.healthypeople.gov/document/tableofcontents.htm, 2001.
33. National Cancer Institute: Questions and answers about smoking cessation, retrieved August 1, 2005, from http://cis.nci.nih.gov/fact/10_19.htm.
34. National Cancer Institute: Cancer facts: chemoprevention, retrieved August 1, 2005, from http://cis.nci.nih.gov/fact/4_2.htm.
35. McLaughlin J, Hrubec Z: Smoking and cancer mortality among US veterans: a 26-year follow-up, *Int J Cancer* 60(2):190-193, 1995.
36. Woodson K, Tangrea J, Barrett M et al: Serum alpha-tocopherol and subsequent risk of lung cancer among male smokers, *J Natl Cancer Inst* 91(20):1738-1743, 1999.
37. Cook N, Lee I, Gaziano J et al: Low-dose aspirin in the primary prevention of cancer: the Women's Health Study: a randomized controlled trial, *JAMA* 294(1):47-55, 2005.
38. Khuder S, Herial N, Mutigi A et al: Nonsteroidal antiinflammatory drug use and lung cancer: a metaanalysis, *Chest* 127(3):748-754, 2005.
39. National Cancer Institute: NIH halts use of COX-2 inhibitor in large cancer prevention trial, retrieved August 1, 2005, from http://www.nci.nih.gov/newscenter/pressreleases/APCtrialCOX2.
40. Rivera M, Detterbeck F, Mehta A: Diagnosis of lung cancer: the guidelines, *Chest* 123(1 Suppl):129S-136S, 2003.
41. Sone S, Li F, Yang Z-G et al: Lack of benefit from semi-annual screening for cancer of the lung: followup report of a randomized controlled trial on population of high-risk males in Czechoslovakia, *Int J Cancer* 73:137-145, 2000.
42. Henschke C, Shaham D, Yankelevitz D et al. CT screening for lung cancer: Past and ongoing studies *Semin Thorac Cardiovasc Surg* 17(2):99-106, 2005.
43. Gilbert S, Luketich J, Christie N: Fluorescent bronchoscopy, *Thorac Surg Clin* 14(1):71-77, 2004.
44. Chiyo M, Shibuya K, Hoshino H et al: Effective detection of bronchial preinvasive lesions by a new autofluorescence imaging bronchovideoscope system, *Lung Cancer* 48(3):307-313, 2005.
45. Gift AG, Jablonski A, Stommel M et al: Symptom clusters in elderly patients with lung cancer, *Oncol Nurs Forum* 31(2):203-212, 2004.
46. Gift AG, Stommel M, Jablonski A et al: A cluster of symptoms overtime in patients with lung cancer, *Nurs Res* 52:393-400, 2003.
47. Given B, Given C, Azzouz F et al: Physical functioning of elderly cancer patients prior to diagnosis and following initial treatment, *Nurs Res* 50(4):222-232, 2001.
48. Sarna L: Functional status in women with lung cancer, *Cancer Nurs* 17(2):87-93, 1994.
49. Vogelzang N, Breitbart W, Cella D et al: Patients, caregiver, and oncologist perceptions of cancer-related fatigue: results of a tripart assessment survey, *Semin Hematol* 34(Supp.2):4-12, 1997.
50. Okuyama T, Tanaka K, Akechi T et al: Fatigue in ambulatory patients with advanced lung cancer: prevalence, correlated factors, and screening, *J Pain Symptom Manage* 22(1):554-564, 2001.
51. Cooley M: Symptoms in adults with lung cancer. A systematic research review, *J Pain Symptom Manage* 19(2):137-153, 2000.
52. McHorney CA, Ware JE, Raczek A: The MOS 36-Item Short-Form Survey (SF-36): psychometric and clinical tests of validity in measuring physical and mental health constructs, *Med Care* 31(3):247-263, 1993.
53. Meyers CA, Byrne KS, Komaki R: Cognitive deficits in patients with small cell lung cancer before and after chemotherapy, *Lung Cancer* 12(3):231-235.
54. Ahles T, Silberfarb P, Herndon J et al: Psychologic and neuropsychologic functioning of patients with limited small cell lung cancer treated with chemotherapy and radiation therapy with or without warfarin: a study by the Cancer and Leukemia Group B, *J Clin Oncol* 16:1954-1960, 1998.
55. Sarna L, McCorkle R: Burden of care and lung cancer, *Cancer Pract* 4(5):245-251.

56. Kurtz ME, Kurtz JC, Stommel M et al: The influence of symptoms, age, comorbidity and cancer site on physical functioning and mental health of geriatric women patients, *Women Health* 29(3):1-12, 1999.

57. Christodolou C, Pavlidis N, Samantas E et al: Prognostic factors in Greek patients with small cell lung cancer. A Hellenic Cooperative Oncology Group study, *Anticancer Res* 22(6B):3749-3757, 2002.

58. Hopwood P, Stephens RJ: Depression in patients with lung cancer: prevalence and risk factors derived from quality-of-life data, *J Clin Oncol* 18(4):893-903, 2000.

59. Kurtz ME, Kurtz JC, Stommel M et al: Predictors of depressive symptomatology of geriatric patients with lung cancer-a longitudinal analysis *Psychooncology* 11(1):12-22, 2002.

60. Montazeri A, Milroy R, Gillis C et al: Quality of life: perception of lung cancer patients *Eur J Cancer* 32A(13):2284-2289, 1996.

61. Lenz ER, Pugh LC, Milligan RA et al: The middle-range theory of unpleasant symptoms: an update, *Adv Nurs Sci* 19(3):14-27, 1997.

62. Given BA, Given CW, McCorkle R et al: Pain and fatigue management: results of a Nursing randomized clinical trial, *Oncol Nurs Forum* 29(6):949-956.

63. National Comprehensive Cancer Network: National Comprehensive Cancer Network Clinical Practice Guidelines: non-small cell lung cancer, v2.2005, retrieved August 1, 2005, from http://www.nccn.org/professionals/physician_gls/PDF/nscl.pdf.

64. National Comprehensive Cancer Network: National Comprehensive Cancer Network Practice Guidelines: small cell lung cancer 2005. Retrieved August 1, 2005, from http://www.nccn.org/.

65. Pope R, Hansell D: Extra-thoracic staging of lung cancer, *Eur J Radiol* 45(1):31-38.

66. Silvestri G, Tanoue L, Margolis M et al: Staging of non-small cell lung cancer: imaging of intrathoracic disease, *Eur J Radiol* 123:147s-156s, 2003.

67. Toloza E, Harpole L, Detterbeck F et al: Invasive staging of non-small cell lung cancer: a review of the current evidence. *Chest* 123(1):157S-166S, 2003.

68. Pfister D, Johnson D, Azzoli C et al: American Society of Clinical Oncology treatment of unresectable non-small cell lung cancer guideline: Update 2003, *J Clin Oncol* 22(2):330-353, 2004.

69. National Cancer Institute: Small cell lung cancer, retrieved August 1, 2005, from http://www.nci.nih.gov/cancertopics/pdq/treatment/small-cell-lung/healthprofessional.

70. Abraham J and Allegra CJ, editors: *Bethesda handbook of clinical oncology*, Philadelphia, 2001 Lippincott, Williams & Wilkins.

71. Bremnes R, Sundstrom S, Aasebo U et al: The value of prognostic factors in small cell lung cancer: results from a randomised multi-center study with minimum 5 year followup, *Lung Cancer* 39(3):303-313, 2003.

72. Kurup A, Hanna N: Treatment of small cell lung cancer, *Crit Rev Oncol Hematol* 52(2):117-126, 2004.

73. Nakamura H, Kato Y, Kato H: Outcome of surgery for small cell lung cancer—response to induction chemotherapy predicts survival, *Thorac Cardiovasc Surg* 52(4):206-210, 2004.

74. Auperin A, Arriagada R, Pignon J et al: Prophylactic cranial irradiation for patients with small-cell lung cancer in complete remission. Prophylactic cranial irradiation overview collaborative group, *N Engl J Med* 341(7):524-526, 1999.

75. Komaki R, Meyers C, Shin D et al: Evaluation of cognitive function in patients with limited small cell lung cancer prior to and shortly following prophylactic cranial irradiation, *Int J Radiat Oncol Biol Phys* 33(1):179-182, 1995.

76. Pignon J, Arriagada R, Ihde D et al: A meta-analysis of thoracic radiotherapy for small-cell lung cancer, *N Engl J Med* 328(19):1425-1426, 1993.

77. Turrisi A, Kim K, Blum R et al: Twice-daily compared with once-daily thoracic radiotherapy in limited small-cell lung cancer treated concurrently with cisplatin and etoposide, *N Engl J Med* 340(4):265-271, 1999.

78. Skarlos D, Samantas E, Kosmidis P et al: Randomized comparison of etoposide-cisplatin vs. etoposide-carboplatin and irradiation in small-cell lung cancer. A Hellenic Co-operative Oncology Group study, *Ann Oncol* 5(7):601-607, 1994.

79. Kosmidis P, Samantas E, Fountzilas G et al: Cisplatin/etoposide versus carboplatin/etoposide chemotherapy and irradiation in small cell lung cancer: a randomized phase III study, *Semin Oncol* 21(3 Suppl 6):23-30, 1994.

80. Hanna N, Einhorn L: Small-cell lung cancer: state of the art, *Clin Lung Cancer* 4(2):87-94, 2002.

81. Ahrendt S, Decker P, Alawi E et al: Cigarette smoking associated with mutation of the K-ras gene in patients with primary adenocarcinoma of the lung, *Cancer* 92(6):1525-1530, 2001.

82. Ross J: Biology of lung cancer. In Hass M, editor: *Contemporary issues in lung cancer*, Boston, 2003, Jones & Bartlett.

83. Ebright M, Zakowski M, Martin J et al: Clinical pattern and pathologic stage but not histologic features predict outcome for bronchioloalveolar carcinoma, *Ann Thorac Surg* 74(5):1646-1647, 2002.

84. Tyson L: Non-small cell lung cancer. In Houlihan N, editor: *Lung cancer*, Pittsburgh, 2004, Oncology Nursing Society.

85. Tyson L: Oncologic urgencies and emergencies. In Houlihan N, editor: *Lung cancer*, Pittsburgh, 2004, Oncology Nursing Society.

86. Mountain C: Revisions in the international system for staging lung cancer, *Chest* 111:1710-1717, 1997.

87. Firat S, Byhardt R, Gore E: Comorbidity and Karnofsky performance score are independent prognostic factors in stage III non-small cell lung cancer: an institutional analysis of patients treated on four RTOG studies. Radiation Therapy Oncology Group, *Int J Radiat Oncol Biol Phys* 54(2):357-364, 2002.

88. VanMeerbeeck J: Staging of non-small cell lung cancer: consensus, controversies and challenges, *Lung Cancer* 34(Suppl 2):S95-107, 2001.

89. Berardi R, Brunelli A, Tamburrano T et al: Perioperative anemia and blood transfusions as prognostic factors in patients undergoing resection for non-small cell lung cancers, *Lung Cancer* 49(3):371-376, 2005.

90. Cangir A, Kutlay H, Akal M et al: Prognostic value of tumor size in non-small cell lung cancer larger than five centimeters in diameter, *Lung Cancer* 46(3):325-331, 2004.

91. Lopez-Encuentra A, Astudillo J, Cerezal J et al: Prognostic value of chronic obstructive pulmonary disease in 2994 cases of lung cancer, *Eur J Cardiothorac Surg* 27(1):8-13, 2005.

92. Rivera M: Multimodality therapy in the treatment of lung cancer, *Semin Respir Crit Care Med* 25(Suppl 1):3-10, 2004.

93. Vaporciyan A, Merriman K, Ece F et al: Incidence of major pulmonary morbidity after pneumonectomy: association with timing of smoking cessation, *Ann Thorac Surg* 73(2):420-425, 2002.

94. Melendez J, Carlon V: Cardiopulmonary risk index does not predict complications after thoracic surgery, *Chest* 114(1):69-75, 1998.

95. Quinn K: Managing patients through thoracic surgery. In Haas M, editor: *Contemporary issues in lung cancer: a nursing perspective*, Boston, 2003, Jones & Bartlett.

96. Eagle K, Berger P, Calkins H et al: ACC/AHA guideline update for perioperative cardiovascular evaluation for noncardiac surgery—Executive summary a report of the American College of Cardiology/American Heart Association Task Force on Practice Guidelines (Committee to update the 1996 guidelines on perioperative cardiovascular evaluation for noncardiac surgery. Retrieved August 1, 2005, from http://circ.aha.journals.org/cgi/content/full/105/10/1257?ck=nck.

97. Spira A, Ettinger D: Multidisciplinary management of lung cancer, *N Engl J Med* 350(4):379-392, 2004.

98. Arriagada R, Bergman B, Dunant A et al: Cisplatin-based adjuvant chemotherapy in patients with completely resected non-small cell lung cancer, *N Engl J Med* 350(4):351-360, 2004.

99. Non-Small Cell Lung Cancer Collaborative Group: Chemotherapy in non-small cell lung cancer: a meta-analysis using updated data on individual patients from 52 randomised clinical trials. *BMJ* 311(899-909), 1995.

100. Blum R: Adjuvant chemotherapy for lung cancer—a new standard of care, *N Engl J Med* 350:404-405, 2004.

101. Berghmans T, Paesmans M, Meert A et al: Survival improvement in resectable non-small cell lung cancer with (neo)adjuvant chemotherapy: results of a meta-analysis of the literature, *Lung Cancer* 49(1):13-23, 2005.

102. Roth J, Atkinson E, Fossella F: Long-term follow-up of patients enrolled in a randomized trial comparing perioperative chemotherapy and surgery with surgery alone in resectable stage IIIA non-small cell lung cancer, *Lung Cancer* 21:1-6, 1998.

103. Rosell R, Gomez-Codina J, Camps C et al: A randomized trial comparing preoperative chemotherapy plus surgery with surgery alone in patients with non-small cell lung cancer, *N Engl J Med* 330(3):153-158, 1994.

104. Dipierre A, Milleron B, Moro-Sibilot D et al: Preoperative chemotherapy followed by surgery compared with primary surgery resectable stage I (except T1N0), II, and IIIa non-small cell lung cancer, *J Clin Oncol* 20:247-253, 2002.

105. Pisters K, Ginsberg R, Giroux D et al: Induction chemotherapy before surgery for early-stage lung cancer: a novel approach. Bimodality Lung Oncology Team, *J Thorac Cardiovasc Surg* 119(3):429-439, 2000.

106. Van Zandwijk N, Smit E, Kramer G et al: Gemcitabine and cisplatin }as induction regimen for patients with biopsy-proven stage IIIAN2 non-small cell lung cancer: a phase II study of the European Organization for Research and Treatment of Cancer Lung Cancer Cooperative Group, *J Clin Oncol* 18:2658-2664, 2000.

107. PORT Meta-Analysis Trialists Group: Postoperative radiotherapy in non small cell lung cancer: systematic review and meta-analysis of individual patient data from nine randomized controlled trials, *Lancet* 352(9124):257-263, 1998.

108. Hegyvary ST: Patient care outcomes related to management of symptoms, *Ann Rev Nurs Res 1993* 11:145-168, 1993.

109. Thomason TE, Bernard SA, Winer EP et al: Cancer pain survey: patient-centered issues in control, *J Pain Symptom Manage* 15(5):275-284, 1998.

110. Wickham R: Nausea and vomiting. In Yarbro CH, Frogge MH, Goodman M, editors: *Cancer symptom management*, ed 3, Sudbury, Mass, 2004, Jones & Bartlett.

111. Passik SD, Kirsh KL, Donaghy K et al: Patient-related barriers to fatigue communication: initial validation of the fatigue management barriers questionnaire, *J Pain Symptom Manage* 24(5):481-493, 2002.

112. Ripamonti C, Fusco F: Respiratory problems in advanced cancer, *Support Care Cancer* 10:204-216, 2002.

113. Preston F, Tang S, McCorkle R: *Symptom management for the terminally ill. A challenge for the living: dying, death, & bereavement*, Sudbury, Mass, 1994, Jones & Bartlett.

114. Press A: Nonsmokers can be cancer victims too, retrieved August 1, 2005, from http://www.cnn.com/2005/HEALTH/conditions/08/10/lung.cancer.reeve.ap/.

CHAPTER 15

Malignant Lymphoma

Kathleen Peranski

Malignant lymphoma is a diverse group of neoplasms that originate in the lymphatic system. Two types of lymphoid tissues exist: central (bone marrow and thymus) and peripheral (blood, spleen, lymph node, and mucosa-associated).[1] Lymph is derived from interstitial fluid and flows through lymphatic vessels so that it is eventually returned to circulatory system by way of the thoracic duct. Along its course, lymph is filtered of particulate through lymph nodes, which are small, encapsulated organs located along the lymphatic vessels. Lymph nodes have a very specific architecture that allows for areas of lymphocyte maturation and differentiation. Lymphocytes are the predominant cell present in lymph nodes and are the cellular element involved in malignant lymphoma.[2]

Lymphocytes originate in the bone marrow, and through the process of maturation and differentiation develop into several different types of mature lymphocytes. At any stage of this maturation and differentiation, the normal cell may transform into a malignant cell, giving rise to a malignancy that is specific to the stage in which the cell becomes transformed.[2]

Based on the characteristics of the malignant lymphocytes, malignant lymphomas are divided into two major subgroups: Hodgkin's disease and non-Hodgkin's lymphoma.[2]

Hodgkin's Disease

Historical Background

In 1832 Thomas Hodgkin described a progressively fatal condition characterized by enormous lymph node swellings that he believed to be one disease.[2] Characteristic cells involved in this disease were identified microscopically by Sternberg and Reed in 1898 and 1902, respectively.[3] The identification of these cells, now known as Reed-Sternberg cells, allowed for the initial classification of Hodgkin's disease. Reed-Sternberg cells are characterized as binucleated or multinucleated in a background of inflammatory cells. It is unusual in that as a malignancy the tumor cells are in the minority, and the normal inflammatory cells predominate.[4] The presence of Reed-Sternberg cells (large, malformed cells with two nuclei) distinguishes Hodgkin's disease from non-Hodgkin's lymphoma.[5] In the past two decades advances in histology and immunohistology have revealed that the Reed-Sternberg cell is of B-cell lineage, and that Hodgkin's disease is not a single disease, but instead two separate diseases.[6] The classic Hodgkin's disease, which accounts for approximately 95% of cases, includes the subset of nodular lymphocyte predominance Hodgkin's disease.[2]

The four stages of Hodgkin's disease are based on factors such as location, whether cancer is found in more than one group of lymph nodes, or on one or both sides of the diaphragm.[5] The potential curability of Hodgkin's disease was first recognized in 1920, when patients with localized tumors treated with radiation were shown to have a 10% survival rate.[7] By the 1960s about one third of patients were being cured with radiation. In 1970, the National Cancer Institution (NCI) reported that patients with advanced Hodgkin's disease could attain complete remission and long-term survival using a combination chemotherapy of nitrogen mustard, Oncovin (vincristine), procarbazine, and prednisone, known as MOPP.[5,7] These advances resulted in a standard approach to the diagnosis and treatment of Hodgkin's disease. Since the mid-1970s, development and research efforts have focused on more accurate ways of staging, initial therapies for various stages, treatment of resistant and relapsed disease, and the long-term effect of treatment regimens.[2]

Epidemiology and Etiology

Lymphomas represent about 4% of new cancer cases diagnosed in the United States each year. It is the fifth most common cancer diagnosis and the fifth leading cause of cancer death. Although the incidence of most cancers is decreasing, lymphoma is one of only two tumors increasing in frequency, although the cause for this increase in unknown.[8] The American Cancer Society (ACS) estimated that 63,740 new cases of lymphoma will be diagnosed in the United States in 2005: of these 7350 will be Hodgkin's disease and 56,390 will be non-Hodgkin's lymphoma.[9] The incidence curve shows two peaks: the first comprises patients in their 20s and 30s, the second is the elderly. This disease is slightly more common in males than females, and in whites than African Americans. It is also found more often among young people who are well educated and within higher socioeconomic brackets.[10]

The cause of Hodgkin's disease remains elusive. Although Epstein-Barr virus (EBV) is not a proven cause of Hodgkin's disease, specimens taken from patients with Hodgkin's disease often contain multiple copies of the EBV genome.[10] No conclusive evidence for a relationship between EBV and Hodgkin's disease exists. People with a history of infectious mononucleosis have a threefold likelihood of developing Hodgkin's lymphoma (HL), supporting a role for the EBV.[8] A strong genetic predisposition to Hodgkin's disease has not been demonstrated, although same-sex siblings of patients are at slightly increased risk.[10]

Prevention, Screening, and Detection

Early detection is important but may be hampered by the vagueness of the common symptoms including fatigue, weight loss, night sweats, and fever.[2] Patients should be encouraged to seek medical attention for persistent common signs and symptoms.

Classification

The World Health Organization (WHO) classification can be found in Box 15-1.

World Health Organization (WHO) Classification 1999 Recommendations

Classical Hodgkin's Lymphoma
Nodular sclerosis
Lymphocyte-rich classical
Mixed cellularity
Lymphocyte depletion

Nodular Lymphocyte Predominant Hodgkin's Lymphoma
Unique form that accounts for only 3% to 8% of cases

Data from Yung L, Linch D: Hodgkin lymphoma, *Lancet* 361:943-51, 2003; Caley B: Hodgkin disease: the other side, *Cure* 4(1):1, 2005; and Cheson B: What's new in lymphoma? *CA Cancer J Clin* 54:260-272, 2004.

Clinical Features

The most common signs of Hodgkin's disease are lymphadenopathy, fever, night sweats, weight loss, pruritus, and alcohol-induced pain.[2] The most frequent indication is a mass or swelling at one of the lymph node sites in the neck, above the clavicle, under the arms, in the elbow region, or near the groin.[8] Mediastinal nodes may become enlarged to greater than 10 cm, and patients may complain of dry cough or shortness of breath, especially when lying down, as well as substernal pain. Unexplained fever of greater than 38° C during the prior month, drenching and recurring night sweats, and unexplained weight loss greater than 10% in less than 6 months usually signifies advanced disease. Other presenting signs include generalized pruritus and pain in the enlarged nodes after the ingestion of alcohol, which has known prognostic significance.[2]

Since the lymphomas also can involve the bone marrow, the first warning may be anemia with bleeding related to a decrease in platelet count or infection as a consequence of insufficient white blood cells.[10]

Other rare occurrences are superior vena cava syndrome (SVCS), upper extremity thrombosis, phrenic nerve or laryngeal nerve entrapment, ureteral obstruction, lymphedema, venous thrombosis of the lower extremities, and splenomegaly.[2]

Diagnosis and Staging

When a patient is first seen with clinical manifestations suggestive of Hodgkin's disease, a thorough history and physical examination must be performed.[2] Diagnosis is confirmed with a biopsy of the enlarged node. An excisional node biopsy is preferred over a needle biopsy for a suspected lymphoma. The former technique is the only way to distinguish between Hodgkin's lymphoma and to diagnose the specific subtype.[10]

An accurate tissue diagnosis is a major determinant of treatment and is also fundamental for staging (Table 15-1).[10] To stage the extent of the disease accurately, the following procedures should be initiated as soon as possible after a definite diagnosis of Hodgkin's disease:[2,10,11]

1. *Detailed history and physical exam* with emphasis on history of "B symptoms" (fever, night sweats, weight loss), palpation of liver and spleen, evaluation of cardiac and pulmonary status
2. *Radiology workup:* Computed tomography (CT) scan of chest, abdomen, pelvis; chest x-ray exam; lymphangiograms
3. *Positron emission tomography* (PET)
4. *Gallium-67 scan*
5. *A laboratory workup:* Complete blood count (CBC), differential, platelet count, erythrocyte sedimentation rate (ESR), liver and renal function tests, lactate dehydrogenase (LDH), $\beta2$-microglobulin ($\beta2M$)
6. *Bone marrow biopsy and aspirate*
7. *Percutaneous needle biopsy*
8. *Staging laparotomy:* Laparotomy includes splenectomy; biopsy of celiac, splenic, hilar, porta hepatic, para-aortic and iliac nodes; wedge and/or needle biopsy of liver; and open iliac bone marrow biopsy if not done previously.[2] A staging laparotomy is rarely done today, in part because non-Hodgkin's lymphoma is usually considered a systemic disease regardless of the stage at the time of diagnosis.[10]
9. *Immunophenotyping*[2,10]

TABLE 15-1   Ann Arbor Staging System with Cotswold Modifications for Hodgkin's Lymphoma[1, 10]

Stage I	Involvement of one lymph node region or lymphoid structure (e.g., spleen, thymus, Waldeyer's ring)
Stage II	Two or more lymph node regions on the same side of the diaphragm
Stage III	Lymph nodes on both sides of the diaphragm
3_1	with splenic hilar, celiac, or portal nodes
3_2	with para-aortic, iliac, or mesenteric nodes
Stage IV	Involvement of extranodal site(s) beyond that designated E (either in bone marrow and organ or the skin)

Modifying Features	
A	No symptoms
B	Fever, drenching night sweats, weight loss greater than 10% in 6 months
X	Bulky disease: greater than 33% widening of mediastinum, greater than 10 cm maximum diameter of nodal mass
E	Involvement of single, contiguous, or proximal extranodal site
CS	Clinical stage
PS	Pathologic stage

Laboratory studies are not indicative of Hodgkin's disease. A CBC is done routinely to evaluate peripheral blood counts for signs of suppression, which may be an indication of lymphoma in the bone marrow. An elevated LDH correlates with a lymphoma that is bulky or growing rapidly.[10]

Routine assessments of liver and kidney function are basic to the workup. The objectives are to determine the ability to tolerate therapy and whether the disease has affected either of these organs.[10]

Additional distinctions in staging are sometimes made. For example, "S" indicates involvement of the spleen. A patient with two groups of positive nodes, one on either side of the diaphragm, would have stage III disease. Spleen involvement would mean the patient has IIIS disease.[10]

A series of new stains and molecular techniques has expanded the classification of the lymphomas. Leukocyte common antigen (LCA), and cluster designations CD20, CD5, CD23, and CD10 are among the stains used today for the lymphoma immunophenotyping. CD15 and CD30 are useful for Hodgkin's disease. CD20 is a B-cell marker, and CD3 is a T-cell marker. Categorization is now based on the way the cells look under the microscope, the way they stain, and their behavior.[10]

During and after treatment, many of the same staging procedures are repeated to document response to treatment and then to document complete remission. When recurrence is suspected, the diagnostic and staging process is repeated. It is important to document disease recurrence by node biopsy and to determine the site and extent of recurrence. These factors are as important for effective treatment of recurrence as they are for the management of new diagnoses.[2]

METASTASIS

Hodgkin's disease spreads contiguously from one lymph node chain to another. Strong evidence indicates that Hodgkin's disease begins in one lymph node, then spreads to the adjacent nodes, until eventually the malignant cells invade the blood vessels and spread to other organs. Involvement of retroperitoneal nodes, lungs, liver, spleen, and bone marrow usually occurs after Hodgkin's disease is generalized. Mesenteric lymph nodes and any organ can be involved in advanced cases.[2]

Treatment Modalities

As a result of the advances in precise staging, knowledge of prognostic factors, the development of supervoltage radiation therapy, and effective combination chemotherapy, survival rates for Hodgkin's disease have improved greatly.[2] If cure is a realistic possibility, there is an impetus for initiating therapy as soon as possible. Hodgkin's disease, regardless of subtype, is

---

BOX 15-2   Prognostic Factors in Localized Hodgkin's disease (EORTC* Criteria)

Very Favorable (6% of patients)
Clinical stage IA, female, <40 years of age, ESR <50 mm, lymphocyte predominant or nodular sclerosis; mediastinal/thoracic ratio <0.35.

Favorable (45% of patients)
Cs I/II A/B; 1–3 sites; mediastinal/thoracic ratio <0.35; <50 years of age; stage A/ESR <50 or stage B/ESR <30 mm/h.

Unfavorable (45% of patients)
Age >50; or A/ESR ≥50 or B/ESR ≥30; or CS II ≥4 sites or mediastinal/thoracic ratio ≥0.35.

From Cancellos GP: Hodgkin disease. In Freireich EJ, Kantarijan HM, editors: *Medical management of hematological malignant disease*, New York, 1999, Marcel Dekker.
*European Organization for Research and Treatment of Cancer.
ESR, Erythrocyte sedimentation rate.

---

potentially curable. Therefore therapy is started promptly, and the regimen is usually an established aggressive approach based on a proven rate of success.[10]

EARLY-STAGE DISEASE

Stages I and/or II, A or B (with or without symptoms), is defined as early-stage Hodgkin's disease. The European Organization for Research and Treatment of Cancer have grouped negative prognostic factors into very favorable, favorable, and unfavorable criteria for use in early-stage Hodgkin's disease (Box 15-2).[2,12]

There are generally three treatment options for early stage Hodgkin's disease: radiation therapy, chemotherapy, or a combination of both. Table 15-2 illustrates standard fields for radiation.[2] Table 15-3 lists chemotherapy regimens.[2,13,14] Approximately 75% of patients with Hodgkin's lymphoma can be cured with modern chemotherapy and radiation. Most patients are treated according to clinical stage and the associated prognostic factors. For patients with limited-stage Hodgkin's lymphoma, combined modality treatment has replaced subtotal nodal irradiation as the preferred treatment option.[15]

Radiation therapy alone is a possibility for patients whose Hodgkin's disease has been designated as stage IA, IB, or IIA. Radiation is associated with a number of unwanted effects, including an increased incidence of secondary malignancies and heart disease.[8,10] Now that chemotherapy has become safer, the chance

---

TABLE 15-2   Standard Radiation for Hodgkin's disease

Mantle field	From mandible to diaphragm; lungs, heart, spinal cord, and humeral heads are shielded
Inverted Y field	From diaphragm to ischial tuberosities, including the spleen if not removed; spinal cord, kidneys, bladder, rectum, and gonads are shielded
Subtotal lymphoid irradiation	Involves mantle zone and uppermost inverted zone
Para-aortic/spleen zone	Does not include the pelvic, inguinal, or femoral nodes
Total lymphoid irradiation	Mantle zone and complete inverted zone

TABLE 15-3 **Chemotherapy Regimens for Hodgkin's lymphoma**

MOPP	Mechlorethamine	MOPPEBVCAD	Mechlorethamine
	Vincristine		Vincristine
	Procarbazine		Procarbazine
	Prednisone		Prednisone
ABVD	Doxorubicin		Epidoxorubicin
	Bleomycin		Bleomycin
	Vinblastine		Vinblastine
	Dacarbazine		Lomustine
MOPP/ABV	Combinations of both		Melphalan
	regimens		Vindesine
Ch1VPP	Chlorambucil	BEACOPP	Bleomycin
	Vinblastine		Etoposide
	Procarbazine		Doxorubicin
	Prednisone		Cyclophosphamide
PABLOE	Prednisolone		Vincristine
	Doxorubicin		Procarbazine
	Bleomycin		Prednisone
	Vincristine	Stanford V	Mechlorethamine
	Etoposide		Doxorubicin
CHOPE	Cyclophosphamide		Vinblastine
	Doxorubicin		Vincristine
	Vincristine		Bleomycin
	Prednisone		Etoposide
	Etoposide		Prednisone

of successful treatment of Hodgkin's disease may be greatest with a combination of chemotherapy and irradiation.[10]

The standard chemotherapy regimen for Hodgkin's disease in the past was MOPP—mechlorethamine + vincristine + procarbazine + prednisone).[10] The new chemotherapeutic combination is ABVD—doxorubicin + bleomycin + vinblastine + dacarbazine. The risk of secondary leukemias is much lower with ABVD.[5,10,15] In older patients, who may have less efficient cardiac and lung function, ABVD is a concern. MOPP is occasionally selected for a patient older than 75, but ABVD is the primary choice for all others.[10,16]

A group of physicians known as the German Hodgkin Lymphoma Study Group developed a treatment called dose-escalated BEACOPP—bleomycin + etoposide + doxorubicin + cyclophosphamide + vincristine + procarbazine + prednisone. BEACOPP is more toxic than ABVD, but the benefits outweigh the side effects, especially for younger patients and those with aggressive disease.[5]

ADVANCED DISEASE

For patients with stages III or IV, the presence of B symptoms, and/or bulky disease (larger than 10 cm at any site, greater than one third the thoracic diameter), ABVD has become the standard chemotherapy. It has a number of advantages including improved compliance because of intravenous administration, less cumulative myelotoxicity, a lower risk of secondary malignancies (acute myeloid leukemia [AML] or solid tumors), and a lower rate of infertility compared with previous regimens such as MOPP. The regimen can induce complete remissions in 80% to 85% of patients, with a 5-year freedom from progressions of 61% and an overall 5-year survival of 73%.[8] For patients with a

bulky mediastinal mass, a combined modality using chemotherapy and radiation may be beneficial.[2] Combination chemotherapy remains the treatment of choice for advanced Hodgkin's disease, and new dose-intense regimens appear to have improved activity.[11]

RELAPSED OR RECURRENT DISEASE

After initial therapy, 40% to 50% of patients with stage III or IV disease, and 20% to 30% with stage I or II disease will have residual or recurrent disease.[12] Patients who relapse after radiation alone are generally treated with standard chemotherapy, with excellent remission rates and 50% to 80% long-term survival rates.[4] For patients relapsing after chemotherapy, several treatment approaches have been used, with varying degrees of success.[2] Patients who relapse now have a more favorable prognosis with the availability of active salvage regimens, autologous stem cell transplantation, and novel biologic agents.[11]

When relapse occurs after chemotherapy, the length of disease-free survival is important in planning future treatment. Patients experiencing relapse after long disease-free survival have a 70% to 90% complete response rate to standard chemotherapy regimens. Those who relapse less than 12 months after initial therapy are less likely to achieve a complete remission using standard-dose chemotherapy.[4] This group should be offered high-dose chemotherapy with or without radiation therapy followed by an autologous bone marrow or stem cell support.[4,5]

The most common high-dose regimen for Hodgkin's is BEAM—carmustine + etoposide + cytarabine + melphalan. Bone marrow or peripheral blood stem cells are removed before high-dose chemotherapy and then replaced afterward to help the patient replace destroyed blood cells.[5,12] Over the past decade,

BOX 15-3   Summary of Complications of Hodgkin's Disease

Secondary malignancies
Acute leukemia
Pulmonary fibrosis
Cardiac dysfunction
Hypothyroidism
Dental caries
Infertility
Psychologic trauma
Myelodysplasia
Non-Hodgkin's lymphoma
Sterility

Data from Yung L, Linch D: Hodgkin lymphoma, *Lancet* 361:943-51, 2003; Caley B: Hodgkin disease: the other side, *Cure* 4(1):1, 2005; and Armitage J: Current approaches to the lymphomas, *Patient Care* 275:65-87, 1999.

the treatment-related morbidity and mortality associated with autologous stem cell transplantation have been significantly reduced, and stem cell transplant is becoming the treatment of choice for most patients with primary refractory or recurrent Hodgkin's lymphoma. With longer follow-up and long-term complications, secondary malignancy has become the leading cause of late treatment failure for patients with Hodgkin's lymphoma.[15]

Prognosis

Hodgkin's disease is a very treatable and highly curable cancer. For patients with stage IA or IIA disease treated with radiation therapy alone, the 20-year survival rate is 70% to 80%, and the overall survival rate after salvage therapy for those with relapse is 80% to 95%. Patients with stage III or IV advanced disease are able to achieve remission after chemotherapy with a complete remission rate of 89% for ABVD. Patients with relapsed or resistant disease have a less favorable prognosis. Stage I or II disease with relapse has a 57% to 62% disease-free survival rate at 10 years. Relapses after chemotherapy with a less than 12 month remission are projected to have less than 17% survival at 20 years.[17]

Even with survival of Hodgkin's disease, patients face possible treatment-related complications, which can occur years later (Box 15-3). The most common long-term complications of Hodgkin's disease are secondary malignancies and ischemic heart disease. The risk of developing other cancers is more than 5 times greater for survivors of Hodgkin's disease than for the general population.[5] Common secondary malignancies include lung cancer, AML, non-Hodgkin's lymphoma, thyroid cancer, and breast cancer.[1,2] AML is most frequently seen. Combined modality therapy is indicated as the risk factor for developing secondary AML.[18] The risk of developing non-Hodgkin's lymphoma is equal whether the patient was treated with chemotherapy, radiation therapy, or a combination of both.[5,18]

MOPP is associated with high rates of infertility. The risk of infertility and options for preserving fertility should be thoroughly discussed before therapy.[5] Hypothyroidism is common after radiation to the lower neck, occurring in 50% of patients receiving neck irradiation. Thyroid function levels should be measured yearly.[1]

TABLE 15-4   Clinical Trials for Hodgkin's disease

THERAPY	PHASE
Velcade (bortezomib) (refractory or recurrent classical Hodgkin's disease)	I
SGN-30 (monoclonal antibody) (refractory or recurrent Hodgkin's disease)	II
Zevalin (ibritumomab) (refractory or relapsed Hodgkin's disease)	II
LMP-2a specific cytotoxic T cells (relapsed Hodgkin's disease)	I

Breast cancer occurs in approximately 20% to 50% of patients, about 15 years after irradiation, and is significantly more common in young girls and women who received mantle radiation.[1,5] Lung cancer is prevalent in patients who smoke, and the risk is about 4 times that of the normal population. It is theorized that radiation potentiates the cellular changes already initiated by smoking.[2] Additional, less common solid tumor sites include the stomach, soft tissues, bones, and skin.[2]

New Treatments

New therapies are directed toward targeted approaches, especially in the non-Hodgkin's lymphoma where malignant cells can be more reliably isolated.[8] The future lies in combining biologic therapies in a manner that will optimize their activity (which reduces dependence on the more toxic and nonspecific cytotoxic drugs), identifying those patients most likely to respond to those therapies, monitoring disease status, and preventing reccurence.[8]

IMMUNOTHERAPY

A monoclonal antibody is a drug that is more likely to spare healthy cells because it is targeted to a particular protein on cancer cells. One of the most promising antigens for targeted immunotherapy is the CD30 antigen, which is highly expressed on Hodgkin's/Reed-Sternberg cells.[1] Two monoclonal antibodies under investigation for their ability to treat Hodgkin's disease are SGN-30 and MDX-060. Both target CD30.[5] In early clinical trials, both of these monoclonal antibodies have produced partial responses and have been well tolerated[1,5,8] (Table 15-4).

CYTOTOXIC DRUGS

Gemcitabine, an analogue of cytarabine, has antitumor activity in Hodgkin's lymphoma. It is well tolerated with a favorable toxicity profile.[1] Pulmonary toxicity of gemcitabine is uncommon and usually mild when given as a single agent.[8]

Non-Hodgkin's Lymphoma
Epidemiology and Etiology

The term non-Hodgkin's lymphoma (NHL) refers to more than a dozen malignancies that arise from a proliferation of B or T lymphocytes at various stages of differentiation.[19] As a group of neoplasms, NHL is morphologically and clinically different from Hodgkin's disease. After the Reed-Sternberg cell was identified as the cell characteristic of Hodgkin's disease, all other lymphomas were classified as non-Hodgkin's. Essentially, NHL became a term to identify diseases with similarities to Hodgkin's but without the characteristic Reed-Sternberg cell.[2] In 2005, there were an estimated 56,390 new cases of NHL, and the ACS further estimated that 19,200 people would die of NHL in 2005; it represents the sixth most common cause of cancer deaths in the United States. [9,20,21] Not surprisingly, NHL ranks fourth in economic impact among cancers owing to the cumulative years of life lost to the disease in the United States.[19] The incidence has increased by 50% during the past 15 years, partly because of an increase in lymphomas related to human immunodeficiency virus (HIV) and an unexplained increase in older adults. Men are at slightly higher risk than women. It is more common in adults than children; however, there is a steady increase from childhood through 80 years of age. The average age at diagnosis is 45 to 55 years.[19,20]

Although the etiology of NHL remains unknown, a variety of factors have been associated with increased risk (Box 15-4).[2,13,22] These include a number of immunodeficiency conditions, autoimmune disorders, infectious diseases, and environmental factors. Immunodeficiency conditions can be divided into congenital and acquired disorders. These disorders have in common defects in immunoregulation, particularly in cell-mediated immunity, resulting in decreased cytokine production, and uncontrolled B-cell proliferation, often associated with EBV genome.[2,23] Lymphomas that develop under these conditions are usually highly aggressive B-cell NHL that are widely disseminated.[24] Ataxia telangiectasia (AT) is an autosomal recessive disorder associated with chronic EBV infections. Patients with AT have an increased risk of developing NHL, Hodgkin's disease, gastric carcinomas, and dysgerminomas.[2,20,21] Approximately 10% of children with AT develop NHL.[2,24] Wiskott-Aldrich syndrome (WAS) is an X-linked recessive disorder that involves a progressive decline in cell-mediated immunity. NHL occurs in approximately 15% of these children, with the central nervous system (CNS) being the primary site in one third of the cases.[2,23,24] Other congenital immune disorders include severe combined immune deficiency (SCID), common variable immunodeficiency (CVID), immunoglobulin (Ig) A (IgA) deficiency, IgM deficiency, hyper-IgM syndrome, and X-linked hypogammaglobulinemia. All of these disorders are associated with a high incidence of NHL. There is also an increased incidence of NHL occurring in patients receiving long-term immunosuppression (e.g., organ transplant recipients), and in patients with rheumatoid arthritis or celiac disease.[2,13,25]

Infectious agents can also contribute to etiology by virtue of chronic stimulation of the immune system. *Helicobacter pylori, Borrelia burgdorfferi*, hepatitis C virus, EBV, human T-cell leukemia virus type 1 (HTLV-1), and human herpes virus 8 (HHV-8) have been linked to NHL. *H. pylori* infection of the stomach leads to chronic inflammation and is associated with the development of mucosa-associated lymphoid tissue (MALT lymphomas).[2,13,23-26] *B. burgdorfferi*, Lyme disease, is associated with some forms of skin lymphomas.[2,13] EBV is associated with many different forms of NHL as well as Hodgkin's disease.[2,20,22] HTLV-1 is implicated in the etiology of adult T-cell lymphoma and leukemias.[2,13,24-26]

HHV-8 was identified as a new herpes virus through the use of polymerase chain reaction-based technique used in studying

---

BOX 15-4   **Risk Factors Associated with Non-Hodgkin's lymphoma**

Immunodeficiency Disorders

Acquired
Immunosuppression after transplantation
Acquired immunodeficiency syndrome (AIDS)

Congenital
Ataxia-telangiectasia
Wiscott-Aldrich syndrome
Severe combined immunodeficiency
Common variable immunodeficiency
IgA and IgM deficiency
Hyper-IgM syndrome
X-linked hypogammaglobulinemia
X-linked lymphoproliferative disorder

Autoimmune Disorders
Hashimoto's thyroiditis
Sjogren's syndrome
Rheumatoid arthritis
Systemic lupus erythematosus

Infectious Agents
Epstein-Barr virus (EBV)
Human T-cell leukemia virus type 1 (HTLV-1)
Human herpes virus-8 (HHV-8)
Helicobacter pylori
Hepatitis C virus

Environmental Factors
Diphenylhydanytoin (Dilantin)
Phenoxyherbicides
Organophosphates
Benzene
Styrene
1-3 Butadiene
Trichloroethylene
Perchloroethylene
Creosote
Lead arsenate
Formaldehyde
Paint thinner
Hair dyes

Others
Immunosuppressive therapy
Chemotherapy
Radiation therapy
Castleman's disease

Kaposi sarcoma tissue. This virus was found to be present in a number of patients with acquired immunodeficiency syndrome (AIDS) who manifested lymphomas located in body cavities (pleural, pericardial, and peritoneal). Today HHV-8 is a recognized risk factor for body cavity–based lymphomas in patients with HIV infection and in multicentric Castleman's disease.[2,23,27,28] Hepatitis C has also been linked to increased risk of NHL.[2,13,23]

Exposure to some chemicals and physical agents has also been suspected in the increased incidence of NHL. Phenytoin (Dilantin) has been studied in both pseudolymphoma and malignant lymphoma.[2,23] Other drugs implicated include aspirin, antibodies, steroids, digitalis, estrogen, and tranquilizers.[2,23] Occupations that place people at higher risk include agriculture, forestry, fishing, construction, and leather workers. The chemicals used in these jobs include chlorophenols and phenoxyacetic acids.[2,23] Additional factors include hair dyes, ultraviolet light, and nutritional factors. The results are conflicting; however, milk, butter, liver, meat, coffee, and cola have been implicated.[2,13,23] NHL has occurred as a secondary malignancy after chemotherapy and radiation therapy for Hodgkin's disease.[2,13,24]

Prevention, Screening, and Detection

Prevention of NHL is not possible because there are no identified preventable risks. Early detection is important but again is hampered by the vagueness of the common symptoms. Patients should be encouraged to seek medical attention for persistent common signs and symptoms.[2]

Classification

Accurate classification of NHL is vital in gauging prognosis and determining therapy.[28] The classification of lymphomas has evolved over the years on the basis of both a better understanding of the clinical aspects of lymphoma and the additional information gained through the application of immunologic and molecular techniques. Three classification systems are currently in use: the Kiel system, the Revised European-American Lymphoma system (REAL), and the International Working Formulation (IWF) system. Currently, the IWF classification system is the most commonly used staging tool in the United States.[28] Lymphoma types are organized into 10 classes with three major categories: low grade, intermediate grade and high grade (Box 15-5).[28]

Low-grade lymphomas, which make up 20% to 40% of NHL, tend to occur in patients with a median age 50 to 60.[22] Low-grade lymphomas present with few symptoms but disseminated disease. Intermediate and high-grade lymphomas present with localized disease. In NHL, the histology of the tumor type seems to be more important to prognosis than the extent of the disease.[22]

Clinical Features

Approximately 90% of patients first arrive to be seen with stage III or IV, including generalized lymphadenopathy and bone marrow involvement. Despite widespread tumor involvement, low-grade lymphoma is often clinically indolent and patients are frequently asymptomatic for years.[29] The various subgroups of lymphoma are associated with specific signs and symptoms. Nodal indolent lymphomas are typically seen in middle-aged or older adults, who complain of painless lymphadenopathy but are otherwise healthy.[13] They often report a long history of waxing and waning adenopathy. B symptoms are uncommon in indolent lymphomas.[13] Most patients have bone marrow involvement when they are first seen. Extranodal indolent lymphomas are found in the stomach, the parotid gland, the thyroid, or the lung. They are usually localized stage I or II disease. Patients may complain of abdominal discomfort relating to splenomegaly and may have neutropenia or thrombocytopenia.[13]

BOX 15-5 **International Working Formulation Classification of Non-Hodgkin's Lymphoma**

Class
Low Grade
A. Small lymphocytic
B. Follicular small, cleaved cell
C. Follicular, mixed small, cleaved and large cell

Intermediate Grade
D. Follicular, large cell
E. Diffuse, small, cleaved cell
F. Diffuse, mixed small, cleaved and large cell
G. Diffuse large cell

High Grade
H. Large cell, immunoblastic
I. Lymphoblastic
J. Small, noncleaved cell Burkitt's

Aggressive lymphomas are more symptomatic at presentation. Patients complain of pain, obstructive symptoms such as swelling in legs or SVCS, or B symptoms. T-cell lymphomas have presenting symptoms of extranodal involvement and severe B symptoms more frequently. Extensive retroperitoneal adenopathy is more common than peripheral adenopathy. The site of disease is often indicative of histology. For example nasopharyngeal lymphoma is usually an EBV-associated T-cell or natural killer (NK)–cell lymphoma. Patients first come to the attention of health caregivers with varying stages of disease; however, more extensive disease is associated with a worse prognosis.[13] Very aggressive lymphomas are more commonly found in younger adults and children, and occasionally in older adults. Bone marrow, peripheral blood, and CNS involvement is common. Very high LDH levels are seen in this type of lymphoma but not in the others.

Diagnosis and Staging

Patients are first seen with localized or general lymphadenopathy, B symptoms, and/or infiltration of the bone marrow. Vague symptoms of back pain or abdominal discomfort may also be present, which could indicate an abdominal mass.[22]

The management of Hodgkin's and non-Hodgkin's lymphoma is dependent on the accurate staging of the disease, evaluation of histology, and other risk factors. The patient's clinical exam should focus on a detailed history and physical examination.[22]

The staging evaluation should include the following: [2,22,30]

1. *Laboratory work:* CBC, differential, blood smear exam, LDH, β2M levels, liver function tests (LFTs), renal function tests, electrolytes, calcium and uric acid levels, hepatitis B and C titers, and HIV, HTVL-1, EBV serology, and bilateral bone marrow aspiration and biopsy
2. *Radiology:* Chest X-ray, CT of the thorax, abdomen, pelvis, and head depending upon the symptoms
3. *PET scan*
4. *Gallium-67 scan* (in intermediate- and high-grade lymphomas)
5. *Magnetic resonance imaging (MRI)*
6. *Bone scans*

Surgical staging is no longer used, and therefore staging is primarily performed with CT scanning or the use of MRI for extranodal sites and bone marrow involvement.[30] The accuracy of CT in the identification of small-volume nodal disease or the presence of disease in the spleen, the liver, or other extranodal sites is unreliable. Also, the role of CT in the assessment of disease activity is poor when residual masses are identified after treatment. Functional imaging techniques such as gallium-67 and, more recently, PET are thought to convey an advantage over anatomic imaging (CT, MRI) both in staging and in the assessment of disease response.[30]

Biopsy of an abnormal lymph node or mass is necessary to diagnose NHL. After a diagnosis of NHL, the clinical stage of disease must be determined. After diagnosis is made through excisional or incisional biopsy, staging and identifying the presence of prognostic factors is essential in determining treatment strategies. The history should focus on the presence of B symptoms, as well as the duration and rate of lymph node enlargement. The physical examination includes assessment of lymph node chains including measurement of enlarged nodes.[2,24] Subsequent diagnostic studies are indicated by specific disease entity or presentation of the disease. Like Hodgkin's disease, no specific laboratory studies are indicative of NHL; however, they do provide additional prognostic and site-specific information.[2,24] In addition to routine blood tests, serum LDH and β2M levels are important indicators of prognosis and indirect indicators of tumor burden.[2,20] Cytogenetic and molecular analyses of bone marrow and peripheral blood are also obtained. With the advent of polymerase chain reaction technology, it is possible to identify specific immunoglobulin gene rearrangements or chromosomal translocations with high accuracy and to evaluate the significance of minimal residual disease in a variety of subtypes of lymphomas. Although it is early to base treatment recommendation on the molecular analysis, in the future these techniques will likely affect treatment strategies.[2,20]

Imaging studies should include routine chest x-ray exam and CT scan of the abdomen and pelvis. Chest x-ray film may reveal hilar or mediastinal adenopathy, pleural effusion, or parenchymal involvement.[2,20] If there is an abnormality on the chest x-ray exam, CT of the chest is indicated. CT of the abdomen and pelvis is necessary to evaluate mesenteric and retroperitoneal involvement.[2,13] Patients with indolent lymphomas should have a lymphangiogram since this procedure is more sensitive in assessing lower abdominal and pelvic adenopathy, an important factor in considering treatment options.[2,13] Gallium scans are positive in nearly all-aggressive, highly aggressive lymphomas and in approximately 50% of indolent lymphomas. They are used to identify initial sites of disease, monitor response to treatment, and detect early recurrence.[2,20]

Bone marrow biopsy should be routine for staging NHL. Many institutions routinely do bilateral biopsies because these have about 15% higher yield than unilateral biopsy specimens.[2,13] A lumbar puncture is recommended in highly aggressive lymphomas, mantle cell lymphoma, HIV-related lymphoma, primary CNS lymphoma, and large cell lymphoma with bone marrow involvement. If liver involvement is suspected, a liver biopsy may be indicated.[2,13] For patients with head and neck involvement or those with a gastrointestinal (GI) primary, an upper GI series with small bowel follow-through and endoscopy

are indicated. Staging laparotomies and splenectomies are no longer routinely performed in patients with NHLs.

Although originally designed for staging of Hodgkin's disease, the Cotswold modification of the Ann Arbor staging system has been routinely applied to NHL (see Table 15-1). The staging system is based on the number of sites of involvement, the presence of disease above or below the diaphragm, evidence of systemic symptoms, and extranodal disease.[2,20] Because of the differences in the patterns of disease spread in Hodgkin's disease and NHL, it has been necessary to identify additional prognostic clinical factors that more accurately reflect NHL.[2,13] Table 15-5 shows two systems currently used to predict the prognosis of patients before initiating therapy: the International Prognostic Index (IPI) and the MD Anderson Tumor Score System. The IPI is based on five parameters: age, performance status, serum LDH, involvement of more than one extranodal site, and stage of disease. A point is assigned to each factor, and then points are summed for a total score according to risk.[2,13,20] The MD Anderson Tumor Score System is also based on five parameters, with a score given for presence or absence of these parameters.

TABLE 15-5   International Index and Tumor Score System

A. International Index

PARAMETER	CRITERIA	SCORE
Age	<60 y	0
	>60 y	1
Ann Arbor stage	I–II	0
	III–IV	1
Serum LDH	Normal	0
	> Normal	1
Performance status	0–1	0
	>1	1
Extranodal sites	0–1	0
	>1	1

TOTAL SCORE	RISK
0, 1	Low
2	Low-intermediate
3	High-intermediate
4, 5	High risk

B. Tumor Score System

PARAMETER	ADVERSE FEATURE
Ann Arbor stage	III–IV
Symptoms	Presence of B symptoms
Tumor bulk	Mass >7 cm or CXR-detectable mediastinal mass
β2M	≥3.0
LDH	≥685

Each adverse feature scores one point. Totals of 3 or greater define poor-risk patients.
β2M, β2-microglobulin; *CXR*, Chest e-ray exam; *LDH*, lactate dehydrogenase.
From Marlton P, Cabanillas F: Therapy of aggressive lymphoma. In Freireich EJ, Kantarjian HM, editors: *Medical management of hematologic malignant diseases*, New York, 1998, Marcel Dekker.

A score greater than 3 identifies the patient as having a poor risk or prognosis and would be treated on investigational protocols. Those with a score of less than 3 have an 80% disease-free survival rate when treated with conventional regimens.[2,13]

METASTASIS

The metastatic process varies with the type of lymphoma: follicular has bone marrow involvement and diffuse disseminates rapidly and involves areas such as the CNS, bone and GI tract.[2]

Treatment Modalities and Prognosis

Treatment approaches to NHLs are based on the specific histology of the neoplasm, stage of disease, the prognosis, and the physiologic status of the patient. Many institutions will use either the IPI or the MD Anderson Tumor Score System, then use these parameters to aid in planning treatment.[2] In general, treatment includes radiation, single-agent chemotherapy, or combination chemotherapy.[22]

INDOLENT NON-HODGKIN'S LYMPHOMA

Controversy surrounds whether treatment of indolent or low-grade NHL can induce long-term disease-free survival and actually alter the disease's natural history. Because the natural history of indolent lymphomas includes very slow growth that rarely invades normal structures, this controversy is understandable. They are very responsive to a variety of treatments; however, multiple relapses are the rule. Patients generally have a long survival after diagnosis, but indolent NHLs are unlikely to be cured with current therapies.[2] Indolent NHLs are unique in that they transform into more aggressive forms, and may undergo spontaneous regression.[2] After transformation, indolent NHLs have a reported survival of less than a year.[2]

Early-stage indolent NHL is generally described as Ann Arbor stages I and II, and are generally uncommon.[2] Radiation therapy to the involved field or total nodal radiation produces up to 85% disease-free survival with follow-up over 10 years.[2] Although these numbers appear to suggest that a limited number of patients may be curable, the survival curves do not reflect relapses over 10 years.[2] Most relapses occur outside of the radiation field. The role of chemotherapy in the treatment of early-stage indolent lymphoma has not been greatly explored. Small studies report fewer relapses by combining radiation and chemotherapy; however, no improved survival has been shown.[2]

The majority of patients with indolent NHL have advanced (stage III or IV) disease at diagnosis. The optimal regimen for these patients remains controversial and ranges from watchful waiting to intensive chemotherapy and autologous bone marrow transplant.[2] Unfortunately, no treatment option has been shown to improve survival. Treatment options tend to be determined by the patient and physician preference or by investigational protocols.[2] Treatment may be deferred until symptoms become bothersome or the disease has transformed into a more aggressive type of lymphoma.[2] Patients may be offered conventional chemotherapy, such as CVP—cyclophosphamide + vincristine + prednisone— or CHOP—cyclophosphamide + doxorubicin + vincristine + prednisone; but there is no convincing survival benefit shown for this group.[2] Interferon has been effective in producing remissions, especially in patients with follicular lymphoma. It has been used mainly with combination chemotherapy, either in the induction phase or as maintenance therapy.

Nucleoside analogues such as fludarabine and cladribine (2-CDA) have been active in treating indolent lymphomas. They are associated with profound immunosuppression, and treatment can be complicated by opportunistic infections such as *Pneumocystis carinii* pneumonia, herpes infections, and fungal pneumonias.[2] Topoisomerase I inhibitors, topotecan, irinotecan (CPT-11), and camptothecine have shown some effectiveness in heavily treated patients, and may have synergy with topoisomerase II inhibitors such as etoposide.[2] These are early phases of studies, and the optimal placement of these newer agents is uncertain. Monoclonal antibodies have also been used in the treatment of NHL. Idec-C2B8 (Rituximab) is a chimeric anti-CD20 antibody. The CD20 antigen is expressed in 95% of B-cell lymphomas. This antibody has minimal toxicity and a short treatment schedule, making it very tolerable for patients.[2] High-dose chemotherapy and autologous or allogeneic bone marrow transplantation has been used as clinical trials with encouraging results.[2]

AGGRESSIVE NON-HODGKIN'S LYMPHOMA

The most common type of aggressive lymphoma is diffuse large B-cell lymphoma. There is more knowledge and there are more treatment options for this group. After diagnosis and staging is determined, a decision is made whether the disease is curable with the CHOP regimen. The IPI or MD Anderson Tumor Score is used for this purpose. If the score for cure with CHOP is greater than 75%, it should be administered. CHOP is well tolerated, simple to administer, and has a disease-free survival rate of 10 years in 82% of stage I patients and 64% in stage II patients.[2] Patients with poor cardiac function require a regimen that does not include anthracyclines.[2] The value of radiation therapy is uncertain. In some cases it is used for consolidation in bulky disease for both early and advanced stages.[2]

Patients with a tumor score greater than 2 or an IPI greater than 3 are considered to have an unfavorable prognosis and would not benefit from the CHOP regimen. The cure rate with CHOP is less than 30%. The best treatment for this group of patients is still undetermined. Varying combinations of chemotherapy have been studied (Table 15-6).[2,31] Currently, a novel approach to treating high-risk patients consists of alternating triple therapy with ASHAP—doxorubicin + methyprednisolone + cytarabine + cisplatin; M-BACOD—methotrexate + leucovorin + bleomycin + doxorubicin + cyclophosphamide + vincristine + dexamethasone; and MINE—mesna + ifofamide + mitoxantrone + etoposide. The results show a benefit superior to that of the CHOP regimen. This group of patients may have high-dose chemotherapy followed by autologous bone marrow transplant. One study showed a 59% 5-year disease free-survival following transplant.[2]

Of patients with aggressive NHL, 40% will not respond to conventional induction therapy, and approximately 50% of those who do respond will relapse.[2] This makes salvage regimens critically important. Most salvage regimens are based on non–cross-resistant agents, or at least different agents than those used initially.[2,23] Table 15-7 displays selected salvage regimens. With the approval of Idec-C2B8 by the FDA for refractory or relapsed B-cell NHL, most protocols now give this monoclonal antibody on day 1 of each cycle of chemotherapy. High-dose chemotherapy with growth factor support is one among many new regimens. Patients who respond to the salvage chemotherapy regimens are often offered autologous bone marrow transplantation.

TABLE 15-6	Chemotherapy Regimens for Non-Hodgkin's lymphoma
CHOP	Cyclophosphamide
	Doxorubicin
	Vincristine
	Prednisone
CHOP-Bleo	Cyclophosphamide
	Doxorubicin
	Vincristine
	Prednisone
MACOP-B	Methotrexate
	Leucovorin
	Doxorubicin
	Cyclophosphamide
	Vincristine
	Prednisone
	Bleomycin
m-BACOD	Methotrexate
	Leucovorin
	Bleomycin
	Doxorubicin
	Cyclophosphamide
	Vincristine
	Dexamethasone
CHOP-Rituximab	Rituximab
	Cyclophosphamide
	Doxorubicin
	Vincristine
	Prednisone

TABLE 15-7	Salvage Chemotherapy Regimens for Non-Hodgkin's lymphoma
ESHAP	Etoposide
	Methylprednisolone
	Cytarabine
	Cisplatin
EPOCH	Etoposide
	Vincristine
	Doxorubicin
	Cyclophosphamide
	Prednisone
DHAP	Cisplatin
	Cytarabine
	Dexamethasone
CEPP	Cyclophosphamide
	Etoposide
	Procarbazine
	Prednisone
IMVP-16	Ifofamide
	Methotrexate
	Etoposide
MIME	Methyl-gag
	Ifofamide
	Methotrexate
	Etoposide
MINE	Mesna
	Ifofamide
	Mitoxantrone
	Etoposide

HIGHLY AGGRESSIVE NON-HODGKIN'S LYMPHOMA

Highly aggressive lymphomas are primarily either T-cell lymphoblastic or B-cell (Burkitt's) lymphomas.[2] The lymphoblastic lymphomas are histologically and cytologically the same as the lymphoblasts of acute lymphoblastic leukemia.[2] Therefore treatment of highly aggressive lymphomas requires an intense chemotherapy regimen similar to those used to treat acute leukemia.[2] The treatment regimen should provide prophylactic treatment to the CNS (methotrexate or cytarabine intrathecally) because lymphoblastic lymphoma is associated with a high risk of CNS involvement. An effective treatment regimen commonly used is hyper-CVAD (cyclophosphamide, mesna, vincristine, doxyrubicin [adriamycin] decadron) alternating with methotrexate-cytarabine. Courses are alternated every 3 weeks for eight cycles.[2] Maintenance therapy consists of 6-mercaptopurine, methotrexate, vincristine, and prednisone. If complete remission is not achieved with initial therapy, the chance of any significant disease-free survival is dismal. After aggressive treatment, more than 90% of patients with good prognostic features can experience a 5-year relapse-free survival.[2] Because of the increased risk of relapse in this patient population, clinical trials are now investigating the use of high-dose chemotherapy with or without total body irradiation with autologous or allogeneic bone marrow support for poor prognosis patients.[2]

Nursing Management

Patients with malignant lymphoma can experience a broad range of physical conditions, from being mildly symptomatic to being acutely ill. Patients with localized or indolent disease may be relatively asymptomatic from the disease and treatment. The majority of these patients are treated as outpatients, and the side effects from their treatments are generally not severe. Patients with extensive or aggressive disease are more often acutely ill and at risk for potentially severe side effects of therapy.[2]

Several potential complications are specific to patients with malignant lymphoma. Nurses should monitor these patients closely to appropriately implement nursing interventions promptly (Table 15-8). Potential complications are lymphadenopathy, myelosuppression, and CNS involvement.[2] Additional complications include side effects related to chemotherapy and radiation therapy. Acute side effects of chemotherapy can be anticipated, including nausea, vomiting, and alopecia, as well as potential mood changes associated with steroid therapies. Oncologic emergencies are being seen more frequently, because patients are living longer and new treatment regimens are causing unforeseen acute reactions. Oncologic emergencies common in patients with lymphoma are SVCS, spinal cord compression, tumor lysis syndrome (TLS), and sepsis.[22,32] Drugs, such as vincristine, can

TABLE 15-8 Sample Nursing Care Plan for Care of the Patient with Lymphoma		
NURSING DIAGNOSIS	**OUTCOME**	**INTERVENTIONS**
Ineffective family/patient coping related to new diagnosis	Patient/family will be able to identify stressors and demonstrate effective use of coping strategies and problem solving behaviors.	Assess family relationships and coping patterns. Along with patient include family/significant other in teaching sessions. Use a multidisciplinary team approach and initiate referrals as necessary.
Risk for infection related to myelosuppression	Patient will remain free from infection.	Monitor for signs and symptoms of infection including temperature greater then 100° F. Instruct patient and family regarding appropriate use of medications that may mask fever and infection. Avoid crowds and people with colds or flu; instruct patient and family about meticulous hand washing.
Altered nutrition related to nausea, vomiting, diarrhea, or mucositis	Patient will maintain weight.	Assess baseline nutritional status. Monitor weights at least weekly, monitor prealbumin levels, provide small frequent meals, consult a nutritionist, and provide favorite foods (except when nauseated).
Altered fluid and electrolyte balance related to nausea, vomiting, and diarrhea	Patient will have normal fluid balance.	Assess for signs of dehydration, dry mucus membranes, or confusion. Monitor daily weights, monitor urine output, offer free amounts of fluids and instruct on use of antiemetics, or antidiarrhea medications.
Potential for injury related to unsteady gait or fatigue	Patient will remain free from injury.	Coordinate activities to allow for rest periods, assess mobility for ambulation and self care activities, and encourage patient to perform active range of motion and moderate exercise. Request physical and/or occupational therapy (PT/OT).
Self-care deficit related to fatigue and altered mobility, related to CNS involvement, fatigue, and altered mobility	Patient's self-care needs will be met while providing for patient dignity and independence.	Assess baseline functional status, assess for comorbidities (such as arthritis), incorporate hobbies and other pleasurable activities into daily routine, and incorporate energy conservation strategies into activities of daily living (ADLs).
Knowledge deficit related to treatment regimens	Patient and family will demonstrate knowledge of treatment regimens and possible side effects.	Assess readiness to learn, educational level, and anxiety. Provide patient and family with information regarding side effects of chemotherapy and radiation therapy. Provide patient with community resources.
Altered sexuality patterns related to disease process and treatment	Patient will maintain satisfying sexual role.	Promote open communication regarding sexual issues, discuss effects of disease and treatment on libido, assess for diminished self-concept, and assess for physical symptoms that may effect libido such as fatigue, anorexia, and pain.
Altered tissue perfusion related to lymphadenopathy	Patient will have normal tissue perfusion.	Assess for signs and symptoms of lymphadenopathy, encourage mobility of affected limb(s), and consult with therapist specializing in lymphadenopathy.

cause neurotoxicity. Side effects of radiation therapy may include fatigue and skin reactions.[22]

Lymphadenopathy is the primary symptom of malignant lymphoma. The enlarged nodes usually are nontender. However, they can cause pain or dysfunction by compressing neighboring tissues or organs. Lymphadenopathy can also cause a decrease in lymph and venous return to the heart. The flow of lymph through the affected lymph nodes is blocked because the disease process has destroyed the architecture of the nodes. Because the lymphatic system is anatomically located near the venous system, enlarged nodes may mechanically obstruct venous blood flow. The blockage of lymph and venous flow creates lymphedema in the tissues distal to the affected node region. When assessing a patient with lymphadenopathy, it is important to note the function of the surrounding tissues and organs and the presence of lymphedema. A plan must be implemented that provides for optimal mobility and drainage of the affected limb.

Myelosuppression is a complication of treatment. Patients are at increased risk for infection, bleeding, and anemia. Myelosuppression in lymphoma can be caused by the disease as well as the treatment regimens. This is significant, because these patients may experience marked and prolonged myelosuppression that results in increased morbidity. The compromised bone marrow function seen in lymphoma produces a more rapid and generally prolonged myelosuppressive period. Patients who are myelosuppressed must be monitored closely for signs and symptoms of infection, bleeding, and anemia. Thorough assessment and prompt treatment are essential to decreasing morbidity and mortality in the myelosuppressed patient.

The degree and duration of myelosuppression may also affect the treatment plan. Treatment may be delayed until bone marrow function recovers, and future chemotherapy doses may be decreased to prevent severe myelosuppression. In both instances, optimal treatment is being compromised and may affect disease response. In addition to protecting patients from

Patient Teaching Priorities

Side Effects of Treatment

Infection: teach proper hand washing techniques, how to minimize exposure to potential pathogens, and self assessment of signs and symptoms of infection

Anemia: educate patients on the importance of adequate rest and sleep, a balanced diet including foods with iron, and moderate exercise

Bleeding: teach patients to report any signs of blood in urine or stools, using an electric razor, use of a soft toothbrush; instruct patient to check with physician before taking any over-the-counter medications

Cardiotoxicity: teach patients and families signs and symptoms of congestive heart failure: weight gain, swollen ankles, shortness of breath, and increased heart rate

Gastrointestinal: teach patient to take antiemetics, have patients remove dentures when not eating to prevent oral irritation (mucositis), and teach patients to avoid favorite foods when nauseated

Neurotoxicity: teach patients that the risk of loss of balance and falling is increased

Data from Daniel BT: Malignant lymphoma. In Otto S, editor: *Oncology Nursing*, St. Louis, 2001, Mosby and Hogan D, Rosenthal L: Oncologic emergencies in the patients with lymphoma, *Semin Oncol Nurs* 14(4):312-320, 1998.

infection, bleeding, and anemia, nurses must assist patients in coping with possible changes in their treatments.

Lymphomatous involvement of the CNS is another potential complication of malignant lymphoma. It is prevalent in aggressive and highly aggressive types of NHL. The involvement can occur as a space-occupying lesion in the brain or the spinal cord, or as an infiltration of the cerebrospinal fluid that causes irritation to the meninges. Cord compression, seizures, altered mental status, or cranial nerve palsies can occur as a result. Therefore, nurses must be alert to subtle changes in patients' neurologic functioning. Nursing care must include assessment of mobility, sensory deficits or enhancements, cognitive abilities, and self-care abilities. Interventions must be appropriate to the patient's level of functioning. The ultimate goal is to assist the patient to achieve optimal functioning.

More than 50% of patients diagnosed with malignant lymphoma today will be alive in 5 years. However, complications can occur years after diagnosis and successful treatment and may have a significant impact on psychosocial functioning. Patients generally have an increased sense of vulnerability or fear of recurrence, as well as distress over changes in their physical condition. Patients may have no apparent bodily changes secondary to disease and treatment but may feel less adequate, physically damaged, and out of control.

Patients and families bring their history, experiences, and preconceived ideas into new situations. For teaching to be effective, these factors need to be identified and incorporated into the teaching plan. Because the malignant lymphomas are such a diverse group of diseases, they are often confusing. This is also a stressful time for patients and families, and it can be difficult for them to comprehend the abstract concepts of the disease and its treatment. Consistent repetition and a variety of teaching methods generally increase the ability to understand new concepts. Community resources can provide educational, emotional, or financial support and assistance. An assessment of patients' support systems, resources, and ability to communicate needs and feelings is important for nurses to be able to assist patients in maintaining or reestablishing roles and identities in school, work, and interpersonal relationships.

Considerations for Older Adults

America is aging. The U.S. Census Bureau estimates that 12.6% of the population is aged 65 years and older, and this percentage is projected to increase to 20.3% by the year 2030. This translates into 70 million people older than 65 by the year 2030.[32] Health care professionals must become adept at managing the complexities associated with older patients, because these patients often are seen with multiple comorbidities and a high rate of disability.[33] Myelotoxicity, cardiotoxicity, mucosal toxicity, and neurotoxicity may appear to occur more frequently in older patients receiving chemotherapy.[33]

Conclusion

To provide the best patient care, nurses must be knowledgeable about the disease process and the principles of chemotherapy and radiation therapy. Nurses need to provide patients and families with information regarding the disease process, the treatment options, the side effects, and the consequences of treatment.[2] Nurses interact with patients before treatment is initiated and throughout the course of care. These interactions provide a strategic opportunity for oncology nurses to promote novel approaches that most likely are to reduce treatment-related morbidities and complications, and improve quality of life (Patient Teaching

Considerations for Older Adults

Hodgkin's Disease and Non-Hodgkin's Lymphoma

- Chemotherapy dose and schedule may be delayed or reduced because of infection, altered tissue perfusion, bleeding, anemia, or compromised cardiac, hepatic, renal, respiratory, gastrointestinal, and/or neuromuscular function.
- Radiation therapy side effects include skin reactions, fatigue, and medication adjustments.
- Financial considerations include transportation to and from clinic, prescriptions, and help at home for personal care and needs.

$\mathcal{P}$atient Teaching Priorities

Hodgkin's Disease and Non-Hodgkin's Lymphoma

- Signs and symptoms of disease: fever, night sweats, weight loss, painless lymphadenopathy, generalized vague gastrointestinal discomfort, back pain
- Signs and symptoms of infection: fever, chills, cough, erythema, malaise
- Sexual dysfunction: infertility, sterility; discuss options for contraception and ovary and sperm banking
- Discuss treatment options: chemotherapy, radiation therapy, surgery, bone marrow transplant (BMT); purpose, schedule, simulation plan for radiation therapy; monitoring weekly blood counts; chemotherapy drug side effects and schedule; BMT types (allogeneic or autologous); before-, during-, and after-transplant care components

Priorities: Side effects of Treatment box).[34,35] This information is necessary for patients and families to make informed choices and to monitor signs and symptoms on a routine basis (Patient Teaching Priorities: Hodgkin's Disease and Non-Hodgkin's Lymphoma box).[2]

Psychosocial issues, such as coping, sexuality, and survivorship, also must be addressed. Malignant lymphomas, particularly Hodgkin's disease, have peak incidences in young to middle adulthood, affecting most patients at a very productive, goal-oriented time of life. Caring for lymphoma patients offers the nurse varied and exciting challenges.[2]

REVIEW QUESTIONS

✓ Case Study

A 50-year-old female comes to be seen because of back pain for several weeks and fullness in the left neck. She also has complaints of weight loss and fatigue. On examination, an enlarged supraclavicular lymph node is palpable.

- Computerized tomograms show lymphadenopathy consistent with lymphoma.
- CBC is within normal limits. Excisional biopsy reveals follicular lymphoma.
- Serum protein electrophoresis normal. Cerebral spinal fluid is normal.
- Staging of the lymphoma is determined at stage III.
- Multidrug chemotherapy is initiated with ifosfamide, methotrexate, vincristine, cytarabine, etoposide, and dexamethasone. This was given for five cycles, and then followed by additional chemotherapy with COMA (cyclophosphamide, vincristine, high-dose methotrexate, and doxorubicin). Currently the patient is in remission.

QUESTIONS

1. What was unusual in regard to this particular patient being diagnosed with Hodgkin's disease?
   a. Incidence peaks in the 20s and 30s.
   b. Incidence peaks in the 60s and 70s.
   c. Incidence gradually increases after age 20, then decreases after age 50.
   d. Incidence has two peaks, between the ages 20 and 29 and again after age 60.
2. According to the WHO classification system, Hodgkin's disease is divided into which two major groups?
   a. Nodular lymphocyte predominance Hodgkin's disease and classical Hodgkin's disease
   b. Mixed cellularity Hodgkin's disease and nodular sclerosis Hodgkin's disease
   c. Lymphocyte depletion Hodgkin's disease and nodular lymphocyte predominance Hodgkin's disease
   d. Nodular sclerosis Hodgkin's disease and nodular lymphocyte predominance Hodgkin's disease
3. What are B symptoms?
   a. Lymphadenopathy, weight loss, and fever
   b. Pruritus, weight loss, and fever
   c. Weight loss, fever, and night sweats
   d. Lymphadenopathy, fever, and night sweats
4. What is the most common presenting symptom of NHL?
   a. Mediastinal lymphadenopathy
   b. Painless generalized lymphadenopathy
   c. Painful lymph nodes
   d. Retroperitoneal lymphadenopathy
5. What is the most common second malignancy that may develop after curative treatment for lymphoma?
   a. Acute nonlymphocytic leukemia
   b. Superior vena cava syndrome
   c. Sterility
   d. Bladder carcinoma
6. What is the recognized treatment of choice for advanced-stage aggressive lymphoma?
   a. Combination chemotherapy
   b. Radiation therapy alone
   c. Single-agent chemotherapy
   d. Surgical intervention
7. Side effects of chemotherapy include which of the following?
   a. Myelosuppression
   b. Mucositis
   c. Nausea and vomiting
   d. All of the above
8. Potential "probable" precursors, which have been found in some patients with Hodgkin's disease although not conclusively tied to its development include which of the following?
   a. Human papilloma virus
   b. Previous mononucleosis

Continued

REVIEW QUESTIONS—CONT'D

c. Previous positive tuberculin (TB) testing

d. Ten childhood streptococcal infections

9. Which of the following describes patients with advanced-stage Hodgkin's disease?

a. Stage I or II, A or B, with or without symptoms

b. Stages III and IV

c. Stage III and IV, the presence of B symptoms, and/or bulky disease

d. All the above

10. One of the symptoms this patient complained of at her initial visit upon was back pain. This is most likely due to what?

a. Urinary tract infection, common initial finding in these patients

b. Superior vena cava syndrome

c. Involvement of the mesenteric lymph nodes

d. Involvement of the retroperitoneal nodes

ANSWERS

1. **D.** *Rationale:* Incidence of lymphoma does occur in two peaks, the first in patients in their 20s to 30s and the second in the elderly. Therefore, for this woman to be diagnosed at the age of 50 did not "fit" with the generally accepted age peaks for incidence.

2. **A.** *Rationale:* Although lymphoma has several different subclasses, in 1999, the WHO recognized classical Hodgkin's lymphoma and nodular lymphocyte predominant Hodgkin's lymphoma as the two major groups.

3. **C.** *Rationale:* Although there are numerous and often vague presentations described by patients during the initial work-up of the disease, classic "B symptoms" consist of weight loss, fever, and night sweats.

4. **B.** *Rationale:* Despite often widespread tumor involvement, low-grade lymphoma often is clinically indolent in patients and frequently asymptomatic for years.

5. **A.** *Rationale:* The risk of developing other cancers is 5 times higher in survivors of Hodgkin's disease than for the general population. Sterility is a side effect of treatment, not a second malignancy. Superior vena cava syndrome is a consequence of the disease in which enlarged lymph nodes can compress cardiac structures. Acute myelocytic leukemia (acute nonlymphocytic leukemia) is a common secondary malignancy seen, in addition to lung cancer, non-Hodgkin's lymphoma, and thyroid and breast cancer. Bladder cancer is not in this group.

6. **A.** *Rationale:* Surgical therapy is not a well recognized option for patients with lymphoma since numerous lymph nodes are usually affected. The greatest number of patients will benefit if exposed to the largest number of agents at full doses as early as possible in the treatment course.

7. **D.** *Rationale:* The most common acute side effects occur as a result damage of the gastrointestinal tract, hair, skin, bladder, peripheral nervous system, and bone marrow.

8. **B.** *Rationale:* The cause of Hodgkin's disease is not known, although patients who have been diagnosed with the disease are often also found to have had mononucleosis and EBV.

9. **C.** *Rationale:* Advanced disease is describes as patients with stage III or IV, the presence of B symptoms, and/or bulky disease, described as larger than 10 cm at any site, greater than one third of thoracic diameter.

10. **D.** *Rationale:* Hodgkin's disease begins in one lymph node and then spreads to adjacent nodes, until eventually the malignant cells invade the blood vessels and spread to other organs. Generalized spread includes retroperitoneal nodes, liver, lung, spleen, and bone marrow. The back pain is most likely due to the retroperitoneal node involvement.

REFERENCES

1. Yung L, Linch D: Hodgkin lymphoma, *Lancet* 361:943-51, 2003.

2. Daniel BT: Malignant lymphoma. In Otto S, editor: *Oncology Nursing*, St. Louis, 2001, Mosby.

3. Stein H: Hodgkin disease: Biology and origin of Hodgkin and Reed-Sternberg cells, *Cancer Treat Rev* 25:161, 1999.

4. Yahalom J, Straus D: Hodgkin disease. In *Cancer management: a multidisciplinary approach*, ed 3, Melville, NY, 1998, PRR.

5. Caley B: Hodgkin disease: the other side, *Cure* 4(1):1, 2005.

6. Stein RS: Hodgkin disease. In Lee GR, Foerster J, editors: *Wintrobe's clinical hematology*, ed 10, Baltimore, 1999, Williams & Wilkins.

7. Lister A: The management of Hodgkin disease, cancer genesis of lymphomas, *Curr Opin Oncol* 11:351, 1999.

8. Cheson B: What's new in lymphoma? *CA Cancer J Clin* 54:260-272, 2004.

9. Jemal A, Tiwari RC, Murray T et al: Cancer statistics, *CA Cancer J Clin* 55(1):8-29, 2005.

10. Armitage J: Current approaches to the lymphomas, *Patient Care* 275: 65-87, 1999.

11. Ekstrand BC, Horning SJ: Hodgkin disease, *Blood Review* 16(2):111-117, 2002.

12. Cancellos GP: Hodgkin disease. In Freireich EJ, Kantarijan HM, editors: *Medical management of hematological malignant disease*, New York, 1999, Marcel Dekker.

13. DeVita VT, Mauch PM, Harros NL: Hodgkin's diease. In DeVita VT, Hellman S, Rosenberg SA, editors: *Cancer: principles and practice of oncology*, ed 5, Philadelphia, 1997, Lippincott-Raven.

14. Van Besien K, Cabanillas F: Clinical manifestations, staging, and treatment of non-Hodgkin lymphoma. In Hoffman R, editor: *Hematology: basic principles and practice*, ed 3, New York, 2000, Churchill Livingstone.

15. Hehn S, Miller T: What is the treatment of choice for advanced stage Hodgkin lymphoma: ABVD, Stanford V, or BEACOPP? *Curr Hematol Rep* 3:17-26, 2004.

16. Fung HC, Nademanee AP: Approach to Hodgkin' lymphoma in the new millennium, *Hematol Oncol* 20(1):1-15, 2002.

17. Duggan DB, Petroni GR: Randomized comparison of ABVD and MOPP/ ABV hybrid for the treatment of advanced Hodgkin disease: report of an intergroup trial, *J Clin Oncol* 21(4):583-585, 2003.

18. DeVita VT, Mauch PM, Harros NL: Hodgkin disease. In DeVita VT, Hellman S, Rosenberg SA, editors: *Cancer: principles and practice of oncology*, ed 5, Philadelphia, 1997, Lippincott-Raven.

19. Portlock CS, Glick J: Hodgkin disease: clinical manifestation, staging, and treatment. In Hoffman R, editor: *Hematology: basic principles and practice*, ed 3, New York, 2000, Churchill Livingstone.

20. Hendrix C, deLeon C, Dillman R: Radioimmunotherapy for non-Hodgkin lymphoma with Yttrium 90 Ibritumomab Tiuxetan, *Clin J Oncol Nurs* 6(3):144-148, 2002.

21. Shipp MA, Harris NL: Non-Hodgkin lymphomas. In Goldman L, Bennett JC, editors: *Cecil textbook of medicine,* ed 21, Philadelphia, 2000, Saunders.

22. Hendrix C: Radiation safety guidelines for radioimmunotherapy with Yttrium 90 Ibritumomab Tiuxetan, *Clin J Oncol Nurs* 8(1):31-34, 2004.

23. Estes J, Clapp K: Radioimmunotherapy with tositomomab and iodine-131 tositumomab for low grade non-Hodgkin lymphoma: nursing implications, *Oncol Nurs Forum* 31(6):1119-1125, 2004.

24. Greer JP, Macon WR, McCurley TL: Non-Hodgkin lymphoma. In Lee GR et al, editors: *Wintrobe's clinical hematology,* ed 10, Baltimore, 1999, Williams & Wilkins.

25. Shipp MA, Mauch PM, Harris NL: Non-Hodgkin lymphoma. In DeVita VT, Hellman S, Rosenberg SA, editors: *Cancer: principles and practice on oncology,* ed 5, Philadelphia, 1999, Lippincott-Raven.

26. Gil-Delagado MA, Khayat D, Johnson SAN: Lymphomas. In Pollock RE, editor: *Manual of clinical oncology,* ed 7, New York, 1999, Wiley-Liss.

27. Sarris A, Ford R: Recent advances in molecular pathology. In Lee GR, Foerster J, editors: *Wintrobe's clinical hematology,* ed 10, Baltimore, 1999, Williams & Wilkins.

28. Lyons SF, Leibowitz DN: The roles of human viruses in the pathogenesis of lymphoma, *Semin Oncol* 25(4):461, 1998.

29. Kosits C, Callaghan M: Rituximab: a new monoclonal antibody therapy for non-Hodgkin lymphoma, *Oncol Nurs Forum* 27(1):51-59, 2000.

30. Neviljon B, Sowers K: Hematologic cancers. In *A nurse's guide to cancer care,* Philadelphia, 2000, Lippincott.

31. O'Doherty M, MacDonald E, Barrington S et al: Positron emission tomography in the management of lymphomas, *Clin Oncol* 14(5):415-426, 2002.

32. Beveridge R: *A guide to selected cancer chemotherapy regimens and associated adverse events,* California, 2002, Amgen.

33. Hogan D, Rosenthal L: Oncologic emergencies in the patients with lymphoma, *Semin Oncol Nurs* 14(4):312-320, 1998.

34. Green J, Hacker E: Chemotherapy in the geriatric population, *Clin J Oncol Nurs* 8(6):591-597, 2004.

35. Miaskowski C, Eilers J, Dodd M: Introduction: shaping oncology nursing care for the future, *Oncol Nurs Forum* 31(4):3-4, 2004.

CHAPTER 16

Multiple Myeloma

Shirley E. Otto

Epidemiology

Multiple myeloma (MM) is a rare malignancy of plasma cells that accounts for only 1% of all malignancies and 14% of malignant hematologic disorders in the United States. The disease accounted for an estimated 15,980 new cases and 11,300 deaths in the year 2005. An increase in the incidence rate over the past decades is partially attributable to an improvement in diagnostic techniques.[1-5]

The median age at diagnosis is 65 years. Multiple myeloma is diagnosed primarily in individuals over 40 years of age, with a peak incidence at about 70 years of age. An equal number of men and women are affected. It occurs 14 times more frequently in African Americans than in whites; however, the death rate among African Americans is approximately twice that of whites.[2,4,6,7]

Etiology and Risk Factors

The etiology of MM is not understood. Basic research in animal models has identified cellular factors such as chromosomal abnormalities, host-genetic factors, chronic antigenic stimulation, viruses, and growth factors as possible contributors to the development of plasma cell dyscrasias. Other host factors, such as advancing age, race, and occupational exposure to ionizing radiation, pesticides (such as dioxin) petroleum products, farming-related chemicals, wood and leather products, may contribute to increasing risk for the disease.[2,4,6-8]

Prevention, Screening, and Detection

No recommendations exist for the prevention or screening of asymptomatic individuals for multiple myeloma. Any persons who have presence of continuous infections, sustained fatigue, and/or bone pain not relieved by usual methods should consult with their physician for a thorough clinical exam. Detection of MM in symptomatic persons is based on a thorough history, physical examination, laboratory findings, and radiographic studies.

Clinical Features

Although some individuals may be asymptomatic, most patients present to the clinician with a history of anemia, anorexia, weight loss, fatigue, recurrent infections, and/or bone pain. Bone pain may be associated with compression fractures of the humerus, the scapula, or the spine. Approximately 30% of patients are first seen with a pathologic fracture, and often patients have multiple osteolytic lesions or the presence of osteoporosis. Depending on the sites of involvement, additional symptoms may include recurrent infection, changes in urinary patterns, and cognitive, sensory, or motor changes. There may be fever, redness, swelling, tenderness, and pus formation associated with bacterial infections. Peripheral neuropathies are often noted. The skin may be pale with petechiae, or ecchymoses may be present.[3,4,6-9]

Diagnosis and Staging

The diagnosis of multiple myeloma is based on findings obtained from laboratory and radiographic studies. Serum and urine electrophoretic and immunologic studies reveal elevations in immunoglobulins (Ig) IgG, IgA, and IgM, and in light-chain levels. The hallmark feature is described as a tall, narrow-based monoclonal spike (M-spike) on electrophoresis of blood serum or urine. Additional laboratory studies and bone marrow biopsy may reveal anemia, thrombocytopenia, and leukopenia in the presence of bone marrow involvement, hypercalcemia in the presence of lytic bone lesions, and proteinuria, hyperuricemia, azotemia, and elevated blood urea nitrogen (BUN), creatinine, and Bence Jones urine protein levels with renal involvement.[2,4,5,7-9]

Radiographic studies typically include skeletal x-ray films, bone surveys, and magnetic resonance imaging (MRI) to detect the presence of osteoporosis, osteolytic lesions, or pathologic fractures. For a diagnosis of multiple myeloma to be made, one or more of the following criteria must be met: (1) plasma cell infiltration of the bone marrow of at least 10%, (2) a monoclonal spike (M-spike) on serum or urine electrophoresis, (3) radiographic confirmation of osteoporosis and osteolytic lesions, and (4) soft-tissue plasma cell tumors. Multiple myeloma may be staged using the Durie-Salmon staging system, which is based on the following factors:[2,4,5,7-11]

- The level of abnormal monoclonal immunoglobulin in the blood or urine
  - Increased immunoglobulins are usually IgG 75% and IgA 15%
  - Stage I = IgG level <5 g/dl; Ig A level <3 g/dl
  - Urinary monoclonal protein value (Bence Jones protein) <4 g/24 h
  - Stage II Intermediate, neither stage I nor III
  - Stage III IgG level >7 g/dl; IgA level >5 g/dl
  - Urinary monoclonal protein value (Bence Jones protein) >12 g/24h
- Serum calcium level
  - Adult normal levels: 9.0-10.5 mg/dl
  - Stage I and stage II
  - Calcium level normal
  - Stage III
  - Calcium level >12 mg/dl
- Hemoglobin level
  - Adult normal levels
  - Male: 14-18 g/dl
  - Female 12-16 g/dl
  - Stage I and stage II
  - Hemoglobin level >10 g/dl
  - Stage III
  - Hemoglobin level <8.5 g/dl

- Lytic bone lesions
  - Stage III
  - Advanced lytic bone lesions

PROGNOSTIC INDICATORS

Recent advances have identified new prognostic markers, such as the complete deletion of chromosome 13 or its long arm, as detected by karyotyping; the t(4;14) or t(14;16) translocation; and increased density of bone marrow microvessels. These complement established markers of adverse outcomes, such as increase in the plasma-cell-labeling index, increased levels of serum β2-microglobulin, low levels of serum albumin, plasmablastic features in the bone marrow, and circulating plasma cells.[2,6,7]

METASTASIS

Multiple myeloma is disseminated via plasma cell proliferation and the hematogenous route to the bone marrow and the bone structure, with respiratory and renal involvement.

Disease-Related Complications and Nursing Care Considerations

HYPERCALCEMIA

Hypercalcemia is usually accompanied by anorexia, nausea, polyuria, polydipsia, constipation, and confusion. Interventions include hydration with isotonic saline and administration of diuretics (furosemide) and corticosteroids (prednisone). Bisphosphonates (pamidronate disodium, etidronate sodium, and zoledronic acid) are administered via intravenous (IV) infusion on a dose and frequency schedule based on the patient's serum calcium level.[2,4,7,8]

Nursing Care Considerations. Administer hydration, diuretics, and bisphosphonates as prescribed in a timely manner. Teach patient about drug-related side effects such as thirst, bone pain, and increased urination. Recommend that fluids be increased and fiber be added to diet such as raw fruits and vegetables that can be peeled. Take stool softener daily and allow time and privacy for bowel elimination.[8,12,13]

HYPERVISCOSITY

Hyperviscosity is characterized by oronasal bleeding, blurred vision, neurologic symptoms, (weakness, imbalance, headache, visual disturbance, irritability) and congestive heart failure. Interventions are related to the specific clinical feature. Plasmapheresis provides prompt relief and should be implemented regardless of the viscosity level. Progression of symptoms such as severe back pain should be investigated for spinal cord compression. Multiple diagnostics such as MRI, myelography, and computed tomography (CT) scans with use of corticosteroids and radiation therapy should be implemented to prevent further bladder or bowel dysfunction, paresthesias of lower extremities, and further neurologic deficits.[2-4]

Nursing Care Considerations. Administer prescribed analgesics in a timely manner. Educate the patient regarding the diagnostics requirements, such as no metal objects for MRI, CT scan, and myelography. These particular diagnostics require specific patient positions during the procedure. Analgesia should be offered to the patient before each lengthy diagnostic exam. Side effects related to neurologic symptoms such as lower extremity numbness, tingling, or loss of balance should be reviewed.

Progressive symptoms may include difficulty emptying bladder or bowel contents.[8,14,15]

ANEMIA

Anemia manifests itself as fatigue, dyspnea, and headache, with hemoglobin levels under 10 g/dl. Interventions include packed red blood cell (RBCs) transfusions and colony-stimulating factors such as epoetin alfa or darbepoetin alfa. The number and frequency of RBC infusions is based on the patient's age and hemoglobin level and patient response. Dose, route, and frequency schedule of colony stimulating–factor drugs are based on the patient's therapeutic response.[2-4,7,16,17]

Nursing Care Considerations. Administer blood products or colony-stimulating factors in a timely manner. Teach patient about side effects related to blood-product transfusions such as fever, chills, rash, or dyspnea, and to report these symptoms promptly to the nurse.[2,13,16-18]

BONE DISEASE

Bone diseases such as osteoporosis, fractures, and bone pain are typical. The treatment(s) is based on the severity of bony destructions. Patients need to be as active as possible to increase solid bone mass. Surgical interventions include fixation of long-bone fractures with an intramedullary rod, or vertebroplasty for patients with compression fracture of the spine. All other lytic bone lesions, pathologic fractures, or severe osteopenia should be treated with intravenous bisphosphonates indefinitely (zoledronic acid 4 mg IV over 15 minutes every 4 weeks; or pamidronate 90 mg IV over 2 hours every 4 weeks). Additional therapy includes analgesics for pain and discomfort, nutritional interventions, and patient teaching strategies that minimize falls or trauma.[2-5,7,19]

Nursing Care Considerations. Administer prescribed medications in a prompt and timely manner. Provide or teach the patient to prevent pain with around-the-clock analgesia; report promptly any increased or unrelieved pain. Teach patient exercise measures such as walking to increase bone mass and relieve fatigue symptoms.[19-21]

RENAL FAILURE

Approximately 20% of patients first come in to be seen with renal insufficiency, and another 20% develop this complication in later stages of the disease. Allopurinol is used to prevent and treat hyperuricemia. Hemodialysis may be required for patients with symptomatic azotemia (excessive amounts of nitrogenous compounds in the blood). Plasmapheresis may be helpful in acute renal failure.[2-5,7]

Nursing Care Considerations. Explain the procedures for hemodialysis and plasmapheresis. Each session will be approximately 60 to 90 minutes. Obtain patient weight daily or weekly, and monitor intake and output. Teach the patient to increase intake of fluids when taking allopurinal.[13,15]

INFECTIONS

Infections most often are seen from recurrent gram-positive organisms (*Streptococcus pneumoniae*, *Staphylococcus aureus*, and *Haemophilus influenzae*). They necessitate prompt and appropriate IV antimicrobial therapy to treat the specific organisms, around-the-clock analgesics for discomfort, and hydration and nutrition for comfort measures.[8,10,18,22,23]

Nursing Care Considerations. Prompt administration of antimicrobials is of the utmost importance to maximize therapeutic benefit. Teach the patient to use around-the-clock analgesia to prevent and manage pain rather than respond to pain intermittently.

PSYCHOSOCIAL

All patients with MM need substantial and ongoing emotional support. They benefit from encouragement to participate in MM support group meetings, seek professional counseling, and/or practice complementary therapies such as meditation, music and art therapy, massage, relaxation or distraction techniques, imagery, spiritual healing and prayer, and/or biofeedback. These will enhance the patient's coping strategies and provide reassurance during the disease and treatment process.[13-15,20,21,24]

Nursing Care Considerations. Assess the patient's strengths and coping strategies. Offer guidance and explanation regarding the varied interventions and contact resources for the patient.

Medical Treatment Modalities, Complications, and Nursing Care Considerations

Treatment of multiple myeloma in the early stages of the disease consists of observation, if patients are asymptomatic. Patients are monitored at intervals with clinical exams and laboratory and radiographic studies for signs of progressive disease such as severe anemia, thrombocytopenia and leukopenia, bone pain, osteolysis, or renal failure. Once progression of disease is documented, active treatment with chemotherapy, peripheral blood stem cell transplantation (PBSCT), biotherapy, and radiation therapy is initiated.

CHEMOTHERAPY

Chemotherapy usually consists of intermittent melphalan and prednisone and results in a 50 % to 60% objective response rate. Responses are generally short-term, and some patients experience progression of the disease with drug resistance. Clinicians have used combinations of prednisone, high-dose melphalan, vincristine, carmustine (BCNU), cyclophosphamide, and doxorubicin. Examples of combination chemotherapy regimens include the following: MP—melphalan + prednisone; VBMCP—vincristine + melphalan + carmustine + cyclophosphamide + prednisone; VBAP—vincristine + carmustine + doxorubicin + prednisone; and VAD—vincristine + doxorubicin + prednisone.[2-5,7]

Nursing Care Considerations. Complications related to the listed chemotherapy drugs include the following: nausea, vomiting, alopecia, constipation, myelosuppression, peripheral neuropathy, peripheral edema, and infusion-related side effects such as vein irritation and/or drug extravasation. Nursing interventions include the following: provide dietary recommendations and antiemetics to reduce nausea and vomiting, and stool softeners for constipation; infuse irritant and vesicant drugs via central venous access; administer colony-stimulating factors on a scheduled frequency for drug-related myelosuppression; and care for hair loss and its effects with gentle shampoos and use of wig or cap/hat. Peripheral neuropathy and peripheral edema necessitates specific patient monitoring to ascertain severity, onset, and duration. Follow the physician-prescribed interventions based on the patient's clinical features.[10,15,16,25-27]

NOVEL AGENTS

New drugs making a significant impact in the treatment of MM and disease remission status include thalidomide, lenalidomide, bortezomib, and arsenic trioxide. In the 1990s, thalidomide demonstrated antitumor activity in relapsed MM and received an orphan drug status from the U.S. Food and Drug Administration (FDA) in 1998 for the treatment of multiple myeloma. Its use in MM is based on several studies showing significant activity in relapsed and refractory myeloma disease. Due to the adverse effects of thalidomide, prescribing thalidomide in the United States requires participation of physicians, pharmacists, and patients in the System for Thalidomide Education and Prescribing Safety (STEPS) program to prevent teratogenicity (severe birth defects). Before the start of thalidomide treatments, female patients are instructed to prevent pregnancy and male patients are instructed not to impregnate their partners by using two reliable forms for birth control at all times.[3,7,9,28-30]

Thalidomide is usually administered orally in a dosage of 400 to 800 mg by mouth (PO) per day over a schedule of selected weeks and is used with dexamethasone. Response rates when thalidomide was used with corticosteroids, as compared with thalidomide alone, increased to approximately 50% and to more than 70% when used in a three-drug combination of thalidomide, dexamethasone, and an alkylating agent (cyclophosphamide or melphalan). Multiple clinical trials are in place to determine the best dose and schedule efficacy, as well as drug combination(s) for induction therapy, first- and second-line therapy, relapsed and/or refractory disease, PBCST, and/or maintenance therapy.[3,25,29-31]

Nursing Care Considerations. Complications related to thalidomide include peripheral neuropathy, deep venous thrombosis, cardiovascular complications (e.g., bradycardia, tachycardia, hypertension, hypotension, peripheral edema), fatigue, sedation, constipation, and skin rash (Tables 16-1 and 16-2).[15,20,25,28,31]

TABLE 16-1	Adverse Effects of Thalidomide
EFFECT	**INTERVENTION**
Birth defects	Physicians, pharmacists, and patients required to follow STEPS program
Peripheral neuropathy	See Table 16-2; nerve conduction studies
Deep venous thrombosis	Therapeutic anticoagulation, international normalized ratio (INR) maintained in the range of 1.2 to 1.5 in patients with uncomplicated disease
Fatigue	Assess fatigue level; encourage patient to perform daily activities; moderate exercise
Constipation	Diet to include fiber sources such as whole grains, fruits, and vegetables; drink adequate fluid amounts; daily activity such as walking or exercise; and take stool softeners.
Neutropenia	Monitor absolute neutrophil count (ANC); consider granulocyte colony–stimulating factor for ANC ≤500 to 1000 mm³
Xerostomia	Increase fluid intake; use mouth moisturizers

Data from References 2, 3, 5, 7, 15, 22, 29, and 31.

TABLE 16-2   Neuropathy Treatment Options

Vitamins and Supplements	Multi-B complex with B₁, B₆, B₁₂ Folic acid, vitamin E, and amino acids (acetyl L-carnitine, alpha lipoic acid)	Take vitamins and/or supplements with food or beverages
	Magnesium and potassium supplements	Alternate foods high in magnesium (help relieve leg and foot cramping) and potassium; include bananas, oranges
Medications	Gabapentin, carbamazepine Antianxiety (amitriptyline, lorazepam, sertraline)	Take all medications as prescribed, usually in divided doses over a 24-hour period.
	Analgesics such as hydrocodone, lidocaine patches, oxycodone, tramadol	Prevent pain by taking analgesics around the clock
Nonpharmacologic	Acupuncture, exercise, massage, relaxation techniques	All techniques help to diminish fatigue
	Creams applied to fingers, toes, and feet, such as cocoa butter and capsaicin	Creams may be purchased in an over-the-counter pharmacy

Data from References 8, 14, 25, 32, 34, and 40.

Lenalidomide, a thalidomide derivative, has shown greater antitumor effects than thalidomide in preclinical studies in myeloma cell lines. Dosages between 25 mg and 50 mg PO daily have shown clinical responses in patients with relapsed or refractory myeloma. Current clinical trials with combinations of lenalidomide and bortezomib along with thalidomide or dexamethasone may provide even greater benefits for patients with multiple myeloma and other hematologic malignancies.[2,3,31,32]

Bortezomib is indicated for the treatment of MM patients who have received at least two prior therapies and have demonstrated disease progression on the last therapy. Secondary treatment guidelines include patients with relapsed and/or refractory myeloma disease. The usual dose and schedule is bortezomib 1.3 mg/m² administered IV on days 1, 4, 8, and 11 of each 21-day cycle. In a phase III study, bortezomib was compared to traditional high-dose dexamethasone. In the bortezomib arm, 45% of second-line patients achieved a complete or partial response compared to 20% in the high-dose dexamethasone arm. In relapsed and refractory myeloma, overall response rates of more than 60% have been achieved with bortezomab in combination with therapies such as liposomal doxorubicin, thalidomide, and melphalan.[7,28,29,33]

Nursing Care Considerations. Complications include peripheral neuropathy, anemia, thrombocytopenia, asthenia, hyponatremia, orthostatic hypotension, skin rashes or hives, and gastrointestinal symptoms such as nausea, vomiting, diarrhea, and constipation. Nursing interventions for thalidomide, lenalidomide, and bortezomib complications include administering colony-stimulating factors for asthenia, anemia, and thrombocytopenia, as well as diphenhydramine or hydrocortisone creams for rashes and hives; frequent monitoring of serum sodium levels at or above the range of 136-145 mEqL, and encouraging intake of sodium rich foods and fluids, such as tomato juice. Gastrointestinal interventions include varied dietary measures (see Chapter 26). Nurses also monitor patients at risk for bradycardia, tachycardia, hypotension, peripheral edema, in addition to those patients on prescribed cardiovascular medications.[10,13,21,24,25]

Arsenic trioxide has been identified as an effective treatment for acute promyelocytic leukemia and is now being investigated in phase II studies for its clinical efficacy in multiple myeloma. Administered as daily IV infusions at 0.15 mg/kg, a phase II study showed a response in 3 to 14 disease-relapsed patients. Myelosuppression is the most common complication and is treated with colony-stimulating factors.[2,3,7]

BIOLOGIC RESPONSE MODIFIERS

Interferon-α has been used alone and in combination with conventional chemotherapy to treat patients with multiple myeloma. Response rates among patients previously untreated and among patients who were refractory to conventional therapy make interferon-α a promising second-line treatment. Clinical options include colony-stimulating factors such as epoetin alfa and darbepoetin for anemia; filgrastim for granulocyte recovery; sargramostin for granulocyte, eosinophil, and monocyte recovery; pegfilgrastim for neutrophil recovery, and oprelvekin to prevent thrombocytopenia following combination chemotherapy and/or high-dose chemotherapy; and allogeneic or autologous stem cell transplantations. These drugs have lessened the myelosuppressive effects related to the associated therapies and have improved the overall survival outcomes.[2-5,7]

Nursing Care Considerations. Complications related to interferon and the colony-stimulating factors include: bone/joint pain, low-grade fever, chills, dyspnea, rash, and fluid retention. The intensity and duration of the side-effects are related to the drug dose(s). Interventions used in the management of these side effects are: acetaminophen for pain or fever; diphenhydramine for rash; oxygen for dyspnea; and based on the patient's fluid retention, diuretic medications as prescribed.[10,13,14,34-36]

PERIPHERAL BLOOD STEM CELL TRANSPLANTATION

Autologous and allogeneic PBSCT is being used in the treatment of selected patients with multiple myeloma—usually those less than 72 years of age, dependent upon stage of disease, and with favorable response to initial chemotherapy. Success has been limited by the inability to eradicate the malignant plasma cell clone. Patients who are eligible for autologous stem cell transplantation (SCT) are initially treated with a chemotherapy regimen that is not toxic to the hematopoietic cells, which ensures adequate mobilization of stem cells. Thalidomide with dexamethasone is being used increasingly for therapy before autologous SCT in the stem cell mobilization and collection process. It has also shown benefit in the stem cell engraftment process. Ongoing randomized clinical trials are exploring thalidomide induction and engraftment effect. Although not curative, autologous SCT improves the likelihood of a complete response and prolongs disease-free survival.[2,4,5,7]

Advantages of allogeneic SCT are that donor cells are not contaminated with myeloma disease cells, and the patient has a graft-versus-myeloma effect. Approximately 5% to 10% of all the patients with multiple myeloma are candidates for allogeneic transplantation. Limitations include age, an HLA-matched sibling donor, and adequate major organ function. There is also the risk of acute or chronic graft-versus-host disease and a high rate of treatment-related deaths. Intensive myeloablative therapy with PBSCT consistently improves the patients' time-to-progression of disease but does not improve overall survival.[2,4,5,7]

Nursing Care Considerations. PBSCT complications effects include myelosuppression with increased risk for infection, anemia, and thrombocytopenia, acute and chronic graft-versus-host disease, sustained fatigue, and chemotherapy-induced nausea and vomiting. (See Chapters 21 and 23).

RADIATION THERAPY

Radiation therapy may be used to treat patients with chemotherapy-resistant disease, to relieve bone pain, and to treat spinal cord compression. It has been estimated that 70% of all patients eventually require and potentially benefit from radiation therapy as a palliative agent. Complications include fatigue and myelosuppression. Although radiation therapy can greatly improve the quality of life for patients with multiple myeloma, the length of survival is not enhanced. Radiation therapy should be used sparingly, since irradiation of multiple sites may impair the process for peripheral blood stem cell mobilization and apheresis in patients who are candidates for high-dose therapy and SCT.[2,3,5,7]

Prognosis

Multiple myeloma is an incurable disease. The course of disease progression for patients is determined by the severity of organ involvement at the time of diagnosis and response to active treatment. Asymptomatic patients may live with the disease for months to years without active treatment. For symptomatic patients requiring treatment, a pattern of response has been described. The medium length of survival after diagnosis is approximately 3 years.

During the initial 2 to 3 years of treatment, patients respond well to the varied therapies. A plateau phase follows when the disease remains stable but does not respond as well as in the initial phase. During the third phase the disease becomes resistant to the varied therapies and progresses at a rapid rate. Survival can range from a few months to more than 10 years, with a median survival of 3 years. The 5-year survival rate for stage I is about 50%, with a median survival of more than 60 months; stage II is about 40%, with a median survival time of 41 months; and stage III survival rate is 10% to 25%, with a median survival of 23 months.[37]

Considerations for Older Adults

The peak incidence of MM occurs at 60 years of age. Major lifestyle changes occurring at that time include occupational issues (such as reduced work hours) and retirement. Because of the reduced energy levels from the disease and/or therapies, social and recreational activities will need to be adjusted so energy can be conserved and the risk of injury minimized. Mental status changes may occur, necessitating supervision in certain tasks such as financial management (payment of household bills or insurance and balancing checkbook), scheduling appointments for health care or car maintenance, and assistance with transportation.[14,17,38,39]

Risk factors for the older adult include a suppressed bone marrow related to age, disease, and/or treatment. The bone marrow recovery response is delayed in the older adult, resulting in chronic anemia, thrombocytopenia, and neutropenia. These changes are evidenced by increased infections, fatigue, and decreased energy levels. Resources should be presented to manage self-care needs for hygiene, nutrition, elimination, and comfort. Maintaining a safe home environment by removing throw rugs, installing safety equipment in bathrooms, and keeping frequently used articles within reach will diminish patient falls. Meal planning and preparation to facilitate nutritious intake and assistance with household chores, shopping, and errands will enable the older adult to lead a more independent life.[14,17,27,36,38,39]

Conclusion

Multiple myeloma is primarily a disease of the adult and elderly population. There is currently no known cure for multiple myeloma, although research is in progress to increase the length of remission, to prevent relapse, and to improve quality of life for these patients. Because of the age of these patients, it is likely that most will have some comorbidities, which can greatly affect not only their response to therapy, but the management of side effects and the extent to which a particular treatment can proceed. For most, the care they receive as the disease progresses will be supportive in nature.

BOX 16-1

CANCER RESOURCES	WEBSITES
American Cancer Society	http://www.cancer.org
American Society of Pain Management Nurses	http://www.aspmn.org
Cancer Research Institute (supports research aimed at developing methods of preventing, treating and curing cancer)	http://www.cancerresearch.org/impower.html
Clinical Trials Listings	http://www.cancer.gov/clinicaltrials
International Myeloma Foundation	http://www.myeloma.org
National Marrow Donor Program (NMDP)	http://www.bmtitfo.org

Over the course of this disease the oncology nurse will be involved in a relationship with this patient and family. As they work to make decisions in the care of these patients, nurses are pivotal in educating the patient and family in their understanding of the disease course and its treatment, side effects management, newer options with their anticipated outcomes and side effects, as well as guiding the formation of reasonable patient expectations. It is essential that the oncology nurse remain abreast of not only the new advances, but the effects and the management of these options in patients who have multiple medical problems.

BOX 16-2   Patient/Family Cancer Resources

American Cancer Society	http://www.cancer.org
Cancer Care, Inc	http://www.cancercare.org
Cancer Fatigue	http://www.cancerfatigue.org
Cancer Symptom Management	http://www.concensus.nih.gov/ ta/022/022_statement.htm
I Have Cancer	http://www.ihavecancer.com
Neuropathy Organization	http://www.neuropathy.org
Pain	http://.pain.com
People Living With Cancer	http://www.plwc.org
Social Security Administration	http://www.ssa.gov

REVIEW QUESTIONS

✓ Case Study

RCD, a 58-year-old male aircraft employee for 30 years was admitted to oncology services with complaints of shortness of breath and chest discomfort upon deep inspiration, pain in right scapula and difficulty using his right arm at work, extreme fatigue, and new onset of numbness in both feet. His social history included smoking history of two packs per day for 40 years; however since experiencing the onset of shortness of breath, he cut back to a few cigarettes a day. His diagnostic workup included CBC, immunoglobulin electrophoresis, urinalysis, serum electrolytes, bone scan, and chest x-ray. Findings included the following: white blood cells (WBC): 12,000; hemoglobin (Hgb) 7.5 g/dl; hematocrit (Hct) 25 %; serum calcium 18 mg/dl; IgA 500 mg/dl; Ig G 2000 mg/dl; multiple lytic bone lesions in scapula, ribs, and right arm; and lesions in both lobes of the right lung. Results of bone marrow aspiration and Bence Jones protein in 24-hour urine specimen were pending; however, a potential diagnosis was multiple myeloma.

Upon confirmation of bone marrow aspiration testing and Bence Jones protein results that were positive for MM, RCD was place on thalidomide 100 mg qid; dexamethasone 20 mg daily for 4 days, starting on day 22 each month; pamidronate 90 mg via IV infusion q 28 days; and oxycodone 5/500, two tablets PO q 4 hours. Instructions regarding the STEPS program for thalidomide and drug side effects were discussed with the couple. While at the infusion clinic, RCD and his wife asked the nurse, "How many people are diagnosed with multiple myeloma? What are the other treatment options if these current drugs do not respond—that is, what is new in research?"

QUESTIONS

1. Multiple myeloma occurs in approximately _____% of the U.S. population.
   a. 1%
   b. 5%
   c. 10%
   d. 15%
2. Multiple myeloma initial clinical features may include Which of the following?
   a. Increased fatigue, bone pain, and constipation
   b. Increased fatigue, bone pain, and dyspnea
   c. Increased fatigue, chest pain, and anorexia
   d. Increased fatigue, abdominal pain, and dyspnea

3. Multiple myeloma disease-related complications include which of the following?
   a. Hypercalcemia, hyperviscosity, renal failure, bone disease, and thrombocytopenia
   b. Hypercalcemia, hyperviscosity, hepatic failure, bone disease, and thrombocytopenia
   c. Hypercalcemia, hyperviscosity, renal failure, bone disease, and anemia
   d. Hypocalcemia, hyperviscosity, renal failure, bone disease, and thrombocytopenia
4. What chemotherapy drugs are commonly used in combination treatment for multiple myeloma?
   a. Melphalan, prednisone, vinblastine, danorubicin, cyclophosphamide, and BCNU
   b. Melphalan, prednisone, vincristine, doxorubicin, cyclophosphamide, and BCNU
   c. Melphalan, prednisone, vinblastine, doxorubicin, ifosfamide, and BCNU
   d. Melphalan, prednisone, vincristine, daunorubicin, ifosfamide, and BCNU
5. Which of the following symptoms is the most important for the patient with multiple myeloma to report to the nurse and/or physician?
   a. Increase in the severity of pain with movement
   b. Presence of edema in the lower extremities
   c. Increase in the level of fatigue with activity
   d. Loss of sensation in the lower extremities, bowel and bladder problems
6. What are some of the novel agents currently used in treatment for multiple myeloma?
   a. Bortezomib, thalidomide, lenalidomide, and arsenic trioxide
   b. Bevacizumab, thalidomide, rituximab, and arsenic trioxide
   c. Bevacizumab, cetuximab, thalidomide, and lenalidomide
   d. Cetuximab, alemtuzumb, thalidomide, and lenalidomide
7. What are some of the possible interventions for hypercalcemia and hyperviscosity?
   a. Transfusion, monitoring blood counts, bleeding precautions, and fall precautions
   b. Hydration, pamidronate, plasmapheresis, corticosteroids, and radiation therapy

Continued

REVIEW QUESTIONS—CONT'D

    c. Vincristine, BCNU, platelet transfusions, and oxygen therapy

    d. Plasmapheresis, strict urinary output, albumin levels, allopurinol, and dialysis

8. Pharmacologic agents currently used in management of peripheral neuropathy associated with the multiple myeloma novel agents include which of the following?

    a. Gabapentin, chlorazine, oxycodone, and amitriptyline

    b. Gabapentin, chlorazine, oxycodone, and lorazepam

    c. Gabapentin, carbamazepine, amitriptyline, and lorazepam

    d. Gabapentin, hydrocodone, aprepitant, and amitriptyline

9. The Durie-Salmon staging system used to classify multiple myeloma includes the following factors:

    a. IgG and IgA levels, Bence Jones protein, serum calcium, lytic bone lesions

    b. IgM, and IgA levels, Bence Jones protein, serum sodium, lytic bone lesions

    c. IgG and IgA levels, Bence Jones protein, serum sodium, lytic bone lesions

    d. IgG and IgM levels, Bence Jones protein, serum potassium, lytic bone lesions

10. What is the overall medium length of survival after diagnosis despite all the innovative therapies used treat multiple myeloma?

    a. 1 Year

    b. 2 Years

    c. 3 Years

    d. 5 Years

ANSWERS

1. **A.** *Rationale:* Multiple myeloma is a rare malignancy of plasma cells that accounts for only 1% of all malignancies, and 14% of hematologic malignancies in the United States. It usually occurs in individuals over the age of 40 years, and the incidence is equal in men and women, but is 14 times more prevalent among African Americans than whites. The peak incidence occurs at about 70 years of age.

2. **B.** *Rationale:* Although a few patients may be asymptomatic, most of those who come to the attention of health caregivers have a history of anemia, anorexia, weight loss, fatigue, recurrent infections, and bone pain, usually associated with compression fractures. Because of the multiple sites that can be involved, additional symptoms are neuropathy, changes in urination, and cognitive and motor changes. If a bacterial infection is present, fever, redness, swelling, and pus may be evident.

3. **C.** *Rationale:* RCD diagnostics included lytic bone lesions, lesions in lung, Hgb of 7.5- anemia, and serum calcium of 18 mg/dl. The physician and nurse discussed complications regarding MM hypercalcemia, fractures (bone disease), and anemia (low hemoglobin).

4. **B.** *Rationale:* Chemotherapy for multiple myeloma consists of intermittent melphalan and prednisone, resulting in a 50% to 60% objective response rate. Responses are usually short-lived after combination administrations of prednisone, high-dose melphalan, vincristine, carmustine (BCNU), cyclophosphamide, and doxorubicin. Daunorubicin and vinblastine are not among these choices.

5. **D.** *Rationale:* Complications of the disease and signs of metastasis are due to dissemination via the plasma cells to bone marrow and bone structure and eventual bone breakdown. Hypercalcemia and hyperviscosity result. Therefore the loss of sensation in the patient's lower extremities with bowel and bladder changes indicates metastatic disease in RCD.

6. **A.** *Rationale:* RCD and wife asked about new research drugs that might be an option if thalidomide is not effective. Thalidomide has been used in multiple myeloma since 1998, showing promise in refractory and relapsed disease. It is usually administered with cyclophosphamide and melphalan. Lenalidomide is a derivative of thalidomide and shows greater antitumor effect potency on myeloma cell lines. Bortezomib is used in patients who show disease progression after receiving at least two prior therapies, and has been used in combination with doxorubicin, thalidomide, or melphalan. The use of arsenic trioxide in multiple myeloma is under investigation.

7. **B.** *Rationale:* Transfusion blood counts, and bleeding and fall precautions will combat anemia and thrombocytopenia. Vincristine, BCNU, platelet transfusions, and O_2 therapy are likely to be used in the "treatment" phase, before the discovery of metastatic disease. Plasmapheresis, strict monitoring of intake and output (I&O), albumin, allopurinol, and hemodialysis are directed at renal failure. Hydration, pamidronate administration, plasmapheresis, use of corticosteroids, and radiation therapy are directed at bone metastasis and impending spinal cord compression.

8. **C.** *Rationale:* Pharmaceutical agents used in management of peripheral neuropathy include gabapentin, carbamazepine, amitriptyline, and lorazepam. Options for managing the effects of peripheral neuropathy include the use of multi-B vitamin complex, folic acid, vitamin E, and amino acids. Foods high in magnesium and potassium are encouraged, such as bananas and oranges.

9. **A.** *Rationale:* Diagnostic work-up of multiple myeloma will reveal elevations on serum and urine electrophoresis of IgG, IgA, and IgM. Additional laboratory studies and bone marrow biopsy may reveal anemia, thrombocytopenia, and leucopenia. Hypercalcemia is attributed to the lytic bone lesions. Renal involvement is determined from elevated Bence Jones urine protein levels, elevated BUN, and creatinine. Hyperuricemia, azotemia, and proteinuria are usually present. RCD had an elevated IgG level of 2000 mg/dl, IgA of 500 mg/dl, lytic bone lesions, and Bence Jones protein level positive for MM.

10. **C.** *Rationale:* The severity and course of multiple myeloma is determined by the severity of organ involvement and the patient's response to treatment. Asymptomatic patients may have the disease for months to years before it is detected. The median length of survival after diagnosis is 3 years. RCD, with stage III disease and metastasis to lung, will potentially have a survival of 3 years.

REFERENCES

1. Jemal A, Murray T, Ward E et al: Cancer Statistics, 2005, *CA Cancer J Clin* 55(1):10, 2005.
2. Kyle RA, Rajkumar SV: Multiple myeloma. In Rakel RE, Bope ET, editors: *Conn's current therapy*, St. Louis, 2005, Saunders.
3. Kyle RA, Rajkumar SV: Drug therapy: multiple myeloma, *N Engl J Med* 351:1860, 2004.
4. Kyle RA and Blade J: Multiple myeloma and related disorders. In Abeloff MD, Armitage JO, Lichter AS et al, editors: *Clinical oncology,* ed 2, New York, 1999, Churchill Livingstone.
5. Munshi NC, Tricot G, Barlogie B: Plasma cell neoplasms. In DeVita VT Jr, Hellman S, Rosenberg SA, editors: *Cancer: principles and practice of oncology*, ed 6, Philadelphia, 2001, Lippincott-Raven.
6. Bloomfield CD: Prognostic factors in multiple myeloma, *Clin Adv Hematol Oncol* 3(3):167, 2005.
7. Deskin R, Jagannath S, Richardson P et al: Multiple myeloma and other plasma cell dyscrasias. In Pazdur R, Coia LR, Hoskins WJ et al, editors: *Cancer management: A multidisciplinary approach,* ed 7, Manhasset, NY, 2004, CMP Healthcare Media, Oncology Publishing Group.
8. Devenney B, Erickson C: Multiple myeloma: an overview *CJON* 8(4):401, 2004.
9. Ferri FF: Multiple myeloma, In Ferri FF, editor: *Ferri's clinical advisor, instant diagnosis and treatment,* St. Louis, 2005, Mosby.
10. Camp-Sorrell D: Myelosuppression. In Itano JK, Taoka KN, editors: *Core curriculum for oncology nursing*, ed 4, St. Louis, 2005, Saunders.
11. Pagana KD, Pagana TJ: *Mosby's diagnostic and laboratory test reference* ed 7, St. Louis, 2005, Elsevier.
12. Itano JK, Taoka KN, editors: *Core curriculum for oncology nursing*, ed 4, St. Louis, 2005, Saunders.
13. Otto SE: *Oncology nursing clinical reference,* St. Louis, 2004, Mosby.
14. Pearce JD: Alterations in mobility, skin integrity, and neurological status. In Itano JK, Taoka KN, editors: *Core curriculum for oncology nursing*, ed 4, St. Louis, 2005, Saunders.
15. Porock D, Beshears B, Hinton P et al: Nutritional, functional, and emotional characteristics related to fatigue in patients during and after biochemotherapy, Oncol *Nurs Forum* 32(3):661, 2005.
16. Crawford J: Improving the management of chemotherapy-induced neutropenia, *Support Oncol* 2(2 Suppl 2):36, 2004.
17. Gillespie TW: Effects of cancer-related anemia on clinical and quality-of-life outcomes, *CJON* 6(4):206, 2002.
18. Hood LE: Chemotherapy in the elderly: supportive measures for chemotherapy-induced myelotoxicity, *CJON* 7(2):185, 2003.
19. Reich CD: Advances in the treatment of bone metastases, *CJON* 7(6):641, 2003.
20. Coleman EA, Hall-Barrow J, Coon S et al: Facilitating exercise adherence for patients with multiple myeloma, *CJON* 7(5):529, 2003.
21. Coon SK, Coleman EA: Keep moving: patients with myeloma talk about exercise and fatigue *Oncol Nurs Forum* 31(6):1127, 2004.
22. Hodgson BB, Kizior RJ: *Saunders nursing drug handbook 2006*, St. Louis, 2006, Elsevier.
23. Schmidt KV: Immunology. In Itano JK, Taoka KN, editors: *Core curriculum for oncology nursing*, ed 4, St. Louis, 2005, Saunders.
24. Oncology Nursing Society: *Chemotherapy and biotherapy guidelines and recommendations for practice*, ed 2, Pittsburgh, 2005, Oncology Nursing Press.
25. Armstrong T, Almadrones L, Gilbert MR: Chemotherapy-induced peripheral neuropathy. *Oncol Nurs Form* 32(2):305, 2005.
26. Bedell C: Pegfilgrastim for chemotherapy-induced neutropenia, *CJON* 7(1):55, 2003.
27. Otto SE: Multiple myeloma, In Otto SE, editor: *Oncology nursing,* ed 4, St. Louis, 2001, Mosby.
28. Colson K, Doss DS, Swift R et al: Bortezomib, a newly approved proteasome inhibitor for the treatment of multiple myeloma: nursing implications, *CJON* 8(5):473, 2004.
29. Tariman JD: Understanding novel therapeutic agents for multiple myeloma, *CJON* 7(5):521, 2003.
30. Tucker S: Thalidomide—defining a role...finally, *Community Oncol* 2(2):113, 2005.
31. Ghobrial IM, Rajkumar SV: Management of thalidomide toxicity, *Support Oncol* 1(3):194, 2003.
32. Marrs J: Updating your peripheral neuropathy "know-how," *CJON* 7(3):299, 2003.
33. Richardson PG, Sonneveld P, Schuster MW et al: Bortezomib or high-dose dexamethasome for relapsed multiple myeloma, *N Engl J Med* 352:2487, 2005.
34. Gralla R: New antiemetic agents, *Clin Adv Hematol Oncol* 3(5):350, 2005.
35. Viale PH: Integrating aprepitant and palonosetron into clinical practice: a role for the new antiemetics, *CJON* 9(1):77, 2005.
35. Yarbro CH, Grogge MH, Goodman M, editors: *Cancer nursing: principles and practice,* ed 6, Sudbury, Mass, 2005, Jones & Bartlett.
37. Jemal A, Murray T, Ward E, et al: Cancer statics, 2005, *CA Cancer J Clin* 55(1):10, 2005. Retrieved July 11, 2005, from http://www.cancer.org.
38. Green JM, Hacker ED: Chemotherapy in the geriatric population, *CJON,* 8(6):591, 2004.
39. Holley S: A look at the problem of falls among people with cancer, *CJON* 6(4):193, 2002.
40. Bashey A, Huston JW: *100 Questions & Answers about myeloma*, Sudbury, Mass, 2005, Jones & Bartlett.

CHAPTER 17

Skin Cancers

Norma Sheridan-Leos

Skin cancer is the most common cancer in the United States.[1] Nonmelanoma skin cancer (NMSC) is the umbrella term used to describe basal cell carcinoma (BCC) and squamous cell carcinoma (SCC).[2] These two cancers were expected to account for more than 1 million new cases of skin cancers in the United States in 2005.[1,3] These cancers are highly curable, and more common among individuals with lightly pigmented skin.[3,4] A diagnosis of BCC or SCC does not raise the kind of alarm signals associated with melanoma. However, if left untreated, SCC and BCC can result in serious morbidity and death.[2] Malignant melanoma is the most deadly type of skin cancer.[3,5] It was estimated that 59,580 new cases of melanoma would occur in the United States in 2005, and that 7770 people would die from the disease.[4] About 1 in 70 people will develop melanoma during their life.[5] The incidence rate is 10 times higher in whites than in African Americans, and malignant melanoma is one of the most common cancers in young adults.[4,6,7] In addition to melanoma and NMSC is Kaposi sarcoma, another type of skin cancer, which commonly occurred in people with AIDS before the widespread use of protease inhibitors.[4]

Nonmelanoma Skin Cancers

BASAL CELL CARCINOMA

Epidemiology

BCC is the most common cutaneous tumor.[4] Comprising 70% of the primary skin cancers, BCC is characterized by a slow-growing lesion that invades local tissue.[2] Metastases and death are rare.[8] BCC is most commonly found on the face, the neck, and the hands and arms, but it can occur anywhere.[9]

The BCCs can grow in size and result in significant cosmetic and functional morbidity.[2,8] Although they can be any size, lesions typically range between 3 and 15 mm in diameter at initial presentation. A large BCC can become very destructive. Larger lesions are more likely to erode into muscle, cartilage, or bone.[2] BCC is derived from the same cell line as SCC, the keratinocytes.[2] These basal cells, or keratinocytes, are situated at the lowest layer of the epidermis, just above the basement membrane that attaches the epidermis to the dermis. When one basal cell divides, one daughter cell advances slowly upward through the epidermis as a keratinocyte, while the other remains a basal cell in the basal layer to reproduce again.[2] Basal cells that fail to mature into keratinocytes retain their capacity for mitotic division, later forming a tumor.

Etiology and Risk Factors

The risk of BCC and SCC increases with age; this type of skin cancer is relatively uncommon (although it is becoming more common) in persons younger than age 40.[2] Individuals who freckle easily or who have fair skin, red or blond hair, and blue or green eyes are at greatest risk for the development of BCC.[7,9] Several inherited syndromes make early onset of BCC more likely; these include albinism, xeroderma pigmentosum, or albinism and nevoid BCC syndrome. Other risk factors include male gender, occupational exposure to carcinogens, immunosuppression, and a family history of BCC.[7] There is growing evidence that psoralen and ultraviolet A (PUVA) therapy for psoriasis increases the risk for NMSC.[2]

SUNLIGHT

Exposure to sunlight (ultraviolet [UV] radiation) causes almost all cases of basal and squamous cells cancer and is a major cause of melanoma.[4,9] Ultraviolet radiation initiates and promotes carcinogenesis by (1) DNA point mutations, (2) oncogene activation, (3) tumor suppressor gene inactivation, (4) cellular proliferation, and (5) inflammation.[10] Disruption of the earth's ozone layer by pollution (the "ozone hole") may cause increased levels of UV radiation.[4] Discussions of and opinions regarding changes in the ozone layer and the relationship of that phenomenon to skin cancer are both complicated and numerous.[11] Further studies are needed to determine the varying effects that ozone layer depletion may have on skin cancer development and trends.[11]

INDOOR TANNING

Some people believe tans that are a result of artificial light (tanning beds and lamps) are "safer tans" and will protect them from skin damage and skin cancer. A study done in 2002 indicates otherwise. Study participants who used tanning devices were 1.5 times more likely to develop BCC and 2.5 times more likely to develop SCC than people who did not use tanning beds and lamps. Adjusting for a history of sunburns, sunbathing, and sun exposure did not change these conclusions.[12]

Prevention and Screening

PRIMARY PREVENTION

The relationship between skin cancer development and UV radiation is well established.[3,8,9] Avoiding direct sunlight by staying indoors or in the shade or by wearing protective clothing is the most effective measure for reducing exposure to UV light; however, there are no randomized trials of sun avoidance to prevent skin cancer.[9,13] Sunscreens with a sun protection factor of 15 that provides both UVA and UVB protection, generously applied and reapplied during outdoor activities, are the most effective.[8] Sunscreen use alone is not considered adequate protection against UV radiation.[3] Sunscreens, no matter how high the protection factor, are secondary to covering up with protective clothing.[14]

SECONDARY PREVENTION

Screening. The relatively slow growth and early visibility of NMSC makes this cancer a posterchild for early detection.[2] The American Cancer Society (ACS) recommends screening for skin cancer by a health care professional every 3 years in persons 20 to 39 years old and annually for people 40 and older.[15]

Classification

There are five types of BCC: (1) nodular (50% to 54% of cases), (2) superficial (9% to 11%), (3) pigmented (6%), (4) morpheaform or sclerotic (2%), and (5) basosquamous.[2]

Clinical Features

Among these five categories, some BCCs are easily recognized and others are less obvious (Clinical Features of Basal Cell Carcinoma box). BCC may start as a translucent growth that has pink and white tones, a shiny border, giving it a "pearly" appearance, and a tendency to crust.[9,15] This "pearl-like lesion" can have an overlying telangiectasis.[2,16] Often these nodules become quite friable and may develop a hemorrhagic ulceration. If left untreated, they can severely damage underlying tissue and the skin.[9]

Diagnosis and Staging

A complete skin examination is the key diagnostic component. Once suspected clinically, BCC must always be definitely diagnosed by histology. If the physical examination is normal, no additional evaluation is generally necessary. Evaluate any suspicious cutaneous lesion or lymph adenopathy with biopsy to rule out metastases or new primary lesions.[16] Typical techniques used to perform the biopsy include a small punch biopsy or shave biopsy.[16] A shave biopsy (top lesion into depth of middermis) is performed using local anesthesia. Punch biopsy (sharp, small circular "punch" similar to a cookie cutter approach) is used if the tumor is suspected to be in the deeper layers of the skin. The tissue sample is examined to determine the clinical diagnosis and identifying features of the various classifications. Specific treatment modalities are recommended based upon the clinical diagnosis, classification, and histopathologic grading.

The American Joint Committee on Cancer (AJCC) recommends stage groupings as shown in Table 17-1.

Clinical staging is based on the physical examination and palpation of lymph nodes. Pathologic staging requires resection of the entire site and confirmation of any lymph node involvement. Underlying bony structures should be imaged, especially if these lesions occur on the scalp. Complete excision of the site and microscopic verification are necessary to determine histologic type.[11] It is important to avoid very thin shave biopsies that do not penetrate through the full thickness of the epidermis; such incomplete specimens will not enable the pathologist to differentiate in situ tumors from invasive ones.[16]

Histologic grading for BCCs and SCCs is similar to the grading system for other cancers. G1 signifies well-differentiated tumor cells, G2 refers to moderately well differentiated cells, G3 signifies poorly differentiated cells, and G4 signifies undifferentiated cells. Confirmation of cutaneous or subcutaneous spread and the extent of disease by biopsy is imperative.[11]

Metastases and Recurrence

Metastatic BCC is extremely rare.[9,17] It usually occurs via hematologic or lymphatic spread. The malignant characteristics of the tumor are based on the destructive growth of the primary tumor rather than on metastasis.[18] A patient who develops one BCC has a 35% to 50% chance of developing a second BCC lesion within the next 3.5 to 5 years, as well as other skin cancers.[8] Close observation of the patient for recurrence is recommended.[19] In one study, tumor location was found to be of prognostic significance: primary lesions on the head or neck were

Clinical Features of Basal Cell Carcinoma (BCC)

Nodular BCC
Bulky, nodular growth is caused by lack of keratinization.
Characteristics include a thinning epidermis, producing a shiny pink, translucent, pearly hue over the lesion.
Early stages resemble a smooth pimple that fails to heal.
As the tumor enlarges, the border edge raises and the center becomes necrotic.
Lesion bleeds easily from mild injury and doubles in size every 6 to 12 months at the rate of 5 mm per year.

Superficial BCC
Tends to develop in multiple sites, growing peripherally across the skin surface, becoming as large as 10 to 15 cm
Appears most frequently on the trunk as a well-demarcated, erythematous, scaly patch with discreet nodules
Often confused with psoriasis

Pigmented BCC
Contains melanin in the epidermis, the dermis, and within the tumor itself

Often mistaken clinically for melanoma
Colors include blue, black, or brown, with a raised pearly border
Found in dark-complexioned persons such as Latin Americans or Japanese (not African Americans)

Morpheaform or Sclerotic BCC
More aggressive lesion that appears as a flat, depressed scar like plaque, pale yellow or white
Margins indistinct, with nodules, ulcerations, or bleeding occurring within the plaque
Often undetected or misdiagnosed, with a lower cure rate than nodular BCC
Basosquamous
Aggressive in growth
Often recurs locally
Type most likely to metastasize

Data from Vargo N: Basal and squamous cell carcinoma, *Semin Oncol Nurs* 19(1):12-21, 2003 and American Cancer Society: *Cancer facts and figures, 2005*, Atlanta, 2005, Author.

| TABLE 17-1 | American Joint Committee on Cancer AJCC-BCC Stage Grouping |

Primary Tumor (T)

TX	Primary tumor cannot be assessed
T0	No evidence of primary tumor
Tis	Carcinoma in situ
T1	Tumor 2 cm or less in greatest dimension
T2	Tumor more than 2 cm but not more than 5 cm in greatest dimension
T3	Tumor more than 5 cm in greatest dimension
T4	Tumor invades deep extradermal structures (i.e., cartilage, skeletal muscle, or bone)

NOTE: In the case of multiple simultaneous tumors, the tumor with the highest T category will be classified and the number of separate tumors will be indicated in parentheses, e.g., T2(5).

Regional Lymph Nodes (N)

NX	Regional lymph nodes cannot be assessed
N0	No regional lymph node metastasis
N1	Regional lymph node metastasis

Distant Metastasis (M)

MX	Distant metastasis cannot be assessed
M0	No distant metastasis
M1	Distant metastasis

STAGE GROUPING

Stage 0	Tis	N0	M0
Stage I	T1	N0	M0
Stage II	T2	N0	M0
	T3	N0	M0
Stage III	T4	N0	M0
	Any T	N1	M0
Stage IV	Any T	Any N	M1

BCC, Basal cell carcinoma.
Used with the permission of the American Joint Committee on Cancer (AJCC), Chicago, Illinois. The original source for this material is the *AJCC Cancer Staging Handbook*, ed 6, New York, 2002 Springer (www.springeronline.com).

more likely to recur than those on the trunk or extremities, particularly those located around the ear.[18]

Treatment Modalities

Treatment for both BCC and SCC depends upon the size and location of the lesion, the histologic type of cancer, extension into nearby structures, the presence of metastases, previous treatment, anticipated cosmetic results, and the patient's age and condition.[8] Multiple modalities exist for the treatment of BCC including surgical excision, cryosurgery, Mohs surgery, laser surgery, electrodesiccation and curettage, radiation therapy, chemotherapy, and biotherapy.[2,8,17] There is no single treatment ideal for all lesions. The goals of therapy are permanent cure, preservation of function,[8] and the best possible cosmetic results.[2] If BCC is located on the face, substantial disfigurement can occur.[18]

SURGERY

Surgical intervention is used to treat approximately 90% of BCCs. The goal is complete removal of the tumor. Most of the procedures require local anesthesia, use minimal equipment, and can be performed in an ambulatory setting.[8]

Excisional Surgery. Surgical excision is an effective form of therapy for BCC, particularly for large lesions or those with poorly defined margins in high-risk sites such as the cheek, the forehead, the trunk, and the leg.[2] Often a simple ellipse with suturing is feasible. In more difficult anatomic locations, the use of skin flaps and grafts may be necessary. For tumors smaller than 2 cm, the minimal margin necessary to eradicate the entire cancer is 4 mm in 95% of cases.[2] Surgical excision may also be indicated when metastasis is present.[11]

Cryosurgery. Cryosurgery involves tissue destruction by freezing. A spray or cryoprobe is used to administer liquid nitrogen. Rapid freezing results in intracellular and extracellular ice crystallization. Cell destruction occurs owing to the rapid freeze and slow thaw cycle.[2,8] This method is useful in small to large nodular and superficial BCCs but is not indicated for deeply invasive tumors or BCCs of the scalp. The advantages of cryosurgery are that it is cost-effective, fast, and easy.[8] It does not cause blood loss or require anesthesia. Disadvantages include patient discomfort with therapy, delayed healing time and, occasionally, hypopigmentation.[8] Cryosurgery should not be used for patients who have recurrent BCC or a history of cryoglobulinemia, cold agglutinin syndrome, or Raynaud's phenomenon.[8]

Electrodesiccation and Curettage. This method of treating BCC is more efficient and cost-effective compared to surgical excision, Mohs surgery, or radiation therapy.[8] However, the success of the procedure depends on the skill of the clinician. Acquiring proper technique and identifying lesions that are appropriate for this treatment takes considerable experience.[2,8] This method uses heat to destroy tissue. After the tumor is marked and anesthetized, a debulking process is used to scrape abnormal tissue, which is then electrodesiccated. Curettage of the base is performed using both a large and a tiny curette to track any extension of the tumor. The procedure is repeated as necessary until a normal plane of tissue is reached.[8] These interventions are useful with small (smaller than 2 cm) to medium nodular and superficial BCCs with well-defined margins. Electrodesiccation and curettage has a lower cure rate than excision and, consequently, is less appropriate for removal of tumors with high risk for metastasis or deep invasion because of their location.[16] BCCs larger than 2 cm in diameter, those located in zones at high risk for recurrence, and all high-risk SCCs are best treated by other methods.[8,11] This method is also not used for lesions adjacent to the lips, the nasal orifices, or the eyelids, because the healing process results in significant retraction of the surrounding tissues.[8]

Microscopically Oriented Histologic Surgery (Mohs) Micrographic Surgery. Mohs micrographic surgery involves surgical removal of the tumor, layer by layer, until all margins are free of the tumor on microscopic examination. Mohs microsurgery permits the best histologic verification of complete removal and allows for maximum conservation of tissue.[2] It is the treatment of choice for invasive SCCs and primary BCCs larger than 2 cm in diameter, having indistinct clinical margins, located on zones of the face with a known high recurrence rate, occurring in a cosmetic or functional area, such as the nose or eyelid, or are aggressive, such as morpheaform BCC.[8,11] A unique feature is that specimens are sectioned and color-coded in a manner that permits microscopic examination of the entire surgical margin simultaneously.[16] This allows for repeated sectioning and microscopic examination until all the cancer is removed; immediate repair can then be performed. Using Mohs surgery, a tumor can be completely excised in 1 day without removing more than 1 to 2 mm of normal skin. Mohs surgery has the highest cure rates for primary and recurrent BCC and SCC.[8]

Lasers. The carbon dioxide laser has the advantage over conventional surgery in that it seals small blood vessels and nerves. It provides a relatively bloodless surgical field and reduced postoperative pain.[11,20]

Postsurgical Care. The appropriate follow-up interval depends on the details of the individual case.[8] Patients with a superficial BCC and little other evidence of sun exposure may only need to be seen once a year, whereas those with high-risk SCC need to be initially seen every 1 to 2 months. Follow-up focuses on identifying recurrent and new primary tumors. A complete skin examination should be done and regional lymph nodes checked for evidence of possible metastasis, particularly if the patient was treated for SCC.[16]

RADIATION THERAPY

BCC and SCC are radiosensitive.[2] The indications for ionizing radiation therapy for these skin cancers are continually being modified, as alternative treatments become readily available. Radiation therapy may be used when surgery is not feasible, surgical destruction is not desirable, or when surgical interventions are contraindicated, as in elderly or debilitated persons who are unable to tolerate a surgical procedure.[2] One benefit of radiation therapy is tissue conservation, particularly on the nose, eyelids, or lips.[8] Dosing depends upon tumor type, size, location, and depth. A single treatment can be as effective as fractionated doses, although most malignancies require treatment over a 5-day period.[2] Disadvantages of this form of therapy are radionecrosis over bony areas, radiodermatitis, further aging of the skin,[8] and reoccurrence after radiation of more aggressive tumors.[2]

Radiation therapy should not be used for the following:[2,8,11]

- Lesions in areas such as the inner canthus, where recurrences might be catastrophic
- Lesions in patients younger than 50 years, who would be subject to long-term sequelae such as carcinogenesis and chronic radiation dermatitis
- Lesions in previously irradiated areas
- Tumors located on the trunk, the extremities, the hands, or the scalp
- Those tumors arising in sweat and sebaceous glands
- Morpheaform basal cell tumors or verrucous squamous cell tumors
- Tumors larger than 8 cm
- Tumors located on the upper lip and growing into the nostril

CHEMOTHERAPY

Topical chemotherapy, using topical 5-fluorouracil (5-FU) (Efudex, Fluroplex), is an effective modality for superficial multicentric BCCs but is ineffective for other histologic types.[8] 5-FU destroys the surface tumor without affecting deeper cells, thus allowing invasion to continue at the base of the tumor.[11] Treatment must continue for 4 to 6 weeks.[8] Patient compliance may be problematic as a result of the severe degree of inflammation usually accompanying treatment.[8]

The newest FDA approved treatment for superficial basal cell cancer is topical imiquimod (Aldara cream). It is used when surgery is not appropriate. It can be used on the body, the neck, the arms, or the legs. It is not used for treatment on the face. Patients may experience skin reactions at the treatment site, such as redness, swelling, a sore or blister, peeling, itching, and burning.[21]

Prognosis

Metastatic disease is rare with BCC; however, if left untreated, the tumor will locally invade vital structures such as blood vessels, lymph nodes, nerve sheaths, cartilage, bone, lungs, and the liver.[2] With early detection and treatment, cure rates are close to 100% in persons with lesions smaller than 1 cm. When surgical intervention is used, the overall 5-year survival rate is approximately 99% for primary lesions and 96% with recurrent lesions. Persons with a history of BCC need defined scheduled follow-up examinations by a physician,[11] an integrated program of skin cancer awareness, and sun protection.[8]

SQUAMOUS CELL CARCINOMA
Epidemiology

Squamous cell carcinoma (SCC) is a tumor of the keratinizing cells of the epidermis.[2,16] SCC is less common than BCC.[4,8] SCC accounts for 20% of all nonmelanoma skin cancers and has a mortality rate of 1% to 2%.[8,17] SCC occurs more frequently in persons with light complexions.[2] Persons at greatest risk sunburn easily, tan poorly, and have red or blonde hair and blue eyes.[4] SCC is also more common in men, and the incidence increases with age. The average age at onset of SCC is approximately 60 years.[1] Unlike BCC, this tumor frequently occurs on the hands and forearms as well as on the head and neck region, especially the ears, the lower lip, the scalp, and the upper face.[11]

Etiology and Risk Factors

Squamous cell carcinoma is most often found in sun-damaged skin previously affected by actinic keratosis.[22] All the predisposing risk factors mentioned in regard to BCC have also been associated with the development of SCC.[4]

Prevention and Screening

Prevention and detection methods are similar for both SCC and BCC. The avoidance of UV light and the use of sunscreens and protective clothing are important.[4] Using sunscreen has been shown to prevent squamous cell cancer.[13] In addition to the head and neck area, the hands and forearms should also be liberally spread with sunscreen.[11]

ACTINIC KERATOSES

Actinic (solar) keratoses are currently believed by many authorities to be an early stage in the development of squamous cell carcinoma.[10,22] Treatment of actinic keratosis may prevent the formation of invasive squamous cell carcinoma and potential metastases.[2,22]

Classification and Clinical Features

Because of the varying general characteristics and the source of tissue presentation, SCC is classified by presenting symptoms, tissue source, and histologic difference. SCC should be suspected whenever clinical features are noted (Clinical Features of Squamous Cell Carcinoma box). Presentations vary: lesions may be superficial, discrete, and hard, and have an

Clinical Features of
Squamous Cell Carcinoma (SCC)

General Characteristics

- Occurs anywhere on sun-damaged skin and on mucous membrane with squamous epithelium
- Appears round to irregularly shaped, with a plaquelike or nodular character covered by a warty scale, indistinct margins, and firm erythematous dome-shaped nodule with core like center that ulcerates
- Dull red in color
- Grows by expansion and infiltration, as well as by tracking along various tissue planes
- Invades below the level of the sweat gland and has a higher degree of malignant potential
- Overall invasiveness and depth of neoplasm are significant when determining risk of recurrence

Ischemic Ulceration

- Occurs in varicose ulcers, chronic ulcers, and poorly healed fistulas or tracks with old scars
- Accompanied by increased drainage, pain, and bleeding

Bowen's Disease

- Associated with arsenic ingestion
- Multiple superficial lesions

- Occurs on sun-exposed and non–sun-exposed areas of the skin, including mucous membrane of vulva, vagina, nose, and conjunctiva
- Multiple superficial lesions; nodular reddish brown plaque with areas of scales and crusts

Actinic Cheilitis

- Rapidly growing, progressive invasive lesion that occurs on the lip, often a result of smoking
- Lower lip is primary site in 95% of patients
- Early appearance is local thickening, progressing to a firm nodular lesion with destructive ulceration
- Diagnosis is frequently missed (as long as 2 years after onset), and lesion is usually 1 to 2 cm in diameter at initial biopsy
- Reported risk of metastasis from SCC of lip has ranged from 5% to 37%

Verrucous

- Well-differentiated lesion frequently seen on glans penis, vulva, scrotum, sole, back, or buttock; appears as a slowly growing, warty lesion. Often very large, Extensive local spread
- Surgical excision is treatment of choice

Data from Vargo N: Basal and squamous cell carcinoma, *Semin Oncol Nurs* 19(1):12–21, 2003; American Cancer Society: *Cancer facts and figures, 2005*, Atlanta, 2005, Author; Gross E: Non-melanoma skin cancer: clues to early detection, keys to effective treatment, *Consultant* 39(3):829, 1999; and Rigel DS, Carucci JA: Self-examination of the skin, *CA Cancer J Clin* 4(50):223-226, 2000.

indurated, rounded base. They may be dull red and contain telangiectasias, or they may be dome-shaped nodules with ulcerations and crusting.[2] If SCC is suspected, special attention should be paid to the regional lymph node chains, particularly if the lesion is located on the hands, the ear, or the lip.[16]

Diagnosis and Staging

Diagnosis and staging for SCC are the same as described earlier in this chapter for BCC.[11]

Metastasis

The frequency of metastasis of SCC of the skin is higher that of than BCC and ranges from 0.5% to 30%.[2] The occurrence and degree of metastasis varies according to morphologic characteristics, and size and depth of penetration of the tumor.[2] Metastasis occurs late via the lymphatics after the tumor has invaded the subcutaneous lymph nodes and the lymphatics of the deeper structure.[2]

Treatment Modalities

Squamous cell carcinoma can be treated by procedures similar to those used with BCC with some alterations. For example, a slightly larger excisional margin should be performed surgically,[8] and it is important to examine the regional lymph nodes for the presence of tumor.[11] The therapeutic approach will depend on the size and location of the carcinoma, the extent of local involvement, and the potential for metastasis. The occurrence of metastasis varies according to morphologic characteristics, size, and depth of penetration of the tumor.[11]

CRYOTHERAPY

Cryotherapy for SCC is useful in selected patients. Lesions with a diameter of 0.5 to 2.0 cm and well-defined borders are amenable to this modality. This technique boasts exceptional cosmetic results and has achieved 5-year cure rates of 90% to 95%.[2]

CHEMOTHERAPY

Topical 5-FU is recommended for treatment of premalignant actinic keratoses (see section on chemotherapy for BCC). An alternative to topical 5-FU is topical masoprocol (Actinex), which was effective in treating actinic keratoses on the head and neck.[11] In advanced SCC, systemic retinoids have produced response rates greater than 70%.[11]

RADIATION THERAPY

Radiation therapy is recommended for treatment of primary SCC using a variety of fractionation regimens (see section on radiation therapy for BCC).

MOHS SURGERY

The treatment of choice for high-risk tumors with no palpable nodes is Mohs surgery (see under surgical intervention for BCC). The 5-year cure rate is 90% for high-risk SCC to 97% for lower-risk SCC.[2]

Prognosis

Squamous cell carcinoma has high cure rates (75% to 80%) when either surgery or radiation is used. Because this lesion has the capacity to metastasize as well as recur, it is generally considered a higher-risk skin cancer.[8] Most deaths resulting from nonmelanoma skin cancer can be attributed to SCC.[2]

Melanoma Skin Cancers
MALIGNANT MELANOMA
Epidemiology

Malignant melanoma was expected to affect an estimated 47,700 people in the United States in 2005 and cause 7700 deaths.[4] The incidence has risen 3% to 7% on average over several decades.[24] It has the fifth highest occurrence of cancers in men and the sixth highest of those in women.[1] In 1930 the lifetime risk of developing invasive melanoma was 1 in 1500; it is currently 1 in 71.[25] Melanoma is a malignant tumor of the melanocytes, cells that are derived from the neural crest. Although most melanomas arise in the skin, melanoma can arise anywhere the cells migrate.[26] This accounts for the fewer than 10% of melanomas that occur in more obscure locations, such as the eyes, the oral and genital mucosa, the esophagus, and the meninges.[11]

COMPARISONS BETWEEN NMSC AND MELANOMA

Similarly to the nonmelanoma skin cancers, malignant melanoma most frequently affects whites; most African Americans are far less likely to develop melanoma.[4,5] When dark-skinned persons and Asians do get melanoma, it tends to occur at sites not exposed to the sun, such as palms, soles, nail beds, fingers, toes, and mucous membranes.[6,11,17] The median age at diagnosis is 53.[27] Unlike BCC and SCC, melanoma may occur in persons in their teens and early 20s or 30s.[17] It has become one of the most common cancers in younger adults. In men, the trunk is the most common site of occurrence; the back and the lower extremities are the most common sites in women.[5,11,26]

Melanoma is most common in parts of the world where fair-skinned people live in very sunny climates.[17] The closer one lives to the equator, the higher the risk for developing melanoma.[7,13,17] The risk of developing melanoma is highest in countries with a high ambient solar radiation. For every 1000 feet above sea level, there is a compounded 4% increase in UV radiation exposure.[11] The risk for developing melanoma for fair-skinned people living in higher elevations in those countries tends to be greater for native-born people than immigrants to that country.[7] The world's highest incidence of melanoma is in Australia and in Israel (approximately 40 cases per 100,00 individuals per year).[17] In the United States, the occurrence of melanoma is greatest in the "Sun Belt" states such as California, Arizona, and Texas (approximately 20 to 30 cases per 100,000 individuals per year).[4,17]

Etiology and Risk Factors

A single blistering sunburn before the age of 20 increases the risk of melanoma later in life.[17] The greatest risk is associated with a history of multiple blistering sunburns in childhood.[5] Unlike the more common skin cancers, which are associated with total cumulative exposure to UV radiation, melanomas are associated with intense intermittent exposure, although the disease also develops in people who have had regular, cumulative exposure.[5,6,13,17] A person's ability to tan seems to be a factor. Persons who burn easily and are poor tanners have an increased risk.[5,11] Persons who are fair-skinned are at higher risk, although malignant melanoma can occur in persons of any skin type.[11,17] Other characteristics,

such as blond or red hair color, are risk factors for the development of both nonmelanoma skin cancers and melanoma.[4,6,11,17] Melanoma is at least 5 times more likely to occur in someone who has already had melanoma.[4] Additional risk factors include immunosuppression, previous hematogenic malignancy, and xeroderma pigmentosum.[17]

MOLES

Typical moles are also called melanocytic nevi. These moles are usually smaller than 6 mm in size, tan to brown in color, and raised above the skin surface. People with more than 25 to 50 melanocytic nevi are at increased risk for melanoma.[5,7,17,28] Atypical moles, also called dysplastic nevi, are generally larger than 6 mm and are irregularly shaped, with various shades of coloration. People with at least one dysplastic nevus have a 6% lifetime risk of developing melanoma.[7,17] The third type of mole is called giant congenital nevi; this is a pigmented lesion present at birth. Only the giant nevi larger than 20 cm are documented as a precursor to melanoma.[5,17]

Prevention, Screening, and Detection
PRIMARY PREVENTION

If melanoma could be prevented it would be of significant public benefit. The major environmental factor associated with melanoma is excessive sun exposure, in particular, excessive intermittent sun exposure.[13] The avoidance of intense sun exposure and the use of protective clothing and sunscreens are important for both adults and children. Children should also be protected from sunburns because an increased risk for melanoma exists in persons who have experienced traumatic sunburns as children.[28]

SECONDARY PREVENTION

Early detection and prompt treatment are essential. Warning signs of melanoma are any unusual skin condition: scaliness, oozing, or bleeding of a mole or other pigmented growth; a change in color or size of a mole or any other pigmented growth or spot; a spread of the pigment beyond the normal border; a change in sensation, itchiness, tenderness, or pain; and the development of a new lesion or nodule. The early warning signs of malignant melanoma can be easily remembered by thinking of the acronym ABCD: asymmetry, border irregularity, color, and diameter greater than 6 mm.[4,5,25] Malignant melanomas are usually asymmetric (i.e., one half of the mole does not match the other half). Early malignant melanomas tend to have irregular borders. The edges become ragged, notched, or blurred, unlike smooth margins. Pigmentation in malignant melanomas is not uniform. Colors may range from various hues of tan and brown to black, with intermingling of red and white.[5] Malignant melanomas are often greater than 5 to 6 mm when first identified. A sudden or continued increase in the size of a mole should be reported.[4,11] A total body skin examination by health care providers is critical for the initial visit and follow-up for people at risk for melanoma.[17] The best outcomes depend on the provider's ability to identify and remove hazardous lesions before they flourish. Although screening for the early detection of melanoma is recommended by many, widespread acceptance of screening is hindered by the lack of a randomized trial showing that screening is effective in saving lives.

Although the efficacy of self–skin screening has not been proven to reduce mortality in a randomized controlled trial, many people do detect their own skin cancers. The only evidence for the effectiveness of skin self-screening currently comes from a single documented case control study reporting that self-examination is associated with lower incidence and mortality from melanoma.[13] However, screenings by individuals, family, and especially care providers are important tools to prevent morbidity due to melanoma.[28]

Classification and Clinical Features

TYPES OF MELANOMA

Early primary melanoma is characterized by a radial growth phase confined to the epidermis, the superficial dermis, or both. This can evolve into advanced melanoma which has a vertical growth phase for invasion of the deep dermis and development of metasta-sis.[17] Early-stage melanoma is curable, but the prognosis for individuals with metastatic disease is dismal, with a 5-year survival rate of only 12%.[29] Melanoma metastasizes to remote sites early, and these metastases are characteristically unresponsive to treatment.[2]

There are four types of malignant melanoma: (1) superficial spreading, (2) nodular, (3) lentigo maligna, and (4) acral lentiginous (Clinical Features of Malignant Melanoma Pigmented Lesions box).[17] The cellular subtypes are considered descriptive and do not have prognostic or therapeutic significance.[26] Superficial spreading malignant melanoma is the most common form.[17] About 70% of all cutaneous melanomas are of this type. These occur more often in women than in men, usually between the ages of 40 and 50.[11] Most lesions occur on the back in men and on the lower legs in women.[11]

Nodular malignant melanoma is the second most frequently occurring melanoma, representing 10% to 15% of cutaneous melanomas.[17] Nodular melanomas may occur anywhere on the body; however, common sites of occurrence are the head, neck, and trunk regions.[11] Most nodular melanomas appear as a blue or black nodule, although 5% have no pigmentation. These amelanotic nodular melanomas are frequently misdiagnosed.

Lentigo maligna melanoma, accounts for 10% to 15% of melanomas. These lesions occur after age 60 and primarily on the sun-exposed areas of the body, most often the head, the neck and the hands.[11] These lesions arise from a precursor lesion known as lentigo maligna.[17] The term "lentigo maligna melanoma" is reserved for invasive lesions.

Acral lentiginous melanoma is the least common; it accounts for less than 10% of all melanomas.[11] This type of melanoma is the most common in African Americans, Hispanics, and Asians. It is frequently found on the palms, the soles, and the periungual and subungual surfaces. It frequently has a short radial growth phase, resulting in late detection and a poor prognosis.[17]

Diagnosis and Staging

Melanoma has two growth phases: radial and vertical.[17] During the radial growth phase, the tumor spreads laterally along the skin surface. During the vertical growth phase the melanoma extends downward through the layers of the epidermis and dermis and into the subcutaneous tissue. As it continues to grow downward, it invades the lymphatic and vascular systems. This results in local and regional disease, as well as spread to distant lymph nodes and visceral organs.[17] When a lesion is suspected to be melanoma, a biopsy should be performed. The technique of choice is a total excisional biopsy.[17] Suspicious lesions should never be "shaved off" or cauterized.[17,26,30] To reduce the possibility of misdiagnosis, review by a qualified pathologist should be considered.[26] Overall prognosis and treatment are based on the stage of disease using the AJCC's staging classification (Table 17-2).

Diagnostic work-up should include a complete physical, with a full skin check to rule out a second primary.[17] Special note should be made of symptoms suggestive of metastatic disease such as abdominal pain, bone pain, weight loss, double vision, headaches, malaise, and seizures. A chest film should be ordered to exclude the possibility of a silent lung metastasis. The liver, the spleen, and regional lymph nodes should be palpated for lymphadenopathy.[11] Further diagnostic testing includes routine laboratory tests, complete blood count (CBC), lactate dehydrogenase, blood urea

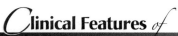

Malignant Melanoma Pigmented Lesions

Superficial Spreading Melanoma
- Variegated in color with areas appearing blue, black, gray, white, or pink
- Irregular, pigmented plaque with areas of regression and notched borders; horizontal or radial extension
- May appear scaly and crusty and itch; frequently arise from existing moles
- Increasingly more common among young adults

Nodular Melanoma
- Often resembles a "blood blister"
- Appears as a symmetric, raised, dome-shaped lesion; vertical growth patterns

- Gray or blue–black in color
- Can be amelanotic

Lentigo Malignant Melanoma
- Appears as a large, flat, irregular lesion resembling a stain
- Variegated in color, ranging from tan to black with areas of regression
- Located on face and neck of elderly, severely sun-tanned whites

Acral Lentiginous Melanoma
- Usually flat and irregular, with an average diameter of 3 cm
- Blue or black discoloration or a tan and brown stain
- Occurs on palms and soles or under nail beds

Data from American Cancer Society: *Cancer facts and figures, 2005,* Atlanta, 2005, Author; Goldstein B, Goldstein AO: Diagnosis and management of malignant melanoma, *Am Fam Physician* 63(7):1359-1368, 2001; Gilchrest B, Eller M, Geller AC et al: Mechanisms of disease: the pathogenesis of melanoma induced by ultraviolet radiation, *N Engl J Med* 340(17):1341-1348, 1999; Margolin KA, Sondak VK: Melanoma and other skin cancer In Pazdur R, Coua LR, Hoskins WJ et al, editors: *Cancer management: a multidisci-plinary approach* Manhasset, NY, 2004, CMP Healthcare Media; and Lamb LA, Halpern AC, Hwu WJ: Diagnosis and management of stage I/II melanoma. *Semin Oncol Nurs* 19(1):22-31, 2003.

TABLE 17-2 AJCC Staging Melanoma Classification

Primary Tumor (T)

TX	Primary tumor cannot be assessed
T0	No evidence of primary tumor
Tis	Melanoma in situ
T1	Melanoma ≤1.0 mm in thickness with or without ulceration
T1a	Melanoma ≤1.0 mm in thickness and level II or III, no ulceration
T1b	Melanoma ≤1.0 mm in thickness and level IV or V or with ulceration
T2	Melanoma 1.01-2.0 mm in thickness with or without ulceration
T2a	Tumor 1.01-2.0 mm in thickness, no ulceration
T2b	Melanoma 1.01-2.0 mm in thickness, with ulceration
T3	Melanoma 2.01-4.0 mm in thickness, with or without ulceration
T3a	Melanoma 2.01-4.0 mm in thickness, no ulceration
T3b	Melanoma 2.01-4.0 mm in thickness, with ulceration
T4	Melanoma greater than 4.0 mm in thickness with or without ulceration
T4a	Melanoma >4.0 mm in thickness, no ulceration
T4b	Melanoma >4.0 mm in thickness, with ulceration

Regional Lymph Nodes (N)

NX	Regional lymph nodes cannot be assessed
N0	No regional lymph node metastasis
N1	Metastasis in one lymph node
N1a	Clinically occult (microscopic) metastasis
N1b	Clinically apparent (macroscopic) metastasis
N2	Metastasis in two to three regional nodes or intralymphatic regional metastasis without nodal metastases
N2a	Clinically occult (microscopic) metastasis
N2b	Clinically apparent (macroscopic) metastasis
N2c	Satellite or in-transit metastasis *without* nodal metastasis
N3	Metastasis in four or more regional nodes, or matted metastatic nodes, or in-transit metastasis or satellite(s) *with* metastatis in regional node(s)

Distant Metastasis (M)

MX	Distant metastasis cannot be assessed
M0	No distant metastasis
M1	Distant metastasis
M1a	Metastasis to skin, subcutaneous tissues or distant lymph nodes
M1b	Metastasis to lung
M1c	Metastasis to all other visceral sites or distant metastasis at any site associated with an elevated serum lactic dehydrogenase (LDH)

CLINICAL STAGE GROUPING

Stage 0	Tis	N0	M0
Stage IA	T1a	N0	M0
Stage IB	T1b	N0	M0
	T2a	N0	M0
Stage IIA	T2b	N0	M0
	T3a	N0	M0
Stage IIB	T3b	N0	M0
	T4a	N0	M0
Stage IIC	T4b	N0	M0
Stage III	Any T	N1	M0
	Any T	N2	M0
	Any T	N3	M0
Stage V	Any T	Any N	M1

Note: *Clinical staging includes microstaging for the primary melanoma and clinical/radiological evaluation for metastases. By convention, it should be used after complete excision of the primary melanoma with clinical assessment for regional and distant metastases.*

Continued

TABLE 17-2   **AJCC Staging Melanoma Classification—cont'd**

PATHOLOGIC STAGE GROUPING

Stage 0	Tis	N0	M0
Stage IA	T1a	N0	M0
Stage IB	T1b	N0	M0
	T2a	N0	M0
Stage IIA	T2b	N0	M0
	T3a	N0	M0
Stage IIB	T3b	N0	M0
	T4a	N0	M0
Stage IIC	T4b	N0	M0
Stage IIIA	T1-4a	N1a	M0
	T1-4a	N2a	M0
Stage IIIB	T1-4b	N1a	M0
	T1-4b	N2a	M0
	T1-4a	N1b	M0
	T1-4a	N2b	M0
	T1-4a/b	N2c	M0
Stage IIIC	T1-4b	N1b	M0
	T1-4b	N2b	M0
	Any T	N3	M0
Stage IV	Any T	Any N	M1

Note: *Clinical staging includes microstaging for the primary melanoma and clinical/radiological evaluation for metastases. By convention, it should be used after complete excision of the primary melanoma with clinical assessment for regional and distant metastases.*

nitrogen, partial thromboplastin time, liver enzyme studies, urinalysis, serum creatinine, and blood chemistries. Other studies, such as computed tomography (CT) scans or magnetic resonance imaging (MRI), are guided by the symptomatology reported by the patient and outcome of the above tests.[11]

MICROSTAGING

In clinically node-negative patients, the degree of microscopic invasion is of critical importance in predicting outcome.[17] Clark's level and Breslow's thickness are two methods to predict prognosis of melanoma, which is related to the depth of invasion of the primary tumor. Clark's level is a qualitative description of the increasing levels of penetration (invasion) through the dermis to the subcutaneous fat (Fig. 17-1), whereas Breslow's thickness is a direct measurement of the primary tumor depth or thickness, using a micrometer in the microscope eyepiece.[5,11] The problem with the Clark system is that the thickness of the skin varies in different parts of the body.[17] Breslow's thickness is the crucial parameter of vertical tumor thickness, from the top of the granular layer to the base of the tumor. Breslow's thickness reflects the observation that prognosis worsens with increasing ranges of tumor thickness. To date, the single attribute best predictive of clinical outcome is the depth of tumor invasion, Breslow's thickness, considered the gold standard for stratifying patients according to risk of metastatic disease.[29,30]

LYMPH NODE INVOLVEMENT

A part of the surgical treatment of melanoma is actually an extension of the diagnostic process of staging the patient's disease. Historically, staging was first done through elective lymph node dissection (ELND).[31] Regional lymph nodes are a common site for the first appearance of metastatic tumor. Therefore, the presence or absence of node involvement is a second powerful predictor of outcome.[5] ELND has limited use in light of the advent of sentinel node biopsy and selective lymphadenectomy.[17]

SENTINEL LYMPH NODE TECHNIQUES

The concept of sentinel lymph node (SLN) biopsy was introduced when work with lymphoscintigraphy demonstrated that lymph node basins draining from a specific site could be defined by injection of a radionuclide. Animal and then human studies demonstrated that there are well-defined pathways from each cutaneous site to a specific regional lymph node or nodes. This rationale assumes that for every site, the lymphatic drainage is not only to a specific basin, but also first to a specific node. Therefore, if the sentinel (first) node is negative, the remaining distal nodes will also be negative.[5] Complete node dissection then would not be indicated.[31] False-negative rates remain under 4% for SLN biopsy.[5,17]

Two techniques are available to identify the sentinel node draining a cutaneous melanoma.[17] The first uses a blue lymphangiogram dye that is injected intradermally at the site of the primary lesion. An incision is made 5 minutes later over the lymph node basin. A blue-stained node is identified and removed. The dye technique identifies the sentinel node 80% of the time. A second technique involves the use of a radiolabeled solution. A handheld gamma detector is used to identify the sentinel node.[5] Since the radiolabeled technique does not provide the visual clues of the blue dye, most surgeons combine the two techniques. The combined use of these techniques has identified the sentinel node in more than 98% of the cases. SLN biopsy has been widely accepted as the preferred method for patients with clinically negative nodes and melanomas 1 to 4 mm thick.[5,17] Compared to ELND, there are far fewer side effects with the SLN technique.[32]

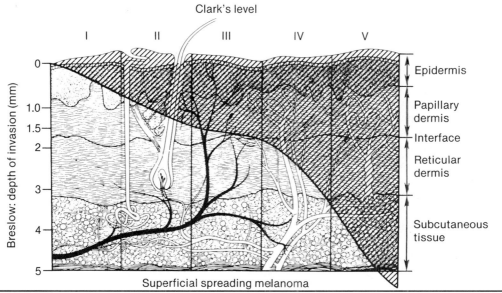

Clark's level

I   II   III   IV   V

Epidermis

Papillary dermis

Interface

Reticular dermis

Subcutaneous tissue

Breslow: depth of invasion (mm)

Superficial spreading melanoma

FIG. 17-1   Anatomic landmarks and Breslow's depth of invasion. (From DiSaia PJ, Creasman WT: *Clinical gynecologic oncology*, ed 5, St. Louis, 1997, Mosby.)

Selected lymphadenectomy is not used in patients with wide excision of the primary melanoma because of the changes in the lymphatic drainage patterns. Any patient who has an involved sentinel node should undergo a full lymph node dissection.[17]

Metastases

Patients with melanoma smaller than 1 mm have a low likelihood of nodal involvement (less than 5%). Melanomas of 1 to 4 mm have a 20% to 25% chance of occult lesions and a high incidence of occult systemic metastasis at the time of diagnosis.[17] Malignant melanoma may spread to any organ or remote viscera. Common sites for disseminated disease are the skin (intracutaneous or subcutaneous metastasis), the bone, the brain, the lung, and the liver.[11]

Treatment Modalities

SURGERY

Surgical resection remains the mainstay of melanoma treatment for stages I and II disease.[26] For stage 1 melanoma, in lesions less than 2 mm thick, a radial excision with margins of 1 cm would be performed. Lymphatic mapping and SLN biopsy in patients who have tumors of intermediate thickness or ulceration could identify any occult nodal disease. In patients with stage 2 disease (melanomas with a thickness between 2 and 4 mm), surgical margins must be 2 cm wide. Lymphatic mapping is done to assess for the presence of occult disease. Stage 3 disease necessitates a wide local excision of the primary tumor with 1- to 3-cm margins, depending on tumor thickness and location. Skin grafting may be necessary.[26] For patients with known disease in the regional lymph node basin, a lymph node dissection is indicated. Even after surgical resection, these patients face a high risk of recurrence.[11] Surgery done for stage 4 disease is palliative in nature.[26]

RADIATION THERAPY

Historically, melanoma was felt to be radioresistant,[11] but studies are under way to challenge this belief.[17] Radiation is given for palliative therapy.[26] It is beneficial for patients who are in pain due to bone metastasis, but full regression of the tumor is rare.[5]

CHEMOTHERAPY

Dacarbazine (DTIC). Primarily used in stage IV with metastatic disease, dacarbazine (DTIC) is the most readily recognized agent approved by U.S. Food and Drug Administration (FDA).[11] Single-agent dosing at 850 to 1,000 mg/m^2 once every week is the standard therapy for advanced melanoma. It has a 10% to 15% response rate when given as a single agent.[17] The adverse side effects of DTIC are myelosuppression and gastrointestinal distress.

Temozolamide (Temodar). This is an oral alkylating agent and an analogue of DTIC that has the ability to cross the blood-brain barrier and is helpful for patients who develop brain metastasis or those who have central nervous system involvement. The drug can cause severe myelosuppression, depending on dose and administration schedule.[11]

Other agents. Nitrosoureas, vinca alkaloids, and cisplatin may be given in combination regimens. These have response rates of 10% to 15% for brief duration.[17]

HYPERTHERMIC REGIONAL PERFUSION

This technique, also called isolated limb perfusion (ILP), was developed in the 1950s to treat various cancers, but is most effective in treating melanoma of the limbs.[17,31] It is the perfusion of chemotherapeutic agents, most often melphalan (Alkeran), directly into an extremity.[11,17] It is most often used for in transit metastasis,[17] involving skin or subcutaneous tissue more than 2 cm from the primary tumor but not beyond the regional lymph nodes.

The limb is usually perfused for 1 hour with a high concentration of drug at 39° to 41° C (102.2° to 105.8° F), using a perfusion pump and extracorporeal circulator.[17] The hyperthermia enhances the cytotoxic effect so that the total dose of drug may be reduced. This delivers a high concentration of drug to areas of local and regional recurrences in an extremity and produces minimal side effects.[11] This procedure is performed in specialized and limited clinical settings.[17]

BIOTHERAPY

Interferon. Since adjuvant chemotherapy has not been beneficial in improving disease-free survival or life expectancy, research has focused on biotherapy, which uses agents normally produced in the body in small amounts that heighten the immune system's ability to recognize and fight cancer. These are referred to as biologic response modifiers (BRM)s. Recombinant interferon-α 2b, a BRM, was first approved as adjuvant therapy to surgery for patients with malignant melanoma. At its inception, its use was indicated in adults 18 years and older who were free of disease postoperatively but likely to experience a recurrence.[17] A multi-center randomized controlled study found there was a prolongation of relapse-free and overall survival for patients who receive high-dose interferon.[26]

Interleukin-2 (IL-2). Recombinant interleukin-2 (IL-2) is a cytokine that stimulates the immune system to produce T cells, lymphokine-activated killer cells, and natural killer (NK) cells that may target and kill cancer cells. Recombinant IL-2 also promotes the creation and release of other cytokines and activates B cells to produce immunoglobulins.[11] High-dose therapy with IL-2 requires intensive inpatient management. The most common side effects are hypotension, acidosis, renal insufficiency, neurotoxicity, and cardiovascular complications that can be life-threatening. A generalized capillary leak syndrome can occur and may lead to multiorgan failure.[17]

LONG-TERM FOLLOW-UP

Patients who have had one melanoma are at increased risk of a second primary lesion and should remain under careful surveillance, with both self–skin examination and professional examination.[4,5] These skin exams should take place every 3 to 6 months for 2 to 3 years, depending upon the thickness of the presenting lesion.[5] Melanoma is not considered cured after a 5-year period with no recurrence. It is common for patients to develop evidence of metastasis 5 to 10 years after the primary lesion was removed, or even more than a decade or two later. In addition, CBC, blood chemistries, and an annual chest film should be done.[5] Those patients with thick melanomas should have blood drawn for alkaline phosphatase and alanine aminotransferase levels to be ascertained. If these are elevated, a CT scan of the liver should be ordered.

Prognosis

The single best predictor of clinical outcome is depth of tumor invasion, the Breslow's thickness. It is considered the gold standard for stratifying patients according to risk of metastatic disease.[11,17] The presence or absence of lymph node involvement is the second most powerful predictor of outcome. In 2005, the 5-year relative survival rate for localized melanoma is 98%, for regional disease it is 60%, and for distant disease 16%.[1] Improvements in survival appears to be related to earlier diagnosis.[24]

KAPOSI SARCOMA
Epidemiology

It was estimated that fewer than 2500 new cases of Kaposi sarcoma (KS) were diagnosed in the United States in 2005. In developed countries, KS occurs most often among immigrant groups from countries where KS is common; in recipients of organ transplantation; and in patients with immune suppression from chemotherapeutic drugs.[4]

Etiology and Risk Factors

The presence of human herpes virus 8 is considered necessary in order for KS to develop. Immune suppression induced by the human immunodeficiency virus (HIV) profoundly increases the risk.[4]

Prevention and Screening

Primary prevention behaviors include sexual abstinence, a monogamous relationship with an uninfected partner, and consistent and correct condom use.[33] Secondary prevention strategy includes the use of highly active antiretroviral therapy (HAART), which reduces the risk of KS among patients infected with HIV and may be effective in treating the tumors.[34]

Classification

Although the histopathology of the different types of KS is the same, the clinical features and the courses of the diseases are different (Box 17-1).[35] KS is divided into five types: (1) classic, (2) African, (3) immunosuppressive treatment–related, (4) epidemic, and (5) nonepidemic gay-related.[36]

BOX 17-1   Kaposi Overview

Classic
- Epidemiology: Considered a rare disease occurring more often in males; usual age of onset 50 to 70 years
- Clinical features: Presents with one or more asymptomatic red, purple, or brown lesion of the lower extremities
- Prognosis: Indolent course for 10 to 15 years
- Staging: Individualized because of the advanced age of the patient; there is no universally accepted staging system
- Treatment: Solitary lesion—radiation therapy or surgical excision. For widespread skin disease radiation therapy is tailored to treat the distribution of disease. Chemotherapy may be of benefit; a few patients have been treated with single-agent vinblastine at weekly doses at 0.1 mg/kg, with good response.

African
- Epidemiology: In the 1950s it was a relatively common neoplasm in native populations of equatorial Africa; occurs more often in males; age of onset is younger than the other types of KS
- Clinical features: May be indolent or aggressive with fungating tumors that invade the tissues

Immunosuppressive Treatment–Related
- Epidemiology: 1969 first described in a renal transplant patient
- Clinical features: Average time to develop is 16 months post-transplant; often localized to the skin, but dissemination to visceral organs can occur
- Treatment: Difficult, requiring a balance in treating the KS and the risk of graft rejection. Some patients have noted spontaneous and lasting remissions following the discontinuation of immunosuppressive therapy; radiation therapy given for disease limited to the skin; chemotherapy with single or multiple agents.

Continued

BOX 17-1 Kaposi Overview—cont'd

Epidemic

- Epidemiology: 1981, first reported in young homosexual or bisexual men as part of the acquired immunodeficiency syndrome (AIDS) epidemic.
- Clinical features: Multifocal widespread lesions at onset may involve skin, oral mucosa, and lymph nodes with lymphadenopathy; disease then becomes disseminated
- Staging incorporates the extent of the disease, severity of immunodeficiency, and presence of systemic symptoms.
- Treatment: Local lesions may be treated with cryotherapy or by surgical excision. Generally responsive to local radiation with doses around 2,000 cGy. Chemotherapy is not used often owing to depressed immunologic state, which limits the use of systemic chemotherapy. If chemotherapy is used, first-line therapy is liposomal anthracycline. Single agents or combinations of doxorubicin, bleomycin, vinblastine, vincristine, and etoposide. Biologic agents—recombinant interferon-α 2a and interferon-α 2b were the first agents approved for the treatment of KS. Today interferon is given in combination with either drugs active against human immunodeficiency virus (HIV) in lower doses than used in the past.

Nonepidemic Gay-Related

- Epidemiology: There have been reports documenting KS in homosexual men who have no evidence of HIV infection.
- Clinical features: Indolent and cutaneous, with a new lesion appearing every few years

Data from Scadden D: Neoplasm in Acquired immunodeficiency syndrome. In Holland JF, Frei E, editors: *Cancer medicine*, ed 6, London, 2003, BC Decker; Safai B: Kaposi's sarcoma and acquired immunodeficiency syndrome. In DeVita VT, Hillman S, Rosenberg S, editors: *AIDS: etiology, diagnosis, treatment and prevention*, ed 4, Philadelphia, 1997, Lippincott-Raven; and National Cancer Institute: Kaposi's sarcoma PDQ(r) treatment, health professional version, September 29, 2003, retrieved June 13, 2005, from www.nci.nih.gov on 6/13/05.

Considerations for Older Adults: All Skin Cancers

SECONDARY PREVENTION

Since life expectancy in the United States is expected to improve, it is likely that older persons will present with a diagnosis of skin cancer. Older persons may be less aware of skin changes and may not realize there has been a change in the skin or in a preexisting mole. This can lead to late-stage disease being found at diagnosis. Studies show that older adults were less likely to report itching and changes in elevation or color of a lesion. Older persons did report ulceration; however, this is a symptom of advanced disease.[37]

A study of melanoma showed middle-aged and older men comprising only 25% of those participating in screening at the Academy of Dermatology national skin cancer screening programs. However, this represented almost half (44%) of those with a confirmed diagnosis of melanoma.[38]

CONSIDERATIONS FOR OLDER ADULTS
Skin Cancers

- The geriatric population has greatest incidence of precancerous and cancerous NMSC skin lesions. Researchers estimate that 40% to 50% of the people in the United States who live to age 65 will have NMSC at least once.
- The average age of onset for squamous cell, lentigo malignant melanoma, and acral lentiginous melanoma is 60 years.
- Age-related sensory and muscle deficits require assistance of another person for monthly skin self- examination.
- Age-related changes in skin characteristics include fair skin and easily bruised superficial tissue.
- Limited access to health care system and limited health care resources may inhibit preventive health care.
- Limited access to medical specialists is common.
- Classic KS has usual age of onset or 50 to 70 years.
- Senior citizen centers should be targeted to reach those who participate in organized activities.
- Melanoma incidence and mortality continues to rise in older adults, particularly men. Specialized educational efforts must be considered for older men and their spouses for early detection.
- Moles that persist into old age have an increased risk of malignant degeneration.

KS Kaposi sarcoma; *NMSC,* nonmelanoma skin cancer.
Data from References 2, 9, 23, 36-38, and 40-42.

TREATMENT ISSUES IN THE OLDER ADULT

There may be misconceptions about treatment for the older adult. As older patients are presumed to be at higher risk of complications from the treatment of skin cancer, they may not receive aggressive curative treatment. A study examining the safety of isolated limb perfusion in the elderly (more than 75 years old), found similar response rates in the elderly with recurrent melanoma without increased toxicity, complications, or long-term morbidity compared to younger patients.[39] Research also shows that patients older than 65 years of age who had only surgical excision of a thick melanoma and did not get adjuvant treatment did significantly worse than historical controls. The authors concluded that treatment for patients older than 65 should be as aggressive as for younger patients, and that older patients should not be denied adjuvant treatment based only on age.[40]

Conclusion

The skin cancers are a major public health problem. To decrease the mortality and morbidity, efforts must be focused on primary and secondary prevention strategies. Nurses can influence the public to practice these strategies to prevent skin cancers. Late-stage malignant melanoma can be a devastating disease; the side effects of treatment can be horrendous. Health care providers need to design better strategies to address treatment-related side effects.

REVIEW QUESTIONS

✓ Case Study

1. Your organization has received a grant to devise and implement a community-wide educational and skin cancer screening program at your hospitals based in Denver, Colorado and Orlando, Florida. You, as an oncology nurse, have been asked to be the lead for this project. Why were Denver and Orlando selected for this project?
   a. The number of Caucasians living in these areas
   b. The elevation of these locations
   c. The higher incidence of skin cancer in these areas
   d. The support there is for these types of educational programs in these communities

2. You have been asked to use decreased mortality as the indicator of success in regard to the screening portion of this grant. What is the primary explanation for the difficulty of measuring decreased mortality as an outcome of skin cancer screening programs?
   a. Fact that optimal follow-up time being 5 to 10 years later
   b. Cost of program set-up and follow-through
   c. Decreased access to healthcare
   d. Failure of participants to do monthly self–skin examinations

3. You are working on a primary prevention program. What is one important fact you know?
   a. Skin cancer may be the ideal cancer for prevention because the risk factors for its development are well known.
   b. Screening for skin cancer is low-cost.
   c. Screening for skin cancer has a minimum false-positive finding.
   d. Many insurers pay for skin cancer screening.

4. What are skin cancer prevention measures that you would educate the public about?
   a. Avoid all sunlight, use sunscreens with a higher than 15 SPF, wear comfortable attire, and perform weekly self–skin exams
   b. Avoid afternoon sunlight, use sunscreens with a higher than 30 SPF, wear comfortable attire, and perform monthly self–skin exams
   c. Avoid intense sunlight, use sunscreens with a 15 SPF, wear protective attire, and perform monthly self–skin exams
   d. Avoid intense sunlight, use sunscreens with a higher than 10 SPF, wear cool attire, and perform weekly self–skin exams

5. During a presentation at a cosmetology program, a student tells you she has been using a tanning salon to get a tan to prevent summer sunburns for the last 3 years. She is blonde, with blue eyes, and usually burns with light tanning. Her grandfather died of melanoma 10 years ago. She is 22 years old. She feels that getting a tan from the tanning salon will decrease her chance of skin cancer later in life. If she cannot get to the tanning salon, she uses a sunless tanning agent to protect her skin. What learning needs does this participant have?
   a. None: she is correct; the tan from the salon is a safer tan than a tan from the sun; this and the sunless tanning agent provides her with protection from sun damage.
   b. Tanning salons do not provide a safe tan; indoor tanning can be a risk factor for skin cancer development.
   c. Tanning salons use the type of ultraviolet light that is less damaging than a natural suntan, but the tan that occurs from indoor tanning does not prevent sunburns.
   d. She has a higher risk for skin cancer; the tanning salon does not prevent damage from the sun, and the use of self-tanning agents will not protect her skin from natural or artificial light.

6. During the skin cancer-screening program, a participant shows you a pathology report from his wife; it indicates she has basal cell carcinoma (BCC). What are types of BCC?
   a. Nodular, superficial, pigmented, keratonic, and verrucous
   b. Nodular, superficial, pigmented, and morpheaform
   c. Composed nevus, seborrheic keratosis, nodular, pigmented, and actinic chelitis
   d. Morpheaform, keratonic, superficial, junctional nevi, and simple lentigo

7. The skin cancers are a major public health problem. To decrease morbidity and mortality of the skin cancers, many health care providers are shifting their efforts to primary and secondary prevention. What is an example of tertiary prevention of skin cancer?
   a. Tertiary efforts would focus on the prevention and detection of additional primary skin cancers.
   b. Tertiary efforts would focus on the siblings of patients diagnosed with skin cancer.
   c. Tertiary efforts would focus on the children of skin cancer survivors.
   d. Tertiary efforts would focus on palliative care for late-stage melanoma patients.

8. What are some of the most important prognostic factors in melanoma?
   a. Clark's level and presence of regional lymph node involvement
   b. Breslow's thickness and presence of node involvement
   c. Location of primary lesion and depth of lesion
   d. Melanoma type, diagnostic evaluation, and treatment modality

9. You are working on a busy medical oncology unit, caring for a male bone marrow transplant patient. He has a history of transplant-related low platelet counts and Raynaud's phenomenon. His hemoglobin and hematocrit levels are stable at low normal value. His posttransfusion platelet count is 75,000, and the absolute neutrophil count (ANC) is 2,000. You are told to send the patient to the dermatology clinic for cryosurgery for the removal of a 2-mm basal cell carcinoma located on the face. What are some considerations before sending the patient?
   a. The patient must give informed consent before the procedure.
   b. Given the low platelet count and Raynaud's phenomenon, cryosurgery might not be the best procedure for the patient.
   c. The patient has a low white cell count and is at risk for infection.
   d. The patient will not heal well after the procedure because of his transplant, and he will require dressing changes when he goes home.

10. You are working in a busy outpatient oncology clinic when a concerned daughter approaches you about the treatment plan for her 69-year-old mother. The daughter is very concerned that a 69-year-old woman cannot possibly undergo both surgery and chemotherapy for skin cancer. As an oncology nurse you know which of the following?
    a. Patients at this age are at risk for complications when both surgery and chemotherapy are used to treat cancer.
    b. The daughter is controlling and the decision for treatment is up to the patient.
    c. Treatment for patients older than 65 should be as aggressive as for younger patients, and older patients should not be denied adjuvant treatment based only on age.
    d. Patients of this age are prone to developing many different types of skin cancer.

ANSWERS

1. **C.** *Rationale:* A and B are risk factors that can lead to the possible development of skin cancer, but choice C combines these risk factors.
2. **A.** *Rationale:* Skin cancers do cause death, but often there is as much as a 20-year time lag from diagnosis to end point. Patients may be "lost" to the study because of attrition, relocation, and comorbidities amongst other reasons.
3. **A.** *Rationale:* The risk factors for skin cancer are well known, allowing for prevention techniques to be identified.
4. **C.** *Rationale:* Self-exams should be done monthly, and protective clothing is the correct response, not comfortable clothing. Avoiding all sunlight is not a practical suggestion.
5. **D.** *Rationale:* She is at risk because of her fair complexion, hair coloring, and family history. Self-tanning agents are simply a color applied to the skin. Tanning salons do not provide "safer" tan; the tan provided increases the risk of skin cancer.
6. **B.** *Rationale:* There are five types of basal skin cancer: nodular, superficial, pigmented, morpheaform, and basosquamous.
7. **A.** *Rationale:* Skin cancers can reoccur. Tertiary efforts focus on cancer survivors.
8. **B.** *Rationale:* Breslow's thickness is the crucial parameter of vertical tumor thickness—from the top to the granular base of the tumor. It is considered the "gold standard" for determining a patient's risk of metastatic disease. Nodal involvement is the second most important prognostic indicator.
9. **B.** *Rationale:* Low platelet count could predispose the patient to bleeding. Although healing could be delayed because of the patient's immunosuppression, cryosurgery is contraindicated in Raynaud's syndrome and should not be used on the face because it can cause hyperpigmentation.
10. **C.** *Rationale:* The treatment plan for a patient should be based on the physical condition of the patient not on the age of the patient.

REFERENCES

1. Jermal A, Taylor M, Ward E: Cancer statistics 2005, *CA Cancer J Clin* 55(1):10-30, 2005.
2. Vargo N: Basal and squamous cell carcinoma, *Semin Oncol Nurs* 19(1): 12-21, 2003.
3. Saraiya M, Glantz K, Briss, PA et al: Interventions to prevent skin cancer by reducing exposure to ultraviolet radiation, *Am J Prev Med* 27(5): 422-466, 2004.
4. American Cancer Society: *Cancer facts and figures, 2005*, Atlanta, 2005, Author.
5. Goldstein B, Goldstein AO: Diagnosis and management of malignant melanoma, *Am Fam Physician* 63(7):1359-1368, 2001.
6. Gilchrest B, Eller M, Geller AC et al: Mechanisms of disease: the pathogenesis of melanoma induced by ultraviolet radiation, *N Engl J Med* 340(17):1341-1348, 1999.
7. Geller AC, Annas G: Epidemiology of melanoma and nonmelanoma skin cancer, *Semin Oncol Nurs* 19(1)2-11, 2003.
8. Nguyen TH, Quynh-Dao D: Nonmelanoma skin cancer, *Curr Treatment Option Oncol* 3:193-203, 2002.
9. National Cancer Institute: Background on skin cancer, Reported by Sarah Schroeder July 1, 2003, retrieved June 13, 2005, from www.cancer.gov.
10. Richmond E, Viner JL: Chemoprevention of skin cancer, *Semin Oncol Nurs* 19(1):62-69, 2003.
11. Langhorne M: Skin cancers. In Otto S, editor: *Oncology nursing*, ed 4, St. Louis, 2001, Mosby.
12. Karagas MR, Stannard VA, Mott, LA et al: Use of tanning devices and risk of basal cell and squamous cell skin cancers, *J Natl Cancer Inst* 94(3):224-226, 2002.
13. U.S. Preventive Services Task Force: Counseling to prevent skin cancer: recommendation and rationale, *Am J Nurs* 104(4)87-91,2004.
14. Hill D: Skin cancer prevention: a commentary, *Am J Prev Med* 27(5):482-483, 2004.
15. American Cancer Society: American Cancer Society guidelines for the early detection of cancer, *CA Cancer J Clin* 51(2):81-88, 2001.
16. Gross E: Non-melanoma skin cancer: clues to early detection, keys to effective treatment, *Consultant* 39(3):829, 1999.
17. Margolin KA, Sondak VK: Melanoma and other skin cancer. In Pazdur R, Coua LR, Hoskins WJ et al, editors: *Cancer management: a multidisciplinary approach* Manhasset, NY, 2004, CMP Healthcare Media.
18. Apgar B: A comparison of treatments for basal cell carcinoma, *Am Fam Physician* 61(5):1460, 2000.
19. Levi F, LaVecchia C, Te C et al: What is the risk of a second invasive cancer following basal cell carcinoma? *Arch Dermatol* 135(12): 1531, 1999.
20. Iyer S, Bowes L, Kricorian G et al: Treatment of basal cell carcinoma with pulsed carbon dioxide laser: a retrospective analysis, *Dermatol Surg* 30(9)1214-1218, 2004.
21. Food and Drug Administration: FDA approves new use of drug to treat superficial basal cell carcinoma, a type of skin cancer *FDA News* P04-66 July 15, 2004, retrieved February 17, 2005, from www.fda.gov.
22. Silapunt S, Goldberg H, Alam M: Topical and light-based treatments for actinic keratosis, *Sem Cutan Med Surg* 22(3)162-170, 2003.
23. Rigel DS, Carucci JA: Self-examination of the skin, *CA Cancer J Clin* 4(50):223-226, 2000.
24. Bedingfield FC: The melanoma epidemic: res ipsa loquitur, *Oncologist* 8(5):459-465, 2003.
25. Rigel DS, Carucci JA: Malignant melanoma: prevention, early detection and treatment in the 21st century, *CA Cancer J Clin* 4(50):215-235, 2000.
26. National Cancer Institute: Melanoma PDQ® treatment, health professional version February 1, 2005, retrieved May 17, 2005, from www.nci.nih.gov on 5/17/05.
27. Edman RL, Klaus SN: Is routine screening for melanoma a benign practice? *JAMA* 284(7):883-886, 2000.
28. Oliveria S, Dusza S, Berwick M: Issues in the epidemiology of melanoma, *Expert Rev Anticancer Ther* 1(3):453-459, 2001.
29. Reed J, Albino A: Update of diagnostic and prognostic markers in cutaneous malignant melanoma, *Dermatol Clin* 17(3):631-643, 1999.
30. Lamb LA, Halpern AC, Hwu WJ: Diagnosis and management of stage I/II melanoma. *Semin Oncol Nurs* 19(1):22-31, 2003.
31. Pitts J, Maloney M: Therapeutic advances in melanoma, *Dermatol Clin* 18(1):157-167, 2000.

32. Oncology Nursing Society: *Sentinel lymph node biopsy: current status,* 1999 Annual Congress-Symposia Highlights:1-2, 1999.

33. Centers for Disease Control and Prevention: Management of possible sexual, injecting-drug-use, or other non-occupational exposure to HIV including considerations related to antiretroviral therapy. Public Health Service Statement *MMWR* September 25, 1998 (RR-17). Reviewed 5/5/05,retrieved June 10, 2005, from www.cdc.gov.

34. Scadden D: Neoplasm in Acquired immunodeficiency syndrome. In Holland JF, Frei E, editors: *Cancer medicine,* ed 6, London, 2003, BC Decker.

35. Safai B: Kaposi's sarcoma and acquired immunodeficiency syndrome. In DeVita VT, Hillman S, Rosenberg S, editors: *AIDS: etiology, diagnosis, treatment and prevention,* ed 4, Philadelphia, 1997, Lippincott-Raven.

36. National Cancer Institute: Kaposi's sarcoma PDQ(r) treatment, health professional version, September 29, 2003, retrieved June 13, 2005, from www.nci.nih.gov on 6/13/05.

37. Christos PJ, Oliveria S, Berwick M et all: Signs and symptoms of melanoma in older populations, *J Clin Epidemiol* 53(10):1044-1053, 2000.

38. Geller AC, Sober AJ, Zhang Z et al: Strategies for improving melanoma education and screening for men age > or = 50 years: findings from the American Academy of Dermatological National Skin Cancer Screening Program, *Cancer* 95(7):1554-1561, 2002.

39. Noorda EM, Vrouenraets BC, Nieweg OE et al: Safety and efficacy of isolated limb perfusion in elderly melanoma patients, *Ann Surg Oncol* 9(10):939-940, 2002.

40. Chang Ck, Jacobs IA, Theodosiou E et al: Thick melanoma in the elderly, *Am Surg* 69(11):988-993, 2003.

41. Tsao H, Bevona C, Goggins W et al: The transformation rate of moles (melanocytic nevi) into cutaneous melanoma, *Arch Dermat* 139(3):282-288, 2003.

42. Swetter SM, Geller AC, Kirkwood JM: Melanoma in the older person, *Oncology* 18(9):1187-1196, 2004.

CHAPTER 18

Pediatric Oncology

Nancy King, Melissa Christensen,
Molly S. Hemenway, Jennifer R. Madden,
Angela Carrie Peltz, and Elizabeth Pounder

Introduction

Approximately 12,000 new cases of cancer in children and adolescents are diagnosed annually in the United States. The most common malignancies of childhood are leukemia (25%), central nervous system tumors (17%), and lymphomas (16%). Other, less common diagnoses include sympathetic nervous system tumors, soft tissue tumors, bone tumors, renal tumors, tumors of the retina, and germ cell tumors. The incidence of cancer is highest in the 0- to 4-year-old and 15- to 19-year-old age groups.[1] In general, boys are more likely to develop cancer than girls, and white children are more prone than black children.

The cause of cancer in children is not fully understood. Malignant cell transformation in children is most likely multifactorial, representing an interplay of genetic, immunologic, environmental, and socioeconomic factors. The role of lifestyle choices and exposures in children is less clear than in adults, where many types of cancer are known to be preventable by lifestyle changes and avoidance of known carcinogens. Consequently, there are no screening tools currently in use for childhood cancers and no known preventive measures other than avoidance of known carcinogens.

The overall survival rate for children with cancer is currently 77%; however, childhood cancer remains the fourth cause of death under the age of 20 years and the primary cause of death from illness in children between the ages of 1 and 15 years in the United States.[1] Treatment for childhood cancer has advanced rapidly, largely as a result of the early creation of interinstitutional study groups for this population. Cooperation between institutions has enabled the development of standards of care for various types of cancer and continues to generate research and education to improve the lives of children affected by cancer.

The Leukemias

Epidemiology

Leukemias are the most common pediatric malignancy, with approximately 3000 new cases diagnosed annually in the United States. The majority of leukemias in childhood are acute leukemias. Acute lymphoblastic leukemia (ALL) is a malignancy of lymphocytes and accounts for approximately 75% of all leukemias diagnosed in children and adolescents.[2] Acute myeloid leukemia (AML) arises from the myelocytic cell line and represents about 20% of childhood leukemias, with approximately 500 new cases diagnosed annually in the United States.[3] Juvenile myelomonocytic leukemia and chronic myelocytic leukemia are both seen in childhood and adolescence, but are rare. The average age at diagnosis is between 2 and 5 years. Boys are affected more often than girls at a ratio of approximately 1.2:1.

White children have a twofold risk of developing leukemia compared to black children.[2]

Etiology and Risk Factors

Chromosomal abnormalities associated with an increased risk of leukemia include Bloom's syndrome and Fanconi's anemia. Blackfan-Diamond syndrome, neurofibromatosis, familial monosomy 7, and *p53* mutation. Children with trisomy 21 have a twentyfold chance of developing leukemia compared to the general population.[4] Immunodeficiency syndromes such as ataxia-telangiectasia and Wiscott-Aldrich also have an increased incidence of leukemia. An identical twin under the age of 7 years has approximately a 20% chance of developing leukemia if the other twin is affected. Siblings of a child with cancer have twice to 4 times the risk compared to the general population; however, reports are rare.[2]

ACUTE LYMPHOBLASTIC LEUKEMIA (ALL)

Etiology

The precise cause of ALL is unknown. Although it is known that exposures to ionizing radiation, benzene, and chemotherapeutic agents have been directly linked to the development of leukemia, exposure of children to these substances is not common. Several of the translocations common in ALL are known to be present prenatally at a rate 100 times that of leukemia. This suggests that although mutagenesis occurs during embryonic development, there must be another triggering event that induces development of the leukemic clone. Postulated, but not yet proven, triggers include maternal dietary intake of compounds such as flavonoids, indoor exposure to pesticides, and low folate intake during pregnancy.[5]

Classification

ALL can develop at any point along the lymphocytic lineage and therefore can be of B- or T-cell origin. Immunophenotyping of lymphoblasts provides an accurate classification system for the subtypes of leukemia. ALL is further classified into risk factors based upon age, presenting symptoms, and cytogenetic findings.

Clinical Features

Presenting signs and symptoms depend upon the degree to which the bone marrow has been replaced or tissues infiltrated by the leukemic cells. The onset of symptoms is often insidious and attributed to more common childhood illnesses. The duration of presenting symptoms can vary from several weeks to several months.

Anemia presents as pallor, lethargy, and fatigue. Petecchiae, ecchymosis, and bleeding are the result of thrombocytopenia, and infection can occur when the circulating neutrophils are diminished. Bone pain and arthralgias are caused by periosteal involvement of the long bones. The liver and the spleen may be enlarged and cause abdominal pain. Nonspecific fever is also common and may indicate infection, or may be a result of cytokine production by the lymphoblasts.

Lymphadenopathy is present in approximately 40% of children with ALL.[2] Acute-onset respiratory distress and superior vena cava syndrome can result from enlarged mediastinal nodes, especially in children with T-cell ALL.

Diagnosis

The diagnosis of leukemia is most commonly made when children have sufficient circulating lymphoblasts in their peripheral blood to be seen on a complete blood count. The definitive test is a bone marrow aspirate and biopsy. The cerebrospinal fluid (CSF) is also sampled to determine the presence of lymphoblasts in the spinal fluid.

Prognostic Indicators

The most significant prognostic factors for childhood ALL are age at diagnosis, the white blood cell (WBC) count at the time of diagnosis, and the presence and extent of central nervous system (CNS) disease. New studies discount sex as a significant predictor for outcome.[6] Cytogenetics and molecular factors are also critical in determining prognosis and treatment. Favorable cytogenetic features include the *TEL/AML* rearrangement, and trisomy of chromosomes 4, 10, and 17. Unfavorable cytogenetic features include the 11q23 abnormality and presence of the Philadelphia chromosome.[7] Hyperdiploidy is generally a favorable prognostic indicator, whereas fewer than 45 chromosomes is unfavorable.[6]

Approximately 3% of children will have evidence of CNS involvement with leukemic blasts seen in the cerebral spinal fluid at diagnosis.[8] Children with CNS disease are usually asymptomatic, but occasionally will first be seen with complaints of headache, cranial nerve palsies, or complaints of vision changes. CNS status is determined by the number of white blood cells on the spinal fluid differential and the number of blasts seen in the cytospin preparation. CNS status is graded from CNS1 (fewer than 5 WBC and no lymphoblasts) to CNS3 (more than 5 WBC and presence of lymphoblasts).

Based upon these factors, ALL is subcategorized by immunophenotype and further categorized into three risk categories: standard risk, high risk, and very high risk. Separate categories apply to infants and to children with mature B-cell leukemia. Table 18-1 displays the subtypes of ALL and associated prognostic factors.

Medical Treatment and Nursing Care Considerations

CHEMOTHERAPY

Current treatment for standard and high risk ALL consists of chemotherapy lasting about 30 months for girls and 36 months for boys. Treatment is longer for males because of their risk for testicular relapse, and because males tend to have a higher incidence of bone marrow and CNS relapse than females for reasons not completely understood.[6] The initial phase of therapy, induction,

lasts for approximately 4 weeks and is intended to eradicate the leukemic blasts and induce remission, defined as less than 5% lymphoblasts in the bone marrow with normal marrow cellularity and resolution of clinical disease. Initial CNS prophylaxis with intrathecal chemotherapy agents is given at time of diagnosis. During induction, the child's bone marrow will be significantly suppressed and the risk for infection is high. Ninety-five percent of children will be in remission by the end of induction; those that are not have a poorer prognosis and require more aggressive chemotherapy.[8]

The second phase, consolidation, aims to solidify the remission and provide prophylaxis against CNS disease. During this phase, the child will require frequent lumbar punctures to administer intrathecal chemotherapy in addition to systemic chemotherapy.

Following consolidation, maintenance chemotherapy is initiated. Additional intensified phases are interspersed in some treatment plans. During maintenance, most children are able to return to their normal activities and generally feel well.

Children with very high-risk disease may require a hematopoietic stem cell transplant to have their best chance for survival. If transplant is indicated and a donor match is available, these children will go to transplant as soon as they are in remission.

Nursing Care Considerations. Immediate care priorities are directed toward stabilizing the newly diagnosed child hemodynamically, maintaining adequate renal function, providing appropriate pain management, and supporting the child and family psychosocially and spiritually. Neutrophils may not function normally, even with an adequate percentage represented in the complete blood count (CBC), leaving persons newly diagnosed with leukemia at very high risk for bacteremia and sepsis. Children who are febrile receive immediate intravenous antibiotics following blood and other symptom-appropriate cultures.

Family education in anticipation of discharge starts at the time of diagnosis. Teaching includes information about the disease and the treatment, home care needs such as central line care and medication administration, and education about infection risk, preventive measures, and response to fever.

RADIATION

Cranial irradiation is used, in addition to intrathecal chemotherapy, only in cases of overt CNS disease and for those at very high risk for CNS relapse.

Disease-Related Complications and Treatment

The most common complication of leukemia therapy is infection resulting from neutropenia and immunosuppression. Preventive measures include teaching parents about neutropenia, preventing exposures to ill contacts, and good general hygiene at home. Children are usually started on combination sulfamethoxazole and trimethoprim to help prevent acquisition of *Pneumocystis jiroveci*. Children may also be prescribed oral antifungal medications to prevent candidal infection, especially when receiving high-dose steroids or prolonged antibiotic courses. Children who are neutropenic and febrile require prompt medical evaluation and initiation of broad spectrum antibiotic therapy. Because neutrophil production is markedly decreased, children may not develop significant redness, infiltrates, or swelling. Consequently, it is important to listen to the child's complaints and the parent's observations, and to assess the child carefully for areas of pain or tenderness.

TABLE 18-1 **Classification of ALL Subtypes**

IMMUNOLOGIC CLASSIFICATION	RISK ASSIGNMENT AND PROGNOSIS	ASSOCIATED PROGNOSTIC FACTORS
Pre–B-cell 80%–85% of childhood ALLs	**Standard** WBC <50,000/mm³ Age between 1 and 10 years No CNS involvement Cure rate 80%–85%	*TEL/AML1* rearrangement, hyperdiploidy (>50 chromosomes), and trisomy 4,10, and 17 are favorable factors
	High Age older than 10 and/or WBC >50,000/mm³ Cure rate 70%	Higher WBC associated with increased incidence of CNS disease
Mature B-cell ~5% of childhood ALLs	Cure rate 80% with aggressive treatment	t(8;14)
Infant	Age less than 1 year (infants less than 6 months have poorest prognosis) Cure rate approximately 50%	11q23 abnormality in 60%–80% of cases *MLL* rearrangement is poor prognostic sign
T-cell 15%–17% of childhood ALLs	Standard Cure rate 80% with aggressive treatment	Associated with males, older age at diagnosis, leukocytosis, and higher incidence of extramedullary disease, especially mediastinal mass Favorable factors: *HOX11* overexpression and t(11;19) with *MLL-ENL* fusion
	High Cure rate 70%	Leukocyte count >100,000 at diagnosis has higher incidence of CNS relapse Poor marrow response at day 7 is unfavorable prognostic factor
	Very high Cure rate 70% with bone marrow transplant	Presence of *BCR/ABL* translocation [Philadelphia chromosome; t(9;22)], *MLL* rearrangement, hypoploidy (less than 44 chromosomes), slow response to induction therapy

ALL, Acute lymphoblastic leukemia; *CNS*, central nervous system; *WBC*, white blood cell count.

Leukemic cells have a short life span. When large numbers of leukemia cells are present at diagnosis, the rapid cell turnover induced when initiating chemotherapy can release large amounts of intracellular components such as potassium, uric acid, and phosphorus into the extracellular space. Tumor lysis syndrome (TLS) is the result of these metabolic abnormalities and can rapidly lead to renal impairment and, ultimately, renal failure. The risk for TLS is highest in children who have very high WBC counts or extensive extramedullary disease. Aggressive treatment with intravenous hydration, alkalinization, electrolyte management, xanthine inhibitors or blockers, and phosphorus binders can prevent renal damage in the majority of cases.

Prognosis

About 85% of children with standard-risk ALL and 65% of those with high-risk disease can expect to achieve cure. Children who enter treatment with CNS3 disease are at increased risk for treatment failure. CNS2 disease may portend an increased risk for relapse, but this may be overcome by intensifying intrathecal chemotherapy.[9]

Despite the best therapy known to date, however, some children do experience relapse of their disease. Common sites of relapse are the bone marrow, the central nervous system and, in males, the testicles. Children who relapse during the first year after completion of chemotherapy have only a 10% to 20% chance of survival, whereas those who relapse after more than a year off therapy have at least a 40% to 65% chance of regaining a curable remission. For these children, hematopoietic stem cell transplant (HSCT) is a viable option if a donor match is available.[8]

ACUTE MYELOID LEUKEMIA

Epidemiology and Risk Factors

As in ALL, boys and whites are more commonly afflicted. AML has a double peak: in children less than 2 years of age and in young adolescents.[10] Children with Down syndrome are at higher risk for AML, as are children with neurofibromatosis, ataxia-telangiectasia, Bloom's syndrome, and Fanconi's anemia. AML as a second malignancy has been seen after treatment with alkylating drugs such as cyclophosphamide, and topoisomerase II inhibitors such as etoposide.

Etiology

Like ALL, the cause of AML is not fully understood, although translocations common to AML can also be seen during fetal development.[5]

Classification

As seen in Table 18-2, there are eight currently known subtypes of AML as classified by the French-British-American (FAB) system. The majority of children will be seen with M1 or M2 subtypes. Infants and children under the age of 2 years primarily are seen with M4 AML, which carries a very poor prognosis. The M5 and M6 subtypes are extremely rare and respond poorly to chemotherapy. M4, M5, and M6 subtypes are best treated by HSCT, initiated as soon as possible. The M7 subtype is seen in children under the age of 3 and children with Down syndrome. Children with Down syndrome generally do well with chemotherapy treatment alone; however, children without Down syndrome have a less favorable outcome, and HSCT is the treatment of choice.

Clinical Features

Children with AML often are more ill when they first come for treatment than children with ALL. They may have a concomitant infection and/or have experienced bleeding episodes around the time of diagnosis. The WBC is generally elevated, averaging 25,000/mm^3. Thrombocytopenia, neutropenia, and anemia are usually quite profound. Bone pain is less commonly seen in AML than in ALL. Children with AML are more likely to have extramedullary disease in the liver, the spleen, the soft tissues, the gums, and the skin. Chloromas, localized masses of leukemic cells, can be found in the orbital area, the soft tissues, the bones, and the central nervous system and may cause pain, soft tissue swelling, and nerve palsies. CNS disease is seen primarily in infants and in children who enter treatment with a WBC greater than 100,000/mm^3.

Diagnosis

The definitive test for AML is a bone marrow aspiration and biopsy. As in ALL, the CSF is also sampled to assess for CNS disease. Immunophenotyping and cytogenetic testing is done to identify the specific subtype and determine treatment.

Medical Treatment and Nursing Care Considerations

CHEMOTHERAPY

In general, AML presents a challenging treatment course. Chemotherapy is aggressive and of short duration, averaging 6 months. Common chemotherapeutic agents include cytarabine, daunorubicin, etoposide, and mitoxantrone.

The M3 subtype is somewhat unique in its presentation. Though highly curable, the mortality risk during induction is high from hemorrhage caused by release of procoagulants from the promyelocytes during lysis. This risk has been significantly decreased by the administration of all-trans retinoic acid (ATRA) during induction. ATRA induces promyelocytes to mature into myelocytes, which do not contain procoagulants.

Nursing Considerations. The child with AML will be profoundly neutropenic for an extended period of time after chemotherapy. Prevention of infection and meticulous assessment for signs of infection are a priority for these patients. Pneumocystis prophylaxis and oral antifungals are usually given in an effort to prevent infections. Treatment with cytarabine, a mainstay of AML therapy, increases the risk of infection with alpha streptococcus. As with ALL, children with AML require prompt assessment and intervention for fevers or other signs of illness.

TABLE 18-2 Classification of AML Subtypes

FAB SUBTYPE	PATHOLOGIC DESCRIPTION	COMMON CYTOGENETIC ABNORMALITIES
M0—Acute nonlymphocytic leukemia (ANL) without maturation	Large agranular, poorly differentiated blasts expressing at least 1 myeloid antigen	Trisomy 8, del(5), del(7)—seen in all subtypes
M1—ANL with poor maturation	Poorly differentiated with occasional Auer rods	t(8;21)
M2—ANL with maturation Most common type of AML	Myeloblasts resemble immature neutrophils, Auer rods may be prominent	t(8;21), inv(16)
M3—Acute promyelocytic leukemia (APL)	Hypergranular blasts with bundles of Auer rods (faggoting) and a grooved or bi-lobed nucleus M3v is a variant that may mimic acute monocytic leukemia	t(15;17)
M4—Acute myelomonocytic leukemia	20%-80% monoblasts M4Eo variant has >5% eosinophilic precursors	t(9;11), inv(16), t(11;19), MLL rearrangements
M5—Acute monocytic leukemia	>80% monoblasts, promonocytes, or monocytes	t(9;11), t(11;19) MLL rearrangements
M6—Erythroleukemia	>50% erythroblasts and >30% myeloblasts	
M7—Acute megakaryocytic leukemia	>30% megakaryoblasts Bone marrow fibrosis common	t(1;22)

AML, Acute myeloid leukemia; FAB, French-American-British.

Treatment of AML causes profound bone marrow suppression. Consequently, children with AML may require blood product support with packed red blood cell and platelet transfusions. Preparation of the child and family for blood product transfusion is essential and includes information about the specific blood product, safety, the possibility of reaction, and expected outcomes.

Children with AML often experience more frequent and prolonged hospitalizations for chemotherapy and fevers. Some treatment protocols necessitate hospitalization until count recovery following high dose chemotherapy regimens because of the high risk of life-threatening sepsis in this population. Nurses are key providers of support to families during these stressful times.

HEMATOPOIETIC STEM CELL TRANSPLANT

HSCT may be an option for children with myeloid leukemia who have a matched sibling donor once remission is achieved. Unrelated donors and partial matched transplants are not used at this time since the success rate with chemotherapy alone surpasses the current success rate with these types of transplants.

Disease-Related Complications and Treatment

Because of the aggressive nature of the treatment, marrow recovery is slow and the risk of fungal infections is high throughout the duration of therapy. Fungal infections are generally acquired from the environment. It is helpful to restrict exposure of profoundly immunosuppressed patients to areas where fungus is likely to breed, such as construction sites and damp or moldy rooms. Use of a respiratory mask when outdoors may also be protective. Fungal infection may be suspected when defervescence does not occur despite broad-spectrum antibiotic therapy. Computed tomography (CT) scans of the sinuses, chest, and abdomen are done for fungal surveillance at this time. Antifungal medications such as amphotericin are usually initiated empirically.

Fungal infections are extremely serious and sometimes fatal. Families dealing with one need support, education, and encouragement. Nursing assessment of the child's condition and response to therapy is crucial, as well as attention to the child and family's emotional and psychologic well-being.

Prognosis

The overall survival rate for AML is 40% to 45%. Children who experience relapse of their disease have a very poor prognosis and require HCST for their best chance of survival.[1]

MYELODYSPLASTIC AND MYELOPROLIFERATIVE DISEASES

Myelodysplastic syndromes (MDSs) are disorders of hematopoiesis characterized by anemia, thrombocytopenia, and neutropenia. Predisposing factors include Down syndrome and other chromosomal abnormalities, Fanconi's anemia, and prior exposure to alkylating chemotherapy agents. Monosomy 7 is frequently seen in MDS. In children, MDS often progresses to AML. HSCT is the treatment of choice.

Myeloproliferative diseases are characterized by overproduction of cells of monocytic and granulocytic lineage. It is seen most commonly in the toddler and older infant age group and presents with splenomegaly, pallor, infection, skin bleeding, and cough.

When the absolute monocyte count exceeds 1×10^9, a diagnosis of juvenile myelomonocytic leukemia (JMML) is made. About 25% of patients with JMML will have monosomy 7; the remainder will have normal karyotypes. HCST is the treatment of choice since JMML does not achieve a durable response to chemotherapy.[3,6]

Chronic myelogenous leukemia (CML) is a myeloproliferative disorder that is characteristically associated with the presence of the Philadelphia chromosome in the leukemic clone. CML is extremely rare in childhood. The treatment of choice is allogeneic HSCT. Hydroxyurea is used to keep white blood cell proliferation in check to allow time for treatment planning. Imatinib mesylate (Gleevec) is a new agent that specifically targets the oncogenic protein tyrosine kinase produced by the Philadelphia chromosome. This drug may be useful in reducing the leukemic blast population in patients who are transplant candidates.[12]

Lymphomas

Lymphomas are malignant tumors of lymphoid origin and can arise any place in the body where lymphoid tissue is present. Lymphomas are classified as either Hodgkin's lymphoma, also referred to as Hodgkin's disease, or non-Hodgkin's lymphoma. Lymphomas represent about 12% of pediatric cancers; non-Hodgkin's lymphoma predominates, accounting for about 60% of all lymphoma cases in children under the age of 15 years.[13]

HODGKIN'S LYMPHOMA

Epidemiology

Hodgkin's lymphoma is a lymphoid malignancy whose unique characteristics include the presence of Reed-Sternberg cells seen in an environment of normal inflammatory cells in the lymph node tissue.[14] Rare before the age of 5, Hodgkin's lymphoma has a double peak, one in the older adolescent/young adult age groups and the other in late adulthood. In children under 10 years of age, Hodgkin's lymphoma occurs almost twice as frequently in boys as in girls; in adolescence the incidence equalizes.[15]

Etiology

The cause of Hodgkin's disease is not known. There is an increased incidence in children with immunologic disorders. The Epstein-Barr virus (EBV) has been implicated as a potential cofactor in the development of Hodgkin's disease; however, the connection is not entirely clear.[14]

Classification

Four histologic types of Hodgkin's disease are currently recognized: nodular sclerosis, mixed cellularity, lymphocyte-predominant, and lymphocytic-depleted. Approximately 70% of adolescents and 40% of younger children will develop the nodular sclerosing form. Mixed cellularity is seen in approximately 30% and is more common in children less than 10 years of age and in those with human immunodeficiency virus (HIV) infection. The lymphocyte-predominant type is seen in only 10% to 15% of cases and is more common in boys. The lymphocyte-depleted subtype is rarely seen in children.[14]

Clinical Features

The most common initial findings are enlarged, painless, firm, nonmobile cervical or supraclavicular lymph nodes. Mediastinal enlargement is seen in about 50% of patients and may compress or deviate the airway, causing symptoms of airway obstruction.[15] Splenomegaly may be present; hepatomegaly is uncommon. Anorexia, fatigue, and weight loss are commonly noted. Bone marrow involvement and metastatic disease in the liver, the lungs, and the bones can also be seen.

Diagnosis

The definitive diagnostic test is a lymph node biopsy. Other diagnostic tests include a chest x-ray to look for mediastinal enlargement and CT scans of the chest, the abdomen, and the pelvis. Positron emission tomography (PET) scans are becoming an increasingly popular modality to look for sites of disease and to follow clinical response. Patients with Hodgkin's lymphoma may have elevated levels of serum copper, fibrinogen, and serum ferritin, as well as elevated sedimentation rates.

Staging

Based upon extent of disease and histology, the patient's disease is staged as I, II, III, or IV and as A or B based upon the absence or presence of B symptoms. B symptoms are defined as unexplained weight loss of more than 10% of body weight over a 6-month period, recurrent or persistent fever above 38° C, and night sweats. B symptoms are seen in about one quarter of patients and are commonly associated with widespread or locally extensive disease. The presence of B symptoms is an unfavorable prognostic factor.[14]

Medical Treatment and Nursing Care Considerations

Treatment of Hodgkin's disease in children and adolescents is the same as for adults. The majority of patients with Hodgkin's disease will be teenagers and young adults. Along with disease and treatment information, nursing measures include support and education to help the young person cope with the impact of treatment, hair loss, and other side effects at a critical time in their emotional and social development.

Prognosis

Patients with stage I and II disease have a 90% chance of disease-free survival; those with more advanced disease do less well, but can achieve a 70% or better chance of survival.[15] Patients who relapse following completion of chemotherapy may be eligible for HSCT.

NON-HODGKIN'S LYMPHOMA

Epidemiology

Non-Hodgkin's lymphoma (NHL) is a disease of lymphoblastic origin and is closely related to leukemia. NHL is differentiated from leukemia by the presence of bulky disease and less than 25% lymphoblasts in the bone marrow. The median age for NHL is 10 years; it is rare in infants and toddlers under the age of 3 years.[16] NHL is 3 times more common in males, and twice as common in whites. The risk is increased in children with immune deficiency syndromes and those receiving immunosuppressive therapy after transplantation.

Etiology

As with Hodgkin's disease, the etiology is not known. EBV has been associated with the African type of Burkitt's lymphoma, but the causal relationship of this or other viral agents to the development lymphoma is not fully understood.[13]

Classification

NHL, like lymphoblastic leukemia, is classified as either B-cell or T-cell and further subclassified by morphology, histology, and immunophenotype (Table 18-3). The B-cell lymphoma group includes precursor B, mature B or Burkitt's, and diffuse large B-cell and mediastinal large B-cell lymphomas. The T-cell lymphoma group includes precursor T, anaplastic large cell, and peripheral T-cell lymphomas.[16]

Clinical Features

In children, the primary site of disease is extranodal, unlike in adults, who more commonly are first seen with nodal disease. In children, NHL is most frequently an abdominal, head, neck, or mediastinal mass. NHLs are aggressive, rapidly growing tumors, and the majority of children will have hematogenous spread of their disease at diagnosis. The CNS can be involved, which leads to cranial nerve palsies.

Diagnosis

Presenting symptoms usually have an abrupt onset as a result of the rapid growth of the tumor mass. Mediastinal, head, and neck masses may first be noted with respiratory symptoms such as cough, snoring, sleep disturbances, or nasal stuffiness, and earache. Superior vena cava syndrome is a serious complication of mediastinal compression. Abdominal tumors may cause abdominal pain mimicking appendicitis, constipation, or intussusception. Children with NHL are at high risk for TLS when therapy is initiated because of the rapid growth rate of these tumors. Some patients may exhibit signs of TLS even before therapy is begun.

The diagnostic work-up includes appropriate radiologic tests based upon symptoms and site of presentation, measurement of serum lactate hydrogenase (which is an indicator of tumor burden), and sampling of the bone marrow and CSF.

TABLE 18-3 Most Common Types of NHL in Children by WHO Classification	
B-CELL	**T-CELL**
Precursor B–lymphoblastic lymphoma	Precursor T lymphoblastic lymphoma
Mature B-cell (Burkitt's) lymphoma	Anaplastic large cell lymphoma
Diffuse large B-cell lymphoma	Peripheral T-cell lymphoma
Mediastinal large B-cell lymphoma	

WHO, World Health Organization.

Staging

Lymphomas are staged as I, II, III, or IV depending upon the amount and location of nodal and extranodal disease, bone marrow involvement, and CNS disease. Table 18-4 describes the staging criteria for NHL.

Medical Treatment and Nursing Care Considerations

CHEMOTHERAPY

Lymphomas are exquisitely sensitive to chemotherapy. B-cell tumors are treated with short-term, intensive treatment lasting about 6 months. Like ALL, treatment is in three phases: induction, consolidation, and maintenance. Common chemotherapeutic agents include vincristine, cyclophosphamide, methotrexate, and doxorubicin. T-cell lymphomas respond best to the same therapy as that used for T-cell leukemia. All lymphomas require CNS prophylaxis therapy as well as systemic treatment.

The agents used in the treatment of lymphoma are strongly associated with the development of mucositis. Attention to oral hygiene is important to prevent superinfection. Mouth care with soft toothbrushes or sponges should be done at least twice daily. Oral rinses made from topical anesthetics may be helpful, but are not always well tolerated because of their tendency to cause a burning sensation or because of taste. Children who develop mucositis may need narcotic pain medications until the lesions begin to heal. During this time, they may be unable to eat or drink adequately and will likely need nutritional and fluid support.

TABLE 18-4	**Murphy Staging System for Non-Hodgkin's Lymphoma**
Stage 1	Single extranodal mass or single regional nodal involvement, excluding the mediastinum and abdomen
Stage 2	Single extranodal mass with regional node involvement
	Two or more nodal areas on the same side of the diaphragm
	Two single extranodal masses with or without regional node involvement on the same side of the diaphragm
	A primary gastrointestinal tract tumor (usually ileocecal) with or without involvement of mesenteric nodes only
Stage 3	Two single extranodal tumors on opposite sides of the diaphragm
	Two or more nodal areas above and below the diaphragm
	Any primary intrathoracic tumor of the mediastinum, the pleura, or the thymus
	Extensive primary intraabdominal disease
	Paraspinal or epidural tumor with or without additional site involvement
Stage 4	Involvement of the bone marrow or the central nervous system (CNS) in addition to any of the above findings

Adapted from Murphy S, Childhood non-Hodgkins lymphoma, *N Engl J Med* 299:1446-1448, 1978.

RADIATION

Although radiation therapy is no longer used routinely for treatment of NHL, lymphomas are radiosensitive, and it is sometimes used in emergent situations where immediate decompression of the airway, the spinal cord, or the superior vena cava is required.

Support of the child's respiratory status through use of positioning and oxygen may be necessary when airway compression is present. Allowing the child to assume a position of comfort will reduce anxiety associated with impaired oxygenation. Sedation is not given to children with airway compression, and children may need additional support during painful or stressful procedures to help them remain calm and prevent additional airway stress. Families can be assured that most lymphomas respond quickly to radiation and the child usually feels rapid relief from his symptoms of air hunger.

Disease-Related Complications and Treatment

Superior vena cava syndrome (SVC) is a potential complication of tumors in the mediastinum. Tumor compression leads to diminished venous return and is characterized by swelling of the head and neck, cyanosis and plethora, distention of the neck veins, and proptosis. Horner's syndrome can also be seen with SVC. SVC is considered an oncologic emergency. Emergent irradiation of the tumor site and initiation of chemotherapy are done to rapidly shrink the tumor. Nursing interventions include maintaining adequate oxygenation, monitoring vital signs closely, and providing comfort measures. Preparation of the family for diagnostic tests, radiation therapy, and initiation of chemotherapy is critical and often must be done in a minimum of time because of the serious nature of this complication.

TLS is a significant risk for children with NHL. The tumor burden is generally high as a result of the rapid proliferation of the lymphoma, and the chemosensitivity of the cells leads to rapid cell lysis.

Abdominal masses may compress the kidneys or obstruct the intestine. Tumor reduction is achieved with chemotherapy and, if necessary to preserve function, radiation is given. Nursing assessment of the child's condition and progress is key. Intake and output are monitored meticulously. Pain control and other comfort measures are provided around the clock.

Prognosis

Survival for children with NHL is greater than 80%.[16] Relapse can occur, but is not common after treatment is completed.

POSTTRANSPLANT LYMPHOPROLIFERATIVE DISORDER (PTLD)

PTLD is a relatively new disease entity that has come to the forefront with the increasing number of solid organ transplants. PTLD is associated with viral infection by EBV in immunocompromised patients and can present as enlarged lymph nodes or as an extranodal mass. The current trend is to treat these patients with decreased doses of immunosuppressants.[17] If this treatment is not successful, chemotherapy like that for mature B-cell lymphoma is given. Newer experience with a monoclonal antibody, rituximab (Rituxan), is also promising, and research is ongoing.[12]

Tumors of the Central Nervous System

Epidemiology

Brain tumors are the second most common type of pediatric malignancy, the most common solid tumor, and the most common cause of death in children with cancer. Tumors of the CNS occur in 3 out of 100,000 children.[18]

Etiology and Risk Factors

The cause of most pediatric brain and spinal cord tumors is not known.[19,20] Risk factors include a few rare genetic syndromes and a history of therapeutic radiation. Advances in neuroimaging, surgical techniques, radiation therapy, and autologous stem cell rescue have increased the 5-year survival over the last 40 years to 70%.[21-25] High-dose chemotherapy has improved tumor-free survival and helped to obviate or delay radiation to the developing brain.[26,27] In spite of these advances, significant numbers of patients have disease progression. Therefore new strategies are being developed to target specific receptors, control signal transduction, and prevent tumor angiogenesis.[28]

Classification

GLIAL TUMORS

Tumors of the glial cells include astrocytoma and ependymoma. Astrocytoma describes the starlike shape of the brain cell involved in this tumor. Astrocytomas can be divided into low-grade and high-grade tumors. Pilocytic astrocytomas, a low-grade type, are the most common glioma in children.[18] High-grade astrocytomas include anaplastic astrocytoma and glioblastoma multiforme (GBM).

Ependymomas arise from the ventricular lining and account for 6% to 12% of all intracranial childhood tumors and 30% of those in children younger than 3 years.[18]

Brain stem glioma, also referred to as diffuse pontine glioma, is a type of GBM that infiltrates the brain stem. Brain stem gliomas are uniformly fatal, conferring a life expectancy of 6 to 18 months. Treatment is palliative, with the goal of reducing symptoms and improving quality of life before death.

PRIMITIVE NEUROECTODERMAL TUMOR (PNET)

Primitive neuroectodermal tumor (PNET) includes medulloblastomas (in the posterior fossa) and supratentorial PNETs. One third of PNETs metastasize through the CSF pathways. The average age for PNETs is 5 years, although the incidence of medulloblastomas peaks at age 7; and 70% occur before the age of 16. Males are more often diagnosed with PNETs than females, and children less than 2 years of age at diagnosis have a worse prognosis than older patients.[28]

A new subset of PNET has recently been classified, atypical teratoid rhabdoid tumor (ATRT). Unfortunately, the prognosis for ATRT is poor in spite of the use of autologous bone marrow transplant.[29]

CRANIOPHARYNGIOMA

This tumor accounts for 5% to 10% of intracranial lesions in children. It is a benign, partly cystic tumor of the sellar region.[18]

INTRACRANIAL GERM CELL TUMORS

CNS germ cell tumors account for about 3% of intracranial masses in children.[15] They are divided into germinomas and nongerminomatous germ cell tumors (NGGCTs). NGGCTs are diagnosed by the presence of tumor markers α-fetoprotein (AFP) and β–human chorionic gonadotropin (β-HCG) found in serum or CSF.

Clinical Features

Symptoms are based on the location of the lesion in the brain and include headache, vomiting, head tilt, ataxia, dysmetria, seizures, vision changes, changes in consciousness, and endocrine abnormalities. Increased head circumference is common in children under the age of 2 years. Older children and adolescents may have initial findings that include school failure and psychiatric diagnoses.

Symptoms of increased intracranial pressure (ICP) occur when ventricular drainage is compromised and include headache and vomiting. Vomiting is an innate life-preserving measure in response to increased ICP that induces dehydration and thereby decreases the ICP.

Diagnosis

Dramatic advances in the outcome of pediatric brain tumors is largely due to the development of modern imaging techniques.[30] Magnetic resonance imaging (MRI) is considered the best method to evaluate full extent of disease, although newer metabolic imaging techniques are being developed that may increase diagnostic sensitivity.[31] Children usually undergo a surgical biopsy or resection of the tumor. A lumbar puncture may be required to assess for metastatic disease in the CSF. Diagnosis is confirmed by pathologic review of the tumor specimen.

Staging

The World Health Organization (WHO) has established a grading system ranging from grade I to grade IV based on the biology of the CNS tumor. Low-grade tumors corresponding to WHO grade I include pilocytic astrocytoma and craniopharyngioma. Ependymoma corresponds to WHO grade II. High-grade tumors are anaplastic astrocytoma (WHO grade III) and GBM (WHO grade IV). Brain tumors are further staged based on the presence and extent of metastatic disease. Table 18-5 describes the metastatic staging system currently used.

TABLE 18-5	Metastatic Staging for Brain Tumor
No metastases	M0
Tumor cells in the CSF	M1
Metastatic lesions in the brain	M2
Metastatic lesions in the spine	M3
Metastatic lesions outside the CNS	M4

CNS, Central nervous system; CSF, cerebrospinal fluid.

Medical Treatment and Nursing Care Considerations

SURGERY

Surgery is the primary treatment for most brain tumors. The goal is complete resection of the mass, where possible. New imaging and surgical techniques have improved surgical outcomes by enabling the surgeon to carefully plan the surgical approach and minimize injury to normal tissues.

Nursing care of the child postoperatively is focused on careful and ongoing neural assessment, comfort measures, and maintenance of an isovolemic state. Overhydration can cause an increase in ICP and can induce a brisk drop in the sodium level, which may precipitate seizure activity.[32]

RADIATION

Although radiation is an effective treatment for many brain tumors, the effects of radiation on a growing, developing brain can be disastrous. Consequently, efforts are made to delay radiation when it is necessary until after the age of 3 years. Radiation is delivered in fractionated doses over a period of several weeks for total doses ranging from 1800 to 6000 cGy, depending upon the area to be treated.

The ability to remain perfectly still is essential to positioning for radiation delivery. Very young children may require sedation or, in some cases, anesthesia for each treatment. Older children with the capacity to understand and cooperate can do well with support and appropriate distraction techniques. Education of parents and children about radiation therapy and its expected effects, side effects, and late effects is an important nursing role.

CHEMOTHERAPY

Chemotherapy is rapidly becoming standard therapy for many types of brain tumors. It is useful in young children to delay radiation therapy. Common chemotherapeutic agents include cisplatin, carboplatin, etoposide, ifosfamide, and the nitrosoureas. Advances in the administration of high-dose chemotherapy followed by HCST has greatly improved the outcome for some types of brain tumors.

Newly diagnosed children receiving chemotherapy must be monitored closely for alterations in neural status from the fluid volumes required for some chemotherapy treatments. Strict adherence to fluid limits is imperative. Symptoms of increased ICP should be treated promptly with mannitol and, if necessary, corticosteroids.

TREATMENT FOR SPECIFIC CNS TUMORS

Glial Tumors. Low-grade astrocytomas that are completely removed do not need further treatment, and are followed by periodic monitoring with MRI.[33] Incomplete resection in locations such as the optic nerves, the hypothalamus, or the brainstem necessitates radiation or low-dose chemotherapy. Grade II astrocytomas, more common in adolescents, have a worse prognosis because of the higher likelihood of upgrading. High grade tumors are initially treated surgically; however, complete resection is often not possible owing to diffuse infiltration of the brain. Current treatment includes induction chemotherapy followed by radiation with or without concurrent chemotherapy. Maintenance chemotherapy follows radiation. Ependymoma is initially treated by surgical resection.

Chemotherapy is used to shrink residual tumor if resection was incomplete and is followed by a second-look surgery. Radiation to the tumor site may follow surgical resection.

PNET. Treatment for PNET consists of surgical resection followed by chemotherapy and radiation. Children with metastatic disease and those with supratentorial PNETs are treated with surgical resection followed by one round of chemotherapy, after which stem cells are harvested and saved in case of relapse. Six weeks of craniospinal radiation with concurrent chemotherapy is given, followed by maintenance chemotherapy for 1 year. Children younger than 3 years receive high dose chemotherapy followed by autologous HSCT.

Craniopharyngioma. Treatment for this tumor includes surgical resection of the solid portion followed by local radiation. The cystic portion of the tumor can be problematic and may be treated with injections of chemotherapy into the cyst through an implanted reservoir.

Intracranial Germ Cell Tumors. Treatment of germ cell tumors consists of three rounds of moderate chemotherapy followed by local and ventricular radiation. Craniospinal radiation is used for metastatic disease. Treatment for NGGCT includes chemotherapy followed by craniospinal radiation, with a boost to the local tumor site.

Disease-Related Complications and Treatment

Increased ICP is the most common complication for children with brain tumors. Symptoms of increased ICP include severe headache and vomiting. Untreated, increased ICP can rapidly progress to decreased levels of consciousness, seizures, and death. Decadron and mannitol are the emergency medications of choice for increased ICP. As tumor swelling and edema decreases, symptoms will resolve.

Prognosis

The prognosis for children with brain tumors has improved significantly over the past decades; however, there is still great room for improvement.

- The prognosis for pilocytic astrocytoma is good, with about 90% survival rate at 5 years; however, the survival rates drop dramatically for the higher-grade tumors, with grade III astrocytoma at about 30% and grade IV tumors at less than 5%.[18] Children with ependymoma have a 60% chance of survival with complete resection, but less than 10% if the tumor is not fully resected or if multiple relapses occur.[18]
- Patients with PNET have an overall survival rate for medulloblastomas that reaches about 80%.[34] Nonmetastatic medulloblastomas in children over the age of 3 years offers the best prognosis (85%). Patients with supratentorial PNETs have a worse survival rate.[35]
- Craniopharyngioma is a completely curable disease; however, many of these patients have quality of life issues as a result of the hypothalamic location. Panhypopituitarism is common, and patients will require replacement of thyroid hormone, cortisol, desmopressin, and growth hormone. Unfortunately, morbid obesity often occurs as a result of hypothalamic dysfunction.
- Germinomas have a prognosis of 80% to 85% survival regardless of metastatic disease.[18]
- NGCCT prognosis for survival is 60% to 70%, but somewhat less for β-HCG–positive tumors.[18]

Bone Cancer

Malignancies of the bone account for 6% of all pediatric malignancies, or 8.7 cases per 1 million children under the age of 20 years. Approximately 650 to 700 new cases of bone cancer are diagnosed each year in the United States. Osteogenic sarcoma (OS) and Ewing's sarcoma are the most common types of bone tumors in children and adolescents. Malignant changes in bone are likely related to rapid bone growth. This may explain why girls tend to have bone malignancies earlier in adolescence than boys, whose growth spurt typically occurs later.[36]

The 5-year relative survival rates for children with bone cancer have improved in the last 20 years from 49% to 63%. Overall, females have a better survival rate than males. There is no significant difference in survival between white and black children.[36]

OSTEOSARCOMA

Epidemiology

OS accounts for 56% of all pediatric bone malignancies. The peak is in the 10- to 14-year-old age group, coinciding with the adolescent growth spurt. It occurs equally between the sexes until late adolescence, when the incidence is higher in males. Black children have a higher overall incidence of osteosarcoma than white children.[37]

Etiology and Risk Factors

OS arises from primitive bone-forming mesenchymal stem cells. The malignant cells produce immature osteoid cells, which form the tumor mass. Identified factors associated with an increased risk of OS are direct ionizing radiation and a few genetic susceptibility syndromes such as hereditary retinoblastoma, Li-Fraumeni syndrome, Rothmund-Thomson syndrome, and Bloom's and Werner's syndromes.[37] Prior irradiation for another solid tumor increases the risk of developing a secondary osteosarcoma. In addition, prior exposure to chemotherapy, especially alkylating agents, may also be associated with secondary osteosarcoma.[38]

Clinical Features

OS can occur in any bone, but most frequently originates in the long bones near the metaphysis. The most common sites are the distal femur, the proximal tibia, and the proximal humerus, as well as the middle and proximal femur. Initial complaints may include a several-month history of localized pain and altered patterns of weight bearing, sometimes following an injury. A tender soft tissue mass may be palpable.[39]

Diagnosis

The diagnostic work-up includes MRI, CT scan, radionuclide bone scan, and biopsy. An MRI study of the entire affected bone should be conducted to check for skip lesions that are metastases not in direct contact with the primary lesion but within the same bone. A CT scan of the chest is essential to check for lung metastases and a bone scan is done to look for bony metastases elsewhere in the body. The diagnosis is confirmed by surgical biopsy.

Staging

The staging system most often used for bone cancer is the Musculoskeletal Tumor Society staging system (MSTS). MSTS categorizes nonmetastatic tumors as grade I (low-grade) or grade II (high-grade), with metastatic disease staged as a grade III. This system is primarily for surgical purposes, and chemotherapy decisions are not based on the classification stage.

Medical Treatment and Nursing Care Considerations

SURGERY

Surgical resection with preoperative and postoperative chemotherapy is the standard of care.[40] Surgical options include amputation and limb salvage techniques for extremities and resection for axial disease, with the goals of complete resection of the tumor and achieving the best possible function. The surgical decision is based upon tumor location, extent, and the patient's age and growth potential.[41] Limb-salvage surgery is the surgical option of choice in 85% of patients. Studies have shown that there is no difference in survival between amputation and limb-salvage surgery.

Nursing care in the postoperative stage is geared toward pain management and rehabilitation. Pain control consists of treatment for both acute surgical pain and the neuropathic pain resulting from the disruption of nerve pathways. Emotional support for the child and family is essential throughout treatment. Alterations in physical appearance and ability may be difficult for the young person, and the adjustment period may be very stressful.

CHEMOTHERAPY

Chemotherapy is given preoperatively to shrink the tumor mass and enable the best possible surgical resection. The second goal of chemotherapy is to prevent metastatic spread of the disease. Methotrexate, cisplatin, and doxorubicin are commonly used drugs. Side effects of these chemotherapeutic agents include nausea, stomatitis, and bone marrow suppression. Cisplatin can cause hearing loss.

Nursing care includes providing adequate nausea control during chemotherapy encounters and teaching the child and family about side effects and home management.

The majority of children diagnosed with OS will be adolescents. Changes in body image can be very distressing. It is helpful to create an atmosphere of trust that enables them to have privacy when they need it, to ask questions, and to explore their feelings about having cancer.

Disease-Related Complications and Treatment

The most common complications of treatment for osteogenic sarcoma are neutropenia and fever. Blood cultures are done to rule out sepsis. Postoperatively, the surgical site and any prosthetic implants must be assessed for infection. Broad-spectrum antibiotics are given until infection is ruled out or adequately treated. Nursing care priorities are directed toward assessing the patient for signs and symptoms of infection, response to therapy, and providing comfort measures.

Hearing loss is a significant risk with cisplatin therapy. Audiometric testing is done at routine intervals throughout chemotherapy. The hearing loss is most commonly in the high-frequency range but can also involve lower frequencies and have an impact on speech perception. Children with hearing loss may need special accommodations in school, and some children require hearing aids. Assessment for changes in the child's attention to conversation, increasing television or radio volumes, or other behaviors that may indicate hearing loss is part of the routine nursing assessment.

Prognosis

The survival rate for nonmetastatic extremity OS is currently approximately 75%.[36] Patients with central axis disease and those with metastatic disease fare less well. Recurrent disease is usually seen as pulmonary metastasis. Isolate pulmonary metastasis may be treated by surgical resection alone. However, most children will have multiple metastasis. With surgical resection and aggressive chemotherapy, survival is approximately 30%.[36]

EWING'S SARCOMA

Epidemiology

Ewing's sarcoma accounts for 34% of bone tumors in the pediatric and adolescent population. As in OS, the peak incidence is during the teen growth spurt. Boys and girls are equally affected.[36]

Etiology and Risk Factors

Ewing's sarcomas arise from neural crest tissue and include Ewing's sarcoma, atypical Ewing's sarcoma, and peripheral PNET of the bone.[36] White children have 6 times the incidence of Ewing's sarcoma as black children.[36]

Classification

Ewing's sarcoma is one of several types of small round blue cell tumors primarily seen in childhood. The family of Ewing's sarcomas is characterized by the presence of the t(11;22) chromosomal abnormality, which is seen in approximately 95% of tumors.[42]

Clinical Features

Ewing's sarcoma is found equally in the central axis, including the vertebral column, the ribs, the sternum, the clavicle, and the pelvis, and the extremities.[36] Most patients with Ewing's sarcoma first complain of localized pain and swelling occurring over a few weeks to months; this pain intensifies over time and becomes worse with exercise and at night. On physical exam, a distinct, tender, fixed, soft tissue mass may be palpable. Patients with juxtaarticular tumors may have loss of movement in the affected joint. Tumors of the vertebral column, the pelvis, and the sacrum cause back pain and symptoms related to tumor compression of the spinal nerves, such as weakness, paresis, and dysfunction of the bladder and bowel.

Staging

Approximately 20% to 30% of patients have documented metastatic disease, and most patients are believed to have subclinical metastatic disease at diagnosis. Metastasis to the lungs will exhibit systemic symptoms upon diagnosis such as fever, fatigue, weight loss, and anemia.[40] At initial presentation, pulmonary or hematopoietic symptoms are rare.[42] The most common site for bone metastasis is the spine.[43] Of those with

primary pelvic tumors, there is a significantly higher incidence of metastatic disease at presentation when compared to other primary sites.[44]

Diagnosis

The initial work-up for metastatic Ewing's sarcoma is the same as for osteosarcoma, with the addition of a bone marrow aspiration and biopsy to determine bone marrow involvement.

Medical Treatment and Nursing Care Considerations

The best outcomes for patients with Ewing's sarcoma are achieved with multimodality treatment including surgery, chemotherapy, and radiation. Bone marrow transplant is being studied as a treatment modality in some centers.

SURGERY

A biopsy is initially performed to obtain the diagnosis. Surgery is later used for local control of the tumor. Complete resection is ideal, but not always achievable or desirable if it will cause significant loss of function. Definitive surgery is most often done after tumor debulking with chemotherapy. Issues surrounding surgical options for tumors of the limbs are the same as for osteosarcoma.

Postoperatively, patients are monitored for signs and symptoms of infection at the surgical site. Healing can be significantly impaired by immunosuppression from chemotherapy. If reconstructive hardware has been placed, a wound infection can lead to infection of the hardware, which then may have to be removed.

CHEMOTHERAPY

Chemotherapy is the mainstay of Ewing's therapy. The addition of ifosfamide and etoposide to other drugs that are used such as vincristine, doxorubicin, and cyclophosphamide has improved response to chemotherapy for patients with nonmetastatic Ewing's sarcoma.[45]

Chemotherapy treatment for Ewing's sarcoma is intensive and highly emetogenic. Survivors of treatment for Ewing's often recall nausea and vomiting as the worst part of their treatment. Administration of antiemetic therapy should come before the scheduled treatment and continue at regular intervals until the nausea resolves.

RADIATION

Radiation therapy is routinely used as a local control measure for patients who have unresectable disease or microscopic disease at the surgical margins. Irradiation may also be helpful as a palliative measure to reduce pain and symptoms in patients who have painful metastatic bone lesions.

In young children, radiation will impair growth in the affected region. Radiation therapy also increases the risk of secondary malignancies. Patient and parent education about the potential late effects of radiation is part of the nursing care plan.

Disease-Related Complications and Treatment

Treatment for Ewing's sarcoma incorporates high total doses of alkylating agents such as ifosfamide and cyclophosphamide. These drugs significantly increase the risk for sterility in males.

Sperm banking is an option that should be offered to pubescent males. Collection must be done before initiation of chemotherapy to obtain adequate and viable sperm. Nurses need to be knowledgeable about sperm banking to be sensitive, effective educators and advocates for teenage males who may find this a difficult subject to discuss.

Prognosis

The overall 5-year relative survival rate for children with Ewing's sarcoma is 58%, with rates for males at 50% and for females at 68%.[43] Large primary tumors, high serum lactate dehydrogenase (LDH) at diagnosis, age greater than 15 year at diagnosis, tumors of the pelvis, the spine, or the skull, and poor responses to induction chemotherapy are unfavorable prognostic factors.[43] Axial primary sites confer a worse prognosis than extremity lesions.[44] With current treatment, long-term survival in patients with nonmetastatic disease now approaches 70%.[40] For patients with metastatic Ewing's sarcoma, the survival rate drops to less than 30%, and those with bone metastases have the worst prognosis, with a survival rate of less than 10%.[42]

Rhabdomyosarcoma

Epidemiology

Rhabdomyosarcoma (RMS) is a soft tissue tumor that develops from embryonic mesenchymal cells. These cells give rise to skeletal muscle, although RMS is also found in tissues of nonstriated origin such as the bladder. RMS is the third most common solid tumor outside of the brain and is the most common soft tissue sarcoma in children.[1]

Almost two thirds of RMS cases develop in children under the age of 6 years. There is a slight predilection for boys over girls, and black girls are less likely to develop RMS than white girls.[46] The most common sites of origin are the parameningeal tissues, the orbit, the extremities, the head and neck areas, the urinary system, and the reproductive organs.

Etiology

The cause of rhabdomyocarcoma is not known. RMS is one of a cluster of tumors associated with Li-Fraumeni syndrome and is also associated with neurofibromatosis, but the majority of RMS cases are not familial.

Classification

RMS is another of the small round blue cell tumors. There are three subtypes of RMS: embryonal (including botyroid and spindle cell variations), alveolar, and pleomorphic. In children, the embryonal and alveolar subtypes are most common. Embryonal tumors are most commonly found in the orbit and the genitourinary tract. Alveolar RMS usually occurs in the extremities, is more often seen in adolescents, and is associated with poor outcomes.

Diagnosis

Early detection and treatment are essential to the best outcomes for children with RMS. Presenting signs and symptoms of this disease depend upon the location of the primary tumor. Most often the presenting sign is a lump that does not disappear and raises concern for the family. Other presenting signs and symptoms of RMS are related to organ dysfunction caused by the tumor.

Staging

RMS is staged according to the tumor, nodes, and metastasis (TNM) pretreatment staging system (see Table 18-6). Tumors are further classified into low-, intermediate-, or high-risk groups. The prognostic factors for a child or adolescent with RMS are related to age, site of origin, resectability of the tumor, presence and extent of metastasis, and the histopathologic and biologic characteristics of the tumor cells.

RMS can metastasize to bone, bone marrow, the lungs, and other muscle tissue. Of affected children, 15% will have metastasis at diagnosis; however, there is usually a single distant site rather than widespread disease.[47]

Medical Treatment and Nursing Care Considerations

SURGERY

The treatment of RMS requires a multimodal approach for optimal management including surgical resection, chemotherapy, and radiation therapy. Surgical resection has the greatest impact on prognosis. Whenever possible, a complete surgical resection is attempted. Where complete resection is not feasible initially, the tumor is debulked as much as possible and then chemotherapy and radiation are given to further reduce the tumor size. A second surgical resection is then performed to remove any residual tumor.

Preoperatively, nurses prepare the child and family for the expected outcome of the procedure, including anticipated changes in the child's physical abilities or appearance. Postoperatively, nursing care is focused on providing adequate pain management, maintaining adequate fluid and electrolyte balance, and helping the child return to normal activity. If a deformity has resulted from the surgical procedure, it is important to help the child and family adapt to the child's new appearance and learn constructive coping skills.

TABLE 18-6	**Staging System for Rhabdomyosarcoma**
Stage 1	Tumor is localized
	Usually involving the head and neck region (excluding parameningeal sites), the orbital region or the genitourinary region (excluding bladder/prostate sites), or the biliary tract (favorable sites)
Stage 2	Tumor is localized but does not originate in any site included in the stage 1 category (unfavorable sites)
	Primary disease is 5 cm or smaller in diameter; and no lymph node involvement by tumor
Stage 3	Tumor is localized in any other primary site
	These patients have primary tumors larger than 5 cm and/or regional lymph-node metastases
Stage 4	Patient has metastatic disease at initial assessment

Adapted from crist WM, Anderson JR, Meza JL et al: Intergroup rhabdomyosarcoma study-IV: results for patients with nonmetastatic disease, *J Clin Oncol*, 19(12): 3091-3102, 2001.

RADIATION

Radiation therapy is very useful as a treatment modality of RMS. It enables control of gross or microscopic disease and is instituted approximately 9 weeks after initiation of chemotherapy. If the tumor involves the CNS, radiation therapy will start immediately. Radiation is generally given in small incremental doses over a period of several weeks. Interstitial implantation of radioactive seeds, or brachytherapy, has been used in some cases in an attempt to deliver targeted radiation to critically located tumors and at the same time preserve organ function and decrease radiation scatter to bordering organs.

Radiation to the abdominal region may cause abdominal pain, diarrhea, cramping, and loss of appetite. Giving parents suggestions for maximizing caloric intake during this time will be helpful. Some children may need to have enteral or parenteral nutrition to support them until they have recovered from the radiation effects.

CHEMOTHERAPY

Chemotherapy usually consists of vincristine, dactinomycin, and cyclophosphamide. Topotecan, irinotecan, and vinorelbine are currently being studied with hopes that they will improve the outcome for metastatic stage IV disease. The role of high-dose chemotherapy followed by autologous transplant is currently under investigation in some clinical trials.

Provision of adequate emetic control during and immediately after chemotherapy is essential since these drugs can cause significant nausea and vomiting. Close attention to intake and output is needed to prevent dehydration from vomiting and hemorrhagic cystitis from cyclophosphamide.

Disease-Related Complications and Treatment

Treatment for RMS predisposes children to significant late effects. Sterility can result from use of alkylating agents and from radiation to the abdomen. Most boys with RMS are too young at diagnosis to bank sperm. Other potential late effects are growth abnormalities from radiation, renal tubular dysfunction from chemotherapy, and an increased risk of second malignancies. Parents need to be educated about the potential for late effects based upon the location of their child's tumor and must have information that will enable them to obtain necessary testing and monitoring for these effects as their child grows up.

Prognosis

Collaborative expertise has led to major advances in treatment, and the 3-year event-free survival (EFS) rate for the child with nonmetastatic RMS is now greater than 70%. The low-risk category has an estimated 3-year EFS rate of 88%.[48] Those classified in the intermediate-risk category have an estimated survival prognosis of 55% to 76%. The high-risk category, which includes those with metastatic RMS or undifferentiated tumor at diagnosis, have a poor 5-year survival rate of 30%.[47]

Neuroblastoma

Epidemiology

Neuroblastoma is a heterogenous small round blue cell tumor that is derived from the primitive cells giving rise to the sympathetic nervous system. Neuroblastoma is almost exclusively a childhood cancer. It is the third most common type of childhood cancer and accounts for about 15% of all pediatric cancer fatalities. This tumor occurs most frequently in children under 10 years of age and is the most common malignancy in infants under 12 months.[49]

Etiology

There is no definitive cause for neuroblastoma. There is an increased incidence in patients with neurofibromatosis, Beckwith-Wiedemann syndrome, and Hirschsprung's disease.[50] It is familial in a very small number of cases. In children less than 1 year of age, spontaneous regression of the tumor occurs frequently.

Classification

Neuroblastoma is one of several pediatric tumors that stain as small round blue cells. It is differentiated from other types of tumors by a characteristic "rosette" pattern in which tumor cells cluster around a pink fibrillar center when stained. Varying degrees of ganglion maturation can often be identified within the tumor. Deletion of a part of chromosome 1p is seen in approximately 30% of patients with neuroblastoma. 1p deletions are highly associated with overexpression, or amplification, of the oncogene MYCN, which is associated with a poor prognosis. Other chromosomal abnormalities include a gain of one to three copies of chromosome 17, seen in approximately 50% of patients, and deletion of 11q.[49]

Clinical Features

Neuroblastomas can arise anywhere along the sympathetic nerve pathway. About half present as an abdominal mass arising from the adrenal gland. Other primary sites include the chest, the neck, the pelvis, the spinal column, and the head. Abdominal tumors are firm, palpable masses that may cross the midline. Intrathoracic masses are most often found incidentally on a chest radiograph that may have been obtained to evaluate symptoms of respiratory distress. Other symptoms depend upon the location of the tumor. Abdominal tumors may cause distention, pain, constipation from tumor compression of the bowel, or diarrhea from vasoactive intestinal peptide secretion. Children who have spinal tumors are first seen with symptoms of cord compression including loss of function in the lower extremities and loss of bowel and bladder control. Metastatic disease is often present at the time of diagnosis.[52] The most common sites of metastasis are the bones, the bone marrow, and the skin. Children may be first seen with symptoms of metastatic disease including severe bone pain, periorbital ecchymosis, fatigue and malaise, or skin nodules.[52]

Diagnosis

Diagnostic work up includes a urine evaluation for homovanillic acid (HVA) and vanillylmandelic acid (VMA), the intermediates of catecholamine metabolism. Neuroblastoma cells do not effectively synthesize catecholamines, and these metabolites are elevated in most patients with neuroblastoma. VMA and HVA levels are useful monitors for response to treatment and for presence of recurrent disease. Radiologic evaluation includes CT scan or MRI, metaiodobenzylguanidine (MIBG) scan, bone radiographs, and a chest radiograph to rule out metastatic disease.

Bilateral bone marrow aspiration and biopsies are done to rule out involvement of the bone marrow.

Staging

Age at diagnosis, extent of disease, and the presence of gene mutations are the primary predictive factors for outcome.[49] Infants with localized primary tumors as defined for stage 1 or 2 and with dissemination limited to liver, skin, or bone marrow are staged in a special category, 4S. Infants with disease classified as low-risk 4S have a high rate of spontaneous regression, and treatment can be deferred if close monitoring of the mass is in place, although those with high-risk 4S disease will require chemotherapy.

The International Neuroblastoma Staging System (INSS) stratifies tumors as stages 1 to 4 and 4S based upon tumor extent, resectability, and metastasis (see Table 18-7). Tumors are further classified into low-, intermediate-, and high-risk groups based upon MYCN amplification, DNA content, patient age, and tumor histology. Hyperdiploid tumors are associated with lower tumor staging, better response to therapy, and better prognosis than diploid tumors. The low-risk stage I and II group has a 90% survival rate with surgery alone. The intermediate-risk group includes those classified as stage III who are over the age of 1 year without MYCN amplification, and infants without MYCN amplification who are in stages 3 and 4. These patients require both chemotherapy and excision surgery.

Medical Treatment and Nursing Care Considerations

SURGERY

Surgical intervention is done to debulk the tumor or, in some cases, completely resect it. Large tumors may be biopsied initially and then treated with chemotherapy and radiation before a second surgical resection. This process can often enable a less invasive or extensive surgical procedure. Surgery is urgent in the case of cord compression to prevent permanent paralysis.

TABLE 18-7	INSS Staging for Neuroblastoma
Stage 1	Tumor is restricted to the area of origin Completely resected
Stage 2	Tumor is localized and may or may not have lymph node disease Not completely resectable at the time of diagnosis
Stage 3	Large tumor that that cannot be resected at the time of diagnosis This tumor crosses the center of the body; patient may have affected lymph nodes unilaterally or bilaterally
Stage 4	Widespread disease with metastatic disease in distant lymph nodes, bone marrow, liver, and/or other organs
Stage 4S	Child is less than 1 year of age Tumor is restricted to area of origin with spread to liver, skin, and/or bone marrow

Adapted from Brodeur GM, Pritchard J, Berthold F et al: Revisions of the international criteria for neuroblastoma diagnosis, staging, and response to treatment, *J Clin Oncol*, 11(8): 1466-1477, 1993.

Postoperative care is focused on pain control, comfort measures, and frequent assessment of the child's condition. Following surgery to relieve cord compression, careful positioning, log rolling, and monitoring of the child's neurologic status is critical.

CHEMOTHERAPY

Chemotherapy is intensive and includes drugs such as cisplatin or carboplatin, doxorubicin, ifosfamide, etoposide, vincristine, and cyclophosphamide. Children often experience dramatic relief of pain from bony metastasis after chemotherapy is instituted.

High-risk groups have the lowest survival rates and require very intensive treatment. Disease control can be achieved using surgery and radiation therapy in addition to aggressive chemotherapy and autologous stem cell rescue; however, the disease recurs in over half of these children. The use of cis-retinoic acid therapy has been found to aid in prevention of tumor recurrence by inducing cellular maturation in any remaining neuroblastoma cells.[52]

Intensive chemotherapy often affects the child's ability to maintain caloric requirements. Nursing care includes monitoring weight and intake, and educating parents on ideas to help maintain the child's nutritional status such as ways to incorporate more calories without increasing the volume of foods and drinks. Some children may need enteral or parenteral nutrition during therapy for neuroblastoma.

RADIATION

Neuroblastoma is radiosensitive, and children will receive radiation to the primary tumor site. Radiation can be used emergently to decrease tumor size or reduce cord compression, or later in the treatment regimen.

Nursing care for the child receiving radiation for is the same as described for the child with rhabdomyosarcoma.

Disease-Related Complications and Treatment

A small number of children enter treatment with a neurologic syndrome called opsoclonus-myoclonus-ataxia syndrome (OMAS), characterized by nystagmus, jerking motions, and ataxia. OMAS is a paraneoplastic syndrome that is believed to be immune-mediated, but the exact mechanisms are not fully understood.[53] Untreated, OMAS can lead to delayed motor, cognitive, and behavioral development. Treatment with intravenous immune gamma globulin in addition to chemotherapy appears to be helpful.

The child with OMAS may have uncontrollable body movements and impaired vision due to nystagmus. Providing the child with a safe environment is essential. Nursing interventions also include assisting the child to find appropriate diversionary activities, monitoring during immune globulin infusions for side effects, and parent support and education.

Prognosis

Age at diagnosis, extent of disease, and the presence of gene mutations are the primary predictive factors for outcome.[50] Children under the age of 1 year have the best outcomes; 80% of patients over the age of 1 have high-risk factors at diagnosis and therefore have a very poor prognosis.[54]

Children in the low-risk category have a 5-year survival rate of approximately 98%. The high-risk group includes those children over 1 year of age and anyone with MYCN amplification classified as stage 4. With multifaceted therapy, a 5-year EFS of approximately 30% can be achieved for this group of patients. Infants with tumors staged as 4S have an overall 3-year survival rate of 93%.[51]

Wilms' Tumor

Epidemiology

Wilms' tumor is a malignant renal tumor accounting for about 6% of all childhood cancers. There are approximately 460 cases diagnosed yearly, and 80% are in children less than 5 years of age.[55] The peak incidence is between 2 and 3 years of age, and there is a slight predominance in females. Although the majority of Wilms' tumors are sporadic, a small percentage are familial.

Etiology

Wilms' tumor is strongly associated with several congenital disorders. Children with Beckwith-Wiedeman syndrome, WAGR (an acronym for the most notable features of the disease, including Wilms' tumor, aniridia, genital and/or urinary tract abnormalities, and mental retardation) syndrome, or Denys-Drash syndrome are at increased risk for the development of Wilms' tumor. Increased risk is also associated with congenital anomalies such as aniridia, hemihypertrophy, cryptorchidism, and hypospadius. Research has identified two loci on chromosome 11 that are key in the development of Wilms' tumor: the Wilms' tumor suppressor gene located at 11p13 and a second Wilms' tumor gene at 11p15. These same loci are also associated with all three congenital syndromes.[56]

Classification

Wilms' tumor is the most common of the pediatric primary renal tumors that also include clear cell sarcoma, rhabdoid tumor of the kidney, and congenital mesoblastic nephroma. Wilms' tumor is classified as having either favorable or unfavorable (anaplastic) histology, a significant factor in prognosis and treatment.

Nephrogenic rests are clusters of primitive nephrogenic cells usually found in the periphery of the kidney. Multiple foci of these rests increase the likelihood of later development of Wilms' tumor.

Clinical Features

Wilms' tumor commonly presents as a firm, one-sided, painless flank mass. Wilms' tumors are often very large at diagnosis and are vascular in nature, encased in a fragile, gelatinous capsule, commonly with a necrotic center. Hemorrhage into the mass may occur and cause acute-onset abdominal pain. Hypertension is present in about 25% of patients; hematuria and vomiting are also common presenting symptoms.

Diagnosis

Wilms' tumor is most commonly found incidentally during bathing by a caregiver or during a routine physical examination. The tumor is usually seen on renal ultrasound, CT, or MRI as a renal mass that is either cystic or solid, encapsulated, spherical, or unilateral. A urinalysis, blood pressure measurement, complete blood count, serum chemistries, chest x-ray, and chest CT are also part of the diagnostic work-up.

Staging

Wilms' tumors are grouped according to the National Wilms' Tumor Study Group criteria from stages I to V and are categorized with either favorable or unfavorable histology. Approximately 85% of Wilms' tumors will have favorable histology, which has an excellent prognosis. Unfavorable histology carries a poorer prognosis and includes those tumors with poor cellular differentiation, or anaplasia, and those with rhabdoid and sarcoid features. Bilateral disease is seen in about 5% of cases.[55]

Metastatic disease at time of diagnosis is uncommon. Approximately 10% to 15% of children have pulmonary disease at diagnosis.[56] Metastasis can occur in the brain, the lungs, the liver, the kidney, and the bone. Tumors may also grow upward through the vena cava into the heart, causing symptoms of vascular compression and cardiac insufficiency.

Treatment

SURGERY

Surgical resection plays a critical role in staging and treatment. It is important to remove the tumor without allowing it to rupture to prevent upstaging due to tumor spill. At the time of surgery, extent of disease is assessed by lymph node sampling and careful examination of the contralateral kidney and the liver. The affected kidney and tumor are completely removed except in cases of bilateral disease. In cases of bilateral disease, the affected kidney is left in place and chemotherapy given to shrink the tumor, enabling a partial resection of the kidney at a later date.

Preoperatively, it is important to prevent accidental rupture of the mass. The nursing care plan includes measures to prevent abdominal injury and limit palpation.

Postoperatively, these children need meticulous monitoring of their vital signs, blood pressure, and urine output. A Foley catheter will be in place; prevention of urinary tract infection during this time is imperative. The abdominal incision will cross the abdomen, and pain management is a top priority. Many institutions are now using epidural analgesia for the first few days following surgical resection for improved pain control.

Postoperative hypertension is a common finding, which usually resolves over time as the remaining kidney recovers from operative manipulation. However, some children will require antihypertensive therapy.

RADIATION

Radiation is given for stages III and IV tumors. Common side effects of abdominal irradiation include anorexia, nausea, vomiting, fatigue, and diarrhea. The skin in the radiation field may become reddened and irritated.

Nursing considerations for the child undergoing abdominal irradiation include helping parents optimize their child's dietary intake to reduce gastrointestinal symptoms and maintain caloric requirements, management of diarrhea, and skin care at the radiation site.

CHEMOTHERAPY

Chemotherapy is used for all tumors stages. Common chemotherapeutic agents include dactinomycin, vincristine, and cyclophosphamide. Doxorubicin is used for higher-stage tumors and metastatic disease. Chemotherapy for nonmetastatic Wilms' tumor lasts 3 to 6 months.

Neuropathic effects from vincristine are a risk during this therapy. Constipation is the most common side effect. Nursing assessment should include ascertaining the child's normal bowel pattern and administering stool softeners or laxatives as needed to prevent or treat constipation.

A thorough neurologic examination for neuropathy should also be done before every chemotherapy administration and anytime the parent or child reports symptoms. Neuropathy can present as tingling in the hands, the fingers, or the feet, difficulty with fine motor tasks such as handwriting or picking up small objects, inability to climb stairs, a slap-footed gait, and ptosis of the eyelids. Foot drop in young children may be mistaken for normal developmental clumsiness.

Protection of the remaining kidney from injury and infection will be a life-long mission for these patients. Families should be counseled on appropriate activities and protective gear for the child who is active in sports. Hard-contact sports are discouraged.

Prevention of urinary tract infection is extremely important for the child with one kidney. Teaching children proper hygiene techniques after using the toilet, avoidance of bubble baths, and maintaining adequate hydration is essential. Parents and patients should know the signs and symptoms of urinary tract infection and report them to their medical care provider promptly.

Prognosis

The prognosis for children with Wilms' tumor is, overall, excellent. Those children with nonmetastatic, favorable histology tumors and those with stage I anaplastic histology can expect a 90% survival rate. Children with stages III and IV tumors have an 80% survival rate. Bilateral stage V disease also carries a very favorable prognosis. Children with diffusely metastatic, anaplastic, and rhabdoid tumors fare less well, with a survival rate of only 56%.[55]

Most relapses occur within 2 years after completion of therapy. The majority of patients can be successfully retreated with additional chemotherapy, surgery, and radiation. Relapses that occur after treatment with radiation or doxorubicin, those occurring in the abdomen, and those occurring less than 12 months after completion of therapy carry a more dismal prognosis.

Hematopoietic Stem Cell Transplant in Children and Adolescents

Hematopoietic stem cell transplant (HSCT) been widely used to treat specific cancers in children, such as leukemia, lymphoma, neuroblastoma, and other solid tumors. HSCT may be also be done for certain types of hematologic disorders such as severe aplastic anemia or sickle cell anemia, hereditary immunodeficiency disorders, and some metabolic and genetic disorders. There is ongoing research to determine the efficacy of HSCT in other types of illnesses such as autoimmune disorders. Advances in transplantation have led to increased use of HSCT as primary treatment for pediatric brain tumors and neuroblastoma, and as salvage therapy for many relapsed solid tumors.

Complications of bone marrow transplantation in children are common and potentially fatal. Complications include infections, organ toxicity, relapse, and graft rejection. Graft-versus-host disease (GVHD) is a complication that may also have a beneficial role. Although the manifestations of GVHD can be life-threatening, recent studies show it may also have some benefit in preventing disease recurrence.[57]

Infections continue to be a major obstacle for pediatric transplant recipients. This population is at an extraordinary risk of life-threatening infections from bacterial, viral, fungal, or parasitic infections, and these patients are at high risk for sepsis. Empiric antibiotics started early in the posttransplant period can decrease the risk of gram-negative and gram-positive bacterial infections. Common viral infections include cytomegalovirus, adenovirus, respiratory syncytial virus, and varicella reactivation or infection. Prophylactic antiviral medications such as acyclovir can be effective in preventing some viral reactivations. The use of intravenous immunoglobulin (IVIG) is useful in reducing the incidence of infection following allogeneic transplant.

Patients are at high risk for fungal infections as a result of immunodeficiency and the high doses of corticosteroids given for GVHD prophylaxis or therapy. Most commonly, fungal infection is caused by a species of *Aspergillus* or *Candida*. Antifungal prophylaxis is initiated soon after HSCT and may include medications such as fluconazole, itraconazole, and micafungin.[58]

Parasitic infections include toxoplasmosis and *Pneumocystis jiroveci* pneumonia (formerly known as *Pneumocystis carinii* pneumonia, or PCP). Pentamidine or trimethoprim-sulfamethoxazole are the prophylactic medications of choice.

Another complication of transplant is hepatic veno-occlusive disease (VOD). This obstructive syndrome is characterized by hepatomegaly, jaundice, and ascites and is due to hepatic venous outflow obstruction from occlusion of the terminal hepatic venules and sinusosoids. The risk of VOD is higher in allogeneic unrelated or mismatched transplant patients compared to autologous recipients. VOD is serious, but recovery can be attained with early diagnosis and treatment.[59,60]

Pulmonary complications in the posttransplant period are significant causes of morbidity and mortality in the pediatric population. Viral, bacterial, and parasitic infections can lead to pulmonary infection and, respiratory failure. A less understood cause of lung disease is idiopathic pneumonia syndrome (IPS). IPS is a syndrome of alveolar injury. These patients have symptoms of pneumonia with negative culture results.[61,62] Chemotherapy and radiation toxicity, GVHD, or an undiagnosed viral infection may contribute to this condition. Rapid diagnosis and treatment is vital. A small number of patients respond to systemic corticosteroids, but the mortality rates continue to be approximately 75%.[63]

Late Effects of Pediatric Cancer Treatment

Three quarters of children diagnosed with cancer today will be long-term survivors. In young adults aged 20 to 34 years, 1 in 570 individuals is currently a long-term survivor.[64] Some therapy-related complications do not manifest until years after therapy, and effects may be heightened in a population that is continuing to grow and develop physically. Guidelines have been developed by the Children's Oncology Group to encourage early intervention and ongoing follow-up.[64] Many pediatric treatment centers offer late effects programs that provide treatment, education, and appropriate referrals to adult medicine providers.

Cardiac function can be affected by anthracyclines and alkylating agents, both of which are used in many childhood cancer therapies. The age at time of administration and the total amount received are the major predictive factors. Anthracyclines affect the growth of cardiac muscle cells, resulting in cell death and a decreased number of myocytes. Compensatory mechanisms may fail with increased stress throughout life, leading to congestive heart failure. Specific cardiac stresses such as pregnancy require close monitoring, and isometric exercises such as weightlifting may have to be avoided. Radiation therapy to the chest has an additive effect to chemotherapy-induced cardiotoxicity. Radiation therapy alone can result in valvular damage, pericardial thickening, and ischemic disease, especially at higher doses.[65] Frequent monitoring of cardiac function with echocardiograms and electrocardiograms is recommended, particularly if the exposure was at an early age or if higher doses were administered.

The endocrine system can be significantly affected by chemotherapy and radiation. It is important that patients with a history of previous radiation have regular endocrine evaluation since certain interventions must be offered within specific time frames, such as administering growth hormone before epiphyseal closure to extend growth. Endocrine evaluation is warranted when pubertal development or gonadal function is affected. Alkylating agents such as cyclophosphamide can affect gonadal development and fertility. The risk is total dose–dependent. Radiation in conjunction with alkylating agents increases the risk of gonadal toxicity. Males are generally more affected because the testes are extremely sensitive to the effects of chemotherapy and radiation. The potential for impaired fertility should be addressed before treatment, as patients reach puberty, or if there is difficulty with reproduction. Sperm or oocyte collection may be an option before treatment, and hormonal therapy may be necessary following treatment.

Radiation therapy can impair growth and development of tissues within the radiation field. Problems may become apparent with growth, such as scoliosis. Linear growth can be affected if parts of the hypothalamic-pituitary axis are in the field of radiation.

Pulmonary toxicity can be more severe in children than adults because alveolar formation and enlargement occurs in infancy and childhood. Pulmonary fibrosis can develop after damage to the pulmonary tissue and may have lasting effects. Bleomycin, most often used in germ cell tumors and Hodgkin's lymphomas, is a significant cause of pulmonary toxicity. Nitrosoureas such as carmustine (BCNU), most often used in brain tumor therapy, are associated with increased risk of pneumonitis. Children treated with these agents should have periodic pulmonary function testing. The risk is related to dose; therefore the frequency of follow-up is dictated by a history of acute damage and the total dose of chemotherapy and radiation administered. Radiation therapy has an additive effect when given in conjunction with these medications. Lung injury after radiation results from direct tissue damage and from constrictive lung disease secondary to chest wall hypoplasia.

Neuropsychologic and neurocognitive deficits have been evaluated in childhood cancer survivors. Severe mental retardation is uncommon, but mild cognitive deficits are common with CNS therapy given to children with leukemia and lymphoma. Radiation to the brain is associated with severe neurocognitive sequelae which negatively impact the intelligence quotient (IQ). Age at the time of CNS radiation and the total dose delivered are the major predictive factors for the extent of neurocognitive deficits. The rate of IQ decline is associated with younger age at treatment, longer time since treatment, and the volume of brain radiation. Loss of IQ is especially challenging as we strive to improve the quality of life of a pediatric brain tumor survivor.[66,67] Brain tumor location and resection can also contribute to cognitive deficits. Survivors should be evaluated with neuropsychologic testing to determine need for educational intervention.

The genitourinary tract can be affected during therapy, but problems can also progress or arise after therapy. Radiation has been associated with tubular damage and hypertension from renal artery stenosis. The use of cyclophosphamide and ifosfamide can cause hemorrhagic cystitis and fibrosis. Even asymptomatic patients have been found to be at increased risk of developing bladder cancer.[64] Patients treated with ifosfamide may require long-term replacement of potassium, calcium, and phosphorus because of renal tubular wasting. Treatment with cisplatin can lead to chronic magnesium wasting, and patients should have annual evaluation of blood pressure, urinalysis to detect hematuria, and renal function tests.

Survivors are also counseled on the potential for secondary malignancies. The overall risk to cancer survivors of developing a secondary malignancy is 3.2% at 20 years.[68] Specific risks are related to the cumulative dose of cytotoxic therapies. AML can occur up to 10 years following therapy with alkylating agents and up to 6 years following therapy with epipodophylotoxins. Secondary solid tumors can occur after radiation therapy. The risk of developing a leukemia diminishes over time; however, the risk of solid tumors after radiation increases with time. The most common tumors are breast cancer after mantle radiation for Hodgkin's disease; brain tumors after cranial radiation; and soft tissue or bone sarcomas. A regimen of annual breast exams, early mammograms, and periodic films of radiated areas may be instituted for patients at higher risk due to younger age of treatment or higher doses of therapy.

Experimental Therapeutics in Pediatric Oncology

So that advances in the treatment and care of pediatric oncology patients can continue to be made, children with refractory or relapsed cancers must be offered the opportunity to participate in phase I and II clinical trials. Research is funded by a variety of different sources including the National Cancer Institute, pharmaceutical companies, and independent foundations. Clinical trials may include new agents based on laboratory science, biologically targeted agents, combinations of new agents and established drugs, or novel uses of established drugs. As is the case in all clinical trials for children, the ethical issues surrounding experimental therapeutics in a vulnerable population must be meticulously addressed and appropriately handled. Multicenter trials enable more patients to be enrolled in studies, and therefore data is gathered more quickly. Two of the primary study groups are the Pediatric Oncology Experimental Therapeutic Investigators Consortium and the Children's Oncology Group.

Parents often express the need to pursue all possible treatments for their child's cancer when the disease no longer responds to standard therapies. It is appropriate to offer families the opportunity to participate in clinical trials as well as offering the option for palliative care. During the experimental therapeutics consultation, available treatment protocols that are available for the child's disease are discussed. The realities of phase I and II clinical trials including the study rationale, treatment schedules, requirements for participation, side effects, and the lack of known benefit to the child are disclosed. Informed consent by the parents or guardians is required for participation in a clinical trial. A child over the age of 7 must assent to the treatment as well.

Nursing Implications and Supportive Care for Children with Cancer and Their Families

Childhood cancer is a family experience, and the stressors inherent in childhood cancer and its treatment make an impact on every member of the family.[69] As an integral part of an interdisciplinary care team, nurses are crucial in their role as physical caretakers. Equally important, however, is the provision of emotional support, education, and advocacy to families throughout the continuum of the disease process.

Children need to have their care approached in a developmentally appropriate manner at all times. Age is not the sole factor for determining appropriate interventions. Cognitive development and past experiences also influence a child's ability to understand and cope. Parents may find it difficult to continue to enforce family expectations for behavior and discipline when their child is seriously ill. Assisting parents to maintain as much normalcy in the child's life as possible can positively influence a child's sense of security.

All children diagnosed with cancer can be expected to experience discomfort at some time during diagnosis and treatment. Pain has been described as the most feared aspect of cancer treatment, but it is frequently underassessed and undertreated in children. Pain can result from tumor invasion and compression; however, pain from procedures such as surgery, intravenous access, lumbar puncture, and bone marrow aspiration is more frequently reported by children and is often largely preventable.[70] Anxiety and fear can intensify the pain experience. A consistent pain scale appropriate to age and cognitive ability should be used at regular intervals throughout diagnosis and treatment. Appropriate pain medications and nonpharmacologic pain reduction techniques are offered whenever there is distress. Analgesic or anesthetic agents, including topical and local anesthetics, should be considered before any painful procedure. Most children tolerate appropriate doses of pain medications well, including narcotics. However, special care must be exercised when administering narcotics to children with brain tumors or other neurologic insults, since they may exhibit an increased sensitivity to narcotics.

Nutrition can be adversely affected by fatigue, persistent nausea, taste changes, mucositis, and the psychologic effects of hospitalization and treatment. Up to 30% of patients will have evidence of malnutrition during their treatment.[71] Maintenance of good nutritional status is important for continued growth, immune function, and healing. A wide variety of food choices, availability of snacks, and foods from home or local restaurants may be helpful in maintaining a child's interest in food. Nutritional intervention with oral, enteral, or parenteral supplementation may be necessary when children are unable or unwilling to take in adequate calories. Using food to disguise medication is discouraged, since it may cause eating aversions.

Education for the family regarding the treatment plan, expected side effects, home care, and late effects starts at the time a diagnosis of cancer is confirmed. Instruction in procedures such as central line care or administering injections may be necessary in order for parents to care for their child after discharge.

Teaching will also include signs of illness in an immunocompromised child, infection prevention, and how to interpret relevant laboratory results such as the absolute neutrophil count. Parents and other caregivers may have a difficult time attending to educational information during this high-stress time. Education plans are most successful when learning needs and styles are carefully assessed and a variety of educational techniques are employed. Frequent review of instructional material or procedures and provision of written information will help ensure that families have the information they need to adequately care for their child.

Psychosocial and spiritual support of the child and family is imperative. Families need to develop coping skills that will allow them to function adequately throughout the treatment process. Nurses are often seen as trusted family advocates during cancer treatment. Referrals to social work, psychology, and chaplaincy services and child life programs can also be very helpful to children and families.

Stress and anxiety are significant risks for children and teens undergoing chemotherapy.[72] Loss of control, fear, pain, and anxiety can all contribute to a decline in a child's sense of well-being. Body image changes from hair loss, weight loss or gain, central venous catheters, and treatment-related scars or deformities are especially difficult for school age children and adolescents. Assisting older children and teens to find appropriate cosmetic aids such as wigs, hats, and make-up may be helpful in helping them regain some of their self-confidence. Assessment for depression is an essential part of patient management both during and after the cancer experience. Nurses play a key role in educating family members about depression and its treatment. Refer children for supportive services when signs and symptoms of depression are present.

Siblings of children with cancer have unique support needs. Siblings report feelings of isolation, deprivation, guilt, and a loss of control.[73] Nurses can provide support and information to families regarding the special needs of siblings as well as offer emotional support and information to the siblings. Many centers offer support opportunities just for siblings such as group events and summer camp programs.

School is an important aspect of children's lives, and cancer therapy may affect a child's ability to attend school regularly. Families may need help obtaining special home services from their school districts such as tutoring or individualized education plans that specifically address a child's needs during and after treatment. Reintegration into the school environment after diagnosis or a prolonged absence is often difficult for children and can provoke questions from both peers and teachers about how best to help the child. A school visit by the nurse along with other involved health care team members may help facilitate the transition back into the classroom.[71]

Conclusion

The treatment of childhood cancer continues to improve, and more children can look forward to a normal, healthy life after cancer treatment. However, challenges still exist, and ongoing research is needed to improve treatment and outcomes for all children. Nurses have the opportunity to make a positive impact on the lives of children with cancer and their families by promoting evidence-based practices and actively participating in research and education.

REVIEW QUESTIONS

✓ Case Study

Joe M. is a 4-year-old white male who has been seen by his primary care physician three times in the last 2 months for recurrent bilateral otitis media despite antibiotic therapy. At his most recent visit, his doctor noted that he seemed pale and was carried in by his mother. She stated that he cries whenever he is asked to get up and walk and constantly rubs at his legs.

On physical exam the physician noted a slightly enlarged liver and scattered petecchial hemorrhages. Joe had full range of motion of his legs, and no tenderness to palpation or swelling was noted; however, Joe did refuse to walk to his mother when placed on the floor. A complete blood count (CBC) showed a hemoglobin of 7.6 gm/dl, platelets of 25,000/mm³, and a WBC count of 6500/mm³. The differential was notable for 10% neutrophils, 40% lymphocytes, and 50% lymphoblasts.

Joe's family was asked to take him to the nearest children's hospital immediately. Upon arrival, his vital signs were the following: temperature 38.9° C., pulse 148, respiratory rate 36, and blood pressure 90/60.

The pediatric oncologist explained to the parents that Joe had leukemia, based upon examination of his peripheral blood. A bone marrow aspiration and biopsy as well as a lumbar puncture with intrathecal chemotherapy was done the next morning along with placement of an implanted venous access device. Joe began chemotherapy once the diagnosis of pre–B-cell ALL was confirmed. His CSF was negative for leukemic cells.

After discharge he returned to the hospital once with fever during a neutropenic episode. His cultures were negative, his fevers resolved within 48 hours, and he was again discharged.

The remainder of his therapy was delivered in the outpatient setting. Joe completed 36 months of chemotherapy and is a healthy, active second-grade student. Joe is scheduled to have his central line removed in 2 weeks. He will continue to visit the clinic every 3 months for a blood test and physical examination.

QUESTIONS

1. What is a priority intervention for Joe upon arrival at the hospital?
   a. Teaching relaxation and distraction techniques to reduce anxiety
   b. Education regarding chemotherapy agents
   c. Discussion with parents on how to maintain normalcy for Joe at home after the diagnosis of cancer
   d. Pain assessment and appropriate intervention

2. Joe is to have a surgical procedure in the morning. Based upon his age, what is likely to be his greatest fear?
   a. Fear of the unknown
   b. Fear of postoperative pain
   c. Fear of body mutilation and punishment
   d. Fear of death

3. Administration of intrathecal chemotherapy is scheduled at the time of the initial spinal tap. Joe's mother asks why Joe will need chemotherapy injected into his spinal canal since they don't know if he has leukemia in his brain. How would you respond?
   a. Explain that intrathecal chemotherapy is given to prevent CNS leukemia.
   b. Explain that most children have leukemia in their spinal fluid at diagnosis.
   c. Reassure her that getting a head start on his treatment now shortens the duration of his therapy.
   d. Assure her there are no side effects from intrathecal chemotherapy.

4. The bone marrow confirms that Joe has pre–B-cell ALL with *TEL/AML1* rearrangement. Based upon all of his risk factors at diagnosis, what risk category does Joe fit into?
   a. High-risk
   b. Very high-risk
   c. Low-risk
   d. Standard-risk

5. Joe was febrile on admission. What interventions will he need?
   a. Blood culture, intravenous (IV) antibiotics
   b. Blood culture, oral antibiotics
   c. Continue his oral antibiotic from home for his otitis media.
   d. His fever is most likely related to his leukemia, so no interventions are necessary.

6. Joe's mother is very anxious about taking Joe home. Which teaching strategy will be most effective at this time?
   a. Verbal explanations on the day of discharge
   b. Computerized teaching module for newly diagnosed families
   c. Use of a written handout
   d. Ask Joe's mom how she learns new information best and what her most pressing concerns about taking care of Joe at home are.

7. Joe presents in the oncology clinic with a platelet count of 25,000/mm³. What would be the most appropriate guidelines for Joe's activities?
   a. Joe should not go outside to play.
   b. Joe should avoid rough play.
   c. Joe should avoid play with other children.
   d. Joe does not need any activity restrictions at this time.

8. Joe was attending a preschool program at the local school while his parents worked. Joe's mother wants to know when he can return to school and what the school needs to know. What would be the best advice?
   a. Joe's schooling should be deferred until he finishes chemotherapy.
   b. Advise Joe's mother to begin home schooling at this time.
   c. Joe should wait until he begins maintenance therapy to resume school; offer to arrange a school visit by Joe's outpatient team.
   d. Joe can return to school immediately.

9. During his diagnosis admission, Joe responded to medication administration with screaming, spitting, hitting, and throwing his toys. How would you intervene to help Joe's parents deal with his behavior?
   a. Explain that children his age often respond to fear, stress, and insecurity with behavior changes. Suggest that the parents continue to calmly enforce family expectation for behavior, reward success with a sticker chart, and ask the child life specialist to work with Joe.

Continued

REVIEW QUESTIONS—CONT'D

   b. Tell the parents to simply ignore the behavior since it will resolve once he has been discharged and he is back in his normal environment.

   c. Instruct the parents to punish Joe by taking away his play privileges.

   d. Make an immediate referral for psychiatric consultation.

10. What pain assessment tool would be the best choice for a 4-year-old child with age-appropriate cognitive development?

   a. 0-10 self-report scale

   b. A tool that allows Joe to pick a picture of a face that corresponds to how he feels

   c. Joe's mother should rate his pain on a 0-10 scale since a 4-year-old is an unreliable reporter of his own pain.

   d. Give Joe a set of words describing pain and ask him to choose the best words for his pain.

ANSWERS

1. **D.** *Rationale:* Assessment for pain is a priority for every child. Joe is exhibiting symptoms of pain in his legs by his refusal to walk, crying with weight bearing, and rubbing his legs. The most likely cause in this case is bone pain caused by the rapid proliferation of leukemic cells in the marrow space, a common finding in children with leukemia. Prompt treatment with an appropriate analgesic is indicated and should continue around the clock until treatment has been initiated for his leukemia. Bone pain usually resolves rapidly once the tumor burden in the marrow begins to decrease.

2. **C.** *Rationale:* Preschool-age children who are ill may believe that medical treatments and procedures are punishments because they misbehaved or did something that was bad. They may also believe they did something to cause their illness. They are concerned about bodily integrity and may have fantastical fears about what will happen to their bodies after a surgical procedure or venipuncture. Their understanding of the body and how it works is limited, but they are capable of understanding simple explanations. Careful preoperative and preprocedural preparation of preschoolers in simple, clear terms is critical to help them understand what will happen to them, how their body will look afterward, how they will feel, and what will be done to help them. It is also important to emphasize to children at this developmental level that illness and treatments are not punishments and that being sick is not their fault or the fault of anyone else. Medical play is a very useful technique for this age group. Placement of bandages over punctures and incisions is often very comforting and reassuring to preschoolers.

3. **A.** *Rationale:* Leukemia cells are carried throughout the body in the blood stream. These cells can be deposited in the CNS tissues where they begin to proliferate. The protective blood-brain barrier limits the amount of systemic chemotherapy that can get across and into the CSF. By giving chemotherapy directly into the CSF through a lumbar puncture, these cells can be eradicated and CNS leukemia can be prevented in most cases.

4. **D.** *Rationale:* Based upon his age of 4 and his WBC of 6500/mm³, he falls into the standard-risk category. The *TEL/AML1* rearrangement is a favorable cytogenetic finding in ALL.

5. **A.** *Rationale:* Although cytokines from leukemia cells can induce fever, children with leukemia have an impaired immune system. Untreated, children with bacterial infections can become septic and deteriorate rapidly. Bacteremia must therefore be ruled out by blood culture, and broad-spectrum IV antibiotic coverage is initiated presumptively.

6. **D.** *Rationale:* Parents of children with cancer require a great deal of information in order to care for their child safely at home. This may include learning skills such as injections, medication administration, and dressing changes that may be previously unknown to the learner. Moreover, stresses associated with having a child diagnosed with cancer can make comprehending and retaining information more difficult. By assessing Joe's mother's learning style, teaching strategies can be more effectively tailored to her needs. Knowing what concerns the mother most about taking Joe home will enable the teacher to create a teaching plan that specifically addresses those issues.

7. **B.** *Rationale:* A low platelet count increases the risk of bleeding after an injury. He should avoid activities where there is greater potential for injury such as wrestling, contact sports, or roughhouse play, but should be allowed to continue his other usual play activities.

8. **C.** *Rationale:* Most children remain quite neutropenic during the induction and intensification phases of leukemia treatment, require frequent clinic visits, and are still recovering their sense of well-being. By the time they begin maintenance therapy, they are less at risk for infection and generally feel well enough to resume most of their usual activities. School is an important part of a child's development, and school attendance should be encouraged. Many treatment centers offer school reintegration programs to address any special needs of the child, provide education about the child's disease and treatment to the school staff, other students, and parents, and answer questions the school may have about having a child with cancer in the classroom.

9. **A.** *Rationale:* Behavioral responses to stress and anxiety are common in preschool-age children. The hospital environment is a strange and unsettling place for young children. Continuing to enforce normal household expectations of behavior maintains a sense of security for young children. Preschoolers like to be successful and respond well to praise and rewards. Sticker charts are a simple and effective reward tool. Child life specialists help children develop coping techniques, express their emotions, and overcome their fears of medical procedures and treatments through play.

10. **B.** *Rationale:* Young children can be very accurate reporters of their pain when an appropriate pain tool is used. Children at this age respond well to tools such as the Wong-Baker Faces Pain Rating Scale or the Oucher Scale that allow them to select a match for how they feel from a series of pictures or drawings of facial expressions. Numerical scales and word association tools require more advanced cognitive skills and are inappropriate to use in young children. Parental assessment of a child's pain is important to elicit, but should not replace the child's own assessment.

REFERENCES

1. Ries LA, Percy CL, Bunin GR: Introduction. In Ries LA, Smith MA, Gurney JG et al, editors: *Cancer incidence and survival among children and adolescents: United States SEER program*, National Cancer Institute, SEER Program, Bethesda, MD, NIH Pub No 99-4649.
2. Landier W: Childhood lymphoblastic leukemia: Current perspectives, *Oncol Nurs Forum* 28(5):823-833, 2001
3. Arndt CAS, Anderson PA: Acute myeloid leukemia. In Behrman RE, Kleigman RM, Jenson HB, editors: *Nelson textbook of pediatrics*, Philadelphia, 2000, Saunders.
4. Ross JA, Spector LG, Robison LL et al: Epidemiology of leukemia in children with Down syndrome, *Pediatr Blood Cancer* 44(1):8-12, 2005.
5. Smith MT, McHale CM, Wiemels JL et al: Molecular biomarkers for the study of childhood leukemia, *Toxicol Appl Pharmacol* 206(2):237-245, 2005.
6. Pui CH, Evans EE: Treatment of acute lymphoblastic leukemia, *N Engl J Med* 354(2):166-178, 2006.
7. Robinson DL: Childhood Leukemia: understanding the significance of chromosomal abnormalities, *J Pediatr Oncol Nurs* 18(3):111-123, 2001.
8. Westlake SK, Bertolone KL: Acute lymphoblastic leukemia. In Baggott CR, Kelly KP, Fochtman D et al, editors: *Nursing care of children and adolescents with cancer*, ed 3, Philadelphia, 2002, WB Saunders.
9. Burger B, Zimmermann Z, Mann G et al: Diagnostic cerebrospinal fluid examination in children with acute lymphoblastic leukemia: significance of low leukocyte counts with blasts or traumatic lumbar puncture, *J Clin Oncol* 21(2):184-188, 2003.
10. Landier W: Myeloid diseases. In Baggott CR, Kelly KP, Fochtman D et al, editors: *Nursing care of children and adolescents with cancer*, ed 3, Philadelphia, 2002, WB Saunders.
12. Ghobrial IM, Habermann TM, Ristow KM et al: Prognostic factors in patients with post-transplant lymphoproliferative disorders (PTLD) in the rituximab era, *Leuk Lymphoma* 46(2):191-196, 2005.
11. Smith M, Hare ML: An overview of progress in childhood cancer survival, *J Pediatr Oncol Nurs*, 21(3):160-164, 2004
13. Hussong MR: Non-Hodgkin's lymphoma. In Baggott CR, Kelly KP, Fochtman D et al, editors: *Nursing care of children and adolescents with cancer*, ed 3, Philadelphia, 2002, WB Saunders.
14. Connors JM: Hodgkin's lymphoma. In Abeloff MD, Armitage JO, Niederhuber JE et al, editors: *Clinical oncology*, ed 3, Philadelphia, 2004, Elsevier.
15. Liebhauser, P: Hodgkin's Disease. In Baggott CR, Kelly KP, Fochtman D et al, editors: *Nursing care of children and adolescents with cancer*, ed 3, Philadelphia, 2002, WB Saunders.
16. Sandlund JT, Behm FG: Childhood lymphoma. In Abeloff MD, Armitage JO, Niederhuber JE et al, editors: *Clinical oncology*, ed 3, Philadelphia, 2004, Elsevier.
17. Gross TG, Bucuvalas JC, Park JR et al: Low dose chemotherapy for Epstein-Barr virus–positive post-transplantation lymphoproliferative disease in children after solid organ transplantation, *J Clin Oncol* 23(27):6481-6488, 2005.
18. Kleihues P, Cavenee WK: *Pathology and genetics: tumors of the nervous system*, Lyons, France, 2000, International Agency for Research on Cancer.
19. Baldwin RT, Preston-Martin S: Epidemiology for brain tumors in childhood—a review, *Toxicol Appl Pharmacol* 199(2):118-31, 2004.
20. Bunin G: What causes childhood brain tumors? Limited knowledge, many clues, *Pediatr Neurosurg* 32(6):321-326, 2000.
21. Habrand JL, De Crevoisier R: Radiation therapy in the management of childhood brain tumors, *Childs Nerv Syst* 17(3):121-133, 2001.
22. Khatua S, Jalali R: Recent advances in the treatment of childhood brain tumors, *Pediatr Hematol Oncol* 22(5):361-71, 2005.
23. Kirsch DG, Tarbell NJ: New technologies in radiation therapy for pediatric brain tumors: the rationale for proton radiation therapy, *Pediatr Blood Cancer* 42(5):461-464, 2004.
24. Maher CO, Raffel C: Neurosurgical treatment of brain tumors in children, *Pediatr Clin North Am* 51(2):327-357, 2004.
25. Suh JH, Barnett GH: Stereotactic radiosurgery for brain tumors in pediatric patients, *Technol Cancer Res Treat* 2(2):141-146, 2003.
26. Dunkel IJ, Finlay JL: High-dose chemotherapy with autologous stem cell rescue for brain tumors, *Crit Rev Oncol Hematol* 41(2):197-204, 2002.
27. Wolff JE, Finlay JL: High-dose chemotherapy in childhood brain tumors, *Oncology* 27(3):239-245, 2004.
28. Gururangan, S, Friedman, HS: Recent advances in the treatment of pediatric brain tumors, *Oncology* 18(13):1649-1661, 2004.
29. Strother, D: Atypical teratoid rhabdoid tumor of childhood: diagnosis, treatment, and challenges, *Expert Rev Anticancer Ther* 5(5):907-915, 2005.
30. Bouffet E: Common brain tumours in children: diagnosis and treatment, *Paediatric Drugs* 2(1):57-66, 2000.
31. Warren KE: Advances in the assessment of childhood brain tumors and treatment-related sequelae, *Curr Neurol Neurosci Report* 5(2):119-26, 2005.
32. Berghmans T, Paesmans M, Body JJ: A prospective study on hyponatraemia in medical cancer patients: epidemiology, aetiology and differential diagnosis, *Support Care Cancer*, 8(3):192-197, 2000.
33. Rashidi M, DaSilva VR, Minagar A et al: Nonmalignant pediatric brain tumors, *Curr Neurol Neurosci Report* 3(3):200-205, 2003.
34. Packer RJ: Progress and challenges in childhood brain tumors, *J Neurooncol* 75(3):239-242, 2005.
35. Jackaki R: Treatment strategies for high-risk medulloblastoma and supratentorial primitive neuro-ectodermal tumor. Review of the literature, *J Neurosurg* 102(1 Suppl):44-52, 2005.
36. Gurney JG, Swensen AR, Bulterys M: Malignant bone tumors. In Ries LAG, Smith MA, Gurney JG et al, editors: Cancer incidence and survival among children and adolescents: United States SEER program 1975-1995, Bethesda, Md, 1999, NIH Pub No 99-4649.
37. Hauben EI, Arends K, Vandenbroucke JP et al: Multiple primary malignancies in osteosarcoma patients. Incidence and predictive value of osteosarcoma subtype for cancer syndromes associated with osteosarcoma, *Eur J Hum Genet* 11(8):611-618, 2003.
38. Newton WA, Meadows AT, Shimada H et al: Bone sarcomas as second malignant neoplasms following childhood cancer, *Cancer* 67(1), 193-201, 1991.
39. Betcher DL, Simon PJ, McHard KM: Bone tumors. In Baggott CR, Kelly KP, Fochtman D et al, editors: *Nursing care of children and adolescents with cancer*, ed 3, Philadelphia, 2002, WB Saunders.
40. Goorin AM, Schwartzentruber DJ, Devidas M et al: Presurgical chemotherapy compared with immediate surgery and adjuvant chemotherapy for nonmetastatic osteosarcoma: Pediatric Oncology Group Study POG-8651, *J Clin Oncol* 21(8):1574-1589, 2003.
41. Grimer RJ: Surgical options for children with osteosarcoma, *Lancet Oncol* 6(2):85-92, 2005.
42. Hendershot E: Treatment approaches for metastatic Ewing's sarcoma: a review of the literature, *J Pediatr Oncol Nurs* 22(6):339-352, 2005.
43. Wilkins RM, Pritchard DJ, Durgart EO et al: Ewings sarcoma of the bone: experience with 140 patients, *Cancer* 58 (11):2551-2555, 1986.
44. Cotterill SJ, Ahrens S, Paulussen M et al: Prognostic factors in Ewing's tumor of bone: analysis of 975 patients from the European Intergroup Cooperative Ewing's Sarcoma Study Group, *J Clin Oncol* 18(17):3108-3114, 2000.
45. Grier HE, Krailo MD, Tarbell NJ et al: Addition of ifosfamide and etoposide to standard chemotherapy for Ewing's sarcoma and primitive neuroectodermal tumor of bone, *N Engl J Med* 348(8):694-701, 2003.
46. Gurney JG, Young SL, Roffers SD, et al: Soft tissue sarcomas. In Ries LA, Smith MA, Gurney JG et al, editors: *Cancer incidence and survival among children and adolescents: United States SEER program 1975-1995*, Bethesda, Md, 1999, NIH Pub No 99-4649.
47. Breneman JC, Lyden E, Paapo AS et al: Prognostic factors and clinical outcomes for children and adolescents with metastatic rhabdomyosarcoma- a report from the Intergroup Rhabdomyosarcoma Study IV, *J Clin Oncol* 21(1):78-84, 2003.
48. Raney RB, Anderson JR, Barr FG et al: Rhabdomyosarcoma and undifferentiated sarcoma in the first two decades of life: A selective review of Intergroup Rhabdomyosarcoma Study Group experience and rationale for Intergroup Rhabdomyosarcoma Study V, *J Pediatr Hematol Oncol* 23(4):215-220, 2001.
49. Maris J: The biologic basis for neuroblastoma heterogeneity and risk stratification, *Curr Opin Pediatr* 17(1):7-13, 2005.
50. Nemecek ER, Sawin RW, Park J: Treatment of neuroblastoma in patients with neurocristopathy syndromes. *J Pediatr Hematol Oncol*, 25(2):159-62, 2003.
51. Dadd G: Neuroblastoma. In Baggott CR, Kelly KP, Fochtman D et al, editors: *Nursing care of children and adolescents with cancer*, ed 3, Philadelphia, 2002, WB Saunders.

52. Matthay KK, Villablanca JG, Seeger RC et al: Treatment of high-risk neuroblastoma with intensive chemotherapy, radiotherapy, autologous bone marrow transplantation, and 13-cis-retinoic acid. Children's Cancer Group, *N Engl J Med* 341(16):1165-1173, 1999.

53. Wilson J: Neuroimmunology of dancing eye syndrome in children, *Devel Med Child Neurol* 48(8):693-696, 2006.

54. Brodeur GM, Maris JM: Neuroblastoma. In Pizzo PA, Poplack DG, editors: *Principles and practice of pediatric oncology*, Philadelphia, 2002, Lippincott, Williams, & Wilkins.

55. Drigan R, Androkites AL: Wilms Tumor. In Baggott CR, Kelly KP, Fochtman D et al, editors: *Nursing care of children and adolescents with cancer,* ed 3, Philadelphia, 2002, WB Saunders.

56. Anderson PM: Neoplasms of the kidney. In Behrman RE, Kleigman RM, Jenson HB, editors: *Nelson textbook of pediatrics*, Philadelphia, 2000, Saunders.

57. Couriel D, Caldera H, Champlin R et al: Acute graft-versus-host disease: pathophysiology, clinical manifestations, and management, *Cancer* 101(9):1936-1946, 2004.

58. Goodman JL, Winston DJ, Greenfield RA et al: A controlled trial of fluconazole to prevent fungal infections in patients undergoing bone marrow transplantation [see comments], *N Engl J Med* 326(13): 845-851, 1992.

59. Kumar S, DeLeve LD, Kamath PS et al: Hepatic veno-occlusive disease (sinusoidal obstruction syndrome) after hematopoietic stem cell transplantation, *Mayo Clin Proc* 78(5):589-598, 2003.

60. Wadleigh M, Ho V, Momtaz P et al: Hepatic veno-occlusive disease: pathogenesis, diagnosis and treatment, *Curr Opin Hematol* 10(6): 451-462, 2003.

61. Shankar G, Cohen DA: Idiopathic pneumonia syndrome after bone marrow transplantation: the role of pre-transplant radiation conditioning and local cytokine dysregulation in promoting lung inflammation and fibrosis, *Int J Exp Pathol* 82(20):101-113, 2001.

62. Roychowdhury M, Pambuccian SE, Aslan DL et al: Pulmonary complications after bone marrow transplantation: an autopsy study from a large transplantation center, *Arch Pathol Lab Med* 129(3):366-371, 2005.

63. Fukuda T, Hackman RC, Guthrie KA et al: Risks and outcomes of idiopathic pneumonia syndrome after nonmyeloablative and conventional conditioning regimens for allogeneic hematopoietic stem cell transplantation, *Blood* 102(8):2777-2785, 2003.

64. Landier W, Bhatia S, Eshelman D et al: Development of risk-based guidelines for pediatric cancer survivors: the Children's Oncology Group long term follow-up guidelines from the Children's Oncology Group Late Effects Committee and Nursing Discipline, *J Clin Oncol* 22(24):4979-4990, 2004.

65. Schwartz C: Long-term survivors of childhood cancer: the late effects of therapy, *Oncologist* 4(1):45-54, 1999.

66. Mullhern RK, Merchant TE, Gajjar A et al: Late neurocognitive sequelae in survivors of brain tumours in childhood, *Lancet Oncol* 5(7):399-408, 2004.

67. Ullrich NJ, Pomeroy SL: Pediatric brain tumors, *Neurol Clin* 21(4): 897-913, 2003.

68. Neglia JP, Friedman DL, Yasui Y et al: Second malignant neoplasms in five-year survivors of childhood cancer: Childhood Cancer Survivor Study, *J Natl Cancer Inst* 93(8):618-629, 2001.

69. Bjork, M., Wiebe, T., Hallstrom, I: Striving to survive: families lived experiences when a child is diagnosed with cancer, *J Pediatr Oncol Nurses* 22(5):265-275, 2005.

70. Ljungman G, Gordh T, Sorenson S et al: Pain variations during cancer therapy in children: a descriptive survey, *Pediatr Hematol Oncol* 17(2):211-221, 2000.

71. Panzarella C, Baggott CR, Comeu M et al: Management of disease and treatment-related complications. In Baggott CR, Kelly KP, Fochtman D et al, editors: *Nursing care of children and adolescents with cancer,* ed 3, Philadelphia, 2002, WB Saunders.

72. Hedstrom M, Ljungman G, von Essen L: Perceptions of distress among adolescents recently diagnosed with cancer, *J Pediatr Hematol Oncol* 27(1):15-22, 2005.

73. Sidhu R, Passmore A, Baker D: An investigation into parent perceptions of the needs of siblings of children with cancer, *J Pediatr Oncol Nurs* 22(5):276-287, 2005.

Cancer Treatment Modalities

CHAPTER 19

Surgery

Joanne Lester

Definition

Surgery, by definition, is the branch of medicine that uses manual and instrumental means to deal with the diagnosis and treatment of injury, deformity, and disease. Surgical oncology is defined as the branch of surgery focusing on the surgical management of malignant neoplasms, including biopsy, staging, and surgical resection.[1] The modality of surgical intervention is an important option in the treatment of cancer. Potentially, surgical oncology procedures may be used to prevent a cancer occurrence in the high-risk patient, to diagnose a primary or metastatic site of malignancy, to provide primary or secondary treatment of an identified malignancy, to provide a route of administration of therapy, to rehabilitate by means of reconstructive interventions, or to offer palliative care through symptom management in advanced cancer. Historically, surgical interventions have evolved from radical en bloc procedures to less invasive, often tissue-sparing procedures, depending on the presentation of the malignancy and the goals of treatment.

Oncology patients typically undergo at least one surgical procedure at some point in the trajectory of their cancer. Nursing fulfills important roles in the care of the surgical oncology patient throughout the entire cancer experience. Nurses' involvement with the cancer patient may lead them to identify risk factors or behaviors that prompt a preventive surgical procedure. They may play a role during the initial assessment and evaluation of symptoms, testing, and diagnosis; throughout the preoperative, perioperative, and postoperative care of primary or secondary surgical procedures; in the identification of need and advocacy for devices to enhance administration of therapy; throughout reconstructive procedures during the rehabilitation phase; or in symptom identification and management during the palliative phase of care. Therefore, it is important that nurses understand the fundamentals of surgical oncology. Nurses must be instrumental in the identification, planning, implementation, and evaluation phases of surgical treatment to provide a comprehensive plan of care and enhance patient outcomes.

Historical Perspective

Surgery in the mid-eighteenth century provided the era of observation and discovery of the clinicopathologic features of malignant tumors that led to today's medical and surgical management of malignancies. Through primitive efforts at eradicating tumors, to advances in pathology, antisepsis, and anesthesia and further advances in multimodality management, surgical oncology remains a vital part of cancer care. Surgery is the oldest cancer intervention, and one that has offered the possibility of cure. Adequate surgical resection continues to bear responsibility for the cure of many cancers today.[2]

Historically, cancer surgery can be traced back over 5000 years to treatment of breast cancer, albeit primitive, in that preanesthesia era. In 1809, Ephraim MacDowell excised a massive ovarian tumor,

which initiated the prospect of successful cancer surgery.[3] Elliot, in 1822, reported microscopic examination of a lymph node related to breast cancer; and Paget, in 1856, published observations from 374 breast cancer cases. In the mid-1800s, the European schools of surgery evolved as surgical scholars replaced barber-surgeons. Morton introduced anesthesia at Massachusetts General Hospital in 1846, and Lister introduced the concept of antisepsis in 1867. These landmark discoveries brought surgery to the forefront in the United States, since patients could now undergo surgery without pain or significant risk of sepsis.[3,4]

Surgical procedures significantly advanced through the work of Halsted in radical mastectomy; Billroth in gastrectomy, laryngectomy, hemipelvectomy, and prostatectomy; and Wier, von Mikuliez and Mayo in colon cancer. In the early 1900s, advances continued through Kocher and Lahey in thyroid surgery; Crile, Senn, and Martin in head and neck surgery; and Clark and Wertheim in uterine malignancies. Further advances in the early-to mid-1900s were developed by Miles in abdominoperineal resection; Graham in pneumonectomy; Whipple in pancreaticoduodenectomy; and Brunschwig in pelvic exenteration. These surgical procedures focused on controlling locally advanced disease identified at the time of diagnosis.[3]

The notion of identifying and surgically removing cancer in an earlier stage was the basis for study of surgical interventions after World War II. The advent of antimicrobials and advances in anesthesia and blood transfusions enabled surgeons to further advance their work. Halsted's concept of the surgical treatment of breast cancer, that is, removal of the entire breast and the regional lymphatics, became the model for other sites of cancer. Surgical procedures for various other cancers expanded this concept, with removal of adjacent structures that may be involved in the spread of cancer. This was the era of the bigger, the better. The more radical the surgical procedure, the better the chance that a cure could be obtained.[3]

In the mid-1950s it was noted that despite the technical advancement of these radical procedures, the mortality rates associated with certain cancer sites were not improving. In addition, many of these radical surgeries created significant morbidity issues even if a cure was obtained. Crile challenged the high mortality risk in pancreaticoduodenectomy and the premise of axillary node dissection in breast cancer. In the later 1950s and 1960s, formal clinical trials emerged in surgical oncology. Fisher incorporated biologic principles and challenged Halsted's hypotheses of radical breast cancer surgery, introducing less aggressive surgical approaches.[3]

Today, with the aid of advanced diagnostics, many cancers are diagnosed in an earlier stage through effective screening and early detection practices. Various clinical innovations guide presurgical staging and planning, making it more possible to distinguish those patients who will benefit from surgical intervention from those who will not. Quality of life issues are now considered, as well as adjuvant therapies that potentially allow a less extensive surgical procedure. Most importantly, clinical trials have provided information that guides evidence-based practice and helps establish standards of care.[3] Historically, the surgical management of cancer has been instrumental in establishing the prevailing treatment of most cancer sites, and stands to continue doing so.

Principles

The principles of surgical oncology are based in the foundations of surgery and oncology, nursing, and medicine. Principles create the basic framework, but rapidly advancing scientific and technologic methods may change the identification or ranking of principles related to new and possibly unidentified needs of the cancer patient. Therefore the surgical oncology team should be familiar with various cancers and their natural history, as well as treatment modalities of surgery, radiation therapy, chemotherapy, and biologic therapies. Nurses, depending on their area of practice, level of expertise, level of education, and practice role, may have to acknowledge and employ varying degrees of theoretic expertise. This may range from the non–oncology nurse who seldom encounters a surgical oncology patient, to a surgical nurse in the operating room, to a nurse who works solely on a surgical oncology unit, or to an advanced practice nurse in a surgical oncology clinic.[5] In addition, various members of the cancer multidisciplinary team may be involved in caring for the surgical oncology patient, exerting their own disciplines' principles of practice, which intertwine with the nursing approach. Although some nursing functions carry over from their own disciplines, in creating a collaborative care environment, the nurse will operate as a member of the surgical oncology team.

PREVENTION AND IDENTIFICATION OF RISK FACTORS

With the advent of widespread education, advances in cancer surveillance, improved understanding of cancer biology, better characterization of premalignant disease, and genetic testing, a clear role for surgical oncology in preventive surgery in the high-risk patient has emerged. Surgery remains one of the best options for many high-risk individuals. However, as in all prevention modalities, the cancer risk must be balanced with the benefit and risk of surgical treatment.[6,7]

The issues surrounding surgical prevention vary widely among different cancer types and etiologies. Not only must the specific cancer be scrutinized, but so must the individual. The age and specific risk related to age must be considered. Survival and quality-adjusted survival curves for the preventive measures should be discussed, measuring the benefits dependent on the age at which the surgical intervention is performed.[8] Certain patients and their family members must consider preventive surgery at an early age, while others may have decades to decide. Various factors regarding current surveillance methods should be considered, including the specificity of the screening tool related to age and individual effects. Routine screening with increased frequency of clinical examinations should be established, stressing the importance of close surveillance. The surgical oncology team has a responsibility to educate and alert the patient and family to hereditary potentials of certain cancers and their possible occurrence in other family members.

The particular organ(s) at risk bears much consideration, with concerns related to the potential morbidity of surgery. In addition, the potential aggressiveness of the cancer, once present, must be weighed against preventive surgery with the knowledge that the cancer may never occur.[6] Quality of life indices must also be considered and discussed with the patient and family. Persons undergoing prophylactic surgery must weigh the potential long-term physical and psychologic consequences against the potential physical, emotional, and economic effects if the cancer does occur.[8] Additional challenges arise in the newly diagnosed patient who also may have an identifiable genetic risk, thus adding prevention to treatment. Although the diagnosed cancer outcome may not be affected by further preventive surgery, increased anxiety related to a potential genetic mutation may be disabling. Unfortunately, there are few circumstances that permit the delay of definitive cancer surgery to wait for genetic testing results, which may take weeks to months to obtain. It is prudent to avoid the combination of cancer-related surgery and prophylactic surgery if the genetic status is unknown.[9] Often, once the cancer is treated, the issues related to prevention resurface and are addressed.

DIAGNOSIS AND STAGING OF CANCER

Cancer, with potential involvement of nearly every organ system in the human body, can present a challenging histologic picture. An accurate histologic diagnosis specific to the origin of the tumor is critical to proper identification of the malignancy, as well as appropriate treatment planning. Attention to tumor cell characteristics may be important, such as differentiation, mitotic rate, and other markers inherent to specific cancers. Consideration must be made of known, clinically evident disease as well as potentially unidentified symptoms or unknown disease. The results of pathology studies must be correlated with the physical examination as well as radiographic and hematologic studies, including tumor markers for certain cancers. Often, the surgical oncology team is challenged to arrive at a diagnosis by process of elimination. Equally so, obvious disease should not be accepted as unambiguous, since each patient is unique, as is every cancer diagnosis and trajectory. The burden often lies with the surgical oncology team to delve into far-reaching areas for an accurate and thorough diagnosis.

Another major role of the surgical oncology team is to obtain adequate tissue for histologic diagnosis. Different surgical approaches may be required for different cancers; therefore it is important for the surgical oncology team to decide on the surgical diagnostic approach and properly educate the patient and their family on the procedure and the intended results. Often, another discipline may be performing the biopsy, such as radiology. If a series of diagnostic procedures may be required to adequately diagnose a suspected malignancy, it is important to share this information. There are a variety of surgical techniques that are used to obtain tissue samples for examination. These include fine-needle aspiration, core needle biopsy, incisional biopsy, and excisional biopsy.[10]

Fine-needle aspiration utilizes a small-gauge needle and syringe with the goal of aspirating cells and tissue fragments from the suspected lesion. This procedure is useful in identifying the presence of malignant cells, but is not as definitive as obtaining larger amounts of tissue. If a malignancy is suspected and the fine-needle aspiration is benign, further tissue sampling should be pursued. If neoadjuvant therapy is planned, additional tissue sampling should be performed in the event that all other pathologic evidence of tumor is destroyed by the neoadjuvant treatment.

Major surgical procedures should not be based only on the histo-logic evidence provided by a fine-needle aspiration.[10]

Core needle biopsy is a common biopsy technique used to obtain small slivers of tissue from the suspected malignancy.[10] This biopsy can be performed utilizing a hand-held, spring-loaded instrument for palpable or nonpalpable lesions. Core needle biopsies are often performed with radiographic guidance in the event that the malignancy is not easily felt. If a core needle biopsy is benign and a malignancy is suspected, further tissue sampling is warranted. Core needle biopsies are often performed instead of more invasive procedures such as incisional or exci-sional biopsies.

An incisional biopsy removes a small wedge of tissue from a large, suspicious mass via a skin incision. Most tumor masses do not require this type of biopsy, although this procedure may be preferred in certain soft tissue and bony masses. An excisional biopsy removes the entire area of suspicion, via a skin incision, with little or no margin of normal tissue surrounding the mass. This biopsy technique is typically performed to identify the histologic features of the mass, not to obtain clear margins. In most cases, further definitive surgery must be performed to adequately stage the tumor and ensure clear margins.[10] Sutures are typically required in both incisional and excisional biopsies. An exception to this may be when tissue is retrieved through endo-scopic procedures, such as bronchoscopy, mediastinoscopy, upper endoscopy, or colonoscopy. These procedures allow either an inci-sional or excisional biopsy through a flexible fiberoptic instrument intended to retrieve tissue from an intraluminal location.

The following principles should be followed in all tissue biopsies: (1) needle tracks or incisions should be placed in an appropriate anatomic position and plane so that the area can be excised with subsequent definitive surgery; (2) during the biopsy, contamination of adjacent tissue planes should be avoided; adequate pressure should be applied to the site for hemostasis in an effort to prevent large hematomas; (3) sufficient tissue rele-vant to the suspect malignancy should be provided to the pathol-ogist; and (4) appropriate tissue handling should occur with accurate tissue markings relative to orientation of the specimen.[10] The surgical oncology team is responsible for educating the patient and the family, for providing emotional support, for iden-tifying and preventatively treating pain, and for creating a safe environment.

Coupled with the pathologic diagnosis is the staging of the cancer, which describes the cancer as it relates to local, regional, and distant extent. Tumors are staged by site, typically using the tumor-nodes-metastasis (TNM) classification system from the American Joint Committee for Cancer Staging and End Results Reports (AJCC SEER). The TNM classification describes the tumor based on size and local extension (T), nodal involvement (N), and distance metastasis (M).[11] Proper staging is important for accurate treatment planning and subsequent disease management and prognosis. Lack of proper staging can compromise the plan of care and the ability to cure a patient. Staging may be performed solely by means of surgery, but most likely will be initiated before surgery and include radiographic and serum and/or tumor marker studies. Thorough surgical staging may spare a patient unneces-sary surgical resection if the disease has advanced, or may iden-tify area(s) that require further resection. It is important for the surgical oncology team to thoroughly understand the etiology, biologic nature, and trajectory of each cancer since appropriate

surgical staging may be necessary before definitive surgery.[12] At times, based on the type of tumor and presentation, referral to a larger institution or cancer center that performs such procedures on a regular basis may be in the patient's best interest. These diffi-cult discussions are the responsibility of the surgical oncology team as it strives to provide the best outcome possible for each individual patient.

TREATMENT

Cancer surgery can be straightforward or complicated, based on the natural history of the individual cancer, each specific pres-entation and evidence of identifiable disease, and the patient's overall health status. Unfortunately, at the initial presentation, patients with solid tumors have a 70% chance of having micrometastasis beyond the primary site. Therefore, it is important for the surgical oncology team to have a clear understanding of current treatment trends for each cancer type. The emergence of nonsurgical therapies may be very effective in improving the cure rate of the 70% of patients who have micrometastatic disease. Therefore multidisciplinary discussions should occur with review of current clinical research trends before initiating definitive surgery.[10,12] As a result, other therapies may be administered before surgery, during surgery, or immediately after surgery, such as neoadjuvant chemotherapy, intraoperative radiation therapy, or use of biologic therapy options.

Neoadjuvant or concurrent therapies have strong biologic rationale and provide promising strategies for many cancers. Administering neoadjuvant therapy may avail the opportunity to study and measure in vivo response of a tumor before, during, and after a specific treatment modality, possibly affording predictors of prognosis and therapeutic response.[13-15] Clinical trials related to the study of gene expression by individual tumors may also be important in the consideration of individualized therapy.[16] However, despite the fact that clinical research results often support combined modality approaches, the incremental gains they produce may be modest compared to the additional toxicities that result. In fact, the optimal sequencing of each treatment modal-ity may be controversial and difficult to determine.[19] Another issue of concern with neoadjuvant therapy is the possibility of chemotherapy-induced sterilization; that is, the elimination of evidence of tumor in adjacent or regional tissues, confusing the identification of the stage of disease at the time of definitive surgery. This potential pitfall may necessitate surgical staging, such as sentinel lymph node biopsy, before delivery of neoadjuvant therapy, in an effort to prevent false-negative results from tissue evaluation and a mistakenly low staging assignment.[18]

The surgical oncology team must individualize care and include the patient and their family in the decision making process, noting the pros and cons of various options. Although improvements in survival may or may not be experienced, decrease of the tumor size itself may occur with neoadjuvant therapy, allowing a less aggressive surgical intervention with improved local control and/or organ preservation.[12,19] It is important to provide up-to-date clinical information to guide patients toward a choice of strategy to appropriately diagnose, stage and treat their cancer. The goals are to maximize their potential for cure, minimize undesirable comorbidities, and provide the satisfaction to patients of being an active partner in their care.[20-22] Unfortunately, the interaction(s) with each individual patient is often not predictable, and so decision making is made more difficult during a time when initiating any type of treatment is imperative in the mind of the patient and family.

The surgical oncology team is also responsible, preoperatively, to determine operative risk. The potential benefits of surgical cancer intervention must be weighed against the surgical risks. The determinants of operative risk include general health status, underlying illness and its severity, disruptive degree of surgery to physiologic functions, complexity of procedure in relation to potential complications, type of anesthesia, and experience of involved team members.[10] A thorough history and physical should be performed before considering any surgical intervention. Further evaluation of identifiable problems is imperative if they pose an added risk to the morbidity or mortality of the planned surgical procedure. Appropriate referrals are the responsibility of the surgical oncology team to clarify and resolve any known health issues before surgery.

REHABILITATION AND RECONSTRUCTION

As a result of improved cancer therapies and treatment modalities, patients are increasingly benefiting from extended years of life or are anticipating cure of their disease. More than 8 million people are *living* with cancer. This growing population of persons that achieve long-term periods of remission, survival, and even cure directs us to the importance of cancer rehabilitation.[23] Rehabilitation to improve physical, psychologic, social, and spiritual outcomes should be considered at the time of diagnosis and throughout the cancer trajectory. Prioritization according to stage of disease, health of the individual, and other related issues must be considered. Rehabilitation should include education for patients and their families on how to deal with acute and chronic functional impairments.[24,25]

Issues regarding surgical rehabilitation must be addressed to improve function and cosmetic appearance secondary to anatomic defects.[10] Although the surgical oncology team may not directly be performing these rehabilitative surgical procedures, discussion should occur along with appropriate referrals, whether preoperative, postoperatively, or long-term. Often, the ability to remediate a loss of function or an anatomic defect is dependent on how the definitive cancer surgery was performed. Breast reconstruction is an integral part of cancer rehabilitation for many women, improving self-esteem and body symmetry.[26] Concerns regarding future fertility options in young women diagnosed with certain cancers may be prudent before any surgical intervention. Cancers that affect the head and neck require significant rehabilitative efforts and discussion at the time of diagnosis, since there may be a significant impact on self-image, self-expression, coping mechanisms, and socialization. For these patients and their families, ongoing counseling and support may significantly improve outcomes.[25]

PALLIATION

The World Health Organization (WHO) defines palliative care as "an approach that improves the quality of life of patients and their families for problems associated with life-threatening illness, through the prevention and relief of suffering .... [It] provides relief from pain and other distressing symptoms .... [It] will enhance quality of life, and may also positively influence the course of illness ..."[27] The surgical oncology team may direct, or provide consultation for, the discussion of surgical interventions for the relief of pain, symptoms, or functional abnormalities to

improve quality of life for cancer patients with incurable disease. At times, the intended procedure may loom larger than the cancer itself, as in instances of advanced disease. Treatment decisions can be difficult for both the surgical oncology team and the patient and family, and there must be frank discussion regarding risks and benefits. Comprehensive care should focus on a balance of offering aggressive care, maintaining optimal symptom management, and providing comfort.[28]

Appropriate purposes for palliative surgery may include the following: (1) relief of symptoms when the extent of tumor is already known; (2) resection of residual tumor after surgery; (3) resection for recurrent or persistent disease when primary treatment has failed; and (4) supportive care with technical intervention required by the multidisciplinary team.[29] The physical and social impact of uncontrolled symptoms and the need to maintain hope have been found to be motivators of palliative surgery. Even when the palliative nature of surgery is clearly discussed, some patients and their families may still hope for cure, whether through surgery or the discovery of a new drug, or just for the prolongation of life.[28]

The impact of palliative surgery on family caregivers is yet another dimension that should be addressed by the surgical oncology team. Caregivers should be assessed for specific psychologic, social, and spiritual needs, and appropriate education and support referrals made as required.[29] Family conferences may prove useful during these difficult times as patients, family members, and health care providers alike struggle with the enormity of these decisions.

Types of Therapies
CATEGORIES OF THERAPIES

The role of surgery in cancer can be divided into six categories: (1) definitive surgery for primary cancer, local therapy, and integration with other adjuvant modalities; (2) surgery for residual disease; (3) surgery for metastatic disease with curative intent; (4) surgery for oncologic emergencies; (5) surgery for reconstruction and rehabilitation; and (6) surgery for palliation.[10] The initial surgical intervention may be planned as a primary cancer intervention, but may instead become a debulking surgery or include identification of metastatic disease. It is important for the surgical oncology team to support the original intent and informed consent of the patient and family when these previously unsuspected findings emerge, and to communicate appropriately. The decision may be made to abbreviate or abort a surgical procedure until further discussion with the patient can occur. New clinical information may change the course or sequence of therapies, or the desires of the patient and family.

Definitive surgery for primary cancer aims to remove the cancer with a margin of clear tissue around the cancer itself.[10] This surgery may also include assessment and/or removal of adjacent or regional structures to verify the stage of disease. The initial surgery alone may be curative in nature, or identify the need for additional surgery. Often, these decisions cannot be made at the time of surgery, but instead, must be made after the final pathology report is received.

Surgery for residual disease, or cytoreductive surgery, may enhance the ability of other interventions to improve the outcome for a specific cancer. Such examples include Burkitt's lymphoma and ovarian cancer, where other cancer modalities, such as chemotherapy, may make an impact on remaining disease that is unresectable.[10] Unfortunately, some cytoreductive surgical procedures may be ineffective, or worsen outcomes, and should possibly be avoided.

Surgery for metastatic disease may be curative in nature, based on the type of cancer, location and number of metastatic deposits, and other available treatment options. The functional sequelae of surgical resection, as in brain metastasis, should also be considered before intervention.[10]

Oncologic emergencies may necessitate surgery related to impending destruction of vital organs, hemorrhage, perforation, obstruction, compression, or abscess formation.[10] In these instances, seldom does the surgical procedure have a direct impact on the primary or metastatic site(s) of cancer, but instead is performed because of a complication of the cancer itself or related treatment modalities. Surgical intervention may promote comfort and ease pain, even if death is imminent. These difficult decisions require thoughtful consideration by the surgical oncology team and appropriate communication with the patient and/or family.

Surgeries for rehabilitation or reconstructive needs and palliative concerns have been addressed in the earlier "Principles" section. An additional identifiable surgical need is the assessment for, advocacy of, and insertion of devices to aid in the administration of therapies either regionally or systemically. The surgical oncology team is often responsible for identifying poor venous access early in the patient's cancer trajectory and should plan and intervene appropriately. Other devices may be inserted at the initial surgery for control of metastatic disease, or may be utilized at a later time with recurrent disease. Adequate patient and family education should occur before the insertion of any device with discussion of the risks, benefits, potential complications, intended duration of treatment, maintenance requirements, and ongoing care. Therapeutic devices include those intended for delivery of drug to a specific organ or region, or catheters that provide venous access for systemic use. Multiple types and brands are available with the ever-continuing development of new products. Some examples are nontunneled catheters, tunneled catheters, implantable ports, intraventricular reservoirs, intrathecal catheters, intraperitoneal catheters, external pumps, and implantable pumps. Although these devices may enhance delivery of drug to a specific area, with significant improvement in symptom management or disease control, they often are frustrating reminders of cancer to patients and their family. The surgical oncology team can be instrumental in preventing complications, providing psychosocial support, educating the patient and family, and assessing disease or symptom response.

INDICATIONS FOR USE

The basic tenets of surgery are based on the principles as outlined above, but new approaches and techniques abound in the surgical oncology arena. Definitive cancer surgery continues to trend toward minimally invasive procedures when possible. Unfortunately, many cancer surgeries still require more radical procedures, although improved equipment, instrumentation, surgical supplies, immunologic therapy, and radiographic guidance have the potential to reduce postoperative morbidity.

Procedures such as **ductal lavage** and **fine-needle aspiration (FNA)** are being studied in cancer prevention and early detection clinical trials. These studies focus on changes in breast epithelial cells in an effort to identify cytologic or molecular changes over

time that correlate with the carcinogenic continuum and cancer development.[18,30] Identifying cancer in its earliest stages not only improves the mortality rate, but potentially decreases the need for more invasive surgical procedures. Preventive surgical applications may also involve discussion regarding fertility-sparing surgery and/or other options depending on a number of variables specific to the patient and type of cancer.

Sentinel lymph node biopsy has been one of the most exciting surgical procedures in the last decade, specifically for breast cancer and melanoma, as studies for other cancer primaries continue. This procedure enables the surgeon to perform intraoperative lymphatic mapping with vital blue dye and/or a radioactive tracer. The sentinel lymph node basin is noted visually; the gamma-ray counter and probe verify in vivo radioactivity. The sentinel node(s) is dissected, with pathologic examination of this first draining lymph node(s) of the tumor. At the time of surgery, if the sentinel node is negative for tumor, most often a lymph node dissection is not necessary. If the sentinel node is positive, a regional lymph node dissection may occur. Clinical trials are currently in progress to measure the value of performing a regional lymph node dissection even when the sentinel node is reactive. This procedure has spared innumerable patients the threat, or actual occurrence, of lymphedema related to extensive node dissection.[31]

Additional examples of **radioguided surgery** being studied are **radioguided parathyroidectomy (RGP)** and **radioimmunoguided surgery-intraoperative radiotherapy (RIGS-IORT)**. Similar to sentinel lymph node biopsy use, RGP patients are injected with a radioactive tracer; the neoprobe is used to localize parathyroid tissue that may otherwise be difficult to identify, thus reducing operative time and frozen section(s) and incurring improved outcomes.[32] Previous studies in colorectal cancer utilized the neoprobe to define areas of residual microscopic disease labeled with radioactive monoclonal antibodies, with intended maximal resection of tumor and possible IORT.[33]

Video-assisted thoracoscopic surgery (VATS), commonly used to diagnose and manage thoracic pathologies, offers a minimally invasive approach. Visualization of the chest is enhanced, offering access for biopsies from the pleura, the diaphragm, and the pericardium. VATS is beneficial for the diagnosis and treatment of metastatic pleural effusions, allowing pleurodesis with the avoidance of frequent thoracentesis.[34]

Light amplification by stimulated emission (LASER) light is an intense, narrow beam that enables the performance of precise surgery to remove precancerous or cancerous tissue, or to relieve symptoms of cancer. It is more commonly used on the surface of the body or the lining of intraluminal organs. Often laser therapy is administered through endoscopic instruments, resulting in less bleeding and damage to normal tissue than traditional surgical procedures. **Laser-induced interstitial thermotherapy (LITT)** or interstitial laser photocoagulation utilizes laser light and heat to kill tumor cells. **Photodynamic therapy (PDT)** utilizes a photosensitizing agent injected in the body, followed by targeted laser therapy to destroy cancer cells. Although laser therapy effects in cancer may not last, it provides yet another alternative in surgical cancer care.[35]

Cryosurgery, or **cryotherapy,** utilizes the cold effect of liquid nitrogen to destroy precancerous or cancerous tissues. It is applied externally on the skin, or internally through a cryoprobe instrument, either at the time of surgery or percutaneously. Cryosurgery provides a less invasive method of targeting and destroying tissue, with decreased bleeding and pain than traditional surgical methods. Although cryosurgery may not be curative for some tumors, it may offer a method of local control with minimal side effects.[36]

Radiofrequency ablation (RFA) is yet another novel approach to eradicating cancerous tissue. RFA destroys tumors in situ by thermal coagulation and protein denaturation. High-frequency alternating current flows from uninsulated electrode tips into surrounding tissue, resulting in friction heating as tissue ions follow the change in direction of alternating current. It is presumed that this heating mechanism forces extracellular and intracellular fluid(s) out of tissue, thus resulting in coagulative necrosis.[37,38]

Laparoscopy is evolving with multiple clinical trials to identify its efficacy and safety in the care of cancer patients, from diagnosis and staging through treatment and palliation. Laparoscopy enables a surgeon to diagnose intraperitoneal and retroperitoneal masses, lymph nodes, and visceral lesions without a large abdominal incision. It also can help stage various intraabdominal cancers, either sparing the patient an extensive, futile surgery, or encouraging the surgeon to be aggressive in a curative fashion.[39] Laparoscopy continues to be studied as a vehicle for definitive surgery, as in laparoscopic radical prostatectomy. Such surgeries offer the advantage of lower morbidity rates, shorter hospital stays, and improved quality of life outcomes. Long-term cancer control and survival rates continue to be monitored for comparison to more aggressive surgery as surgeons strive to improve cancer care and cause less trauma to the patient.[40]

Biologic therapies and other **adjuvant therapies** play an interesting role in the surgical management of the cancer patient. Human granulocyte colony-stimulating factor (G-CSF) used with neoadjuvant or concurrent radiation therapy or chemotherapy can dramatically decrease neutropenia-related infections and complications. The use of preoperative recombinant human erythropoietin or iron in anemic surgical patients may enhance the ability to sustain red blood cell levels, provide autologous blood, and/or reduce the need for allogeneic blood transfusions.[41] Novel use of these and other agents in the cancer patient is the responsibility of the surgical oncology team.

NURSING CARE CONSIDERATIONS

Nurses, as key members of the surgical oncology team, play vital roles in the education, support, and care of cancer patients and their families. From prevention and early detection to diagnosis and staging, during preoperative, perioperative, and postoperative care, and through rehabilitation and palliative care, nurses continually contribute valuable interventions and insight. The patient and family, as well as the surgical oncology team, benefit from information they provide and teach that is crucial for successful communication and treatment.

Evidence-based practice standards, guidelines, and clinical pathways are necessary to guide practice and improve outcomes of cancer care. Nurses need to take an active part in researching, creating, and implementing such tools for improved patient and family delivery of care as well as for staff competency and satisfaction. The National Comprehensive Cancer Network (NCCN) provides clinical guidelines that focus on various cancers and common symptoms associated with cancer. The National Cancer Institute (NCI), American Cancer Society (ACS), Oncology Nursing Society (ONS), and a host of other cancer-related organizations have joined with NCCN in efforts to coordinate cancer

care worldwide.[42] The process of care from initial entry to outcome is measured by means of quality indicators, with resulting changes in practice as needed.

Advanced practice nurses (APNs) can enhance the surgical oncology team through collaborative as well as independent roles. As administrators, APNs can create a multidisciplinary environment conducive to meeting the needs of patients and families. As educators, APNs can enhance teaching moments throughout the cancer trajectory, for nursing staff as well as the patient and family. APNs functioning as expert clinicians are vital in coordinating medical and nursing problems toward solutions, using advanced assessment and communication skills. As researchers, APNs fulfill an important role in advancing nursing science based on theory, as well as procuring grant funds to investigate patient and family care issues. Finally, as consultants, APNs provide expertise in the management of cancer patients and families, coordinating the various multidisciplinary resources available for improved care.[43]

Nursing care of the surgical oncology patient employs all the skills and knowledge of the nurse caring for any oncology patient or any type of cancer. The preoperative phase includes a thorough assessment including medical and surgical history, psychosocial history, nutritional status, medications, laboratory and imaging studies, and teaching needs. With assessment for potential perioperative or postoperative complications, appropriate nursing management of comorbid diseases such as diabetes, heart disease, mental illness, respiratory disease, and gastrointestinal malfunction, as well as of safety issues, must occur concomitantly with cancer care. This overall assessment and plan of care should operate throughout the patient's cancer trajectory, with subsequent revisions secondary to changes in treatment, condition, or cancer status. The perioperative phase is typically confined to issues related to surgery, anesthesia, blood products, fluid and electrolyte balance, cardiac hemostasis, and safety. Postoperatively, managing potential alternations in respiratory, cardiovascular, and gastrointestinal function and fluid volume, as well as pain, infection, and bleeding, are crucial in preventing postoperative complications.[44] Discharge planning that involves self-care objectives and potential independence is important, in conjunction with appropriate patient and family education, to provide care for alterations related to surgery.

After the immediate surgical phase, nursing considerations shift to rehabilitative and/or palliative care for the patient and family. Psychosocial needs, whether perceived or actual, and related to coping mechanisms, communication skills, lifestyle changes, body image alterations, sexuality dysfunction, and disease recurrence, present challenges for the surgical oncology team. Physical needs related to surgery, potential long-term side effects, concomitant disease, multimodality therapy, and/or progressive or recurrent cancer require strong assessment and interventional skills. Quality of life issues must be addressed to guide clinical decision making with optimal outcomes. Often the patient and family are the center of the decision making at this phase. Cancer survivors require interventions related to their long-term rehabilitation, as well as healthy lifestyle and general health surveillance measures. Cancer patients facing death from their primary disease or concomitant illness may have varying needs based on their own personal belief systems, ethics and end-of-life desires. The surgical oncology team plays a vital role in providing palliative care through continued assessment and evaluation of potential surgical interventions to relieve symptoms and/or pain.

Considerations for Older Adults

Surgery in older adults is often modified or withheld because of perceptions of physical intolerance, or because the overall life expectancy is considered too short. Although mortality rates do not differ between the younger and older cancer patient, psychologic well-being has been shown to influence functional recovery when variables such as age, comorbidities, site of cancer, and symptom severity were controlled. The older patient with cancer should be carefully assessed and scrutinized preoperatively, and then treated in the manner that would be offered to any patient, regardless of age. Attention to routine screening and early detection practices remain important in the older person in the effort to detect and diagnose cancer at an earlier stage. Elective management of early-stage cancer is far preferable to emergent surgery without adequate preoperative assessment, planning, and education. Many of the surgical techniques for limited disease are well tolerated since they offer a less invasive approach, cause less physical and psychosocial trauma, and require shorter periods of anesthesia.[45-49]

REVIEW QUESTIONS

✓ Case Study

MA, a 44-year-old white, premenopausal female reports a lump in her left breast at her annual gynecologic visit. A clinical examination is not performed; the annual mammogram is normal with slight asymmetry. Six months later, MA notes that the mass is larger and seeks a surgical opinion.

MA and her husband visit the surgeon; physical examination and FNA are performed. The following plan is formulated: bilateral modified radical mastectomies because of family history (maternal grandmother, age 82, unilateral breast CA) and to improve chance of cure.

MA's husband arranges a second opinion. You are the breast nurse educator, part of the surgical oncology team. The nurse practitioner's clinical exam confirms a palpable mass in the lower outer quadrant (LOQ) of left breast, approximately 1.5 × 1.5 cm.; the right breast is normal. Bilateral axillae are negative to palpation. Bilateral mammogram show these results: normal right breast; 1.7 × 1.5 cm spiculated lesion in LOQ left breast. The surgical oncologist concurs; a core needle biopsy is performed. The plan is as follows: surgery, followed by possible postoperative radiation and systemic therapies. The surgical alternatives are delineated:

1. Left lumpectomy with sentinel lymph node biopsy (SLNB) and possible axillary node dissection (AND); *OR*
2. Left total mastectomy, (+/− reconstruction) with SLNB and possible AND.

QUESTIONS

1. You are nurse practitioner (NP) caring for MA 6 months ago. What actions do you take?
   a. You perform clinical breast examination (CBE) as routine annual care.
   b. You reassure MA that premenopausal women have lumpy breasts.
   c. You address an identified change, and perform CBE at the annual visit.
   d. You remind yourself how many times women have lumps and they turn out to be nothing.
2. Surgeon #1 recommended modified radical mastectomy. What is the rationale?
   a. Unsure.
   b. The more radical, the better.
   c. Most women are cured with a mastectomy.
   d. This woman needs to do everything possible to cure her breast cancer.
3. Surgeon #1 also recommended bilateral mastectomies. What is the rationale?
   a. This is a wise choice because of family history.
   b. No one should have to do this twice.
   c. This surgical option is up to MA.
   d. The more tissue removed, the better the cure rate.
4. You are nurse practitioner (NP) caring for MA now. MA asks why a second biopsy is recommended. What is your answer?
   a. The first surgeon may have been wrong.
   b. I don't know; we need to ask the doctor.
   c. The FNA is often correct, but the core needle biopsy will give us more information about the tumor before starting treatment.
   d. Our hospital will not use another doctor's information.
5. MA's husband asks about axillary node dissection compared to sentinel lymph node biopsy. What do you respond about the rationale for each?
   a. Axillary nodal status and pathologic size of tumor determine the stage; SLNB offers a less-invasive option than AND with potentially less long-term side effects.
   b. It is better to remove all the axillary lymph nodes during surgery.
   c. SLNB removes only one node; AND removes all of the nodes.
   d. Don't worry, the surgeon will do what he has to do.
6. MA asks the NP about taking her birth control pill (BCP) the morning of surgery. What do you say?
   a. No, since you cannot eat or drink after midnight.
   b. Yes, but limit your water to a sip.
   c. Why are you taking BCPs?
   d. We need to discuss an alternative to BCPs.
7. MA's blood pressure (BP) is 178/102. Recheck 1 hour later is 172/98. What do you conclude and/or do?
   a. BP is elevated as a result of anxiety.
   b. Refer MA to primary care provider (PCP) to ascertain stability before surgery
   c. Prescribe an antihypertensive to decrease BP preoperatively.
   d. Do not worry about it; MA will be fine the morning of surgery.
8. MA is confused during this consult: less surgery, but chemotherapy? What do you say when discussing this with her?
   a. Chemotherapy is recommended to treat possible micrometastasis.
   b. If the SLNB is negative, chemotherapy will not be necessary.

Continued

REVIEW QUESTIONS—CONT'D

    c. If a mastectomy is performed, chemotherapy will not be necessary.

    d. If all of your lymph nodes are removed, chemotherapy will not be necessary.

9. MA is confused about needing both radiation therapy and chemotherapy. What do you say when discussing this with her?

    a. Radiation therapy treats the remaining breast tissue after a lumpectomy.

    b. Radiation therapy is not necessary, just chemotherapy.

    c. Radiation therapy will replace chemotherapy.

    d. Radiation therapy is easier than chemotherapy.

10. MA is tearful about possible changes in breast appearance, potential loss of hair, loss of BCP, and potential onset of menopause after chemotherapy. How do you respond?

    a. We will continue to help you and your husband with sexuality concerns, physical changes, and coping skills.

    b. Don't worry, you'll be fine.

    c. This is a serious problem.

    d. We need to do these things so you do not die.

ANSWERS

1. **C.** *Rationale:* CBE is performed annually by age 40, and/or for symptom(s). Correlate mammogram and CBE.

2. **A.** *Rationale:* Breast cancer is suspect for micrometastasis, requiring consideration of systemic treatment. Surgical treatment can often be achieved with lumpectomy.

More extensive surgery does not necessarily improve survival of MA's current cancer.

3. **C.** *Rationale:* Only 5% to 10% of breast cancers are hereditary, occurring most often in premenopausal women with a family history of first-degree relatives with breast and/or ovarian cancer, and/or bilateral breast cancer, at an early age. Concepts of genetics should be discussed; decisions can be made after definitive breast cancer surgery.

4. **C.** *Rationale:* FNA enables cytological examination only; core needle enables pathologic examination.

5. **A.** *Rationale:* The axillary node status must be confirmed pathologically. SLNB may actually remove more than one node, but does not remove all the nodes as in AND.

6. **D.** *Rationale:* BCPs are discontinued at time of diagnosis because they are hormonal agents. Discuss the importance of temporary birth control precautions and long-term options.

7. **B.** *Rationale:* The surgical team can prescribe an antihypertensive, but the PCP has long-term history of care. Further preoperative work-up is indicated.

8. **A.** *Rationale:* Adjuvant chemotherapy is recommended in premenopausal women with pathologic stage T1C invasive cancer. Neither mastectomy or AND affect systemic treatment.

9. **A.** *Rationale:* Lumpectomy requires postoperative radiation therapy for maximal local control of tumor.

10. **A.** *Rationale:* Ongoing care of the patient and family is important throughout the cancer trajectory.

REFERENCES

1. Houghton Mifflin Company: *The American heritage dictionary of the English language*, ed 4, Boston, Mass, 2004, Houghton Mifflin.

2. Lopez MJ: The evolution of radical cancer surgery, *Surg Oncol Clin North Am* 14(3):xiii-xv, 2005.

3. Lawrence W, Lopez MJ: Radical surgery for cancer: a historical perspective, *Surg Oncol Clin North Am* 14(3):441-446, 2005.

4. Winchester DP, Trabanino L, Lopez MJ: The evolution of surgery for breast cancer, *Surg Oncol Clin North Am* 14(3):479-498, 2005.

5. Hughes E: Principles of post-operative patient care, *Nurs Stand* 19(5):43-51, 2004.

6. Bertagnolli M: Surgical prevention of cancer, *J Clin Oncol* 23(2):324-332, 2005.

7. Haber D: Prophylactic oophorectomy to reduce the risk of ovarian and breast cancer in carrier of *BRCA* mutations, *N Eng J Med* 346(21):1660-1662, 2002.

8. Grann V, Jacobson J, Thomason D et al: Effect of prevention strategies on survival and quality-adjusted survival of women with *BRCA 1-2* mutations: an updated decision analysis, *J Clin Oncol* 20(10):2520-2529, 2002.

9. Stolier AJ, Fuhrman GM, Mauterer L et al: Initial experience with surgical treatment planning in the newly diagnosed breast cancer patient at high risk for *BRCA-1* or *BRCA-2* mutation, *Breast J* 10(6):475-480, 2004.

10. Rosenberg S: Principles of surgical oncology. In DeVita VT, Hellman S, Rosenberg S, editors: *Cancer: principles and practices of oncology*, Philadelphia, 2005, Lippincott, Williams & Williams.

11. Fleming I: *American joint commission for cancer staging manual*, ed 5, Philadelphia, 1998, Lippincott-Raven.

12. Eberhardt WE, Hepp R, Stamatis G: The role of surgery in stage IIIA non-small cell lung cancer, *Hematol Oncol Clin North Am* 19(2):303-319, 2005.

13. Choy H: Recent advances in combined modality therapy for solid tumors, *Semin Oncol* 30(4):1-2, 2003.

14. Honig A, Rieger L, Sutterlin M et al: Preoperative chemotherapy and endocrine therapy in patients with breast cancer, *Clin Breast Cancer* 5(3):198-207, 2004.

15. Chakravarthy B, Pietenpol JA: Combined modality management of breast cancer: development of predictive markers through proteomics, *Semin Oncol* 30(4):23-36, 2003.

16. Nogaret JM, Bernard-Marty C, Mancini I et al: Breast cancer treatment in 2004: towards a tailored approach, *Rev Med Brux* 25(4):A394-A403, 2004.

17. Robins HI, Peterson CG, Nehta MP: Combined modality treatment for central nervous system malignancies, *Semin Oncol* 30(4):11-22, 2003.

18. Newman, L: Current issues in the surgical management of breast cancer: a review of abstracts from the 2002 San Antonio breast cancer symposium, the 2003 Society of Surgical Oncology annual meeting, and the 2003 American Society of Clinical Oncology meeting, *Breast J* 10(1):22-25, 2004.

19. Suntharalingam M: The role of concurrent chemotherapy and radiation in the management of patients with squamous cell carcinomas of the head and neck, *Semin Oncol* 30(4):37-45, 2003.

20. Selman TJ, Luesley DM, Murphy DJ et al: Is radical hysterectomy for early stage cervical cancer an outdated operation? *Br J Obstet Gynaecol* 112:363-365, 2005.

21. Hughes S, Steller, MA: Radical gynecologic surgery for cancer, *Surg Oncol Clin North Am* 14(3):607-631, 2005.

22. Harris D, Dawson R, Moseley L et al: Patient satisfaction after surgery for GI malignancy, *Gastrointest Nurs* 2(10):25-31, 2004.

23. Holley S, Borger D: Energy for living with cancer: preliminary findings of a cancer rehabilitation group intervention study, *Oncol Nurs Forum* 28(9):1393-1396, 2001.

24. Wolfe, SL: Quality of life through rehabilitation at end of life, *Cancer Pract* 10(4):174-178, 2002.

25. Cady J: Laryngectomy: beyond loss of voice – caring for the patient as a whole, *Clin J Oncol Nurs* 6(6):1-5, 2002.

26. Thomas S, Greifzu SP: Oncology today: breast reconstruction, *RN* 63(4):45-47, 2000.

27. World Health Organization: WHO definition of palliative care, retrieved October 7, 2005, from http://www.who.int/cancer/palliative/definition/en/.

28. Ferrell BR, Chu D, Lawrence W et al: Patient and surgeon decision making regarding surgery for advanced cancer, *Oncol Nurs Forum* 30(6):E106-E114, 2003.

29. Borneman T, Chu D, Lawrence W et al: Concerns of family caregivers of patients with cancer facing palliative surgery for advanced malignancies, *Oncol Nurs Forum* 30(6):997-1005, 2003.

30. Baltzell K, Eder S, Wrensch M: Breast carcinogenesis – can the examination of ductal fluid enhance our understanding? *Oncol Nurs Forum* 32(1): 33-39, 2005.

31. Hsueh EC, Hansen N, Giuliano A: Intraoperative lymphatic mapping and sentinel lymph node dissection in breast cancer, *CA Cancer J Clin* 50(5):279-291, 2000.

32. Nichol PF, Mack E, Bianco J et al: Radioguided parathyroidectomy in patients with secondary and tertiary hyperparathyroidism, *Surgery* 134(4):713-719, 2003.

33. Nag S, Martinez-Monge R, Neiroda C et al: Radioimmunoguided-intraoperative radiation therapy in colorectal carcinoma: a new technique to precisely define the clinical target volume, *Int J Radiat Oncol Biol Phys* 44(1):133-137, 1999.

34. Cerfolio, RJ, Bryant AS, Sheils TM et al: Minimally invasive techniques: video-assisted thoracoscopic surgery using single-lumen endotracheal tube anesthesia, *Chest* 126:281-285, 2004.

35. Butani A, Arbesfeld DM, Schwartz RA: Premalignant and early squamous cell carcinoma, *Clin Plastic Surg* 32(2):223-235, 2005.

36. Chen WR, Carubelli R, Liu H et al: Laser immunotherapy: a novel treatment modality for metastatic tumors, *Mol Biotechnol* 25(1):37-44, 2003.

37. Bojarski, JD, Dupuy DE, Mayo-Smith WW: CT imaging findings of pulmonary neoplasms after treatment with radiofrequency ablation: results in 32 tumors, *AJR Am J Roentgenol* 185(2):466-471, 2005.

38. Thanos L, Mylona S, Kalioras V et al: Palliation of painful perineal metastasis treated with radiofrequency thermal ablation, *Cardiovasc Intervent Radiol* 28(3):381-383, 2005.

39. Lefor AT: The role of laparoscopy in the treatment of intra-abdominal malignancies, *Cancer J* 6(2):S159-S168, 2000.

40. Touijer AK, Guillonneau B: Laparoscopic radical prostatectomy, *Urol Oncol* 22(2):133-138, 2004.

41. Monk TG: Preoperative recombinant human erythropoietin in anemic surgical patients, *Crit Care* 8(2):S45-S48, 2004.

42. Carlson RW, Anderson BO, Burstein HJ et al: The NCCN breast cancer clinical practice guidelines in oncology, *J Nat Compreh Cancer Net* 3(3): 238-289, 2005.

43. Scarpa R: Advanced practice nursing in head and neck cancer: implementation of five roles, *Oncol Nurs Forum* 31(3):579-583, 2004.

44. Stevenson RD, McNeill JA: Surgical management of testicular cancer, *CJON* 8(4):355-360, 2004.

45. Hodgson NA, Given CW: Determinants of functional recovery in older adults surgically treated for cancer, *Cancer Nurs* 27(1):10-16, 2004.

46. Kemeny MM: Surgery in older patients, *Semin Oncol* 31(2):175-184, 2004.

47. Clark AJ, Stockton D, Elder A et al: Assessment of outcomes after colorectal cancer resection in the elderly as a rationale for screening and early detection, *Br J Surg* 91(10):1345-1351, 2004.

48. Zack E: Sentinel lymph node biopsy in breast cancer: scientific rationale and patient care, *Oncol Nurs Forum* 28(6):997-1007, 2001.

49. Nikoletti S, Kristjanson LJ, Tataryn D et al: Information needs and coping styles of primary family caregivers of women following breast cancer surgery, *Oncol Nurs Forum* 30(6):987-996, 2003.

CHAPTER 20

Radiation Therapy

Juli Aistars

Radiation therapy is one of the four major modalities used to treat cancer. Currently, about 60% of cancer patients will receive radiation at least once during the course of their illness. It is given alone or in combination with surgery, chemotherapy, or biotherapy. Radiation may be used to cure cancer by eradicating disease, or for long-term control when cure is not possible. About 50% of radiation treatment given is for palliation of symptoms to relieve pain, bleeding, obstruction, or neurologic compromise. Optimizing a person's quality of life is a major consideration in treatment decisions.[1,2]

Definitions

Radiation therapy is the use of ionizing radiation in the treatment of patients with benign and malignant diseases. The intent is to deliver a precisely measured dose of radiation to a defined tumor volume with minimal damage to adjacent healthy tissue.[1,3]

Radiation oncology is the medical discipline concerned with the causes, prevention, and treatment of cancer involving special expertise in the therapeutic use of radiation therapy, either alone or in conjunction with surgery, chemotherapy, biotherapy, heat, or oxygen.[3]

Historical Perspective

Wilhelm Roentgen described the x-ray in 1895 when he passed a current through a Crookes' tube covered by black cardboard and produced a ray on paper. One year later, Henri Becquerel discovered the natural radioactivity of uranium. While in pursuit of the source of this new energy, Marie and Pierre Curie discovered radium in 1898.[3,4] The groundwork was laid for the development of therapeutic radiation as a viable cancer treatment.

In 1922, deep-therapy x-ray machines were available for treating patients.[5] In France, Coutard presented evidence that advanced laryngeal cancer could be cured without disastrous side effects by dividing the total dose into daily fractions. By 1934, he had developed a fractionated scheme based on clinical observations that remains the basis for radiation therapy today.[3,5]

In the 1950s, the Cobalt-60 machine and the linear accelerator were introduced. The rad was adopted as the unit of absorbed dose. By the end of this decade, clinical trials were underway studying radiation combined with other therapies. The 1970s brought advances in machine design, refinement of planning and treatment techniques, and application of computer science. During the 1980s and 1990s, various treatment methods such as hyperthermia, intraoperative radiation, and alternative fractionation schemes were studied in clinical trials. The term *Gray (Gy)* replaced the *rad* as the international standard measure of radiation dose. The development of multileaf collimation (MLC), three-dimensional conformal radiation therapy (3D CRT) treatment planning and intensity-modulated radiation therapy (IMRT) minimized toxicities without compromising treatment goals. In the past 20 years, technologic progress has come primarily in the form of treatment planning advances.[3-7]

Principles of Radiation Therapy

Radiation is categorized as electromagnetic (radio waves, microwaves, visible light, x-rays, and gamma rays) or particulate (electrons, protons, neutrons, negative pi-mesons, and heavy ions). X-rays, gamma rays, and electrons are the most commonly used types of ionizing radiation. Whereas x-rays are produced electrically by a machine, gamma rays are emitted naturally during radioactive decay. Radiation can be described as packets of energy in the form of photons (x-rays and gamma rays) or particles (electrons).[2,7]

Radiation kills cells primarily by damaging the DNA. Because cells are mostly water, the majority of the damage is indirect; it is caused when ionizing radiation interacts with the cell's water to produce free radicals. These are highly reactive and can cause breakage of DNA strands.[8]

The radiosensitivity of cells is influenced by many factors. Tissues containing a majority of mitotic cells are more sensitive to radiation than tissues containing slowly dividing or non-dividing cells. The cell is most sensitive to radiation during the M (mitosis) phase of the cell cycle when division occurs, and late G_2 (gap 2) phase, when protein and RNA synthesis occurs. The cell is most radioresistant during the S phase (synthesis), when DNA is duplicated. The presence of oxygen enhances radiation damage by interfering with repair processes. Poorly differentiated tumors are more radiosensitive because of their high mitotic rate. Larger tumors have a greater volume of hypoxic tissue, rendering them more radioresistant. Tumors arising from radiosensitive tissues are usually more sensitive to the effects of radiation (see Table 20-1).[1]

The radiocurability of tumors depends on their radiosensitivity as well as the normal tissue tolerance. The therapeutic ratio is a measure of radiocurability and is dependent on the overlap of the normal tissue tolerance dose and the dose required to destroy the tumor. This ratio can be improved by precise treatment planning that targets the tumor while sparing normal tissue.[1]

Fractionation, or dividing the total dose into equal daily fractions, takes advantage of the *"four R's"* of radiobiology. **Repair** is the ability of cells to recover from sublethal damage. Initially, both normal and tumor cells can recover, but as the radiation dose accumulates, the ability of the tumor cells to repair damage decreases. **Redistribution** is based on the sensitivity of the cell to radiation at different phases of cell division. Dividing the radiation dose into smaller daily doses disrupts the cellular life cycle, causing a greater number of cells to enter the more radiosensitive mitotic phase. Tumor cells may be more susceptible to redistribution than normal cells. **Repopulation** refers to regeneration of cells after radiation damage. Cellular repopulation that occurs between radiation fractions is greater in the normal tissue than in

TABLE 20-1	Various Tumors and Tissues in Decreasing Order of Radiosensitivity	
TUMORS	RELATIVE RADIOSENSITIVITY	TISSUES OF ORIGIN
Lymphoma, leukemia, seminoma, dysgerminoma	High	Lymphoid, hematopoietic (marrow), spermatogenic epithelium, and ovarian follicular epithelium
Squamous cell cancer of oropharynx, glottis, bladder, skin, and cervical epithelia; adenocarcinoma of alimentary tract; breast	Fairly high	Oropharyngeal stratified epithelium, sebaceous gland epithelium, urinary bladder epithelium, optic lens epithelium, gastric gland epithelium, colon epithelium, breast epithelium
Salivary gland tumor, hepatoma, renal cancer, pancreatic cancer, chondrosarcoma, osteogenic sarcoma	Fairly low	Mature cartilage or bone tissue, salivary gland epithelium, renal epithelium, hepatic epithelium, chondrocytes, osteocytes
Rhabdomyosarcoma, leiomyosarcoma, ganglioneurofibrosarcoma	Low	Muscle tissue and neuronal tissue

Reprinted with permission from Rubin P: *Clinical oncology: a multidisplinary approach for physicians and students*, ed 8, Philadelphia, 2001, WB Saunders.

the tumor. **Reoxygenation** is based on the fact that the presence of oxygen enhances the effect of ionizing radiation, particularly when x-rays or gamma rays are the source. As the tumor shrinks, the oxygen-deprived core is exposed to the oxygen-rich blood supply, increasing the tumor's sensitivity to radiation.[1,6,7]

Radiation causes side effects when normal tissue in the treatment field is affected, particularly tissues that proliferate rapidly such as skin, the gastrointestinal tract, and hematopoietic cells in the bone marrow. Nonproliferating cells such as mature neurons, bone, cartilage, and muscle are less sensitive to radiation. The response of normal tissue to ionizing radiation depends on the total dose, the daily dose, the number of treatments, and the volume of the treatment field.[6]

The radiation dose is expressed as the absorbed energy per unit mass. The gray (Gy) is the standard unit for reporting dose. One Gy equals 100 centigray (cGy). The cGy is equivalent to the rad.[4]

Administration of Radiation Therapy

Radiation therapy can be delivered by various methods. External beam radiation or teletherapy is delivered by a machine such as the linear accelerator, placed at some distance from the target site. It is generally a local treatment, but it can also be administered to the whole body in select cases. Stereotactic radiosurgery is a precisely targeted external beam radiation treatment that is given in one session when used to treat brain lesions. Brachytherapy entails placement of a sealed radioactive source in or near the tumor or tumor bed, either permanently or temporarily. Radiation can also be administered by injection or oral ingestion of radioactive materials.[9]

Radiosensitizers and radioprotectors are agents that can alter the tissue response to radiation. Radiosensitizers are agents that enhance radiation damage to tumor cells when they are present at the same time radiation is administered. Examples are 5-fluorouracil (5-FU), paclitaxel (Taxol), and the nitroimidazoles.[1] Concurrent external radiation and 5-FU prior to surgery is one of the standard treatment protocols for colorectal cancer.

Sulfhydryl-containing compounds are radioprotectors that act as "radical scavengers," interacting with ionized particles to prevent DNA damage to healthy tissue. Amifostine was the first FDA-approved radioprotector and has been studied in a number of trials as a protector of normal tissue against both radiation and chemotherapy in head and neck, lung, and rectal cancers.[1]

Nursing Management in Radiation Therapy

Regardless of how radiation is administered, the role of the nurse includes patient and family education, assessment and management of symptoms, coordination of care, and providing emotional support throughout treatment. Patients need information regarding what to expect during planning and treatment, the onset and duration of possible side effects, self-care measures, and follow-up care. Published studies have consistently demonstrated that the provision of information about presentation, prevalence, and duration of side effects reduces the patient's anxiety level and enhances self-care.[10] Patients should be informed not only about what will happen but also about what they will see, feel, and hear. The results of a study conducted by Poroch showed that patients who received structured sensory and procedural information exhibited less anxiety and greater satisfaction with treatment than those in the control group receiving standard information.[11]

Johnson and colleagues studied patients undergoing radiation and found that concrete, objective information based on self-regulation theory enhanced their ability to maintain usual activities.[12] Two additional studies demonstrated that preparatory information significantly increased satisfaction with care in patients receiving radiation therapy.[13,14] Teaching methods are tailored to the learner. The use of printed materials, audiotapes, videotapes, CD-ROMs, verbal instruction, and/or demonstration is based on the patient's learning style and personal preference. Educational materials such as booklets and videotapes are available through the National Cancer Institute (NCI), the American Cancer Society (ACS), the American Society for Therapeutic Radiology and Oncology (ASTRO), and the Oncology Nursing Society (ONS).

There are also many patient-centered websites related to specific cancers or symptoms.

Although patients are becoming more adept at obtaining information about their illness and treatment, fears of radiation "burns" and "becoming radioactive" are still expressed. Allowing the patient to verbalize fears and providing education may alleviate these concerns. Anxiety related to the diagnosis of cancer and fear of recurrence and death is a normal response, even in early-stage cancers. Fostering an environment where the patient and family feel comfortable expressing their feelings and concerns can mitigate anxiety.

Unlike chemotherapy toxicities, most expected side effects of radiation therapy are site-specific. They are dependent upon the area of the body treated, the volume of tissue in the treatment field, the total dose, the fractionation schedule, the number of treatments, and the method of radiation delivery.

External Radiation Therapy

External radiation is the most common treatment method in radiation therapy. It may be used alone or in combination with other cancer treatments.

CONSULTATION AND TREATMENT PLANNING

Patients who are candidates for radiation are typically referred to the radiation facility by one of their physicians. They meet with the radiation oncologist and the radiation oncology nurse to determine if radiation is indicated. Patients may choose to have family members or significant others present at the time of consultation. If the patient is not capable of making informed decisions, a person who is authorized to do so must be available. The radiation oncologist reviews the diagnosis and staging, the extent of disease, treatment options, and the goal of treatment. He or she addresses the patient's or family members' questions or concerns. The patient's general condition and comorbidities are considered when making treatment decisions. The radiation oncologist may make recommendations at the time of consultation. However, in some cases further collaboration with other physicians, additional imaging studies, or presentation before a tumor board may provide valuable information before deciding on a course of treatment. The physician obtains written, informed consent from the patient or patient's representative before proceeding with treatment planning.

Radiation therapy requires comprehensive planning and quality assurance (QA). Treatment planning is a team effort involving the radiation oncologist, physicists, dosimetrists, and other specialty physicians who may be involved, such as a neurosurgeon. The plan is dependent on the reproducibility of the patient's position on a daily basis. Various immobilization devices such as casts, masks, bite-blocks, pull-ropes, and arm boards are used to ensure consistent positioning (Figs. 20-1 and 20-2). Patient imaging studies such as computerized tomography (CT), magnetic resonance imaging (MRI), positron emission tomography (PET), or the combination PET/CT are used to plan treatment. This data is transferred to the treatment planning system, and the treatment volume and organs at risk are identified. Dose distributions are computed, and any necessary blocks are produced.[15] QA is a series of checks throughout planning and treatment that are specific to each patient to ensure that treatment is being delivered as planned.

Once the plan is complete, it is tested by simulation, usually a day or two after the first planning appointment. Treatment will typically begin the day following simulation. However, for certain

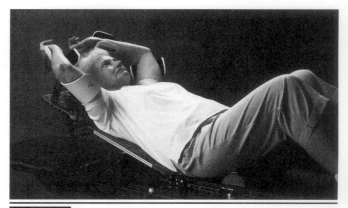

FIG. 20-1 One type of breastboard used to immobilize a patient during radiation treatment for breast cancer. (Courtesy of Medtec, Orange City, IA.)

treatments such as radiation for bone metastases, planning and treatment can be done on the same day. The simulator uses a diagnostic x-ray tube that duplicates a radiation treatment machine in terms of its geometric, mechanical, and optical properties. During simulation, the radiation beams are defined and guided to meet the prescribed therapy goals. The orientation and size of beams, the placement of blocks, and skin markings (usually replaced by tiny permanent tattoos) allow for reliable reproduction of treatment geometry on a daily basis.[15]

The radiation oncology nurse plays a critical role during consultation. Patients and families are often anxious and fearful at this stage. To allay anxiety, the nurse informs them what to expect during treatment planning, treatment, and follow-up. Some basic questions that should be addressed are the following: How long will I be in the department for treatment planning sessions and daily treatments? How many treatments will I receive? Is there any special preparation for treatment planning? What should I wear? Can I take my regular medications? Will I feel anything? What will be expected of me during planning and treatments? Let the patient know if oral or intravenous contrast will be used, or if any tubes or catheters will be necessary for planning. Inform them of any markings or tattoos that they may expect. The patient should be aware of any immobilization devices to be used.[15] Be cognizant of the patient's state of mind and learning style. Keep the information as simple as possible and provide a written copy. Support the patient and family emotionally as needed. Initiate appropriate referrals before treatment begins.

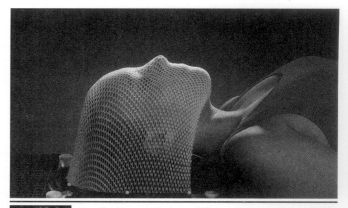

FIG. 20-2 A uniframe used to immobilize a patient during radiation treatment for head and neck cancer. (Courtesy of Medtec, Orange City, IA.)

TREATMENT DELIVERY

External radiation is given daily, Monday through Friday, for 2 to 8 weeks. Palliative treatments, such as for bone metastases, may be delivered at higher daily doses over 2 to 3 weeks. The typical treatment time is 2 to 5 minutes. The length of the appointment is approximately 10 minutes, allowing for patient set-up and positioning. A radiation therapist delivers the treatment as prescribed by the radiation oncologist. The typical daily fraction is 180 to 300 cGy.

The linear accelerator is the most commonly used treatment machine in external radiation (see Figure 20-3). This machine treats with x-rays for intermediate to deep penetration, with low to moderate skin dose; or electrons for shallow penetration, resulting in a high skin dose. The head, or gantry, rotates around the patient. Multiple energies are available for treatment. The depth penetration selected depends upon the location of the tumor.[15]

Patient safety and comfort are an important consideration with treatment positioning. In select cases, it may be appropriate to invite the patient and family to see the treatment room and associated equipment before treatment begins.[15] The radiation therapist can provide a tour, answer questions, and address concerns.

Patients see the physician and the radiation oncology nurse at least once per week throughout treatment. At this visit, the patient's general status and response to treatment is assessed and appropriate interventions are implemented. Patients with special issues such as language barriers, noncompliance, cognitive dysfunction, or severe toxicities may be evaluated more frequently.

General Side Effects

Side effects are categorized as acute or late. Acute side effects occur during therapy or within 2 to 3 months of completion. Late side effects may occur months to years later.[16]

SKIN

Ionizing radiation causes skin reactions by damaging the mitotic ability of stem cells within the rapidly proliferating, radiosensitive, basal layer of the epidermis.[17] Depending upon treatment goals, a brisk skin reaction may be the anticipated outcome, such as in the treatment of superficial skin cancers or the chest wall. However, a radiation-induced skin reaction can greatly affect quality of life and treatment outcomes if it becomes a source of significant pain or discomfort, limits daily activities, or interrupts treatment.

Factors that have an impact on the severity of radiodermatitis include the type of energy used (electrons or photons), tangential fields, proximal skin surfaces in the treatment field, gel-like (bolus) sheets placed on the skin during treatment, general skin condition, moist areas causing friction such as the axilla, age, nutritional status, smoking, concurrent chemotherapy, and underlying medical conditions such as scleroderma or lupus.[16-17] Skin reactions experienced during the course of radiation can range from erythema or hyperpigmentation, to **dry desquamation,** when basal-layer stem cells become depleted; or **moist desquamation,** when stem cells are eradicated from the basal layer, causing ulceration.[17] Skin changes may be seen within the first 2 to 4 weeks of treatment, and usually peak in the third to sixth week. Healing begins 1 to 2 weeks after completion of therapy. Although skin care protocols vary among institutions, an example of typical patient instructions is shown in Box 20-1. A recent literature review cites two studies that provide some evidence that the presence of deodorant or other products on the skin in the treatment area does not influence the onset or severity of skin reactions. If further research confirms this conclusion, patients can be allowed to use their own skin care products at their convenience, causing less disruption to their usual hygiene routine.[17a]

Skin assessments are performed weekly, evaluating the appearance of the skin as well as the presence of pain, itching, or tenderness. The NCI 4-point scale is often employed in the radiation oncology setting (NCI scale version 3.0).[18] Identified shortcomings of this scale include the lack of information about associated symptoms. A pilot study evaluated the reliability and validity of a skin toxicity assessment tool (STAT) in patients with breast cancer receiving radiation therapy. This instrument was found to be reliable, valid, and easy to use. It is unique in that it addresses subjective symptoms such as pain, itching, and tenderness.[19]

Before treatment, patients and families are advised of potential skin reactions, expected onset, and anticipated healing, as well as self-care measures. Skin-care protocols vary widely. There is currently minimal evidence to support the use of any particular skin care product. Aquaphor (Beiersdorf, Hamburg, Germany), TheraCare (Emumagic, Nevis, MN), Biafine (OrthoNeutrogena, Los Angeles, CA), and RadiaPlex Gel (Medical, Inc., Irving, Texas) as well as aloe vera gels, are commonly used in the prevention and/or treatment of erythema or dry desquamation. In a phase III study by Heggie and colleagues in 2002, aqueous cream and aloe vera gel were compared in patients with breast

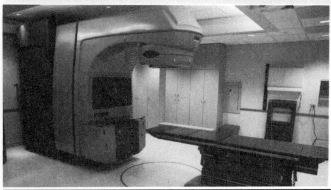

FIG. 20-3 Varian linear accelerator. (Courtesy of Northwest Community Hospital, Arlington Heights, IL.)

BOX 20-1 Self-Care Guidelines to Minimize Radiation Skin Reactions

- Wash treated area gently with lukewarm water and mild soap; pat dry
- Avoid applying tape, rubbing, or scratching in treatment area
- Wear loose-fitting, soft clothing over the treated skin
- Use only an electric razor if shaving in the treated area
- Avoid swimming in chlorinated water
- Avoid sun exposure or extremes of heat or cold in treated area
- Use only skin care products recommended by the radiation staff
- Do not apply skin care products 4 hours prior to each treatment
- For treatment of breast:
  - Do not wear a bra when possible
  - Avoid underwire bras
  - Avoid use of deodorant on the treated side

cancer who were receiving radiation. Aloe vera did not significantly reduce skin damage; aqueous cream was better than aloe vera gel in reducing dry desquamation and pain.[20]

Roy and colleagues conducted a randomized trial to evaluate the effects of washing the skin with soap and water on skin toxicity.[21] Study trends showed more severe skin reactions in the nonwashing arm. Olsen and others conducted a prospective randomized blinded clinical trial comparing aloe vera gel and mild soap (Dove) to mild soap alone in preventing skin reactions in patients undergoing radiation therapy. Results showed no difference up to a dose of 2700 cGy. At higher doses, skin erythema was seen at 5 weeks in the aloe arm, compared to 3 weeks in the soap-only arm, thereby implying a protective effect to adding aloe.[22] Another study compared Biafine to best supportive care (Aquaphor or aloe vera gel) in patients with breast cancer who were receiving adjuvant radiation. The trial did not demonstrate a statistically significant difference in skin toxicity between the two treatment arms.[23]

When moist desquamation occurs, supportive care includes pain control and minimizing the risk of infection. Research has established that creating a moist environment promotes wound healing.[17] Some examples of products used are as follows: normal saline compresses, Domeboro's soaks, Silvadene cream, and hydrocolloid dressings. Late skin side effects, such as telangiectasis (dilated vessels visible on the skin), fibrosis, and necrosis rarely develop with improved methods of treatment planning.[16]

FATIGUE

Cancer-related fatigue (CRF) is the most commonly reported side effect of cancer treatment, occurring in up to 90% of patients. Prospective studies have shown that fatigue increases over the course of radiation. When receiving radiation therapy, fatigue gradually increases as treatment progresses, peaks in the last week of treatment, and slowly returns to pretreatment levels 3 months after treatment ends.[24] Patient education regarding fatigue is essential in allaying the fears that this symptom heralds the return or spread of cancer. The fact that fatigue is likely to occur and strategies for preventing or coping with it are discussed with the patient and family before treatment begins. The National Comprehensive Cancer Network (NCCN) has published guidelines, which are available online, for screening, assessment, and management of CRF.[25] Studies demonstrate that exercise, energy conservation, and treatment of anemia can be of great benefit in managing fatigue.[26-29] Although nutritional support and supplements are often recommended, one study has found no correlation between fatigue and nutritional status.[30] In advanced cancer, corticosteroids and psychostimulants appear to increase energy. Other interventions include treatment of underlying depression or anxiety and control of symptoms such as pain, nausea, emotional distress, or sleep disturbance.[25] Since fatigue is such a prevalent problem during radiation therapy, it should be assessed, monitored, and managed both during and after treatment.

BONE MARROW SUPPRESSION

Patients at highest risk for bone marrow suppression are those receiving concurrent chemotherapy and radiation, total body irradiation, extended-field radiation with greater than 15% of active bone marrow in the field, and splenic radiation. Blood counts are monitored based on individual patient risk factors. The patient and family are educated regarding possible decreased blood

counts that could place them at risk for infection, bleeding, or fatigue. When chemotherapy and radiation are combined, growth factors or blood transfusions may be indicated.[31] Patients and families are educated regarding known causes of decreased blood counts and self-care measures such as prevention of infection and bleeding precautions. Radiation and/or chemotherapy may be discontinued temporarily until blood counts recover.

Site-Specific Side Effects

HEAD AND NECK

Head and neck cancers comprise about 5% of the cancers diagnosed each year in the United States. This includes cancers of the oral cavity, the oropharynx, the nasal cavity, the paranasal sinuses, the nasopharynx, the larynx, the hypopharynx, and the salivary glands. Surgery combined with radiation is the treatment of choice, with chemotherapy added for advanced disease or as a radiosensitizer.[32] Effective treatment of head and neck cancers requires a multidisciplinary approach by including medicine, surgery, nursing, dietary, social services, occupational and physical therapy, and psychology.[33] Toxicities are both severe and chronic, including stomatitis, xerostomia, taste changes, dental caries, osteoradionecrosis, and hypopituitarism. A feeding tube is recommended in patients who are nutritionally compromised before treatment begins or when the treatment protocol is likely to cause a significant decrease in oral intake since these patients are at risk for weight loss, aspiration, and dehydration.

Oral Mucositis. Oral mucositis is a common complication in patients receiving radiation for head and neck cancer. The risk increases with higher radiation doses, altered fractionation schedules, combined modality treatment; and patient-specific factors such as age, comorbidities, and the condition of the oral mucosa.[34-36] Oral mucositis is characterized by inflammation and ulceration resulting from destruction of epithelial stem cells occurring in a multiphase process. It has a major impact on daily functioning, well-being, quality of life, cost of medical care, and treatment outcomes.[34,36] Four stages are identified as vascular, epithelial, ulcerative, and healing. With head and neck radiation, oral mucositis typically occurs in the floor of the mouth, the buccal regions, the tongue, and the soft palate. It is clinically evident by the second week of radiation, peaks from weeks 5 to 6, and can last for several weeks following treatment.[36]

Shih and colleagues conducted a comprehensive review of published papers relevant to the prevention, palliation, or reduction of radiation-induced oral mucositis. Antimicrobial, coating, and antiinflammatory agents did not decrease the severity of mucositis. Two studies in this review concluded that cytokine granulocyte-macrophage colony-stimulating factor (GM-CSF) in mouthwashes may facilitate healing.[35] There are a variety of agents that prevent and treat oral mucositis. Over the past several years, randomized clinical trials have failed to demonstrate consistent findings. Bland rinses such as 0.9% saline solution or saline and sodium bicarbonate mixtures are widely employed. Mucosal protectants include sucralfate suspension, Gelclair (OSI Pharmaceuticals, Melville, NY), and the radioprotector, amifostine. Multiagent rinses, also known as "magic mouthwash," are commonly used, but evidence to support their efficacy is lacking. Chlorhexidine, an antiseptic agent, lidocaine used as a topical anesthetic, and growth factor mouthwash formulations have shown some benefit, but the results are not consistent.[37]

There is currently no recommended "gold standard" product in management of oral mucositis related to radiation. Evidence does support some type of oral care protocol including regularly scheduled dental care, regular oral assessment, and the initiation of an oral care program before treatment begins.[35,37] The most widely used oral assessment tool in clinical practice is the Oral Assessment Guide (OAG).[36] It is easy to use, reliable, and reproducible. An important component of any oral care program must include patient education and compliance with a self-care program. Patients and families can use the OAG for daily assessment of the oral cavity. Providing the necessary tools such as a dental mirror, penlight, dental floss, and a soft toothbrush can greatly enhance patient compliance.[37] Frequent oral assessment promotes the early identification and treatment of bacterial and fungal infections. Measures to relieve discomfort include minimizing use of dentures and topical or systemic pain relief. When oral infection occurs, prompt treatment with antifungals or antibiotics is indicated.

Xerostomia, or dry mouth, is one of the most severe symptoms experienced by patients receiving radiation to the oral cavity and neck. Saliva plays an important role in the preservation of oral-pharyngeal health. Impaired salivation can predispose the patient to mucositis, dysphagia, dental caries, poor denture fit, oral pain, taste changes, and fungal infection. These complications can affect overall nutritional status. The major salivary glands are the parotid (located below and in front of each ear), submandibular (located in the lower jaw), and sublingual glands (located beneath the tongue). These glands are responsible for 70% to 80% of salivary flow. Radiation-induced xerostomia is influenced by treatment field, dose, use of IMRT, and concomitant chemotherapy.[32] Within 1 week of the start of irradiation, salivary output can decrease by 60% to 90%, with anticipated total recovery if the total dose is less than 2600 cGy.[33]

Randomized trials have shown that the radioprotectant amifostine given intravenously or subcutaneously before treatment significantly reduced the incidence of grade II or higher xerostomia from 78% to 51% in a randomized trial.[38] Johnstone and others demonstrated that acupuncture alleviates xerostomia for many patients, some for greater than 3 months.[39] The advent of IMRT, a three-dimensional treatment planning and dose delivery technique, has significantly reduced radiation exposure to salivary glands, resulting in sparing of salivary output.[33] Other self-care measures that have shown efficacy are frequent sips of water; avoidance of mouthwashes with alcohol; eating soft, moist foods; and avoidance of alcohol and smoking.[16]

Artificial saliva substitutes and lubricants (Biotene mouthwash or Oralbalance gel; Laclede Research Laboratories, Gardena, CA) have been proven effective for some patients in clinical trials. The use of a humidifier at night is helpful, since salivary output is lower during sleep. Salivary output can be stimulated with the use of sugar-free chewing gums, candies, and mints. Oral candidiasis is common with dry mouth and is treated with antifungals such as Diflucan (Pfizer Inc., New York, NY).[33] Avoid using oral troches in patients with xerostomia, because saliva is needed to dissolve the troche.[32] The oral cavity should be inspected weekly. The patient is educated on the signs and symptoms of a candidal infection and encouraged to inspect the mouth daily. If xerostomia is expected to be a permanent side effect, this is included in patient education.[40]

Taste changes occur because radiation to the head and neck region reduces the number of taste buds and damages the microvilli.

The sweet taste buds are the least affected. Patients report 50% taste loss when they have received 3000 cGy. A dose of 6000 cGy can cause a permanent loss of taste. Patients may report a peculiar taste in their mouth with foods, describing a cardboard or metallic taste. Taste buds contain rapidly proliferating cells located on the tongue, the soft palate, the glossopalatine arch, and the posterior areas of the pharynx. Taste alterations can persist 7 years or longer.[41] Anorexia and weight loss may coincide with taste changes.

Teaching patients that taste alterations are treatment related and usually temporary may alleviate anxiety. Mouth care is performed before and after meals, and smoking should be avoided. Seasoning or marinating food and experimentation with different foods are ways to deal with taste changes. Serving food at room temperature may blunt peculiar tastes. Small, frequent meals can help maintain adequate caloric intake.[41] Megastrol acetate 400 mg twice daily may help stimulate appetite, especially in the presence of greater than 5% weight loss. Increasing fluids to 2 to 3 liters per day can prevent dehydration. A study by Ripamonti and others discussed administering zinc sulfate 25 mg 4 times a day to a small sample of patients. Patient's serum levels of zinc, taste perception, and taste bud anatomy were normalized.[42]

Tooth decay and caries may occur as a late effect of radiation when the oral cavity is in the treatment field. In chronic xerostomia, saliva is unable to restore oral pH and regulate bacterial populations. This leads to an environment conducive to colonization of caries-associated bacteria and enamel demineralization.[33] Dental caries may set in 3 to 6 months after radiation is completed.[32]

Patients are advised to have a comprehensive dental evaluation before treatment begins. Any restorative work and a cleaning should be done at this time. If extractions are necessary, this should be completed at least 10 to 14 days before radiation begins to allow time for healing.

Osteoradionecrosis, a serious late complication of head and neck irradiation, affects the mandible and can occur with dosages in excess of 6000 cGy. It is characterized as a dissolution of the bone and can be progressive, necessitating surgical intervention, hyperbaric oxygen (HBO) treatments, or both. The efficacy of HBO is based on uncontrolled studies. Risk factors include continued tobacco or alcohol use and poor nutritional status.[43]

Nursing management encompasses teaching and reinforcing good oral hygiene, the avoidance of alcohol or smoking, properly fitting dentures, maintaining adequate nutritional status, and education regarding the importance of dental care prior to radiation treatment and frequent dental follow-up after radiation treatment.[16]

Hypopituitarism is also a late effect of radiation to the head and neck. It can occur if the pituitary gland is in or near the treatment field, but it is more likely to occur with treatment of brain tumors. Signs and symptoms are fatigue, weight loss or gain, muscle weakness, dry skin and hair, and a decrease in libido. The symptoms can develop several years after radiation therapy. Patient education for those at risk should include typical onset, signs, and symptoms. Adrenal insufficiency is treated with adrenocorticosteroid replacement. Hormone replacement therapy is initiated for sex hormone deficits.[9]

CHEST

Radiation therapy is given to the chest for lung cancer, non-Hodgkin's and Hodgkin's lymphomas, esophageal cancer, and metastatic spread to the mediastinum.

Esophagitis can occur approximately 2 to 3 weeks after the start of treatment. The patient may complain of "a lump in the throat" sensation. A dietary consult is initiated for any patient at risk of esophagitis. A soft or bland diet that provides a high-calorie, high-protein intake is recommended. Viscous lidocaine used alone or in combination with an antacid and an antihistamine, taken 15 minutes before meals, can be used to alleviate dysphagia. Systemic analgesics may be necessary. A clinical trial published in 2001 showed that the radioprotector amifostine given 15 minutes before each radiation treatment can reduce the incidence of esophagitis in patients with lung cancer.[44]

Nonproductive cough may develop or worsen when radiation is used to treat lung cancer. Ensuring an adequate fluid intake, humidification, avoiding irritants such as smoke, and use of cough medications are some ways to manage a cough.

Radiation pneumonitis usually occurs 1 to 3 months after treatment. It is caused by a decrease in surfactant in conjunction with endothelial cell and vessel permeability. It occurs in 5% to 15% of patients treated for lymphoma or lung cancer and in less than 1% of patients treated for breast cancer. Symptoms include cough, fever, and dyspnea. Treatment includes bed rest and administration of oxygen, bronchial dilators, steroids, and antibiotics. A physical and/or occupational therapy consult may be indicated.[16]

Radiation fibrosis is a late effect that occurs 6 to 12 months after radiation therapy to the lung. Symptomatology depends upon the size of the field treated. If large fields are treated, the patient may exhibit shortness of breath. Risk factors are low performance status, compromised pulmonary function before treatment, smoking history, large radiation doses, or concomitant treatment with chemotherapy.[16] Treatment is limited to supportive care.

The clinical trial that found that amifostine reduced the severity of esophagitis also demonstrated that amifostine reduced the incidence of both pneumonitis and lung fibrosis without compromising treatment of the tumor.[44]

BREAST/CHEST WALL

Skin reactions are site-specific side effects that may occur when the breast or chest wall is treated. Acute skin reactions include erythema, tanning, dry desquamation, and moist desquamation.[18] Late skin effects secondary to radiation occur months to years later and may include hyperpigmentation, depigmentation, atrophy, telangiectasia, fibrosis, and necrosis. Some of the late complications are related to microvascular changes.[17]

The management of acute skin reactions is similar to other treated areas (see "Skin" under "General Effects"). Pain secondary to skin reactions is managed with antiinflammatory drugs, mild analgesics, or topical anesthetics to the treatment area.

ABDOMEN

The abdomen is treated in stomach and pancreatic cancers. With testicular seminoma, the nodes in the paraaortic region in the abdominal area are sometimes treated.

Nausea and vomiting usually occurs within a few hours of treatment if radiation fields include the whole abdomen, extended pelvic fields, the epigastric or paraaortic region or, in rare cases, the chemoreceptor trigger zone in the brain.[16] Radiation-induced nausea and vomiting (RINV) occurs in 40% to 80% of patients who receive radiation, particularly to the upper torso or whole body.[45,46] Patient-specific risk factors include age, gender, alcohol intake, previous experience with nausea and vomiting,

and anxiety level. Preventing RINV is highly efficacious compared to allaying the symptoms. Trials have shown that 5-HT$_3$–receptor antagonists are more effective than placebo or antiemetic combinations such as metoclopramide with dexamethazone and lorazepam.[45] Based on research studies, ganisetron and ondansetron with or without a steroid are indicated for treatment of RINV, depending on the level of risk.[45,46] Prophylactic treatment of RINV will improve quality of life and compliance to therapy, decrease costs, and influence patient survival.[45]

There are various nonpharmacologic techniques for management of RINV including biofeedback, relaxation techniques, and guided imagery.[16] Dietary interventions of small, frequent meals, avoiding foods that increase nausea such as fried, rich, or spicy foods, minimizing fluids with meals, and serving food at room temperature all can aid in relieving RINV. A dietary consult should be initiated for all patients at risk for RINV.

PELVIS

Radiation is used to treat the pelvis for gynecologic, prostate, testicular, or rectal cancers, as well as lymphomas.

Diarrhea can result from denuding the bowel lining, with subsequently decreased absorption of fluids and increased motility.[31] Malabsorption of nutrients and bile salts also contributes to diarrhea, which can start by week 2 or 3 of treatment and usually resolves 2 to 3 months after treatment.[16] Diarrhea can be defined as an increased number of stools or watery stools with cramping. Patients with colostomies will have an increase in the amount and change in the consistency of the stool. Radiation treatments may be interrupted for a period to allow the bowel to recover, if severe diarrhea persists that is unresponsive to intervention.

The patient's baseline bowel pattern is assessed before treatment. Patients with diarrhea may benefit from a low-residue diet. Reductions in dietary fats, spicy foods, and milk products may minimize diarrhea. Antidiarrheal medications such as diphenoxylate atropine or loperamide HCL can be helpful. The discomfort of proctitis and hemorrhoidal irritation is decreased with sitz baths and hemorrhoidal preparations.[47-49] Psyllium preparations such as Metamucil and Benefiber can slow diarrhea by increasing stool bulk.[50] When the prostate is treated, patients are instructed to fill the bladder by drinking one to two glasses of noncaffeinated fluid before treatment so that the bladder pushes the small bowel out of the treatment field.

Cystitis can occur if the bladder is in the treatment field. Symptoms may appear after 3 to 5 weeks of radiation and could include dysuria, urinary frequency, urgency, nocturia, and urinary hesitancy.[16] Hematuria rarely occurs.

Patients should maintain fluid intake at 1 to 2 liters per day, stopping fluids a few hours before bedtime and avoiding caffeinated beverages. Smoking and spicy foods can irritate the lining of the bladder. A bladder infection may need to be ruled out with dysuria, since symptoms of radiation-induced cystitis can mimic a urinary tract infection (UTI). A UTI requires treatment with appropriate antibiotics. Analgesic medications such as ibuprofen and phenazopyridine hydrochloride can provide pain relief. These may tint the urine orange-red. To minimize nocturia and incomplete bladder emptying, α_1-blockers such as terazosin may be used.[51]

Erectile dysfunction can occur after irradiation of the prostate as a result of fibrosis of the pelvic vasculature and damage to pelvic nerves. It manifests as a decline in the ability to attain and maintain an erection and may be irreversible. Urologic consultation, including pharmacologic interventions, devices, and prostheses, may be of benefit to restore erectile function.[51]

Vaginal stenosis can develop when the treatment field encompasses the vaginal vault. It may manifest as dyspareunia and difficult pelvic examinations. Vaginal stenosis can be minimized with the use of a vaginal dilator for 15 minutes, 3 times a week for at least 1 year. If the patient is sexually active, the dilator can be used less often. Vaginal dryness can be relieved with lubricants such as KY or Astroglide and vaginal moisturizers such as Replens.[52]

Sterility may occur when the ovaries or testicles are in the treatment field. Hot flashes, amenorrhea, decreased libido, and osteoporosis can result from ovarian failure. The ovaries can be shielded from the radiation by surgically moving the ovaries out of the treatment field (oophoropexy). The testicles are shielded from radiation if possible. If exposure is unavoidable, spermatogenesis will be affected and can result in permanent sterility.[9] Nursing management involves identifying patients at risk of sterility, and providing necessary information and counseling regarding options and resources.

BRAIN

Radiation to the brain is indicated for benign and malignant brain tumors as well as metastatic lesions. In small cell lung cancer, for example, the goal of whole brain radiation is to increase the disease-free interval before the exacerbation of micrometastases.

Cerebral edema occurs as tissues around the brain tumor become swollen and inflamed. Symptoms are headache, nausea, vomiting, seizures, vision changes, motor function disabilities, slurred speech, and changes in mental status. Steroids may have been previously prescribed for symptom management or are started at the time of radiation. Instruct the patient and family on the signs and symptoms of cerebral edema and the side effects and precautions in the use of steroid medication.[16] It should be emphasized that steroid medications require a gradual downward dose tapering and cannot be abruptly discontinued. Steroid usage can cause increase risk of oral candidiasis, therefore daily mouth inspections are imperative.

Alopecia occurs on the scalp in the area of the radiation port. Hair loss can be very distressing and a constant reminder of the cancer. With doses over 5000 cGy, hair loss may be permanent. Regrowth of hair starts 2 to 3 months after the end of treatment. The texture and color of the hair may change when regrowth occurs.[31]

Patients are advised to wash hair with a gentle shampoo. A randomized controlled clinical trial by Westbury and colleagues concluded that normal hair washing during cranial radiotherapy did not increase skin toxicity.[53] Metz and colleagues used tempol, a nitroxide radioprotector, directly applied to the scalp before radiation and found that it did prevent hair loss but that the solution pooled at the base of the scalp. Further study is being conducted using tempol in gel form.[54] The nurse can provide resources for obtaining wigs, head coverings or scarves, as well as emotionally support patients by allowing them to express their feelings and concerns regarding the affect alopecia may have on their body image.

Scalp irritation may include redness, dryness, and itching. The patient can protect the scalp by covering the head outdoors.

Hair coloring or permanents should be avoided during treatment and for a few weeks afterwards since they may irritate the scalp.

Cognitive dysfunction is a late effect of brain irradiation. With an increase in long-term survival of patients treated for brain tumors and metastases, even subtle changes may diminish quality of life. A need exists for neuropsychologic testing, cognitive and vocational rehabilitation, and psychologic counseling for patients with cognitive dysfunction after treatment with chemotherapy or radiotherapy.[55]

Internal Radiation Therapy

BRACHYTHERAPY

Brachytherapy has been used since the early 1900s and is performed by placing radioactive materials in or near the treatment volume. Brachytherapy allows the delivery of a high dose of radiation to a specific tumor volume, with a rapid falloff in dose to adjacent normal tissues.[56] It is often combined with external beam radiation and other treatments to achieve local tumor control while minimizing normal tissue injury.[57] Methods include interstitial implants or intracavitary implants. Interstitial implants may be in the form of needles, seeds, wires, or catheters. The radioactive source may be placed directly into the body cavity via an applicator.[56]

Brachytherapy is administered by high-dose rate (HDR) or low-dose rate (LDR). In HDR, one or more doses may be given over a few minutes and separated by at least 6 hours. LDR is administered continuously over several days after the patient is admitted to the hospital. Permanently sealed radioactive sources are left in the tissue indefinitely. Brachytherapy is used in cervical, endometrial, head and neck, breast, brain, prostate, and lung cancers.

In *gynecological cancers*, among the applicators used to insert sources in the uterus and vagina are the Fletcher-Suit (Fig. 20-4), the Henschke, interstitial implants with needles for LDR radiation delivery, and a vaginal cylinder for HDR radiation delivery. Sources used are cesium-137 and iridium-192. The patient with an LDR implant is radioactive and therefore stays in the hospital, and radiation precautions are observed. These patients are placed on low-fiber diets and receive diphenoxylate atropine to prevent a bowel movement. Postoperative pain is managed with oral and intravenous medications. HDR procedures are done on an outpatient basis. Patients receive instructions on possible side effects, when to call the doctor, and self-care measures. Fatigue and dysuria may be experienced regardless of the type of implant used. A water-based lubricant is recommended to combat vaginal dryness. Routine vaginal dilatation is recommended for up to 1 year to prevent vaginal stenosis if the patient is not sexually active.[52]

In *breast cancer*, surgically implanted catheters have been used in the past to deliver LDR and HDR radiation for partial breast irradiation. This method has been largely replaced by the MammoSite radiation system, which entails placement of a balloon catheter in the lumpectomy cavity either at the time of surgery or a few weeks later with treatment delivered by HDR twice a day for 5 days.[58] Patient education includes possible side effects, signs and symptoms of infection, when to call the physician, and self-care including a daily dressing change.

Brachytherapy for *head and neck cancer* is often combined with chemotherapy and external radiation therapy. Temporary interstitial or intracavitary implants are used, and radioisotopes

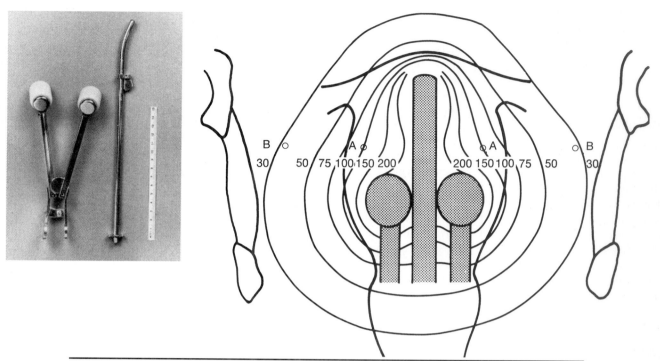

FIG. 20-4 The Fletcher-Suit applicator is one of many kinds of applicators used to deliver intracavitary irradiation for carcinomas of the cervix and the endometrium. The long central tandem is placed in the uterine cavity. (To the right is a section of tubing used to hold the radioactive sources and place them in the hollow tandem.) The movable sleeve on the tandem marks the cervical os, permitting localization of the os on x-ray film as a reference point for computerized dosimetry. The colpostats are placed in the lateral fornices. The entire apparatus is held in place with vaginal packing. After the applicator is in place, x-ray films are taken to confirm the accuracy of placement. Computerized dosimetry is then done to determine the best loading pattern and the time required for treatment. Finally, the radium or cesium sources are put into place. (Photograph courtesy Virginia Mason Medical Center, Seattle, WA; drawing from DiSaia P, Creasman W: *Clinical gynecologic oncology*, ed 4, St Louis, 1993, Mosby.)

may include cesium-137, iridium-192, radium-226, and cobalt-60, delivered by LDR in the inpatient setting or HDR in the outpatient setting. Nursing care includes minimizing airway obstruction, pain control, frequent oral care, and facilitating communication. Nasogastric or gastric tube feedings are given to provide a high-protein, high-calorie liquid diet.[56] Multidisciplinary care may include dietary and occupational therapy consults.

For *prostate cancer*, permanent implants of iodine-125 seeds may be used alone or in combination with external beam radiation. This source of radiation is implanted deep in the body cavity and also has a short half-life; therefore exposure to others is minimized. Patients with prostate seeds are instructed to filter urine for dislodged radioactive seeds, to use a condom when having sexual intercourse, and to avoid close contact with pregnant women and children for a designated period. Postoperative complications are pain, cystitis, hematuria, infections, and fatigue.[51]

In *malignant brain tumors*, a stereotactic technique has been used to implant radioactive sources into brain tissue via ribbons using iridium-192 delivered by LDR. Another method is permanent implants of iodine-125 or gold-198.[56] A more advanced technique is the Gliasite radiation system, where a balloon is placed in the surgical cavity and a radioactive isotope is instilled into the balloon. This procedure is safe, well-tolerated and currently being performed on an outpatient basis.[59] Possible side effects, self-care activities and radiation precautions are reviewed with the patient and family.

In *lung cancer*, sources are implanted for 2 to 7 days (LDR), or HDR is administered via catheters implanted directly into the tumor

via bronchoscopy.[56] Nursing management includes patient education about the procedure, possible side effects, and self-care.

NONSEALED RADIOACTIVE THERAPY

Iodine-131, an unsealed isotope, is used for *benign and malignant thyroid conditions*. This procedure is not encountered frequently, but it requires specialized nursing care. It consists of the oral ingestion of a radionuclide such as Iodine-131. Because of the dose that is used, hospitalization and radiation precautions are standard. The most common side effects are sialadenitis, nausea, and temporary bone marrow suppression. During and immediately after treatment with iodine-131, pregnancy should be prevented.[60] Since body fluids are contaminated, patients and families must be educated on radiation safety precautions.

Radiation Safety

With external beam radiation, there is minimal risk of exposure to radiation. Nursing care and radiation safety precautions required for implants are dependent on the type of radioactive isotope, the dose, and the method of administration. The nurse's knowledge of radiation biology can reduce anxiety and fear of exposure when caring for these patients.

Isolation precautions and film badges are necessary when caring for patients receiving radiation from sealed or unsealed sources.[56] The inpatient staff nurse provides daily care of implant patients or patients treated with Iodine-131. One aspect of the radiation oncology nurse's role is as a resource for the nursing

TABLE 20-2   Comparison of Radiation Safety Precautions for Sealed and Unsealed Radioactive Sources

SEALED SOURCES	UNSEALED SOURCES
Private room	Private room
No minors or pregnant visitors allowed	No minors or pregnant visitors allowed
Adult visitors may spend 15 minutes per day at a distance of 10 feet	Adult visitors may spend 15 minutes per day at a distance of 10 feet
Staff and visitors to keep lead shield in room between themselves and the patient as much as possible	Staff and visitors to keep lead shield in room between themselves and the patient as much as possible
Radiation monitoring badges must be worn by nursing personnel	Radiation monitoring badges must be worn by nursing personnel
No special precautions for handling excreta, dishes, dressings, bed linens	Body fluids are a source of radioactive contamination
	Cover pillows, phone headsets, and floor with waterproof material
	Bed linens and gowns must be placed in separate plastic bags and saved for the radiation safety officer (RSO)
Foley catheter for cervical implants	Must use toilet if possible, flush toilet 3 times
Regular dishes	Only disposable dishes and eating utensils
	Dishes and utensils placed in plastic bags and saved for RSO
Patient may be limited to bed rest depending on location of implant	Patient may be up in room
Check for dislodgement of source.	
If source becomes dislodged, it is handled with long forceps and placed in a lead container.	
Never touch the source	
When implant is removed, patient is no longer radioactive	Patient is surveyed by RSO to determine when radioactivity is at safe level for discharge

staff regarding information about the type of radiation, potential side effects, nursing care, and protection of staff and visitors.

ALARA (as low as reasonably achievable) is the acronym for a guideline used for radiation protection of staff involved in the care of patients receiving radiation. It is a regulatory requirement of all radiation safety programs. The techniques used to keep exposure ALARA are time, distance, and shielding. See Table 20-2 for standard radiation safety precautions based on ALARA.

TIME

The amount of exposure is directly related to time spent near the radioactive source. The nurse provides needed nursing care while minimizing the time spent in close contact with the patient receiving gamma radionuclide therapy. The patient and family are educated regarding the need for these precautions and the time family members are allowed to be in the room, excluding children under 18 or pregnant visitors.

DISTANCE

The amount of radiation exposure is inversely related to the distance from the radioactive source (inverse square law). If the distance from the source is doubled, the amount of exposure is reduced by one fourth.

SHIELDING

The amount of radiation exposure can be decreased by using a shield placed between the source and those susceptible to exposure. The correct material for the shield depends on the type of emitters (e.g., lead for high-energy gamma sources).

All staff members who may potentially be exposed to radiation must wear film badges. These are read periodically, usually once a month. The institution's radiation safety officer monitors occupational exposure rates of all employees with potential radiation exposure. Film badges are usually worn between the waist and collar, where the highest dose is likely to be received.

Other Treatment Options in Radiation Therapy

STEREOTACTIC RADIATION THERAPY (SRS)

SRS is a minimally invasive procedure that delivers a large dose of external beam radiation to a precisely targeted area of the brain with minimal damage to surrounding tissue, used for treating vascular lesions, malignant and benign brain tumors, and brain metastases. It can be used alone, after surgery, and in combination with whole-brain radiation.[61]

There are three current methods of ensuring accurate precision with SRS. One is use of a metal ring head frame[62]; another is the Gamma Knife (Electa Instruments, Stockholm, Sweden), which has been considered the gold standard for many years. The CyberKnife (Accuray, Sunnyvale, CA) is a radiosurgical system using a linear accelerator and robotic arm that can treat larger tumors, including tumors in extracranial sites, and has the advantage of not requiring a head frame. It is capable of precisely targeting a tumor from any direction. A custom-fit facemask is used to stabilize the patient's head.[61] SRS can be performed as a 1-day outpatient procedure that requires merging of a CT scan and MRI for treatment planning. CyberKnife may entail up to five outpatient treatments.

The nurse's role includes patient and family education about the procedure, preprocedural preparation, review of lab values, assessment and monitoring, discharge instructions, and collaborating in the details of SRS planning.[62] Nursing care may also involve procedures such as insertion of an intravenous catheter, pain assessment and control, symptom monitoring, and emotional support of patients and families.

INTENSITY-MODULATED RADIATION THERAPY

IMRT is an advanced form of 3D CRT treatment planning in which varying intensities of small subdivisions of beams are used to custom design optimal radiation dose distributions. The tumor is "painted," allowing high doses to the tumor volume and sparing of normal tissue. Patient immobilization is critical to the success of IMRT. Special treatment planning software is required. IMRT is expensive, and treatment planning is time consuming. It is used selectively in cases where treatment outcomes can be significantly affected. Minimal side effects are anticipated since less normal tissue is included in the treatment volume. Nursing care would include patient education and management of side effects similar to that for standard external beam radiation.[63]

INTRAOPERATIVE RADIATION THERAPY (IORT)

Intraoperative radiation therapy (IORT) is the delivery of radiation therapy during a surgical procedure. It provides direct visualization and treatment of tumors at the time of surgery by use of a targeting cone placed directly at the tumor site. The cone helps to displace normal tissue and minimize toxicities. A single dose delivered during surgery is equal to several weeks of daily radiation. With the development of the mobile linear accelerator, patients do not have to be transported to the radiation department. IORT is used to treat gastric, pancreatic, colorectal, bladder, cervical, and retroperitoneal sarcomas. High-dose rate IORT (HDR-IORT) has been used for advanced head and neck cancers.[64] Side effects may include nausea, vomiting, and anorexia.

RADIOPHARMACEUTICALS

Strontium-89 and samarium-153 can offer effective pain relief for multiple sites of malignant bone lesions,[65] used alone or in combination with external radiation. Strontium-89 has been shown to be as effective as wide-field radiotherapy in patients with prostate cancer, with reduced toxicity.[66] Samarium is less penetrating than strontium, minimizing exposure of healthy tissue.[65] Both radiopharmaceuticals are given as an intravenous injection in the outpatient setting. Pain relief is usually noted within 1 to 2 weeks after an initial "pain flare" within 72 hours after injection.

Nursing management includes patient education regarding the procedure, radiation safety, possible side effects, self-care, and expected pain relief (Box 20-2). Continuing current pain medications and use of nonsteroidal antiinflammatory drugs (NSAIDs) offer effective pain relief during the "pain flare." Baseline CBC is obtained and monitored every 2 weeks for 8 weeks since myelosuppression, especially thrombocytopenia, is an expected side effect. Radiation precautions for body fluids is necessary for approximately 7 days.

PHOTODYNAMIC THERAPY (PDT)

PDT, or photodynamic therapy, is used to treat bladder, skin, head and neck, endobronchial, and esophageal cancers. It is used primarily to alleviate obstruction of lumens such as the esophagus and the bronchi of the lung. PDT is a selective therapy that targets cancer cells and causes minimal damage to surrounding healthy tissue. It is a two-step procedure involving the administration of a photosensitizing agent such as porfimer sodium in the outpatient area followed 48 hours later by exposure to a nonthermal laser in the operating room.

Before PDT, patients and family are educated on the process and self care measures necessary after the procedure. Possible site-specific side effects include mucositis, pharyngitis, nausea and vomiting, constipation, bleeding at the site, infection, dysphagia, and bronchitis. Immediately after the procedure, the patient is monitored closely to ensure a patent airway and provide adequate pain control.

Photosensitivity can begin as early as 5 minutes after porfimer sodium injection and lasts 4 to 6 weeks. The patient must wear protective clothing and avoid direct sunlight or strong indoor lighting. A photosensitivity reaction is characterized by swelling, redness, or blistering, which cannot be prevented with sunscreen. Psychologic support is ongoing throughout the procedure.[67]

RADIOIMMUNOTHERAPY (RIT)

Zevalin (Biogen Idec, Inc., Cambridge, MA) was the first FDA-approved radioimmunotherapy (RIT) agent used to treat patients with relapsed or refractory non-Hodgkin's lymphoma (NHL). RIT delivers radiation to the cancer cells by attaching radionuclides to monoclonal antibodies to form radioimmunoconjugates that target a specific antigen expressed on tumor cells (CD20). Because of this specificity, RIT should be less toxic to normal tissues. Rituximab (Rituxan, Genentech Inc., San Francisco CA, and Biogen Idec Inc.) is administered on day 1, followed by imaging studies to verify the biodistribution. Rituximab is repeated on days 7, 8, and 9, followed within 4 hours by a therapeutic dose of yttrium-90 ibritumomab tiuxetan. Imaging studies are repeated at 48 to 72 hours, and 90 to 120 hours.[68]

BOX 20-2 **Patient and Family Instructions after Samarium Injection**

- You may experience a "pain flare" or increase in pain 24 to 72 hours after injection.
- You can expect pain relief as soon as 1 week after injection.
- Pain relief can last an average of 4 months.
- Drink extra fluids during the first 12 hours after injection.
- Urinate as often as possible, flushing the toilet 2 to 3 times after urinating.
- If you have a Foley catheter, you will need to change the bag 48 hours after injection and return the original bag to the radiation department.
- Wash your hands frequently.
- If blood or urine gets on your clothes, store them for 2 weeks before washing and wash them separately.
- Do not have intimate sexual contact with your partner for 12 hours after injection.
- For about 8 weeks after injection, tell any health care professionals that you have had samarium.
- Blood counts recover in about 8 weeks.
- You will need a complete blood count (CBC) drawn at 2, 4, and 6 weeks after the injection.
- Call your radiation or medical oncologist if you have an increase in pain unrelieved by pain medications.

Because yttrium-90 emits only beta particles with a half-life of 2.7 days, risk of radiation exposure to others is low. A study monitoring family members who had taken no special precaution except avoidance of contact with the patient's body fluids and wastes revealed their exposure to radiation after 7 days was similar to background radiation.[68]

The nurse coordinates and maintains the patient's strict schedule over the 1-week period as well as educates the patient and family about the treatment regimen and possible side effects. Because decreased blood counts are common, infection and bleeding precautions are included in patient education. Family members and visitors must avoid contact with the patient's body fluids. An infusion reaction to rituximab can occur. During rituximab infusion, the patient is monitored for an infusion reaction characterized by hypotension and hypoxia. Blood counts are taken at least weekly.[68]

Iodine-131 tositumomab (Bexxar; Corixa Corp., Seattle, WA) is also used in radioimmunotherapy to treat NHL. Bexxar emits both beta and gamma radiation. Lugol's solution is given orally before and after the procedure to block uptake by the thyroid. Radiation precautions are instituted to protect medical personnel, family members, and others from exposure (see "Radiation Safety"). Adverse effects are similar to those for Zevalin, and nursing care would be similar except for the difference in radiation precautions. Written and oral instructions regarding precautions are provided to the patient and family.[68] These include separate sleeping arrangements, separate bathroom, segregating utensils and laundry, minimizing time spent in public places, avoiding contact with children and pregnant women, and avoiding sexual contact for up to 7 days.[69]

Conclusion

Increased knowledge and understanding of the basic biology of ionizing radiation and how it interacts with living tissue has lead to many technological and treatment-planning advances since radiation was first used to treat patients. With increasingly aggressive cancer therapies that include radiation, patients are at risk for multiple toxicities. The nurse has established an important role in radiation oncology that has evolved and changed over the years. Assessing and monitoring the patient throughout treatment, instructing the patient and family on what they can expect and self-care, managing early and late toxicities, initiating appropriate referrals and providing emotional support are responsibilities that are within the scope of the radiation oncology nurse. The nurse also supports clinical trials, utilizes research, and may even conduct nursing research to improve patient outcomes. The overall goal is to provide quality nursing care that is evidence-based and outcome-focused.

CONSIDERATIONS FOR OLDER ADULTS

In the United States, the majority of people with cancer are 65 years of age or older.

There are biologic changes that happen with aging that can influence the older person's response to treatment. They tend to have more comorbid conditions and are felt to have a shorter life expectancy.[70]

Hematopoietic: There may be a decreased response to erythropoietin, preexisting anemia, diminished bone marrow reserve, and immune deficit.[70]

Fatigue: They may have preexisting fatigue that can compound cancer-related fatigue.

Gastrointestinal: Older people have decreased parotid function, so they are more susceptible to xerostomia and mucositis.[71]

Psychosocial Factors: Transportation issues and the person's self-care ability during treatment are more likely to be a concern in the elderly. In a study by Goodwin et al, 10-year survival in cancer patients over 65 could be predicted by diagnosis, comorbidities, functional status, level of physical activity, socioeconomic and cognitive status, type of treatment, and availability of social support. Decisions regarding radiation treatment in the elderly may be influenced by correctable factors such as lack of transportation.[72]

Patient Education: Impaired cognitive function, sensory changes and impaired vision can influence the patient teaching plan.

Medications: When prescribing medications to patients 65 years of age or older, factors to consider include declining organ function, increased incidence of comorbid conditions, and polypharmacy. Drug interactions in the elderly are more likely, and they are less able to tolerate side effects of medications. The 5HT3 antiemetics, for example, are better tolerated than prochlorperazine because of increased likelihood of extrapyramidal side effects in the elderly population.[46]

The National Comprehensive Cancer Network has published practice guidelines for senior adult oncology.[73] Table 20-3 provides an example of factors that are assessed in the older patient. This assessment will provide important information that is helpful in guiding treatment decisions and identifying the need for social work or dietary referrals.

Data from Avritscher EB, Cooksley CD, Elting LS: Scope and epidemiology of cancer therapy-induced oral and gastrointestinal mucositis, *Semin Oncol Nurs* 20(1):3-10, 2004; Goodwin JS, Hunt WC, Samet JM: Determinants of cancer therapy in elderly patients, *Cancer* 72(2):594-601, 1993; and Balducci L: NCCN practice guidelines in oncology: senior adult oncology. Retrieved June 24, 2005, from http://www.nccn.org/professionals/physician-gls/PDF/senior.pdf.

TABLE 20-3 Comprehensive Geriatric Assessment

PARAMETER	ASSESSMENT
Function	• Activities of daily living (ADLs)—Eating, dressing, continence, grooming, transferring, using the bathroom • Instrumental activities of daily living (IADLs)—Using transportation, managing money, taking medications, shopping, preparing meals, doing laundry, doing housework, using telephone • Performance status
Comorbidity	• Number of comorbid conditions • Seriousness of comorbid conditions (comorbidity index)
Socioeconomic issues	• Living conditions • Presence and adequacy of caregiver • Income • Access to transportation
Geriatric syndromes	• Dementia—Mini-Mental Status (MMS), other • Depression—Geriatric Depression Scale (GDS) • Delirium—For minimal infection or medication • Falls (≥1 per month) • Osteoporosis (spontaneous fractures) • Neglect and abuse • Failure to thrive • Persistent dizziness
Polypharmacy	• Number of medications • Drug-drug interactions
Nutrition	• Nutritional risk—Mini-Nutritional Assessment (MNA)

Reproduced with permission from the NCCN Senior Adult Oncology Guideline, *The Complete Library of NCCN Clinical Practice Guidelines in Oncology [CD-ROM]*. Jenkintown, Pennsylvania: © National Comprehensive Cancer Network, May 2005. To view the most recent and complete version of the guidelines, go online to www.nccn.org.

REVIEW QUESTIONS

✓ Case Study

Robert Smith is a 77-year-old man who comes to the outpatient radiation department for consultation for a recently diagnosed poorly differentiated squamous cell carcinoma of the tongue. He gives a history of a sore on the right side of the tongue for 3 weeks. He was seen by an ear, nose, and throat (ENT) physician, who biopsied the lesion. A CT scan of the soft tissues of the neck revealed one mildly prominent lymph node. The stage is T3, N1, M0. Past history includes bilateral femoral bypass for peripheral vascular disease, angioplasty for coronary artery disease (CAD), and hypertension. He is a retired engineer. Smoking history includes 1 ½ pack of cigarettes per day for 62 years. Alcohol use has decreased, but he still has about 10 whiskey-based drinks per week. His wife died during surgery for lung cancer 2 years ago. Mr. Smith lives alone, but his daughter and son-in-law live nearby and are supportive. He has 3 grandchildren in their 20s who see him often. His appetite is poor, and he has lost 8 pounds over the past month. He states, "I'm just not hungry. Sometimes I'm too tired to eat." The ENT physician proposed surgery before radiation and chemotherapy. He also suggested a gastrostomy tube for nutritional support. Mr. Smith declined both the surgery and the feeding tube, saying, "What's the point—I'm 77 years old. I might as well enjoy the time I have left without being hooked up to a tube all the time." The radiation oncologist recommends radiation to the tongue tumor and bilateral neck nodes (6000 cGy in 30 treatments) with concurrent cisplatinum once a week.

A radioactive implant may be considered after radiation and chemotherapy are completed.

QUESTIONS

1. When is a dietary consult indicated in Mr. Smith's case?
   a. As long as he is eating, it is not necessary
   b. At consultation
   c. When the patient loses 5% of his baseline weight
   d. When Mr. Smith asks questions about his diet
2. Based on the nurse's assessment, she determines that Mr. Smith is anxious about the possibility of a gastrostomy tube because of his limited understanding of the rationale and how it will affect his lifestyle. Which of the following actions is most likely to increase Mr. Smith's compliance with the placement of the gastrostomy tube?
   a. Assure Mr. Smith that he will need the gastrostomy tube to get through treatment successfully.
   b. Involve Mr. Smith and his family in a discussion of the rationale for the gastrostomy tube, an explanation of how it is inserted, and self care.
   c. Provide a referral to a surgeon for placement of a gastrotomy tube.
   d. Explain to Mr. Smith and his family that most patients receiving head and neck treatment never need to use the gastrostomy tube, but it is more difficult to insert it once treatment has started.

3. What late effect of radiation is the nurse addressing when she suggests a dental consult?
   a. Fibrosis of the gums
   b. Facial paralysis
   c. Temporomandibular joint disease (TMJ)
   d. Dental caries

4. What immobilization device would be appropriate in the treatment of tongue cancer?
   a. A full-body cradle
   b. A band around the feet
   c. An aquaplast mask(uniframe)
   d. Pull-ropes to immobilize arms during treatment

5. When educating the patient, you will tell him that the most common site-specific acute side effect related to radiation that he will experience is:
   a. Neutropenia
   b. Fatigue
   c. Mucositis
   d. Hair loss

6. In treating the side effect in question 3, the published scientific evidence includes which of the following?
   a. Oral rinses with an antacid every 2 hours
   b. Amifostine given subcutaneously 15 minutes before radiation treatment
   c. Rinsing the mouth with water before each radiation treatment
   d. Fluoride treatments twice a day prescribed by a dentist

7. What would the nurse include in patient education that would help minimize mucosal damage while allowing Mr. Smith to be an active participant in his care?
   a. Emphasizing the importance of excellent oral hygiene including frequent mouth care and inspecting the oral mucosa daily for signs of infection
   b. Assure him that he will not be radioactive with external beam radiation
   c. Use fluoride treatments as directed by his dentist
   d. Fluids and foods should be served hot

8. If Mr. Smith has a head and neck implant after external radiation and chemotherapy, the following radiation precaution will be observed by the nursing staff:
   a. Dishes and utensils will be disposable.
   b. Children under 18 will be allowed to visit for only 5 minutes.
   c. No one will be allowed to enter the room.
   d. A personal radiation badge will be worn by all staff caring for Mr. Smith.

9. Is Mr. Smith a good candidate for IMRT instead of standard external beam radiation therapy?
   a. Yes
   b. No

10. Because side effects will be worse if Mr. Smith continues to smoke, the nurse does the following:
    a. Tells his son-in-law to make him quit
    b. Insists that Mr. Smith quit smoking
    c. Talks to Mr. Smith about the relationship between smoking and tongue cancer and how smoking can influence side effects
    d. Nothing—Mr. Smith knows that he needs to quit

ANSWERS

1. **B.** *Rationale:* Since the patient has a poor appetite and has lost 8 pounds over the past month, it has already been established that his intake is inadequate. Drinking alcohol and smoking cigarettes will further compromise his nutritional status by increasing the severity of treatment side effects. He has refused a feeding tube. Once he has lost 5% of his baseline weight, it will be more difficult to correct the weight loss. The nurse consults the dietitian before treatment begins to evaluate his caloric intake and make dietary recommendations with the goal of stabilizing his weight. The dietitian would also recommend a feeding tube and explore Mr. Smith's readiness to decrease tobacco and alcohol use.

2. **B.** *Rationale:* It is not sufficient to tell Mr. Smith that he needs a gastrostomy tube. Telling him he can't be treated without one is inaccurate and takes one more choice away from him at a time when he is already feeling a lack of control. The statement in "d" is not true except for the fact that it may be more difficult to insert the tube once treatment has begun. Research has shown that preparing a patient for a procedure with both factual and sensory information will decrease anxiety and increase satisfaction. Mr. Smith's family is supportive and should be involved in patient education. These outcomes are likely to have a positive effect on compliance.

3. **D.** *Rationale:* Fibrosis of the gums, facial paralysis, and TMJ are not caused by radiation to the head and neck. Dental caries is a late effect of radiation involving the oral cavity and can occur several months after radiation is completed. The xerostomia Mr. Smith will experience during his treatment may be permanent. Plaque formation can cause inflammation and recession of the gums. Decreased, thickened saliva promotes plaque formation, leading to dental caries.

4. **C.** *Rationale:* A full-body cradle can be frightening and anxiety provoking. Since the whole body is not being treated, it is unnecessary in this case. A band around the feet will not affect the mobility of the head. To treat the oral cavity, the head and neck must be immobilized with an aquaplast mask that is customized to the patient and attached to the table in the same position every day to ensure reproducibility of the treatment position.

5. **C.** *Rationale:* Mr. Smith's scalp is not being treated, so alopecia will not occur from radiation. Blood counts may be decreased from chemotherapy but not from radiation to the oral cavity, since no bone marrow is in the treatment field. Fatigue is the most common side effect from radiation, but it is a general, not site-specific side effect. The mucosa of the oral cavity is dividing rapidly and is directly in the radiation field when treating the oral cavity, making it highly susceptible to radiation damage.

6. **B.** *Rationale:* Fluoride treatments are used to prevent dental caries. Oral rinses with an antacid or water have not been shown to prevent mucosal damage. Several studies have been published demonstrating the efficacy of amifostine in protecting the oral mucosa.

7. **A.** *Rationale:* Assuring him he will not be radioactive is important but will not affect damage to the oral mucosa. Fluoride treatment will prevent dental caries but will not minimize mucositis. Serving foods and fluids hot can
Continued

REVIEW QUESTIONS—CONT'D

contribute to damage to the oral mucosa. If the mouth is kept clean and free of debris, mucositis can be minimized. Also, daily inspection of the oral mucosa is critical for prompt treatment of oral infections.

8. **D.** *Rationale:* Since this type of implant is a sealed source, dishes and utensils do not have to be disposable. Children under 18 are not allowed to visit at all because of potential exposure. Adult visitors are allowed 15 minutes per day at a distance of 10 feet from the patient. The amount of radiation exposure to staff is monitored by the personal radiation badge and read each month. If the occupational exposure exceeds recommended limit for the year, the staff member would not be allowed to care for these patients.

9. **A.** *Rationale:* IMRT is ideal for head and neck patients, since the patient can be immobilized adequately and accurate reproducibility of treatment can be accomplished. Considering his age and comorbid conditions, it would decrease potential for side effects since less normal tissue would be in the treatment field.

10. **C.** *Rationale:* No one, including Mr. Smith's son-in-law or the nurse, can coerce him to quit smoking. The nurse can't assume that Mr. Smith knows that he needs to quit or that he knows how to quit. She or he starts by exploring his knowledge of the relationship between smoking and tongue cancer and how smoking can influence his response to treatment.

REFERENCES

1. Rubin P, Williams JP: Principles of radiation oncology and cancer radiotherapy. In Rubin P, editor: *Clinical oncology: a multidisciplinary approach for physicians and students,* ed 8, Philadelphia, 2001, WB Saunders.
2. Hilderly LJ: Principles of teletherapy. In Dow KH, Bucholtz J, Iwamoto RR et al: *Nursing care in radiation oncology,* ed 2, Philadelphia, 1997, WB Saunders.
3. Halperin EC, Schmidt-Ullrich RK, Perez CA et al: The discipline of radiation oncology. In Perez CA, Brady LW, Halperin EC et al, editors: *Principles and practice of radiation oncology,* ed 4, Philadelphia, 2004, Lippincott, Williams & Wilkins.
4. Mieszkalski GB, Brady LW, Yaeger TE et al: Basis for current major therapies for cancer: radiotherapy. In Lenhard RE, Osteen RT, Gansler T, editors: *The American Cancer Society's Clinical Oncology,* Atlanta, 2001, American Cancer Society.
5. Hilderly LJ: Radiation oncology: historical background. In Dow KH, Bucholtz J, Iwamoto RR et al: *Nursing care in radiation oncology,* ed 2, Philadelphia, 1997, WB Saunders Company.
6. Gosselin-Acomb TK: Principles of radiation therapy. In Yarbro CH, Frogge MH, Goodman M, editors: *Cancer nursing: principles and practice,* ed 6, Boston, 2005, Jones & Bartlett.
7. Connell PP, Martel MK, Hellman S: Principles of radiation oncology. In DeVita VT, Hellman S, Rosenberg SA, editors: *Cancer: principles and practice of oncology,* ed 7, vol 1, Philadelphia, 2005, Lippincott, Williams & Wilkins.
8. McBride WH, Withers HR: Biologic basis of radiation therapy. In Perez CA, Brady LW, Halperin EC et al, editors: *Principles and practice of radiation oncology,* ed 4, Philadelphia, 2004, Lippincott, Williams & Wilkins.
9. Iwomoto RR: Radiation therapy. In Otto S, editor: *Oncology Nursing,* St. Louis, 2001, Mosby.
10. Wengstrom Y, Forsberg C: Justifying radiation oncology nursing practice—a literature review, *Oncol Nurs Forum* 26(4):741-750, 1999.
11. Poroch, D: The effect of preparatory patient education on the anxiety and satisfaction of cancer patients receiving radiation therapy, *Cancer Nurs* 18(3):206-214, 1995.
12. Johnson JE, Fieler VK, Wlasowicz GS et al: The effects of nursing care guided by self-regulation theory on coping with radiation therapy, *Oncol Nurs Forum* 24(6):1041-1050 1997.
13. D'Haese S, Vinh-Hung V, Bijdekerke P et al: The effect of timing of the provision of information on anxiety and satisfaction of cancer patients receiving radiotherapy, *J Cancer Educ* 15(4):223-227, 2000.
14. Haggmark C, Bohman L, Ilmoni-Brandt K et al: Effects of information supply on satisfaction with information and quality of life in cancer patients receiving curative radiation therapy, *Patient Educ Couns* 45(3): 173-179, 2001.
15. Behrend SW: Radiation treatment planning. In Yarbro CH, Frogge MH, Goodman M, editors: *Cancer nursing: principles and practice,* ed 6, Boston, 2005, Jones & Bartlett.
16. Bruner DW, Haas ML, Gosselin-Acomb TK, editors: *Radiation oncology nursing practice and education,* ed 3, Pittsburgh, 2005, Oncology Nursing Society.

17. Harper JL, Franklin LE, Jenrette JM et al: Skin toxicity during breast irradiation: pathophysiology and management, *South Med J* 97(10): 989-993, 2004.
17a. Aistars, J: The validity of skin care protocols followed by women with breast cancer receiving external radiation, *Clin J Oncol Nurs* 10(4): 487-492, 2006.
18. National Cancer Institute: *Common terminology criteria for adverse advents* (v. 3.0). Bethesda, Md, 2003.
19. Berthelet E, Truong PT, Musso K et al: Preliminary reliability and validity testing of a new skin toxicity assessment tool (STAT) in breast cancer patients undergoing radiotherapy, *Am J Clin Oncol: Cancer Clinical Trials* 27(6):626-631, 2004.
20. Heggie S, Bryant GP, Tripcony L et al: A phase III study on the efficacy of topical aloe vera gel on irradiated breast tissue, *Cancer Nurs* 25(6): 442-450, 2002.
21. Roy I, Fortin A, Larochelle M: The impact of skin washing with water and soap during breast irradiation: a randomized study, *Radiother Oncol* 58:333-339, 2001.
22. Olsen DL, Raub W, Bradley C et al: The effect of aloe vera gel/mild soap versus mild soap alone in preventing skin reactions in patients undergoing radiation therapy, *Oncol Nurs Forum* 28(3):543-547, 2001.
23. Fisher J, Scott C, Stevens R et al: Randomized phase III study comparing best supportive care to biafine as a prophylactic agent for radiation-induced skin toxicity for women undergoing breast irradiation: radiation therapy oncology group (RTOG) 97-13, *Int J Radiat Oncology Biol Phys* 48(5):1307-1310, 2000.
24. Irvine DM, Vincent L, Graydon JE, et al: Fatigue in women with breast cancer receiving radiation therapy, *Cancer Nurs,* 21(2):127-135, 1998.
25. Mock V, Barsevick A, Escalante CP, Hinds P: NCCN clinical practice guidelines in oncology: cancer-related fatigue. Retrieved June 24, 2005, from http://www.nccn.org/professionals/physician/PDF/fatig.
26. Nail LM: Fatigue in patients with cancer, *Oncol Nurs Forum* 29(3): 537-544, 2002.
27. Stricker CT, Drake D, Hoyer KA, Mock V: Evidence-based practice for fatigue management in adults with cancer: exercise as an intervention, *Oncol Nurs Forum* 31(5):963-976, 2004.
28. Sarna L, Conde F: Physical activity and fatigue during radiation therapy: a pilot study using actigraph monitors, *Oncol Nurs Forum* 28(6): 1043-1046, 2001.
29. Barsevick, AM, Dudley W, Beck S et al. A randomized clinical trial of energy conservation for patients with cancer- related fatigue, *Cancer* 100(6):1302-1310, 2004.
30. Beach P, Siebeneck B, Buderer NF et al: Relationship between fatigue and nutritional status in patients receiving radiation therapy to treat lung cancer, *Oncol Nurs Forum* 28(6):1027-1031, 2001.
31. Maher KE: Radiation therapy: toxicities and management. In Yarbro CH, Frogge MH, Goodman M, editors: *Cancer nursing: principles and practice,* ed 6, Boston, 2005, Jones & Bartlett.
32. Bruce SD: Radiation-induced xerostomia: how dry is your patient? *Clin J Oncol Nurs* 8(1):61-67, 2004.

33. Ship JA, Hu K: Radiotherapy-induced salivary dysfunction, *Semin Oncol* 31(6 Suppl 18):29-36, 2004.

34. Sonis ST: Oral mucositis in cancer therapy, *J Support Oncol* 2 (6 Suppl 3):3-8, 2004.

35. Shih A, Miaskowski C, Dodd M et al: Continuing education. A research review of the current treatments for radiation-induced oral mucositis in patients with head and neck cancer, *Oncol Nurs Forum* 29(7):1063-1080, 2002.

36. Dodd MJ: The pathogenesis and characterization of oral mucositis associated with cancer therapy, *Oncol Nurs Forum* 31(4 Supp):5-11, 2004.

37. Eilers J: Nursing interventions and supportive care for the prevention and treatment of oral mucositis associated with cancer treatment, *Oncol Nurs Forum,* 31(4 Supp):13-23, 37-39, 2004.

38. Brizel DM, Wasserman TH, Henke M et al: Phase III randomized trial of amifostine as a radioprotector in head and neck cancer, *J Clin Oncol,* 18(19):3339-3345, 2000.

39. Johnstone PA, Niemtzow RC, Riffenburgh RH: Acupuncture for xerostomia: clinical update, *Cancer* 94(4):1151-1156, 2002.

40. Maher, K. Xerostomia. In Yarbro CH, Frogge MH, Goodman M, editors: *Cancer symptom management,* ed 3, Boston, 2004, Jones & Bartlett.

41. Sherry VW: Taste alterations among patients with cancer, *Clin J Oncol Nurs* 6(2):73-77, 105-106, 2002.

42. Ripamonti C, Zecca, Brunneli C et al: A randomized, controlled clinical trial to evaluate the effects of zinc sulfate on cancer patients with taste alterations caused by head and neck irradiation, *Cancer* 82(10):1938-1945, 1998.

43. Mendenhall WM: Mandibular osteoradionecrosis, *J Clin Oncol* 22(24):4867-4868, 2004.

44. Antonadou D, Coliarakis N, Synodinou M et al: Randomized phase III trial of radiation treatment +/- amifostine in patients with advanced-stage lung cancer, *Int J Radiat Oncol Biol Phys* 51(4):915-922, 2001.

45. Horiot JC: Prophylaxis versus treatment: is there a better way to manage radiotherapy-induced nausea and vomiting? *Int J Radiat Oncology Biol Phys* 60(4):1018-1025, 2004.

46. Feyer P, Maranzano E, Molassiotis A et al: Radiotherapy-induced nausea and vomiting (RINV): antiemetic guidelines, *Support Care Cancer* 13:122-128,1018-1025, 2005.

47. Anthony L: New strategies for the prevention and reduction of cancer treatment-induced diarrhea, *Semin Oncol Nurs* 19(4 Suppl 3):17-21, 2003.

48. Stern, J, Ippoliti C: Management of acute cancer treatment-induced diarrhea, *Semin Oncol Nurs* 19(4 Suppl 3):11-16, 2003.

49. Gwede CK: Overview of radiation and chemoradiation-induced diarrhea, *Semin Oncol Nurs* 19(4 Suppl 3):6-10, 2003.

50. Murphy J, Stacey D, Crook J et al: Testing control of radiation-induced diarrhea with a psyllium bulking agent: a pilot study, *Can J Oncol Nurs* 10(3):96-100, 2000.

51. Iwamoto RR, Maher KE: Radiation therapy for prostate cancer, *Semin Oncol Nurs* 17(2):90-100, 2001.

52. Gosselin TK, Waring JS: Nursing management of patients receiving brachytherapy for gynecological malignancies. *Clin J Oncol Nurs* 5(2):59-59-63, 2001.

53. Westbury C, Hines F, Hawkes E et al: Advice on hair and scalp care during cranial radiotherapy: a prospective randomized trial, *Radiother Oncol* 54(2): 09-116, 2000 (abstract).

54. Metz JM, Smith D, Mick R et al: A phase I study of topical Tempol for the prevention of alopecia induced by whole brain radiotherapy, *Clin Cancer Res* 10(19): 6411-6417, 2004

55. Remer S, Murphy ME: The challenges of long-term treatment outcomes in adults with malignant gliomas, *Clin J Oncol Nurs* 8(4):368-376, 2004.

56. Dunne-Daly C: Principles of brachytherapy. In Dow KH, Bucholtz JD, Iwamoto RR, editors: *Nursing care in radiation oncology,* ed 2, Philadelphia, 1997, WB Saunders.

57. Devine P, Doyle T: Brachytherapy for head and neck cancer: a case study, *Clin J Oncol Nurs* 5(2):55-57, 2001.

58. Gordils-Perez J, Rawlis-Duell, Kelvin JF: Advances in radiation treatment of patients with breast cancer, *Clin J Oncol Nurs* 7(6):629-636, 2003.

59. Chan TA, Weingart JD, Parisi M et al: Treatment of recurrent glioblastoma multiforme with GliaSite brachytherapy, *Int J Radiat Oncol Biol Phys* 62(4):1133-1139, 2005.

60. Stajduhar KI, Neithercut J, Chu E et al: Thyroid cancer: patients' experiences of receiving iodine therapy, *Oncol Nurs Forum* 27(8):1213-1218, 2000.

61. Quinn AM: CyberKnife: A robotic radiosurgery system, *Clin J Oncol Nurs* 6(3):149-156, 2002.

62. Law E, Mangarin E, Kelvin JF: Nursing management of patients receiving stereotactic radiosurgery, *Clin J Oncol Nurs* 7(4):387-392, 2003.

63. Hong TS, Ritter MA, Tome WA et al: Intensity-modulated radiation therapy: emerging cancer treatment technology, *Br J Cancer* 92(10):1819-1824, 2005.

64. Beddar AS, Kubu ML, Domanovic MA et al: A new approach to intraoperative radiation therapy, *AORN* 74(4):500-505, 2001.

65. Reich, CD: Advances in the treatment of bone metastases, *Clin J Oncol Nurs* 7(6):641-646, 2003.

66. Blum RH, Novetsky D, Shasha D et al: The multidisciplinary approach to bone metastases, *Oncology,* 17(6):845-857, 2003.

67. Bruce S: Photodynamic therapy: another option in cancer treatment, *Clin J Oncol Nurs* 5(3):95-99, 2001.

68. Byar K: Educating patients about radioimmunotherapy with yttrium 90 ibritumomab tiuxetan (Zevalin), *Semin Oncol Nurs* 20(1):20-25, 2004.

69. Riley MB, Byar K: The rationale for and background of radioimmunotherapy: an emerging therapy for B-cell non-Hodgkin's lymphoma, *Semin Oncol Nurs* 20(1):1-7, 2004.

70. Denduluri N, Ershler WB: Aging biology and cancer, *Semin Oncology* 31(2):137-148, 2004.

71. Avritscher EB, Cooksley CD, Elting LS: Scope and epidemiology of cancer therapy-induced oral and gastrointestinal mucositis, *Semin Oncol Nurs* 20(1):3-10, 2004.

72. Goodwin JS, Hunt WC, Samet JM: Determinants of cancer therapy in elderly patients, *Cancer* 72(2):594-601, 1993.

73. Balducci L: NCCN practice guidelines in oncology: senior adult oncology. Retrieved June 24, 2005, from http://www.nccn.org/professionals/physician-gls/PDF/senior.pdf.

CHAPTER 21

Chemotherapy

Shirley E. Otto

It is estimated that 1,372,910 people in the United States were newly diagnosed as having cancer in 2005. More than half of these people will receive systemic chemotherapy as a form of treatment because of disease recurrence, as secondary therapy after a local treatment, or for treatment of hematologic disease. The primary focus of chemotherapy is to prevent cancer cells from multiplying, invading adjacent tissue, or developing metastasis.[1-4]

Definition

Chemotherapy is the use of cytotoxic drugs in the treatment of cancer. It is one of the four treatment modalities (the others being surgery, radiation therapy, and biotherapy) that provide cure, control, or palliation. Chemotherapy is a systemic treatment, rather than localized therapy, as are, for example, surgery and radiation therapy.[2,3,5,6] Chemotherapy may be used in six ways:

1. *Adjuvant therapy*—a course of chemotherapy used in conjunction with another treatment modality (surgery, radiation therapy, or biotherapy) and aimed at treating micrometastases.
2. *Neoadjuvant chemotherapy*—administration of chemotherapy to shrink a tumor before it is removed surgically.
3. *Primary therapy*—the treatment of patients who have localized cancer for which an alternative but less than completely effective treatment is available.
4. *Induction chemotherapy*—drug therapy given as the primary treatment for patients who have cancer for which no alternative treatment exists.
5. *Combination chemotherapy*—administration of two or more chemotherapeutic agents to treat cancer; this allows each medication to enhance the action of the other or to act synergistically with it (an example of combination chemotherapy is the widely known MOPP regimen of nitrogen mustard, vincristine [Oncovin], procarbazine, and prednisone, which is used to treat patients with Hodgkin's disease).
6. *Myeloblative therapy*—dose-intensive therapy used in preparation for peripheral blood stem cell transplantation.

Historical Perspective

Research for chemotherapy began in the early 1900s, when Paul Ehrlich used rodent models of infectious diseases to develop antibiotics. Further developments led to the use of rodents to test potential cancer chemotherapeutic agents. An additional discovery in drug development was made as the result of servicemen's exposure to mustard gas during World Wars I and II. This exposure led to the observation that alkylating agents caused marrow and lymphoid suppression in humans. This experience resulted in the use of these agents to treat Hodgkin's and other lymphomas; the therapy was first attempted at Yale's New Haven Medical Center in 1940. Because of the secret nature of the gas warfare program, the work was not published until 1946. Chemotherapy as a treatment

modality was introduced in the late 1950s and became established in medical practice in the 1970s.[1,2,6]

Since the start of cytotoxic drug research, thousands of chemical agents have been tested for their ability to destroy cancer cells. More than 400 cytotoxic agents are available for commercial or experimental use with approval by the federal Food and Drug Administration (FDA). Research continues to contribute discoveries in the area of chemotherapy as a cancer treatment modality, and as a result of this intensive investigation, new areas have been tapped for further study, such as the use of chemotherapeutic agents as radiosensitizers, chemoprotectants, and compounds to reduce multidrug resistance.[1-3,6]

Principles of Chemotherapy

CELL GENERATION CYCLE

The cell cycle is the sequence of events that results in replication of DNA and equal distribution into daughter cells, a process called **mitosis.** Normal cells and cancer cells go through the same division cycle, which is characterized by the following phases: G_0—resting or dormant phase; G_1—phase in which protein synthesis takes place in preparation for the S-phase–DNA synthesis; and G_2—phase for further protein synthesis in preparation for the M phase—mitosis and cell division. The generation time, or the time it takes a cell to complete the phase or cycle, varies from hours to days. Chemotherapeutic drugs are most active against frequently dividing cells, or in all the phases of the cell cycle except G_0. Normal cells with rapid growth changes that are most commonly affected by chemotherapeutic agents include bone marrow (platelets and red and white blood cells), hair follicles, the mucosal lining of the gastrointestinal (GI) tract, and skin and germinal cells (sperm and ova). Chemotherapy is given according to schedules that have proved most effective for tumor kill and that are planned to allow normal cells to recover.[1-3,6]

TUMOR GROWTH

The regulatory mechanism that controls the growth of cancer cells differs from that of normal cells. Unlike normal cells, cancer cells grow by means of a pyramid effect; however, they grow at the same rate as the tissue from which they originated (e.g., breast cancer develops at the same rate of growth as normal breast tissue development). The time required for a tumor mass to reach a certain size is called **doubling time.** Tumors probably have undergone approximately 30 doublings from a single cell before they are clinically detected. Between the seventh and tenth doubling time, the possibility arises for the tumor to shed cells, a process called **micrometastasis.** During the early stages of tumor growth, doubling time is more rapid than at later stages; this pattern of growth is called **Gompertzian function.** Tumor cells are more sensitive than normal cells to chemotherapy agents that are toxic to rapidly dividing cells. The roles of tumor growth and cell kinetics are important in understanding the action of cytotoxic therapy. Hematologic diseases, such as leukemia and lymphoma, have many rapidly dividing cells. When chemotherapy is initiated, there is the potential for rapid, extensive cellular destruction because of the nature of the bone marrow stem cells and the rapidly dividing cancer cells.[1-3,5,7]

Factors Influencing Chemotherapy Selection and Administration

BLOOD–BRAIN BARRIER

The blood-brain barrier (BBB) is made up of cellular structures that can inhibit certain substances from entering the brain or central nervous system tumors and acts as a screening device, thereby protecting the brain and cerebrospinal fluid from harmful agents. The barrier is formed by continuous supporting cells, particularly astrocytes, and the endothelial cells of brain capillaries, which form intertwining junctions. The passage of substances across the lipid membranes of endothelial cells depends on molecular weight, lipid solubility, and ionization state. Large, water-soluble (e.g., glucose) charged particles and compounds bound to plasma proteins are unable to penetrate the BBB; conversely, small, water-soluble chemotherapeutic drugs (carmustine, lomustine, cytarabine), normally excluded from the brain by the BBB, may reach enhancing areas of the tumor (Fig. 21-1).[3,6]

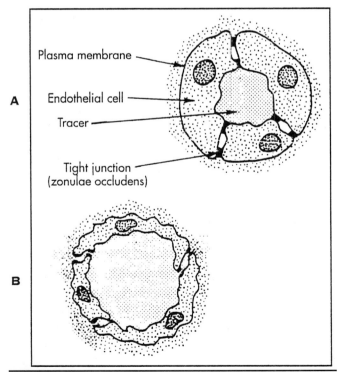

FIG. 21-1 Schematic representation of the blood-brain barrier. **A,** Normal cerebral capillary showing tight junctions. **B,** Blood-brain barrier opening created by widening of the interendothelial tight junctions. When the endothelial cells shrink in a hypertonic environment, the permeability of the junctions increases. (From Groenwald SL and others: *Cancer nursing: principles and practice,* ed 4, Sudbury, Mass, 1997, Jones & Bartlett. Reprinted with permission.)

Chemotherapy drug administration via the intrathecal route (Ommaya reservoir) effectively bypasses the BBB and permits delivery of drugs directly into the CSF. This intrathecal method (Ommaya reservoir or lumbar puncture) both allows access to the CNS for drug (analgesia and chemotherapy) administration and permits sampling of the CSF. Intrathecal drug administration provides more consistent drug levels in the CSF, thereby increasing cell kill in primary or metastatic tumors located in the brain.

CHEMOPREVENTION

Chemoprevention via a pharmacologic intervention refers to the concept of reducing cancer risk in individuals who are highly susceptible to certain cancers by prescribing certain natural or chemical synthetic products or chemotherapy drugs that may reduce or suppress the process of carcinogenesis. Carcinogenesis is a stepwise process that begins at the genetic level and progresses with cellular changes that initiate and promote the development of a malignancy. Chemoprevention seeks to arrest the process of carcinogenesis before the tumor develops.[6,8]

Chemoprevention trials generally are conducted in noncancer populations more than in populations at high risk for the development of cancer. The population of trial subjects includes those at high risk for specific cancers (e.g., breast, prostate, and colorectal cancers, melanoma) as well as subjects from the general population. "Designer estrogens" appear to be the new focused attention of the clinical researchers. These selective estrogen-receptor modulators appear to act as potent estrogen agonists in some tissues but as estrogen antagonists in other tissues. "Aromatase inhibitors" are the second group of drugs gaining research attention because of their selectivity in depriving the "breast cancer tumor" of estrogen, thereby exhibiting cell kill. Finasteride (which inhibits the conversion of testosterone to its active metabolite dihydrotestosterone) has been used in the largest phase III trial (Prostate Cancer Prevention) ever conducted in the United States.[8]

CHRONOTHERAPY OR CIRCADIAN RHYTHM

Circadian rhythm is a term used to describe a regular, repeated fluctuation in biologic functions during a 24-hour period. The term often is used in conjunction with the term **diurnal,** which refers to "events happening in the daytime." In the many ongoing physiologic mechanisms that occur in the human body, many variables are affected by circadian rhythms. These **circadian variables** can influence drug absorption, metabolism, distribution, and elimination. They can be manipulated to allow for both dose intensification of the drug and reduction of cytotoxic side effects. Previous studies have revealed time-dependent variations for both toxic side effects and therapeutic drug efficacy. Circadian variations are evident in several human parameters, such as DNA synthesis in the intestinal mucosal tissue, the skin, the bone marrow, and spleen, testis, and thymus tissue.[3,7]

CYTOPROTECTANTS

This new category of drugs has emerged in the past decade. Cytoprotectants are used to prevent or decrease specific system effects (e.g., cardiotoxicity, nephrotoxicity, bladder toxicity, and hemopoietic toxicity) related to certain drug therapies. These drugs selectively protect normal tissues from the cytotoxic effects of drugs or irradiation while preserving their antitumor effects. *Usual* administration and monitoring guidelines for cytoprotectants include:

- Follow the specific manufacturer's guidelines related to preparation, reconstitution, and timed infusion administration components.
- Administer the cytoprotectant *30 to 60 minutes before* the chemotherapy and radiation therapy treatment.
- Refer to the manufacturer's product literature regarding drug specificity side effects such as nausea, vomiting, transient hypotension, warm flushed feeling, diarrhea, and joint pain.

The current cytoprotectant drugs and their respective system toxicity include the following:

- Carvedilol (Coreg), used to prevent or decrease anthracycline-associated cardiotoxicity
- Dexrazoxane (Zinecard), used to prevent or decrease doxorubicin-associated cardiotoxicity
- Mesna (Mesnex), used to prevent or decrease hemorrhagic cystitis induced by ifosfamide (Ifex) and cyclophosfamide (Cytoxan).
- Amifostine (Ethyol) is used as a pancytoprotectant and to decrease cumulative renal toxicity associated with repeated administration of cisplatin in patients with ovarian and non–small cell lung cancer.

Cytoprotectants offer many patients with cancers, such as breast, non–small cell lung, head and neck, or ovarian cancer, or those patients requiring chemotherapy dose-intensification therapy for peripheral blood stem cell or marrow transplantation, an improved quality of life.[2,5,6,9]

LIPOSOMES

Advances in liposome technology used for drug delivery purposes have made it possible to manipulate chemotherapy drugs and tailor them to penetrate specific target tissues. This novel system will allow better administration of poorly soluble cancer drugs, thus enhancing drug delivery and uptake in the tumor, boosting dose intensity, and subsequently improving antitumor response, overcoming drug resistance and decreasing chemotherapy toxicities.[6]

Chemotherapy drugs currently used for patients with AIDS-related Kaposi's sarcoma, breast, and ovarian cancers are Doxil—doxorubicin HCL liposome; DaunoXome—daunorubicin liposome; DepoCyt—cytarabine; and Abelecet—amphotericin. Several liposomal formations undergoing phases I and II evaluations include liposomal vincristine, platinum, mitoxantrone, all-trans retinoic acid (ATRA) and lurtotecan. Mucositis, nausea, vomiting, lumbar pain, skin rash, and headache were the most frequent reported side effects. Drug-related myelosuppression and vesicant extravasation that are usually associated with antitumor antibiotics (daunorubicin, doxorubicin) were not as evident or cumulative with the above-mentioned drugs. Administration guidelines include the following: *DO NOT* mix with other drugs or use an in-line filter; follow manufacturer's preparation and infusion time guidelines; premedications are not necessary; and if an untoward clinical event occurs during drug administration, stop the infusion immediately.[6,9]

RADIOSENSITIZERS

Radiosensitizers are compounds that enhance the sensitivity of tumors to the effects of radiation, but not to normal tissue. This concept includes administering concomitant chemotherapy at cytotoxic doses followed by radiotherapy that allows for better control on micrometastases and better local control on the tumor because of radiosensitization by the chemotherapy drugs. The combination of radiation therapy and chemotherapy promises benefits for patients such as reducing radioresistance. Clinical trials are under way for various malignancies using concomitant chemotherapy and radiation therapy. Chemotherapeutic agents that have demonstrated efficacy as radiosensitizers include amifostine, cisplatin, docetaxel, fludarabine, 5-fluorouracil (5-FU), gemcitabine, hydroxyurea, and paclitaxel.[10]

Chemotherapy Drug Classification

Chemotherapeutic agents are classified according to their pharmacologic action and their interference with cellular reproduction. Following are the basic groups and their potential action:

Cell cycle phase-specific drugs are active on cells undergoing division in the cell cycle. Examples include antimetabolites, vinca plant alkaloids, and miscellaneous agents such as asparaginase and dacarbazine. These drugs are most effective against actively growing tumors that have a greater proportion of cells cycling through the phase in which the drug attacks the cancer cell.

Cell cycle phase–nonspecific drugs are active on cells in either a dividing or resting state; examples include alkylating agents, antitumor antibiotics, nitrosoureas, hormone and steroid drugs, and miscellaneous agents such as procarbazine. These agents are active in all phases of the cell cycle and may be effective in large tumors that have few active cells dividing at the time of administration.

The mechanism of most chemotherapeutic drugs is targeting of the cell DNA in some manner. This action may result in direct interference with the DNA, inhibition of enzymes related to RNA or DNA synthesis or both, and/or destruction of the cells' necessary proteins.

Alkylating agents are cell cycle phase–nonspecific. They act primarily to form a molecular bond with the nucleic acids, which interferes with nucleic acid duplication, preventing mitosis. This category of drugs has a phase activity similar to that observed in radiation therapy, with two peaks of maximum lethal activity: one in G_2 to M phase; and one near the G_1 to S phase boundary.

Antibiotics (antitumor agents) are cell cycle phase–nonspecific. These drugs disrupt DNA transcription and inhibit DNA and RNA synthesis.

Antimetabolites are cell cycle phase–specific. They exhibit their action by blocking essential enzymes necessary for DNA synthesis or by becoming incorporated into the DNA and RNA, so that a false message is transmitted.

Hormones are cell cycle phase–nonspecific. These chemicals, secreted by the endocrine glands, alter the environment of the cell by affecting the cell membrane's permeability. By manipulating hormone levels, tumor growth can be suppressed. Hormone therapies are not cytotoxic, and therefore not curative. Their purpose is to prevent cell division and further growth of hormone-dependent tumors.

Antihormonal agents derive their antineoplastic effect from their ability to neutralize the effect of or inhibit the production of natural hormones used by hormone-dependent tumors.

Nitrosoureas are cell cycle phase–nonspecific. They have the ability to cross the BBB. Their action is similar to that of the alkylating agents; synthesis of both DNA and RNA is inhibited.

Corticosteroids exert an antiinflammatory effect on body tissues (e.g., they reduce intracranial or spinal cord compression and suppress lymphocytes). They may also promote a feeling of well-being and increase the appetite.

Vinca plant alkaloids are cell cycle phase–specific. They exert a cytotoxic effect by binding to microtubular proteins during metaphase, causing mitotic arrest. The cell loses its ability to divide and dies.

Miscellaneous agents may be cell cycle phase–specific or cell cycle phase–nonspecific or both. These drugs act by a variety of mechanisms. For example, L-asparaginase is unique because it is an enzyme product that acts primarily by inhibiting protein synthesis.[1,3,9,11]

CELL KILL HYPOTHESIS

A single cancer cell is capable of multiplying and eventually killing the host. Every tumor cell must be killed to cure cancer. With each course of the drug therapy, a given dose of chemotherapeutic drug kills only a fraction, not all, of the cancer cells present (Fig. 21-2). Repeated courses of chemotherapy must be used to reduce the total number of cancer cells. This cardinal rule of chemotherapy—*the inverse relationship between cell number and curability*—was established by Skipper and colleagues in the early 1960s.[1-3]

FACTORS CONSIDERED IN DRUG SELECTION

- Patient's eligibility for chemotherapy (confirmed diagnosis; age; bone marrow, nutritional, cardiac, hepatic, respiratory, and renal status; previous therapies)
- Cancer cell type (e.g., squamous cell, adenocarcinoma)
- Rate of drug absorption (e.g., treatment interval and routes—oral, intravenous, intraperitoneal)
- Tumor location (many drugs do not cross the BBB)
- Tumor load (larger tumors are generally less responsive to chemotherapy)
- Tumor resistance to chemotherapy (tumor cells can mutate and produce variant cells distinct from the tumor stem cell of origin)

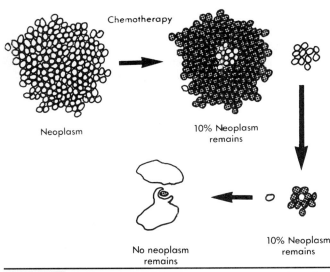

Chemotherapy

Neoplasm

10% Neoplasm remains

No neoplasm remains

10% Neoplasm remains

FIG. 21-2 Cell kill hypothesis. (From Goodman MS: *Cancer: chemotherapy and care*, Evansville, IN, Bristol Laboratories, Bristol-Myers Co.)

CHEMOTHERAPY DOSING LISTINGS

- *Standard-dose therapy*—Usual adult dose administered for most patients with cancer
- *High-dose therapy*—An increased drug dose is given to achieve tumor cell death; usually results in severe side effects such as myelosuppression.
- *Dose intensity*—Specific drugs are administered at a greater dose than standard therapy and at shorter intervals, such as every 21 days rather than every 28 days.
- *Dose density*—This refers to increased drug doses and combinations of varied drugs and is sometimes stated as *doublet* or *triplet therapy* in cancer protocols.[12]

COMBINATION CHEMOTHERAPY

Chemotherapeutic drugs are most often given in combination because this enhances the effect of the drugs on the tumor cell kill. Considerations for drugs used in combination include verified effectiveness as a single agent, increased tumor cell kill, increased patient survival, presence of a synergistic action, varied toxicities, different mechanisms of action, and administration in repeated courses to minimize the immunosuppressive effects that might otherwise occur. Combination chemotherapy provides additional benefits that are not possible with single-drug treatment, such as maximal cell kill within the range of toxicity tolerated by the host for each drug, a broader range of coverage of resistant cell lines in a heterogeneous tumor population, prevention, or slowing of the development of new resistant lines.[1-3]

Chemotherapy Administration
CALCULATION OF DRUG DOSAGE

The drug dosage for cancer chemotherapy is based on body surface area (BSA) in both adults and children. The dosages of some drugs are calculated proportionally to the patient's BSA. BSA is calculated in square meters (m^2). A nomogram is used to correlate height with weight to determine the BSA. Ensure that an accurate patient height and weight is obtained on a scheduled frequency. The drug dose is ordered in milligrams per square meter. All drug calculations should be verified by a second person to ensure dose accuracy.[13]

DRUG RECONSTITUTION

All staff who reconstitute drugs should do so under a class II biologic safety cabinet. When the drugs are prepared and reconstituted, aseptic technique must be used in accordance with manufacturer's current recommendations. All syringes of reconstituted drugs are immediately labeled with the name of the drug.

Recent concerns voiced by the **National Patient Safety Agency** have to do with drug preparation, labeling, and administration of certain drugs, such as those for intrathecal administration. Preparation of these medications should be done in the pharmacy as close as possible to the time of administration. Drugs should be labeled with the appropriate short expiration time (e.g., 4 hours), delivered, and administered in a designated (ideally separate) location, and at a specified time of the day or week.[14]

Special considerations for intrathecal drugs should also include wrapping such drugs within a sterile bag that is then wrapped in a sterile towel or container and labeled: "FOR INTRATEHECAL USE ONLY." Wraps or packages must be removed *immediately* before drug injection ONLY by the person administering the drug.

Establish a list of drugs that can be administered intrathecally, designate specific locations where intrathecal drugs may be administered, and ban ALL other drugs from these locations during the times of intrathecal drug administration. At least TWO qualified health professionals should independently verify and document drug, dose, route, date, and time of the pharmacy drug preparation, and verify correct patient identification before each intrathecal drug administration.[14,15]

ADMINISTRATION GUIDELINES[8,9,15,16]

Routes

Oral. Emphasize the importance of the patient's complying with the prescribed schedule. Plan for drugs with emetic potential to be taken with meals; whereas drugs that require hydration (e.g., cyclophosphamide [Cytoxan]) must be taken early in the day.[17]

Subcutaneous and intramuscular. Demonstration and return demonstration may be needed if the patient is giving self-injections. Injection sites should be rotated for each dose and a log kept of the drug dosing schedule.

Topical administration. Cover surface area with a thin film of medication; instruct the patient to wear loose-fitting cotton clothing. Wear gloves and wash hands thoroughly after procedure. Caution the patient not to touch the ointment.

Intraarterial. This method requires catheter placement in an artery near the tumor. Because of arterial pressure, the drug is administered in a heparinized solution through an infusion pump. Throughout the infusion, monitor vital signs, the color and temperature of the extremity, and the site for potential bleeding. Instruct the patient and family in the care of the catheter and infusion pumps (e.g., routine filling and maintenance of the infusion pump) if chemotherapy is to be given at home.[18,19]

Intracavity. Instill the drug into the bladder through a catheter, or into the pleural cavity via a chest tube. Follow prescribed premedication dosage to minimize local irritation.

Intraperitoneal. Deliver the drug into the abdominal cavity through the implantable port or the external suprapubic catheter (e.g., Tenckhoff catheter). Use dry heat to warm the infusate solution to body temperature before administration. Monitor the patient for abdominal pressure, pain, fever, and electrolyte imbalance after the infusion; measure abdominal girth.[15,20,21]

Intrathecal. Reconstitute all intrathecal medications with preservative-free sterile normal saline or sterile water. Medication may be infused through an Ommaya reservoir or implantable pump, if available, or through lumbar puncture. Usually the volume of medication given via an Ommaya reservoir or lumbar puncture is 15 ml or less. Maintain sterile technique throughout the procedure. The medication should be injected slowly. If chemotherapeutic drugs (cytarabine or methotrexate or both) are given in high doses, monitor the patient closely for potential neurotoxicity. *Usually* a physician administers intrathecal drugs via an Ommaya reservoir or lumbar puncture. (*See reconstitution guidelines earlier in text.*)[14,15,22]

Intravenous route. Drugs administered by intravenous (IV) route may be given through central venous catheters or peripheral venous access. Methods of administration include IV push (bolus), piggyback (secondary setup), or continuous infusion. Follow agency guidelines on how often continuous chemotherapeutic infusions are to be monitored.

Vein Selection and Venipuncture. Many chemotherapeutic agents irritate the veins and surrounding tissues.

Venipuncture sites must be changed on a planned basis every 48 hours to reduce the possibility of phlebitis and infiltration. Peripheral sites should be changed daily before administration of vesicants. Veins suitable for venipuncture feel smooth and pliable, not hard or sclerotic. Select a vein that is large enough to allow adequate blood flow around the IV device. Observe and palpate the extremity. Use distal veins first, and choose a vein above areas of flexion; subsequent venipuncture should be done proximal to previous sites. Veins commonly used include the basilic, cephalic, and metacarpal veins (Fig. 21-3). Large veins on the forearm are the preferred site. If a drug extravasates in this area, maximum soft-tissue coverage is present to prevent functional impairment. Do not use the antecubital fossa and the wrist because extravasation in these areas can destroy nerves and tendons, resulting in loss of function.[8,15,22]

Procedure for Administering Chemotherapeutic Drugs. Verify the patient's identification, drug, dose, route, and time of administration against the physician's order. Review drug allergy history with the patient. Anticipate and plan for possible side effects or major system toxicity (Table 21-1). Review appropriate laboratory data and other tests. Verify informed consent for treatment. Select the appropriate infusion therapy equipment and supplies. Calculate and/or verify the drug doses and verify such

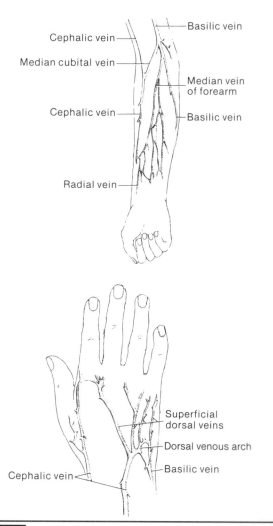

FIG. 21-3   Venous anatomy. (From Perry AG, Potter PA: *Clinical nursing skills and techniques*, ed 6, St. Louis, 2006, Mosby.)

TABLE 21-1 Major System Toxicity or Dysfunction and Nursing Care Considerations

TOXICITY/DYSFUNCTION	NURSING CARE CONSIDERATIONS
Cardiac Toxicity Drugs associated with potential for cardiac toxicity: chlorambucil, cyclophosphamide, dactinomycin, daunorubicin, doxorubicin, mitoxantrone, and high-dose ifosfamide, paclitaxel	Verify baseline cardiac studies (e.g., electrocardiogram [ECG], ejection fraction, cardiac enzymes) before drug administration. Monitor cardiac status and report symptoms regarding tachycardia, shortness of breath, distended neck veins, gallop heart rhythm, and ankle edema. Monitor and record total cumulative dose of drug in the patient's medical record. Verify physician order for potential administration of dexrazoxane or carvedilol.[23-25]
Hematopoietic Toxicity *Anemia* Hemoglobin: Male, 14-18 g/dl; Female, 12.5-16.0 g/dl Hematocrit: Male, 42%-52%; Female, 37%-47% *Leukopenia* Most myelosuppressive agents produce white blood cell (WBC) nadir 7-14 days after drug administration; myelosuppression will be severe and prolonged with increased dosages: for example, with cytarabine 3-6 g; busulfex 2-6 g; cyclophosphamide 2-3 g; methotrexate 6-8 g; etoposide 2-3 g. *Thrombocytopenia* Drugs associated with a delayed cumulative effect: mitomycin and all nitrosoureas Normal platelet count 150,000-400,000/mm³	Monitor hematocrit and hemoglobin level, especially during drug nadir. Ensure prompt administration of prescribed red blood cell infusion(s).[26-28] Monitor absolute neutrophil count. Obtain and monitor vital signs; report promptly temperature 100.4° F or higher. Follow prescribed orders to obtain blood cultures from venous access site and an additional peripheral site. Initiate promptly all prescribed antimicrobials, antiviral, and/or antifungal medications.[2,29-31] Ensure aseptic technique is used for all nursing interventions associated with venous access device. Monitor and report any signs of bleeding such as blood in emesis or urine, tarry stools, or bleeding gums. Ensure prompt platelet infusion when prescribed. Avoid invasive procedures, injections, use of suppositories or rectal thermometer; vaginal or rectal exam; patient use of sharps such as razor, and going barefoot.[30]
Hepatic Toxicity Drugs associated with potential for hepatic toxicity: asparaginase, busulfan, carmustine, chlorambucil, cytarabine, doxorubicin, 5-fluorouracil, lomustine, mercaptopurine, methotrexate, mitoxantrone, mithramycin, mitomycin, paclitaxel, and streptozotocin	Monitor liver function studies, such as lactic dehydrogenase (LDH), bilirubin, prothrombin time, and liver function tests (SGOT, SGPT). Report to the physician signs of jaundice, tenderness over the liver, and urine and stool color changes.[18,32]
Hypersensitivity Reaction Drugs associated with potential for hypersensitivity: asparaginase, bleomycin, docetaxel, doxorubicin (local erythema), etoposide, paclitaxel, and teniposide	Review the patient's allergy history. Monitor for symptoms of hypersensitivity and anaphylaxis, such as agitation, urticaria, rash, chills, cyanosis, bronchospasm, abdominal cramping, and hypotension; onset may be rapid or delayed; advise the patient to report subjective symptoms promptly.[15,33]
Metabolic Alterations *Hypercalcemia* Serum calcium 8.5-10.5 mg/dl *Hyperglycemia* Blood glucose fasting 65-110 mg/dl *Hyperkalemia* Potassium 3.5-5.0 mEq/L *Hypernatremia* Sodium 135-145 mEq/L	Monitor serum level; observe for anorexia, constipation, nausea, vomiting, polyuria, and mental status change. Monitor serum and urine levels; observe for symptoms of thirst, hunger, glucosuria, and weight loss. Monitor serum level: observe for symptoms of confusion, complaints of numbness or tingling, weakness, and cardiac dysrhythmias. Monitor serum level and weight loss; observe for symptoms of thirst, dry mucous membranes, poor skin turgor, rapid and thready pulse, restlessness, lethargy.

Continued

TABLE 21-1	Major System Toxicity or Dysfunction and Nursing Care Considerations—cont'd
TOXICITY/DYSFUNCTION	**NURSING CARE CONSIDERATIONS**
Hyperuricemia Creatinine 0.7-1.4 mg/dl Serum protein 6.3 - 8.6 gm/dl Uric acid: Male, 3.4-7.0 mg/dl; Female, 2.4-5.7 mg/dl Potential with treatment of highly proliferative tumors, such as leukemia and lymphoma	Monitor serum and urine levels; daily intake and output. Initiate prescribed drug therapy (e.g., allopurinol) to inhibit the formation of uric acid before administration of chemotherapy drug. Alkalize urine to pH >7.0 by administration of IV $NaHCO_3$ (sodium bicarbonate). Provide vigorous hydration, such as oral and IV fluid intake (2000-3000 ml), beginning 12-24 h after initiation of chemotherapy.[9,34]
Hypocalcemia Serum calcium 8.5-10.5 mg/dl	Monitor serum level; observe for symptoms of muscle cramping, tingling of extremities, and tetany.
Hypomagnesemia Magnesium 1.6-2.6 mg/dl	Monitor serum level; observe for symptoms of personality changes, anorexia, nausea, vomiting, lethargy, weakness, and tetany.
Hyponatremia Sodium 135-145 mEq/L	Monitor serum level; observe for symptoms of rales, shortness of breath, distended neck vein, weight gain, edema of sacrum or lower extremity, increasing mental status changes.
Neurotoxicity Drugs associated with potential for neurotoxicity: ifosfamide, vinblastine, vincristine, high peak plasma levels of etoposide, 5-fluorouracil; high-dose and/or intrathecal administration of cytarabine, carboplatin, cisplatin, and methotrexate	Monitor and report symptoms of weakness, numbness, and tingling sensation of hands, arms, and feet; also monitor and report symptoms of hoarseness, jaw pain, hallucinations, mental depression, decreased or absent deep tendon reflexes, slapping gait or foot drop, severe constipation, and paralytic ileus.[9,15,35-37]
Ototoxicity Drug associated with potential for ototoxicity: cisplatin	Verify physician order for administration of amifostine (Ethyol). Verify baseline audiogram. Monitor and report symptoms of tinnitus, hearing loss, and vertigo.[15,37]
Pulmonary Toxicity Drugs associated with potential for pulmonary toxicity: bleomycin, busulfan, carmustine	Verify baseline respiratory function. Individuals older than age 70 years have increased risk. Monitor respiratory status and report symptoms of dyspnea, dry cough, rales, tachypnea, and fever.
Renal System Toxicity Drugs associated with potential for renal system toxicity: carmustine, cisplatin, cyclophosphamide, ifosfamide, methotrexate, mitomycin C, streptozotocin, and thiotepa	Assess 24-h urine creatinine clearance before treatment, 2-3 L for 24 h before and after therapy. Verify baseline renal function. Encourage adequate fluid intake, such as 2-3 L for 24 h before and after therapy. Monitor intake and output, weight changes. Report diminished output to physician, e.g., >500 ml in 24 h. Administer mesna concomitant with ifosfamide, and high-dose cyclophosphamide.[8,9]
Reproductive System Dysfunction Drugs associated with potential for reproductive system dysfunction: busulfan, chlorambucil, cyclophosphamide, mechlorethamine, melphalan, thalidomide, thiotepa, vinblastine, and vincristine Antihormal agents: fenretinide, finasteride, flutamide, goserelin, letrozole, leuprolide, tamoxifen.	Assess for nature and frequency of sexual dysfunction. Counsel patients regarding avoidance of pregnancy and sperm banking before chemotherapy administration; provide information on contraceptives. Inform the patients of potential for temporary or permanent infertility and loss of libido. Women may experience symptoms including amenorrhea, "hot flashes," insomnia, dyspareunia, and vaginal dryness.[15,27]

SGOT, Serum glutamic-oxaloacetic transaminase; *SGPT*, serum glutamate pyruvate transaminase.
From Otto SE, editor: *Pocket guide to intravenous therapy*, ed 5, St. Louis, 2005, Mosby.

drug(s) doses, concentration, and infusion solution with volume before drug administration. Verify patient identification with two health professionals, and check drug(s), dosages, volume, route, date, time against drug administration record. Explain the procedure to the patient and family, and answer questions regarding potential side effects and self-care measures. Ensure prescribed premedications such as antiemetics have been administered. Monitor the patient at scheduled intervals throughout the course of drug administration. Dispose of all used supplies and unused drugs in approved, puncture-proof, leak-proof containers outside of patient area.[15]

Documentation recommendations include the following: site assessment before and after infusion or injection of chemotherapeutic drug; establishment of blood returns before, during, and after IV and intraarterial infusion of chemotherapy; and establishment of catheter or device patency before, during, and after infusion of chemotherapy (e.g., intraperitoneal, intrathecal administration). In addition, at minimum, the record should include the chemotherapy protocol, the chemotherapy agent, the drug dose, the route, the time administered, premedications, postmedications, other infusions, and supplies used for the chemotherapy regimen.

It is also vital to note and record any complaints offered by the patient of discomfort or symptoms experienced before, during, or after the chemo infusion.

Equally important is the record of patient and family education, detailing potential side effects and toxicities; self-care management of side effects; and the schedule of follow-up blood work, tests, and procedures.[8,22,15]

Safe Handling of Chemotherapeutic Agents

Clinical studies have indicated that many chemotherapeutic agents are carcinogenic, mutagenic, and teratogenic, or any combination of the three. Exposure to these chemotherapeutic agents can occur by inhalation, absorption, or digestion. Safe handling guidelines should be followed when implementing policy and procedure within each agency that prepares, administers, stores, or disposes of either supplies or unused chemotherapeutic agents.[21]

DRUG PREPARATION

To ensure safe handling, all chemotherapeutic drugs should be prepared according to the package insert in a class II biologic safety cabinet (BSC). Venting to the outside, where feasible, is desirable. Personal protective equipment includes disposable surgical latex gloves and a gown made of lint-free, low-permeability fabric with a closed front, long sleeves, and elastic or knit cuffs. Eye-protective splash goggles or a face shield must be worn when these drugs are prepared if a BSC is not used. Consider the use of multiple latex-free products for personnel who experience latex allergies. Gloves should be changed between preparation and administration of the drug and at least every 30 minutes during preparation and administration.[8,15,21,22]

DRUG ADMINISTRATION

Wear protective equipment (gloves, gown, eyewear; Fig. 21-4). Explain to the patient that chemotherapeutic drugs are harmful to normal cells and that protective measures used by personnel minimize their exposure to these drugs. Administer drugs in a safe,

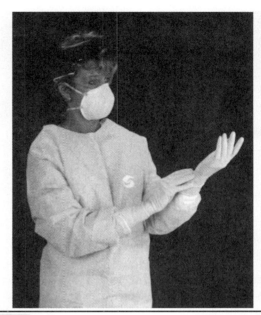

FIG. 21-4 Woman wearing gloves, gown, eyewear, and mask. (Courtesy Biosafety Systems, Inc., San Diego, CA.)

unhurried environment. Place a plastic-backed absorbent pad under the tubing during administration to catch any leakage.[8,13,15,21,22]

DISPOSAL OF SUPPLIES AND UNUSED DRUGS

Place all unused supplies or drugs in containers in a leak-proof, closeable, puncture-proof, appropriately labeled container; keep these containers in every area where drugs are prepared or administered so that waste materials need not be moved from one area to another. Dispose of containers filled with chemotherapeutic supplies and unused drugs in accordance with regulations of hazardous wastes (e.g., in a licensed sanitary landfill) or incinerate at 1832° F (1000° C).[8,13,21,22]

MANAGEMENT OF CHEMOTHERAPY SPILLS

Chemotherapy spills should be cleaned up immediately by properly protected personnel trained in the appropriate procedures. A spill should be identified with a warning sign so that other people will not be contaminated. The following are recommended supplies and procedures for managing a chemotherapy spill on hard surfaces, linens, personnel, and patients: a respirator mask for airborne powder spills, plastic safety glasses or goggles, heavy-duty rubber gloves, absorbent pads to contain liquid spills, absorbent towels for cleanup after spill, small scoop to collect glass fragments, two large waste disposal bags, a protective disposable gown, containers of detergent solution and clear tap water for cleaning up the spill, puncture-proof, leak-proof closeable container approved for chemotherapy waste disposal, and an approved, specially labeled, impervious laundry bag (Fig. 21-5). Placement of eyewash faucet adapters or fountain should be in or near work area.[8,13,15,21,22]

Procedure for Spill on Hard Surface, Linen, Personnel, or Patient. Restrict the area of the spill. Obtain the drug spill kit. Put on a protective gown, gloves, and goggles and, if a powder spill is involved, a respirator mask. Open waste disposal bags (NOTE: it is important that these be *double* bags).

Spill on hard surface: Place absorbent pads gently on the spill, being careful not to touch them, then place the saturated

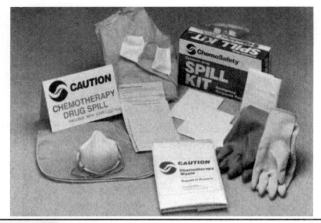

FIG. 21-5 Chemotherapy spill kit. (Courtesy Biosafety Systems, Inc., San Diego, CA.)

absorbent pads in the waste bag. Clean the surface with absorbent towels, using detergent solution, and rinse it clean with clean tap water and wipe dry.

Spill on linen: Remove soiled, contaminated linen from the patient's bedside. Place the linen in an approved, specially marked, impervious laundry bag. The contaminated linen should be washed twice by the laundry, and laundry personnel should wear surgical latex gloves and gown when handling this material. Clean the contaminated area with absorbent towels and detergent solution.

Spill on personnel or patient: Immediately remove any contaminated protective garments or linen. Wash the affected area of skin with soap and water. Follow procedures for contaminated linen. Notify the physician if the drug spills on the patient. Place all contaminated materials (e.g., gown, gloves, saturated absorbent pads, towels) in double-bagged waste disposal bags. Discard the waste bags and contents in an approved container, and then wash hands thoroughly with soap and water.

Eye exposure: Immediately flood the affected eye with water for at least 5 minutes; follow agency guidelines regarding follow-up care with a clinical eye exam.

Caring for Patients Receiving Chemotherapeutic Drugs

All personnel who handle blood, vomitus, or excreta from patients who have received chemotherapy within the previous 48 hours should wear disposable surgical latex gloves and gowns, which are discarded appropriately after use. Linen contaminated with chemotherapeutic drugs, blood, vomitus, or excreta from a patient who has received these drugs within the prior 48 hours should be placed in a specially marked, impervious laundry bag according to procedures for drug spills on linen.[8,13,21,22]

EXTRAVASATION MANAGEMENT

Vesicant extravasation is the accidental leakage of a drug into the subcutaneous tissue that causes pain, necrosis, or sloughing of tissue. A **vesicant** is an agent that can produce a blister, tissue destruction, or both. An **irritant** is an agent that can cause aching, tightness, and phlebitis at the injection site or along the vein line with or without an inflammatory reaction. A **flare** is a local allergic reaction without pain that usually is accompanied by red blotches along the vein line. Local allergic symptoms subside within 30 minutes with or without treatment.[8,9]

Injuries that may occur as the result of extravasation include tissue sloughing, infection, pain, and loss of mobility in an extremity. The degree of tissue damage is related to several factors, including drug vesicant potential, drug concentration, amount of drug extravasated, duration of tissue exposure, venipuncture site and device, needle insertion technique, and individual tissue responses. **Delayed extravasation** is one in which symptoms occur 48 hours or more after the drug is administered.

Treatment strategies for managing extravasation involve using specific antidotes and following guidelines for immediate intervention to minimize tissue damage. Preventing extravasation and instituting prompt intervention are key to successful extravasation management. The nurse should know which drugs have vesicant potential, and test the vein or ensure catheter lumen patency with normal saline. Observe the IV site before, during, and after drug administration, and validate a dark, brisk blood return before, during, and after drug administration. (See Table 21-2 for a list of chemotherapeutic drugs with vesicant potential.)

Tissue destruction from drug extravasation may be subtle and progressive. Initial symptoms include pain or burning at the IV site, progressing to erythema, edema, and superficial skin loss. Tissue necrosis may not develop for 1 to 4 weeks after extravasation. Documentation of extravasation management should include the following: date and time; needle product, catheter size, and insertion site, or type of venous access device; drug sequence; approximate amount of drug extravasated; nursing management of extravasation; photographic documentation; patient's complaints and/or statements; appearance of site; notification of physician; follow-up measures; and nurse's signature.[8,9,15]

ANAPHYLAXIS

Nursing personnel administering chemotherapy in all settings should be alert and prepared for the possible complications of anaphylaxis. The drugs and supplies needed to manage these complications must be readily available. The nurse must be informed and prepared for the specific drugs known to pose a risk of anaphylaxis. Test dosing before infusing the drug, as well as following infusion precautions, reduces the incidence of anaphylaxis. Emergency medications and supplies for managing anaphylaxis include the following:

- Injectable aminophylline, diphenhydramine hydrochloride (Benadryl), dopamine, epinephrine, heparin, hydrocortisone
- Oxygen setup, tubing cannula, or mask and airway device
- Suction equipment
- IV fluids (isotonic solutions)
- IV tubings and supplies for venous access

Prompt, effective nursing intervention for anaphylaxis reduces complications. The nurse must be alert to the signs and symptoms of an anaphylactic response to a chemotherapeutic drug. Patients may exhibit all of some of these symptoms: anxiety, hypotension, urticaria, cyanosis, respiratory distress, abdominal cramping, flushed appearance, and chills. The calm, reassuring presence of the nurse will facilitate the management of these symptoms, which proceeds as follows:

- Immediately stop the drug infusion.
- Maintain an IV line with isotonic saline.
- Position the patient for comfort and to promote perfusion of the vital organs.

TABLE 21-2	Chemotherapeutic Drugs with Vesicant Potential
GENERIC NAME	**TRADE NAME**
Dactinomycin	Actinomycin D, Cosmegen
Daunorubicin	Cerubidine, Daunomycin
Doxorubicin	Adriamycin
Epirubicin	Pharmorubicin
Esorubicin	4-Deoxydorubicin
Idarubicin	Idamycin
Mechlorethamine	Nitrogen mustard, Mustargen
Mitomycin C	Mutamycin
Menogaril	Tomosar
Paclitaxel	Taxol
Oxantrazole	Piroxantrone
Plicamycin	Mithracin
Vinblastine	Velban
Vincristine	Oncovin
Vindesine	Eldisine
Vinorelbine	Navelbine

From Otto SE, editor: *Pocket guide to intravenous therapy*, ed 5, St. Louis, 2005, Mosby.

- Notify the physician, nursing agency, or emergency medical services.
- Maintain the airway, and anticipate the need for cardiopulmonary resuscitation.
- Monitor vital signs according to agency policy.
- Administer appropriate medications with an approved physician's order.
- Follow the nursing agency's protocol for follow-up care.
- Document the incident in the patient's medical record.

An anaphylactic episode is upsetting to both the patient and family. Follow-up care is required to diminish anxiety and to monitor for delayed side effects. Instruct the patient and family in the pertinent drug side effects, when and where to call for assistance, and what symptoms require immediate health care intervention (e.g., shortness of breath, rash on the body that increases in size and intensity, flushed appearance, fever, chills, abdominal cramping, feeling of anxiousness).[8,15,19,33]

Alternative Care Settings

Improved drug delivery, cost containment, and consideration of quality of life have affected trends in chemotherapy administration. Options for giving chemotherapy in outpatient settings include ambulatory care centers, physicians' offices, extended care facilities, and home health agencies. Principles of chemotherapy administration and standards of care for patients must be maintained by the staff regardless of the setting. Home health care has expanded extensively to include more care options for oncology patients.[13,28,32,37-39] Criteria specific to home administration of chemotherapy include the following:

1. A caregiver is available who is able and willing to assist.
2. The patient's physical condition is stable and within the range of home care capabilities.
3. Living conditions are stable and suitable (cleanliness, plumbing, refrigeration, telephone).
4. The patient has access to emergency assistance.

Patients and family members who are involved in the infusion of chemotherapeutic drugs and/or the management of side effects require procedural information in verbal, written, demonstration, and return demonstration forms. Following are suggested nursing interventions to facilitate education of the patient and family in drug administration in the home:

- Assess the patient's ability and willingness to learn, the availability of a caregiver, the home environment, the patient's ability to assume self-care, and compliance with the treatment regimen.
- Describe the purpose, the schedule, and the procedure of the chemotherapeutic regimen.
- Explain to the patient the possible side effects of chemotherapeutic drugs (e.g., nausea and vomiting, anorexia, stomatitis, constipation, diarrhea, alopecia, skin and hematopoietic changes).
- Instruct the patient or caregiver in dealing with specific side effects.
- Review symptoms, such as temperature elevation over 100.4° F (38° C), severe constipation or diarrhea, persistent bleeding from any site, sudden weight gain or loss, shortness of breath, pain which is not relieved by prescribed medications, and severe nausea and vomiting more than 24 hours after treatment. *Emphasize* the importance of promptly reporting these symptoms to the physician.
- Instruct the patient or caregiver in the management of infusion devices.
- Validate the aseptic technique and skills of the patient or caregiver for prescribed self-administration and discontinuation of chemotherapeutic drugs.
- Explain the safe handling precautions for administration and disposal of chemotherapeutic drugs.
- Provide information and a list of resources for the obtaining, storing, and disposing of drugs and supplies. Also provide a schedule of follow-up tests and care.
- Record the drug, the dose, the route, and the time given in the home, and provide this information to the agency responsible for care management.
- Discard all unused drugs and used supplies in a recommended puncture-proof, leak-proof, closeable container. Return this container to the appropriate agency for disposal (Fig. 21-6).
- Use plastic sheeting to protect bedding or furniture if incontinence is anticipated.
- Carefully handle linen contaminated by chemotherapeutic drugs and excreta. Machine wash these items twice, separately from all other linen.

It is recommended that the patient receive the first chemotherapy dose in an acute care or outpatient setting.

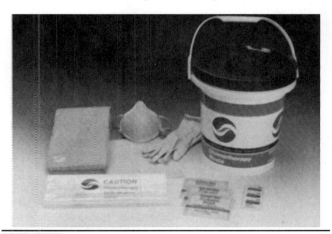

FIG. 21-6   Home health care kit. (Courtesy Biosafety Systems, Inc., San Diego, CA.)

NURSING CARE CONSIDERATIONS

Nursing management of the patient receiving chemotherapy requires multiple assessment and intervention strategies. Nursing care begins with a thorough understanding of five primary elements: the patient's condition; the goal of therapy; dosage, route and schedule of the drug; principles of administration; and potential side effects. Additional nursing management includes monitoring the response to therapy, reassessing and documenting signs and symptoms, and communicating pertinent information to other members of the health care team. Continual psychosocial evaluation and patient teaching components require astute nursing interventions. Many resources are available, both locally and nationally. The Oncology Nursing Society, the American Cancer Society, the National Cancer Institute, and the Leukemia Society all provide lay and professional educational materials.[4,23,26,29,35,36,40,41]

Chemotherapeutic drugs may cause adverse side effects, major system toxicity, and dysfunction. Side effects and toxicities vary in severity according to the patient's individual response to the drug therapy. The most frequent side effects are myelosuppression, nausea, and vomiting. Myelosuppression can be a dose-limiting toxicity. The chemotherapeutic drugs work by destroying or suppressing new leukocytes, platelets, and erythrocytes. These effects are monitored by reviewing the blood counts at scheduled intervals. The time or level at which a blood count reaches its lowest point is the **nadir.** The nadir varies with individual drugs but usually occurs between 7 and 21 days after administration.

Nausea and vomiting often are the most distressing side effects of chemotherapy. Nausea can be acute, anticipatory, delayed, or persistent. Acute nausea and vomiting occur within 1 to 2 hours of treatment and last approximately 24 to 48 hours. Anticipatory nausea and vomiting occur before the treatment. Nausea and vomiting after the initial 24 hours of treatment may be referred to as *delayed* or *persistent*. Assessing and reporting the frequency, severity, and pattern of nausea and vomiting are critical to the patient's recovery process.[9,10,42,43]

The incidence of these side effects is related to the emetic potential of the chemotherapy agent: the dose; the route, schedule, and duration; and combinations of drug administration (Table 21-3). The combination of antiemetic drugs, each with a separate mechanism of action, round-the-clock administration, and higher dosages has proved more effective than single-agent dosing and as-needed (PRN) schedules. (See Table 21-4). With the development and use of the serotonin (5-HT3) antagonists and NK-1–receptor antagonists (e.g., aprepitant [Emend], OKdolasetron [Anzemet], granisetron [Kytril], ondansetron [Zofran], and palonosetron [Aloxi]), great strides have been made in effective antiemetic therapy. Practice guidelines help to increase efficacy in treatment outcomes, and promote cost-effectiveness. The usual dosing schedule is less frequent (30 minutes before chemotherapy, and after infusion). The dose frequency varies depending upon initial drug dose and route. Side effects thus far are mild, including headache, constipation, and transient elevation of liver enzymes.[9,10,42,43]

The nurse's responsibilities include evaluating the patient's response to the drugs, teaching the patient or caregiver self-management interventions, and monitoring laboratory data and signs and symptoms reported by the patient. Pertinent information related to the major system toxicities (i.e., cardiac, hematopoietic, hepatic, hypersensitivity, neurologic, ototoxicity, pulmonary, reproductive, renal) and to metabolic alterations (see Table 21-1) imposes dose-limiting restrictions on many of the drugs. If symptoms occur and the chemotherapeutic drug dose or schedule (or both) is not altered or evaluated, the potential for irreversible side effects grows. All the toxicities listed in Table 21-1 require astute observation and prompt intervention by all members of the health care team. Additional circumstances that may affect the patient's response to a drug include the setting in which the drug is administered (acute care or home care), the needs posed by activities of daily living, and lifestyle changes.[23,26,28-30,33,35,40,41,44]

Considerations for Older Adults

The physiologic changes that occur with biologic aging are an important consideration in the treatment of cancer and chemotherapy pharmacokinetics. The inability of an older person's hematopoietic system to respond as readily as that of a younger person partly determines the selection of chemotherapeutic agents and dose intensities, which in turn imposes an increased risk of infection. A gradual wasting of body muscle mass and an increase in fat can influence drug distribution and decrease liver function and renal excretion after drug metabolism and excretion.

TABLE 21-3 Emetic Potential of Common Chemotherapeutic Drugs		
MILD POTENTIAL	**MODERATE POTENTIAL**	**SEVERE POTENTIAL**
Bleomycin	Amifostine 340-500 mg/m²	Carmustine <250 mg/m²
Busulfan	Cytarabine <1 g/m²	Cisplatin <50 mg/m²
Chlorambucil	Cyclophosphamide IV >750 mg/m²	Cyclophosphamide 750-1500 mg/m²
5-Fluorouracil	Doxorubicin 20-60 mg/m²	Dacarbazine >500 mg/m²
Hydroxyurea	Epirubicin <90 mg/m²	Dactinomycin <1.5 mg/m²
Mercaptopurine	Idararubicin	Irinotecan
Methotrexate (>50 mg or <250 mg/m²)	Ifosfamide	Mechlorethamine
Paclitaxel	Mitoxantrone <15 mg/m²	Melphalan
Teniposide	Oxaliplatin	Methotrexate >1 g/m²
Thiotepa		Mitoxantrone >15 mg/m²
Topotecan		Procarbazine (PO)
		Streptozotocin

IV, Intravenous route; *PO,* by mouth.

TABLE 21-4   Selected Parenteral Antiemetic Regimens (Adult)

DRUG	DOSAGE	SCHEDULE
Metoclopramide (Reglan)	1-3 mg/kg IV	30 min before and 90 min after chemotherapy, then every 4 h PRN
Dexamethasone (Decadron)	20 mg IV	30-40 min before chemotherapy
Lorazepam (Ativan)	1.5 mg/m² IV	30 min before chemotherapy
Or		
Diphenhydramine (Benadryl)	50 mg IV	30 min before chemotherapy
(The above drugs are used in varying doses and schedules depending upon severity of emetic episode.)		
Aprepitant (Emend)	125 mg PO	
	80 mg PO	60 minutes before chemotherapy on day 1 once daily in AM on days 2 and 3
Dolasetron (Anzemet)	1.8 mg/kg IV	30 min before chemotherapy
	100 mg PO	60 min before chemotherapy
Granisetron (Kytril)	10 mcg IV	30 min before chemotherapyOK mcg
	2 mg PO	60 min before chemotherapy
Ondansetron (Zofran)	0.15 mg/kg IV in 30-50 ml; infused over 15-30 min (IV dose 16-32 mg/day) 4-8 mg PO tid	30 min before chemotherapy, then at 4 and 8 h after initial dose
Palonosetron (Aloxi)	IV 0.25 mg	Give IV 30 minutes before chemotherapy

IV, Intravenous route; *PO,* by mouth; *PRN,* as needed.
Data from *Physician drug reference,* Montvale, NJ, 2005, Medical Economics Data, Medical Economic Co, and Bethesda, MD, 2003, American Hospital Formulary Service; Hodgson BB, Kizior RJ: *Saunders nursing drug handbook 2006,* St. Louis, 2006, Elsevier.

Cardiovascular changes must be considered when cardiotoxic chemotherapeutic agents or surgery are the possible cancer treatment modalities.[35-37,43,45-48]

Additional considerations include the following:

- Anticipate potential sedative effects related to antiemetic therapy and analgesics.
- Monitor serum electrolytes values closely; the potential exists for concomitant diseases such as hypertension, or diabetes.
- Query the patient and/or the caregiver regarding all current medications (prescribed and over-the-counter) that may interfere with increased toxic effects of the chemotherapy drugs.
- Age-related neuromuscular sensory deficits may include but are not limited to visual, hearing, and fine motor skills, mobility status, and bowel and bladder elimination and/or continence.

Conclusion

Although great strides have been made in the areas of advanced protocols and combination chemotherapy to treat oncology diseases, the management of side effects, and the safe administration of chemotherapy, chemotherapy administration is a significant aspect of the oncology nurse's role. It carries with it great responsibilities for the nurse in terms of patient care, patient and family communication and education, and collaboration and coordination between multiple departments, and a heightened potential for harm, not only to the patient, but also to the nurse and the health care institution. The oncology nurse is called upon to remain current in his or her knowledge of chemotherapy drugs and their purpose, safe dosage parameters, potential reactions, and state-of-the-art management of side effects, extravasation, and anaphylaxis.

REVIEW QUESTIONS

✓ Case Study

Martha RN has changed clinical practice settings, from working in home care to a 28-bed inpatient unit that cares for patients with multiple cancer diagnoses receiving chemotherapy as well as peripheral blood stem cell transplantation. She is reviewing the chemotherapy protocols for chemotherapy drug preparation, administration, and disposal; to ensure she has all the necessary supplies for IV drug administration (doxorubicin and cytarabine, intrathecal methotrexate) to TK, a 72-year-old male with acute myelogenous leukemia (AML). TK was previously prescribed allopurinal and instructed to drink at least 8 to 10 once glasses of water per day. He has a Hickman catheter (HC) for multiinfusion therapy and will have

a lumbar puncture to receive an additional dose of intrathecal methotrexate.

Martha introduces herself to TK, ensures proper patient identification, and begins explaining that she will administer his chemotherapy. As she begins, she reviews with him the exact drugs he will receive, discusses possible drug side effects, explaining that she will continually monitor him throughout the course of the infusion, and pointing out symptoms which he should immediately report to her or another nurse.

Upon verification of TK's identity and correlation of drug(s), dose(s), and routes with his medication record, she verifies blood return status, flushes the HC with normal saline, and then administers doxorubicin by IV push. Following the

Continued

doxorubicin, she again flushes the HC and initiates a 12-hr infusion of cytarabine.

She answers TK's questions regarding how the different drugs work via the varied doses, routes, drug schedule, and certain cancer types. Martha RN also explains that later in the afternoon she will assist the physician in giving methotrexate via a lumbar puncture, emphasizing that TK is required to remain in bed for a short period following that procedure.

QUESTIONS

1. What are included among factors considered in chemotherapy drug selection for cancer treatment?
   a. Cancer cell type, bone marrow status, tumor burden, and tumor resistance
   b. Cardiac, hepatic, renal, and sexuality status
   c. Patient's age, diagnosis, pain status, and tumor burden
   d. Rate of drug absorption, nausea potential, renal status, and tumor burden
2. Interventions necessary to minimize complications related to hyperuricemia include which of the following?
   a. Moderate hydration, alkalize urine to pH >7, administer allopurinol
   b. Vigorous hydration, alkalize urine to pH >7, administer dexrazoxane
   c. Vigorous hydration, alkalize urine to pH >7, administer allopurinol
   d. Limit hydration, alkalize urine to pH >7, administer dexrazoxane
3. Why are chemotherapy drugs often given in combination?
   a. To reduce emetogenic potential
   b. To prevent micrometastasis
   c. To reduce the length of clinic appointments
   d. To increase tumor cell kill
4. What are clinical features that may occur during a hypersensitivity or anaphylaxis event?
   a. Anxiety, cyanosis, dyspnea, and urticara
   b. Anxiety, chills, fever, and hives
   c. Anxiety, facial edema, hoarseness, and fatigue
   d. Cyanosis, dyspnea, hives, and alopecia
5. Concepts of liposomal chemotherapy drug administration include which of the following?
   a. Inhibiting certain substances from entering the brain or central nervous system tumors
   b. Not using an in-line filter, enhanced delivery of drugs to specifically targeted tissues
   c. Reducing drug-related myelosuppression and incidents of extravasation
   d. Liposomal agents can be mixed and administered with other drugs
6. What is the goal of neoadjuvant chemotherapy administration?
   a. To treat remaining the remaining cancer cells or micrometastasis
   b. To shrink a tumor before it is removed surgically or treated with radiation therapy
   c. To treat patients who have localized disease and no lymph node involvement
   d. It is administered during remission to prevent the cancer disease from recurring.
7. Chemotherapy drug extravasation has potentially serious consequences. What are some prevention and management strategies?
   a. Know drugs with vesicant potential; test vein with normal saline carefully; observe drug administration; validate blood return before, during, and after.
   b. Since tissue destruction may occur up to 4 to 6 weeks following drug administration, patient complaints during and immediately after infusion are not important.
   c. Nonvesicant drugs can cause aching, tightness, or flare along the vein line that does not subside.
   d. Once extravasation is suspected, documentation of the type or size of needle or access device is not an issue.
8. "Circadian variables" in the concept of circadian rhythm include which of the following?
   a. Drug absorption, distribution, dose modification, and metabolism
   b. Drug absorption, metabolism, drug administration, and elimination
   c. Drug absorption, metabolism, distribution, and elimination
   d. Drug absorption, distribution, dose intensification, and elimination
9. Chemoprevention trials are conducted for varied cancers, drugs, and/or participants. Which of the following is the largest chemoprevention trial conducted to date?
   a. Chemoprevention trial for colorectal cancer
   b. Chemoprevention trial for melanoma
   c. Chemoprevention trial for prostate cancer
   d. Chemoprevention trial for lung cancer
10. How are chemotherapy dosing guides used in multiple cancer protocols are administered?
   a. Standard-dose, dose intensification, drug resistance, and palliation
   b. Standard-dose, high-dose, dose intensity, and dose density
   c. Drug resistance, high-dose, dose intensity, and dose density
   d. Standard-dose, high-dose, drug resistance, and chemoprevention

ANSWERS

1. **A.** *Rationale:* The patient's age, comorbidities, and clinical picture regarding renal and hepatic function are concerned with drug metabolism, clearance, and the rate of drug absorption. One's sexuality is not a factor in drug selection. TK has AML, and the drugs selected are based on that disease protocol.
2. **C.** *Rationale:* To minimize hyperuricemia, 2000 ml hydration was initiated with allopurinol.
3. **D.** *Rationale:* When drugs are examined as potential agents for combination chemotherapy regimens, consideration is given to synergistic effects, varied toxicities, differing mechanisms of action, and immunosuppressive effects.

Once combination protocols are formulated, this method enhances the effect of the drugs on the tumor cell kill.

4. **A.** *Rationale:* Signs and symptoms of anaphylaxis to a chemotherapeutic drug include anxiety, hypotension, urticaria, cyanosis, respiratory distress, abdominal cramping, flushed appearance, and chills.

5. **B.** *Rationale:* Liposomal therapy has allowed for agents to be developed that target specific tissues, avoiding organ toxicities. Liposomal agents should not be administered concomitantly with other agents, nor should an in-line filter be used. The most common side effects are mucositis, headache, lumbar pain, and nausea and vomiting. Extravasation and severe myelosuppression are not common.

6. **B.** *Rationale:* The purpose of "neoadjuvant chemotherapy" is shrink the tumor before it is surgically excised or radiated.

7. **A.** *Rationale:* Agents known as irritants can cause aching, tightness, or phlebitis at the injection site or along the vein line, accompanied by inflammation. A flare is a local reaction which is usually painless and appears blotchy along the vein line. These usually subside within a short time with or without treatment. Extravasation documentation should include the type, size of needle or access device, insertion site, time, date of administration, all agents administered- their sequence, volume, and dosage, an estimate of the amount of fluid extravasated, patient complaints, nursing management and photographic record of the extremity or area.

8. **C.** *Rationale:* The term *circadian rhythm* refers to regular, repeated fluctuation in biologic function during a 24-hour period. There are many human bodily functions that operate in a circadian manner, which influence drug absorption, metabolism, distribution, and elimination. Circadian rhythm would be taken into consideration if dose intensification or dose modification was being considered, but circadian rhythm does not cause dose intensification or dose modification. Circadian rhythm may influence the timing of drug administration, but not the manner in which it is administered.

9. **C.** *Rationale:* To date, finasteride for prostate cancer has been the largest chemoprevention trial in U.S. history.

10. **B.** *Rationale:* Doses are based on the disease, patient BSA, and effectiveness of treatment protocols.

REFERENCES

1. Chu E, DeVita Jr. VT: *Physicians' cancer chemotherapy drug manual 2005,* Sudbury, 2005, Jones & Bartlett.
2. Chu E, DeVita Jr. VT: Principles of cancer management: chemotherapy. In DeVita VT Jr., Hellman S, and Rosenberg SA, editors: *Cancer principles and practice of oncology,* ed 7, Philadelphia, 2004, JB Lippincott.
3. Ghobrial IM, Witzig TE, Adjei AA: Targeting apoptosis pathways in cancer therapy *CA Cancer J Clin* 55(3):178, 2004.
4. Jemal A, Murray T, Ward E et al: Cancer Statistics, 2005, *CA Cancer J Clin* 10(1):10, 2005.
5. Lee W, Lockhart AC, Kim RB et al: Cancer pharmacogenomics: powerful tools in cancer chemotherapy and drug development, *Oncologist* 10(2):104, 2005.
6. Page R, Takimoto C: Principles of chemotherapy. In Pazdur R, Coia LR, Hoskins, WJ et al, editors: *Cancer management: a multidisciplinary approach,* ed 7, Manhasset, NY, 2004, CMP Healthcare Media.
7. Gopal R: How to maintain multidisciplinary treatment schedules, *Support Oncol* 3(3):248, 2005.
8. Otto SE: *Oncology nursing clinical reference,* St. Louis, 2004, Mosby.
9. Hodgson BB, Kizior RJ: *Saunders nursing drug handbook 2006,* St. Louis, 2006, Elsevier.
10. Vallerga AK, Zarling DA, Kinsella TJ: New radiosensitizing regimens, drugs, prodrugs, and candidates, *Clin Adv Hematol Oncol* 2(12):793, 2004.
11. Cunningham RS: Using clinical practice guidelines to improve clinical outcomes in patients receiving emetogenic chemotherapy, *Oncol Support Care Q* 3(1):4, 2004.
12. Blayney DW, McGuire BW, Cruickshank SE et al: Increasing chemotherapy dose density and intensity: phase I trials in non-small cell lung cancer and non-Hodgkin's lymphoma, *Oncologist* 10(2):138, 2005.
13. Oncology Nursing Society: *Access device guidelines,* Pittsburgh, 2004, Oncology Nursing Press.
14. National Patient Safety Agency, retrieved July, 2005, from http://www.npsa.nhs.uk/display?contentld=2396.
15. Polovich M, White JM, Kelleher LO, editors: *Chemotherapy and biotherapy guidelines and recommendations for practice,* ed 2, Pittsburgh, 2005, Oncology Nursing Press.
16. Stuart OA, Knight C, Sugarbaker PH: Avoiding carcinogen exposure with intraperitoneal paclitaxel, *Oncol Nurs Forum* 32(1):44, 2005.
17. Birner A: Safe administration of oral chemotherapy, *CJON* 7(2):158, 2003.
18. Cahill BA: Management of patients who have undergone hepatic artery chemoembolism, *CJON* 9(1):69, 2005.
19. Huddleston R, Berkheimer C, Landis S, et al: Improving patient outcomes in an ambulatory infusion setting, *J Infus Nurs* 28(3):170, 2005.
20. Robinson W, Omar H, Blades N: Toxicity of intraperitoneal chemotherapy may be related to age in women treated for optimally debulked ovarian cancer, *Community Oncology* 2(3):271, 2005.
21. US Department of Labor, Office of Occupational Medicine, Occupational Safety and Health Administration: Controlling occupational exposure to hazardous drugs, Washington, DC, OSHA, retrieved July 17, 2005, from http://www.osha-slc.gov/SLTC/hazardousdrugs/index.html.
22. Otto SE, editor: *Pocket guide to infusion therapy,* ed 5, St. Louis, 2005, Mosby.
23. Loerzel VW, Dow KH: Cardiac toxicity related to cancer treatment, *CJON* 7(5):557, 2003.
24. Schmidt KV: Immunology. In Itano JK, Taoka KN, editors: *Core curriculum for oncology nursing,* ed 4, St. Louis, 2005, Saunders.
25. Simpson C, Herr H, Courville KA: Concurrent therapies that protect against doxorubicin-induced cardiomyopathy, CJON 8(5):497, 2004.
26. Capo G, Waltzman R: Managing hematologic toxicities, *Support Oncol* 2(1):65, 2004.
27. Donovan HS, Ward S: Representations of fatigue in women receiving chemotherapy for gynecologic cancers, *Oncol Nurs Forum* 32(1):113, 2005.
28. Gillespie TW: Effects of cancer-related anemia on clinical and quality-of-life outcomes, *CJON* 6(4):206, 2002.
29. Bedell C: Pegfilgrastim for chemotherapy-induced neutropenia, *CJON* 7(1):55, 2003.
30. Camp-Sorrell D: Myelosuppression. In Itano JK, Taoka KN, editors: *Core curriculum for oncology nursing,* ed 4, St. Louis, 2005, Saunders.
31. Sonis ST: Oral mucositis in cancer therapy, *Support Oncol* 2(6 Suppl 3): 3, 2004.
32. Oeffinger KC, Hudson MM: Long-term complications following childhood and adolescent cancer: foundations for providing risk-based health care for survivors, *CA Cancer J Clin* 54(4):208, 2004.

33. Bonosky K, Miller R: Hypersensitivity reactions to oxaliplatin: what nurses need to know *CJON* 9 (3):325, 2005.

34. Pagana KD, Pagana TJ: *Mosby's diagnostic and laboratory test reference* ed 7, 2005, St. Louis, Elsevier.

35. Armstrong T, Almadrones L, Gilbert MR: Chemotherapy-induced peripheral neuropathy, *Oncol Nurs Form* 32(2):305, 2005.

36. Marrs J: Updating your peripheral neuropathy "know-how," *CJON* 7(3):299, 2003.

37. Pearce JD: Alterations in mobility, skin integrity, and neurological status. In Itano JK, Taoka KN, editors: *Core curriculum for oncology nursing*, ed 4, St. Louis 2005, Saunders.

38. Glajchen M: The emerging role and needs of family caregivers in cancer care, *Support Oncol* 2(2):145, 2004.

39. Martin S, Larson E: Chemotherapy-handling practices of outpatient and office-based oncology practices, *Oncol Nurs Forum* 30(4):575, 2003.

40. Conte PF, Guarneri V: Safety of intravenous and oral bisphosphonates and compliance with dosing regimens *The OncologistVolume* 9(9 Suppl 4):1-20, 2004.

41. Harris DJ, Knobf MT: Assessing and managing chemotherapy-induced mucositis pain, *CJON* 8(6):622, 2004.

42. Crawford J: Improving the management of chemotherapy-induced neutropenia *Supportive Oncology* 2(2 Suppl 2):36, 2004.

43. Gralla R: New antiemetic agents, *Clin Adv Hematol Oncol* 3(5):350, 2005.

44. Hockett KC: Stevens-Johnson syndrome and toxic epidermal necrolysis: oncologic considerations, *CJON* 8(1):27, 2004.

45. Green JM, Hacker ED: Chemotherapy in the geriatric population, *CJON* 8(6):591, 2004.

46. Holley S: A look at the problem of falls among people with cancer, *CJON* 6(4):193, 2002.

47. Hood LE: Chemotherapy in the elderly: supportive measures for chemotherapy-induced myelotoxicity, *CJON* 7(2):185, 2003.

48. Reich CD: Advances in the treatment of bone metastases, *CJON* 7(6):641, 2003.

CHAPTER 22

Biotherapy

Carol Pappas Appel

The rapid introduction of novel agents and approaches and an improved understanding of the biology of cancer have opened an exciting era in cancer therapy. Traditionally, surgery, radiation therapy, and chemotherapy, either singly or in combination, have been the mainstays of cancer therapy. Over the past 25 years, biotherapy has emerged as an important modality for treating cancer. It has revolutionized bone marrow or stem cell transplantation and the delivery of chemotherapeutic drugs at higher doses and at more frequent intervals. Biotherapy has changed the way cancers are treated, targeting cancer cells and protecting normal cells in the process, thereby minimizing treatment side effects. In combination with chemotherapy and radiation therapy, biotherapy has changed the face of cancer treatment in the twenty-first century.

Oncology nurses caring for patients receiving biotherapy need a basic understanding of the immune system, the rationale for biotherapy, and the primary clinical agents currently in use.

Biotherapy Defined

Biotherapy may be defined as treatment with agents derived from biologic sources and/or affecting biologic responses. Many agents were derived from the mammalian genome.

The explosion of biotherapy research and technologic advances has led to the use of numerous agents, both commercially and in clinical trials. Earliest agents included nonspecific immunomodulating agents such as bacillus Calmette-Guérin (BCG), *Corynebacterium parvum*, and cytokines, which act as messengers between cells and are naturally occurring substances, as are interferons, interleukins, monoclonal antibodies, and hematopoietic growth factors. Cytokines are protein products from cells that serve as cell modulators and stimulate or amplify the immune response. More specifically, lymphokines are products of lymphocytes, and monokines are products of monocytes. In general, biologic response modifiers (BRMs) can be classified into three major divisions: agents that augment, modulate, or restore the host's immunologic mechanisms; agents that have direct antitumor activity (cytotoxic or antiproliferative mechanisms); and agents that exert other biologic effects (those that affect differentiation or maturation of cells, that interfere with the ability of a tumor cell to metastasize, or that affect initiation or maintenance of neoplastic transformation).[1,2]

Historical Perspective

The immunotherapy of cancer can be divided into two approaches, active and passive. Active immunotherapy consists of giving a tumor-bearing host agents that are designed to elicit an immune response capable of retarding or eliminating tumor growth. The two types of active immunotherapy are *specific* and *nonspecific*. **Active specific immunotherapy** is immunization with tumor cells or tumor cell extracts, such as proteins or gangliosides administered as tumor antigens, or vaccines. The use of monoclonal antibodies as vaccines was an area of intense investigation. Active nonspecific immunotherapy is an attempt to boost overall immunity through the use of adjuvants such as bacterial extracts. The latter approach was based on the observation that adjuvants administered in animal systems could cause tumor regression. It was also based on the idea that those with tumors have diminished defense mechanisms. **Passive immunotherapy** is the administration or transfer of previously sensitized immunologic reagents such as antisera (which contain sensitized antibodies) or immune-reactive cells to a tumor-bearing host. These reagents directly or indirectly mediate antitumor responses. **Adoptive immunotherapy** refers to the passive transfer of sensitized cells such as lymphocytes or macrophages.[1,2]

Principles

Early trials failed to establish immunotherapy as a major modality as a result of the lack of purity and definition of immunotherapeutic agents, the lack of analogy between animal-model and human systems, the variability of experimental procedures, and inadequate administration of immunotherapeutic agents. Technologic advances in the 1980s and 1990s led biologic therapy to emerge as a major modality in cancer treatment. Recombinant DNA technology allowed production of large quantities of purified products. Fluorescent in situ hybridization (FISH) technology also opened the way to the modern era of biotherapy.

Biotherapy encompasses more than just the immune system. It includes treatments affecting other biologic responses such as growth and differentiation factors, chimeric molecules, and agents that may affect the ability of tumor cells to metastasize.[1,2]

Major Agents in Use

INTERFERONS

Interferon (IFN) has proved effective in the treatment of several malignancies and viral diseases. IFNs are divided into three major classes, according to antigenic type: alpha (α), beta (β) and gamma (γ). IFN-α and IFN-β are produced primarily by leukocytes and fibroblasts respectively: IFN-γ is made primarily by T lymphocytes. The IFNs may be called a family of glycoprotein hormones possessing pleiotrophic biologic effects. All IFNs mediate their cellular effects after binding to a specific receptor. IFN-α and IFN-β share a receptor, whereas IFN-γ uses a separate one. The IFNs have a wide range of biologic effects including antiviral, antiproliferative, and immunomodulatory.[1,2]

The antiviral activity of IFN renders uninfected cells resistant to attack by the offending virus as well as by a variety of other viruses. Internalization of the IFN-receptor complex causes a sequence of events that results in the production of antiviral proteins and enzymes. Both in vitro and in vivo experimentation have demonstrated the antiproliferative effects of IFN. IFN extends all phases of the cell cycle and lengthens overall cell generation time. The proteins also may inhibit DNA and protein synthesis to block the growth of tumor cells. Cellular protoonco-genes play an important role in the regulation of cell growth, and IFNs are known to inhibit expression of protooncogenes.

A variety of immunomodulatory effects have been described for the IFNs; these differ for the different classes of IFN. IFN increases the killing potential of natural killer (NK) cells by recruiting pre-NK cells and enhancing the cytotoxic activity of activated cells. Low doses of IFN appear to stimulate antibody production, whereas higher doses have a suppressive effect. IFN-γ appears to be a potent activator of macrophage function compared to IFN-α or IFN-β; however, all three are capable of inducing tumoricidal activity and increasing phagocytosis. IFNs are also capable of affecting the production of other lymphokines that regulate immune responses.[1,2]

In 1986, two recombinant IFN-α products, Intron A (IFN-α2b) and Roferon A (IFN-α2a), were approved for treatment of hairy cell leukemia (HCL) and Kaposi sarcoma. Since then, Intron A has been used as an adjuvant treatment in patients with melanomas at high risk for recurrence. These are patients with a deep primary lesion (more than a 4-mm thickness) or any patient with primary or recurrent nodal involvement. Median disease-free survival was extended from 1 to 1.7 years, overall survival from 2.8 to 3.8 years, and 5-year survival from 37% to 46%. In solid tumors, IFN has also demonstrated efficacy in such tumors as melanoma, renal cell cancer, ovarian carcinoma (via the intraperitoneal route), and superficial bladder cancers.

A variety of hematologic malignancies have been treated with IFN-α including, chronic myelogenous leukemia, Philadelphia-negative myeloproliferative disorders such as essential thrombocythemia and polycythemia vera, cutaneous T-cell lymphomas, multiple myeloma, and chronic lymphocytic leukemia.

Interferon continues to be explored as a single agent and in combination with other BRMs and chemotherapeutic agents. A phase II and III trial of IFN-α2a with and without 13-cis retinoic acid (13-CRA) in patients with progressive metastatic renal cell cancer found a benefit in progression-free and overall survival in patients treated with (IFN-α2a) plus (13-CRA). Unfortunately, this improvement in survival was coupled with an increase in toxicity. Molecular studies of resistant and sensitive cells may lead to a better selection of patients for immunotherapy treatment in the future.[3]

Randomized trials evaluating the role of IFN-α2 in the treatment of follicular lymphoma showed a survival advantage and a prolonged remission rate when intensive chemotherapy was given in conjunction with IFN-α2.[4]

The most common routes of administration for IFNs are intramuscular (IM), subcutaneous (subQ), and intravenous (IV), but they are also given intralesionally, intraperitoneally, intravesically, intraarterially, and intrathecally.

The toxicity of IFN has been well established. In general, side effects are similar for all classes of IFN. High-dose IFN therapy can be very debilitating. Nearly all patients report fatigue (approximately 25% reporting grade III fatigue), flulike symptoms, and gastrointestinal symptoms as the most frequently cited reasons to discontinue therapy. Side effects are generally reversible on cessation of therapy. Because IFN is generally given as long-term therapy, side effects can be divided into acute and chronic (those occurring as therapy progresses).

Nearly all patients beginning therapy with IFN have flulike symptoms. Although severe at first, adjustment to these symptoms over time prevents dose limitations. Symptoms include chills followed by fever spikes up to 104° F (40° C), headaches, myalgias, arthralgias, and malaise.

Chronic side effects tend to increase in intensity and maintain their level of intensity after patients have been undergoing therapy for several weeks. Fatigue and anorexia with weight loss can become dose limiting. IFN therapy may have to be held or the dose reduced, if the side effects become too severe. Patients also experience lethargy, lack of concentration, neutropenia, mild thrombocytopenia, elevated transaminases, proteinuria, and asymptomatic hypotension; other side effects are nausea, vomiting, diarrhea, altered taste, depression, decreased libido, memory changes, electroencephalogram (EEG) abnormalities, peripheral neuropathies, rashes, exacerbation of psoriasis, reactivation of herpes simplex, inflammation at injection sites, and minor alopecia. In addition, altered laboratory values include hypercalcemia, hyperkalemia, and elevated blood urea nitrogen (BUN) and lactate dehydrogenase (LDH) levels. In general, low-dose IFN therapy is reasonably well tolerated. It is usually recommended that IFN be administered before bedtime to allow patients to sleep through the side effects. Since the most common life-threatening toxicity is cardiac failure, patients with strong history of cardiovascular disease should not be considered for IFN therapy.[1,2]

LYMPHOKINES—INTERLEUKINS

Interleukin-2 (IL-2) is a glycoprotein produced by activated T-helper or CD_4 cells. IL-2 is a potent modulator of immune responses. The first response is the activation of T cells by antigen or mitogen, and the second is through interactions with IL-1. Like many polypeptide hormones, IL-2 exerts its biologic effects by binding to membrane-bound receptors on certain immune cells. IL-2 supports the growth and maturation of subpopulations of T cells both in vitro and in vivo, stimulates cytotoxic T cells, stimulates the proliferation and activity of NK cells, and develops the capacity in lymphoid cells incubated with IL-2 to lyse fresh tumor cells. These cells, known as **lymphokine-activated killer (LAK)** cells, have served as the basis for adoptive immunotherapy regimens. IL-2 also enhances antibody responses by activating other lymphocytes to produce lymphokines important to B cell function (IL-4 and IL-6), stimulates the expression of its own cell surface receptor, and induces the release of other lymphokines, such as IFN-γ and granulocyte-macrophage colony-stimulating factor (GM-CSF), that can mediate physiologic effects. Both in vitro and in vivo studies have demonstrated that IL-2 can reverse immune deficiency.

IL-2 was approved for treatment of both renal cell cancer and melanoma. The approved regimen used high doses of IL-2 by IV bolus every 8 hours for up to 14 doses. Given in this manner, side effects can be severe, and most patients are unable to receive all 14 of the planned doses. Although responses to high-dose IL-2 therapy are seen, severe systemic toxicities make it difficult to tolerate. The range and severity of toxicity seen with IL-2 are related to and influenced by dose, schedule, and concomitant use of adoptive immunotherapy, other BRMs, and chemotherapy.[1,2]

While IL-2 may directly cause some side effects, the induction of other cytokines by IL-2 also plays a role. Most IL-2–related side effects disappear once therapy is completed. IL-2 is administered on a cyclic basis. This gives patients the opportunity to recuperate between cycles or courses, although cumulative toxicity does occur with repeated cycles. Patients have exhibited a marked decline in performance status over time, and more severe toxicity and impairment have been observed as the number of total doses increase.

As with other BRMs, patients receiving IL-2 have flulike symptoms including chills, fevers, headaches, myalgias, arthralgias, and general malaise. Pretreatment with acetaminophen and nonsteroidal antiinflammatory drugs (NSAIDs) helps control some of these side effects. With continuous infusions of IL-2, these medications are often necessary around the clock to control fevers. The major cardiovascular and pulmonary toxicity associated with IL-2 administration stems from capillary leak syndrome. Treatment includes judicious use of IV fluids, along with the use of low-dose vasopressors (dopamine or neosynepherine) to maintain renal perfusion while reducing the risk of pulmonary edema and cardiac dysrhythmias.

Other side effects associated with IL-2 include nausea, vomiting, diarrhea, and anorexia. The aggressive use of multiple antiemetics and antidiarrheal agents is essential to minimize weight loss and malnutrition. Mucositis, glossitis, and xerostomia can further damage nutritional status. Central nervous system (CNS) toxicity includes confusion, lethargy, decreased concentration, extreme somnolence, depression, hallucination, paranoia, and combativeness and, if therapy is not discontinued, may lead to coma and death.

Skin changes occurring with IL-2 therapy include erythema, erythematous rash, pruritus, dryness and, occasionally, dry desquamation, either alone or in combination. Skin biopsies performed on rashes resulting from IL-2 therapy show whether they are related to the proinflammatory cytokine activities caused by IL-2's increased production of IFN-α and TNF. Biopsy results that lack eosinophils suggest that these skin rashes were not due to hypersensitivity reactions.[1,2,5]

Abnormal laboratory values include neutropenia, thrombocytopenia, anemia, and marked eosinophilia with rebound lymphocytosis and elevated hepatic enzymes and bilirubin, as well as decreased magnesium, calcium, phosphorus, and albumin. Replacement therapy compensates for decreased values, and the continued monitoring of liver function studies after completion of therapy is recommended.

Although agents such as IL-2 and IFN have shown significant toxicity and only modest benefit, scientists have been expanding their knowledge of immune system–tumor interactions. This understanding provides novel targets for manipulation of anticancer immune responses, and several new agents and approaches are currently under investigation.

HEMATOPOIETIC GROWTH FACTORS

Hematopoietic growth factors (HGFs) are a family of glycoproteins responsible for the proliferation, differentiation, and maturation of hematopoietic cells in vitro. They also stimulate functions of certain mature leukocytes. The classic growth factors, known as colony-stimulating factors (CSFs), are GM-CSF, granulocyte colony-stimulating factor (G-CSF), and erythropoietin. All are now produced in recombinant form.

To understand HGFs, one needs a basic understanding of hematopoiesis, the production and development of blood cells. This process normally occurs in the bone marrow, where cells of various lineages proliferate, differentiate, and mature. Most blood cells have a relatively short life span; to offset continual turnover, therefore, they must be constantly produced. Baseline levels of granulocytes and macrophages are maintained within a narrow range. However, the body has a remarkable ability to increase production in response to stresses such as infection and inflammation. Factors thought to be important in the control of hematopoiesis are the bone marrow microenvironment, cell-to-cell interaction, and humoral substances.

The process starts with a multipotent or pluripotent stem cell. These cells have the capacity for self-renewal and the ability to form multilineage colonies, although they are relatively quiescent under normal circumstances. Cells become successively more proliferative during differentiation, and their capacities to renew themselves and to form multilineage colonies becomes more restricted. CSFs appear more important in the stress response, and they seem to help control the number of effector cells in the immune response.[1,2]

Sargramostim (Leukine; GM-CSF) is a glycoprotein that shortens time to neutrophil recovery following chemotherapy administration. Early studies evaluated its application in patients with acquired immunodeficiency syndrome (AIDS), myelodysplastic syndrome (MDS), and aplastic anemia. The duration of neutropenia appeared shorter after chemotherapy administration, and leukocyte recovery was enhanced after transplantation, compared with controls. Overall, no significant effects were seen related to platelet recovery. GM-CSF received U.S. Food and Drug Administration (FDA) approval for the acceleration of myeloid recovery in patients with non-Hodgkin's lymphoma (NHL), acute lymphoblastic leukemia (ALL), and those patients undergoing autologous bone marrow transplantation (BMT) for Hodgkin's disease.[6]

Clinical trials are continuing to find that GM-CSF has additional benefits over those previously identified. At a dose of 250 mcg/m^2/day (rounded to the nearest vial size), GM-CSF may decrease the course of chemotherapy-induced mucositis, stimulate dendritic cells, and possess immunologic tumor-control capabilities. GM-CSF has been found to enhance proliferation of endothelial cells and keratinocyte growth, and may have a role in promoting wound healing. Ongoing studies are evaluating the use of GM-CSF as a vaccine adjuvant against infectious diseases and malignancies, and as immunotherapy in the treatment of various malignancies, such as melanoma, breast cancer, and neuroblastoma. The most commonly observed side effects with GM-CSF include bone pain, mild rash, transient low-grade fevers, and injection site reactions.[6]

Early clinical trials of **filgrastim (Neupogen; G-CSF)** focused on its use after chemotherapy. These trials demonstrated a shorter duration of severe neutropenia after G-CSF therapy. Patients who received G-CSF had fewer days of antibiotic therapy and a reduced incidence and severity of mucositis, and were more likely to be able to stay on their chemotherapy schedules than other patients. Patients exhibited a dose-dependent increase in leukocyte counts, mainly because of an increase in the absolute number of neutrophils. Counts fell rapidly once therapy was stopped. G-CSF has also been investigated in neutropenia arising from other causes, such as HCL and MDS. Filgrastim received FDA approval in 1991. Its initial indication was to reduce the incidence of infection in patients with nonmyeloid malignancies who were receiving myelosuppressive anticancer drugs associated with a significant incidence of severe neutropenia with fever. In 1994, filgrastim received approval for use in BMT in nonmyeloid malignancies. This revolutionized autologous BMT and allowed individuals to undergo this intensive therapy on an almost completely outpatient basis. Indeed, the prophylactic use of filgrastim can reduce the incidence of febrile neutropenia and decrease hospitalizations, as well as the need for intravenous antibiotics. It facilitates the time of delivery of chemotherapy doses. The daily recommended dose of filgrastim is 5 mcg/kg (rounding to the nearest vial size) until postnadir absolute neutrophil count (ANC) recovery to normal or near-normal levels. The first dose should be given 1 to 3 days after completion of chemotherapy, and treatment should continue through postnadir recovery. Its only drawback is in the necessity for daily dosing because of the rapid clearance in the kidneys.[7]

Scientists discovered that by attaching a polyethylene glycol molecule to the filgrastim protein, the duration of action increased to permit once-per-cycle dosing. This new product, **pegfilgrastim (Neulasta),** is also eliminated by the kidneys, but increases filgrastim's molecular size, which impairs renal clearance and prolongs circulation time and duration of action. The major route of elimination is through receptors on neutrophils, so the serum concentration of pegfilgrastim remains elevated until the ANC has recovered sufficiently to produce enough mature neutrophils to clear the drug.[8]

The recommended dose of pegfilgrastim is 6 mg per chemotherapy cycle to be administered subQ 1 to 3 days after chemotherapy. Evidence supported the use of pegfilgrastim in chemotherapy regimens given every 3 weeks. Phase II clinical trials demonstrated the efficacy of pegfilgrastim in dose-dense chemotherapy regimens.

The side effects of pegfilgrastim are essentially the same as those found with filgrastim; bony aches and pains are usually controlled with acetaminophen or NSAIDs.[8]

Erythropoietin is also a natural body glycoprotein essential for the growth of erythroid progenitor cells. Erythropoiesis is regulated by erythropoietin in response to changes in tissue oxygenation. Secreted primarily by the kidneys, erythropoietin acts on specific target cells in the bone marrow to increase the rate of production and release of red blood cells. Recombinant human erythropoietin, **epoetin alfa (Epogen, Procrit),** was initially approved in 1989 as treatment for chronic anemia in end-stage renal disease.[9,10]

In 1993, epoetin alfa received approval for the treatment of anemia in cancer patients undergoing chemotherapy. Cancer-related anemia is commonly associated with fatigue and a decreased quality of life. Treatment of the anemia to achieve optimal hemoglobin levels in patients who are receiving chemotherapy can alleviate common symptoms of anemia and give patients meaningful survival. Epoetin alfa can be administered safely and effectively once weekly to anemic patients receiving concomitant chemotherapy.[10-13] In a more recent study, patients with breast cancer receiving chemotherapy were randomly assigned to receive epoetin alfa 40,000 units weekly or according to standard of care. Patients on the epoetin alfa arm had improved quality of life, maintained their hemoglobin levels, and had reduced transfusion requirements when compared to the standard-of-care arm.[14]

A second randomized double-blind study comparing epoetin alfa with placebo in anemic patients receiving chemotherapy again demonstrated significantly improved hemoglobin levels and reduced transfusions in the patients receiving epoetin alfa when compared with the placebo group, supporting the use of weekly doses to treat cancer-related anemia.[15] With greater clinical experience, trial designs have focused on fine-tuning the use of epoetin alfa to achieve clinical outcomes such as reduced transfusion requirements and improved quality of life.

Currently, the field of hematopoietic support for anemia of cancer continues to evolve. The next generation of erythropoietin, **darbepoetin alfa (Aranesp),** has now been approved for the treatment of chemotherapy-induced anemia in patients with nonmyeloid malignancies. Darbepoetin alfa is a recombinant human erythropoietin with a longer half-life than epoetin alfa, which allows for less frequent dosing. Patients are able to undergo treatment of their anemia with a single subQ injection once every 2 weeks. Of particular benefit with dose-dense regimens, patients are no longer inconvenienced by weekly injections. As with all erythropoietic therapies, there is an increased risk of thrombotic events. The most commonly reported side effects in clinical trials were fatigue, edema, nausea, vomiting, diarrhea, fever, and dyspnea. Patients are usually started on a dose of 150 to 200 mcg subQ every 2 weeks. Doses can be increased based on response to therapy, in much the same fashion as epoetin alfa.

Guidelines have been developed by a number of groups, including the American Society of Clinical Oncology (ASCO), the American Society of Hematology (ASH), and the National Comprehensive Cancer Network (NCCN), to name a few. These guidelines determine the optimum treatment indications, doses and time intervals for the use of epoetin alfa and darbepoetin alfa.[11-13]

Oprelvekin, or **IL-11 (Neumega),** is another hematopoietic growth factor that stimulates the growth and development of megakaryocytes and platelets. It is used to prevent severe chemotherapy-induced thrombocytopenia and to reduce the need for platelet transfusions following myelosuppressive chemotherapy in patients with nonmyeloid malignancies.[1,2]

MONOCLONAL ANTIBODIES

An antigen is any substance that the body recognizes as foreign and attacks with an immune response. The humoral immune response produces immunoglobulins against the invading antigen from B cell–derived plasma cells. These immunoglobulins, or antibodies, react specifically with the antigenic determinants or epitopes of the inducing antigen. The antigenic determinants are parts of the antigen recognized by the antibodies. Each antigen has any number of epitopes, depending on the complexity of its structure. Individual B cells produce an antibody specific for single antigenic determinants; therefore, when an antigen invades the body, a variety of antibodies against it are produced. These cells are called monoclonal antibodies, or MoAbs.[1,2]

Numerous clinical trials have been conducted with native MoAbs–those not bound to drugs, toxins, or isotopes—for a large number of malignancies. An unconjugated antibody may demonstrate an anticancer effect in several ways. One is to mediate an antitumor cytotoxic effect through complement-dependent cytotoxicity or antibody-dependent cellular cytotoxicity. The constant region of the immunoglobulin reacts with either the first component of the complement system or with immune effector cells; the end result is tumor cell lysis.

Tumor cells express a variety of receptors that play an important role for their growth and proliferation. A second biotherapeutic approach uses MoAbs directed against cell surface receptors involved in proliferation, such as the epidermal growth factor receptor (EGFR). The intent is to block or downgrade the number of available receptors, thereby inducing an antiproliferative effect. An extensively studied approach is the use of anti-idiotype antibodies. Idiotypes are the variable regions of the immunoglobulin molecule that contain the antigen-combining region. A malignant B-cell clone produces cells that express and occasionally secrete a specific antibody. Infusions of antibodies directed against a B-cell lymphoma idiotype may suppress that clone back to its baseline. Another approach, actually a method of passive immunization, uses antibodies as surrogate tumor antigens to stimulate an immune response against the tumor.[1,2]

In 1997, the first MoAb was approved by the FDA specifically for the treatment of human malignancy. Rituxan (chimeric anti-CD20 MoAb rituximab) targets the CD20+ antigen found on the surface of normal pre-B and B cells including the malignant B cells of over 95% of non-Hodgkin's lymphomas. Since the CD20 antigen is not found on the surface of stem cells or committed progenitor cells, it is not myelosuppressive. Rituximab may mediate antibody-dependent cell-mediated cytotoxicity by human NK cells and activate complement-dependent cytolysis. It induces apoptosis in some antigen-positive cell lines and sensitizes lymphoma cells to the cytotoxic effects of certain chemotherapeutic agents.[16-18]

Rituximab has been studied in numerous clinical trials as both a single agent and in combination with chemotherapies (cyclophosphamide + doxorubicin + vincristine + prednisone, or R-CHOP), radioimmunotherapies (R-Zevalin), and other biotherapies (R-IFN) in the treatment of a variety of NHLs and chronic lymphocytic leukemia and small lymphocytic lymphoma (CLL and SLL).[19-23]

Initial trials were done in patients with relapsed or refractory disease. Response rates were significant and side effects relatively minor, compared with other treatment modalities.[24]

Recently, rituximab in combination with CHOP chemotherapy is now used as frontline therapy for newly diagnosed NHLs.[20,21] Response rates increased to 95% to 100% when rituximab was combined with CHOP.[20,21] Other trials explored rituximab in the setting of high-dose chemotherapy with autologous stem cell rescue, to purge the CD20 cells before stem cell collection, and after marrow recovery as consolidation therapy.[25]

The second MoAb to be approved was trastuzumab (Herceptin), the first for use in solid tumors. This agent was first used in a group of patients with breast cancer whose tumors overexpress the HER2/neu receptor. HER2/neu is a member of the epidermal growth factor (EGF) tyrosine kinase receptor family. Overexpression of the *erb*B-2 protooncogene results in overexpression of the HER2/neu receptor on the cell surface. This causes increased cell proliferation. Trastuzumab is a recombinant DNA MoAb that selectively binds to the HER2 protein. In patients who overexpress HER2 proteins, weekly administration of trastuzumab resulted in objective tumor responses in women with metastatic breast cancer (MBC).[26] Subsequent trials of trastuzumab in combination with chemotherapy yielded significantly higher response rates. Current trials have shifted trastuzumab-chemotherapy combinations to first-line treatment of patients with HER2/neu-positive MBC, and even in combination with chemotherapy as neoadjuvant treatment in operable breast cancer patients with HER2/neu-positive disease.[27,28] Trastuzumab weekly as opposed to every 2 week as opposed to every 3 weeks is also being studied for optimum response rates, as well as time to progression and overall survival benefits.[29] Scientists are now looking at other solid tumors that overexpress HER2 protein such as ovarian cancer, combining trastuzumab with chemotherapy (docetaxel) or with other biotherapeutic agents (IL-2).[30] Phase II clinical trials of gemcitabine with trastuzumab for the treatment of HER2-positive metastatic pancreatic cancer is underway. Approximately 20% of pancreas cancers overexpress HER2 and tend to offer a poorer prognosis.[31]

In the last several years, a number of other MoAbs have been developed for treatment of both solid and hematologic cancers. Gemtuzumab ozogamicin (Mylotarg) is a MoAb-targeted chemotherapy that binds specifically to the CD33+ antigen found on the surface of myeloid leukemia cells in more than 30% of patients with AML. Efficacy and tolerability of gemtuzumab have been documented in first-relapse AML, particularly in patients 60 years of age or older, who have no other treatment options. The approved treatment dose is 9 mg/m^2 IV infusion run over 2 hours, every 14 days, for 2 cycles.[32]

Denileukin diftitox (Ontak), another MoAb, is a fusion protein; the receptor-binding domain of IL-2 is fused to the diphtheria toxin to make a combination MoAb/vaccine. It targets activated T cells expressing CD25, the alpha chain of the IL-2 receptor. When denileukin diftitox is taken up into these cells, toxin is released, resulting in inhibition of protein synthesis and cell death. The advantage of this approach is in the ability of this protein to maximize tumor targeting while minimizing potential side effects to normal cells. Denileukin diftitox is used in the treatment of persistent or recurrent cutaneous T-cell lymphoma and other NHLs whose malignant cells express the CD25 component of the IL-2 receptor. Overall response rates of 45% have been seen with this treatment. Dosages of 9 to 18 mcg/kg/day IV for 5 days every 21 days are prescribed.[33,34]

Alemtuzumab (Campath) is a MoAb directed against the CD52 cell-surface antigen. CD52 is expressed on normal and malignant B and T lymphocytes. Alemtuzumab is indicated for the treatment of B-cell chronic lymphocytic leukemia in patients who have been treated with alkylating agents and have failed fludarabine therapy. Patients who were refractory to fludarabine are also eligible for this therapy. Alemtuzumab is effective as a single agent in CD52+ malignancies. Phase II trials with fludarabine induction followed by alemtuzumab consolidation as first-line therapy for B-cell CLL are also underway. Eradication of minimal residual disease in B-cell CLL by alemtuzumab is achievable, leading to improved overall and treatment-free survival. Treatment consists of a 3 mg initial intravenous dose infused over 2 hours daily until tolerated without reactions. Premedication is necessary to prevent acute reactions. Doses are escalated to 30 mg IV3 times/week for 12 weeks. Alemtuzumab is thought to cause a tremendous cytokine release during drug administration, which can severely suppress the immune system, leaving patients at risk for infection. Antiinfection prophylaxis to reduce the risk of bacterial, viral, or fungal infections should also be ordered.[35,36]

Two of the most recently approved MoAbs target colorectal cancers. Bevacizumab (Avastin) is a recombinant human MoAb designed to directly target vascular endothelial growth factor (VEGF), a ligand that attaches to the VEGF receptor (VEGFR), stimulating angiogenesis. Angiogenesis occurs when VEGFR-1 and VEGFR-2 bind to endothelial cell receptors; this contributes to endothelial cell survival by stimulating proliferation, migration, and inhibition of endothelial apoptosis. Activated endothelial cells secrete plasminogen activator, causing basement membrane breakdown. The endothelial cells migrate to the surrounding tissue and secrete substances leading to the formation of new blood vessels. Bevacizumab attaches to VEGF so that the receptors on endothelial cells are unable to attach to VEGF. Since they cannot attach, the receptors cannot stimulate the growth and survival of endothelial cells, which inhibits the angiogenesis-signaling cascade. In colorectal cancer, increased VEGF expression has been correlated with vascularity, invasiveness, metastasis, and poor prognosis.[37] Bevacizumab was approved in combination with 5-FU–based chemotherapy as first-line therapy for patients with metastatic colorectal cancer (MCRC). In randomized studies, the addition of bevacizumab to 5-FU + leucovorin (LV) significantly increased survival and progression-free survival compared to 5-FU + LV alone. Bevacizumab was well tolerated, with toxicities including bleeding, thrombosis, hypertension, diarrhea, and proteinuria.[38,39] Bevacizumab was added to irinotecan + 5-FU + LV (IFL) in first-line treatment for MCRC. Survival increased by 5 months in patients who received bevacizumab in addition to the chemotherapy. The addition of bevacizumab to oxaliplatin + 5-FU + LV (FOLFOX-4) also resulted in prolonged survival. Studies were also evaluated comparing IFL to FOLFOX-4, either first-line or second-line, with first-line therapy to include bevacizumab. Results suggested that first-line therapy with bevacizumab and two active chemotherapies, followed by a third active chemotherapy upon disease progression, optimizes overall survival.[39-42] Bevacizumab is given intravenously at 5mg/kg every 2 weeks. Clinical trials are ongoing, evaluating bevacizumab in multiple cancers, including lung, head and neck, breast, and renal cell cancers.[43]

The second MoAb recently approved for second-line treatment of MCRC is cetuximab (Erbitux). Cetuximab is a chimeric immunoglobulin G1 MoAb that targets the extracellular domain of epidermal growth factor receptor (EGFR) with high specificity and affinity. It competes for the binding site, inhibiting endogenous ligand binding and thereby inhibiting subsequent EGFR activation. Studies demonstrating activity in MCRC initially selected only those patients whose tumors expressed EGFR by immunohistochemistry (IHC).[41,42,44] Recent information suggests that cetuximab shows activity in tumors that don't express EGFR by IHC.[45] Clinical trials evaluated cetuximab as a single agent and cetuximab in combination with irinotecan. Cetuximab was approved by the FDA in both settings as second-line therapy for MCRC. Doses of 400mg/m^2 intravenously over 2 hours as an initial dose, followed by 250mg/m^2 IV over 1 hour weekly, are used in both single-agent and combined therapy settings. The most significant side effect is the development of an acneiform rash. Limiting sun exposure and practicing good skin hygiene usually suffice, but occasionally the rash becomes severe enough to require dose reduction or even discontinuation of cetuximab altogether.[46] Clinical trials using cetuximab and carboplatin in the treatment of nasopharyngeal cancers—recurrent or metastatic—are ongoing.[47]

RADIOIMMUNOTHERAPY

Radioimmunotherapy combines radioactive isotopes such as iodine-131 (I-131) and yttrium-90 (Y-90) with a MoAb. The radioisotope is carried to the tumor by the MoAb that attaches to a specific antigen present on the tumor cell surface. Once at the tumor site, radiation is targeted to tumor with the surrounding normal cells receiving less radiation than if they were exposed to external beam radiation therapy. Cancer cells are destroyed by the combination of targeted radiation therapy, the biologic effects of the MoAb, and the cross fire effect of the radiation on nearby tumor cells to which the antibody didn't bind.[16]

Two such agents have been approved for use in treating NHL. Y-90 ibritumomab tiuxetan (Zevalin) consists of a murine MoAb (the parent to rituximab) to the CD20 antigen stably bound to tiuxetan, which chelates the radionucleotide Y-90. It is indicated for the treatment of patients with relapsed or refractory low-grade, follicular, or transformed B-cell NHL, including patients with rituximab-refractory NHL. It is given with rituximab in a single treatment course on 2 days, 1 week apart. On the first day it is given with a tracer indium-111 to assess its biodistribution. Once that is determined, the biotherapeutic dose of Y-90 ibritumomab tiuxetan is injected slowly over 10 minutes. Dosage is based upon the patient's platelet count.[48,49]

In that Y-90 emits only beta radiation, it doesn't penetrate outside the patient's body, so fewer safety precautions are necessary. For the first 3 days after treatment, patients are taught to wash hands thoroughly and clean spilled urine and dispose of any materials contaminated with body fluids. Patients are also reminded to use condoms for 1 week after treatment and avoid pregnancy for 1 year after treatment.[48,49]

Tositumomab I-131 (Bexxar) is an anti-CD20 MoAb conjugated with I-131, which emits beta and gamma rays. It is used in the treatment of B-cell lymphoma in combination with radiation therapy. Treatment is well tolerated, with the most common side effects including hematologic toxicity, fatigue, fever, nausea, vomiting, rash, pruritus, and infection.[16]

EPIDERMAL GROWTH FACTOR RECEPTOR–TYROSINE KINASE INHIBITORS

EGFR is a growth-promoting protein found on the surface of many different types of tumor cells, including lung, breast, and colon cancers. EGFR-tyrosine kinase inhibitors (TKIs) are responsible for activating multiple downstream signaling pathways governing tumor growth.

Clinical trials of targeted EGFR-TKIs have demonstrated benefits in patients with advanced solid tumors and have been associated with unique clinical features and safety profiles when compared with conventional cytotoxic therapies. EGFR-TKIs may provide important treatment options for patients with advanced solid tumors whose disease has progressed while receiving chemotherapy, or for patients who cannot tolerate the toxicities associated with chemotherapy.

EGFR-TK plays a pivotal role in the development of many of the most common solid tumors. EGFR, also known as erbfl1 or HER1, is present in most cell types, with the exception of hematopoietic cells. In tumor cells, normal regulations that limit EGFR-TK enzyme activity and the subsequent transduction of growth signals are lost. A variety of tumor cell responses result from aberrantly activated EGFR-TK, including stimulation of cell growth, promotion of cell motility, alteration of adhesion and invasiveness, prolongation of cell survival, and stimulation of angiogenesis.[50]

Two new EGFR-TKIs have been approved for the treatment of patients with advanced non–small cell lung cancer (NSCLC). Gefitinib (Iressa) and erlotinib (Tarceva) are biologically-based, molecular targeted therapies with a novel mechanism of action. They selectively inhibit the EGFR-TK activity. Both agents are oral and are taken once daily. Treatment is well tolerated. Clinical trials of gefitinib resulted in durable tumor responses and improvement in lung cancer–related symptoms. Study subjects were pretreated with platinum- and docetaxel-based chemotherapy regimens. Results suggest that nonsmokers and women are more likely to respond to therapy with gefitinib or erlotinib. Current trials are trying to determine sequencing of EGFR-TKIs, either before chemotherapy or in tandem with first-line chemotherapy regimens. Side effects of treatment include skin toxicities, specifically a pustular or papular eruption with an acneiform distribution. The rash tends to improve over time, even with continued use of the gefitinib or erlotinib. Other side effects include diarrhea, managed with over-the-counter antidiarrheal medications, and ophthalmologic toxicity, including conjunctivitis, keratitis, dry eyes, and corneal erosion, also treatable with nonprescription eye drops.[51-56]

ANGIOGENESIS INHIBITORS

Angiogenesis is the process of blood vessel formation. Uncontrolled angiogenesis is pathologic and leads to the development and progression of malignant tumors. Angiogenesis inhibitors are a class of drugs that inhibit the formation of blood vessels, thus cutting off the supply of nutrients and oxygen to malignant tumors, resulting in their death.

Thalidomide (Thalomid) is an angiogenesis inhibitor. It inhibits basic fibroblast growth factor (bFGF) and VEGF production, thus reversing the angiogenic switch. Without adequate blood supply, tumor cells die. Thalidomide is also a cytotoxic agent that inhibits processing of mRNA that encodes peptide molecules, TNF-α, and angiogenic VEGF. Early research in the 1990s was done on thalidomide because of the discovery in the 1960s that thalidomide caused disruption of limb growth in fetuses of pregnant women who took the drug. Scientists began exploring the drug for its antiangiogenesis potential. Most clinical work focused on malignancies characterized by high plasma levels of bFGF and VEGF that result from neovascularization in the bone marrow. Myelomas and brain tumors were also studied because these tumors overexpress VEGF. The potential mechanisms of action of thalidomide include inhibition of angiogenesis, alteration of adhesion molecule expression, selective inhibition of TNF-α production, induction of T-helper cell type 2 cytokine production, inhibition of IL-6, IL-10, and IL-12, increase in the synthesis of IL-2 by mononuclear cells, and stimulation of T lymphocytes.[57]

Because of the known teratogenicity of thalidomide, the System for Thalidomide Education and Prescribing Safety (STEPS) program was developed to control and monitor access to the drug. Patients and their partners are required to use two effective forms of birth control and are surveyed on a regular basis. Prescriptions for the therapy must come from health care providers who have been educated and entered into the program as prescribers. An authorization number must be obtained before a prescription can be filled. Thalidomide is taken orally at doses of 200 mg/day, and escalated if tolerable. It is approved for use in multiple myeloma, and is also being used and studied for the treatment of advanced renal cell, prostate, ovarian, and breast cancers. Side effects to treatment include sedation, lightheadedness, peripheral neuropathy, constipation, and skin rash. Deep venous thrombosis

(DVT) can also be a serious complication, so patients are placed prophylactically on anticoagulation, either with warfarin or low-molecular-weight heparin. Thalidomide is usually taken at bedtime, and a good bowel regimen is initiated with therapy initiation. Prothrombin time (PT) and/or international normalized ratio (INR) is monitored if the patient is on warfarin therapy. Peripheral neuropathy is cause for discontinuation of the therapy, because it is not reversible.

With careful follow-up and education, it is hoped that patients can avoid the severe consequences of thalidomide therapy while gaining response over their cancers.[57]

Considerations for Older Adults

Biotherapeutic agents are generally well tolerated by geriatric patients. With the exception of high-dose IL-2, all are given on an outpatient basis. Many of the newest targeted therapies are oral and have very few side effects. However, because many elderly patients live alone and may have limited resources, it is very important to assess their functional status, economic status, and support systems before initiating treatment. For elderly patients receiving IFN or other self-injection biotherapy, it is critical to assess both their ability and their willingness to learn, as well as any physical capabilities that may inhibit their ability to learn.

Hepatic and renal function should be assessed before and during treatment with most biologic agents. Elderly patients may be at greater risk for cardiac complications, necessitating dose reductions or discontinuation of treatment. CNS-associated side effects, including confusion, memory loss, and diminished thought processes, must also be closely monitored. Fatigue is a significant side effect of biologic agents, and the elderly are at particular risk because of an already diminished functional status. Skin toxicities may be more prevalent in the geriatric patient because of decreased tissue, skin, and mucous membrane integrity. As with all cancer treatment, it is important to evaluate the patient's medication profile to detect drugs that may be contraindicated and may cause additional toxicity.

Conclusion

There are a number of investigational biologic therapies in phases I, II, and III trials at this time. As we learn more about the drugs that are currently in use, we gain further understanding about how tumors grow and develop, how they spread, and how they die. A number of cancer vaccines are being studied in a variety of cancers, including breast, cervical, lung, prostate, and renal cell cancers, as well as melanoma, myeloma, and NHL. Though it is unlikely that a prophylactic cancer vaccine will be developed, these therapeutic cancer vaccines hold promise as forms of active immunotherapy, inducing the host to mount an immune response against its own tumor cells.[58,59] Further research into dendritic cells, which are potent antigen-presenting cells in the immune system, will help us to understand their role in the development of acquired immunity, surveillance in monitoring for viral and bacterial infections, and the processing of cancer cells for apoptosis.[60]

Oncology nurses who care for patients receiving biotherapy are on the cutting edge of cancer therapy. They must stay abreast of the continual changes, be knowledgeable about therapeutic agents and modalities, and develop standards of care to manage toxicities. The possibilities for nurses in the exciting, rapidly changing world of biotherapy are on the rise and equally exciting.

REVIEW QUESTIONS

✓ Case Study

DR is a 76-year-old male who in 1998 was diagnosed with Duke's C rectal cancer. He underwent resection of the tumor with formation of a left upper quadrant colostomy. He completed adjuvant chemotherapy with 5-FU + leucovorin as well as local radiation therapy. He was followed on a regular basis by both medical and radiation oncology teams. In July 2004, on routine follow-up, he was found to have an elevated carcinoembryonic antigen (CEA) level of 45. Computed tomography (CT) scan work-up revealed liver and lung metastases, none greater than 2 cm in greatest diameter.

He was an active gentleman who lived alone but had strong family support in the immediate area. He had no comorbidities, and his ECOG performance status was 0. After a detailed discussion regarding risks and benefits, as well as side effects to therapy, he decided to begin treatment with oxaliplatin + 5-FU + leucovorin (FOLFOX-4) plus bevacizumab therapy. He had a Mediport placed before the initiation of treatment. He received his treatment over 3 days along with growth factor support in the form of pegfilgrastim 6 mg subQ and darbepoetin alfa 200 mcg subQ, according to ASCO, ASH, and NCCN guidelines. This was decided upon because of his pretreatment neutrophil and hemoglobin levels, which were below normal secondary to his earlier radiation and chemotherapies. He was treated on an every 2-week basis and tolerated therapy well without significant side effects. He did complain about fatigue, but insisted it was not significant enough to interfere with his activities of daily living. He continued to live alone and care for his home independently. After six cycles of treatment, CT scan restaging was done, and his tumors appeared to be responding to therapy. He continued treatment at full doses.

Upon completion of the tenth cycle of treatment, he developed grade 4 diarrhea, necessitating hospitalization for 5 days. He also complained of peripheral neuropathy, and further treatment was discontinued. He decided to take a break from additional treatment and spent the next month vacationing with friends out of state. Three months later, after returning home, he began experiencing increasing fatigue. He was found to have rising liver function tests, which prompted CT scan reevaluation. Although the disease in his lungs had remained stable, the liver lesions had progressed. At this time, he was fully recovered from the side effects of the FOLFOX-4 + bevacizumab therapy. He was still living independently and had an ECOG performance status of 0. He again decided to begin treatment after discussion regarding his options. Mr. R. was offered irinotecan + cetuximab on a weekly basis. After receiving his first dose of treatment, he had a significant drop in both neutrophil and platelet counts. He continued to receive weekly cetuximab infusions, but was only able to tolerate irinotecan on an every 2-week basis, despite dose reductions and growth factor support. After 8 weeks of therapy, liver function tests had normalized and CT scan reevaluation showed regression of liver lesions and stable lung lesions. He continued to experience fatigue, but had developed strategies to manage it. These included taking breaks between activities such as showering and dressing and eating breakfast, taking a short walk around the block with a neighbor each afternoon, taking a short nap after his walk, and most importantly, agreeing to allow his family to provide healthy meals for his lunch and dinner that could be prepared by Mr. R. with a minimal amount of effort. Throughout the course of these treatments, he was able to maintain his weight and nutritional status. This allowed him to maintain his activity schedule and his energy level.

The combination of these strategies allowed him to maintain his independence while providing his family with a way to assist him and be part of his support system. He also made a point of spending time each day with one or more of his eight grandchildren. According to Mr. R., this was his way of "keeping my mind sharp." This was of utmost importance to him and his family.

QUESTIONS

1. Which of the following factors places Mr. R. at increased risk of developing febrile neutropenia with FOLFOX-4 + bevacizumab chemotherapy?
   a. Bevacizumab therapy
   b. Age (>65 years old)
   c. Presence of lung metastases
   d. ECOG performance status 0

2. Which of the following statements *best* describes the mechanism of action of bevacizumab?
   a. Bevacizumab is a monoclonal antibody that is directed to the CD52 cell-surface antigen, which is indicated for the treatment of metastatic colorectal cancer.
   b. Bevacizumab targets the extracellular domain of epidermal growth factor receptor (EGFR), competing for the binding site, thereby inhibiting subsequent epidermal growth factor receptor (EGFR) activation.
   c. Bevacizumab is a monoclonal antibody designed to directly target vascular endothelial growth factor (VEGF) by attaching to the VEGF receptor (VEGFR) so that receptors on endothelial cells are unable to bind to VEGF, inhibiting the angiogenesis-signaling cascade.
   d. Bevacizumab is a monoclonal antibody that selectively binds to the HER2 protein and limits cancer cell proliferation in patients with tumors that overexpress the HER2/neu receptor.

3. Which of the following statements is true of interferon?
   a. It increases the killing potential of natural killer (NK) cells.
   b. It is approved for the treatment of metastatic colorectal carcinoma (MCRC).
   c. It has no antiviral activity.
   d. It regulates the production of T helper cells

4. Interleukin-II, given in high dose fashion, causes which of the following side effects?
   a. Acneiform rash
   b. Profound myelosuppression
   c. Capillary leak syndrome
   d. Hand-foot syndrome

5. In a recent study of breast cancer patients receiving chemotherapy randomly assigned to receive either epoetin alfa or standard-of-care treatment, patients on the epoetin alfa arm experienced which side effect?
   a. Decreased quality of life
   b. Elevated platelet counts
   c. Elevated hemoglobin
   d. Increased transfusion requirements
6. Rituximab is a chimeric monoclonal antibody (MoAb) that does which of the following?
   a. Selectively binds to HER2 protein
   b. Targets the CD20+ antigen on malignant B cells
   c. Is an effective therapy for the treatment of metastatic melanoma
   d. Targets the extracellular domain of epidermal growth factor receptor (EGFR)
7. Which of the following is a monoclonal antibody?
   a. Gemtuzumab ozogamicin
   b. Thalidomide
   c. Erlotinib
   d. Oprelvekin
8. Radioimmunotherapy combines radioactive isotopes and _____.
   a. Monoclonal antibodies
   b. Interferons
   c. Tumor-specific vaccines
   d. Hematopoietic growth factors
9. Which of the following is true about epidermal growth factor receptor–tyrosine kinase inhibitors (EGFR-TKIs)?
   a. EGFR-TKIs activate multiple downstream signaling pathways governing tumor growth.
   b. EGFR-TKIs block angiogenesis.
   c. Side effects of EGFR-TKIs include hand/foot syndrome and neutropenia.
   d. Trastuzumab and alemtuzumab are two approved EGFR-TKIs.
10. Which of the following is true of thalidomide?
   a. It is an angiogenesis inhibitor.
   b. It is an EGFR-TKI.
   c. It is given intravenously over 2 hours, every 21 days.
   d. It is contraindicated in patients receiving warfarin therapy.

ANSWERS

1. **B.** *Rationale:* Neutropenia is not a side effect of bevacizumab; patients who are over the age of 65 while receiving chemotherapy are at risk for febrile neutropenia—Mr. R is 76 years old; presence of lung metastases does not increase the risk of neutropenia; and, patients with a poor performance status (ECOG >2) are at risk for neutropenia—Mr. R has an ECOG performance status of 0.

2. **C.** *Rationale:* Bevacizumab is a recombinant human monoclonal antibody designed to directly target VEGF. In colorectal cancer, increased VEGF expression has been correlated with vascularity, invasiveness, metastasis, and poor prognosis. Bevacizumab is approved in combination with 5-FU–based chemotherapy as first-line therapy for patients with metastatic colorectal cancer.

3. **A.** *Rationale:* Interferon increases the killing potential of natural killer (NK) cells by recruiting pre-NK cells and enhancing the cytotoxic activity of activated cells.

4. **C.** *Rationale:* The major cardiovascular and pulmonary toxicity associated with IL-2 administration stems from capillary leak syndrome. Treatment includes judicious use of IV fluids, along with the use of low-dose vasopressors (dopamine or neosynepherine) to maintain renal perfusion while reducing the risk of pulmonary edema and cardiac dysrhythmias.

5. **C.** *Rationale:* Epoetin alfa causes elevation in hemoglobin levels.

6. **B.** *Rationale:* Rituximab targets the CD20+ antigen found of the surface of normal pre-B and B cells, including the malignant B cells of over 95% of non-Hodgkin's lymphomas.

7. **A.** *Rationale:* Gemtuzumab ozogamicin is a MoAb-targeted chemotherapy. Thalidomide is an angiogenesis inhibitor. Erlotinib is an EGFR-tyrosine kinase inhibitor. Oprelvekin is a hematopoietic growth factor.

8. **A.** *Rationale:* Radioimmunotherapy combines radioactive isotopes such as I-131 or Y-90 with a monoclonal antibody. The radioisotope is carried to the tumor by the monoclonal antibody that attaches to a specific antigen present on the tumor cell surface. Once at the tumor site, radiation is targeted to tumor with the surrounding normal cells receiving less radiation than if they were exposed to external beam radiation. Yttrium-90 ibritumomab tiuxetan and tositumomab I-131 are two examples of radioimmunotherapeutic agents.

9. **A.** *Rationale:* Aberrantly activated EGFR-tyrosine kinase stimulates cell growth, promotion of cell motility, alteration of adhesion and invasiveness, prolongation of cell survival, and stimulation of angiogenesis. EGFR-TKIs are responsible for activation of multiple downstream signaling pathways governing tumor growth.

10. **A.** *Rationale:* Mechanisms of action of thalidomide include inhibition of angiogenesis, alteration of adhesion molecule expression, selective inhibition of TNF-a production, induction of T helper cell type 2 cytokine production, inhibition of IL-6, IL-10, and IL-12, increase in the synthesis of IL-2 by mononuclear cells, and stimulation of T lymphocytes.

REFERENCES

1. Rieger PT: Biotherapy. In Rieger PT, editor: *Biotherapy: a comprehensive overview*, Sudbury, Mass, 2001, Jones & Bartlett.
2. Rosenberg SA, editor: *Principles and practice of the biologic therapy of cancer*, Philadelphia, 2000, Lippincott, Williams & Wilkins.
3. Aass N, De Mulder PHM, Mickisch GHJ et al: Randomized phase II/III trial of interferon alfa-2a with and without 13-*cis*-retinoic acid in patients with progressive metastatic renal cell carcinoma: the European Organization for Research and Treatment of Cancer Genito-Urinary Tract Cancer Group (EORTC 30951), *J Clin Oncol* 23(18):4172-4178, 2005.
4. Rohatiner AZS, Gregory WM, Peterson B et al: Meta-analysis to evaluate the role of interferon in follicular lymphoma, *J Clin Oncol* 23(10):2215-2224, 2005.
5. Newton S, Jackowski C, Marrs J: Biotherapy skin reactions, *Clin J Oncol Nurs* 6(3):181-182, 2002.
6. Buchsel PC, Forgey A, Grape FB et al: Granulocyte-macrophage colony stimulating factor: current practice and novel approaches, *Clin J Oncol Nurs* 6(4):198-204, 2002.
7. Amgen, Inc: Neupogen [package insert], Thousand Oaks, Calif, 2002, Author.
8. Bedell C: Pegfilgrastim for chemotherapy-induced neutropenia, *Clin J Oncol Nurs* 7(1):55-64, 2003.
9. Hood LE: Chemotherapy in the elderly: supportive measures for chemotherapy-induced myelotoxicity, *Clinical Journal of Oncology Nursing* 7(2), 185–190, 2003.
10. Buchsel PC, Murphy BJ, Newton SA: Epoetin alfa: current and future indications and nursing implications, *Clin J Oncol Nurs* 6(5):261-267, 2002.
11. Rizzo JD, Lichtin AE, Woolf SH et al: Use of epoetin in patients with cancer: evidence-based clinical practice guidelines of the American Society of Clinical Oncology and the American Society of Hematology, *J Clin Oncol* 20(19):4083-4107, 2002.
12. Crawford J, Althaus B, Armitage J et al: Myeloid growth factors: clinical practice guidelines in oncology, *J NCCN* 3(4):540-555, 2005.
13. Lyman GH: Guidelines of the National Comprehensive Cancer Network on the use of myeloid growth factors with cancer chemotherapy: a review of the evidence, *J NCCN* 3(4), 557-571, 2005.
14. Chang J, Couture F, Young S et al: Weekly epoetin alfa maintains hemoglobin, improves quality of life, and reduces transfusion in breast cancer patients receiving chemotherapy, *J Clin Oncol* 23(12):2597-2605, 2005.
15. Witzig TE, Silberstein PT, Loprinz CL et al: Phase III randomized, double-blinded study of epoetin alfa compared with placebos in anemic patients receiving chemotherapy, *J Clin Oncol* 23(12):2606-2617, 2005.
16. Sorokin P: New agents and future directions in biotherapy, *Clin J Oncol Nurs* 6(1):19-24, 2002.
17. Kosits C, Callaghan M: Rituximab: a new monoclonal antibody therapy for non-Hodgkin's lymphoma, *Oncol Nurs Forum* 27(1):51-59, 2000.
18. Davis TA, Grillo-Lopez AJ, White CA et al: Rituximab anti-CD20 monoclonal antibody in non-Hodgkin's lymphoma: safety and efficacy of re-treatment, *J Clin Oncol* 18(17):3135-3143, 2000.
19. Martinelli G, Laszlo D, Ferreri AJM et al: Clinical activity of rituximab in gastric mantle zone non-Hodgkin's lymphoma resistant to or not eligible for anti-*Helicobacter pylori* therapy, *J Clin Oncol* 23(9):1979-1982, 2005.
20. Hainsworth JD, Litchy S, Morrissey LH et al: Rituximab plus short-duration chemotherapy as first-line treatment for follicular non-Hodgkin's lymphoma: a phase II trial of the Minnie Pearl Cancer Research Network, *J Clin Oncol* 23(7):1500-1506, 2005.
21. Lenz G, Dreyling M, Hoster E et al: Immunochemotherapy with rituximab and cyclophosphamide, doxorubicin, vincristine, and prednisone significantly improves response and time to treatment failure, but not long-term outcome in patients with previously untreated mantle cell lymphoma: results of a prospective randomized trial of the German low grade lymphoma study (GLSG), *J Clin Oncol* 23(9):1984-1992, 2005.
22. Keating MJ, O'Brien S, Albitar M et al: Early results of a chemoimmunotherapy regimen of fludarabine, cyclophosphamide, and rituximab as initial therapy for chronic lymphocytic leukemia, *J Clin Oncol* 23(18):4079-4088, 2005.
23. Wierda W, O'Brien S, Wen S et al: Chemoimmunotherapy with fludarabine cyclophosphamide and rituximab for relapsed and refractory chronic lymphocytic leukemia, *J Clin Oncol* 23(18):4070-4078, 2005.
24. Rummel MJ, Al-Barton SE, Kim SZ et al: Bendamustine plus rituximab is effective and has a favorable toxicity profile in the treatment of mantle cell and low-grade non-Hodgkin's lymphoma, *J Clin Oncol* 23(15):3383-3390, 2005.
25. Khouri IF, Saliba RM, Hosing C et al: Concurrent administration of high-dose rituximab before and after autologous stem-cell transplantation for relapsed aggressive B-cell non-Hodgkin's lymphomas, *J Clin Oncol* 23(10):2240-2246, 2005.
26. Baselga J, Carbonell X, Castaneda-Soto NJ et al: Phase II study of efficacy, safety, and pharmacokinetics of trastuzumab monotherapy administered on a 3-weekly schedule, *J Clin Oncol* 23(10):2162-2171, 2005.
27. Burstein HJ, Winer EP: HER2 or not HER2: That is the question, *J Clin Oncol* 23(16):3656-3658, 2005.
28. Buzdar AU, Ibrahim NK, Francis D et al: Significantly higher pathologic complete remission rate after neoadjuvant therapy with trastuzumab, paclitaxel, and epirubicin chemotherapy: results of a randomized trial in human epidermal growth factor receptor 2-positive operable breast cancer, *J Clin Oncol* 23(16):3676-3684, 2005.
29. Dressler LG, Berry DA, Broadwater G et al: Comparison of HER2 status by fluorescence in situ hybridization and immunohistochemistry to predict benefit from dose escalation of adjuvant doxorubicin-based therapy in node-positive breast cancer patients, *J Clin Oncol* 23(19):4287-4297, 2005.
30. Marty M, Cognetti F, Maraninchi D et al: Randomized phase II trial of the efficacy and safety of trastuzumab combined with docetaxel in patients with human epidermal growth factor receptor 2-positive metastatic breast cancer administered as a first-line treatment: The M77001 study Group, *J Clin Oncol* 23(19):4265-5274, 2005.
31. Vogel CL, Tan-Chiu E: Trastuzumab plus chemotherapy: convincing survival benefit or not? *J Clin Oncol* 23(19):4247-4250, 2005.
32. Shannon-Dorcy K: Nursing implications of Mylotarg: a novel antibody-targeted chemotherapy for CD33+ acute myeloid leukemia in first relapse, *Oncol Nurs Forum* 29(4):E52-58, 2002.
33. Saxon M: Denileukin diftitox, *Clin J Oncol Nurs* 4(6):289-294, 2000.
34. Walker PL, Dang NH: Denileukin diftitox as a novel targeted therapy in non-Hodgkin's lymphoma, *Clin J Oncol Nurs* 8(2):169-174, 2004.
35. Moreton P, Kennedy B, Lucas G: Eradication of minimal residual disease in B-cell chronic lymphocytic leukemia after alemtuzumab therapy is associated with prolonged survival, *J Clin Oncol* 23(13):2971-2979, 2005.
36. Seeley K, DeMeyer E: Nursing care of patients receiving Campath, *Clin J Oncol Nurs* 6(3):138-143, 2002.
37. Franson PJ, Lapka DV: Antivascular endothelial growth factor monoclonal antibody therapy: a promising paradigm in colorectal cancer, *Clin J Oncol Nurs* 9(1):55-60, 2005.
38. Kabbinavar FF, Schulz J, McCleod M: Addition of bevacizumab to bolus fluorouracil and leucovorin in first-line metastatic colorectal cancer: results of a randomized phase II trial, *J Clin Oncol* 23(16):3697-3712, 2005.
39. Hurwitz HI, Fehrenbacher L, Hainsworth JD: Bevacizumab in combination with fluorouracil and leucovorin: an active regimen for first-line metastatic colorectal cancer, *J Clin Oncol* 23(15):3502:3508, 2005.
40. Sobrero A, Bruzzi P: Bevacizumab plus fluorouracil: the value of being part of a developing story, *J Clin Oncol* 23(16):3660-3662, 2005.
41. Wilkes GM: Therapeutic options in the management of colon cancer: 2005 update, *Clin J Oncol Nurs* 9(1):31:44, 2005.
42. Kelly H, Goldberg RM: Systemic therapy for metastatic colorectal cancer: current options, current evidence, *J Clin Oncol* 23(20):4553:4560, 2005.
43. Herbst RS, Onn A, Sandler A: Angiogenesis and lung cancer: prognostic and therapeutic implications, *J Clin Oncol* 23(14):3243-3256, 2005.
44. Vallbohmer D, Zhang W, Gordon M: Molecular determinants of cetuximab efficacy, *J Clin Oncol* 23(15):3536-3544, 2005.
45. Chung KY, Shia J, Kemeny NE: Cetuximab shows activity in colorectal cancer patients with tumors that do not express the epidermal growth factor receptor by immunohistochemistry, *J Clin Oncol* 23(9):1803-1810, 2005.
46. Thomas M: Cetuximab: Adverse event profile and recommendations for toxicity management, *Clin J Oncol Nurs* 9(3):332-338, 2005.
47. Chan ATC, Hsu MM, Goh BC: Multicenter, phase II study of cetuximab in combination with carboplatin in patients with recurrent or metastatic nasopharyngeal carcinoma, *J Clin Oncol* 23(15):3568:3576, 2005.
48. Hendrix C: Radiation safety guidelines for radioimmunotherapy with yttrium 90 ibritumomab tiuxetan, *Clin J Oncol Nurs* 8(1):31-34, 2004.

49. Hendrix CS, de Leon C, Dillman RO: Radioimmunotherapy for non-Hodgkin's lymphoma with Y90 ibritumomab tiuxetan, *Clin J Oncol Nurs* 6(3):144-148, 2002.

50. Krozely P: Epidermal growth factor receptor tyrosine kinase inhibitors: evolving role in the treatment of solid tumors, *Clin J Oncol Nurs* 8(2): 163-168, 2004.

51. Shah NT, Kris MG, Pao W: Practical management of patients with non-small cell lung cancer treated with gefitinib, *J Clin Oncol* 23(1):165-174, 2005.

52. Janne PA, Engelman JA, Johnson BE: Epidermal growth factor receptor mutations in non-small cell lung cancer: implications for treatment and tumor biology, *J Clin Oncol* 23(14):3227-3234, 2005.

53. Pizzo B: New directions in oncology nursing care: focus on gefitinib in patients with lung cancer, *Clin J Oncol Nurs* 8(4):385-392, 2004.

54. Cella D, Herbst RS, Lynch TJ: Clinically meaningful improvement in symptoms and quality of life for patients with non-small cell lung cancer, *J Clin Oncol* 23(13):2946-2954, 2005.

55. Giaccome G: Epidermal growth factor receptor inhibitors in the treatment of non-small cell lung cancer, *J Clin Oncol* 23(14):3235-3242, 2005.

56. Kobayashi S, Boggon TJ, Dayaram T: EGFR mutation and resistance of non-small cell lung cancer to gefitinib, *N Engl J Med* 352(8):786-792, 2005.

57. Goldman DA: Thalidomide use: past history and current clinical implications for practice, *Oncology Nursing Forum* 28(3):471-477, 2001.

58. King SE: Therapeutic cancer vaccines: an emerging treatment option, *Clin J Oncol Nurs* 8(3):271-278, 2004.

59. Hohenstein M, King SE, Fiore JM: Patient-specific vaccine therapy for non-Hodgkin's lymphoma, *Clin J Oncol Nurs* 9(1):85-90, 2005.

60. DeMeyers ES, Buchsel PC: A dendritic cell primer for oncology nurses, *Clin J Oncol Nurs* 9(4):460-464, 2005.

CHAPTER 23

Bone Marrow and Stem Cell Transplant

Claire Keller

Hematopoietic stem cells are found in the bone marrow, the spongy tissue found in the inner cavities of bone and in the poeripheral blood. Stem cells eventually proliferate into mature erythrocytes, leukocytes, and platelets (see Chapters 13 and 31 for further information). Hematopoietic stem cell transplantation (HSCT) is the process of replacing diseased or damaged bone marrow with normally functioning bone marrow. HSCT is used in the treatment of a wide variety of malignant and nonmalignant diseases. According to the International Bone Marrow Transplant Registry (IBMTR), 30,000 autologous and 15,000 allogeneic transplants were performed worldwide in 2002.[1]

Historical Perspective

The first known documented cases of human HSCT occurred as early as the nineteenth century. Medical practitioners experimented with bone marrow as a treatment modality for poorly understood diseases for which there was no existing treatment. Bone marrow was injected into or sometimes even fed to patients. Some positive results occurred; however, these benefits were sporadic, and the reasons for improvement were poorly understood. These primitive attempts were for the most part abandoned.

Later in the twentieth century, an interest in HSCT again arose as an experimental approach for the treatment of some hematologic diseases. A variety of approaches were used, and many important discoveries were made. Developments in antibacterial, fungal, and viral therapies, blood-banking techniques, chemotherapeutic regimens, growth factors, graft-versus-host disease (GVHD) prophylaxis and treatment, and tissue typing have made HSCT a more effective, viable treatment option. Table 23-1 summarizes the highlights of these significant developments.

Types of Hematopoietic Stem Cell Transplantation

There are two major types of transplant: autologous and allogeneic. The type of transplant is identified by the recipient's relationship to the donor. An autologous transplant is a transplant in which the patient's own bone marrow or stem cells are collected (harvested), placed in frozen storage (cryopreserved), and reinfused into the patient after the conditioning regimen. Therefore, the patient is his own donor. An **allogeneic transplant** is a transplant in which the patient receives someone else's bone marrow or stem cells. There are several types of allogeneic transplant, with each type named according to the donor: **syngeneic**—the donor is the patient's identical twin; **related**—the donor is related to the recipient, usually a sibling; **unrelated**—the donor is no relation to the recipient.

Sources of Stem Cells

AUTOLOGOUS PERIPHERAL BLOOD STEM CELLS

Although stem cells have been traditionally harvested from bone marrow cavities, functional hematopoietic stem cells can also be found circulating in peripheral blood. Peripheral blood stem cells (PBSCs) can be effectively transplanted, as evidenced in 1986 when the first successful PBSC transplants were reported.[2] Today the collection of PBSCs for hematopoietic support after high-dose chemotherapy (HDCT) has become standard practice in the treatment of a variety of diseases (Table 23-2). Advocates of PBSC transplant cite early engraftment as a cost-saving measure because of shortened length of stay and the need for fewer blood products and antibiotics.[2,3] Bone marrow harvest for autologous transplant has largely become a thing of the past. Few centers collect bone marrow except when unable to obtain an adequate cell dose during apheresis.[4]

The process of PBSC collection consists of two phases: mobilization and apheresis.

Mobilization. Peripheral blood in its steady state does not contain adequate numbers of stem cells to allow for efficient collection. Bone marrow contains up to 100 times the number of stem cells found in peripheral blood.[4] To collect an adequate number of stem cells in the least number of apheresis sessions, it is necessary to stimulate the production of PBSCs through a process called **mobilization.** The most significant mobilization occurs when chemotherapy and growth factors are used together rather than when either is used alone.[2-4] It has been reported that the combined use of chemotherapy and growth factors for mobilization also enhances engraftment.[2] When chemotherapy and growth factors are used together, there is an increase in the number of stem cells in the blood and a lengthening in the time they are present.[2]

In current clinical practice, administration of chemotherapy combined with cytokines (granulocyte colony-stimulating factor [G-CSF] or granulocyte-macrophage CSF [GM-CSF]) is the preferred technique to mobilize autologous PBSCs. Cyclophosphamide is the most frequently used chemotherapeutic agent in autologous PBSC mobilization, though agents specific to the underlying malignancy are also used.[2,4] Chemotherapy is used to treat the disease and to take advantage of the accelerated hematopoiesis that occurs during the recovery period that follows myelosuppressive treatment.[2,4] There are two primary disadvantages to chemotherapy-induced mobilization: it can result in neutropenic fever and infection, and it is difficult to predict when the patient will be ready to begin apheresis.[5]

TABLE 23-1 Significant Historical Events in Hematopoietic Stem Cell Transplantation (HSCT)

YEAR	RESEARCHER	SIGNIFICANT FINDING
1896	Quine	Attempted bone marrow transplant (BMT) by injecting or feeding bone marrow to patients; poor results
1939	Osgood et al	Attempted to cure aplastic anemia by massive intravenous (IV) injections of marrow cells
1950	Relders et al	Attempted BMT in dogs; adequate doses of bone marrow, but inadequate radiation exposure did not allow for sufficient immunosuppression for engraftment
1951	Lorenzo et al	Demonstrated that guinea pigs and mice exposed to lethal radiation could be protected by infusion of bone marrow
1955	Lindsley et al	Radiation protection described earlier was result of growth of donor bone marrow
1956	Ford et al	Cytogenetic techniques used to show that radiation protection resulted from transfer and survival of donor marrow cells
1957	Thomas et al	Large quantities of bone marrow could be safely infused IV; one patient showed transient engraftment Estimated necessary dose of marrow cells and warned against graft-versus-host disease reactions
1959	Thomas et al	Demonstrated that IV infusion of marrow from identical twin could protect against lethal radiation doses in patients with refractory leukemia
1964	Mathe	First to achieve enduring bone marrow graft in patient with leukemia
1968	Epstein et al	Detected DL-A antigen in dogs and showed that marrow grafts between litter mates were almost always successful
1968	Gatti et al	Performed first marrow transplant from a matched sibling for an infant with immunodeficiency
1975	Thomas et al	Performed series of successful transplants using HLA-A identical siblings

TABLE 23-2 Diseases Treated with Hematopoietic Stem Cell Transplant

TYPE	DISEASE
Malignant	Acute myelogenous leukemia (AML)
	Acute lymphocytic leukemia (ALL)
	Juvenile myelomonocytic leukemia (JMML)
	Chronic myelogenous leukemia (CML)
	Myelodysplastic syndrome (MDS)
	Hodgkin's disease
	Non-Hodgkin's lymphoma (NHL)
	Multiple myeloma
	Renal cell carcinoma
	Neuroblastoma
	Testicular cancer
	Ewing's sarcoma
	Rhabdomyosarcoma
	Wilms' tumor
	Malignant melanoma
	Lung cancer
	Brain tumors
	Ovarian cancer
Nonmalignant	Aplastic anemia
	Myelofibrosis
	Wiskott-Aldrich syndrome
	Severe combined immunodeficiency syndrome (SCIDS)
	Mucopolysacharoidosis
	Osteopetrosis
	Lipid storage diseases
	Thalassemia
	Paroxysmal nocturnal hemoglobinuria

Apheresis. The PBSCs are collected by a process called **apheresis,** using standard, commercially available cell separators. The cell separators are programmed to collect either lymphocytes or low-density leukocytes. The remaining blood components are returned to the patient. Apheresis is performed for 1 to 3 days. Each session is 3 to 4 hours long, but the duration is based on the rate of blood flow through the central venous catheter. A flow rate of 50 to 70 ml/min is considered optimal.[6] A single, large-volume collection can decrease collection time while providing a safe, cost-effective harvest method.[6,7]

To collect PBSCs, a large-bore, double-lumen central venous catheter is required. This is necessary to provide adequate blood flow through the cell separator. A variety of catheters are in use; generally at least a 12-French size is needed to maintain blood flow. Catheters that have narrower lumens or those constructed of soft material such as silicone may not be able to provide adequate flow rates. Complications related to the central venous catheters have been reported, including thrombosis, occlusion, malpositioning, and infection. These complications contribute to the morbidity and cost of the procedure. The "ideal" apheresis catheter has not yet been found. Current technology does not allow one to identify the circulating stem cells. Several techniques are in development to help determine if an adequate number of stem cells have been collected to ensure engraftment. The easiest and most widely available is to measure the number of mononuclear cells in the apheresis product. Mononuclear cell counts of 4 to 5×10^8/kg patient body weight routinely contain adequate stem cells for engraftment. Another method is to measure the population of cells that express CD34+ using flow cytometry. It is believed that stem cells are found within the group of cells carrying the CD34+ antigen. Currently this is one of the most widely used methods to estimate the number of stem cells in the apheresis product. A CD34+ dose of 5×10^6 is generally considered an adequate dose to provide optimal engraftment.[2]

Side effects of apheresis are minimal but include transient hypocalcemia from the anticoagulant used in the apheresis process, fatigue, anemia, and thrombocytopenia. After each collection the stem cells are placed in a blood bag and cryopreserved using dimethylsulfide (DMSO) as a cryoprotectant. The cells are kept frozen at $-120°$ C.[8]

ALLOGENEIC PERIPHERAL BLOOD STEM CELLS

In recent years, many centers have turned to PBSCs as the source of stem cells for allogeneic transplants. The advantages of using allogeneic PBSCs, compared to bone marrow and umbilical cord blood, include faster engraftment and decreased transplant-related mortality, the ability to obtain a larger number of stem cells, the possibility of faster reconstitution of the immune system, and comparable rates of GVHD.[9]

Allogeneic PBSC collection consists of two phases: mobilization and apheresis.

MOBILIZATION

Mobilization of PBSCs is necessary in the normal donor, since there is not an adequate number available in the peripheral circulation in its steady state.[9] With normal donors, only the use of growth factors—specifically, G-CSF—is considered safe for mobilization. An adequate number of CD34+ cells are available in the circulation after 4 to 5 days of G-CSF administration.[9] Reported side effects include bone pain, headache, fatigue, nausea, and insomnia.[9] These side effects can be managed with oral analgesics in most cases and resolve on their own after the G-CSF is discontinued. Long-term effects of normal donors receiving G-CSF are not known, but it has been speculated that the risk for leukemia may increase by as much as tenfold.[9]

APHERESIS

As with autologous PBSCs, allogeneic PBSCs are collected by apheresis, using standard, commercially available cell separators. The cell separators are programmed to collect either lymphocytes or low-density leukocytes.[6] In normal donors, peripheral lines in the antecubital veins are most commonly used for venous access; in some cases a temporary central line may be needed. An adequate number of CD34+ cells can be collected in one or two sessions, in most cases. The most significant side effect is a 30% to 50% drop in platelet count. The platelet count may take a week or more to recover, and donor follow-up is important.[6,7]

BONE MARROW HARVEST

Harvesting is the process of obtaining bone marrow for transplantation. Bone marrow harvests are becoming less frequent, because many centers have turned to PBSCs or umbilical cord blood (UCB) for autologous and allogeneic transplants. This procedure occurs in the operating room, typically with the patient under general anesthesia. Bone marrow is obtained by performing multiple punctures with a large-bore needle into the patient's posterior and occasionally the anterior iliac crests. Usually two physicians work simultaneously, one on either side of the patient. Multiple punctures are necessary because each aspiration obtains only 2 to 5 ml of bone marrow.

The amount of bone marrow collected depends on the size of the recipient and the donor, as well as the type of bone marrow transplant (BMT)—autologous or allogeneic. Usually, 10 to 15 ml/kg body weight will yield the amount of stem cells needed.

Therefore, a 50-kg patient would contribute approximately 500 to 750 ml bone marrow, and if obtaining about 5 ml/aspiration, approximately 100 to 150 aspirations are required to obtain the desired total of 500 to 750 ml marrow. This is only about 5% of the body's total marrow volume. Ideally, this amount of marrow should contain 1 to 4×10^8 nucleated cells.[6] Once collected, the marrow is mixed with a heparinized solution, filtered to remove bone fragments and fat, and placed in a blood bag.

At this point the marrow can be treated or purged. Purging is the process of removing residual malignant cells from the marrow for autologous transplant. It is performed using monoclonal antibodies or chemotherapeutic agents. The benefit of purging is controversial. Though purging has been shown to decrease the tumor cell contamination, it usually delays engraftment and results in an increased risk of complications. Marrow collected for allogeneic HSCT may also be treated. One such treatment is that of T-cell depletion, which is the process of removing T lymphocytes from the marrow to prevent acute GVHD. If an ABO incompatibility exists, the red blood cells (RBCs) may also be removed from the allogeneic marrow.

When an allogeneic HSCT is to be done, the marrow is transfused into the recipient as soon as possible after the harvest. The marrow is typically brought to the cell processing laboratory and then brought to the patient's room for infusion. For an autologous HSCT, the collected marrow is mixed with the preservative DMSO, placed in a blood bag, and cryopreserved. It is thawed and transplanted at a later date.

After bone marrow harvest, postoperative recovery time is minimal. Pressure dressings are applied to the iliac crests.

Nursing responsibilities after bone marrow harvest include routine postoperative care such as maintaining comfort and mobility, providing care of the dressing, and monitoring vital signs and blood counts.[6] Postoperatively, site discomfort will last for approximately 1 week, and is typically relieved with acetaminophen. The donor's psychologic and emotional needs must be met. There will be anxiety over whether the HSCT will be successful. Donors should be encouraged to ventilate their feelings and be offered support.

UNRELATED DONORS

Another donor option is identifying an unrelated donor. The National Marrow Donor Program (NMDP) was established in 1987 for the purpose of obtaining donors for those in need. The registry contains more than 5.5 million available bone marrow donors, all of whom have had tissue typing completed and have expressed a desire to donate bone marrow. In 1999, the NMDP developed a central registry of cord blood banks to enable transplant centers to search cord blood banks more efficiently. Ethnic minorities remain underrepresented in the registry. The NMDP continues to place major emphasis on the recruitment of minority donors. The registry search determines which listed donors have compatible typing with potential recipient patients. There are several other donor registries that contain approximately 4.5 million donors located throughout the world and are available for searches. It is not inconceivable that a patient in the United States could receive bone marrow from a donor located somewhere in Europe, Asia, Africa, or anywhere else in the world. When chosen, the identities of both the donor and the recipient remains anonymous, as well as the geographic location of the donor. More than 20,000 unrelated HSCTs have been made possible as a result of efforts of the NMDP.[10]

CORD BLOOD TRANSPLANTATION

As with bone marrow, umbilical cord blood (UCB) is rich in stem cells. It is now possible to collect and store cord blood for use in place of bone marrow or PBSCs. The first successful UCB transplant was performed in 1988 on a child with Fanconi's anemia.[11] Cord blood transplants have been successfully performed in patients with leukemia, aplastic anemia, Fanconi's anemia, immunodeficiency, and genetic and metabolic disorders.[11]

The New York Blood Bank Center has banked more than 29,000 cord blood samples.[12] In addition, there are many smaller umbilical cord blood banks across the country and around the world. Because of the relatively low number of stem cells in cord blood, the majority of cord blood transplants have been in children. Cord blood is often selected for unrelated transplants because a greater human leukocyte antigen (HLA) mismatch is tolerated, the units are readily available, and there appears to be a decrease in the incidence and severity of GVHD.[11,13] Until recently, cord blood has not been widely used in adults because the cell dose is limited by size of the cord blood unit, which may have an insufficient cell dose for larger patients. Several studies using two cord blood units in larger children and adults have shown this to be safe and may overcome the low cell dosage barrier that limits the use of cord blood in these populations.[14-17]

Collecting UCB is a simple procedure and poses no risk to the donor. After the placenta is delivered, the umbilical cord is clamped and the blood withdrawn from the umbilical vein, using a needle and syringe. It is then cryopreserved in the same manner as PBSCs or bone marrow.[18]

HUMAN LEUKOCYTE ANTIGEN TYPING

Tissue typing of the patient and potential donors is the first step in identifying whether a patient has a compatible donor. To determine a person's tissue type, a small amount of peripheral blood is drawn, and antigens on the surface of the leukocytes are analyzed. These antigens make up the HLA system, which plays a role in immune surveillance by constantly identifying "self" from "not-self." There is a pair of antigens at several sites called **loci** on the white blood cells (WBCs). Three of these loci, the HLA-A, HLA-B, and HLA-DR, are important in determining the compatability between a patient and a potential donor. The most desirable match is one in which the antigens of both the patient and the potential donor match at all three loci, which minimizes the risk of GVHD and graft rejection.[19]

The antigens which comprise the HLA system are inherited from one's parents. Each offspring receives a set of antigens, referred to as a **haplotype,** from each parent (Fig. 23-1). Thus, the best

chance of finding a matched donor occurs among full siblings. Statistically, each sibling has a 1 in 4 (25%) chance of receiving the same haplotypes from the same parents. It is possible but unlikely that parents or children of a patient will match, because they are usually only a one-haplotype (half) match. In general, relatives outside the immediate family have approximately the same chance of matching as someone from the general population. Overall, the chances of matching someone in the general population are approximately 1 in 20,000, depending on how common the individual's haplotypes are.

Historically HLA-A and HLA-B (class I) antigens were identified by serologic testing, using a small blood sample and a typing tray containing known antisera. HLA-DR (class II) antigens were identified using DNA technology. Most clinical laboratories now use a method of amplification of specific HLA genes from DNA, using polymerase chain reaction typing methods to identify both class I and class II antigens.[20]

Mismatched donors are used in allogeneic transplants, for which no true match exists. Mismatches currently considered for transplant are one antigen mismatches for bone marrow and PBSC and two antigens for UCB. The mismatch can occur at either the A, the B, or the DR locus. A higher number of mismatches will produce a higher incidence of GVHD, graft rejection, and patient mortality.[20]

Mismatching does not refer to ABO incompatibility. Corrections can be made to overcome ABO incompatibility. For example, a patient with blood type O can receive a transplant from a donor with blood type A. When an ABO incompatibility occurs, the donor's erythrocytes can be removed from the bone marrow before transplant. These erythrocytes are not infused, and side effects from the ABO incompatibility are minimized. Seroconversion will occur over time, and the blood type of the recipient will eventually change to that of the donor.

Indications for Hematopoietic Stem Cell Transplantation

Hematopoietic stem cell transplantation is a treatment modality for a variety of malignant and nonmalignant diseases (see Table 23-2). Most HSCTs are performed for malignancies. The type and stage of disease, patient age and performance status, and donor availability determine the type of transplant, as well as the chance of survival. Table 23-3 identifies approximate 3-year disease-free survival (DFS) for autologous and allogeneic transplants.

Allogeneic transplant is used in the treatment of hematologic malignancies, marrow failure, severe combined immunodeficiency syndrome (SCIDS), and some inherited metabolic disorders. Currently, most allogeneic transplants are performed for acute myelogenous leukemia (AML), acute lymphocytic leukemia (ALL), myelodysplastic syndrome (MDS), and non-Hodgkin's lymphoma (NHL).[21,22]

Autologous BMT is used primarily for the treatment of diseases in which the patient's own bone marrow contains adequate stem cells that can eventually generate functioning erythrocytes, leukocytes, and platelets. For example, autologous HSCT is not a viable option for the treatment of aplastic anemia because the patient's own bone marrow is lacking stem cells; however, it can be a treatment option for patients with limited disease in their bone marrow. The diseases most commonly treated with autologous HSCT are multiple myeloma and NHL.[22]

	Mother				Father		
	M-1		M-2		F-1		F-2
A	1		2		3		9
B	5		7		12		13
DR	1		2		4		5

	Child #1		Child #2		Child #3		Child #4	
	M-1	F-1	M-1	F-2	M-2	F-1	M-2	F-2
A	1	3	1	9	2	3	2	9
B	5	12	5	13	7	12	7	13
DR	1	4	1	5	2	4	2	5

FIG. 23-1 Human leukocyte antigen (HLA) inheritance.

TABLE 23-3   Survival Rates: Approximate 3-Year Disease-Free Survival of Patients Receiving Transplant

DISEASE	DFS (%)
Autologous Transplants	
AML (1st CR)	40-50
AML (2nd CR)	30-40
ALL (1st CR)	40-50
ALL (2nd CR)	30
CML (chronic)*	10
Hodgkin's disease	20-60
Non-Hodgkin's	40-60
Multiple myeloma	50-60
Allogeneic Transplants	
AML (1st CR)	50-65
AML (>1st CR)	25-35
ALL (1st CR)	40-60
ALL (2nd CR)	30-60
CML (chronic)	65
CML (accelerated)	30-45
CML (blastic)	15
Hodgkin's disease	25-55
Non-Hodgkin's	20-65
Multiple myeloma*	30
Aplastic anemia	60-80
MDS	30-60

ALL, Acute lymphocytic leukemia; *AML*, acute myelogenous leukemia; *CML*, chronic myelogenous leukemia; *CR*, complete remission; *DFS*, disease-free survival; *MDS*, myelodysplastic syndrome.
*Limited number of patients and follow-up

Autologous HSCT is being used increasingly for the treatment of hematologic malignancies. Since 1990 the number of autologous BMTs has outpaced the number of allogeneic HSCTs.[1]

A concern associated with autologous transplant and PBSC transplant is the potential for contamination with tumor cells. A variety of purging techniques have been developed. A lack of prospective clinical trials, a lack of sensitive and specific assays to measure residual tumor, and the concern that stem cells can be damaged during the purging process have kept marrow purging controversial.

HEMATOLOGIC MALIGNANCIES

Leukemia

Acute lymphocytic leukemia. Allogeneic HSCT has been performed on patients with ALL in remission and in relapse. Survival for patients transplanted in first remission is comparable to survival with conventional chemotherapy.[23,24] However, performing an allogeneic HSCT in first remission is beneficial for patients who are seen at diagnosis with a high WBC count, the Philadelphia chromosome, or other chromosomal abnormalities. Allogeneic HSCT for ALL in second or subsequent remission has shown a survival advantage over conventional chemotherapy.[25] Autologous HSCT and PBSC transplant may also be done if no suitable donor is available.

ALL is the most common leukemia among children; 60% to 70% of these children are cured with conventional chemotherapy. For most children with ALL, HSCT is not considered unless the child relapses while in treatment. HSCT in first remission is indicated only if the Philadelphia chromosome or other chromosomal abnormality is present.[25] For patients who do not have a suitable donor, autologous HSCT has been done, but these patients have a relapse rate of 70% to 75%.

Acute myelocytic leukemia. Survival rates of AML patients following allogeneic HSCT are 35% to 60%, compared with conventional chemotherapy survival rates of 20% to 50%. Timing of transplant remains controversial, but survival is best when the patient is transplanted in first remission.[23] For patients without suitable donors, autologous transplants done during first remission offer survival rates of 40% to 50%. The relapse rate is higher after autologous HSCT, but complications of allogeneic HSCT (e.g., GVHD) result in similar DFS rates.[23,26]

Chronic myelogenous leukemia. Transplant remains the only curative treatment for chronic myelogenous leukemia (CML), although the number of transplants for CML in early stage have decreased with the introduction of imatinib mesylate.[21,22,27] The disease phase at the time of transplantation is the factor most strongly associated with treatment success.[21] Patients who have a HSCT in the chronic phase have higher rates of success. The best results, survival rates of 70%, are seen in young patients, transplanted in chronic phase within a year of the diagnosis.[21] Patients transplanted more than 1 year after diagnosis have survival rates of 60%.[21] To date, no randomized prospective studies comparing imatinib mesylate to allogeneic HSCT have been performed.[27] Timing of transplant has become more controversial in the imatinib mesylate era. Many centers recommend a trial of imatinib mesylate for patients newly diagnosed with CML, with assessment of response at 6 months. Patients with a partial response or no response would then proceed to transplant. Of patients receiving imatinib mesylate in accelerated phase, 10% relapse directly into blast crisis.[27]

For patients without a suitable donor, autologous HSCTs for CML are under investigation. In some studies, PBSCs are collected while the patient is in chronic phase. Patients undergo transplant when they progress to accelerated phase. Although this treatment is not curative, chronic-phase CML has been successfully restored for 4 months to 1 year. Other investigators are looking at autologous transplantation with imatinib mesylate given during mobilization.[27]

Juvenile myelomonocytic leukemia. Juvenile myelomonocytic leukemia (JMML) replaces the older terminology of juvenile chronic myelogenous leukemia (JCML) and chronic myelomonocytic leukemia (CMML). JMML is a disease of infants and young children, a third of whom are diagnosed during the first year of life, and most before age five.[28] JMML frequently presents like acute leukemia but cannot be effectively treated with chemotherapy. Allogeneic HSCT provides event-free survival of 50%, offering the best hope for survival, but relapse rates exceed 30%.[28]

Lymphoma. HSCT in the malignant lymphomas, Hodgkin's and non-Hodgkin's, is widely used as a salvage treatment. Because of the high chemotherapy and radiation sensitivity of these tumors, patients with lymphoma are optimal candidates for HSCT.[23]

Autologous and allogeneic transplants are used, although autologous HSCTs are done most frequently because of the lack of donor availability and decreased complications. Autologous HSCT also allows for treatment of older patients, which is especially important in non-Hodgkin's lymphoma.

The best results have been seen in lymphoma patients treated in second remission or in relapse who have disease that is still responsive to chemotherapy.[23] In Hodgkin's disease, HSCT is usually indicated for patients who fail to achieve a complete response to three or four courses of chemotherapy or who are in early relapse after initial complete response.[23] In non-Hodgkin's lymphoma, HSCT is usually indicated for patients who have relapsed after an initial complete response or who remain responsive to chemotherapy but have residual disease.[23] For patients with residual disease or highly aggressive non-Hodgkin's lymphoma, HSCT should be carried out as a consolidation procedure.[23]

Other Hematologic Malignancies

Myelodysplastic syndrome. MDS consists of a number of disorders characterized by peripheral cytopenias. Allogeneic HSCT is the only curative treatment for patients with MDS. Results are better in patients without excess blasts: cure rates of 60% to 70% have been reported in this population. Patients with excess blasts have a survival rate of 25% to 40%.[29]

Multiple myeloma. HSCT is now considered standard therapy for multiple myeloma.[21] Overall survival rates for patients undergoing allogeneic transplant who fail first-line chemotherapy average 30% to 35%. Allogeneic HSCT is not an option for many patients with multiple myeloma because of their advanced age and the lack of suitable donors. Early transplant-related mortality is high following allogeneic transplant.[21] Autologous HSCT can be tolerated by patients up to age 65. Favorable results reported with autologous HSCT showed that patients most likely to benefit have primary resistant or responding disease with low β-microglobulin and lactate dehydrogenase (LDH) levels.[30] Sequential autologous transplant and autologous transplant followed by an allogeneic nonmyeloablative transplant are under investigation.

SOLID TUMORS

Autologous HSCT is most often done for patients with solid tumors. Solid tumors are the malignancies most frequently treated with dose-intensive strategies. For HSCT to be effective, the disease must be responsive to treatment. Although HSCTs are currently being performed to treat a variety of solid tumors, many are still considered investigational. Tumors for which HSCT has shown some positive responses are Ewing's sarcoma, malignant melanoma, rhabdomyosarcoma, testicular cancer, Wilms' tumor, ovarian cancer, renal cell carcinoma, and small cell lung cancer.

Breast Cancer. There has been a great deal of controversy surrounding HSCT for breast cancer. There is no definitive evidence that high-dose chemotherapy with HSCT support offers a survival advantage over conventional therapy in metastatic or high-risk breast cancer.[31-34] A number of clinical trials suggested that increased dose intensity could produce better response rates and prolong the median time to progression, but did not demonstrate survival benefits.[31-34] Some centers continue to perform autologous HSCT for breast cancer.

Neuroblastoma. Neuroblastoma is the most frequent pediatric solid tumor treated with HSCT. Approximately 60% of patients have advanced disease and only a 10% chance of cure with conventional therapy. Studies of autologous HSCT in these patients suggests an overall 5-year DFS of 20% to 40%. Again, the small number of patients and the brief follow-up make these results encouraging but inconclusive. Further clinical trials are needed to determine if autologous HSCT provides optimal treatment.

NONMALIGNANT DISEASES

Aplastic Anemia. Allogeneic HSCT is responsible for approximately an 80% overall survival rate in patients with aplastic anemia. Patients who have had blood product transfusions before HSCT have a higher rate of graft rejection. Therefore, at the time of diagnosis, HLA typing is done on the entire family. All patients younger than age 45 should be considered for HSCT. Although patients are immunosuppressed because of the disease, a conditioning regimen is usually administered. This is especially important for patients who have received transfusions because of the increased possibility of rejection.

Severe Combined Immunodeficiency Syndrome. The earliest successful HSCTs were in patients with SCIDS. Most patients with SCIDS die within 1 year of diagnosis, and because this disease occurs so early in life, a matched sibling donor may be unavailable. Therefore, the use of a haplo-identical parent and, in some patients, matched unrelated donors is considered. Approximately 70% of patients receiving a matched HSCT will be cured. The survival rate is slightly lower for patients receiving a haplo-identical parent match because of the increased incidence of graft rejection and GVHD. Because the disease has already immunosuppressed the patient, no conditioning regimen is usually given.

Hematopoietic Stem Cell Transplantation Process

PRETREATMENT WORK-UP

An extensive evaluation is performed on the HSCT recipient before transplant. This is done to establish the recipient's physical and psychosocial status. For allogeneic transplants, the donor is also thoroughly assessed. The assessment is done on an outpatient basis and includes a variety of tests, procedures, and consultations (Box 23-1). A team approach is usually used and typically includes psychology, social work, surgery, chaplaincy, and radiology in addition to nursing and medicine.

The patient's family and significant others are also included in this process. These evaluations alert the HSCT team to potential problems, such as physical hindrances, negative coping mechanisms, or financial difficulties. It also ensures that the patient has adequate support systems to help him throughout the rigorous HSCT process.

CONDITIONING REGIMENS

The conditioning regimen is the process of preparing the patient to receive bone marrow or stem cells. It accomplishes two vital functions, obliterating the malignant disease and destroying the patient's preexisting immunologic state, to allow for the proliferation of the transplanted stem cells. In effect, conditioning regimens destroy the patient's own bone marrow. The proliferation of new erythrocytes, leukocytes, and platelets cannot occur unless new functioning stem cells are given to the patient. On completion of the conditioning regimen, the patient must receive a transplant or die. The conditioning regimen consists of high-dose chemotherapy (HDCT) with or without total-body irradiation (TBI). Cyclophosphamide, carmustine, etoposide, busulfan, and cytarabine are all common chemotherapeutic agents used in conditioning regimens. The regimen chosen depends on the disease, previous radiation or chemotherapy, and the response.

BOX 23-1   Pretransplantation Evaluation

Hematopoietic Stem Cell Recipient
History and physical examination
Bone marrow biopsy and aspiration with cytogenetics
Chemistry profile
Complete blood count, platelets and reticulocyte counts
ABO and Rh typing and transfusion history
Coagulation profile
Serum immunoelectrophoresis
Quantitative immunoglobulins
Hepatitis screen
Titers: CMV, HIV, HSV, EBV, VZV
History of previous infections
Renal evaluation, urinalysis, creatinine clearance
Chest x-ray film
Electrocardiogram, echocardiogram
Pulmonary function testing
Sinus x-ray film
Audiology consult
Physical therapy consult
Dental consult–nutritional status assessment
Dietary consult
Social work consult
Psychology or psychiatry consult
Surgery consult, insertion of multilumen catheter

Hematopoietic Stem Cell Donor
History and physical examination
Chemistry profile
Complete blood count, platelet count
ABO and Rh typing
Hepatitis screen
Titers: CMV, HIV, HSV, West Nile virus
Chest x-ray film
Electrocardiogram
Urinalysis

CMV, Cytomegalovirus; *EBV*, Epstein-Barr virus; *HIV*, human immunodeficiency virus; *HSV*, herpes simplex virus; *VZV*, varicella-zoster virus

In addition to severe myelosuppression, patients may experience additional side effects including nausea and vomiting, mucositis, alopecia, fever, diarrhea, and bleeding. Most of these are immediate responses to the chemotherapy and radiation and may continue for several weeks after transplantation. Side effects management focuses on control of symptoms, prevention of further complications, and patient comfort. Long-term effects, such as cataracts and gonadal dysfunction, also can occur and are discussed in the section on complications.

NONMYELOABLATIVE CONDITIONING REGIMENS

Nonmyeloablative conditioning regimens are also considered. Nonmyeloablative regimens are used for allogeneic and autologous transplant in a wide range of malignant and nonmalignant diseases.[35,36] Most of the nonmyeloablative transplants are performed on adults with hematologic malignancies, although there has been an increased use in children, particularly for conditions such as congenital immunodeficiencies and chronic granulomatous disease.[37] This may provide an alternative in patients who could not tolerate the toxicities associated with traditional allogeneic transplant. Appropriate patients are those over the age of 55 or those with preexisting organ damage.[37,38] Nonmyeloablative transplants have also been called minitransplants, as well as low-intensity transplants; however, "reduced-intensity transplant" is the preferred terminology. Nonmyeloablative transplant is based on the view that the immune-mediated graft-versus-tumor effect provides the disease cure, not the conditioning regimen itself.[35,36,39] The best outcomes are seen in less aggressive diseases and lower proliferation rates, which allows for more time for a graft-versus-malignancy effect to take place.[40] Regimens which remain under investigation include fludarabine, single-dose TBI, or a combination of both, and have shown engraftment similar to conventional allogeneic transplants.[38] Due to the wide range of diseases being treated with transplant, optimal regimens will vary.[38,41]

TRANSPLANTATION OF MARROW, STEM CELLS, AND CORD BLOOD

After completion of the conditioning regimen, the bone marrow, peripheral stem cells, or cord blood must be infused. If the patient received prior chemotherapy protocols, a rest period of 24 to 72 hours is allotted before transplant owing to the drug's half life. Most patients describe the actual transplantation of marrow as quite anticlimactic compared to the donor search, the extensive pretreatment work-up, and the toxic conditioning regimen.

For autologous transplant, the frozen stem cells are brought to the recipient's room for transplant. The bag of cells is thawed in a normal saline bath, drawn up in large syringes, and given through a rapid intravenous (IV) push via central venous catheter. The bag of cells can also be hung and transfused. The process takes approximately 20 to 30 minutes, depending on the volume of cells being transplanted. Patients may experience minimal shortness of breath from the rapid infusion of the stem cells, as well as nausea and vomiting from the dimethylsulfoxide (DMSO) preservative. DMSO gives off a strange, garliclike odor as it is excreted through the patient's respiratory system for 24 to 48 hours after autologous transplant.

For allogeneic transplant, stem cells are infused on the same day as they are collected. This procedure resembles an RBC transfusion in that the bag of marrow is hung and transfused via the patient's central venous catheter. Unfiltered tubing must be used to prevent precious stem cells from becoming trapped and not administered. The total time of infusion is dose dependent, usually lasting between 1 and 5 hours. Possible side effects from an allogeneic transplant are similar to RBC transfusion reactions including shortness of breath, chills, fever, rash, chest pain, and hypotension. Reactions are more likely to occur with ABO-incompatible marrow. Reactions are treated with diphenhydramine, hydrocortisone, epinephrine, and oxygen therapy as necessary.

The allogeneic transplant of cord blood is similar to the transplant of frozen bone marrow or stem cells. The bags are thawed and the small volume of cord blood is infused via rapid IV push or hung as a brief infusion. DMSO is used as a cryoprotectant for cord blood, and patients may experience side effects as mentioned above. Diphenhydramine and/or hydrocortisone may be used to prevent or minimize these reactions.

Emergency equipment is always available at the patient's bedside. The physician should be available throughout the entire transplant. The nursing responsibilities include closely monitoring vital signs, assessing anaphylaxis reactions, and patient/family education. The patient and family and/or significant others have been thoroughly educated before the procedure; however, further questions are inevitable, as well as high levels of anxiety in both the patient and loved ones. Patients may view their transplant day as a "birthday" of sorts, because in their eyes they are given a new chance at life.

ENGRAFTMENT PERIOD

The engraftment period is the time immediately after transplant, when the transfused stem cells migrate, by some unknown phenomenon, to the recipient's bone marrow space and begin to regenerate. The time to engraftment varies depending upon the source of the stem cells. Bone marrow typically takes 2 to 3 weeks. PBSCs may engraft as early as 5 days; however, the average is 11 to 16 days after stem cell reinfusion. Cord blood takes an average of 26 days but may take as long as 42 days to engraft. During engraftment the patient experiences severe pancytopenia and immunosuppression. Immediate complications include infection and bleeding, and patient care focuses on prevention and early treatment. Patients typically receive antibiotics and blood components during this time.

Immediately after transplant, one goal is to shorten the length of the pancytopenic period and curtail these complications. Hematopoietic growth factors aid in this process (see Chapter 24).[42] These include, but are not limited to, GM-CSF and G-CSF, which affect the function of mature myeloid cells and the body's ability to stimulate the proliferation of myeloid precursor cells at various stages of differentiation.

G-CSF has been shown to accelerate neutrophil engraftment in both allogeneic and autologous transplants.[43]

Studies of erythropoietin in transplant patients continue. A review of the studies has shown a decrease in the need for RBC transfusions in the allogeneic population.[43] The efficacy of erythropoietin following autologous transplant remains to be seen.[43] Balancing the benefit of erythropoietin against the cost of therapy remains a significant issue.[43]

Complications of Hematopoietic Stem Cell Transplantation

Transplant recipients experience toxic complications associated with the procedure. Most complications result from the effects of the conditioning regimen. The major complications characteristic of transplant are infections, pneumonitis, veno-occlusive disease, GVHD, recurrence of original disease, and graft failure.

INFECTION

Infection is the most common posttransplant complication. Alterations in the integrity of physical barriers and severe granulocytopenia from the pretransplant regimen set up an environment for serious bacterial and fungal infections. One half of all infections occur in the first 4 to 6 weeks after transplant. Usually the causative agents are from the patient's own microflora, particularly from the gastrointestinal (GI) tract and integumentary system. Common agents are gram-positive and gram-negative bacteria such as *Staphylococcus, Streptococcus, Klebsiella*, and *Pseudomonas*. Fungal infections were considered less common than bacterial infections; however, these are increasing in incidence, and account for 10% to 15% of systemic infections.[44]

The use of prophylactic fluconazole has decreased the incidence of candidiasis; leaving aspergillus has the most common posttransplant fungal infection.[45] A number of *Candida* species have become resistant to fluconazole.[44,46] A number of emerging fungal species such as *Fusarium, Alternaria,* and *Scedosporium* are being recognized.[45,47,48]

Viral infections occur at varying times after HSCT. Herpes simplex virus (HSV) reactivation generally occurs in the early posttransplant period, but its incidence can be dramatically decreased in seropositive patients who receive prophylactic acyclovir.[49] Cytomegalovirus (CMV) infection generally occurs 3 to 6 months after transplant. With new early detection techniques available and the preemptive approach of treating with ganciclovir at reactivation, the incidence of CMV disease has decreased.[46,49,50] Varicella-zoster virus (VZV) is usually not seen until a later point during the first year after transplant.[49] Viral infections, CMV and VZV in particular, are also associated with the incidence of chronic GVHD and can occur at any time during its course.

During the first 6 weeks after HSCT, prevention of infection is crucial. Maintaining protective environments, providing good hygiene, frequently monitoring vital signs, and head-to-toe assessments are essential. The greater the speed of marrow recovery, the lower the incidence of bacterial and fungal complications. Therefore the use of growth factors to stimulate engraftment has become routine.

PULMONARY COMPLICATIONS

Interstitial pneumonia accounts for 40% of transplant-related deaths.[51] During the early posttransplant neutropenic period, bacterial infections account for 20% to 50% of pulmonary infections.[52] Interstitial pneumonia typically occurs within the first 100 days after transplant. The risk factors for developing pneumonia include use of immunosuppressants, lung damage, use of TBI, and presence of opportunistic organisms.[52]

Interstitial pneumonia can be caused by an infection or TBI, or it can be idiopathic. The most common viral cause is CMV. It is important that all patients and donors are screened for CMV before transplant so patients at risk can receive the appropriate treatment. Screening consists of serologic testing for CMV antibodies. In an allogeneic transplant a seropositive donor can transmit CMV to a seronegative recipient. Patients who are CMV seropositive or have a seropositive donor generally receive ganciclovir as prophylaxis. Ganciclovir is initiated after the patient is well engrafted. Lung damage can also be caused by carmustine and TBI, although this does not usually manifest until 3 to 4 months after transplant. When recognized early and treated with steroids, the damage is reversible.

VENO-OCCLUSIVE DISEASE

Veno-occlusive disease (VOD) of the liver occurs in approximately 20% of patients undergoing allogeneic HSCT and 10% of patients undergoing autologous HSCT. Mortality rates of up to 50% have been reported.[53] VOD is a complication of the conditioning regimen; the risk is greater for those patients receiving TBI. VOD is the occlusion of the central veins of the liver resulting in venous congestion and stasis; this results in damage to the hepatic cells. The onset of VOD is usually within the first 3 weeks after HSCT, but may occur later. VOD is usually diagnosed by its classic symptoms of weight gain greater than 5% over baseline, hepatomegaly, right upper quadrant pain, total serum bilirubin level above 2 mg/dl, and ascites. Risk factors include a history of hepatitis, elevated transaminase at the time of transplant, mismatched or unrelated transplant, and the use of methotrexate as GVHD prophylaxis.[53,54]

Treatment is aimed at maintaining intravascular volume to minimize further liver damage and maintain renal perfusion. Other treatment approaches remain controversial. Low-dose heparin infusions have been used for prophylaxis and treatment; some studies show favorable results in decreasing the incidence of VOD, but results are inconclusive.[55] Ursodeoxycholic acid used as prophylaxis for VOD has been shown to be safe and effective in some studies.[54] Recombinant tissue plasminogen activator (rTPA), a thrombolytic agent, has been used to treat VOD, and early studies show it to be effective in about 50% of patients; however, unacceptable rates of bleeding have been reported.[55] Infusions of antithrombin III (AT III) concentrate in patients with documented AT III deficiency have been used to treat VOD and appear to be a promising inervention.[56] Defibrotide has no intrinsic anticoagulation properties and is well tolerated. Results from compassionate use studies have reported survival rates of 42%.[55,57]

GRAFT-VERSUS-HOST DISEASE

Graft-versus-host disease is a complication that can occur after allogeneic transplantation. It is an immune-mediated reaction of the newly grafted stem cells to the body of the recipient.[58] The source of stem cells can affect the incidence of GVHD. Stem cells from UCB appear to cause less GVHD. There does not appear to be a significant difference in the incidence of acute GVHD with the use of allogeneic PBSCs, but the incidence of chronic GVHD is higher, and it is more difficult to treat.[59] Following nonmyeloablative transplants, manifestations of acute GVHD commonly are delayed beyond 100 days and may emerge as more typical manifestations of chronic GVHD.[60]

Two types of GVHD have been identified: acute and chronic. They are distinguished from each other by the target organs, the pathologic features, and the timing after BMT. Chronic GVHD may or may not occur after acute GVHD. A patient may also develop chronic GVHD without ever having had acute GVHD.

Acute GVHD. Acute GVHD is typically defined as occurring before 100 days after HSCT. There is a 30% to 60% incidence in HLA-matched sibling donor transplants and greater than 75% incidence in HLA-mismatched related donor transplants and unrelated donor transplants.[58] The risk factors related to the incidence of acute GVHD are advanced patient age (over 45 years), HLA mismatch, and donor-recipient gender mismatch.[58] The skin, the GI tract, and the liver are the primary target organs of acute GVHD. The occurrence of acute GVHD also prolongs immunodeficiency and increases the risk of infection.

Skin involvement is characterized by a maculopapular rash that can proceed to a desquamating dermatitis. A biopsy of the skin is necessary to confirm the diagnosis and rule out other causes for the rash. In the first 20 days after HSCT, this can be difficult because of changes in the skin related to the conditioning regimen. The GI involvement is typically characterized by nausea, vomiting, and diarrhea. Again, a biopsy of the GI mucosa is the only definitive way to make a diagnosis. The pathologic changes seen in the GI tract are similar to those seen in the skin. In both the skin and the GI mucosa, secondary infections can occur because the acute GVHD has altered their integrity. Liver involvement is characterized by jaundice, elevated liver function studies, and hepatomegaly.

Acute GVHD can range from mild to life-threatening and is graded to distinguish its severity (Table 23-4). In its mildest form, acute GVHD typically can be controlled and actually benefits those patients receiving transplants for malignancies, since patients with acute GVHD have a decreased incidence of disease recurrence.

Because acute GVHD can be a life-threatening complication, means of preventing its occurrence are routinely administered. The most common medications used to prevent GVHD are cyclosporine, corticosteroids, mycophenolate mofetil (MMF), tacrolimus, and methotrexate (MTX).[58] All these agents provide immunosuppression after HSCT and are given according to a scheduled regimen. Because GVHD is immune-mediated, suppressing immune reactions after HSCT should prevent its occurrence. The T cells have been identified as the primary culprit in GVHD. Depleting the marrow of T cells before infusion into the recipient has greatly reduced the incidence and severity of acute GVHD. However, the incidence of graft rejection and relapse is also significantly increased.

Treatment for acute GVHD centers around increasing immune suppression. Often, first-line therapy for GVHD is glucocorticoids in moderate to high doses.[58] Antithymocyte globulin (ATG) is often used as second-line therapy. Increasing the doses of cyclosporine or tacrolimus may also be beneficial, but serum drug levels must be closely monitored. MMF shows promise in the treatment of GVHD. About 50% of patients with grade II or III GVHD respond to treatment. The mortality rate can be as high as 50%.

Chronic GVHD. Chronic GVHD is a systemic alloimmune and autoimmune disorder.[59,61] The onset of chronic GVHD is arbitrarily defined as occurring 100 days after transplant; however, it can also occur at 70 days or years after transplant.[60] It affects as many as 50% to 60% of transplant patients and is life-threatening in about 5% of cases.[58] Chronic GVHD is characterized by scleroderma-like features and persistent immunodeficiency. It is a systemic multiorgan syndrome that resembles

TABLE 23-4	Acute Graft-Versus-Host Disease (GVHD) Severity Grading		
STAGE	SKIN	LIVER	GI TRACT
+	Maculopapular rash over <25% of body surface	Bilirubin 2-3 mg/dl	Diarrhea >500 ml/day
++	Maculopapular rash over 25%-30% of body surface	Bilirubin 3-6 mg/dl	Diarrhea >1000 ml/day
+++	Generalized erythroderma	Bilirubin 6-15 mg/dl	Diarrhea >1500 ml/day
++++	Generalized erythroderma with bullous formation (>2-cm vesicle) and desquamation	Bilirubin >15 mg/dl	Severe abdominal pain with or without ileus

collagen-vascular diseases.[61] Chronic GVHD can be **progressive,** a continuation of acute GVHD, **quiescent,** occurring after acute GVHD has resolved, or it can be **de novo,** occurring without any acute GVHD preceding it.[60,61] The risk factors related to incidence are advanced age of recipient (over 45 years), occurrence of preceding acute GVHD, T cell–replete marrow, and female donor to male recipient.[61]

Almost every organ in the body can be affected by chronic GVHD. The basic effect is that of dermal thickening, fibrosis, and dryness. Bacterial, fungal, and viral infections are common in patients with chronic GVHD and are the most frequent cause of death.[61] Late interstitial pneumonitis occurs frequently. Mortality is highest in patients with progressive acute to chronic GVHD and those with multiorgan involvement.[61] Currently, standard treatment for chronic GVHD is prednisone and cyclosporine; it is effective in approximately 50% of cases.[61] Other approaches have been used such as tacrolimus, MMF, phototherapy and extracorporeal photopheresis (ECP), ATG, and thalidomide.[60] Patients who fail to respond to prednisone have poor outcomes.[60]

RECURRENCE

Disease recurrence remains the most significant problem after transplantation. It is the major factor related to patient mortality more than 3 months after HSCT. Relapse is more frequent after autologous HSCT, presumably because of hidden malignant cells in the transplanted stem cells. In allogeneic transplantation the presence of GVHD is associated with decreased incidence of recurrence. Some patients have been successfully retransplanted. Factors associated with better survival after a second transplant are a diagnosis of CML, AML in remission, good performance status, and duration of posttransplant remission longer than 1 year.

GRAFT FAILURE

Graft failure or rejection after transplant is a relatively rare occurrence, but an incidence of 5% to 15% has been reported.[62] **Graft failure** is defined as failure of marrow recovery to occur or the loss of marrow function after an initial period of recovery.[62] An increased risk of graft failure is seen in patients who receive T cell–depleted marrow, a low marrow cell dose, or HLA-mismatched marrow or who have extensive marrow fibrosis before HSCT. Patients with aplastic anemia who have been previously transfused or receive only cyclophosphamide for their conditioning regimen are at an increased risk for graft failure.

LATE EFFECTS

Long-term effects of HSCT can occur several months to several years after transplant. Late effects are a common concern, since more patients survive disease-free for as long as 20 years after HSCT. The more common effects are cataracts, hypothyroidism, growth failure, gonadal dysfunction, and secondary malignancies. The late effects of HSCT are of particular concern in the pediatric population and for patients with the possibility of cure with less intensive treatment.

Cataracts. Cataracts are of concern primarily in patients who receive TBI. Because radiation is now given in fractionated doses, the incidence of cataracts has decreased. Patients receiving TBI in a single dose have an 80% incidence of cataracts as opposed to a 20% incidence when TBI is given in fractionated doses.[61,63] Patients receiving conditioning regimens of chemotherapy only do not have significant risk of developing cataracts.[63]

Gonadal Dysfunction. Sexual development is impaired in both men and women. Older patients (over 40 years) are less likely to recover their reproductive functioning.[64,65] After TBI, most women (75%) experience ovarian failure and require hormone replacement.[61,64,65] After TBI, most men will recover production of testosterone but have absent or abnormal spermatogenesis.[64,65] If TBI is not used as part of the conditioning regimen, both men and women have a better chance of recovering gonadal functioning. There are several reports of patients having children after transplant.[64,65]

Growth Failure. Impairment of growth is a common problem in children after transplantation. Again, the incidence is high in those children who received TBI.[61,64,65] Of children who received TBI, 50% to 60% have decreased growth hormone, causing a retardation of both spinal growth and the pubertal growth spurt.[64,65] Administration of growth hormone has shown some effect on growth velocity, especially if given during the prepubertal period where some catch-up in growth can occur.[65,66]

Hypothyroidism. The incidence of hypothyroidism is also related to preparation with TBI. Thyroid function is affected in as many as 60% of patients receiving single-dose TBI and as many as 25% of those receiving fractionated TBI.[64,65] Patients who have received conditioning regimens of chemotherapy only usually have normal thyroid function; however, the cyclophosphamide + busulfan regimen has been reported to affect thyroid function 11% of the time.[64,65]

Secondary Malignancy. New malignancies may develop 6 months to years after HSCT. A 4% to 6% incidence of secondary malignancies has been reported in long-term survivors of allogeneic HSCT.[61] TBI, immunosuppression, immunodeficiency, viral infection, chronic immune stimulation, and genetic predisposition are factors that have been identified with increased risk of second malignancy after HSCT.[61] Radiation appears to be the most important risk factor.[65] Lymphoproliferative disorders such as ALL, and non-Hodgkin's lymphoma are among the most frequently reported new malignancies and develop more often in donor cells.[67] The appearance of leukemia is most often a recurrence of the original disease. Overall, HSCT recipients have sixfold to sevenfold the tumor incidence of nontransplanted individuals.[63]

Quality of Life and Survivorship. Interest on the part of researchers in quality of life after HSCT has increased in recent years. A number of studies have been done to assess quality of life at various intervals after transplant. A number of tools have been used to collect this information. Some examples are Medical Outcomes Study-Short Form, City of Hope Quality of Life Bone Marrow Transplant, and Functional Assessment of Cancer Therapy Bone Marrow Transplant. There is a need for more research in this area to develop better tools and determine the best times to measure quality of life throughout the transplant process.[63,68] Many HSCT survivors report relatively normal physical and social functioning and perception of quality of life; however, deficits such as low self-esteem, psychologic distress, occupational disability, and impaired social, marital, and family relationships are also reported.[61]

Accreditation

In 1996, the Foundation for the Accreditation of Cellular Therapy (FACT) established standards encompassing all aspects of hematopoietic stem cell collection, processing, and transplant.

FACT was created by the International Society for Hematotherapy and Graft Engineering (ISHAGE) and the American Society of Blood and Marrow Transplantation (ASBMT). The major goal of FACT is to promote quality transplant programs. Accreditation is voluntary; however, third-party payers are looking at FACT accreditation as a standard for reimbursement. As of June 2005, more than 120 transplant centers in the United States were FACT-accredited.[69]

Future Directions and Advances in Hematopoietic Stem Cell Transplantation

According to data from the IBMTR, the number of patients undergoing HSCT continues to increase annually. Future advances will include the use of cord blood stem cells for gene therapy, because they are more efficient at taking up genes than are stem cells from other sources; fetal therapy; transplanting stem cells in utero for patients with congenital diseases such as SCIDS; and expansion of stem cells in the laboratory so fewer stem cells will be needed. The donor pool will continue to expand as the number of donors in the NMDP registry increases.

Outpatient resources and transplantation via the outpatient mode will continue to expand. Third-party reimbursement, length of hospital stay, and financial resources for medications used in transplant recovery will continue to undergo scrutiny.

Ongoing research will continue to look for better conditioning regimens and more effective treatments for infection and GVHD. Manipulation of the immune response against tumor cells following transplant using cellular therapy and cytokines is being explored. Use of peripheral blood CD34+ cells for gene therapy is also under investigation, as is combining immunotherapy with transplant. Expansion of hematopoietic stem cells in vitro is under active investigation. Successful expansion of stem cells could enhance engraftment, reduce the risk of infection, and potentially increase the number of available donors.[70]

Considerations for Older Adults

HSCT has become an accepted treatment option for many older patients; however, it is not appropriate therapy for all older patients. Care must be taken to look at individual cases. HSCT is an intensive treatment with relatively high comorbidity and mortality. Patients must be evaluated for any comorbidities, organ dysfunction, and previous treatments received, as well as emotional health and support systems to ensure that they have a reasonable chance for a positive outcome. Nonmyeloablative transplant has made this therapy available to patients who, in the past, would not have been able to undergo transplant; however, it is still a procedure with significant risks, and the decision to transplant should not be made lightly.

Conclusion

Hematopoietic stem cell transplantation, regardless of the source of stem cells, offers cure and new hope for the future to many patients with life-threatening diseases. Continued expansion of the donor pool and ongoing research exploring better conditioning regimens, hematopoietic growth factors, and antibiotic, antifungal, and antiviral drugs will be ongoing challenges. Financial reimbursement issues will continue to be a challenge; managed care is already having an impact. Many insurance companies are already expecting transplant centers to negotiate a fixed price; this will increase competition among transplant centers, because the lowest bidder will get the contracts and therefore the patients. Many third-party payers already require transplant centers to sign contracts as "centers of excellence" or preferred providers. Patients will no longer be able to choose a transplant center. There will be ongoing debate about which indications for transplantation are experimental. Transplantation is constantly changing, but this challenging practice environment will continue to provide opportunities for skilled nurses.

REVIEW QUESTIONS

✓ Case Study

Bob, a 38-year-old married father of three, was diagnosed 2 years ago with CML in chronic phase. At the time of diagnosis Bob started a course of imatinib mesylate. Bob's disease remained stable until 2 months ago, when he was noted to be in accelerated phase. At the time of diagnosis, Bob's three siblings were HLA-typed; none were found to be a match. A preliminary search of the NMDP found several potential matches at that time. At the time Bob's disease accelerated, a formal search of the registry was initiated and an HLA-identical match was found. During Bob's pretransplant work-up he was found to have slightly elevated liver function tests and had a history of hepatitis B.

Bob received a nonmyeloablative conditioning regimen of fludarabine and low-dose TBI. Bob engrafted on day 23 after transplant, following an uneventful transplant course, and was discharged from the hospital. Bob developed a fever 2 weeks later and was readmitted to the hospital. He was started on broad-spectrum antibiotics; however, his fever did not resolve. Five days later Bob was started on amphotericin because of his persistent fevers. During this time Bob developed a maculopapular skin rash and diarrhea. At the time it was unclear if these symptoms were evidence of GVHD or a reaction to antibiotics. The nursing staff began a skin care regimen consisting of steroid creams and barrier creams to the perirectal area to prevent skin breakdown. A skin biopsy revealed grade II GVHD of the skin. Bob was started on a course of glucocorticoids and cyclosporine to treat the GVHD. Bob's fevers persisted, and the nursing and medical staff were concerned that Bob had developed an infection. However, all diagnostic testing and cultures remained normal. Bob became discouraged as the fevers persisted.

Bob's wife returned to their home in another state. It was necessary for her to return to work for Bob's health care insurance to continue. The nurses and social workers met with the medical team to address Bob's psychosocial issues. At the insistence of the nursing staff, a care conference with the entire team and family was held. The conference provided an opportunity for Bob and his wife to ask questions about his condition and prognosis and for the team to assist in identifying another family member who was able to come and stay with Bob. Two weeks later, Bob was discharged with his GVHD well controlled.

QUESTIONS

1. The donor in an autologous stem cell transplant is which of the following?
   a. A close relative
   b. The patient
   c. A donor from the registry
   d. The donor's parent

2. Nonmyeloablative conditioning regimens are generally used for which patients?
   a. All patients under consideration for transplant
   b. Only young, healthy patients
   c. Patients with organ damage or over 55
   d. Patients from New Jersey

3. What is the most important factor in identifying a potential stem cell donor?
   a. Donor size
   b. Degree of HLA match
   c. Blood type of donor
   d. Donor ethnicity

4. Currently, what is the only "cure" for CML?
   a. Allogeneic transplantation
   b. Autologous transplantation
   c. Interferon
   d. Imatinib mesylate

5. What is the primary purpose of the pretransplant work-up?
   a. To identify potential donors
   b. To determine the patient's physical and emotional readiness for transplant
   c. To allow an opportunity for the patient and donor to meet
   d. To diagnose the patient's underlying disease

6. How is *mobilization* defined?
   a. Stimulating the production of PRBCs before collection
   b. Moving the patient to the transplant center
   c. The process of collecting the PBSCs
   d. The process of collecting bone marrow

7. What is the most common posttransplantation complication?
   a. Graft rejection
   b. Infection
   c. Pneumonitis
   d. Veno-occlusive disease

8. Medications used in prevention of GVHD include which of the following?
   a. Cyclosporine, methotrexate, tacrolimus, and steroids
   b. Cyclosporine, tacrolimus, cytoxan, and steroids
   c. Cyclosporine, tacrolimus, cytarabine, and steroids
   d. Cyclosporine, tacrolimus, foscarnet, and steroids

9. GVHD of the skin poses what potential risks to the patient?
   a. Increased risk of infection.
   b. There are no risks.
   c. The risk is only cosmetic.
   d. There is no risk unless the liver and the gut are also involved.

10. When educating the patient and family about gut GVHD, it is important to include what information?
    a. GVHD of the gut is not a serious complication.
    b. GVHD of the gut is a potentially serious complication and must be controlled with systemic therapy.
    c. GVHD of the gut will go away on its own.
    d. GVHD of the gut does not increase the risk of infection.

ANSWERS

1. **B.** *Rationale:* In an autologous transplant the patient receives his or her own stem cells. They are typically cryopreserved while the patient is receiving the preparative regimen.

2. **C.** *Rationale:* Nonmyeloablative transplants are generally considered for patients over the age of 55 or with organ impairment such as elevated liver enzymes, or comorbidities such as diabetes, or mild heart disease.

3. **B.** *Rationale:* The most important factor in identifying potential donors is the degree of HLA match. HLA mismatch increases the risk of posttransplant complications such as graft failure, GVHD, and infection.

4. **A.** *Rationale:* Currently, only allogeneic transplant can cure CML. Other treatments can induce a remission, but do not eliminate the disease.

5. **B.** *Rationale:* The pretransplant work-up is a complex evaluation designed to determine if the patient is physically and emotionally able to withstand the rigors of the transplant process.

6. **A.** *Rationale:* Mobilization is the process by which stem cells are mobilized from the bone marrow into the peripheral blood circulation for collection.

7. **B.** *Rationale:* Infection is the most common complication following stem cell transplantation. Following transplant the patient is usually significantly immunosuppressed and at high risk for viral, bacterial, and fungal infections.

8. **A.** *Rationale:* Immunosuppressant medications are used following allogeneic transplant to prevent and/or treat GVHD. Medications such as cyclosporine, methotrexate, tacrolimus, and steroids are typically used.

9. **A.** *Rationale:* GVHD, regardless of site, increases the risk of infection. Skin breakdown due to GVHD provides a portal of entry for infectious organisms.

10. **B.** *Rationale:* GVHD of the gut requires aggressive treatment to prevent it from progressing. Systemic immunosuppressants are typically used.

REFERENCES

1. International Bone Marrow Transplant Registry: Current use and outcome of blood and marrow transplantation: part 1 of the 2003 BMT summary slide set, 2003, retrieved June 30, 2005, from http://ibmtr.org/summarysldset/summet1_files/
2. Kessenger A, Sharp JG: The whys and hows of hematopoietic progenitor and stem cell mobilization, *Bone Marrow Transpl* 31:319, 2003.
3. Takeyama K, Ohto H: PBSC mobilization, *Transfus Apheresis Sci* 31:233, 2004.
4. Ng-Cashin J, Shea T: Mobilizations of autologous peripheral blood hematopoietic cells for support of high-dose cancer therapy. In Blume KG, Forman SJ, Appelbaum FR, editors: *Thomas' hematopoietic cell transplantation*, ed 3, Malden, Mass, 2004, Blackwell Science.
5. Ford CD, Chen KJ, Reilly WF et al: An evaluation of predictive factors for CD34+ cell harvest yields form patients mobilized with chemotherapy and growth factors, *Transfus* 43:622, 2003.
6. Confer DL: Hematopoietic cell donors. In Blume KG, Forman SJ, Appelbaum FR, editors: *Thomas' hematopoietic cell transplantation*, ed 3, Malden, Mass, 2004, Blackwell Science.
7. Moog R: Apheresis techniques for collection of peripheral blood progenitor cells, *Transfus Apheresis Sci* 31:207, 2003.
8. Rowley SD: Cryopreservation of hematopoietic cells. In Blume KG, Forman SJ, Appelbaum FR, editors: *Thomas' hematopoietic cell transplantation*, ed 3, Malden, Mass, 2004, Blackwell Science.
9. Schmitz N: Peripheral blood hematopoietic cells for allogeneic transplantation. In Blume KG, Forman SJ, Appelbaum FR, editors: *Thomas' hematopoietic cell transplantation*, ed 3, Malden, Mass, 2004, Blackwell Science.
10. National Marrow Donor Program: History of marrow and blood cell transplants, March 2005, retrieved June 30, 2005, from http://www.marrow.org/NMDP/history_of_transplants.html.
11. Grewal SS, Barker JN, Davies SM et al: Unrelated donor hematopoietic cell transplantation: marrow or umbilical cord, *Blood* 101:4233, 2003.
12. National Cord Blood Program: Homepage, June 16, 2005, retrieved June 30, 2005, from http://www.nationalcordbloodprogram.org/.
13. National Marrow Donor Program: Likelihood of finding an unrelated donor or cord blood unit, January 2005, retrieved June 30, 2005 from http://www.marrow.org/PHYSICIAN/likelihood_of_finding.html.
14. Wagner JE, Barker JN, DeFor TE et al: Transplantation of unrelated donor umbilical cord blood in 102 patients with malignant and non-malignant diseases: influence of CD34 cell dose and HLA disparity on treatment-related mortality and survival, *Blood* 100:1611, 2002.
15. Barker JN, Weisdorf DJ, DeFor TE et al: Transplantation of 2 partially HLA-matched umbilical cord blood units to enhance engraftment in adults with hematologic malignancy, *Blood* 105:1343, 2005.
16. Barker JN, Weisdorf DJ, DeFor TE et al: Rapid complete donor chimerism in adult recipients of unrelated umbilical cord blood transplantation after reduced-intensity conditioning, *Blood* 102:1915, 2003.
17. Laughlin MJ, Eapen M, Rubinstein P et al: Outcomes after transplantation of cord blood or bone marrow from unrelated donors, *N Engl J Med* 351:2265, 2004.
18. Broxmeyer HE, Smith FO: Cord blood hematopoietic cell transplantation. In Blume KG, Forman SJ, Appelbaum FR, editors: *Thomas' hematopoietic cell transplantation*, ed 3, Malden, Mass, 2004, Blackwell Science.
19. Karanes C: Unrelated donor stem cell transplant: donor selection, *Pediatr Transpl* 7(suppl 3):59, 2003.
20. Mickelson E, Petersdorf EW: Histocompatibility. In Blume KG, Forman SJ, Appelbaum FR, editors: *Thomas' hematopoietic cell transplantation*, ed 3, Malden, Mass, 2004, Blackwell Science.
21. International Bone Marrow Transplant Registry: Current use and outcome of blood and marrow transplantation: part 2 of the 2003 BMT summary slide set, 2003, retrieved June 30, 2005, from http://www.ibmtr.org/summarysldset/summet2_files/.
22. National Marrow Donor Program: Changing trends in diseases and patients treated, January 2005, retrieved June 30, 2005, from http://www.marrow.org/PHYSICIAN/changes_trends.html.
23. National Marrow Donor Program: Transplant outcomes data by disease and disease stage, January 2005, retrieved June 30, 2005, from http://www.marrow.org/PHYSICIAN/transplant_outcomesdata.html.
24. Kiehl MG, Kraut L, Schwerdtfeger R et al: Outcome of allogeneic hematopoietic stem-cell transplantation in adult patients with acute lymphoblastic leukemia: no difference in related compared with unrelated transplant in first complete remission, *J Clinic Oncol* 22:2816, 2004.
25. Hoelzer D, Gokbuget N, Ottmann et al: Acute lymphocytic leukemia, *Hematology (Am Soc Hematol Educ Program)* 162:162-192, 2002.
26. Giles FJ, Keating A, Goldstone AH et al: Acute myelocytic leukemia, *Hematology (Am Soc Hematol Educ Program)* 73:73-110, 2002.
27. Maziarz RT, Mauro MJ: Transplantation for CML: yes, no, maybe so.... and Oregon perspective, *Bone Marrow Transpl* 32:459, 2003.
28. Locatelli F, Nollke P, Zecca M, et al: Hematopoietic stem cell transplantation (HSCT) in children with juvenile myelomonocytic leukemia (JMML): results of the EWOG-EBMT trial, *Blood* 105:410, 2005.
29. Greenberg PL, Young NS, Gattermann N: Myelodyplastic syndromes, *Hematology (Am Soc Hematol Educ Program)* 136:136-161, 2002.
30. Hahn T, Wingard JR, Anderson KC et al: The role of cytotoxic therapy with hematopoietic stem cell transplant in the therapy of multiple myeloma: an evidence-based review, *Biol Blood Marr Trans* 9:37, 2003.
31. Gerrero RM, Stein S, Stadtmauer EA: High-dose chemotherapy and stem cell support for breast cancer: where are we now, *Drugs Aging* 19:475, 2002.
32. Dicato M: High-dose chemotherapy in breast cancer: where are we now, *Semin Oncol* 29:16, 2002.
33. Roche H, Viens P, Biron P et al: High-dose chemotherapy for breast cancer: The French PEGASE experience, *Cancer Control* 10:42, 2003.
34. Tartarone A, Romano R, Galasso R et al: Should we continue to study high-dose chemotherapy in metastatic breast cancer patients? A critical review of published data, *Bone Marrow Transpl* 31:525, 2004.
35. Slavin S: Reduced-intensity conditioning or nonmyeloablative stem cell transplantation: introduction, rationale and historic background, *Semin Oncol* 31:1, 2004.
36. Djulbegovic B, Seidenfeld J, Bonnell C et al: Nonmyeloablative allogeneic stem-cell transplantation for hematologic malignancies: a systematic review, *Cancer Control* 10:17, 2003.
37. Schwartz JE, Yeager AM: Reduced-intensity allogeneic hematopoietic cell transplant: graft versus tumor effects with decreased toxicity, *Pediatr Trans* 7:168, 2003.
38. Maloney DG, Sandmaier BM, Mackinnon S et al: Non-myeloablative transplantation, *Hematology (Am Soc Hematol Educ Program)* 2002: 392-421, 2002.
39. Olszewski S: Nonmyeloablative bone marrow transplants, *Clin J Oncol Nurs* 7:675, 2003.
40. Anagostopoulos A, Giralt S: Critical review on non-myeloablative stem cell transplantation, *Crit Rev Oncol Hematol* 44:175, 2002.
41. Antin JH: Stem cell transplantation – harnessing of graft-versus-malignancy, *Curr Opin Hematol* 10:440, 2003.
42. West F, Mitchell SA: Evidence-based guidelines for the management of neutropenia following hematopoietic stem cell transplant, *Clin J Oncol Nurs* 8:601, 2004.
43. Finke J, Mertelsmann R: Recombinant growth factors after hematopoietic cell transplantation. In Blume KG, Forman SJ, Appelbaum FR, editors: *Thomas' hematopoietic cell transplantation*, ed 3, Malden, Mass, 2004, Blackwell Science.
44. Brown JMY: Fungal infections in BMT patients, *Curr Opin Infect Dis* 17:347, 2004.
45. Jahagivdar B, Morrison V: Emerging fungal pathogens in patients with hematologic malignancies and marrow/stem cell transplant recipients, *Semin Respir Infect* 17:113, 2002.
46. Nichols WG: Combating infections in hematopoietic stem cell transplant recipients, *Exper Rev Anti-infect Ther* 1:57, 2003.
47. Hamza NS, Ghannoum MA, Lazarus HM: Choices aplenty: antifungal prophylaxis in hematopoietic stem cell transplant recipients, *Bone Marrow Transpl* 43:377, 2004.
48. Wingard JR: The changing face of invasive fungal infections in hematopoietic cell transplant, *Curr Opin Oncol* 17:89, 2005.
49. No Author: Prevention and treatment of viral infections in stem cell transplant recipients, *Brit J Hematol* 118:44, 2002.
50. Meijer E, Boland GJ, Verdonck LF: Prevention of cytomegalovirus disease in recipients of allogeneic stem cell transplant, *Clin Micro Rev* 16:647, 2002.
51. Wah TM, Moss HA, Robertson RJH et al: Pulmonary complications following bone marrow transplantation, *Brit J Radiol* 76:373, 2003.
52. Paul K: Non-infectious lung complications after transplant, *Ann Hematol* 8(suppl 2):11, 2002.
53. Wadleigh M, Ho V, Momtaz P et al: Hepatic veno-occlusive disease: pathogenesis, diagnosis and current treatment, *Curr Opin Hematol* 10:451, 2003.

54. Barker CC, Butzner JD, Andersen RA et al: Incidence, survival and risk factors for the development of veno-occlusive disease in pediatric hematopoietic stem cell transplant, *Bone Marrow Transplant* 32:79, 2003.

55. Kumar S, DeLeve LD, Kamath PS et al: Hepatic veno-occlusive disease (sinusoidal obstruction syndrome) after hematopoietic stem cell transplantation *Mayo Clin Proc* 78:589, 2003.

56. Arai S, Lee L, Vogelsang G: A systematic approach to hepatic complications in hematopoietic stem cell transplantation, *J Hematother Stem Cell Res* 1:202, 2002.

57. Corbacioglu S, Greil J, Peters C et al: Defibrotide in the treatment of children with veno-occlusive disease (VOD): a retrospective multicentre study demonstrates therapeutic efficacy upon early intervention, *Bone Marrow Transpl* 33:189, 2004.

58. Pallera A, Schwartzberg L: Managing the toxicity of hematopoietic stem cell transplant, *J Support Oncol* 2:223, 2004.

59. Pavletic S, Smith L, Bishop: Prognostic factors of chronic graft-versus-host disease after allogeneic blood stem-cell transplantation, *Am J Hematol* 78:265, 2005.

60. Farag SS: Chronic graft-versus-host disease: where do we go from here? *Bone Marrow Transpl* 33:569, 2004.

61. Wingard JR, Vogelsang GB, Deeg HJ: Stem cell transplantation: supportive care and long term complications, *Hematology (Am Soc Hematol Educ Program)* 422:2002.

62. Wilson C, Sylvanus T: Graft failure following allogeneic blood and marrow transplant: evidence-based nursing case study review, *Clin J Oncol Nurs* 9:151, 2005.

63. No Author: Non-endocrine late complications of bone marrow transplantation in childhood: part II, *Brit J Hematol* 118:23, 2002.

64. No Author: Endocrine late effects after bone marrow transplant, *Brit J Hematol* 118:58, 2002.

65. Sanders JE: Endocrine complications of high-dose therapy with stem cell transplantation, *Pediatr Trans* 8(suppl 5):39, 2004.

66. Socie G, Tichelli A: Long-term care after stem-cell transplantation, *Hematol J* 5(suppl 3):S39, 2004.

67. Forrest DL, Nevill TJ, Naiman SC et al: Second malignancy following high-dose therapy with autologous stem cell transplantation: incidence and risk factor analysis, *Bone Marrow Transplant* 32:915, 2003.

68. Byar KL, Eilers JE, Nuss SL: Quality of life five or more years post-autologous hematopoietic stem cell transplant, *Cancer Nurs* 28:148, 2005.

69. Foundation for the Accreditation of Cellular Therapy: FACT general information, retrieved July 14, 2005, from http://www.unmc.edu/Community/fahct/About_FACT.htm.

70. Devine SM, Lazarus HM, Emerson SG: Clinical application of hematopoietic progenitor cell expansion: Current status and future prospects, *Bone Marrow Transpl* 31:241, 2003.

CHAPTER 24

Complications of Cancer and Cancer Treatment

Jamie S. Myers

Oncologic complications occur frequently in patients with cancer and may be a direct result of the disease. In these cases, presentation of the oncologic complications may be what precipitates the work-up and diagnosis of the malignancy. However, they are more frequently an indication of progressive or advancing disease. Oncologic complications also occur as a result of treatment for cancer. Acute, life-threatening oncologic complications are often referred to as oncologic emergencies.

Oncologic emergencies may be categorized in different ways. Woodard and Hogan[1] group them as follows: neurologic, cardiopulmonary, metabolic, hematologic, infectious, gastrointestinal, genitourinary, and infusion-related. They define oncologic emergencies as "clinical situations in which the condition is secondary to a malignancy or its treatment, and when there are potentially immediate catastrophic consequences in the absence of successful intervention" (Box 24-1).

The Oncology Nursing Society (ONS) *Core Curriculum for Oncology Nursing*[2] divides oncologic emergencies into two main categories: metabolic and structural. This chapter is organized according to the ONS categories (Box 24-2).

Management of an oncologic complication depends on many important factors related to the patient and the underlying disease (Box 24-3). These factors must be given thorough consideration before the initiation of treatment.

Once the oncologic complication is analyzed, decisions about the aggressiveness of treatment can be made. Aggressive treatment may be appropriate when the potential exists for a cure or prolonged survival. However, in advanced disease, palliative treatment may be given to reduce symptoms and restore functional status. Finally, withholding treatment and providing supportive care may be the most appropriate decision in the presence of disseminated metastatic disease.[3] Quality of life should always be the driving force in any decision regarding care of the patient with cancer. The overall goal is to prevent, reverse, or minimize life-threatening oncologic complications through prophylactic measures, early detection, and effective management.

Use of critical care interventions for patients with cancer has increased for a variety of reasons: new hope for cure or long-term remission, increased ability to treat certain complications, and consumer demands. Because of the urgent nature of oncologic complications, prevention, early recognition, adequate decision making, and prompt treatment are of paramount importance when delivering care to patients with cancer. Nurses are in a key role to accurately assess patients who are at high risk for complications.

Assessment is essential, because a change in the patient's condition may be subtle or dramatic. Two key concepts when caring for people with cancer are (1) the identification of patients at risk for developing an oncologic complication and (2) the involvement of the family and significant others. The patient and family require considerable education and support. Time limitations for patient and family education present a great challenge. Explanations of tests, procedures, and the rationale for changes in patient care or setting must be kept simple. Treatment options and goals of therapy must be explained and discussed. This is especially important when the realistic outcome is palliation. Nurses with demonstrated expertise in oncology are a vital component in the care of the patient with an oncologic emergency.

Structural Oncologic Complications

CARDIAC TAMPONADE

Definition

Neoplastic cardiac tamponade is the compression of the cardiac muscle by pathologic fluid accumulation under pressure within the pericardial sac. Fluid accumulates because of pericardial constriction by a tumor or postirradiation pericarditis.[4-6] Compression of the myocardium interferes with dilation of the heart chambers, which prevents adequate cardiac filling during diastole. This in turn reduces blood flow to the ventricles and reduces stroke volume, which results in decreased cardiac output. Other pressures changes that then occur include an elevated central venous pressure (CVP) and a lowered left atrial pressure (Fig. 24-1). Two compensatory mechanisms, initiated by adrenergic stimulation, attempt to counteract these pressures to increase cardiac output and maintain peripheral perfusion.[7] An increase in heart rate (tachycardia) helps maintain cardiac output at low stroke volumes and increases systolic emptying. Peripheral vasoconstriction maintains arterial pressure and venous return. If cardiac output is not increased by compensatory mechanisms, this can cause circulatory collapse, which is fatal if untreated.[3]

Etiology and Risk Factors

A variety of nonmalignant or malignant conditions may be responsible for the development of cardiac tamponade. *Nonmalignant causes* include the following[4,5]:

- Cardiovascular causes: heart surgery, chest trauma, aneurysm, rupture of the great vessel, cardiac procedures (angiography, insertion or removal of pacer wires), or insertion of central venous catheter
- Infectious pericarditis: bacterial, fungal, viral, or tubercular infections
- Connective tissue disorders: systemic lupus erythematosus (SLE), scleroderma, or rheumatoid disease

---

BOX 24-1 **Categories of Oncologic Emergencies**

Neurologic
Spinal cord compression
Intracranial malignancy
Seizures

Cardiopulmonary
Superior vena cava syndrome
Cardiac tamponade
Massive hemoptysis
Airway obstruction
Large pleural effusion

Metabolic
Hypercalcemia
Tumor lysis syndrome
Hyponatremia
Hypoglycemia
Adrenal failure

Hematologic
Thrombocytopenia
Thrombosis
Increased viscosity syndromes

Infectious
Neutropenic sepsis
Vascular access device–related sepsis

Gastrointestinal
Obstruction
Hemorrhage

Genitourinary
Obstruction
Hemorrhage

Infusion-Related
Allergic reactions
Extravasation

Data from Woodard WL III, Hogan DK: Oncologic emergencies: implications for nurses, *J Intravenous Nurs* 19(5):257, 1996.

- Myxedema
- Uremia
- Pharmacologic therapy: anthracyclines (doxorubicin, daunomycin, and others), anticoagulants (heparin, sodium warfarin), hydralazine (Apresoline), or procainamide (Procaine SR, Pronestyl)

Malignant causes include the following[4,5]:
- Neoplastic pericarditis with effusion: primary tumors of the pericardium (mesotheliomas, sarcomas, malignant teratomas) or metastatic tumors of the pericardium (lung cancer, breast tumors, leukemias, lymphomas, melanomas, and sarcomas)
- Neoplastic constrictive pericarditis (metastatic tumor infiltration)
- Radiation pericarditis (exposure of the heart to 400 Gy or more)

BOX 24-2 **ONS Core Curriculum: Oncologic Emergency Categories**

Structural
Cardiac tamponade
Increased intracranial pressure (ICP)
Spinal cord compression (SCC)
Superior vena cava syndrome (SVCS)

Metabolic
Disseminated intravascular coagulation (DIC)
Hypercalcemia
Hypersensitivity reaction (HSR) (anaphylaxis)
Sepsis
Syndrome of inappropriate antidiuretic hormone secretion (SIADH)
Tumor lysis syndrome (TLS)

Data from Gobel BH: Metabolic emergencies, and Hunter JC: Structural emergencies. In Itano JK, Taoka KN, editors: *Oncology Nursing Society core curriculum for oncology nursing*, ed 4, Philadelphia, 2005, Saunders.

BOX 24-3 **Management Factors in the Evaluation and Treatment of an Oncologic Emergency**

Symptoms and Signs
Are the symptoms and signs caused by the tumor or by complications of treatment?
How quickly are the symptoms of the oncologic emergency progressing?

Natural History of the Primary Tumor
Is there a previous diagnosis of malignancy?
What is the disease-free interval between the diagnosis of the primary tumor and the onset of the emergency?
Has the emergency developed in the setting of terminal disease?

Efficacy of Available Treatment
No prior therapy versus extensive pretreatment
Should treatment be directed at the underlying malignancy and/or the urgent complication?
Will the patient's general medical condition influence the ability to administer effective treatment?

Treatment and Goals
Potential for cure
Is prompt palliation required to prevent further debilitation?
What is the risk-versus-benefit ratio of treatment?
Should treatment be withheld if the patient is terminal with minimal chance of response to available antitumor therapies?

From Glover D, Glick JH: Oncologic emergencies. In Holleb AI, Fink DJ, Murphy GP, editors: *American Cancer Society textbook of clinical oncology*, ed 2, Atlanta, 1995, American Cancer Society. Reprinted with permission of the American Cancer Society, Inc.

Pericardial effusion with tamponade is a life-threatening problem whether the cause is malignant or nonmalignant. Cancer is the leading cause of cardiac tamponade in the United States.[8] Malignant pericardial tamponade occurs in approximately 5% to 15% of patients with a neoplasm that involves the heart.[9]

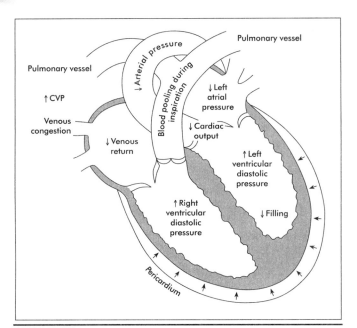

FIG. 24-1 Cardiovascular effects of increased intrapleural pressure. Intraventricular diastolic pressure rises as a result of higher intrapericardial pressure. This prevents adequate filling of the ventricle, causing venous congestion, decreased cardiac output, lowered left atrial pressure, and elevated central venous pressure (*CVP*). ↑, Increased; ↓, decreased. (From Dietz KA, Flaherty AM: Oncologic emergencies. In Groenwald SL and others, editors: *Cancer nursing: principles and practice*, ed 2, Boston, 1990, Jones & Bartlett. Reprinted with permission.)

The high estimates of this complication are based on compilations of autopsy data regarding cardiac (including pericardial) metastasis, which range from 0.1% to 21%.[10] The majority of these patients are asymptomatic, with only 20% to 30% showing clinical evidence of cardiac disease before death.[11]

Most cases of neoplastic cardiac tamponade represent metastatic invasion of the pericardium. Pericardial metastasis is unusual without documentation of other metastases. Only rarely is the cause primary disease of the myocardium (mesothelioma, angiosarcoma, fibrosarcoma, and malignant teratoma).[9] Any cancer has the potential for metastatic spread to the pericardium via direct tumor extension, lymphatic invasion, or hematogenous dissemination. Patients with pericardial effusions are at risk for tamponade. Pericardial effusions caused by metastatic disease are present in 5% to 50% of patients with cancer.[12] However, cancers that pose the greatest risk for the development of neoplastic cardiac tamponade include lung cancer, breast cancer, lymphoma, and leukemia, which accounts for 80% of this complication.[13] Other malignant causes are melanoma, gastrointestinal (GI) cancers, and sarcomas. Approximately 5% of patients who receive radiation therapy to the mediastinum (400 Gy or more) develop acute pericarditis with or without pericardial effusion during treatment, or chronic constrictive pericarditis up to 20 years after treatment. More than 90% of the cases occur in the first year after radiation treatment.[14]

Pathophysiology

The heart and a portion of the great vessels are encased in a thin, tough, double-layered fibrous sac called the pericardium, which contains little elastic tissue. The inner layer, or sheath, is

known as the visceral pericardium. It is a delicate serous membrane that lines the interior of the fibrous sac and is continuous with the surface of the heart.[14] The outer layer of the pericardium is called the parietal pericardium. This sheath is fibrous and provides strength and protection. The left sternal portion is in direct contact with the chest wall. Between the two layers of the pericardium is a cavity that contains 10 to 20 ml of a clear serous lubricating fluid, originating from the lymphatic channels surrounding the heart, and serving to cushion the myocardium.[14]

The pathophysiology of pericardial tamponade is a progressive accumulation of fluid in the pericardial sac (Fig. 24-2), which leads to compression of the heart, hampering dilation of its chambers and thus limiting diastolic atrial filling. The intrapericardial pressure rises, and bilateral ventricular stroke volume decreases. Initially the sac will stretch to accommodate increases in fluid, and compensatory mechanisms—an increased heart rate (tachycardia) and increased peripheral vascular tone (peripheral vasoconstriction)—maintain adequate cardiac output. However, as these temporary adaptive responses begin to fail, a vicious cycle of increased fluid with decreased atrial pressure, decreased cardiac output, and decreased venous return will progress to circulatory collapse and, if untreated, to shock, cardiac arrest, and death.

The severity of cardiac tamponade depends on the amount of fluid in the pericardium, the rate of accumulation, and the degree of pericardial and organic compromise. Usually there will be no change in cardiac activity with the addition of 50 ml or less of fluid in the pericardial space. Gradual fluid accumulation permits the pericardium to stretch and accommodate. As much as 2 L or more can accumulate without producing signs of cardiac compromise.[9] However, 100 to 200 ml of fluid may cause severe cardiac impairment if the accumulation occurs rapidly.[9] Whether gradual or acute, the fluid accumulation that leads to cardiac tamponade in the presence of malignant disease is the result of one of the following mechanisms[12]:

- Direct tumor (primary or metastatic) extension and blockage of the lymphatic drainage
- Malignant lymphatic engorgement and impairment of drainage
- Tumor (primary or metastatic) implantation in or around the pericardium with inflammation and fluid production
- Radiation-induced pericarditis of the pericardium with fluid accumulation

Retrograde lymphatic dissemination is thought to be the main pathway of pericardial metastasis, creating fluid seepage through the visceral pericardium and into the pericardial space.[10] Neoplastic cardiac tamponade related to malignant pericardial effusion, whether resulting from a constricting tumor, lymphatic dissemination, or postirradiation pericarditis, is a medical emergency and must be recognized and treated promptly.

Clinical Features

Patients with neoplastic cardiac tamponade manifest a wide variety of nonspecific clinical signs and symptoms. These are directly related to the amount and rapidity of onset of fluid accumulation and the resultant disruption of normal hemodynamics.[10] Small or slowly developing effusions may be asymptomatic. As fluid increases, the most common symptoms are dyspnea, tachycardia, retrosternal chest pain (usually relieved by sitting up and leaning forward), and a nonproductive cough.[10,15] Other symptoms can include fatigue, weakness, dizziness, palpitations,

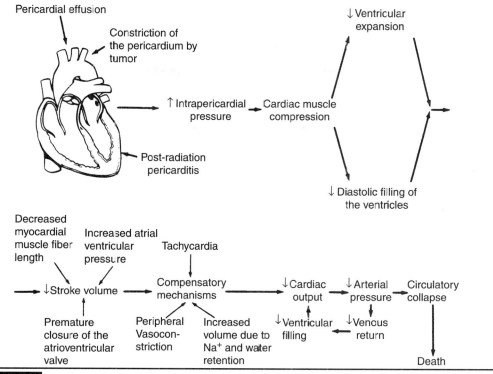

FIG. 24-2   Development of neoplastic pericardial tamponade. (From Yasko JM, Schafer SL: Neoplastic pericardial tamponade. In Yasko JM, editor: Guidelines for cancer care: Symptom management, Reston, VA, © 1983. Reprinted with permission of Prentice-Hall, Inc, Upper Saddle River, NJ.)

and orthopnea.[10] Tamponade due to radiation pericarditis may also cause fever and pleuritic chest pain.[16] The progression of pericardial effusion to cardiac tamponade can be categorized into three stages (Table 24-1).

Other classic signs of cardiac tamponade are pulsus paradoxus and jugular venous distention from increased venous pressure (see "Diagnosis" section).[16,17] Beck's triad has also been considered a hallmark of cardiac tamponade.[5] These three signs include an elevated CVP, distant or muffled heart sounds (resulting from the encasement of the heart by fluid), and arterial hypotension. The point of maximal impulse may shift laterally from the fifth intercostal space as a result of cardiac enlargement.[18] As with the other symptoms described, no one cardinal sign is consistently present and a sufficient clinical indicator to diagnose cardiac tamponade.

Diagnosis

Identification of neoplastic cardiac tamponade depends greatly on a clinical diagnosis based on a detailed history and thorough physical examination. The presence or absence of any of the signs and symptoms depends on the stage of cardiac tamponade. A current or past history of cancer and cancer treatments should be noted. For a patient with no known history of cancer, other possible diagnoses must be ruled out, such as right ventricular heart failure, hydropericardium, rapid blood volume expansion, congestive heart failure (CHF), and pulmonary edema. Patients with cancer may also be at risk for cancer-related or treatment-related processes, such as radiation fibrosis, heart muscle metastases, coronary artery occlusion, or drug-induced CHF.

Two clinical findings that are classic features of cardiac tamponade are pulsus paradoxus and hepatojugular reflux. Testing for these two manifestations can be performed at the bedside.

Pulsus paradoxus (Fig. 24-3) is an abnormal finding of a weaker pulse during inspiration, resulting from a greater than normal (10 mm Hg) decrease in systolic blood pressure during the inspiratory phase of normal respiration. Cardiac tamponade constricts the myocardium, and during inspiration the diaphragm exerts additional pressure on the pericardial sac. The left ventricle receives less blood, and stroke volume is decreased, which is seen as a decrease in systolic blood pressure during inspiration. The arterial pulse may also be absent during inspiration.[19]

Pulsus paradoxus can be determined in one of two ways (see Fig. 24-3). Patients with an indwelling arterial catheter can have their blood pressure monitored during inspiration. Patients without invasive equipment can have their blood pressure evaluated by routine sphygmomanometry. A blood pressure cuff is placed around the arm and inflated to greater than 20 mm Hg above systolic pressure. The cuff is deflated slowly until the first systolic sound (Korotkoff sound) is auscultated, and the reading is noted. This occurs during expiration, and the sounds disappear during inspiration. The cuff is further deflated until sounds can be heard throughout the respiratory cycle (expiration and inspiration). This reading is also noted. The difference in mm Hg between the two readings is the value of the paradox. If the difference is more than 10 mm Hg between the two readings, pulsus paradoxus is present.[4,20]

The assessment for pulsus paradoxus may be inaccurate. Mechanical ventilation can artificially mimic paradoxic pulse.

TABLE 24-1   Stages of a Progressive Pericardial Effusion

STAGE I		STAGE II		STAGE III	
CLINICAL FINDINGS	PATHOPHYSIOLOGIC CORRELATES	CLINICAL FINDINGS	PATHOPHYSIOLOGIC CORRELATES	CLINICAL FINDINGS	PATHOPHYSIOLOGIC CORRELATES
Subjective					
Asymptomatic	Hemodynamic compensatory mechanisms effective	Dyspnea, shortness of breath with exertion, fatigued, lightheaded	Decreased cardiac output and arterial blood pressure	Dyspnea, short of breath at rest, orthopnea	Decreased cardiac output
		Fullness, heaviness felt in chest	Compression of heart	Cough, hoarseness, dysphagia	Impingement of effusion on bronchi, esophagus, and laryngeal nerves
		Abdominal discomfort	Increased right ventricular pressure causes venous stasis in liver and splanchnic veins	Retrosternal chest pain	Compression of heart Progressive hypoxia
				Anxiety, apprehension	
Objective					
Mild tachycardia (100 beats/min)	Maintaining cardiac output	Tachycardia (>100 beats/min)	Maintaining cardiac output	Tachycardia (>100 beats/min)	Decreased cardiac output
		Occasional pulsus paradoxus	Inspiratory fall in arterial systolic pressure	Pulsus paradoxus	Inspiratory fall in arterial systolic pressure
		Mild peripheral edema and abdominal distension	Venous/visceral congestion	Jugular venous distension, ascites	Venous congestion
				Hypotension	Decreased systolic pressure and increased diastolic pressure
				Impaired consciousness	Progressive hypoxia
				Pale, cyanotic appearance	Peripheral vasoconstriction
				Muffled heart sounds, friction rub	Distension of pericardial cavity

Data from Mangan CM: Malignant pericardial effusions: Pathophysiology and clinical correlates, *Oncol Nurs Forum* 19(8):1217, 1992.

If hypotension is present, pulsus paradoxus may not be found by auscultation. In this situation the inspiratory decline in blood pressure can be noted by close examination of the carotid or femoral pulse. Pulsus paradoxus may disappear during extreme tamponade, when the systolic pressure may decrease below 50 mm Hg. Finally, other conditions may be manifested with pulsus paradoxus. These include obesity, severe obstructive respiratory disease, acute cor pulmonale, right ventricular infarction, and hypovolemic shock.[19]

Hepatojugular reflex is an elevation in jugular venous pressure by 1 cm or more. Testing for this abnormal condition is accomplished by placing the patient in the supine position with the head of the bed elevated to a level where jugular venous pulsations are visible. Pressure is then exerted continuously over the right upper quadrant of the abdomen for 30 to 60 seconds, and jugular pressure is observed. An increase in the pressure represents a positive reflex arising from venous congestion associated with a prolonged elevation of the CVP.[4]

Tests ordered by the physician will include a chest x-ray film, electrocardiogram (ECG), and an echocardiogram. A routine chest x-ray film is not a specific diagnostic tool, because it cannot differentiate among possible causes of an enlarged heart shadow. Fluid accumulation of 100 ml will not change the cardiac silhouette on a film, but this amount of fluid can produce tamponade if onset is rapid. More than 250 ml fluid within the pericardial sac will enlarge the cardiac silhouette. A "water bottle heart" is seen

Clinical Features of
Neoplastic Cardiac Tamponade

Clinical Signs

Tachycardia
Low systolic blood pressure
Tachypnea with normal breath sounds
Vasoconstriction
Thready, diminished pulse pressure or pulsus paradoxus
Increased central venous pressure (CVP)
Arterial hypotension
Cardiomegaly
Precordial dullness to percussion
Distant, weak heart sounds
Pericardial friction rub
Engorged neck veins
Ascites
Hepatomegaly
Hepatojugular reflux

Peripheral edema
Cool, clammy extremities or peripheral cyanosis
Oliguria secondary to decreased renal perfusion
Apprehension, anxiety
Clouded sensorium or impaired consciousness

Symptoms

Dyspnea or shortness of breath
Retrosternal chest pain
Diaphoresis
Anxiety
Cough
Hoarseness, hiccups
Nausea, vomiting
Abdominal pain

Data from Beauchamp KA: Pericardial tamponade: an oncologic emergency, *Clin J Oncol Nurs* 2:85, 1998.

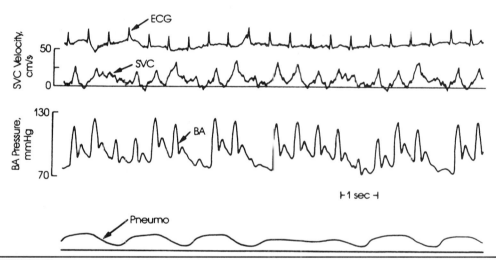

FIG. 24-3 Simultaneous recording of electrocardiogram (*ECG*), blood flow velocity in the superior vena cava (*SVC*), brachial arterial (*BA*) pressure, and the pneumogram (*Pneumo*) in a patient with cardiac compression and paradoxic pulse (pulsus paradoxus). A downward deflection of the pneumogram denotes inspiration, when SVC blood velocity rises and arterial pressure falls (paradoxic pulse). Arterial pressure is maintained during prolonged expiratory pause. (From Braunwald E: Pericardial disease. In Braunwald E and others, editors: *Harrison's principles of internal medicine*, ed 11, New York, 1987, McGraw-Hill. Reproduced with permission of the McGraw-Hill Companies.)

on the x-ray film as a result of the disappearance of the normal contours between the great vessels and the cardiac chambers.[10] More than half the patients with cardiac tamponade have cardiac enlargement, mediastinal widening, or hilar adenopathy.[11] Lung fields on chest x-ray films are usually normal because pulmonary bed capacity has not been impaired.

The ECG provides a limited amount of useful information. Elevated ST segments, nonspecific T-wave changes, decreased QRS voltage, and sinus tachycardia may be seen.[19] **Electrical alternans,** which is the alternation of amplitude and direction of the P wave

and QRS complexes on every other beat, is the most specific—although infrequent—abnormality in patients with neoplastic cardiac tamponade. This heart block, appearing at every other beat, is thought to result from variations in cardiac position at the time of electrical depolarization. In rare cases, atrial fibrillation has been present.[18]

Two-dimensional echocardiography is the most specific and sensitive technique for establishing the presence of pericardial effusion.[4,20,21] This noninvasive, reliable test should be done whenever possible if cardiac tamponade is suspected. The presence, location, and approximate quantity of fluid can be determined by the cardiac ultrasound. Normal findings on the echocardiogram show the posterior left ventricular wall in contact with the posterior pericardium and pleura and the anterior right ventricular wall in close approximation to the chest wall.[22] In tamponade, echo-free spaces that separate the moving walls from the immobile pericardium indicate the presence of fluid. Criteria have been developed to categorize the severity of the effusion: small (less than 10 mm of echo-free space), moderate (10 to 20 mm), severe (more than 20 mm).[23,24] The spaces appear first posteriorly and then anteriorly. The absence of pericardial fluid usually rules out cardiac tamponade. Findings consistent with tamponade include swinging of the heart, right atrial compression, right ventricular collapse with inspiration, and left ventricular diastolic compression.[25] Although an echocardiogram cannot determine the cause of the pericardial fluid's presence, it is extremely helpful in the evaluation of an effusion, as well as in site selection for pericardiocentesis.

Recent advances in echocardiography have added new dimensions to diagnostic testing, including transesophageal echo (TEE), stress echo, and intraarterial echo. TEE has been used in critically ill patients as a diagnostic tool in hypotensive crisis. Pericardial tamponade has been correctly diagnosed in these patients. The esophagus is the closest structure to the heart. Positioning the TEE scope with its transducer in that location permits high-resolution images of the cardiac structure. The TEE scope is a modification of the endoscope, and its tip can be moved antegrade, retrograde, and laterally to obtain tomographic views of cardiac structures using a biplane or omniplane transducer. This procedure can be done at the bedside, in the operating room, or as an outpatient procedure.

Other testing that may be performed during a diagnostic work-up for neoplastic cardiac tamponade includes cardiac catheterization, various types of scanning, and laboratory blood work. Catheterization of the heart can confirm a diagnosis of tamponade and determine the size and exact location of the pericardial fluid. In the presence of tamponade, intracardiac pressure is increased, and diastolic pressures are abnormal but almost equal in all chambers of the heart (10 to 25 mm Hg), as measured during catheterization.

Recent improvements in technology have assisted in the diagnosis of cardiac tamponade. Computed tomography (CT) and magnetic resonance imaging (MRI) have been useful in the assessment of a thickened pericardium and the diagnosis of constrictive pericarditis with effusion as opposed to radiation fibrosis. The CT scan of the chest can be used to visualize and confirm lesions that are difficult to detect as well as to define fluid loculations, mediastinal or hilar lymphadenopathy, pleural masses, and parenchymal disease.[21]

Laboratory blood tests ordered during the diagnostic work-up for neoplastic cardiac tamponade may include hematocrit, potassium (K^+), calcium (Ca^{++}), and arterial blood gases (ABGs). These tests are not conclusive for cardiac tamponade, but they can support a differential diagnosis. Pericardial fluid sent for cytologic examination has been diagnostic in about 80% of patients, but there are a significant percentage of false-negative reports. Certain malignancies make cytologic diagnosis more difficult. Late effusive constrictive pericarditis in lymphoma patients treated with radiation and mantle radiation-related effusion in Hodgkin's disease may present with negative cytologic evaluations.[12]

Testing for neoplastic cardiac tamponade varies greatly in scope and depth, as determined by the patient's clinical appearance, including tolerance for various procedures. Time is of the essence. Clinically evident neoplastic effusions are usually large enough to be evaluated by echocardiography.[26]

Treatment Modalities

Neoplastic cardiac tamponade is a life-threatening situation that requires immediate medical intervention as soon as the diagnosis is confirmed. The immediate goal of treatment is the removal of pericardial fluid to relieve impending circulatory collapse. After symptomatic relief of tamponade, the longer-range goal is management of the underlying disease and prevention of reaccumulation.

PHARMACOLOGIC THERAPY

Mild neoplastic cardiac tamponade may be treated with drug therapy using corticosteroids and diuretics. Supportive measures during cardiac tamponade are aimed at maintaining blood pressure and cardiac functioning. Common prescriptions include prednisone (40 to 60 mg/day) with furosemide (Lasix, 40 mg/day) or Aldactazide (spironolactone and hydrochlorothiazide, 25 to 200 mg/day). Radiation pericarditis is often effectively treated with high-dose steroids or nonsteroidal antiinflammatory drugs (NSAIDs). However, when these drugs are discontinued, the pericarditis often recurs. If an effusion recurs or tamponade becomes acute, more aggressive treatment is indicated. Infusions of blood products and intravenous (IV) fluids will expand volume and increase ventricular filling pressures. Vasoactive drugs (e.g., nitroprusside, isoproterenol, dopamine) may be useful.[4] Isoproterenol can increase heart rate and contractility, and low-dose dopamine may improve contractility. However, α-adrenergic medications will likely increase afterload and adversely affect cardiac output. The use of diuretics at this point will decrease volume and further impair ventricular filling.[10]

FLUID REMOVAL

Immediate withdrawal of fluid from the pericardium is done for both therapeutic and diagnostic reasons. Indications include a slow leak, diagnostic confirmation, rapid relief of acute tamponade, or symptomatic relief when deterioration of the patient's condition is evidenced by cyanosis, dyspnea, changes in mental status, or shock.[27] Another indicator for an aggressive approach to relieve tamponade is the "rule of 20," or a decrease in pulse pressure of more than 20 mm Hg, pulsus paradoxus greater than 20 mm Hg, and CVP greater than 20 cm water before intervention. Temporary measures such as administration of volume expanders, vasoactive drugs, and oxygen therapy are often continued before and during surgical intervention.

Pericardiocentesis is a percutaneous needle pericardiotomy with aspiration. It is considered an emergency treatment option for cardiac tamponade. It is ideally performed with guidance by cardiac catheterization or two-dimensional echocardiogram. Unguided approaches should only be done in extreme-emergency situations.[9]

The technique most often used for pericardiocentesis is the introduction of a large-bore needle into the pericardial space through a small stab incision by a subxiphoid approach. The needle is angled toward the left shoulder. The safety of this procedure depends on attention to the underlying disease and the amount and exact location of the fluid present. An echocardiogram done before pericardiocentesis can be of great assistance in site selection. There is less risk with larger volumes of fluid accumulation because of the increased distance between the pericardium and the surface of the heart. To reduce the risks associated with pericardiocentesis, the procedure is performed with continuous monitoring of CVP and ECG using the V lead directly attached to the metal hub, or shaft, of the needle.[25]

The complications rate of pericardiocentesis range from 10% to 25% and include puncture of the right atrium or ventricle, laceration of the coronary artery, accidental introduction of air into the chambers of the heart, dysrhythmias, vasovagal reaction with bradycardia, and infection.[11] Although the subxiphoid approach avoids the pleural space, pneumothorax or other injury to the lungs can occur.[28] Throughout the procedure, equipment must be available for emergency surgery and cardiopulmonary resuscitation.

Successful penetration of the pericardial sac during peri-cardiocentesis is often confirmed by a palpable "pop." This is accompanied by an increase in the QRS-complex voltage on the ECG, resulting when the pericardium is touched. If there is an acute elevation of the ST and PR segments, premature atrial contractions (PACs), or premature ventricular contractions (PVCs), there has been contact between the needle and the myocardium, and the needle should be withdrawn. After confirmation of needle loca-tion, fluid is aspirated slowly over 10 to 30 minutes. Although there is dramatic improvement in the patient with the removal of 25 to 50 ml fluid, as much of the fluid as possible should be removed.[29]

Pericardial effusion fluid can be classified as a transudate (low-protein fluid leaked from blood vessels due to nonmalig-nant mechanical factors such as cirrhosis) or an exudate (protein-rich fluid leaked from blood vessels with increased permeability). Malignant effusions are typically exudates from the irritation of serous membrane caused by sloughed cancer cells or tumor implants.[11] Fluid return from the pericardium is normally clear and straw-colored. In the presence of a malignancy, it is often bloody. This fluid should be immediately tested for hematocrit and fibrinogen to distinguish between a bloody effusion and penetration of the heart. Bloody effusions have lower levels of hematocrit and fibrinogen than circulating blood.

Although malignant effusions are usually serosanguineous, clear fluid does not rule out a neoplastic disease. Fluid studies include specific gravity, protein, cell count, stains, cultures, and cytologic analysis. Cytologic examination of pericardial fluid is essential to assist with diagnosis.[4] With metastatic cancer the cytologic identification is 80% to 90% accurate, with essentially no false-positive results.[12] The results with lymphomas, sarco-mas, and primary mesotheliomas of the pericardium are much less accurate. Although a positive cytologic examination may define the histopathology of the neoplastic disease, it may not identify the primary site.

Pericardiocentesis is usually effective in relieving signs and symptoms of neoplastic cardiac tamponade, but fluid generally reaccumulates in 24 to 48 hours. In some instances the elevated venous pressure associated with cardiac tamponade may remain despite pericardiocentesis. This situation may result from supe-rior vena cava syndrome (SVCS), CHF, effusive-constrictive pericardial disease caused by radiation therapy (400 Gy or more), tuberculosis, or extensive malignancy. This condition can be confirmed by measuring simultaneous pressures in the pericar-dial sac and the right atrium. Therefore, further local or systemic therapy is required after any pericardiocentesis. The choice of

treatment depends on the etiology and extent of the underlying disease and the patient's overall condition.

Multiple taps and placement of an indwelling catheter have been helpful in controlling fluid accumulation; however, these measures are temporary. Long-term catheter placement is contraindicated because of the high risk of infection. A short-term indwelling pericardial catheter with multiple holes for drainage can be easily inserted with an introducer over a flexible guide-wire. Once it is in place, a stopcock is placed at the distal end of the catheter. The catheter is drained each shift and may be irrigated daily with a small volume (5 to 10 ml) of saline or heparinized saline (100 units/ml). Irrigation may be useful if the tamponade is caused by a coagulopathy. In the presence of neoplastic fluid it is probably not necessary, because fibrinogen levels of the fluid are low. Complications may include catheter infection, catheter blockage, dysrhythmias, and infective pericarditis.[18]

Percutaneous balloon pericardiotomy is done following the pericardiocentesis. A guide wire is inserted into the pericardium. A balloon catheter is then placed, and the balloon inflated to create a window through which fluid may drain more freely into the pleural space. Adhesions may form between the parietal and visceral pericardium. This prevents reaccumulation of fluid.[9]

Subxiphoid pericardiotomy (pericardial window) is indi-cated when pericardiocentesis cannot be performed, and may be performed under local or general anesthesia.[17,21] A small segment of the pericardium is resected (2 to 4 cm) and fluid withdrawn. It is the preferred surgical procedure.[21]

Surgical pericardiectomy involves a thoracotomy or median sternotomy under general anesthesia. Video-assisted thorascopic surgery (VATS) is recommended for this procedure.[21] A large portion of the pericardium is resected, thus allowing continued drainage into the pleural space. This aggressive measure is reserved for patients for whom a significantly long-term survival is anticipated.[13] The postoperative complications are more signifi-cant than the subxiphoid approach.

Total pericardiectomy is the treatment of choice for patients with radiation-induced effusive-constrictive pericardial disease, or fibrosis, and also for those with pericardial mesothelioma. It is usually contraindicated in patients with extensive metastatic disease.

Surgical procedures are usually effective in controlling pericardial effusions by allowing the pericardial fluid to drain into the pleural cavity, which provides greater surface area for resorption. Several potential complications are associated with these procedures, including the usual risks associated with general anesthesia and the possibility of dysrhythmias, bleeding, infection, and hemothorax. Pulmonary edema can occur with postoperative diuresis in patients who were heavily hydrated before surgery. Figure 24-4 illustrates pericardiectomy through the median sternotomy approach.

Sclerotherapy is routinely performed following pericardio-centesis to prevent fluid reaccumulation. Rates of reaccumula-tion range form 44% to 79%.[21] A short-term catheter is left in place to facilitate continued short-term drainage until drainage has slowed enough to allow the successful instillation of a scle-rosing agent. Instillation of such agents irritates the pericardial sac, causing the two linings to adhere to one another and obliter-ate the pericardial space where fluid accumulates. Complications may include localized pain, fever, PVCs, atrial dysrhythmias, pericarditis, and myelosuppression.[18] Sclerosing is considered successful when there is no drainage for a 24-hour period.

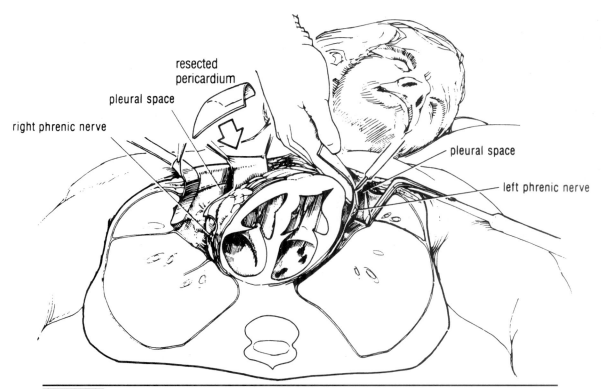

right phrenic nerve

pleural space

resected
pericardium

pleural space

left phrenic nerve

FIG. 24-4   Pericardiectomy through a median sternotomy approach. (From Miller SE, Campbell DB: Malignant pericardial effusions. In Polomano RC, Miller SE, editors: *Understanding and managing oncologic emergencies,* Monograph, Columbus, Ohio, 1987, Adria Laboratories.)

Agents that may be used include bleomycin, tetracycline, doxorubicin, 5-fluorouracil (5-FU), methotrexate, nitrogen mustard, radioactive phosphorus, talc, and thiotepa radioactive gold or phosphorus, quinacrine, thiotepa, doxycycline, cisplatin, and minocycline.[13] Bleomycin is preferred by some because of efficacy as well as decreased incidence of retrosternal pain.[21]

RADIATION THERAPY

Radiation therapy may be the treatment of choice for neoplastic cardiac tamponade of gradual onset caused by a radiosensitive tumor of the lung or breast or a hematopoietic malignancy.[21] Generally, external beam radiation therapy (200 to 400 Gy) is delivered to a port that includes the heart and pericardial structures and the lower mediastinum. Careful assessment of any previous radiation therapy is important to establish tissue tolerance. Cardiac tolerance is 350 to 400 Gy, beyond which a complication of pericarditis may develop.[14]

CHEMOTHERAPY

Systemic chemotherapy may be given to responsive tumors such as lymphoma, breast cancer, or small cell carcinoma of the lung.[21] This may be the initial treatment of a pericardial effusion when it is slow and the patient is asymptomatic. However, in acute neoplastic cardiac tamponade, systemic chemotherapy is done when the patient is clinically stable after pericardiocentesis.

Nursing Considerations

Nursing interventions for the patient with neoplastic cardiac tamponade are multifaceted and highly variable, depending upon the patient's condition. Onset of tamponade may be impending and insidious or rapid and life-threatening. Knowledge of the patient's current and past history, coupled with astute physical assessment skills, is necessary.

Patients may be on a medical oncology unit or in the critical care area. Close monitoring of vital signs is of paramount importance. Nursing care is directed at maintaining optimal cardiopulmonary function and preventing circulatory collapse through immediate identification and treatment of neoplastic cardiac tamponade.

Hemodynamic and cardiovascular status are assessed by monitoring blood pressure, pulse, CVP, cardiac output, and increased jugular pressure. Cardiac monitoring will note abnormalities associated with cardiac tamponade: ST segment elevation, T-wave inversion, and electrical alterations. Administer vasoactive drugs as ordered. Be prepared for cardiac arrest and emergency resuscitation. Observe breathing patterns to note abnormalities associated with cardiac tamponade: pulsus paradoxus, respiratory alkalosis, Kussmaul's sign, and hypoxemia. Note serum electrolytes, particularly Ca^{++} and K^+, because of the risk of cardiac dysrhythmias. Repositioning the patient may enhance circulation; however, it must be done slowly to allow compensation for decreased cardiac output. Measures to reduce workload of the heart can include assistance with all activities, scheduled rest periods, and comfort measures such as analgesics, relaxation techniques, and antianxiolitics. Assess the patient for complications of bleeding, infection, atelectasis, pneumothorax, and pleural effusion.

Prognosis

Overall median survival for patients with pericardial effusion due to malignancy is estimated as less than 6 months. Patients who respond to treatment and exhibit total control of the effusion may average a 9-month survival, depending on the histology of the disease.[21] Survival of the patient with neoplastic cardiac tamponade depends on the cause of the primary malignancy, the stage of cancer at the time of intervention, tumor responsiveness to radiation therapy or chemotherapy, hemodynamic significance of the tamponade, effectiveness of therapy, and general medical condition of the patient. The mortality rate for cardiac tamponade has been reported to be 25%. However, this rate increases to 65% if the tamponade goes unrecognized.[14] Although the overall prognosis of the patient may be poor, the spectacular response that is usually seen with the removal of pericardial fluid warrants aggressive action.

INCREASED INTRACRANIAL PRESSURE

Definition

Increased intracranial pressure (IICP) is also referred to as intracranial hypertension. IICP results when the volume of any of the three components within the skull and meninges is increased. These components include the brain, cerebrospinal fluid (CSF), and cerebral blood volume.[6] IICP, if not successfully treated, can lead to brain herniation and death.

Etiology and Risk Factors

The most common oncologic etiology for IICP is brain metastasis.[30] Of cancer patients, 20% to 40% develop brain metastases.[31] Metastatic brain tumors are 4 to 5 times more common than primary lesions.[32] Lung and breast cancers are the solid tumors that most frequently metastasize to the brain in adults.[33] Colon, breast, and renal cell carcinomas often spread to the brain as single lesions. Lung cancer and melanoma often produce multiple intracranial metastases.[30] The most common site for brain metastasis is the corticomedullary junction, probably because of the amount of blood flow. Brain tumors cause IICP by obstruction of CSF or cerebral blood flow, increasing the volume of brain tissue and edema.[32]

Other causes of IICP that may occur in oncology patients are hematomas, hemorrhage, cerebral irritation, or infection with exudate. Patients with thrombocytopenia or platelet dysfunction are at risk for cerebral bleeding. Those receiving radiation therapy to the brain may experience cerebral irritation. Patients with lymphoma, leukemia, or central nervous system (CNS) tumors and those who have an Ommaya reservoir are at some risk for CNS infection. Syndrome of inappropriate diuretic hormone (SIADH) and CNS infections can cause cellular or cytotoxic edema resulting in IICP. Head and neck cancer can produce IICP from compression of the internal jugular veins. SIADH can cause severe hyponatremia, and IICP can develop from increased intracellular fluid in brain cells as a result of increased extracellular hypoosmolality.[20] CSF resorption has been decreased in conjunction with the use of retinoic acid in promyelocytic leukemia.[30] CSF production may be increased in patients with choroid plexus papillomas, particularly if multifocal.[30]

Pathophysiology

The skull and meninges form a rigid covering that contains the brain tissue (80%), blood (10%), and CSF (10%).

Normal intracranial pressure (ICP) is 4 to 15 mm Hg or 80 to 10 cm of water. Brain metastases cause vasogenic cerebral edema by disrupting the blood-brain barrier. This allows fluid and protein to leak out of the capillaries into the extracellular space, primarily in the white matter of the brain.

The Monro-Kellie hypothesis states that the cranial contents are maintained in a dynamic equilibrium. An increase in the volume of any one component must cause a decrease in volume of the other two.[30] This volume decrease is called compensation. Compensatory mechanisms include movement of the CSF from around the brain tissue to the spinal cord, decreased CSF production by the choroid plexus, increased CSF absorption by arachnoid villi, or shunting of venous blood to other sites.[32] The compensatory mechanisms will eventually be depleted, and very small increases in the volume of the cranial contents will cause significant IICP. Autoregulation is the ability to maintain a constant rate of cerebral blood flow regardless of variations in systemic arterial pressure and venous drainage.[32] This occurs through constriction or dilation of cerebral blood vessels. Autoregulation failure occurs with the exhaustion of the compensatory mechanisms, as well as severe hypotension or hypertension. Slight increases in systemic blood pressure will then cause IICP. Diminished cerebral blood flow leads to tissue hypoxia and reduced removal of carbon dioxide and lactic acid. Build-up of these metabolic by-products causes vasodilation, leading to edema and exacerbating the IICP.[32]

Because cerebral veins have no valves, anything that restricts cerebral venous outflow can cause an increased cerebral volume. Actions that increase intrathoracic or intraabdominal pressures can restrict outflow; these include the Valsalva maneuver, bending over, coughing, sneezing, extreme neck flexion or extension, hip flexion, lying on the abdomen, and positive end-expiratory pressure (PEEP) treatments.[30]

When compensatory mechanisms and autoregulation fail, IICP can displace brain tissue from one cranial compartment to another. This herniation moves brain tissue from the area of high pressure to an area of lower pressure, compressing other neural tissue, blood vessels, and CSF pathways, and increasing edema. Depending on the location and severity of the herniation, the patient can suffer loss of consciousness, and respiratory and cardiac arrest.[32]

Clinical Features

General symptoms of IICP include headache, nausea, vomiting, change in level of consciousness, impaired cognitive function, changes in personality, hemiparesis, language difficulty, dysphagia, ataxia, and seizures. Melanoma is the systemic cancer with the highest incidence of intracranial metastases.[34] Seizures are common with metastases from melanoma because of their hemorrhagic nature, and they are the presenting symptom in 15% to 20% of patients.[32] Headaches are commonly most severe on waking, possibly a result of carbon dioxide retention during sleep that causes cerebral vessel dilatation and enhances cerebral edema. Another explanation may be the decreased venous drainage caused by maintaining a supine position.[30] Visual findings of IICP include blurring, changes in pupil size and light accommodation, visual field deficits, and papilledema (a late sign).[30] Advanced IICP can cause hemiparesis, hemiplegia, decreased reflexes, and decorticate and decerebrate posturing. Cushing's triad, another late sign of IICP, is a combination of hypertension, bradycardia, and irregular or slow respirations.[35] Posturing and Cushing's triad are generally associated with the terminal phase of herniation.[32]

Diagnosis

Patients with cancer who develop neurologic changes should be evaluated immediately for brain metastasis. Both CT scanning with contrast and gadolinium contrast-enhanced MRI are used to evaluate brain metastases.[31] MRI has been found to be the most sensitive tool and is the preferred diagnostic method.[30,35] However, CT may be used initially to quickly image acute hemorrhage, hydrocephalus, or a tumor with edema and focal mass effect.[35] PET scanning is useful in differentiating between recurrent tumor and radiation necrosis.[33] Lumbar puncture should be avoided with IICP because of the risk of exacerbation and herniation.[33]

Treatment Modalities

Rapid reduction of cerebral edema and decompression of the ICP is the immediate treatment goal.

PHARMACOLOGIC MANAGEMENT

Corticosteroids can rapidly decrease peritumoral edema. Improvement in symptoms may be seen within 24 hours. Steroids are continued for at least 3 to 7 days until definitive treatment can be initiated and take effect, or as long as needed to manage the symptoms of IICP.[31] Patients at risk for herniation are started on high dosages, such as 100 mg dexamethasone IV. Maintenance dosages may be as high as 30 mg 4 times a day.[34] Corticosteroids are thought to decrease capillary permeability and promote extracellular fluid resorption.[34] If the differential diagnosis before tissue evaluation is suspected to be CNS lymphoma, corticosteroids may induce apoptosis and obscure the morphology of the cells.[30,36]

Osmotic diuretics (such as mannitol) may also be needed; these decrease cerebral edema by increasing plasma osmolarity and drawing extracellular fluid back into the plasma, where it can be excreted by the kidneys.[33] A typical starting dosage of mannitol is 1 mg/kg IV followed by 0.25 to 0.50 g/kg every 3 to 6 hours.[30,35,37] **Loop diuretics** (such as furosemide) are used to decrease CSF production and enhance the excretion of sodium and water from the brain. Side effects of diuretics may include dysrhythmias and fluid and electrolyte imbalances. Diuretics may be combined with fluid restrictions. Electrolytes and hemodynamics must be closely monitored. Repeated osmotic diuresis may lead to a rebound increase in IICP.[35]

Anticonvulsants (such as phenytoin, carbamazepine, phenobarbital, and valproic acid) are given to manage seizures when appropriate.[34]

Mechanical hyperventilation may be used to reduce the PCO_2 to about 25 mm HG. This induces cerebral vasoconstriction and reduces the cerebral vasculature volume which, in turn, reduces IICP.[33,30] Cerebral perfusion is decreased if PCO_2 levels are lowered too much. Corticosteroids and osmotic diuresis are to be used in conjunction with this therapy since the results are transient.[30,35]

SURGERY

Emergent surgical intervention is needed for the patient with life-threatening IICP. When IICP is due to cerebral edema obstructing the flow of CSF, insertion of a ventriculoperitoneal shunt or a temporary ventriculostomy can provide immediate drainage of CSF and relief of IICP while interventions are initiated to treat the underlying cause of the edema.[32] However, shunting is avoided in leptomeningeal tumors to prevent peritoneal seeding.[30] A ventricular drain may be used to divert CSF directly to an ICP monitor.[37] Partial or complete resection of tumor is necessary for rapidly enlarging brain lesions. This is most quickly accomplished by a craniotomy. Remaining tumor can then be treated with radiation therapy or chemotherapy, depending on the histology and tumor responsiveness. Resection provides the benefit of tissue diagnosis, in addition to reducing tumor volume. Risks of surgery include postoperative edema, further neurologic deficit, bleeding, and infection.[32]

RADIATION AND CHEMOTHERAPY

Radiation and chemotherapy are primarily used to treat brain metastases and primary tumors that can cause IICP, as well as leptomeningeal carcinomatosis.[30] They are most effective for tumors with histologic features that are sensitive to radiation and chemotherapy (e.g., lymphoma, small cell lung carcinoma [SCLC], choriocarcinoma).[31] Acute symptoms of IICP must be addressed immediately with medications to decrease edema and surgical intervention. Once the acute symptoms are controlled, radiation or chemotherapy can be used to address the underlying cause of IICP (see Chapter 6).

Nursing Considerations

As with most oncologic emergencies, the prompt recognition of the signs of IICP is critical to initiating the appropriate interventions before the damage is irreparable.

Once a diagnosis is made, assess airway and maintain patency. Be prepared to transfer the patient to the intensive care unit (ICU), if necessary, for mechanical ventilation and hemodynamic monitoring. Assess baseline neurologic status and reassess every hour as needed. Be alert for mental status changes and seizure activity. Administer steroids and anticonvulsants as prescribed. Position the patient with the head of bed elevated 30 to 45 degrees, and prevent extreme neck flexion, extension, or rotation. Monitor intake and output. Monitor serum electrolytes, osmolality, and creatinine level. Administer steroids, osmotic agents, and diuretics as prescribed. If possible, avoid activities that aggravate IICP, such as endotracheal suctioning. Provide as calm and quiet an environment as possible. Prepare the patient and family for procedures or surgical intervention. Provide education about radiation or chemotherapy as needed.

Prognosis

Prognosis for the patient with IICP initially depends on the severity and rapidity of the symptoms, as well as the early recognition and prompt initiation of appropriate treatment. Ultimate survival depends on the type and stage of cancer and response to overall treatment of the underlying disease. Patients with untreated brain metastases survive an average of 1 month.[21]

SPINAL CORD COMPRESSION

Definition

A neoplasm in the epidural space can encroach on the spinal cord or cauda equina and result in spinal cord compression (SCC).[35,38] SCC is a medical emergency requiring early detection and prompt treatment. Although it is rarely fatal, it can result in permanent neurologic deficits such as paralysis and loss of bowel and bladder control.

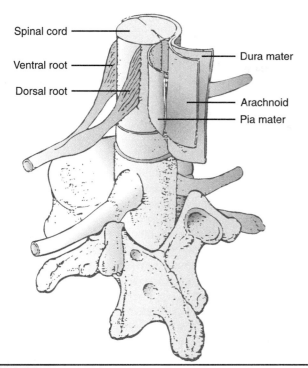

FIG. 24-5   The spinal meninges. (From Hickey JV: The clinical practice of neurological and neurosurgical nursing, ed 3, Philadelphia, 1992, Lippincott.)

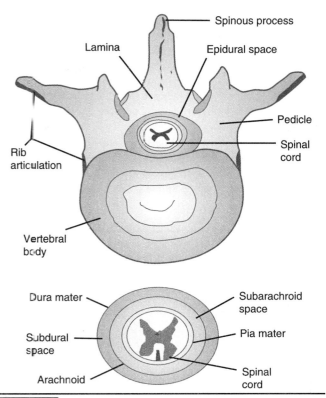

FIG. 24-6   Cross section of vertebra and spinal cord.

Etiology and Risk Factors

Spinal cord compression is the second most common neurologic complication of cancer following brain metastasis.[39] It occurs in 5% to 10% of patients with cancer.[35,40] Primary tumors of the spinal cord account for a very small percentage of SCC. Metastatic disease is the most common cause. Patients with cancer that metastasizes to the bone and those with existing bony disease are at the greatest risk for SCC. Lung, breast, and prostate cancers are associated with about 50% to 60% of SCC cases.[35,38] Other cancers commonly associated with SCC include multiple myeloma, lymphoma, melanoma, renal cancer, and sarcoma.[35,38] The median interval between diagnosis of malignancy and the advent of SCC ranges between 6 to 12.5 months.[40]

Pathophysiology

The adult human vertebral column, or backbone, is a versatile arrangement of 33 vertebrae joined in series and supported by ligaments. The 33 vertebrae include 7 cervical, 12 thoracic, 5 lumbar, 5 sacral, and 4 coccygeal. The sacral and coccygeal vertebrae are fused into the sacrum and the coccyx, respectively. The vertebrae support the body by strength and rigidity while also providing flexibility and mobility. In addition, the column surrounds and protects the spinal cord, which is enlarged in the cervical and lumbar areas. The cord itself is covered by three protective meninges (called leptomeninges), or membranes (Figs. 24-5 and 24-6).

These **meninges** originate as coverings for the brain and extend downward over the spinal cord. The outermost membrane is the **dura mater** (hard mother), which is made up of dense fibrous connective tissue. The space between the walls of the vertebral column and the outer surface of the dura mater is referred to as the **epidural, or extradural, space.** Within that space

can be found blood vessels and connective and adipose tissue. No lymph nodes are located within this space. The **subdural space** follows next, between the inner surface of the dura mater and the underlying arachnoid membrane. Below the arachnoid membrane is the **subarachnoid space.** It lies between the arachnoid membrane and the innermost membrane, the **pia mater** ("gentle mother"), which is closely attached to the spinal cord. The subarachnoid space contains liquid referred to as spinal fluid. However, it is more accurately called **cerebrospinal fluid (CSF),** because the subarachnoid space begins in the brain and continues down the cord.[7]

Metastatic disease to the vertebrae typically occurs in the anterior extradural space and causes SCC from compression to the cord as opposed to tissue invasion.[35] Tumor involvement of the spinal cord may be classified according to the cell of origin (primary spinal cord tumors as opposed to metastatic disease) and the site of anatomic presentation related to the spinal dura (Table 24-2).[41] Primary tumors arising in the spinal cord are intramedullary and directly invade and destroy the cord.[32] Primary tumors of the meninges or nerve roots are extramedullary. Most oncologic SCC is caused by metastatic disease. Twenty-five percent spreads to the extradural space and can displace the spinal cord, irritate spinal nerve roots, or obstruct the flow of CSF[32]; 75% cause vertebral destruction and collapse that forces bony fragments into the extradural space (Fig. 24-7).[39]

The epidural space may be invaded by tumor in a variety of ways. Hematogenous spread of malignant cells, through Batson's paraspinal venous plexus and to the vertebral body, is the most frequent route.[39] It is estimated to lead to 85% of oncologic SCC. Tumor growth from the marrow invades the bone matrix and destroys the vertebral body. Vertebral body destruction allows tumor to directly invade the extradural space and compress the cord. Vertebral body destruction may also allow vertebral body collapse, forcing bony fragments into the extradural space and mechanically compressing the cord. Paraspinal tumors grow through the intervertebral foramen to cause cord compression.[39] Non-Hodgkin's lymphomas cause SCC in this way in about 10% of cases.[34]

Ascending and descending nerve fiber tracts are located in the white matter of the spinal cord (outer portion). Damage to ascending tracts causes pain or sensory deficits or both. Descending tract damage causes motor deficits, bowel and bladder dysfunction, and impaired sexual function. Neurologic deficits are caused by three different processes:

- Direct compression of the spinal cord or cauda equina by the tumor itself

TABLE 24-2   Anatomic Presentation of Spinal Cord Tumors

EXTRADURAL	INTRADURAL
Metastatic solid tumors (breast, lung, prostate)	Extramedullary
Sarcoma	
Lymphoma	Schwannoma
Myeloma	Meningioma
Chordoma	Intramedullary
	Ependymoma
	Astrocytoma
	Oligodendroglioma
	Hemangioblastoma
	Mixed glioma

Modified from Belford K: Central nervous system cancers. In Groenwald SL, Frogge MH, Goodman M et al, editors: *Cancer nursing: principles and practice*, ed 4, Boston, 1997, Jones & Bartlett; and data from Maher DeLeon ME, Schnell S, Rozental JM: Tumors of the spine and spinal cord, *Semin Oncol Nurs* 14:43, 1998.

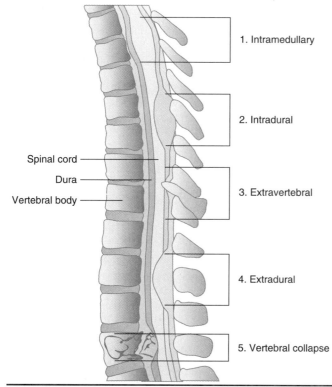

1. Intramedullary
2. Intradural
Spinal cord
Dura
Vertebral body
3. Extravertebral
4. Extradural
5. Vertebral collapse

FIG. 24-7 Malignant invasion of the spinal cord.

- Interruption of the vascular supply to the neural structure by the tumor
- Compression caused by vertebral collapse resulting from a pathologic fracture or dislocation. The bone may extrude onto the cord and produce pressure that compresses the nerve roots. The severity of the compression can increase in the presence of edema from obstruction of the venous plexus, which supplies the spinal cord.

Clinical Features

The clinical presentation of SCC is similar in all patients, regardless of the origin of the tumor. Symptomatology is directly related to the location of the compression. The distribution of spinal metastases with SCC correlates with the number of vertebrae and size of the epidural space in each segment, with 10% in the cervical area, 70% in the thoracic, and 20% in the lumbosacral.[40,42,43] Lumbosacral presentation is typically associated with cancers of the colon and the prostate.[40] Lung and breast cancers are more likely to compress the thoracic spine.[42]

The cardinal signs and associated symptoms of SCC are well documented and usually follow an established pattern of appearance, which includes pain, motor weakness, sensory loss, and finally autonomic dysfunction (see Clinical Features box).

Back pain is the presenting complaint in 96% of patients.[35,42,43] It is related to SCC and may occur weeks or months before neurologic deficits occur. However, fast-growing tumors can rapidly progress to cause irreversible paraplegia in a matter of hours to days after neurologic deficit appears.[34] The pain is either localized or radicular. Localized pain, along the spinal axis, is classically the initial symptom and results from stretching of the periosteum of the afflicted bone, vertebral collapse, invasion of spinal tracts, tension on spinal nerve roots, or tumor attachment to the proximal dura.[31] Pain that is radicular in nature is caused by nerve root compression from a pathologic fracture and compression of the vertebrae. The distribution of radicular pain depends on the level of spinal involvement. It may move along the dermatomal distribution and is aggravated by movement such as coughing, sneezing, straining as with the Valsalva maneuver, or, straight leg raising.[35] Thoracic radicular pain, which is most common, radiates in a band around the chest or abdomen.

The pain associated with SCC is usually intense, persistent, and progressive, although thoracic compression is often felt as

Clinical Features of Spinal Cord Compression

Clinical Signs
Muscle weakness (unsteadiness, foot drop, paralysis)
Sensory impairment (paralysis, loss of bowel and bladder control, paraplegia)

Symptoms
Pain
Tingling and/or numbness in extremities
Diminished pain and temperature sensation
Sexual dysfunction

Data from Fuller BG, Heiss J, Oldfield EH: Spinal cord compression. In DeVita VT Jr, Hellman S, Rosenberg SA, editors: *Cancer: principles and practice of oncology*, ed 5, Philadelphia, 1997, Lippincott-Raven.

a constriction.[43] Any pain of SCC may be accompanied by vertebral tenderness on percussion at or near the level of compression. It is often unilateral when the compression is in the cervical or lumbosacral area, and is usually bilateral in the thoracic region. The pain is usually worse at night, because the spine lengthens when recumbent and the abdominal contents place pressure against the spine and cord.[35,42] A key to early detection is a detailed assessment for any changes in pain. Patients may have been suffering with pain from bony metastasis for a time. With the onset of SCC, the pain often changes its location and intensity.

Weakness typically precedes sensory loss and is the second most common symptom after pain.[35] Weakness is only a presenting complaint in 2% of cases. However, 75% to 86% of patients have subtle evidence of motor defect on initial clinical examination.[42] Initially, motor symptoms are asymptomatic. The time frame for motor weakness to develop following the onset of SCC is variable and ranges from hours to days, weeks, or months.[3] The location of weakness is usually restricted to the lower extremities but may vary based on the location of the tumor. Common patient complaints include stiffness and heaviness of the affected extremity. The weakness may manifest itself as an unsteady gait or ataxia with a favoring or dragging of the affected extremity or extremities. Patients experience difficulty walking or climbing stairs.[40] Symptoms often associated with weakness include hyperreflexia, spasticity, and a positive Babinski's sign.[32]

Sensory loss usually follows motor weakness but precedes actual motor loss. These sensory losses progress in the same pattern as motor symptoms. Symptoms of sensory loss include numbness, tingling, paresthesia, and feelings of coldness in the affected area. Loss of sensation first to light touch, then to loss of pain, and followed by loss of thermal sensation, occur in 80% of patients. Concurrent loss of proprioception, deep pressure and vibratory senses, and position sense indicates a severe compression. Sensory deficit typically occurs 1 to 5 levels below the area of compression.[35,43] After the release of SCC, neurologic functions return in the reverse order of how the dysfunctions appeared. If the motor weakness and sensory loss progress rapidly to motor loss, the prognosis is poor.

Autonomic dysfunction appears if the compression progresses. Urinary disturbances include hesitancy and retention, followed by overflow and incontinence. Early changes may be as subtle as an increased postvoiding residual volume. Lack of urge to defecate and inability to bear down are initial bowel disturbances, which may lead to constipation, obstipation and, finally, incontinence. Loss of sphincter control is a later sign and is associated with a poorer prognosis. Sexual dysfunction may be manifested as impotence.[35] Horner's syndrome can accompany paraspinal cervical or upper thoracic compression. Absence of sweating below the level of compression is typically associated with severe leg weakness or paraplegia.[35]

Diagnosis

When SCC is suspected in any patient, a diagnosis should be confirmed immediately because of the potential for rapid progression and possible permanent neurologic dysfunction. A good history and physical examination should be accompanied by thorough neurologic testing. Physical findings include percussion tenderness at the level of compression. If radicular pain is present, it will increase with spinal movement on straight leg raises. Motor and sensory involvement is manifested by hyperactive reflexes, positive Babinski's signs, variable spastic weakness, and bilateral sensory loss below the level of the compression. Absence of sweating below the level of involvement may be noted. Bowel and bladder dysfunction should also be assessed. Corresponding subjective data should be elicited, because differences can be significant.

Testing for a patient with suspected SCC begins with plain x-ray films. Plain films are positive in 85% of patients with SCC.[42,43] Radiographic findings reveal osteolytic lesions with loss of a pedicle, vertebral body destruction, or collapse of vertebral body. Intervertebral disks are not affected by neoplastic disease because they have an insufficient blood supply. However, a deficiency with plain x-ray films is that if the tumor grows paraspinally, with invasion of the epidural space through the foramina, the bone film may appear normal. This is common with lung tumors and lymphoma. Secondly, a tumor can be present for 6 months without showing changes on x-ray films. Greater than 50% of bone destruction can occur before a positive plain film.[38,43] A bone scan is often more sensitive and may be positive 6 months before plain films. Osteoblastic lesions show new bone formation that may extend into the epidural space.

The diagnostic method of choice to evaluate SCC is the MRI scan.[35,40,42,43] It can identify compression, soft-tissue lesions, and cord lesions, as well as bone destruction. MRI also distinguishes between extradural, intradural, and extramedullary lesions. The major benefits of MRI are as follows:

- It is sensitive to neurologic tissue.
- It is noninvasive.
- It is helpful in patients with severe contrast allergies.
- It images the entire spine, providing various views.
- It is helpful in patients with brain metastasis.
- It may show multiple epidural deposits of tumor that may not be obvious on initial myelogram.
- It avoids the risk of neurologic deterioration after lumbar puncture.
- New open MRI machines have provided an option for people with claustrophobia and those who are too large to fit into a closed machine.

The disadvantages of MRI are the following:
- The patient must lie still in one position, which may be difficult for someone with central back pain.
- Claustrophobia has been a common problem.

Myelography is reserved for cases where MRI does not explain neurologic deficits or when MRI is contraindicated.[40] Myelography is an invasive examination. It requires a needle puncture to withdraw CSF and instill contrast media into the subarachnoid space. Two lumbar punctures may be needed to visualize upper and lower margins of the block. CSF sampling can be done to rule out meningeal carcinomatosis or when unable to do MRI because of lack of access, severe scoliosis, presence of hardware such as a pacemaker, or the patient's inability to tolerate lying in one position for the procedure.[51,44] CSF protein elevations greater than 100 mg/ml have been noted in most patients with SCC. Glucose is normal, cell count is unremarkable, and cytology studies are usually normal. A 16% to 24% risk of neurologic deterioration has been reported if the lumbar puncture is done below the tumor site.[11] There is risk of neurologic deterioration with a complete subarachnoid block.[39] Other risks include infection and bleeding.[43]

CT may identify early destructive lesions not seen on plain films, differentiate tumor from osteoporosis, and define paraspinal tumors that may extend epidurally. It is also useful in predicting epidural tumor extension for patients with severe osteoporosis owing to demonstration of metastatic disruption of the bony cortex around the spinal canal.[42]

Treatment Modalities

The choice of treatment for patients with SCC depends on the primary tumor, the rapidity of onset of the compression, and the level, severity, and duration of the blockage. The most frequent treatment modalities for SCC are steroids, radiation therapy, and surgery. The goals of therapy are to preserve or restore neurologic function, maintain spinal stability, control tumor growth, and relieve pain.[35,42] Symptom relief from metastatic disease facilitates the improvement of quality of life.

STEROIDS

The use of corticosteroids is indicated for cord and nerve root compression; however, there is controversy over the appropriate dosage and schedule.[35] Rapidly progressive symptoms are typically treated with high-dose steroids, such as dexamethasone, 100 mg by IV bolus. This is followed by 16 to 24 mg orally 4 times a day until definitive treatment is begun and symptoms resolve. Steroid administration is frequently begun before the completion of the diagnostic work-up to rapidly decrease pain and swelling. A slower progression of symptoms may be managed with an initial IV bolus of 10 mg, followed by 4 mg orally every 6 hours. Most patients will receive pain relief within a few hours. Dosages are carefully tapered by reducing the dose by one third every 3 to 4 days after treatment is initiated.[34] Patients are closely observed for neurologic deficits during the taper so that higher dosages may be resumed if needed. Rapid withdrawal can precipitate symptoms of acute adrenal insufficiency.[32] Patients are also observed for the short-term side effects and toxicities associated with steroid use, such as fluid retention and blood glucose level and mood alterations. Patients who require long-term steroids for symptom control are at risk for GI bleeding, opportunistic infections, and osteoporosis. Recent studies have indicated that a higher percentage of patients treated with steroids remain ambulatory at long-term follow-up.[35,42]

RADIATION THERAPY

Radiation is the treatment of choice for SCC in most cases and is typically started within 24 hours of diagnosis.[35] Radiation portals are planned to extend two vertebral bodies above and below the site of cord compression. Adjacent sites of bony disease and paravertebral masses are also included in the treatment field.[35,43] Standard doses range from 3000 cGy over 10 fractions to a total dose of 2500 to 4000 cGy in 10 to 20 fractions over 2 to 4 weeks.[35,42,43] Controversy exists over the benefits of using higher treatment fractions for the first 3 days of therapy. Smaller fractions may be used for patients with the best long-term prognosis to decrease damage to the spinal cord.[34] Radiation therapy has been shown to reduce pain, compression, and tumor size in 70% to 80% of patients.[42] It improves motor function and reverses paralysis in 11% to 16% of cases and can prevent local recurrence.[39] Image-guided and intensity-modulated radiosurgery is being investigated as a treatment of cord compression with encouraging results.[45]

SURGERY

Surgery has been replaced by radiation therapy in all but the following situations[35,40,42 43]:

- Spinal instability or bony collapse into spinal canal
- Rapid neurologic deterioration
- The cause for SCC is questionable, or there is no known primary malignancy
- Prior maximum-tolerance radiation at the site of compression precludes further irradiation
- Neurologic deterioration occurs during radiation therapy
- Radioresistant tumor

Surgical stabilization of the spinal column requires intact bone above and below the site of compression. Most tumors appear in the vertebral body and invade the epidural space anteriorly. A posterior decompression laminectomy relieves compression of the spinal cord by removing the spinous processes and the lamina one level above and below the compression. It allows relaxation of the cord, but cannot remove tumor that is anterior to the cord. Posterior laminectomy may cause spinal instability and is reserved for posterior tumors.[43]

Anterior decompression with spinal stabilization is performed for tumors in the vertebral body that produce anterior compression. Anterior decompression allows total removal of the involved vertebral body. A thoracotomy or retroperitoneal approach is used. The vertebral body is replaced with methylmethacrylate and supplemented with metal prostheses that are attached to the adjacent vertebrae.[43] The mortality rate for aggressive resection ranges from 6% to 10%. The complications rate is as high as 48%.[35,43]

There is current controversy over the best surgical approach. Definitive studies are needed. Researchers at Memorial Sloan Kettering have had initial positive results with a posterolateral transpedicular approach (PATA). The procedure has been particularly effective for extensive epidural disease in patients for whom the anterior approach is contraindicated.[46,47]

Surgical interventions for SCC are not appropriate for multiple levels of disease, for complete paralysis, or for those who are poor risks for anesthesia.[39]

CHEMOTHERAPY

Chemotherapy has a role as adjuvant therapy in the treatment of SCC. In most instances, it is combined with radiation therapy to treat SCC resulting from lymphoma.[7] Chemotherapy may be given concomitantly or after radiation therapy as systemic treatment for the primary underlying malignancy. Chemosensitive tumors include lymphoma, myeloma, and breast, prostate, and germ cell tumors.[43]

PREVENTION

Research has demonstrated a role for bisphosphonates in decreasing the skeletal complications of bony metastases. Both zoledronic acid and pamidronate have been shown to reduce skeletal-related events (SREs) in patients with breast cancer and multiple myeloma.[48] Zoledronic acid has shown efficacy in reduction of SREs in prostate cancer.[49] SREs are defined as bone pain, surgery or radiation therapy to the bone, changes in antineoplastic therapy to address bone pain, hypercalemia of malignancy, and SCC.

Nursing Considerations

Spinal cord compression (SCC) is a true oncologic emergency requiring immediate attention. The primary aspect of nursing care is early detection, because response to therapy is directly related to the patient's functional status at diagnosis. An in-depth history and data collection are essential in those patients who are at risk for SCC. Nursing assessment should focus on pain, motor and sensory status, and bowel and bladder functions. The nursing care of these patients is extremely variable, depending on the presence and severity of the compression and the medical treatment. Very subtle changes in patient status are significant and should be reported. Education of both patient and family to recognize and report symptoms of back pain is critical.

Components of assessing the patient's level of function and mobility include checking the presence of sensory loss and paresthesia by noting sensation and deep tendon reflexes in the extremities. Monitor serum calcium levels for potential increase from immobility. Determine motor weakness and dysfunction by checking gait, range of motion (ROM), and coordination. Check for evidence of venous thrombosis by assessing for redness, swelling, warmth, positive Homan's sign (pain on dorsiflexion), venous streaking, and erythema. Implement a pain management program as indicated. Establish an activity regimen according to the patient's physical status and physician order. Passive ROM exercise and assistance with transfer and ambulation may be required. Obtain consultation or referral to rehabilitative services as needed. Encourage and assist patients to perform self-care whenever possible. Encourage and assist with pulmonary hygiene. Consider need for incentive spirometry, ultrasonic nebulizer, and percussion and drainage. Assess skin integrity with special attention to areas over bony prominences; note any redness, discoloration, swelling, or breakdown. Institute appropriate skin care protocol. Assess bowel, bladder, and sexual function. Initiate bowel training program as necessary. Obtain order for indwelling urinary catheter if repeated catheterization is necessary to relieve distention or continued urinary residual. A bladder training program may also be of value. Discuss the potential impact of disease and treatment on sexuality and sexual function. Be respectful of social, cultural, and religious factors that may influence the patient's perceptions of sexuality, sexual function, and sexual identity, and ensure confidentiality.

Nursing care of a patient with SCC is complex and challenging, reflecting the extreme variability among patients. Situations exist along a continuum from early detection and alarm through emergency and rehabilitation. The role of the oncology nurse in coordinating care is crucial.

Prognosis

The degree of neurologic dysfunction at the time of diagnosis is the greatest predictor of outcome. Of patients with little or no ambulatory dysfunction, 80% will remain ambulatory.[40,42,43] Of patients with partial paralysis, 20% to 60% will regain function.[42,43] Only 5% of patients with paraplegia improve.[35,42,43] Patients with favorable histologic characterization (lymphoma, myeloma, breast and prostate cancers, seminoma, SCLC) and those with a slower progression of symptoms have a better chance of functional improvement with treatment.[40] Prompt recognition and treatment cannot be overstressed for patients with SCC. Patient and family education is also vital to facilitate the early reporting of the signs and symptoms associated with SCC. Paraplegia and incontinence are preventable when treatment is begun in time.[39] For patients with untreated SCC, 1-month survival is estimated.[40] Median overall survival is estimated between 3 and 16 months.[40,43]

Therapy-sensitive tumors—that is, lymphoma or myeloma—typically outperform solid tumors.[35,40,43] Approximately 50% of patients surviving 1 year remain ambulatory.[43]

SUPERIOR VENA CAVA SYNDROME

Definition

The superior vena cava is a major venous vessel that returns blood to the right atrium of the heart from the head, the upper thorax, and the upper extremities. Obstruction of the venous flow through this vessel results in impaired venous drainage, with engorgement of the vessels from the head and the upper body torso. As the venous pressure rises in the superior vena cava, blood is shunted to collateral venous pathways to facilitate return to the right atrium. The result is a characteristic constellation of physical findings known as superior vena cava syndrome (SVCS).[50,51]

Etiology and Risk Factors

The causes ascribed to SVCS have changed over the years as information has increased regarding the cancer process. William Hunter first described SVCS in 1757 in a patient with a syphilitic aneurysm.[51] Over the years, benign conditions such as aortic aneurysms, thyroid goiter, tuberculous mediastinitis, and infectious diseases were most frequently considered to be the cause of SVCS.[51] Some benign etiologies for SVCS are listed in Box 24-4. Cancer is responsible for the majority of cases.[50,52] Any tumor, primary or metastatic, can block the blood flow of the superior vena cava (SVC). Three fourths of all malignant cases of SVCS are caused by bronchogenic cancer, particularly SCLC.[50,52] Squamous cell cancer of the lung is the second most common lung histologic type to cause SVCS.[10] Lung cancers occurring on the right side are 4 times more likely to be associated with SVCS because of the proximity to the SVC.[50] Lymphomas account for approximately 15% to 20% of SVCS cases. This includes both Hodgkin's disease and non-Hodgkin's lymphoma (usually involving right-sided perihilar adenopathy).[53] Other mediastinal presentations of malignancies associated with SVCS have been Kaposi's sarcoma, thymoma, and germ cell tumors. Breast cancer is the most common metastatic disease to cause SVCS.[10] Other metastatic diseases causing SVCS include esophageal, colon, and testicular cancers. Fibrous mesothelioma has also been associated with SVCS.[53] SVCS may be the presenting symptomatology in patients with lung cancer.[53]

Innovations in therapeutic interventions for cancer have added two new causes. Venous thrombosis related to indwelling central

---

BOX 24-4	Nonmalignant Causes of SVCS

Aortic aneurysm
Infectious agents
Substernal thyroid
Central venous catheters
Mediastinal fibrosis
Thrombosis of the SVC

SVC, Superior vena cava; *SVCS,* superior vena cava syndrome.
Data from Miaskowski C: Oncologic emergencies. In Miaskowski CM, Buchsel P, editors: *Oncology nursing assessment and clinical care,* St. Louis, 1999, Mosby; and Yahalom J: Oncologic emergencies. In DeVita VT, Hellman S, Rosenberg SA, editors: *Cancer: principles and practice of oncology,* ed 7, Philadelphia, 2005, Lippincott, Williams & Wilkins.

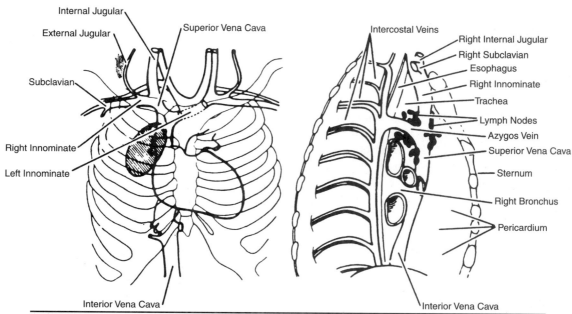

FIG. 24-8 Schematic representation of the thorax, frontal and lateral views. Shaded areas indicate typical site of obstruction. (From Lockich J, Goodman R: Superior vena cava syndrome, *JAMA* 231:58, 1975. Copyright 1975, American Medical Association.)

venous catheters has been observed in patients with SVCS. Several authorities ascribe this to be the most common nonmalignant cause of SVC obstruction.[3,7] Radiation-induced fibrosis can result in the narrowing of the SVC and produce the same clinical picture. SVCS occurs in approximately 3% to 4% of patients with cancer. Most patients with SVCS are in the fourth to seventh decades of life. The ratio of men to women is approximately 3:1.[53] However, as lung cancer incidence and death rates change, especially among women, so will the incidence, age, and gender distribution of SVCS.

Pathophysiology

The SVC is a thin-walled, low-pressure vessel about 7 cm in length (Fig. 24-8). It extends from the junction of the right and left innominate veins to the right atrium. Location in the thorax is to the right of the arteries of the trachea and the right mainstem bronchus, and posterior to the sternum. The thorax is a rigid anatomic compartment with little ability for expansion. In its space within the thorax and mediastinum, the SVC is extremely vulnerable to displacement and compression because it has a thin wall and low venous pressure, and is surrounded by the rigid structures of the sternum, the trachea, the vertebrae, the lymph nodes, the aorta, the pulmonary artery, and the right bronchus.[50,51] Therefore obstruction of the SVC can be a consequence of three physiologic events[14]:

1. External compression by an extrinsic mass, solid tumor, or enlarged lymph node
2. Intravascular obstruction by tumor or thrombosis
3. Intraluminal reaction to tumor invasion or inflammation

Impedance of venous flow through the SVC and subsequent development of SVCS depends on several factors: the degree and location of the blockage, the growth rate of the tumor, patency of the azygos vein, and proliferation of collateral circulation. The azygos vein (see Fig. 24-8) plays a pivotal role in the flow of blood through the SVC, entering it just above the pericardial reflection and making it a major tributary. The azygos vein system is the most important alternative pathway for collateral circulation.

Other collateral systems include the internal mammary, lateral thoracic, paraspinous, and esophageal venous networks.[50]

Impairment of the venous circulation through the SVC reduces blood flow to the right atrium, which results in venous hypertension with venous stasis and a decrease in cardiac output. If untreated, the syndrome progresses from vascular congestion to thrombosis, cerebral edema, pulmonary complications, and death (in weeks to months).[53] Death may occur from brain stem herniation or tracheal obstruction.[18]

Clinical Features

The clinical picture seen in SVCS is directly related to obstruction of venous drainage in the upper body (see Fig. 24-8). Compression of intrathoracic structures, vascular congestion, and venous hypertension present distinguishing clinical features. If the onset is gradual, collateral circulation develops and can compensate for the obstruction of blood flow.[14] The onset is usually insidious, but when fully developed, it requires immediate attention. The most frequent symptom of SVCS is dyspnea, occurring in 63% of patients. Other common complaints include a feeling of fullness in the head with facial swelling (50%), cough (24%), and chest pain (15%).[50-52] The classic clinical picture of SVCS includes facial swelling, periorbital edema, and engorgement of veins across the upper torso. There is disagreement in the literature about the symptoms that occur early as opposed to those that occur late in the course of SVCS. The onset and severity of signs and symptoms vary directly with the underlying disease and related pathophysiology. The presentation may be unilateral or bilateral. Because pressures in the head are higher in the supine than in the standing position, a person with early SVCS may initially have signs and symptoms only in the morning.[50] Most signs and symptoms will be exacerbated by bending forward or the supine position.[50] Early detection of SVCS hinges on a careful in-depth history and physical assessment. The clinical features of SVCS are listed in the Clinical Features box.[3,7,10]

Clinical Features of Superior Vena Cava Syndrome

Clinical Signs	Symptoms
Edema of the face, the neck, the upper thorax, the breasts, and the upper extremities	Respiratory compromise (dyspnea, shortness of breath, tachypnea, cough, orthopnea)
Periorbital edema and/or edema of the conjunctivae, with or without protrusion of the eye	Feeling of facial fullness
Horner's syndrome (sinking of eye with ptosis of eyelid)	Headache
Plethora (fullness) of the face	Visual disturbances
Increased pressure of the jugular veins	Dizziness
Dilation and prominence of collateral vessels in upper thorax and neck	Hoarseness
Telangiectasia (capillary dilation)	Chest pain
Compensatory tachycardia	Stokes' sign (tightness of shirt collar)
	Swelling of fingers (difficulty removing rings)

Data from Stewart IE: Superior vena cava syndrome: an oncologic complication, *Semin Oncol Nurs* 12:312, 1996; and Haapoja IS, Blendowski C: Superior vena cava syndrome, *Semin Oncol Nurs* 15:183, 1999.

Progression of symptoms may lead to severe respiratory obstruction, paralyzed vocal cord, cyanosis of the upper torso, "wet brain syndrome" (manifested by drowsiness, stupor, unconsciousness, and seizures), and possible coma.

Diagnosis

The diagnostic evaluation of a patient with SVCS depends greatly on the patient's physical condition. If SVCS onset is insidious, the diagnostic work-up can proceed slowly, and treatment will not be initiated until a diagnosis is confirmed. If the onset is rapid and symptoms are acute, historically, a definitive diagnosis was deferred and treatment (usually radiation therapy) begun immediately. In the past SVCS was considered one of the rare occasions when treatment could be started even before a tissue diagnosis was confirmed. In this life-threatening situation, chest radiography, the results of which rarely appear normal, and clinical presentation were considered diagnostic. A tissue biopsy to determine a primary lesion and further work-up for metastases proceeded during the course of treatment.

Current literature recommends confirmation of tissue diagnosis before initiation of treatment whenever possible.[51] The diagnosis may be obtained via bronchoalveolar lavage or thoracostomy rather than initiating immediate radiation therapy. Emergency radiation therapy is considered appropriate without a tissue diagnosis when there is altered mental status and risk of brain damage from IICP, severe upper airway compression, or cardiovascular collapse.[11]

Chest films are abnormal in more than 80% of patients with SVCS.[51,52] In 50% of patients, findings are a lung or mediastinal mass, most frequently on the right side because the SVC enters from the right. Also, 25% of patients may have mediastinal widening and pleural effusion.[53] CT scan and MRI may further define the lesion and its location.[54] Important information obtained by radiography includes more detailed information about the SVC and its tributaries as well as the source, size, and exact location of the mass in relation to the azygos vein. This information also provides the anatomic detail necessary to establish the portals for radiation therapy. Accomplishing CT and MRI may be complicated by the patient's inability to tolerate the supine position. MRI has a 96% sensitivity rate for SVCS but requires longer scanning time and is more costly.[54]

Contrast venography may be used to assess the percentage of SVC obstruction and can be valuable when surgical bypass is being

considered. Radionuclide venography using technetium 99m is an alternative method; however, images may be less well defined.[51]

Further diagnostic procedures must be evaluated for the risk versus the benefit they offer to the patient. Biopsy of palpable superficial lymph nodes, sputum for cytology, and bone marrow biopsy are associated with low risk and may provide information about the primary tumor. Invasive procedures such as bronchoscopy, mediastinoscopy, thoracoscopy, thoracotomy, or supraclavicular lymph node biopsy may be necessary but are associated with a risk of thrombosis or bleeding as a result of increased venous pressure. Improved techniques are decreasing the incidence of complications.[51] Percutaneous transthoracic CT-guided fine-needle biopsy has demonstrated a 75% sensitivity rate and may be a safe and effective alternative to open biopsy or mediastinoscopy.[51] Immediate radiation therapy may impede later tissue biopsy because of radiation-induced tissue changes.

Treatment Modalities

Four therapeutic modalities should be considered in the treatment of SVCS: radiation therapy, chemotherapy, surgery, and pharmacologic therapy. The goals are relief of symptoms and reduction of the obstructing lesion. Cure may be the goal when the primary diagnosis is SCLC, non-Hodgkin's lymphoma, or a germ cell tumor, which account for nearly half the malignant causes of SVCS.[51]

The choice of treatment depends on the rate of onset, the causative process (benign or malignant), and the type of mass (intraluminal or extraluminal). The goals of therapy for acute onset of symptoms related to SVCS are maintaining a patent airway and cardiac output.[14]

RADIATION THERAPY

Radiation therapy has been the treatment of choice for SVCS because of its local therapeutic response and minimal toxicities. Treatment is begun immediately in acute and life-threatening situations. The total dose, dose fractionation, size, and type of field depend on tumor histologic type, patient condition, radiologic response, and symptom relief. Delivery of radiation begins initially with high-dose fractionation at 3 to 4 Gy/day for the first 3 days.[51] This is typically followed by a series of lower, fractionated doses. However a standard strategy for amount of daily fractions and total doses varies in the literature.[51] Short courses of hypofractionated radiation are also being studied.[51]

Tumor reduction usually occurs with radiation therapy, especially in patients with lymphoma and SCLC. Subjective improvement has been noted in 3 to 4 days in 75% of patients, regardless of tumor histologic type. Within 7 days, 91% obtain relief. Objective response—a decrease in facial swelling and plethora, reduction of venous engorgement, and shrinkage of tumor mass—is evident in 7 to 14 days.[10]

CHEMOTHERAPY

The use of chemotherapy to treat SVCS has come to the forefront of the treatment regimen. It is an effective primary treatment when the cause of SVCS is SCLC, lymphoma, or a germ cell tumor.[51] Chemotherapy as a single modality may be used if the mediastinal area has a previous maximum radiation dose or when reduction of tumor mass will provide a smaller radiation treatment field.

The choice of chemotherapeutic agents is based on the malignant cause of SVCS. More than 80% of patients with SCLC respond to platinum-based regimens. Relief of symptoms may be seen in 7 to 10 days, with complete resolution of symptoms in about 2 weeks.[51] After the selection of agents, consideration must be given to intravenous administration. Edema and dilation of the veins in the upper extremities lead to impaired circulation. Limited venous access, poor drug distribution, and increased risk of venous irritation and extravasation of medications may contraindicate use of the upper extremities for therapy. In some situations the lower extremities may be used to administer chemotherapy by a central IV catheter placed in the femoral vein.[10]

SURGERY

Specific surgical approaches to SVCS include stent placement or SVC bypass. The placement of a wire stent may open more than 90% of occluded SVCs and result in immediate and long-term palliation.[53] Use of a stent may be indicated when other treatments for SVCS are unusable or ineffective.[54] The most common situation is recurrence of SVCS after maximum-tolerance radiation or when the acuity of the symptoms contraindicates any delay in treatment-related response. Stent placement is contraindicated when there is tumor invasion of the SVC.[54]

The stainless steel stent was designed by Gianturco and is usually referred to as the **Gianturco expandable wire stent (GEWS)** or **Gianturco Z stent.** Other products available are the balloon-expandable Palmaz stent, and the self-expandable **Wallstent.**[51] These products are constructed of stainless steel wire in a cylindrical shape and of similar function.[54] The stent is placed using a small balloon catheter inserted percutaneously with fluoroscopy with the patient under local anesthesia. The catheter is introduced into the vessel with the stent in a compressed form. When the stent is released, it expands and dilates the narrowed venous lumen. If the expansion is insufficient, the balloon is used to enlarge the stent to the desired diameter. Fibrinolytic therapy (with agents such as streptokinase, urokinase, or tissue-type plasminogen activator [TPA]) may be necessary before the procedure. Heparinization will be required during the procedure. The need for anticoagulants afterward is controversial, but may be recommended for 3 to 4 months for patients requiring preprocedure thrombolysis or in whom there is significant postprocedural residual stenosis.[10] A period of about 4 weeks is necessary for the stent to become incorporated into the endothelium of the venous wall. The stent may remain patent for long periods because of its relatively low thrombogenicity. Symptom relief may occur very quickly after stent placement (within 24 to 72 hours).[54]

One study described patient characteristics yielding best response to stent placement: those with postirradiation fibrosis or slowly progressive pressure from a recurrent extrinsic tumor had longer relief of symptoms and greater palliation than patients whose symptoms resulted from direct tumor invasion. Complications from stent placement may include hematoma formation, SVC perforation, infection, and transient renal insufficiency.[14] Rare adverse events may occur, such as stent migration into the right ventricle, stent fracture, and pulmonary edema from a rapid increase in blood flow to the lungs.[54]

Bypass of the SVC is used very judiciously because postoperative morbidity is high. Bypass surgery is indicated when the tumor could be completely removed if the SVC were excised with it, when venous return is inadequate despite collateral circulation, or when the obstruction results from venous thrombosis, fibrosis, or a benign cause. The operative procedure is delicate and precise, and is similar to arterial graft placement. The graft may be constructed using a synthetic Dacron prosthesis or the patient's own saphenous vein. The graft creates a new vessel, which rechannels blood flow around the obstruction. One end of the graft is sutured to the right atrium, and the other is sutured to either the internal jugular or innominate vein.

Patency of the bypass graft depends on the size of the anastomotic site, internal venous pressure, and blood flow. External rigidity of the graft is helpful to prevent collapse but is not required. Postoperatively, patients usually receive anticoagulation therapy and aspirin for an indefinite period to assist with graft patency.[3] When patency is maintained for several weeks, it increases the likelihood of long-term function. Reports demonstrate patency beyond a year.

PHARMACOLOGIC THERAPY

The increased use of indwelling central venous catheters has contributed to a rise in the incidence of SVCS. Whatever the cause, irritation and inflammation of the SVC related to an intraluminal or extraluminal lesion produce platelet aggregation, leading to clot formation. Fibrinolytic therapy with streptokinase, urokinase, or TPA has been used to treat intraluminal thrombosis. Fibrinolytic therapy is contraindicated with brain or spinal cord metastases, bleeding disorders, or history of stroke.[53]

Fibrinolytic therapy is appropriate when initiated within 5 to 7 days of the SVCS symptoms.[51] Anticoagulation is the preferred therapy if more than 5 to 7 days have elapsed. Inpatient heparinization is followed by long-term administration of oral warfarin (Coumadin).

Anticoagulation therapy is indicated for SVCS because of venous stasis. It may be used alone to resolve thrombus obstruction secondary to a central venous catheter or following initial fibrinolytic therapy. It is also used as a maintenance treatment to reduce the extent of the thrombus and prevent its progression. Removal of the central venous catheter should be followed by anticoagulation to avoid embolization. Low-dose warfarin (Coumadin, 1 mg/day) may be used prophylactically in patients with central lines.[54]

During the administration of radiation therapy or chemotherapy, anticoagulants may be given concomitantly as a preventive treatment. Other medical interventions may be instituted as adjunctive therapy for SVCS. Diuretics may be given to reduce edema of the head and neck, which could improve cerebration and breathing. Caution should be used when giving diuretics, because venous return to the heart is low, and hypovolemia resulting from diuresis may induce decreased venous return, dehydration, thrombosis, and shock.[14] Corticosteroids may be administered during active treatment to reduce inflammation related to the obstruction, the radiation, or the chemotherapy and the resulting tumor necrosis. Their use remains controversial.[54] Oxygen therapy may be necessary for the management of respiratory complications and maintenance of oxygen saturation and patient comfort.

Nursing Considerations

The nursing care of patients with superior vena cava syndrome (SVCS) begins with astute assessment skills, identification of those patients considered to be at risk, and close observation and baseline data collection. Documentation of vital signs, mental status, appearance, and level of activity are essential to facilitate detection of changes. Subtle changes in subjective complaints or objective parameters should be reported to the physician. Once a diagnosis of SVCS has been established, the role of the nurse is imperative as she or he observes for signs and symptoms of respiratory distress (i.e., dyspnea, shortness of breath, tachypnea, air hunger, stridor, orthopnea). Observe ventilatory movements (rate and depth), patency of airway, use of accessory muscles, clubbing of fingernails, and discoloration of nail bed or mucous membranes. Palpate the chest for fremitus, crepitus, deviation of the trachea, or nonsymmetric chest expansion. Auscultate for breath sounds. Monitor laboratory and other respiratory function tests, complete blood count (CBC), electrolytes, ABGs, chest x-ray films, and scans. Provide oxygen and mechanical ventilation as indicated. Administer respiratory medications, steroids, and analgesics as prescribed.

Assess patient for changes in cardiac function. Observe for signs of impedance of venous blood flow from the upper torso (i.e., plethora of the face; thoracic and neck vein distention; facial, trunk, and arm edema, especially in the morning; dyspnea, tachypnea, cough; cyanosis; mental status changes). Monitor ECGs. Position patient for comfort and enhancement of venous drainage from upper torso (elevate and support upper extremities; avoid elevation of lower extremities; avoid constrictive clothing). Avoid invasive or constrictive procedures involving upper extremities. Maintain a cool room temperature. Prevent activities that increase intrathoracic or intracerebral pressure (e.g., Valsalva maneuver, vomiting, bending over, stooping). Provide measures to decrease anxiety. Antianxiolitic medications may be needed.

As the acute phase of SVCS passes, the patient will be ready to become more involved in self-care, and anticipatory guidance can be given to facilitate continued therapy and detection of any changes in the patient's condition.

Prognosis

Patients usually respond to treatment for SVCS, showing regression of the tumor. The signs and symptoms of SVCS are largely reversible and subside in 3 days to 2 weeks.[18] SVCS recurs in only 10% to 20% of patients.[11]

The prognosis of patients with SVCS strongly correlates with the prognosis of the underlying disease. Some patients have not responded to treatment. This has been attributed to their generally poorer condition, the presence of thrombosis in the SVC, and metastatic disease. The best responses are seen in patients with lymphoma and SCLC. Other types of lung cancer have fewer

long-term responses. Although a diagnosis of SVCS may not offer long-term survival, with prompt diagnosis and treatment, it can be managed and therefore improves the patient's quality of life.

Metabolic Oncologic Complications
DISSEMINATED INTRAVASCULAR COAGULATION

Definition

Disseminated intravascular coagulation (DIC) is considered to be a bleeding disorder. In the past it was referred to as a "consumptive coagulopathy."[55] Bleeding disorders are classified as congenital or acquired. DIC is one of the acquired disorders. It is not a disease entity but rather an event that can accompany various disease processes. DIC is an alteration in the blood-clotting mechanism, with abnormal acceleration of the **coagulation cascade,** resulting in thrombosis. Hemorrhage occurs simultaneously as a result of the depletion of clotting factors.

Etiology and Risk Factors

This disorder is not a primary, independent disorder. An underlying pathology, benign or malignant, is responsible for DIC. The pathology creates the triggering mechanism or initiating event necessary for the activation of thrombin, which is responsible for the cascade of blood clot formation and clot dissolution, thus producing DIC. A variety of pathologies involve a triggering event, which can cause either endothelial tissue injury or blood vessel injury.

Endothelial injuries include the following[55]:
- *Shock or trauma*—head injury, burns
- *Infections*—aspergillosis, gram-positive sepsis, or gram-negative sepsis
- *Obstetric complications*—abruptio placentae, amniotic fluid embolism, eclampsia
- *Malignancies*—acute promyelocytic myelogenous leukemia (APML), acute myelogenous leukemia (AML), mucin-producing adenocarcinomas (cancers of the lung, colon, breast, and prostate)

Blood vessel injuries include the following:
- *Infectious vasculitis*—Rocky Mountain spotted fever, certain viral infections, severe glomerulonephritis
- *Vascular disorders or interventions*—aortic aneurysm, giant hemangioma, angiography
- *Intravascular hemolysis*—hemolytic transfusion reaction, multiple whole-blood transfusions, massive trauma, extracorporeal circulation devices (e.g., cardiopulmonary bypass machine, aortic balloon pump), heat stroke, peritoneovenous shunting
- *Miscellaneous*—pancreatitis, liver disease (e.g., obstructive jaundice, acute hepatic failure), snakebite

In patients with cancer the incidence of DIC is less than 10% to 15%. It is usually related to the disease process or the treatment of the cancer and often occurs concomitantly with sepsis.[3,7]

Oncology-related DIC occurs with the most frequency in patients with APML. Approximately 85% to 90% of the patients with APML will develop DIC.[48,56] The next most common cancers associated with DIC are the mucin-producing adenocarcinomas (lung, breast, stomach, pancreas, and prostate).[53] However, the most common cause of DIC is sepsis.[57] Independent risk factors include older age, male gender, advanced disease, and the presence of necrosis.[58]

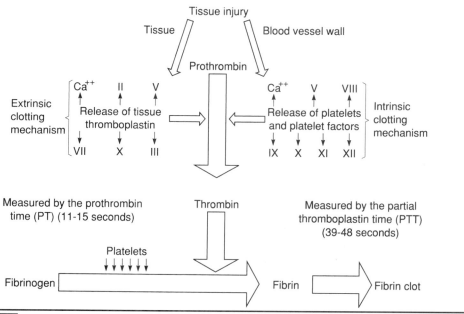

FIG. 24-9   Formation of a blood clot. (From Yasko JM, Schafer SL: Disseminated intravascular coagulation. In Yasko JM, editor: *Guidelines for cancer care: symptom management,* Reston, VA, Reston, (c) 1983. Reprinted by permission of Prentice-Hall, Inc, Upper Saddle River, N.J.)

Pathophysiology

Body hemostasis depends on an intricate balance between blood clot formation and blood clot dissolution. The fibrin blood clot is the end product of the blood-clotting mechanism. Normally, this mechanism is initiated when tissues sustain an injury. Disruption of the vascular endothelium exposes collagen fibers to blood. Smooth muscle spasm then occurs, releasing serotonin. Vasoconstriction follows, which slows the flow of blood and causes circulating platelets to change shape and adhere to the rough surface of injured vessels within 1 to 2 seconds. More platelets aggregate and form a loose plug at the site of injury, creating a seal on the vessel wall to control bleeding. The injured vascular tissue also releases a phospholipid called **thromboplastin,** which initiates the clotting reaction.

The fibrin blood clot is formed through a series of sequential reactions that are protein activated (Fig. 24-9). This protein activation occurs through two different cascades of reactions known as the intrinsic and extrinsic pathways, which operate jointly to form the blood clot. The **intrinsic pathway** is activated by injury to the blood vessel wall. The **extrinsic pathway** is activated after tissue injury. Central to each pathway is the conversion of prothrombin to thrombin through a series of reactions involving various blood factors (phospholipids, proteins, calcium). The thrombin then acts as a catalyst to convert fibrinogen (a monomer) to fibrin (a polymer). The fibrin polymers form a mesh of fibrin strands, which trap platelets, red blood cells (RBCs), and leukocytes, making an occlusive clot.

The series of reactions that forms the clot is balanced by a series of reactions that limits the size of the clot and later dissolves it. Therefore clot dissolution occurs in conjunction with clot formation. When the clot is no longer needed, it is converted from a polymer back to a monomer by **fibrinolysin** (plasmin). Fibrinolysin is formed in the presence of thrombin during coagulation when preactivators come in contact with a tissue enzyme

known as **kinase.** Fibrinogen and fibrin are broken down by fibrinolysis, resulting in **fibrin degradation products (FDPs)** or **fibrin split products (FSPs).** As these fragments circulate, they interfere with the formation of fibrin and coat the platelets, thus decreasing their adhesive ability. The result is anticoagulation along with the process of fibrinolysis: the body forms **antithrombins,** natural anticoagulants that also interfere with thrombin (clotting) activity. Hemostasis is therefore balanced between fibrin clot formation (**coagulation**) and clot dissolution by fibrinolysis (**anticoagulation**).

DIC is a disruption of body hemostasis. One of the triggering mechanisms from the underlying pathology initiates the process (Fig. 24-10). Release of tissue factor (TF), a transmembrane glycoprotein, stimulates the coagulation cascade, which results in the formation of thrombin and fibrinolysin (plasmin).[57] TF is present on the surface of endothelial cells, macrophages, and monocytes. Exposure to cytokines (such as interleukin), tumor necrosis factor, and endotoxin may stimulate its release.[57] Thrombin acts to convert fibrinogen to fibrin to form clots. At the same time, fibrinolysin degrades some of the fibrin into a soluble monomer form; this initiates clot dissolution. The remaining portion of fibrin is an insoluble polymer, which continues to form clots. These clots may be deposited in the extremities or in organs such as the lungs, the kidneys, and the brain. Capillary clots slow the blood flow, resulting in tissue ischemia, hypoxia, and necrosis. The clots also trap circulating platelets in the microvasculature, which results in thrombocytopenia. As the fibrinolysin continues to degrade fibrin, the by-products, FDPs, are produced. These FDPs disrupt the conversion of fibrin to a polymer; coat platelets, decreasing their adherence; and degrade factors V, VIII, and X, which leads to capillary hemorrhage.

Patients with hematologic malignancies are at risk for DIC because of disseminated disease, risk for infection, and rapid cell turnover. Patients with leukemia often have some of the characteristics of DIC without having the complete DIC syndrome.

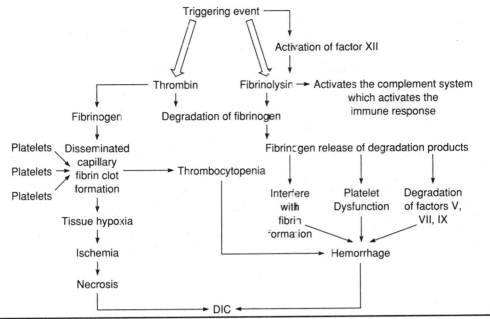

FIG. 24-10 Pathophysiology of disseminated intravascular coagulation (DIC). (From Yasko JM, Schafer SL: Disseminated intravascular coagulation. In Yasko JM, editor: *Guidelines for cancer care: symptom management,* Reston, Va, © 1983. Reprinted by permission of Prentice-Hall, Inc, Upper Saddle River, NJ.)

Occurrence of DIC in patients with leukemia is 1% to 2%. APML typically causes a low-grade or chronic form of DIC that is characterized by thrombotic complications such as deep venous thrombosis.[59] The blast cells in APML are hypergranular and release a procoagulant substance similar to thromboplastin (factor VIII) that stimulates the clotting cascade. This release may occur at any time, such as at diagnosis or after chemotherapy. The increased incidence of DIC in APML has also been explained by the increased expression of annexin II on APML cells. Annexin II, a phospholipid-binding protein on endothelial cell surfaces, binds to plasminogen and increases the production of plasmin. This leads to unopposed fibrinolysis and bleeding.[55-57]

Solid tumors (mucin-producing adenocarcinomas) also tend to produce the more chronic form of DIC. They develop new blood vessels with abnormal endothelial linings that are thought to activate the procoagulant system. Necrotic tissue or tissue enzymes may also be released into circulation and stimulate coagulation.[57] Many solid tumors are associated with an increased production of clotting factors that increase the incidence of thromboses.[56]

More acute forms of DIC are caused by extensive disease, tumor lysis syndrome, and sepsis. Endotoxins associated with sepsis are thought to activate factor XII and initiate coagulation. Gram-positive organisms, human immunodeficiency virus, varicella, hepatitis, and cytomegalovirus are also known to trigger the clotting cascade.[60]

If the underlying pathology with its triggering mechanism is not treated or otherwise eliminated, it will promote further coagulopathy. The term **consumptive coagulopathy** has been used to describe this increased use (consumption) of platelets and clotting factors, leading to a continuation of thrombocytopenia and a further decrease of clotting factors and resulting in bleeding. Thus the abnormal activation of thrombin in DIC results in a cyclic paradox of thrombosis or hemorrhage or both (see Fig. 24-10).

Clinical Features

The onset of DIC may be acute, chronic, or somewhere in between. The clinical manifestations and laboratory findings depend on the triggering event and the body tissues involved. The presenting signs and symptoms result from disseminated clotting and bleeding, which may be overt or occult. Bleeding usually predominates.

Signs of bleeding are multiple and may be seen from any body orifice. Bleeding may range from oozing to frank bleeding or hemorrhage. Patients may have overt oozing from venipuncture sites, mucous membranes, needle puncture sites, or incisions. Petechiae, ecchymoses, purpura, or hematomas may be evident. Profound menstrual or GI bleeding may occur, as well as epistaxis or hemoptysis. The possibility of occult internal or intracerebral bleeding is equally critical. Abdominal distention, blood in stools, blood in urine or skin, and scleral changes may be observed. Other signs of occult bleeding may be mental status changes, orthopnea, and tachycardia.[57]

Clotting resulting from fibrin deposits in the microcirculation will impede blood flow. Early signs of clotting may include oliguria, hypoxemia, and cool and mottled extremities.[61] Progression can cause severe tissue ischemia and lead to tissue necrosis. Multiple system changes may be observed. A major concern for a person experiencing DIC is the possibility of irreversible end-organ damage. The systems with the most risk of microvascular thrombosis include the cardiac, pulmonary, renal, hepatic, and central nervous systems.

Observation of the skin may show acrocyanosis, also known as **Raynaud's sign** (generalized sweating with symmetric mottling of the nose, the fingers, the toes, and the genitalia), and other ischemic changes, which can lead to superficial gangrene. Pulmonary signs, such as severe, sudden dyspnea at rest with tachypnea and progressive rales and rhonchi, are similar to those observed with acute respiratory distress syndrome (ARDS).

The GI tract may have an ischemic insult appearing as an ulceration, and tubular necrosis of the kidney may lead to renal failure. If microcoagulation occurs in the brain, multifocal cerebrovascular accidents (CVAs, or strokes), mental change, delirium, and coma may result. The associated symptoms of bleeding or clotting will vary depending on the system sustaining the ischemic insult or bleeding. Complaints include malaise, weakness, air hunger, altered sensorium, visual changes, and headaches. The presence and magnitude of these disturbances depend on the extent of the clotting and bleeding.

Diagnosis

Laboratory findings substantiate a diagnosis of DIC (Table 24-3). No single blood test can confirm or exclude a diagnosis of DIC. Instead, screening has traditionally been accomplished by measuring platelet count, prothrombin time (PT), partial thromboplastin time (PTT), and fibrinogen level. More recently, if abnormal results are obtained, the diagnosis is confirmed by the level of FDPs and D-dimer (a neoantigen formed when plasmin digests fibrin).[62] D-dimer is abnormal in 93% of cases, and FDP titer is abnormal in 75%. Antithrombin III (now referred to as antithrombin, AT) levels will be abnormal in 89% of cases.[62]

Platelet count is decreased. This indicates **thrombocytopenia,** which is the cardinal laboratory finding. More than 90% of patients with DIC have abnormal platelet count and PT. In about 50% of these patients, the platelet count is less than 50,000/mm³ (normal: 150,000 to 400,000/mm³).

The PT is prolonged (normal: 10 to 13 seconds). This arises from the extrinsic coagulation system, reflecting decreased levels of clotting factors II, V, and X and of fibrinogen.

Fibrinogen level is decreased (normal: 200 to 400 mg/dl), resulting from the consumption of fibrinogen by thrombin-induced clotting and excessive fibrinolysis. Fibrinogen levels less than 150 mg/dl are found in 70% of patients with DIC.

The PTT is prolonged (normal: 39 to 48 seconds), and is a measure of the intrinsic coagulation system.

The FDPs or FSPs are increased (normal: below 10 mcg/ml), and are 100% sensitive for DIC, but only 50% specific. The D-dimer level will be decreased. It is less sensitive than FDP, but 100% specific. Together, the FDP and D-dimer have 95% to 100% specificity and sensitivity.[57,62]

Factor assays, especially V and VIII, are decreased.

Protamine sulfate precipitation test (thrombin activation test) is strongly positive (normal: negative).

Antithrombin III levels are decreased (normal: 89% to 120%).[60]

Additional tests are being developed to determine accelerated coagulation (fibrinopeptide A, prothrombin activation peptides or fragments, thrombin-antithrombin complexes) and accelerated fibrinolysis (plasminogen, α_2-antiplasmin). As availability increases, these tests may help support the diagnosis and monitoring of DIC.[57]

Laboratory tests for DIC can be complicated by underlying conditions. Patients with liver disease have abnormal clotting studies and, often, thrombocytopenia. Laboratory findings in these patients show prolonged PT and decreased fibrinogen levels. Fibrinogen levels, usually elevated in the presence of sepsis, pregnancy, or malignancy, may fall within the normal range if DIC is concurrently present. Serum creatinine and liver transaminases are elevated with extensive clotting. Hemolysis will elevate reticulocytes and blood urea nitrogen (BUN) as hemoglobin decreases.[59] Finally, multiple transfusions may cause alteration in the levels of clotting factors or platelets.

Treatment Modalities

The primary goal of therapy in DIC is to eliminate or alter the triggering event. Sepsis is treated with antibiotics. Surgery, chemotherapy, and radiation therapy are used to treat the underlying malignancy. All-trans retinoic acid has been shown to rapidly reverse DIC in patients with APML.[58,63] Fluid replacement is used to manage hypotension and proteinuria. If the DIC is chronic, only supportive measures may be necessary until the DIC is resolved. Depending on the progression of the DIC, the success of treating the triggering event, and the predominant signs and symptoms, therapy is directed at stopping the intravascular clotting process and controlling the bleeding. When bleeding is severe, blood component therapy is necessary to achieve hemostasis. It is used to correct the clotting deficiencies caused by the consumption of blood components during the DIC process. Common blood products used in treating DIC are as follows:

Platelets contain platelet factor III, which strengthens the endothelium, prevents petechial hemorrhage, facilitates the conversion of prothrombin to thrombin, and functions as a mechanical plug by adhering to the vessel wall. The amount and frequency of platelet replacement is dependent upon the patient's platelet count and physical condition. Spontaneous hemorrhage is of concern, especially when the platelet count falls below 15,000/mm³. Usually, 6 to 10 units are given and will raise the platelet count by 30,000 to 50,000/mm³.

Fresh-frozen plasma (FFP) is used for volume expansion. It contains clotting factors V, VIII, and XIII, and antithrombin III. Usually, 2 to 4 units of FFP are given once or twice a day. Each unit of infused FFP raises each clotting factor by 5%.

Packed red blood cells (PRBCs) are used to increase RBCs and clotting factors. PRBCs are used instead of whole blood to reduce the development of antibodies and fluid overload.

TABLE 24-3	DIC Lab Values	
TEST	**NORMAL VALUE**	**DIC VALUE**
PT	10-13 sec	>15 sec, usually prolonged
PTT	39-48 sec	Usually prolonged
Platelets	150,000–400,000 mm³	<150,000 mm³, decreased
Factor assay		Decreased factors VI, VIII, IX
Fibrinogen	150-350 mg/dl	<100-150 mg/dl, decreased
FDPs	10-40	>40, increased
D-Dimer	<250 ng/ml	>500, increased
Antithrombin	85-125	<85, decreased

PT, prothrombin time; PTT, partial thromboplastin time; FDPs, fibrin degradation products.
Data from Shelton BK, Baker L, Stecker S: Critical care of the patient with hematologic malignancy, *AACN Clin Issues: Adv Pract Acute Crit Care* 7:65, 1996; Yasko JM, Schafer SL: Disseminated intravascular coagulation. In Yasko JM, editor: *Guidelines for cancer care: symptom management,* Reston, VA, 1983, Prentice-Hall; and Glover DJ, Glick JH: Oncologic emergencies. In Holleb AI, Fink DJ, Murphy GP, editors: *American Cancer Society textbook of clinical oncology,* Atlanta, 1991, American Cancer Society.

Usually, 2 units are given when the hematocrit drops below 25%. Each unit of PRBCs should raise the hemoglobin count by 1.

Cryoprecipitate contains fibrinogen (approximately 200 mg/unit) and factor VIII. It is used for patients with severe hypofibrinogenemia. Usually, 2 units of cryoprecipitate is administered every 6 hours when the fibrinogen level falls below 50 mg/dl. A total of 10 units of cryoprecipitate is administered. Each unit of cryoprecipitate increases the level of fibrinogen and factor VIII by 2%.

Heparin therapy, which inhibits thrombin formation, is controversial in DIC. Research is lacking to support the risk/benefit ratio. The anticoagulation effects of heparin result from the prevention of the platelet aggregation that triggers the intrinsic pathway of the coagulation cascade. Heparin interferes with thrombin and stops the conversion of fibrinogen to fibrin, preventing clot formation. It does not lyse clots already formed; those require thrombin to activate fibrinogen.

Dosages of heparin have included 2500 to 5000 units subcutaneously every 8 to 12 hours, 50 units/kg of body weight by IV bolus every 4 to 6 hours, or 100 to 200 units/kg every 24 hours by IV infusion. Current recommendations are to use low-dose continuous infusion heparin for patients with the more chronic form of DIC (5 to 15 units/kg per hour).[56,63] Effective heparin therapy produces cessation of clot formation, a rise in platelet count and fibrinogen levels, and a decrease in the level of FDPs. PTT is monitored to assess the patient's response to heparin. A therapeutic level is reached when the patient's PTT is 1.5 to 2 times the normal level. Heparin is contraindicated in patients with any intracranial insult such as bleeding or CVA. It is also avoided in patients who have had recent surgery.[57]

Failure to respond to heparin therapy has been attributed to a depletion of **antithrombin III** (AT-III). AT-III is a blood component factor that inhibits the competitive action of thrombin during heparin therapy. Therefore, in patients with low AT-III levels and no response to heparin therapy, AT-III may be administered along with heparin; however, this form of therapy is not yet considered standard of care.[59]

Finally, in addition to the control of clotting, medical attention is given to the control of bleeding. Usually, heparin therapy produces anticoagulation and, at the same time, controls fibrinolysis. In 5% of patients, however, fibrinolysis continues, and uncontrolled bleeding results. In these patients, **antifibrinolytic therapy** may be administered, using a drug called **e-aminocaproic acid (EACA)**. EACA interferes with the intrinsic fibrinolytic process, which can lead to further clot formation. Therefore EACA is used only when intravascular clotting is effectively controlled or the primary etiology is related to hyperfibronolysis, such as in prostate cancer.[56,63] The usual dosage is 5 to 10 g given IV by slow bolus, followed by 2 to 4 g every 1 to 2 hours for 24 hours or until bleeding stops. Patients receiving EACA must be closely monitored for hypotension, hypokalemia, cardiac dysrhythmias, and increased intravascular coagulation. A newer, more potent fibrinolytic inhibitor, tranexamic acid, has less toxicity than EACA and is sometimes used with APML.[57] Both EACA and tranexamic acid are controversial because they can cause widespread fibrin deposition that can lead to ischemia and organ failure.[60]

Nursing Considerations

The nursing management of patients with disseminated intravascular coagulation (DIC), as the condition itself, is extremely complex. Depending on the onset and severity of DIC, the nurse's role can range from watchful waiting to intensive participation in treatment. Nursing care focuses on minimizing the multitude of potentially life-threatening problems associated with DIC. Care is directed toward astute and ongoing assessment to detect bleeding (overt or occult) or thrombosis, provision of care for bleeding or thrombosis, prevention of further complications, and support of other needs.

Assessment of organ systems for evidence of bleeding and thrombosis involves the following:

- *Integumentary*: Observe skin for evidence of bleeding (e.g., petechiae, ecchymosis, purpura, pallor, frank blood, oozing). Closely examine the mouth, including the mucous membranes of the palate and gums; the sclera; the nose; the ears; the urethra; the vagina; and the rectum. Check all venipuncture and puncture sites and wound sites.
- *Pulmonary*: Auscultate lungs for crackles, wheezes, and stridor. Observe for dyspnea, tachypnea, cyanosis, hemoptysis, and chest pain.
- *Cardiovascular*: Monitor for tachycardia, hypotension, and changes in peripheral pulses. Assess for palpitations and angina.
- *Renal*: Measure intake and output. Observe for peripheral edema and oliguria.
- *Gastrointestinal*: Palpate abdomen for pain. Measure abdominal girth daily. Test all exretia (i.e., urine, stool, sputum, vomitus) for blood.
- *Neurologic*: Observe for irritability or changes in mental status. Assess frequently for headache, blurred vision, and vertigo.

Monitor laboratory values closely for abnormalities indicative of bleeding or infection, including CBC, platelet count, PT, and fibrinogen level. Avoid administration of aspirin or aspirin-containing products. Discourage activities that increase ICP or intraabdominal pressure (e.g., Valsalva maneuver). Administer stool softeners as ordered. Attempt to prevent further clotting by doing the following:

- Provide adequate hydration.
- Avoid constrictive clothing and devices.
- Use prescribed elastic support hose.
- Discourage leg dangling, sitting for long periods, and crossing legs.
- Elevate legs at intermittent intervals to prevent venous stasis when sitting or lying.
- Perform ROM exercises for legs.
- Encourage deep breathing and coughing.
- Administer heparin therapy as ordered using an infusion-controlling device.

Make all attempts to maintain skin integrity. Limit venipunctures; however, if necessary, use small-gauge needles. Avoid subcutaneous and intramuscular injections. If necessary, apply pressure to site for 5 minutes. Avoid rectal manipulation (i.e., rectal suppositories, thermometers, and digital rectal exams). Use electric razors instead of straight-edged razors. Avoid use of indwelling catheters, but if necessary, keep them well lubricated and without tension. Avoid vaginal manipulation (e.g., tampons, douches). Perform frequent gentle oral hygiene with soft-bristled toothbrush or sponge Toothettes. Avoid mouthwashes with high alcohol content.

The management of a patient with DIC is complex and difficult. The experience is often terrifying for the patient and family, and frustrating for the nurse. The patient's condition can change rapidly. Everyone must be alert to and prepared for all possible sequelae of DIC.

Prognosis

The prognosis of the patient with DIC depends on the underlying cause, the degree of disruption in the coagulation system, and the effects of bleeding and clotting. Most patients with cancer who develop DIC experience hemorrhage. A smaller number demonstrate thromboembolism. The estimated mortality rate for DIC is 54% to 68%. Mortality from DIC has decreased in the past decade. This is attributed to new antileukemia agents, combinations of anticancer therapies, and advances in blood component therapies. Prognostic factors including increasing age, severity of laboratory abnormalities, and number of clinical manifestations increase the mortality from DIC. In the patient with DIC, a minor injury can have a fatal consequence. The most common cause of death in DIC is intracranial hemorrhage.

HYPERCALCEMIA

Definition

Hypercalcemia is a metabolic condition that occurs when the serum calcium level rises above the normal level of 9 to 11 mg/dl. Hypercalcemia is a frequent complication of certain types of malignancies and metastatic disease. It is a potentially life-threatening problem, because the onset is variable and may go unnoticed until the problem becomes severe. Lack of intervention can lead to renal failure, coma, or cardiac arrest. With prompt recognition and adequate treatment, this condition can be reversed.

Etiology and Risk Factors

A variety of conditions can cause hypercalcemia (Box 24-5), with 90% of hypercalcemia caused by primary hyperparathyroidism (65%) or malignancy (35%).[64] Hypercalcemia is one of the most common oncologic emergencies, occurring in 10% to 20% of oncology patients.[65,66] Malignancies associated with this condition include cancers of the breast and the kidneys; squamous cell cancers of the lung, the head, the neck, or the esophagus; lymphoma; leukemia; and multiple myeloma. Solid tumors, lung cancer, and breast cancer account for 80% of malignancy-related hypercalcemia. The remaining 20% include causes from multiple myeloma, leukemia, and lymphoma. Patients with metastatic cancers being treated with estrogens or antiestrogens may experience progression of hypercalcemia, possibly from hormonal stimulation of the tumor.[64] Bony metastasis from any malignant primary tumor may also be a causative condition. Nonmalignant conditions that can induce or worsen hypercalcemia include primary hyperparathyroidism, thyrotoxicosis, prolonged immobilization, vitamins A and D intoxication, renal failure, and diuretic therapy with thiazide preparations. Dehydration, volume depletion, and hypoalbuminemia may contribute to or aggravate hypercalcemia.

Pathophysiology

Calcium is an essential inorganic element in the body. Most of it (99%) is found in skeletal tissue, providing strength and durability. The remaining 1% is in the serum. One half of the serum calcium (0.5%) is ionized, and one half (0.5%) is bound to circulating albumin. Serum calcium levels include both the ionized portion and the protein-bound portion. Under normal conditions the ionized calcium is in equilibrium with the protein-bound calcium. Changes in serum albumin level directly affect serum calcium levels.

Serum calcium levels in the presence of hypoalbuminemia may not be representative of the true value for ionized calcium. Reduction of serum albumin, which is often seen in very ill or

---

BOX 24-5   Causes of Hypercalcemia

Endocrine Disorders
Primary hyperparathyroidism
Multiple endocrine adenomatosis
Familial hyperparathyroidism
Familial hypocalciuric hypercalcemia
Hyperthyroidism
Hypoadrenalism
Pheochromocytoma

Malignancy
Humoral hypercalcemia of malignancy (HHM)
Parathyroid hormone–related protein (PTHRP)
1,25-dihydroxyvitamin D
Transforming growth factor (TGF-α)
Interleukin-1 (IL-1)
Granulocyte-macrophage colony-stimulating factor (GM-CSF)
Tumor necrosis factor (TNF-α and TNF-β)
Prostaglandin E_2 (PGE$_2$)
Interferon
Local osteolytic hypercalcemia (LOH)

Medications
Thiazide diuretics
Theophylline
Lithium
Estrogens and antiestrogens

Granulomatous Disorders
Sarcoidosis
Tuberculosis
Coccidioidomycosis
Histoplasmosis
Beryliosis
Candidiasis
Cryptococcosis
Leprosy

Immobilization

Renal Disease

Diet
Milk-alkali syndrome
Vitamin A or D intoxication

Other
Paget's disease
Adolescence
Parenteral nutrition

Data from Kovacs CS et al: Hypercalcemia of malignancy in the palliative care patient: a treatment strategy, *J Pain Symptom Manage* 10:224, 1995; and Mundy GR, Guise TA: Hypercalcemia of malignancy, *Am J Med* 103:134, 1997.

elderly patients, may result in a greater proportion of ionized calcium because of the unavailability of albumin for binding. Therefore the severity of hypercalcemia in a patient with hypoalbuminemia may be underestimated. Box 24-6 provides a formula to correct for decreased serum albumin. Only the ionized portion of calcium is capable of physiologic function. Calcium is responsible for bone and tooth formation, normal clotting mechanism, and cellular permeability. Calcium ion concentration regulates the contractility of the cardiac, smooth, and skeletal muscles and the excitability of nerve tissue.

Normal serum calcium levels are maintained in a state of equilibrium through a dynamic relationship among all three forms of calcium (stored, ionized, and albumin bound), with a constant shifting from one form to another. Homeostasis is maintained through several body processes: GI calcium absorption, renal calcium resorption, and a balance of bone resorption of calcium and deposition of calcium through new bone formation. A balance is maintained between osteoclast (bone resorption) and osteoblast (bone formation) activity.[64] Metabolism of calcium is controlled by a negative feedback mechanism between calcium ion concentration and three hormones: parathyroid hormone (PTH, parathormone), activated vitamin D (1,25-dihydroxyvitamin D), and calcitonin.

A decrease in serum calcium stimulates an increase in PTH secretion (Fig. 24-11). PTH enhances calcium absorption from the GI tract and renal tubular resorption of calcium with increased excretion of phosphorus. Calcium ions and phosphorus ions have a directly inverse relationship: when the amount of one is increased, the amount of the other is decreased. PTH also promotes osteoclastic activity. Osteoclasts are multinucleated bone cells that function to remove damaged bone tissue. This results in the destruction of bones, releasing calcium into the bloodstream.

Vitamin D is activated by PTH and increases calcium absorption from the GI mucosa. Calcitonin is released by the thyroid gland in response to an increased serum calcium level and inhibits bone resorption of calcium. The effect of calcitonin is short-lived.

In general, hypercalcemia is the result of increased bone resorption of calcium, which exceeds renal ability to excrete the calcium overload. Hypercalcemia resulting from malignancies occurs through several different mechanisms, depending on the location and action of the cancer cells, as follows:

- Direct bony destruction by tumor cells, which causes osteoclastic activity, resulting in the release of calcium from bone into the serum
- Prolonged immobilization, which increases osteoclastic activity
- Ectopic PTH production by tumor cells, which enhances calcium resorption; secretion continues despite an elevated serum calcium level
- Metabolic substances produced by the tumor, such as osteoclast-activating factor (OAF), prostaglandin, or prostaglandin-like substances, all of which enhance osteoclastic activity

Other contributing conditions include the following:

- Dehydration or volume depletion or both
- Hypervitaminosis of A and D (excessive use of vitamin A and D supplements)
- Excessive use of calcium supplements
- Hyperparathyroidism
- Prolonged use of thiazide diuretics

Historically, malignancy-related hypercalcemia has been closely associated with tumor invasion into the bone by direct tumor extension or metastasis. However, 15% of hypercalcemia in malignancy occurs in patients without bony metastases. SCLC and prostate cancer, even though they commonly metastasize to the bone, are not frequently associated with hypercalcemia.[19] For these reasons, researchers continued investigating the pathophysiology of hypercalcemia in malignancy. The skeletal process, **local osteolytic hypercalcemia (LOH)**, is no longer considered the most common mechanism of hypercalcemia. Approximately 80% of hypercalcemic malignancies have been found to be caused by humoral factors associated with the presence of malignant cells.[66] One of these, PTH-related peptide (PTHrP), is produced ectopically by malignant cells and is responsible for 80% to 90% of hypercalcemia of malignancy.[65,66] The humoral agents have a normal physiologic function in the body but can be induced by and released from malignant cells. They cause hypercalcemia by

---

BOX 24-6   Calculation of Estimated Ionized Serum Calcium

Formula to correct for changes in serum albumin concentrations (allow 0.8 mg/dl for each g/dl change in serum albumin):
Corrected serum calcium = actual serum calcium (mg/dl) + ([4.0 - serum albumin (g/dl)] × 0.8)

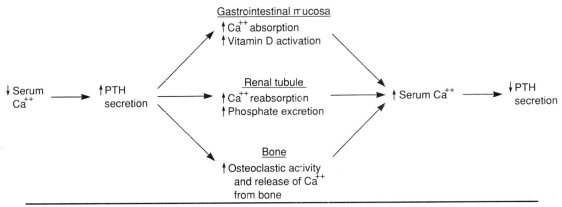

FIG. 24-11 Effects of parathyroid hormone (PTH) on serum calcium levels.

stimulating osteoclastic activity and bone resorption, inhibiting bone formation, and increasing the renal tubular reabsorption of calcium. The various humoral factors are thought to act synergistically. In addition to PTH-rP, humoral factors associated with hypercalcemia include OAFs, transforming growth factors (TGFs), hematopoietic colony-stimulating factors (CSFs), prostaglandins (E series), and 1,25-dihydroxyvitamin D.[64]

Clinical Features

Hypercalcemia disrupts normal cellular functions and adversely affects various organs. Clinical manifestations vary tremendously, depending on the level of serum calcium, the rate of onset, the underlying cause, and the patient's general condition. Patients may be asymptomatic or mildly symptomatic or may have severe problems (Table 24-4). Onset may be insidious or acute. Diagnosis may be difficult because of multisystem involvement making it resemble other disorders, including side effects of chemotherapy and radiation therapy.

Signs and symptoms are directly related to cellular activity of the involved body system (see Table 24-8). Normal cell membranes are lined with calcium ions, which control the permeability of the cell. This gating mechanism allows sodium ions to enter the cell and depolarization to occur. Increased calcium ions decrease cellular permeability and subsequently alter cellular function. This decreases neuron permeability, resulting in a depressive effect on the CNS and peripheral nervous system (PNS).

Symptoms may include restlessness, agitation, lethargy, and confusion, which may progress to coma. Skeletal muscles become hypotonic, with decreased or absent deep tendon reflexes, ataxia, and fatigue. The smooth muscle action of the GI system slows, leading to decreased motility, anorexia, nausea, vomiting, constipation, possible abdominal distention and, later, ileus. Impaired cardiac muscle conduction and contractility can result in dysrhythmias or even cardiac arrest.

Compensatory renal mechanisms increase urinary calcium resorption, leading to an inability to concentrate urine. This causes a syndrome similar to nephrogenic diabetes insipidus and is manifested by polyuria and polydipsia. The polyuria and hypercalciuria result in dehydration and a decrease in glomerular filtration rate (GFR). Dehydration from this eventuality or from nausea and vomiting produces a further decline in the GFR of the kidney. The lowered GFR in turn increases reabsorption of sodium in the proximal tubules in an attempt to retain water. Because sodium and calcium work in tandem, calcium is also resorbed. This can

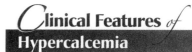

Clinical Signs
Lethargy
Change in mental status (restlessness, confusion, stupor, coma)
Vomiting
Dysrhythmias
Polyuria
Electrocardiogram (ECG) changes
Renal calculi
Renal failure

Symptoms
Anxiety
Fatigue and weakness
Anorexia
Nausea
Polydipsia
Constipation

Data from Barnett ML: Hypercalcemia, *Semin Oncol Nurs* 15:190, 1999.

TABLE 24-4   Degrees of Hypercalcemia: Signs and Symptoms*

BODY SYSTEM AFFECTED	MILD (<12 mg/dl)	MODERATE (12-15 mg/dl)	SEVERE (>15 mg/dl)
Gastrointestinal	Anorexia, nausea, vomiting, vague abdominal pain	Constipation, increased abdominal pain, abdominal distention	Atonic ileus, obstipation
Neurologic	Restlessness, difficulty in concentrating, depression, apathy, lethargy, clouding of consciousness	Confusion, psychoses, somnolence	Coma, death
Muscular	Easily fatigued, muscle weakness (generalized or involving shoulders and hips), hyporeflexia	Increased muscular weakness, bone pain	Profound muscular weakness, ataxia, pathologic fractures
Renal	Nocturia, polyuria, polydipsia	Renal tubular acidosis, renal calculi	Oliguric renal failure, renal insufficiency, azotemia
Cardiovascular	Hypertension (may or may not be present)	Cardiac dysrhythmias, ECG abnormalities (shortening of QT interval on ECG, coving of ST-T wave, widening of T wave)	Cardiac arrest, death

*Signs and symptoms regardless of serum calcium levels may vary from person to person.
From Poe CM, Radford AI: The challenges of hypercalcemia in cancer, *Oncol Nurs Forum* 12(6):29, 1985.

further potentiate the hypercalcemia. Elevation of serum calcium levels produces a supersaturation of calcium and then precipitation. Precipitation in the kidneys can lead to calcium renal stones and possible renal failure, as evidenced by an elevated BUN and creatinine level.

The clinical syndrome of hypercalcemia is complex because of the extreme variability in its manifestation of signs and symptoms. In addition, the symptomatology does not always correlate with serum calcium levels. These must be closely correlated with an in-depth history, physical examination, and laboratory profile. Because of its frequency in patients with cancer, hypercalcemia of malignancy should be one of the first differential diagnoses in patients who develop a change in mental status. Box 24-7 defines Chvostek's and Trousseau's signs.

Diagnosis

The diagnostic work-up for hypercalcemia begins with laboratory determination of the serum calcium level. Normal values are 9 to 11 mg/dl. Ionized serum calcium levels provide the most accurate values when albumin levels are below normal. If ionized levels are unavailable, the serum calcium and albumin levels can be used to calculate the ionized calcium (see Box 24-2).

Urinary calcium may also be measured. Hypercalciuria may be detected before an elevation in serum calcium. Other serum laboratory testing should include phosphorus, alkaline phosphatase, BUN, creatinine, electrolytes, and PTH levels. Patients with no bony involvement (e.g., squamous cell cancer of the head and neck) and whose tumor is producing PTH-like substances may have a normal serum phosphorus level. Hypercalcemia resulting from direct bony involvement (e.g., breast cancer, myeloma, renal cell carcinoma) often results in increased serum phosphorus levels.[29,64] Furthermore, within this subset of patients, only those with breast cancer and bone metastasis usually have an elevated alkaline phosphatase.[64] Serum albumin should be tested, because patients may be more hypercalcemic than serum levels indicate as a result of hypoalbuminemia, as discussed earlier.

Radiographic examinations can be helpful in differential diagnosis. A chest x-ray film may suggest tumor, sarcoidosis, or bony changes associated with hyperparathyroidism. Plain x-ray film or a radioisotope bone scan may demonstrate bone metastases or multiple myeloma. ECGs may show tachycardia, increased PR segment, shortened QT interval, and widening of the T wave. However, these changes may be subtle and difficult to detect.

Treatment Modalities

Decisions concerning whether and how to treat hypercalcemia caused by malignancy depend on the clinical situation. The degree of serum calcium elevation, the symptomatology, the patient's condition, and the ability to treat the underlying disease are determining factors in the decision-making process. Untreated cancer-induced hypercalcemia is typically progressive, and death is usually inevitable. Death from hypercalcemia may be a reasonable way to die for the patient with advanced cancer, because most people become comatose and do not experience pain. However, death may not be rapid, and unpleasant symptoms (e.g., anorexia, nausea, vomiting, sedation, confusion) may occur. Patients with advanced disease must be evaluated carefully. Although the only effective long-term treatment for hypercalcemia is antineoplastic therapy directed at the underlying malignancy, very potent, well-tolerated therapies now exist to readily correct hypercalcemia. If quality of life will not be improved, the decision may be to provide no treatment.

When a decision is made to treat the hypercalcemia, the medical treatment is based on two principles: reduction of bone resorption of calcium and promotion of urinary excretion of calcium.[64] Urgency of treatment is based on the degree of serum elevation and whether the patient is symptomatic. In general, a corrected serum calcium level greater than 13 to 14 mg/dl requires immediate intervention, regardless of symptoms. Asymptomatic patients with calcium levels between 12 and 13 mg/dl may be treated more conservatively. Symptomatic patients require intervention, regardless of the calcium level.

HYDRATION AND DIURESIS

Adequate hydration is usually the primary treatment for hypercalcemia and may be all that is needed for mild hypercalcemia.[65,66] Increase fluids orally, and intravenously rehydrate the patient and dilute the urine, which prevents supersaturation with calcium ions. Large volumes of isotonic saline restore plasma volume and promote urinary calcium excretion through sodium diuresis. Calcium loss follows sodium loss. Fluid volume in the range of about 5 to 8 L daily is common for the first 24 hours, followed by 3 L daily thereafter. Infusions of large volumes of fluids may necessitate CVP monitoring to avoid fluid overload. Accurate recordings of intake, output, and weight and laboratory studies should be done to prevent hyponatremia, hypomagnesemia, and hypokalemia.

Once the patient is rehydrated, loop diuretics (furosemide [Lasix] and ethacrynic acid [Edecrin]) are sometimes used to enhance the excretion of calcium. However, they must be used with caution and careful monitoring, because extracellular fluid loss may exacerbate hypercalcemia by causing the resorption of calcium instead of the desired effect. Loop diuretics may also exacerbate serum depletion of magnesium and potassium. During diuresis, serum levels of potassium and magnesium should be monitored closely and cardiac medication given cautiously. Thiazide diuretics are to be avoided, because they decrease renal excretion of calcium.

PHARMACOLOGIC THERAPY

Bisphosphonates, compounds that are selectively concentrated in bone and inhibit the action of osteoclasts, have become the treatment of choice following hydration.[65,66] Agents that have been studied include clodronate, ibandronate, pamidronate, and zoledronic acid.[66] **Pamidronate**, a second-generation bisphosphonate, has been used as first-line therapy for moderate to severe hypercalcemia. The standard dose is 60 to 90 mg and may be administered in 250-ml normal saline over 2 hours. Reduction of serum calcium levels is seen in 24 to 48 hours with a peak effect in 7 days.[67] The infusion may be repeated weekly, if needed, to maintain normocalcemia until

---

BOX 24-7   Definitions

Chvostek's sign—elicited by tapping the cheek below the temple near the facial nerve. Positive if lip or nose twitches.

Trousseau's sign—elicited by using a blood pressure cuff to occlude arterial flow in the arm for 1 to 5 minutes. Positive if the thumb adducts and the fingers extend.

Data from Stuckey LA: Acute tumor lysis syndrome: assessment and nursing implications, *Oncol Nurs Forum* 20:49, 1993.

definitive treatment for the underlying malignancy is effective. The most common side effects include flulike syndrome (managed with acetaminophen) and venous irritation (if peripheral IV route is used). Other side effects can include nausea, anorexia, taste alterations, and decreased serum phosphate, potassium, and magnesium. Pamidronate may be used in combination with calcitonin. Calcitonin has a more rapid onset of action (4 to 6 hours), but the inhibition of bone resorption is not long lasting. A usual dosage is 4 international units/kg intramuscularly or subcutaneously every 12 hours.[68] As with pamidronate, one benefit of calcitonin is its safety in patients with renal failure. By using them together, there is a rapid initial drop in serum calcium levels from the calcitonin that is then maintained by the pamidronate.[65]

Zoledronic acid has since replaced pamidronate as the bisphosphonate of choice for hypercalcemia. Zoledronic acid is a third-generation bisphosphonate and contains a nitrogen ring. Research demonstrated greater efficacy at achieving normal calcium levels and longer duration of effect as compared to pamidronate.[69] Serum calcium levels are expected to fall within 12 hours of initiation of therapy. Full calcium normalization is achieved within 4 to 10 days and maintained for 4 weeks.[54,70] The approved dose is 4 mg administered over 15 minutes IV. Side effects may include hypophosphatemia, transient arthralgias, myalgias, and low-grade fever.

Like pamidronate, zoledronic acid has also demonstrated efficacy in the prevention of skeletal complications from bone metastases, including bone pain, pathologic fractures requiring radiation therapy or surgery, and spinal cord compression. Studies have demonstrated efficacy in multiple myeloma as well as solid tumors.[49,71]

Before the availability of pamidronate, **etidronate** (Didronel) had shown efficacy in more than 80% of patients with cancer-induced hypercalcemia. Lowered serum calcium was seen in 3 to 5 days after a regimen of 7.5 mg/kg per day IV for 4 to 5 days. The daily dose of etidronate is diluted in 250 ml normal saline and administered over at least 2 hours. IV administration can be followed with oral doses of 20 mg/kg per day for 7 to 10 days, which may be continued for up to 3 months. Etidronate is contraindicated in patients with a serum creatinine level greater than 5 mg/dl or those with renal failure. Hyperphosphatemia may result from etidronate therapy.

Gallium nitrate (gallium) is an antineoplastic agent noted to have hypocalcemic effects by directly inhibiting bone resorption without causing toxicity to bone cells. It is a very potent antihypercalcemic agent, but it must be administered over 24 hours daily for 5 days at a dose of 100 to 200 mg/m^2 mixed in 1 L of 0.9% normal saline or 5% dextrose in water. Adequate hydration must be maintained throughout the treatment period. Nephrotoxicity is the major side effect of gallium nitrate. The requirement of continuous infusion potentially limits its usefulness, especially in the outpatient setting.[65] Its use is limited to patients whose condition is refractory to bisphosphonates.[66]

The use of **oral phosphates** is somewhat limited. It has been shown that patients with renal failure or serum phosphorus levels greater than 3.8 mg/L will not benefit from the use of phosphates. However, patients with low serum phosphorus levels may benefit from oral phosphorus administered in doses of 0.5 g 4 times a day. The mechanism of action, although uncertain, appears to be the reduction of bone resorption of calcium and impairment of the absorption of calcium from the intestine. Diarrhea can result at

these high oral doses and may hamper the use of oral phosphorus. Large IV doses may cause precipitation of calcium in the heart, the lung, or soft tissues, which can lead to renal failure; therefore, they are rarely indicated.

Glucocorticoids have been used to treat hypercalcemia associated with breast cancer, myeloma, and lymphoma. Prednisone, 40 to 60 mg/day, has been given. Glucocorticoids block bone resorption, increase calcium excretion, and decrease GI absorption. Steroids may have some direct effect on the tumor itself, but the exact mechanism is unknown. Increasing the dosage of the steroids does not increase their effectiveness. The effect of steroids may be delayed by a week. If used, they may be combined with calcitonin because of its more rapid effect on calcium levels. Chronic use of glucocorticoids enhances immunosuppression, which can result in osteolytic activity. Steroids are not recommended for long-term maintenance, in view of the possible toxicities associated with chronic administration.

NSAIDs such as indomethacin (Indocin) or aspirin appear to inhibit prostaglandin synthesis and thus mediate bone resorption. Although their role in treating hypercalcemia is minor, they may be of value in patients with refractory hypercalcemia who are unable to tolerate other agents, or if NSAIDs are part of a regimen for cancer pain control. The usual dosage of indomethacin is 75 to 100 mg/day in divided doses. Gastric upset is a frequent side effect of this drug. They are rarely used today.

Plicamycin (mithramycin) has calcium-lowering effects that may not appear for 24 to 48 hours. The usual dosage is a slow infusion of 15 to 25 mcg/kg/day. Disadvantages of plicamycin are venous irritation, myelosuppressive effects, liver toxicity, and potential danger in patients with renal failure. The results are extremely unpredictable. It is not recommended as first-line therapy.

Chemotherapy may be used to treat patients with underlying hematologic malignancies such as multiple myeloma or lymphoma. In patients with breast cancer, chemotherapy or hormonal therapy may produce a remission. However, the initial use of hormonal therapy, especially tamoxifen (Nolvadex), may worsen the hypercalcemia. Some patients receiving hormonal therapy for breast cancer metastasis to the bone may experience episodes of increased serum calcium. This is often referred to as a "flare," which is indicative of tumor response to the hormone. These patients need to be monitored closely.

A new agent in development is **osteoprotegerin (OPG)**. Like the bisphosphonates, OPG inhibits bone resorption through its action against osteoclasts, in this case through inhibition of osteoclast differentiation.[66] Receptor activator of nuclear factor-kappaB (RANK) is a receptor expressed on chondrocytes, mature osteoclasts, and osteoclast precursors. The RANK ligand (RANKL) binds to RANK and increases osteoclast formation, thereby increasing bone resorption. RANKL is also known as osteoclast differentiation factor. OPG acts as a soluble decoy receptor and has shown potent hypocalcemic effects in preclinical trials.[66]

Part of the assessment in the treatment of increased serum calcium is to evaluate the other medications the patient is receiving. Many medications are known to precipitate hypercalcemia, such as estrogens, antiestrogens, thiazide diuretics, high doses of vitamins A and D, and calcium supplements. Whenever possible, these medications should be discontinued. However, it is not always necessary to stop antiestrogens in patients receiving them for treatment of cancer. Tumor flare, a temporary increase in tumor growth after initiating antiestrogens, is typically self-limiting.

Temporary discontinuation of the antiestrogen during antihypercalcemic therapy is based on the degree of serum elevation and symptoms.[64] Patients on digitalis must be carefully monitored, because aggressive therapy for hypercalcemia can significantly lower potassium and magnesium levels, placing the digitalized patient at increased risk for dysrhythmias. Table 24-5 outlines medications used to treat hypercalcemia.

MOBILIZATION

Immobility should be avoided, because it will increase resorption of calcium from the bones. Activity should be appropriate for the patient's physical condition. Weight bearing through standing and ambulation produces physical stress at the ends of long bones, resulting in osteoblastic activity. Osteoblasts synthesize the collagen and glycoproteins to form a matrix and develop into osteocytes, which are mature bone cells. Muscle activity produces acid end products needed to assist in the production of acid urine. Physical therapy may be helpful to establish a program of active exercises with resistance. A pain management program may be necessary to support activities.

DIETARY MANIPULATION

Dietary intake of calcium has very little role in the hypercalcemia of malignancy. Patients with cancer typically have reduced GI absorption of calcium so dietary restriction is unfounded. The only exception to this is in patients with elevated levels of 1,25-dihydroxyvitamin D (lymphoma), which enhances intestinal calcium absorption.

DIALYSIS

Patients who are in renal failure secondary to hypercalcemia but who have a relatively good prognosis with their malignancy could benefit from renal dialysis. Saline diuresis is precluded in these patients so that dialysis will remove both excess calcium and phosphate. Serum phosphate levels should be measured and phosphates replaced as necessary.

Nursing Considerations

Nursing care of the patient with hypercalcemia is directed at early detection and support through treatment. A thorough nursing assessment should include a history of the patient's cancer and cancer treatment, and a review of all medications. Drugs that may cause or potentiate hypercalcemia, such as lithium carbonate, thiazide diuretics, vitamins A and D, and large doses of calcium supplements, should be reported and discontinued. Drugs whose action may be altered by high serum calcium, such as digitalis and some antihypertensive agents, should also be noted. Physical examination results should be correlated with potential symptomatology of hypercalcemia. This is often difficult because of the varying possibilities and degrees of clinical manifestations. However, the initial assessment will dictate the intensity of nursing care.

Assess for signs and symptoms of alterations in fluid volume. Excess fluid is manifested by rales, shortness of breath, neck vein distension, weight gain, and edema of the sacrum and the lower extremities. Fluid deficit is indicated by dry mucous membranes, poor skin turgor, weight loss, rapid and thready pulse, orthostatic hypotension, and restlessness. Auscultate lungs for breath sounds

TABLE 24-5   Medications to Treat Hypercalcemia

MEDICATION	MODE OF ACTION	DOSE	TOXICITY	COMMENTS
Furosemide	Blocks resorption of calcium at loop of Henle	80-100 mg q 1-2 hr	Dehydration Electrolyte loss	May need CVP monitoring Only given after patient is rehydrated
Pamidronate	Bisphosphonate inhibits osteoclast activity	60-90 mg in 250 ml over 2 hr	Flulike syndrome Nausea Phlebitis	First-line therapy after hydration
Zoledronic acid (Zometa)	Bisphosphonate inhibits osteoclast activity	4-8 mg in 30 ml over 15 min	Skeletal pain	First-line therapy after hydration
Etidronate	Bisphosphonate	7.5 mg/kg/day in 250 ml or more over 2-3 hr, then 20 mg/kg/day PO for 30 days	Nausea, vomiting Taste changes	Contraindicated in renal failure
Gallium nitrate	Inhibits bone resorption	100-200 mg/m^2/day × 5 days	Renal toxicity	Contraindicated in decreased renal function
Calcitonin	Inhibits bone resorption Increases urinary excretion	4 international units/kg q 12 hr, may increase to 8 international units/kg	Nausea, vomiting Rash	Short-lived effectiveness Used in combination with pamidronate or glucocorticoids
Prednisone	Inhibits bone resorption Decreases GI absorption	40-100 mg/day IV	Hyperglycemia Na and H$_2$O retention	Used primarily for hematologic and breast cancers
Phosphates	Prevents GI absorption Inhibits bone resorption	0.5-3 g/day PO	Diarrhea	Used to correct hypophosphatemia
Plicamycin	Kills osteoclasts	15-25 mcg/kg over 4-6 h × 3 d	Marrow suppression Hepatic toxicity Renal toxicity Nausea, vomiting	Unpredictable response Third-line agent, rarely used

CVP, Central venous pressure; GI, gastrointestinal; IV, intravenously; PO, by mouth.
Data from Barnett ML: Hypercalcemia, Semin Oncol Nurs 15: 190, 1999; and Heatley S, Coleman R Product focus. The use of bisphosphonates in the palliative care setting, Int J Palliative Nurs 5:74, 1999.

and monitor intake and output closely. Maintain intravenous fluids as ordered. Obtain daily weight. Monitor laboratory values (e.g., serum BUN, creatinine, sodium, and potassium levels). Administer diuretics as ordered. Thiazide diuretics are contraindicated, because they inhibit urinary excretion of calcium and therefore may potentiate hypercalcemia. Obtain urine pH. An acidic urine should be maintained to prevent calcium precipitation, which can lead to renal calculi. Administer oral potassium as ordered (hypokalemia frequently occurs in the presence of hypercalcemia).

Assess patient for changes in cardiac status. Monitor for presence of dysrhythmias, bradycardia, and tachycardia. Observe ECG for shortened QT intervals or prolonged PR intervals. Monitor effects of digitalis and digoxin, if given to patient, because hypercalcemia potentiates their action. The dosage is usually reduced in the presence of hypercalcemia.

Assess patient for presence of spinal cord compression (signs and symptoms: pain, sensory loss or paresthesia, motor weakness or dysfunction, changes in patterns of elimination). Establish an activity and exercise regimen according to patient's physical ability. If not contraindicated, institute weight-bearing activity, such as assisting patient to stand at the bedside for short periods at least 4 to 6 times a day. Footboards and tilt tables may be used for bedfast patients. Consult physical therapy and occupational therapy for evaluation and assistance. Assess immobile patients for evidence of venous thrombosis in lower extremities (i.e., redness, swelling, warmth, positive Homans' sign, pain upon dorsiflexion). Monitor skin integrity and provide appropriate skin care. Provide pain control as needed. Assess level of consciousness and check for changes in mentation and behavior. Monitor status of bowel elimination daily. Avoid administration of antidiarrheal agents, because calcium is excreted via stool. Teach the patient and family about changes caused by hypercalcemia, potential for recurrence, and appropriate measures to be taken.

Hypercalcemia is one of the most common oncologic problems seen in patients with cancer. Therefore, nurses practicing in all areas of cancer care should be educated regarding this problem. Nursing assessment of patients with cancer, especially those cancers typically associated with hypercalcemia (i.e., breast, lung, head and neck, lymphoma, myeloma, bony metastases), should focus on the potential manifestations of this problem.

Prognosis

Cancer-induced hypercalcemia is a common complication of certain cancers and has the potential to be life-threatening. Clinical manifestations and onset vary greatly, but the course is usually progressive and can worsen quickly. Hypercalcemia is reversible in 80% of episodes if it is recognized and prompt aggressive therapy initiated. It has been shown that the more severe the hypercalcemia, the poorer the prognosis, and vice versa. Without prompt treatment, it is associated with a 50% mortality rate. After the diagnosis of hypercalcemia, median survival is 3 months.[72] No treatment of hypercalcemia alone, with the possible exception of intravenous bisphosphonates, has been demonstrated to improve the increased mortality rate associated with this complication.[73]

HYPERSENSITIVITY REACTION TO ANTINEOPLASTIC AGENTS

Definition

Severe hypersensitivity reactions (HSRs), or anaphylaxis, is defined as a life-threatening immunologic response to a foreign

TABLE 24-6	Antineoplastic Agents Associated with HSR	
HIGH RISK	**MODERATE RISK**	**LOW RISK**
L-Asparaginase	Anthracyclines	Cytosine arabinoside
Doxetaxel	Bleomycin	Cyclophosphamide
Paclitaxel	Carboplatin	Chlorambucil
Procarbazine	Cisplatin	Dacarbazine
Teniposide	Etoposide	5-Fluorouracil
Rituximab	Melphalan	Ifosfamide
	Methotrexate	Mitoxantrone
	Herceptin	Aldesleukin
		Gemcitabine
		Hydroxyurea
		Interferons
		Mechlorethamine
		6-Mercaptopurine
		Mitomycin
		Pentostatin
		Pegaspargase
		Vinca alkaloids

HSR, Hypersensitivity reaction.
From Weiss RB: Miscellaneous toxicities. In DeVita VT Jr, Hellman S, Rosenberg SA, editors: *Cancer: principles and practice of oncology,* ed 5, Philadelphia, 1997, Lippincott-Raven.

substance or antigen. Antineoplastic agents, like other drugs, may be recognized by the body's immune system as "not-self." This may initiate a type I reaction, characterized by the release of histamine and other inflammatory mediators that induce the symptoms of an anaphylactic reaction such as respiratory distress and cardiovascular failure.

Etiology and Risk Factors

Risk factors associated with an increased incidence of HSR include age, gender, genetic makeup, nutritional status, stress level, and hormonal and environmental factors.[74] Additional risk factors include the route of administration (e.g., IV, oral, topical, or intramuscular), duration of administration (e.g., IV push versus slow infusion), and the immunologic characteristics of the drug. The nitrosoureas (e.g., carmustine, lomustine) are the only class of antineoplastic agents that has never been documented to induce a HSR. An increased risk of HSR is known to occur with drugs that are proteins, such as L-asparaginase (up to 33%); drugs prepared in antigenic diluents, as are the taxanes and podiphyllotoxins; as well as heavy metal compounds like cisplatin and carboplatin (Table 24-6).

Pathophysiology

The Gell and Coombs classification includes four categories of immunologic reactions (Table 24-7). Most antineoplastic HSRs are thought to be type I reactions. However, there have been case reports of types II, III, and IV as well.[74]

Type I reactions occur in three phases. In the first phase, **sensitization,** the patient is exposed to the foreign substance or antigen, in this case the antineoplastic agent. This exposure causes the formation of specific IgE antibodies that attach to the receptors on basophils and mast cells. Once the patient receives the second exposure to the antigen, called the **activation phase,**

TABLE 24-7	Hypersensitivity Reaction Classifications		
TYPE	**MECHANISMS**	**SIGNS AND SYMPTOMS**	**EXAMPLES**
I. Anaphylactic or anaphylactoid	Antigen-antibody reaction Mediator release from basophils and mast cells Direct binding of antigen to mast cells IgE antibody	Urticaria, bronchospasm, hypotension, angioedema cramping, respiratory and cardiovascular collapse	Anaphylaxis to medication, bee stings, food
II. Cytotoxic	Antibody binding to cell surface IgM and IgG antibodies	Hemolysis	Hemolytic anemia, hemolysis from transfusion
III. Immune complex–mediated	Immune complex formation by antigen-antibody interaction, or anaphylactoid reaction from complement activation	Tissue injury; manifestations depending on location of sickness, immune complex deposits	Systemic lupus, rheumatoid arthritis, horse serum Arthus reaction
IV. Cell-mediated (delayed hypersensitivity)	Sensitized T lymphocytes interact with antigen and release lymphokines	Mucositis, pneumonitis, contact dermatitis, granulomas, homograft rejection	Tuberculosis, poison ivy, granulomas, mechlorethamine sensitivity from topical application

Data from Craig JB, Capizzi RL: The prevention and treatment of immediate hypersensitivity reactions from cancer chemotherapy, *Semin Oncol Nurs* 1:285, 1985; Gell PHG, Coombs RRA: Clinical aspects of immunology, Oxford, 1975, Blackwell Scientific; and Labovich TM: Acute hypersensitivity reactions to chemotherapy, *Semin Oncol Nurs* 15:222, 1999.

the antigen attaches to the IgE molecules on the mast cell surfaces. An influx of calcium into the cells induces the mast cells to degranulate. This results in the release of preformed chemical mediators (i.e., histamine, heparin, chondroitin sulfate, chemotactins) into the surrounding tissue and serum. Newly formed mediators are also released. These include prostaglandins and leukotrienes (also called SRSAs—slow-reacting substances of anaphylaxis).[74]

Histamine release stimulates H_1 and H_2 receptors (located in the myocardium, vessel walls, and smooth muscle lining of the lung, the ureters, the bladder, and the GI tract) that are responsible for many of the clinical features described later in the text and in Table 24-8. The final phase of the HSR, **effector,** involves the immediate neuromuscular and vascular responses seen in the organs targeted by the chemical mediators. Mast cells are concentrated in the skin, the vasculature, the connective tissue, and the GI tract.

L-Asparaginase has been associated with the highest risk of HSR. Incidence has been documented in up to 35% of cases, with an overall risk of 5% to 8% per dose. Incidence may increase up to 33% after the fourth dose.[75] Reactions occur more frequently with significant time lapse between treatments (weekly or monthly as opposed to daily during clinical trials). Intramuscular administration may reduce the severity of reactions and is the recommended route of administration.[75] HSRs may be reduced in treatment plans that include prednisone and vincristine.[75] Reactions to L-asparaginase may occur several hours after administration.[76] L-Asparaginase is a polypeptide of bacterial origin. It is derived from *Escherichia coli.* Since the development of L-asparaginase, a substitute derived from *Erwinia chrysanthemia* (a plant pathogen) has been created. It has been the accepted substitute for L-asparaginase for more than 20 years. No HSR occurs in 75% of patients treated.[75] However, the antileukemia efficacy may be inferior.[77] Most recently, pegaspargase (Oncaspar) has been made available and approved by the U. S. Food and Drug Administration (FDA). Pegaspargase is prepared from *E. coli* asparaginase, but is delivered in strands of polyethylene glycol

(PEG) that allow it to escape detection by the immune system and a longer circulation time. Of the three options, it is most likely the least immunogenic.[77]

Cisplatin is associated with an increased incidence of HSRs after prolonged use. Some studies indicated significant HSR occurrence with six or more doses. Incidence was more pronounced during early clinical trials before the advent of premedication with corticosteroids and antiemetics. The highest rate of reactions has been documented with multiple-dose intravesicular administration for bladder cancer (10% to 25%). **Carboplatin** has been associated with HSRs in patients treated repeatedly with the agent (median of 10 treatments). Incidence in patients with ovarian cancer has been reported as high as 12%.[77] Similarly, **oxaliplatin** is also associated with HSRs after repeated dosing (incidence about 10% to 12% with median administration of 10 doses).[77,78]

Bleomycin-related life-threatening events may actually be due to a massive release of endogenous human leukocyte pyrogens from the white blood cells as opposed to a true HSR. It has been customary to administer a small test dose of bleomycin and observe the patient for reactions, before administering the full prescribed dose. However, practice patterns are now moving away from the test dose while maintaining close observation of the patient for signs of HSR. Risk may be increased for patients with lymphoma or those receiving IV administration.

Biologic agents as an entire group are not commonly associated with HSRs. However, the monoclonal antibodies (MoAbs) are conjugated from murine cells and are known to cause reactions including fever, chills, asthenia, bronchospasm, hypotension, and angioedema. These are minimized by premedication with acetaminophen and diphenhydramine.[75] Patients receiving interleukin (IL)-2 therapy may develop an increased sensitivity to radiologic contrast dye as well as to other antineoplastic agents, such as cisplatin.

Procarbazine and **methotrexate** have induced interstitial pneumonitis and vasculitis, typical of a type III reaction.[77]

TABLE 24-8	Chemical Mediator Manifestations					
HISTAMINE	**HEPARIN**	**CHONDROITIN SULFATE**	**CHEMOTACTIN**	**PROSTAGLANDIN**	**LEUKOTRIENE**	
H_1 Receptor						
Pruritus	Coagulopathies	Edema	Eosinophilia	Vasodilatation	Vasodilatation	
Vasodilatation		Pruritus	Neutrophilia	Smooth muscle contraction	Bronchoconstriction	
Smooth muscle contraction		Hypotension	Platelet aggregation	Viscous mucus production	Mucus production	
Vascular permeability		Bronchoconstriction		Hypotension	Hypotension	
Coronary artery vasospasm		Vascular permeability		Platelet aggregation	Platelet aggregation	
Vagal nerve irritation		Smooth muscle contraction				
Increased mucus viscosity		Nerve fiber stimulation				
Bronchospasm						
Edema						
Hypotension						
Tachycardia						
H_2 Receptor						
Increased heart contractility						
Increased heart rate						
Vasodilatation						
Goblet cell/bronchial gland mucus secretion						

Data from Craig JB, Capizzi RL: The prevention and treatment of immediate hypersensitivity reactions from cancer chemotherapy, *Semin Oncol Nurs* 1:285, 1985; and Gell PHG, Coombs RRA: *Clinical aspects of immunology*, Oxford, 1975, Blackwell Scientific.

A significant number of HSRs related to antineoplastic agents are considered to be anaphylactoid instead of anaphylactic. **Anaphylactoid** reactions occur when the patient has not been previously exposed to the antigen. In these cases, the same mediators are released and the same clinical features are observed, because the antigen binds directly to the mast cell surfaces inducing mediator release or triggers an uncontrolled activation of the complement cascade to produce inflammation and the immune response.[74]

An example of an anaphylactoid HSR can occur with the administration of **paclitaxel** (Taxol). During clinical trials, up to 41% incidence of HSRs was seen. Further study indicated that paclitaxel was probably not the antigen. Taxol is prepared in a diluent made up of 50% dehydrated alcohol and 50% Cremaphor El. Cremaphor El is a polyoxyethylated castor oil vehicle that is known to induce HSRs (also seen in tenoposide, vitamin K, and cyclosporine). **Paclitaxel**-related HSRs have been significantly reduced (1% to 3%) with the advent of appropriate premedication.[48,75,79] Table 24-9 lists a standard regimen for paclitaxel premedication. Recent research has shown that IV dexamethasone 30 minutes before paclitaxel administration is just as efficacious as the oral regimen used previously (20 mg orally 12 hours

TABLE 24-9	Premedication Regimen for Paclitaxel Infusion
Corticosteroid	Dexamethasone, 10-20 mg IV
H_1 antagonist	Diphenhydramine, 25-50 mg IV
H_2 antagonist	Cimetidine, 300 mg IV, or Ranitidine, 150 mg IV, or Famotidine, 20 mg IV

IV, Intravenously.
Labovich TM: Acute hypersensitivity reactions to chemotherapy, *Semin Oncol Nurs* 15:222, 1999; and Quock J, Dea G, Tanaka M: Premedication strategy for weekly paclitaxel, *Cancer Invest* 20:666, 2002.

and 6 hours before paclitaxel).[75,80,81] A newer formulation of paclitaxel is now available, Abraxane. It is a cremaphor-free, protein-stablilized, nanoparticle formulation.[82] Premedication is not required. Incidence of HSRs during clinical trials were 1% or less.[83]

Doxetaxel (Taxotere), an analogue to paclitaxel, has also been associated with HSRs.[80] Doxetaxel is prepared in polysorbate 80 (Tween 80). Standard adjunct medication consists of oral

TABLE 24-10 Clinical Signs and Symptoms of HSR

MOST COMMON	LESS COMMON
Agitation	Nausea
Urticaria	Vomiting
Angioedema	Diarrhea
Upper airway edema	Abdominal cramping and/or bloating
Dyspnea	Rhinitis
Wheezing	Headache
Flushing	Substernal pain
Dizziness	Back pain
Hypotension	Seizure
	Sneezing
	Genital burning
	Metallic taste

HSR, Hypersensitivity reaction.
Data from Craig JB, Capizzi RL: The prevention and treatment of immediate hypersensitivity reactions from cancer chemotherapy, *Semin Oncol Nurs* 1:285, 1985; Labovich TM: Acute hypersensitivity reactions to chemotherapy, *Semin Oncol Nurs* 15:222, 1999; and Lieberman P, Kemmp SF, Oppenheimer J et al: The diagnosis and management of anaphylaxis: an updated practice parameter. *J Allergy Clin Immunol* 115(3 Pt 2):S483, 2005.

BOX 24-8 Protocol for HSR Interventions

Stop the infusion
Call for help
Stay with the patient
Assess airway patency—prepare for possible intubation
Monitor blood pressure, pulse, and oxygenation, and prepare for possible cardiopulmonary resuscitation
Administer epinephrine
- 0.3-0.5 mg, 1:1000 subQ if no significant respiratory distress
- 0.1 mg/kg, 1:10,000 IV if bronchospasm or stridor (over no less than 3-5 min)
Administer isotonic fluids (normal saline or lactated Ringer's) to maintain blood pressure
Administer diphenhydramine 50 mg IV
Administer Solu-Medrol 125 mg IV

IV, Intravenously; *subQ,* subcutaneously.
Data from Labovich TM: Acute hypersensitivity reactions to chemotherapy, *Semin Oncol Nurs* 15:222, 1999; and Lieberman P, Kemmp SF, Oppenheimer J et al: The diagnosis and management of anaphylaxis: an updated practice parameter, *J Allergy Clin Immunol* 115(3 Pt 2):S483, 2005.

dexamethasone the day before, the day of, and the day following treatment. In this instance, premedication and postmedication serves both to prevent HSRs as well as fluid retention.[75,80] Alterations in the premedication regime are made when the drug is given in low weekly doses.

Clinical Features

The signs and symptoms from an antineoplastic-related HSR typically occur within minutes of initiating the agent IV and peak within 15 to 30 minutes. Reactions to oral agents may take 2 hours. Reactions may be further delayed up to several hours, depending on drug metabolism. Once the effects of interventions wear off, recurrence of the HSR may be seen up to 8 to 24 hours later.

The most common effects include dyspnea, agitation, and hypotension. The patient may complain of a feeling of heat, chest or back pain, and trouble breathing. A more complete list of clinical features is listed in the Table 24-10.

The most common cause of death is asphyxiation secondary to laryngeal edema and spasm, which can occur within minutes. Cardiovascular collapse and shock can occur without any cutaneous or respiratory symptoms.[74]

Diagnosis

The diagnosis of antineoplastic-related HSR is made primarily by clinical assessment of the patient. Signs and symptoms of HSR typically occur within minutes of drug administration and are described in the preceding material. Serum levels may be drawn to ascertain with certainty the evidence of a type I reaction, but are not commonly done. Plasma histamine levels may be detectable for 1 hour after symptoms occur. Urine histamine levels will remain elevated and can be detected in a 24-hour urine collection. Prostaglandin D_2 may also be measured in the urine and serum. Serum tryptase is also released from mast cells. These serum levels peak within 1 to 1.5 hours after the onset of symptoms and may remain elevated for up to 5 hours.[69,74] Skin testing or the radioallergosorbent test (RAST) may also be used to evaluate hypersensitivity to a few specific drugs.[69,74] Elevated cardiac enzymes and abnormal ECG readings may be seen from histamine-induced coronary artery vasospasm.[74]

A careful history must be taken to identify patients at high risk for HSR. History should include any prior exposure to the agents being administered, any prior antineoplastic-related or other HSRs and the specific agents involved, and any history of drug sensitivity or atopy (hereditary allergy).

Treatment Modalities

The primary treatment for HSR is prevention. By taking a careful history, the oncology nurse identifies patients who are high risk for HSR. Knowledge of the antineoplastic agents most likely to be associated with HSR and familiarity with appropriate premedication regimens are also valuable prevention tools. In addition, the oncology nurse carefully monitors the patient for signs of HSR, including blood pressure, pulse, and oxygen saturation. Emergency equipment and medications must be readily available, including oxygen supplies, cardiac monitor and defibrillator, intubation supplies, epinephrine 1:1000 or 1:10,000, diphenhydramine 50 mg, corticosteroids such as Solu-Medrol 125 mg, and other drugs such as aminophylline and dopamine sulfate. Antineoplastic agents likely to cause HSR are given in conjunction with patent IV access and compatible fluids.

In the event that the patient begins to experience symptoms implicating HSR, administration of the antineoplastic agent is stopped immediately. IV fluids are continued at a rate consistent with maintaining adequate blood pressure. Administration of oxygen may be necessary to maintain a saturation above 92%. The patient should be continuously assessed for a patent airway.

It is recommended that standing orders be available for medication administration (Box 24-8). Many sources recommend the administration of **epinephrine** 1:1000, 0.3 to 0.5 ml every 5 to 20 minutes subcutaneously to slow the absorption of the antineoplastic agent as well as to counteract the effects of the HSR through bronchodilation, peripheral vasoconstriction, and increasing cardiac contractility and heart rate.[74,84] Epinephrine also reduces mast cell degranulation.[69,74] In the event of airway compromise or shock, 0.1 mg/kg may be given IV over a minimum of 3 to 5 minutes. **Diphenhydramine** is an H_1 antagonist that counteracts the dyspnea and wheezing caused by bronchospasm. H_2 antagonists (e.g., cimetidine, ranitidine, famotidine) may also be used, but are typically second-line therapy.[84] Combinations of diphenhydramine and ranitidine have also been used as second-line therapy.[84] **Aminophylline** or nebulized β-adrenergic agonists, such as **albuterol,** may be used when diphenhydramine is ineffective. Vasopressors, such as dopamine sulfate, may be needed if hypotension persists despite fluid administration. Corticosteroids, such as **Solu-Medrol,** may block the production of prostaglandins and leukotrienes and enhance the efficacy of epinephrine.[74] They may also prevent delayed or recurrent symptoms. Patients taking β-adrenergic blockers, angiotensin-converting enzyme (ACE) inhibitors, monoamine oxidase inhibitors (MAOIs), or some tricyclic antidepressants may be difficult to treat for HSRs. These agents interfere with the effectiveness of epinephrine and the body's compensatory mechanisms.[74] IV glucagon (1 to 2 mg over 5 minutes or 1 mg in 1000 ml of dextrose 5% in water [D5W] at 5 to 15 ml/min) has been proven effective for people taking β-blockers.[85]

Many patients begin to have resolution of symptoms as soon as the antineoplastic administration is stopped. Others require some or all of the interventions described above. In this author's experience, HSRs to paclitaxel have been successfully managed with the administration of Solu-Medrol 125 mg IV and diphenhydramine 50 mg IV, in addition to oxygen per nasal cannula.

There has been controversy about the further use of an antineoplastic agent for a patient who has experienced a serious HSR. However, this philosophy is changing in certain circumstances. For example, 90% of paclitaxel-related HSRs are resolved by the immediate discontinuation of the infusion. Infusions are successfully resumed in approximately 30 minutes. The rationale for reinitiation of the infusion is based on the premise that the initial HSR depletes the immune system of the mediators of hypersensitivity and prevents further reaction during the subsequent infusion.[80] Recent research has shown that patients may be successfully rechallenged with paclitaxel by intensifying the premedication regimen and slowing the infusion time for the treatment. This success may be due in part to the fact that paclitaxel induces an anaphylactoid response. Non–IgE-mediated reactions may be more amenable to desensitization and premedication. Desensitization regimens have also been employed for carboplatin and oxaliplatin.[77,78] Successful rechallenge may be related to the specific agent involved, the mechanism of the HSR, the administration schedule, and the use of premedication. There are some reported instances where rechallenge was not successful.[75]

Nursing Considerations

The importance of chemotherapy certification is clearly supported by the risk of chemotherapy-induced hypersensitivity reactions (HSR). Nurses administering chemotherapy must be knowledgeable about the agents most likely to cause HSR, and be skilled in recognizing and treating HSRs when they occur. The nursing history should include information about any previous allergies or reactions to medications. Baseline vital signs and mental status should be assessed and recorded. Emergency equipment and medications, as well as standing orders for HSR, should be readily available.

In the event of an HSR, the infusion is to be stopped immediately. Maintain airway patency. Deliver high-flow oxygen at a rate to maintain oxygen saturation. Administer emergency medications as described in Box 24-8. Prepare to assist with intubation if required. Continuously monitor blood pressure and pulse if patient becomes symptomatic. Once stable, monitor every 15 minutes 4 times, then every hour 4 times, and then every 4 hours. Deliver prescribed IV fluids at 200 ml/hr or more to maintain blood pressure. Initiate vasopressors as prescribed if blood pressure does not respond to fluid challenge. Use Trendelenburg position, if patient can tolerate it despite respiratory symptoms. Include education about the signs and symptoms and management of HSR when teaching the patient and family about chemotherapy. Education may include the following: review any premedication regimens; discuss the rationale for vital signs monitoring; and describe the interventions that are used in the event an HSR occurs. Evaluate patient and family for level of anxiety and usual coping strategies. Carry out all interventions in a confident, efficient, and calm manner, and explain each step to the patient and family as it occurs.

Prognosis

The outcome of a HSR reaction depends on a variety of factors. Immediate recognition and appropriate treatment are key factors to preventing a fatal event. Other variables include the amount of antigen absorbed and the degree of hypersensitivity manifested by the patient to the antineoplastic agent.

SEPTIC SHOCK

Definition

Shock comprises a group of diverse life-threatening syndromes that result from different pathophysiologic circumstances: decreased cardiac function, hemorrhage, trauma, antigen-antibody reaction, and sepsis. The three major classifications of shock are hypovolemic, cardiogenic, and distributive or vasogenic. **Hypovolemic shock** is a result of decreased intravascular volume. **Cardiogenic shock** results from the heart's impaired ability to pump blood adequately. **Distributive shock** or **vasogenic shock** is the result of an abnormality in the vascular system. Included under distributive shock are neurogenic, anaphylactic, and septic shock. The progression of septic shock produces a severe maldistribution of blood flow in the microcirculation. This leads to inadequate tissue perfusion, cellular ischemia, cellular hypoxia, and organ or system failure.

Sepsis and its sequelae are a complex compilation of related pathophysiologic processes. In 1991 the American College of Chest Physicians and the Society of Critical Care Medicine held a consensus conference to define the terms associated with sepsis and organ failure.[86] (Box 24-9). Sepsis was defined as the systemic inflammatory response to infection that is manifested by two or more of the following: temperature above 38° C or less than 36° C; heart rate greater than 90 beats/min; respiratory rate greater than 20/min or $Paco_2$ less than 32 mm Hg; and WBC above $12,000/mm^3$, less than $4000/mm^3$, or greater than 10% bands. Sepsis is classified as severe when it is associated with organ dysfunction, hypoperfusion, or hypotension. **Septic shock** is defined as sepsis-induced hypotension (despite fluid resuscitation) and organ perfusion abnormalities. Septic shock can lead to irreversible multiorgan dysfunction syndrome (MODS) and death.

Definitions

Infection = microbial phenomenon characterized by an inflammatory response to the presence of microorganisms or the invasion of normally sterile host tissue by those organisms.

Bacteremia = the presence of viable bacteria in the blood.

Systemic inflammatory response syndrome (SIRS) = the systemic inflammatory response to a variety of severe clinical insults. The response is manifested by two or more of the following conditions: (1) temperature >38° C or <36° C; (2) heart rate >90 beats/min; (3) respiratory rate >20 breaths/min or $Paco_2$ <32 mm Hg; and (4) white blood cell count >12,000/mm³, <4,000/mm³, or >10% immature (band) forms

Sepsis = the systemic response to infection, manifested by two or more of the following conditions as a result of infection: (1) temperature >38° C or <36° C; (2) heart rate >90 beats/min; (3) respiratory rate >20 breaths/min or $Paco_2$ <32 mm Hg; and white blood cell count >12,000/ mm³, <4,000/ mm³, or >10% immature (band) forms.

Severe sepsis = sepsis associated with organ dysfunction, hypoperfusion, or hypotension. Hypoperfusion and perfusion abnormalities may include, but are not limited to, lactic acidosis, oliguria, or an acute alteration in mental status.

Septic shock = sepsis-induced with hypotension despite adequate fluid resuscitation along with the presence of perfusion abnormalities that may include, but are not limited to, lactic acidosis, oliguria, or an acute alteration in mental status. Patients who are receiving inotropic or vasopressor agents may not be hypotensive at the time that perfusion abnormalities are measured.

Sepsis-induced hypotension = a systolic blood pressure <90 mm Hg or a reduction of ≥40 mm Hg from baseline in the absence of other causes for hypotension.

Multiple organ dysfunction syndrome (MODS) = presence of altered organ function in an acutely ill patient such that homeostasis cannot be maintained without intervention.

From Bone RG, Balk RA, Cerra FB et al: Definition for sepsis and organ failure and guidelines for the use of innovative therapy sepsis, *Chest* 101(6):1646, 1992.

Etiology and Risk Factors

Septic shock is the most common cause of noncoronary intensive care unit (ICU) deaths in the United States.[87] The incidence of septic shock has increased steadily over the past 20 years. Mortality rate ranges from 10% to 90%.[88] The incidence of sepsis in cancer patients is estimated at 45%, with greater than 30% mortality.[88]

Patients with cancer are frequently immunosuppressed. Neutropenia is caused by most antineoplastic agents as well as radiation therapy to the long bones, the pelvis, and the sternum. Some antineoplastic drugs (asparaginase and vinca alkaloids) can alter the ability of neutrophils to migrate and phagocytize bacteria. Patients with Hodgkin's disease may have impaired cellular immunity (macrophages and T lymphocytes). Patients with chronic lymphocytic leukemia (CLL) may have impaired antibody function that decreases the ability to attach to pathogens and enhance phagocytosis via the monocytes and macrophages. Macrophage function is also decreased in patients who have had a splenectomy.[89] Elevated serum levels of interleukins 6 and 8 (IL-6, IL-8) have recently been associated with increased probability of infection; however, studies are preliminary at this time.[89]

Septic shock can be caused by bacterial, fungal, viral, and protozoal organisms. Gram-negative bacteria (e.g., *E. coli, Klebsiella pneumoniae, Pseudomonas aeruginosa*) have historically been the primary organisms associated with septic shock. More recently there has been an increase in septic shock induced by gram-positive organisms (e.g., *Staphylococcus aureus, Staphylococcus epidermis*). This may be attributed to the increased use of long-term central venous access and the mucosal toxicity of cytotoxic regimens.[28] Another hypothesis is the prevalence of methicillin-resistant strains of *Staphylococcus. Candida* is the fungal organism most commonly associated with sepsis.[87] Because of the immunosuppression in cancer patients, endogenous flora is frequently the source of infection. The organism is not identified in 20% to 30% of cases because of previous exposure to antibiotics.[50] The most common sites of infection are the lung, the abdomen, and the urinary tract.

A particular infectious, life-threatening condition seen in patients with cancer is **neutropenic enterocolitis,** also called **typhilitis,** an inflammation of the small intestine or colon. The exact pathologic etiology is unclear. However, it is proposed to be initiated by direct cytotoxic damage from chemotherapy, radiation therapy, or neoplastic infiltration. Disruption of mucosal integrity, alteration of normal gut flora, and lack of neutrophil response lead to invasion of the GI tract by bacteria, viruses, and fungi. The implicated organisms include gram-negative bacilli such as *Klebsiella, Pseudomonas, E. coli, Candida*, and *Clostridium septicum*. Although *C. septicum* is not a type of flora that is normally found in the gut, it may appear after the use of multiple antibiotics, which alter the normal gut flora. Neutropenic enterocolitis can lead to septic shock. Mortality rates have been estimated to be greater than 50%.

The factors that predispose a patient with cancer to infection and sepsis can be categorized according to the precipitating event, site of infection, and the pathogen (Table 24-11). Each of the events that may initiate an infection leading to septic shock is a consequence of the underlying cancer or its treatment. All four treatment modalities (i.e., surgery, radiation therapy, chemotherapy, biotherapy) can result in profound suppression of host defense mechanisms. Monitoring the patient for effects of tumor growth and side effects of therapy is crucial to preventing septic shock.

Pathophysiology

The presence of an invading pathogen (i.e., bacteria, fungus, virus, protozoa) should stimulate an immune response from the patient. In patients who are immunocompromised, infection may become established, and the release of inflammatory mediators can lead to life-threatening complications that induce MODS. As bacterial pathogens are phagocytized, endotoxins (gram-negative bacteria) and exotoxins (gram-positive bacteria) are released into the bloodstream (Fig. 24-12). The macrophages respond by releasing vasoactive mediators (i.e., histamine, kinins, interleukins, and tumor necrosis factor).[91] IL-1 and tumor necrosis factor-alpha (TNF-α) are potent mediators of inflammation. Their release stimulates the release of additional inflammatory mediators such as IL-6, IL-8, thromboxanes, leukotrienes, platelet activating factor, prostaglandins, and complement.[90]

The inflammatory cascade leads to fever, chills, vasodilation, and hypotension. The vascular endothelium is altered by endotoxins

TABLE 24-11   Factors Predisposing Cancer Patients to Infection

PRECIPITATING EVENT	COMMON SITE OF INFECTION	COMMON ORGANISM
Local Effects of Tumor Growth or TX		
Skin or mucous membrane breakdown	Cancer or TX of skin, head and neck, gastrointestinal (GI) tract, female genital tract	Locally colonizing organisms
Obstruction of natural passages	Solid tumors or TX of cancer (especially pulmonary, biliary, and urinary tracts)	Locally colonizing organisms
Alterations in microbial flora	All cancer sites or TX of cancer (especially pulmonary, GI)	Locally colonizing organisms
Stasis of blood and body fluids secondary to obstruction or inactivity	All cancer sites or TX of cancer	Locally colonizing organisms
Central nervous system (CNS) dysfunction (brain or spinal cord tumors, metabolic abnormalities)	Pulmonary (aspiration pneumonia)	
Urinary tract	Locally colonizing organism	
Hyposplenism secondary to neoplastic infiltration or splenectomy	Disseminated	Bacteria: Streptococcus pneumoniae, Neisseria meningitidis, Escherichia coli, Haemophilus influenzae, Clostridium difficile, Staphylococcus species
Granulocytopenia (neutropenia) prevalent with acute leukemia	Skin lesions, thrombophlebitis, pulmonary (pneumonia), sinuses, pharynx, esophagus, colon, perianal area	Gram-negative bacilli: E. coli, Pseudomonas aeruginosa, Klebsiella pneumoniae, Staphylococcus aureus Yeasts: Candida Filamentous fungi: Aspergillus species, agents of mycosis
Cellular immune dysfunction (T-cell immune alteration) prevalent with T-cell lymphoma	Disseminated	Bacteria: Listeria monocytogenes, Salmonella species, Mycobacterium species, Nocardia steroides Fungi: Cryptococcus neoformans, Histoplasma capsulatum, Coccidioides immitis Viruses: Varicella zoster, cytomegalovirus, herpes simplex Protozoa: Pneumocystis carinii, Toxoplasma gondii, Cryptosporidium Helminths: Strongyloides stercoralis
Humoral immune dysfunction (B-cell immune alteration) prevalent with multiple myeloma	Disseminated	S. pneumoniae, H. influenzae
Iatrogenic factors (invasive procedures, devices, equipment)	Skin	Staphylococcus epidermis
Diagnostic procedures	Mucous membranes	Locally colonizing organisms
Genitourinary tract manipulations		
Bone marrow aspirations		
Biopsies		
Placement of shunts, stents, and tubes		
Venipuncture		
Long-term venous access devices		
Respiratory-assist devices		
Nosocomial Sources		
Air	Pulmonary	Aspergillus species
Surface contact	Skin and mucous membranes	S. aureus

TABLE 24-11   Factors Predisposing Cancer Patients to Infection—cont'd

PRECIPITATING EVENT	COMMON SITE OF INFECTION	COMMON ORGANISM
Food (fresh fruits and vegetables)		Bacteria, fungi
Water (stagnant sources)	Disseminated	P. aeruginosa, Serratia marcescens
Medical personnel (illness, organism transmission or cross-contamination, poor handwashing)	Various	Locally colonizing organisms
Extended prophylactic broad-spectrum antibiotics	Disseminated	Bacteria

Data from Mutnick AH, Bergquist SC, Beltz E: Bacteremia and sepsis. In Herfindal ET, Gourey DR, editors: *Textbook of therapeutics: drug and disease management,* Baltimore, 1996, Williams & Wilkins; and Talan DA: Sepsis and septic shock, *Emerg Med* 29:54, 1997.

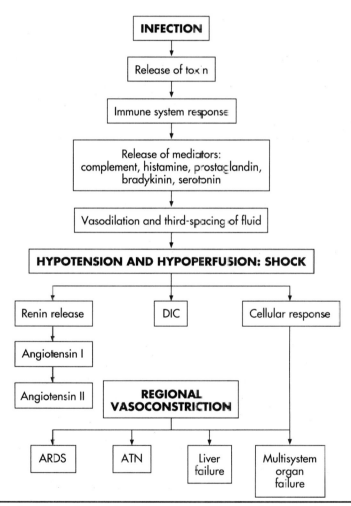

FIG. 24-12 Pathophysiology of septic shock. *ARDS,* Acute respiratory distress syndrome; *ATN,* acute tubular necrosis. (From McMorrow ME, Cooney-Daniello M: When to suspect septic shock, RN 54(10):32, 1991. [Published in RN; copyright© 1991, Medical Economics, Montvale, N.J. Reprinted by permission.])

and exotoxins. The endothelial alteration causes microthrombi to form and activates the complement, coagulation, and fibrinolytic systems. Bradykinin, histamine, and serotonin release increases capillary permeability. The patient in septic shock may exhibit hypovolemia, hypotension, hypoxia, tissue ischemia, DIC, ileus, oliguria, and liver failure (Fig. 24-13).

Clinical Features

The first signs of progressive sepsis may be fever, shaking chills, and mild hypotension. The early phase of septic shock has been referred to as the warm, or hyperdynamic, phase. It is characterized by vasodilation, decreased peripheral vascular resistance, and increased cardiac output. The patient may appear warm and flushed.

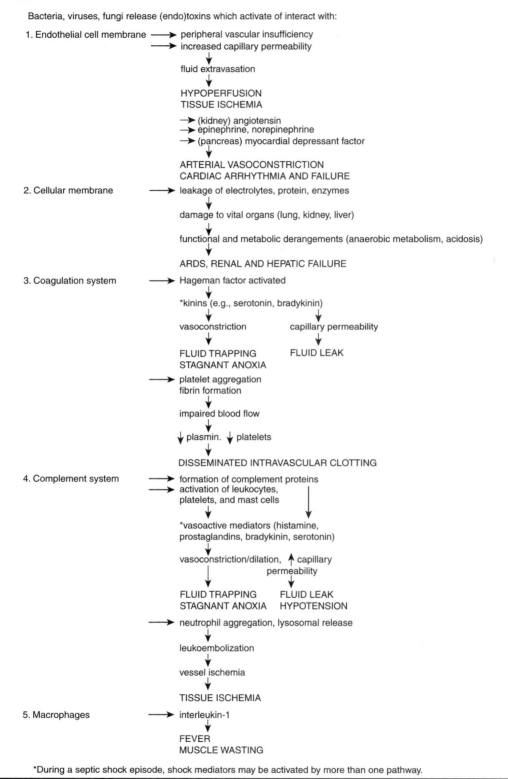

Bacteria, viruses, fungi release (endo)toxins which activate of interact with:

1. Endothelial cell membrane ⟶ peripheral vascular insufficiency
⟶ increased capillary permeability

fluid extravasation

HYPOPERFUSION
TISSUE ISCHEMIA

⟶ (kidney) angiotensin
⟶ epinephrine, norepinephrine
⟶ (pancreas) myocardial depressant factor

ARTERIAL VASOCONSTRICTION
CARDIAC ARRHYTHMIA AND FAILURE

2. Cellular membrane ⟶ leakage of electrolytes, protein, enzymes

damage to vital organs (lung, kidney, liver)

functional and metabolic derangements (anaerobic metabolism, acidosis)

ARDS, RENAL AND HEPATIC FAILURE

3. Coagulation system ⟶ Hageman factor activated

*kinins (e.g., serotonin, bradykinin)

vasoconstriction   capillary permeability

FLUID TRAPPING   FLUID LEAK
STAGNANT ANOXIA

⟶ platelet aggregation
fibrin formation

impaired blood flow

↓ plasmin. ↓ platelets

DISSEMINATED INTRAVASCULAR CLOTTING

4. Complement system ⟶ formation of complement proteins
⟶ activation of leukocytes,
platelets, and mast cells

*vasoactive mediators (histamine,
prostaglandins, bradykinin, serotonin)

vasoconstriction/dilation, ↑ capillary
permeability

FLUID TRAPPING   FLUID LEAK
STAGNANT ANOXIA   HYPOTENSION

⟶ neutrophil aggregation, lysosomal release

leukoembolization

vessel ischemia

TISSUE ISCHEMIA

5. Macrophages ⟶ interleukin-1

FEVER
MUSCLE WASTING

*During a septic shock episode, shock mediators may be activated by more than one pathway.

FIG. 24-13 Pathophysiology of septic shock. *ARDS,* Acute respiratory distress syndrome. (From Harnett S: Septic shock in the oncology patient, *Cancer Nurs* 12(4):191, 1989.)

The respiratory rate is rapid, which leads to alkalosis. The patient may be nauseated, have diarrhea, and be mildly confused. As septic shock progresses, capillary leakage causes fluid to third space (when fluid becomes trapped in the interstitial spaces), cardiac output decreases, and peripheral vascular resistance increases. The patient develops oliguria and metabolic acidosis. Peripheral vasoconstriction leads to ischemia and decreased blood flow to vital organs. Bleeding occurs in the patient with DIC. Peripheral edema becomes more severe. The patient becomes cold, clammy, and cyanotic. Confusion progresses to coma. Without successful intervention, symptoms progress to the cold phase, also known as late or refractory shock. At this point the condition is irreversible. Circulatory and respiratory collapse ultimately occur. (See Clinical Features box.)

Clinical Features of
Stages of Shock

Stage One: Hyperdynamic Stage (Early Shock, Warm Shock)

Decreased tissue perfusion: 10% reduction in blood volume

Usually lasts less than 24 hours

Feelings of anxiety, apprehension, nervousness

Complaints of nausea

Altered mental status, restlessness, irritability, disorientation, inappropriate euphoria

Temperature normal, below normal, or above normal

Skin warm and flushed because of arteriole dilation

Peripheral cyanosis

Tachycardia and bounding peripheral pulses

Normal or slightly elevated blood pressure with a widening pulse pressure

Tachypnea, hyperventilation

Rales and decreased breath sounds

Respiratory alkalosis: decreased oxygen pressure

Renal output normal or elevated (polyuria)

Blood urea nitrogen (BUN) and creatinine may be slowly increasing

Hyperglycemia

Urine may test positive for sugar (glycosuria)

Urine specific gravity normal

No signs of bleeding

Coagulation profile normal

Stage Two: Normodynamic Stage (Intermediate Shock, Cool Shock)

Decreased tissue perfusion: 15% to 20% reduction in blood volume

Usually lasts a few hours

Complains of thirst

Altered mental status: lethargy, confusion

Skin pale, cool, and clammy because of peripheral vasoconstriction and diversion of blood to vital organs

Peripheral edema possible because of increased secretion of antidiuretic hormone and aldosterone leading to sodium and water retention

Temperature normal or subnormal

Tachycardia continues

Blood pressure decreases with a narrow pulse pressure because of decrease in cardiac output

Respirations slow and shallow

Respiratory acidosis

Renal output decreased (oliguria)

Urine specific gravity elevated

Abdominal distention because of air swallowing and decreased peristalsis

Hemorrhagic lesions may be apparent

Stage Three: Hypodynamic Stage (Late Shock, Refractory Shock, Irreversible Shock, Cold Shock, "Classic" Shock)

Decreased cardiac output, decrease in blood volume

Altered mental status, stupor, coma

Skin cold, possible cyanosis of digits and mottling

Temperature subnormal

Tachycardia

Weak or absent pulses because of decreased myocardial contractility: "pump failure"

Hypotension

Respiratory depression

Pulmonary edema, or "shock lung," because of decreased oxygen pressure and decreased pulmonary microcirculation, and acute respiratory distress syndrome (ARDS)

Metabolic acidosis because of anaerobic metabolism and increased levels of lactic acid

Hypoglycemia

No renal output (anuria)

Renal failure: acute tubular necrosis (ATN)

Hemorrhagic lesions

Data from Astiz ME, Rackow EC: Seminar. Septic shock, *Lancet* 351(9114):1501, 1998; and Shelton BK: Sepsis, *Semin Oncol Nurs* 15:209, 1999.

RESPIRATORY FEATURES

Hyperventilation and respiratory alkalosis may occur both with and without fever. Alveolar capillary leakage leads to pulmonary edema and hypoxemia. ARDS occurs most frequently in patients with gram-negative infections. The development of ARDS increases morbidity to 80% to 90%. Concomitant thrombocytopenia raises the morbidity rate even higher.[87]

CARDIOVASCULAR FEATURES

Systemic vascular resistance drops dramatically as a result of vasodilation. Hypotension is associated with the release of complement, TNF-α, and IL-1. Metabolites of nitric oxide are also related to the decrease in vascular resistance. Cardiac output increases in an attempt to compensate. Systemic vascular resistance ultimately increases, with vasoconstriction leading to ischemia and decreased organ perfusion. Elevated lactic acid levels occur, with hypoperfusion of vital organs and hypoxemia. This is a poor prognostic sign.[87]

HEMATOLOGIC FEATURES

Gram-negative sepsis is also associated with the development of DIC. The release of bacterial toxins stimulates the clotting cascade that exhausts clotting factors and leads to simultaneous hemorrhage and thrombosis. (See previous discussion of DIC.) DIC is almost always associated with septic shock and may be one of the presenting signs.[88]

OTHER FEATURES

Septic shock due to GI pathogens may also be accompanied by jaundice, stress ulcers, and bleeding. Renal symptoms of oliguria and proteinuria may progress to acute tubular necrosis (ATN) and renal failure.[87]

Diagnosis

The diagnosis of septic shock depends on astute observations of the patient. Sepsis may or may not have been confirmed. An initial finding could be as subtle a sign as the patient complaint of "just not feeling right." Physical assessment of all systems should be correlated with a brief recent history highlighting any changes and noting any possible sources of infection. Continuous assessment and monitoring of the patient is essential. This includes taking vital signs, observing tissue perfusion, watching for signs of bleeding, checking mental status, and assessing heart, lung, and kidney function.

In the neutropenic patient, fever may be the only sign of an infection. Elevated temperature is produced in the body by the monocytes, not the neutrophils. Some monocytes migrate into body tissue, where they become macrophages. The monocyte secretes an endogenous pyrogen that affects the thalamus, resulting in a rise in temperature. Fever in a neutropenic patient should be treated as an emergency. In a profoundly neutropenic patient, death can occur within 24 to 72 hours if appropriate antibiotic therapy is not initiated. Mortality rates within the first 48 hours of infectious symptoms can exceed 50%.[92]

Once fever is noted, cultures should be obtained from all potential sites of infection before the initiation of antibiotics. Blood cultures are drawn peripherally, as well as centrally if the patient has a central line. Two sets of blood cultures are typically done, 15 minutes apart, to increase the chances of collecting the offending organism. Blood cultures may be repeated with each temperature spike until the organism is identified. When drawing blood from a central line for culture, the initial 5 to 6 ml should not be wasted, but used for the culture. Wasting the initial aspirate decreases the chances of collecting the pathogen. Sputum, urine, stool, central line exit sites, and any other areas where skin integrity is not intact should be cultured.

A CBC is done to evaluate WBC and neutrophil levels. Chest x-ray is performed to evaluate lung status and rule out the lung as the site of infection. CT of the abdomen and pelvis or ultra-sonography may be used to rule out intraabdominal infections or abscesses. Blood gases are done to evaluate any respiratory compromise. Coagulation panels are done to rule out or confirm DIC. Additional lab results may include elevated serum glucose, cortisol, catecholamine, and lactate levels.

Treatment Modalities

The identified stage of septic shock will dictate the necessary medical interventions. Prompt medical treatment is essential to prevent progression of shock syndrome to the irreversible stage and subsequent death. Recognition of the signs and symptoms of shock and the determination of sepsis are the first medical interventions.

As with most oncologic emergencies, prevention is the ideal treatment for septic shock. Measures to protect immunocompro-mised patients from infection are critical. Some of these include meticulous handwashing, low-bacterial diets, and avoidance of crowds. Patients in the acute care setting should have private rooms with limited visitors. Hematopoietic growth factors are used to promote neutrophil recovery after antineoplastic therapy. Patients with prolonged neutropenia and candidates for bone marrow or stem cell transplant may benefit from antimicrobial prophylaxis.[88]

The patient in septic shock requires intervention in a critical care setting. Hemodynamic monitoring is necessary, as is the vigilant nursing care that can be provided in the ICU. The goals of treatment are to maintain blood pressure and tissue perfusion while treating the underlying pathogen. Broad-spectrum antibiotics

should be initiated within an hour of drawing blood cultures. The choice of empiric antibiotic treatment is based on the suspected site of infection and most likely pathogen. High-risk patients currently receive two or more drugs to cover both gram-positive and gram-negative bacteria. Aminoglycosides (such as gentamicin or tobramycin) are included to cover gram-negative bacteria. If the skin is the suspected source of infection, penicillin or a first-generation cephalosporin may be used. Vancomycin is used when central venous access devices are the suspected source of infection and for methicillin-resistant strains.[93] Some of the recommended combinations are listed as follows (see Boxes 24-10 and 24-11 for categories of β-lactams and generations of cephalosporins):

BOX 24-10 **β-Lactam Antibiotics**

Penicillins
Cephalosporins
Carbapenems
Monobactams

Data from Holten KB, ONusko EM: Appropriate prescribing of oral beta-lactam antibiotics, *Am Fam Physician* 62 (3): 2000; retrieved July, 10, 2005, from http://www.aafp.org/afp/2000080/611.html.

BOX 24-11 **Generations of Cephalosporins**

First Generation
Cefadroxil
Cefazolin
Cephalexin
Cephapirin
Cephradine

Second Generation
Cefaclor
Cefotetan*
Cefuroxime
Cefamandole
Cefoxitin*
Cefonicid
Cefprozil

Third Generation
Cefdinir
Cefotaxime
Ceftriaxone
Cefixime
Cefpodoxime
Ceftibuten
Cefoperazone
Ceftazidime
Ceftizoxime

Fourth Generation
Cefepime

*Cephamycins (closely related to β-lactam antibiotics).
Data from *AHFS Drug Information 1999*, Bethesda, Md, 1999, American Society of Health System Pharmacists.

- A fourth-generation cephalosporin (e.g., cefepime) or an antipseudomonal penicillin with an aminoglycoside[88]
- An antipseudomonal β-lactam and an aminoglycoside[93]
- Ceftazidime and an aminoglycoside with or without vancomycin, or piperacillin-tazobactam, an aminoglycoside, and imipenem or meropenem[87]
- An extended-spectrum penicillin (piperacillin, mezlocillin) or a third-generation cephalosporin and an aminoglycoside[91]
- For suspected anaerobes (GI and/or genitourinary [GU]): extended-spectrum penicillin or a third-generation cephalosporin and an aminoglycoside combined with metronidazole or a penicillinase-inhibitor β-lactam combination such as piperacillin-tazobactam or ticarcillin-clavulanate with an aminoglycoside or imipenem and an amiglycoside[91]
- Vancomycin, a carbapenem (imipenem or meropenem), and an aminoglycoside (substitute a quinolone for significant renal impairment)[94]
- An aminoglycoside, an antipseudomonal penicillin, and cefepime, ceftazidime, or carbapenem[92]

Once culture and sensitivity results are obtained, the empiric therapy can be altered to include the most appropriate agents for the pathogens identified. If no pathogen is identified and the patient remains febrile despite broad-spectrum antibiotics, antifungal and/or antiviral agents, or both, must be added.

Fluid replacement with crystalloids or colloids is done to correct hypovolemia. If the patient remains hypotensive, vasopressors such as dopamine or dobutamine are initiated to maintain perfusion of vital organs. Norepinephrine may also be used. Electrolyte imbalances should be corrected and urinary output maintained at 50 ml/hr. Blood products may be needed for the patient with DIC or GI bleeding. Oxygen will be needed to help maintain oxygenation. Ventilatory assistance should be initiated early for patients with respiratory compromise. Almost 85% of patients with septic shock will require ventilator support for 7 to 14 days.[95]

Any loculated sites of infection or drainable abscesses should be surgically drained.[87] Aggressive nutritional support is necessary for the patient with metabolic abnormalities and helps prevent tissue breakdown. TNF has been associated with cachexia. Glucose administration must be closely monitored, because glucose uptake may be impaired because of insulin inhibition caused by hormones responding to the stress response. Protein and nutrient supplements are needed to meet the high energy demands of septic shock and to promote the healing process. Several studies have indicated that corticosteroids are not beneficial in the management of septic shock and may actually be detrimental to the outcome.[87,90] One study indicated a benefit from combination therapy with hydrocortisone and fludrocortisone in patients with septic shock and insufficient adrenal reserve.[96]

Low levels of activated protein C may be associated with a poor outcome in the management of sepsis. This is a regulator of coagulation and inflammatory responses during sepsis. Trials are being conducted with a recombinant human activated protein C, drotrecogin alfa (Xigris). Initial results indicate a reduction in the relative risk of death in severe sepsis and an increase in short-term survival.[89,94] Drotrecogin alfa works as an antiinflamatory agent. It has demonstrated improved organ perfusion, most likely via antithrombotic and profibrinolytic activity. Risk of bleeding makes its use controversial for patients with significant thrombocytopenia, gastrointestinal lesions, or other potential sources of bleeding.[89]

Much study is being done to identify interventions to counteract the inflammatory response to septic shock. Some agents under study include IL-1 receptor antagonists, anti-TNF antibodies, platelet-activating factor (PAF)–receptor antagonists, bradykinin antagonists, ibuprofen, bactericidal permeability-increasing protein, cationic antimicrobial protein, and N-acetylcysteine.[90,91,87]

Nursing Considerations

The nursing care of a patient with sepsis varies with the identified stage of septic shock. Infection and sepsis have a high correlation with neutropenia. Patients at highest risk are those whose neutrophil count is less than 100/mm[3] for more than 3 weeks. Therefore the first nursing goal in the management of septic shock is prevention of infection. The following general measures outline the nursing care for the patient with neutropenia. Complete reverse isolation, although it reduces exogenous colonization, is no longer recommended for patients with neutropenia, because endogenous flora are the major source of infection. Thus current practice is to use protective isolation.

An elevated temperature and changes in blood pressure, pulse, and respiration may be the only sign of an impending infection, since neutropenic patients have a diminished inflammatory response. Observe for other general signs and symptoms of infection or sepsis: nausea, abdominal discomfort, changes in renal status, irritability, and changes in mental status. Assess blood counts daily or every other day to determine the onset of infection, recovery of the bone marrow, status of renal function, and possible need to change antibiotic regimen. This should include CBC with differential, platelet count, and chemistry panel. Prevent cross-contamination by providing care first to patients with neutropenia before caring for other patients. Do not care for both patients with neutropenia and patients with infection. Wash hands consistently and thoroughly after each patient contact. Screen personnel and visitors. Patients should not be exposed to anyone with an infection, recent vaccination, or recent exposure to a communicable disease (e.g., bacterial infections, herpes, colds, influenza, chickenpox, measles). Limit the number of visitors. Provide a neutropenic diet (microbiotic diet) that eliminates unpared fresh fruits and raw vegetables. All food items should be cooked. Avoid the placement of fresh fruits, flowers, or plants in patient's room. Change water to prevent stagnation (e.g., denture cups, water pitchers, humidifiers, respiratory equipment, irrigation containers).

Inspect the patient's body daily with attention to the mouth, all orifices, all skin folds, and any site of an IV catheter insertion, a tube insertion, or a wound. Instruct the patient and provide assistance in meticulous skin and mouth care. Provide lubrications to prevent dryness and cracking. Female patients should also keep the vaginal area clean and lubricated. Prevent trauma to the skin and mucous membranes by avoiding intramuscular or subcutaneous injections whenever possible; rectal manipulations, as with enemas, suppositories, or thermometers; urinary catheterization; or douching and using tampons with the female patient. If urinary catheterization is necessary, maintain a closed sterile drainage system. Avoid rectal trauma by preventing constipation with dietary measures or stool softeners.

Auscultate lungs to assess respiratory status. Observe ventilatory function for difficulties: shallow respirations, tachypnea, dyspnea, frothy secretions, and jugular vein distention. Obtain or assist with measurement of ABGs. Monitor CVP. Administer crystalloids, colloids, and blood products as ordered to maintain circulating fluid volume. Encourage mobility and frequent deep breathing and coughing. Provide nutritional support. Parenteral nutrition may be needed to meet increased caloric needs. Obtain dietitian consultation. Measure weight daily. Monitor laboratory values to assess for protein wasting, with particular attention to serum albumin level. Encourage fluid intake up to 300 ml/day, unless contraindicated. Obtain specimens for cultures and sensitivities as ordered. Blood samples are taken peripherally as well as from each port of central lines. Initial blood draw from central line is to be used for a specimen rather than wasting it, since this may be the best chance at organism identification. Administer antibiotics as ordered. Observe the patient closely for possible toxicities; nephrotoxicity and neurotoxicities are prevalent with the use of aminoglycosides (e.g., tobramycin, gentamicin). Control fevers with antipyretic medications.

The nursing management of a patient with septic shock is extremely complex and challenging. It requires astute assessment and, often, quick decision making. Because septicemia is the triggering event, infection prophylaxis is crucial.

Prognosis

Survival of patients with septic shock depends on preventing or reversing the process of shock and on the status of the underlying disease (i.e., nonfatal, ultimately fatal, rapidly fatal). Less than 5% of deaths are due to cardiac failure; 25% to 33% of patients die from hypotension that cannot be corrected with fluids and vasopressors.[90] The presence of ARDS raises morbidity to 80% to 90%.[87] Once the patient develops MODS, there is very little chance of reversal. Prompt recognition and treatment of septic shock can mean the difference between life and death.

SYNDROME OF INAPPROPRIATE ANTIDIURETIC HORMONE SECRETION

Definition

The syndrome of inappropriate antidiuretic hormone secretion (SIADH) is an endocrine paraneoplastic syndrome that causes a disorder of water balance.[97] Antidiuretic hormone (ADH), also called arginine vasopressin, regulates the body's water balance. SIADH is characterized by elevated serum blood levels of ADH, excessive water retention, hypoosmolality, and hyponatremia.[97]

Etiology and Risk Factors

This syndrome develops in 1% to 2% of patients with cancer.[51] Approximately two thirds of patients with documented SIADH have a neoplasm. The most common malignant disease associated with this syndrome is lung cancer, and about 80% of these cases are small cell carcinoma.[53] In fact, 50% of patients with SCLC have impaired water excretion. As many as 10% to 15% of these patients develop clinically evident SIADH.[53] SIADH may be the presenting symptom in patients with SCLC.[7] Other cancers associated with SIADH include cancer of the esophagus, the duodenum, the pancreas, the prostate, the head and neck, and the bladder; acute myelogenous leukemia; lymphoma; thymoma; mesothelioma; carcinoid tumors; CNS metastases; and non-SCLC.[65] Several chemotherapeutic agents, including cisplatin, cyclophosphamide, melphalan, vinblastine, and vincristine, have been associated with the development of SIADH.[65] Other agents, such as antidepressants, antibiotics, opioids, chlorpropamide, nicotine, and ethanol have also been linked with SIADH.[65]

The incidence of SIADH is rising because of the increased incidence of SCLC and other cancers associated with the ectopic production of ADH.

Nonmalignant conditions that can account for SIADH are CNS disorders, pulmonary infections, asthma, and the use of positive-pressure respirators.[97]

Pathophysiology

All body fluids are solutions containing various concentrations of solute (salt) and solvent (fluid or water). The concentration of salt in body fluid creates an osmotic pressure. Measurement of osmotic pressure (or concentration of a solution) is referred to as **osmolality** or **osmolarity.** It is expressed in osmols (Osm) or milliosmols (mOsm) per kilogram of either water (osmolality) or solution (osmolarity). In a steady state, normal osmolality is maintained at a constant level of 280 to 300 mOsm/kg of body weight. The osmolality and volume of the extracellular fluid and the urine are maintained by a balance of fluid intake and urinary excretion.

Fluid intake is maintained by the thirst mechanism located in the hypothalamus (Fig. 24-14). Lack of water increases the osmolality of the extracellular fluid, which activates the sensation of thirst. Fluid intake is then increased to restore the fluid balance. If excess fluid is ingested, it is excreted to maintain the balance.

The second aspect of the osmolality-regulating system is urinary excretion. The amount of urine excreted by the kidneys depends on how much fluid is resorbed and circulated throughout the body. This regulation of fluid intake and output through the kidneys is controlled by the presence of ADH in the kidneys.

ADH is produced by the hypothalamus and transported to the posterior pituitary, where it is stored. Changes in ADH production and secretion (increase or decrease) are controlled by receptors in the kidneys, the heart, and the brain in response to extracellular or intravascular volume (see Fig. 24-14). ADH secretion is extremely sensitive and responds to a 1% to 2% change in osmolality.

When plasma osmolality is increased or plasma volume is decreased, ADH is secreted from the pituitary gland. Once in the kidneys, ADH increases the permeability of the distal tubule and the collection duct, which allows more water resorption. This enhanced amount of water enters the vascular system, diluting solutes, lowering plasma osmolality, and resulting in concentrated urine excretion. Decreased plasma or blood volume also stimulates ADH secretion. A moderate increase in ADH occurs with a 10% blood loss, and a 25% blood loss can produce 20 to 50 times the normal rate of ADH secretion. This response maintains arterial blood pressure.

If plasma osmolality is decreased, as in the presence of excessive water intake, ADH secretion is halted. This decreases the permeability to water of the renal distal tubule and the collecting duct, allowing more water to be excreted as dilute urine. An increase in plasma or blood volume also stops the release of ADH. Drinking alcohol inhibits ADH secretion. In summary, the thirst mechanism and the ADH feedback mechanisms (see Fig. 24-14) regulate body fluids and maintain a constant osmolality.

A variety of conditions can disrupt the body fluid regulating system and cause SIADH. The following three pathophysiologic mechanisms are responsible for SIADH:

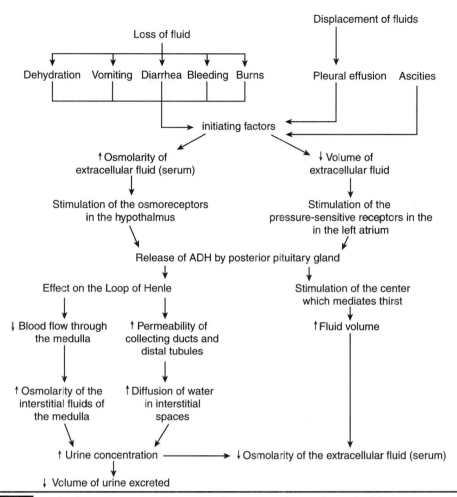

FIG. 24-14 Feedback mechanism regulating the release of antidiuretic hormone *(ADH)*. (From Yasko JM: Syndrome of inappropriate antidiuretic hormone secretion. In Yasko JM, editor: *Guidelines for cancer care: symptom management*, Reston, Va, © 1983. Reprinted by permission of Prentice-Hall, Inc., Upper Saddle River, NJ.)

- Inappropriate secretion of ADH from the supraoptic-hypophyseal system. This mechanism results from CNS disorders such as head trauma, CVA (stroke), meningitis, brain abscess, CNS hemorrhage, CNS tumors (both primary and metastatic), encephalitis, and Guillain-Barre syndrome. Postoperative patients, patients in shock, patients experiencing status asthmaticus, pain, or high stress levels, and patients on positive-pressure breathing may also experience SIADH through this mechanism. These conditions increase intrathoracic pressure or decrease venous return to the heart. Cardiac output decreases, leading to decreased plasma volume, and stimulating ADH secretion.
- ADH or an ADH-like substance is secreted by cells outside the supraoptic-hypophyseal system, referred to as **ectopic secretion.** Ectopic production of the endocrine peptide, ADH, has been demonstrated in a variety of malignancies and is the primary etiology for cancer-related SIADH. Cells in the atrium of the heart may also secrete a peptide, atrial natriuretic peptide, that can increase sodium excretion.[74,97] Infections within the pulmonary system such as those caused by bacteria or viruses may bring about ectopic release of ADH. This may also be

one process leading to the SIADH seen in patients with a malignancy.
- The action of ADH on the renal distal tubules is enhanced. Various drugs can stimulate or potentiate the release of ADH. These include narcotics such as morphine, nicotine, tranquilizers, barbiturates, general anesthetics, potassium supplements, thiazide diuretics, hypoglycemic agents such as chlorpropamide (Diabinese), clofibrate (Atromid-S), acetaminophen (paracetamol, Tylenol), isoproterenol, and five antineoplastic agents: cisplatin (Platinol), cyclophosphamide (Cytoxan), vinblastine (Velban), vincristine (Oncovin), and melphalan (Alkeran). Cyclophosphamide has a direct effect on the renal tubule and is also associated with vigorous hydration that can lead to SIADH.[53]

Patients with cancer may have SIADH resulting from any one of these three mechanisms. Intrathoracic or mediastinal tumors can increase intrathoracic pressure, resulting in a decreased venous return and decreased cardiac output, which stimulates the release of ADH. Patients with SCLC (50%), pancreatic cancer, lymphomas, and thymomas have demonstrated synthesis and secretion of ADH or an ADH-like substance from the neoplastic tissue.

Patients receiving any of the chemotherapy agents just listed have the potential to develop SIADH.

The syndrome is associated with water excess and results from the ectopic production of ADH, which increases the permeability of the kidney to water, promoting water resorption and decreasing urine output. This may be associated with hyponatremia. Hyponatremia may be caused by excessive loss of sodium or excessive gain of water. It is always a result of a relatively greater water concentration than sodium concentration.

However, hyponatremia is not solely diagnostic of SIADH. Some other disorders may also stimulate SIADH. In hypothyroidism and hypoadrenocorticism, the hormone deficiency is responsible, but the exact mechanism is unknown.[50] SIADH can also be seen with hyponatremia secondary to sodium depletion (e.g., renal disease, vomiting, diarrhea, diabetic acidosis), hypokalemia, glucocorticoid deficiency, third spacing, and dilutional hyponatremia related to CHF, renal failure, or ascites related to liver disease.

Two other particular situations will elicit hyponatremia. First, hyponatremia also occurs when nonsodium solutes accumulate in the extracellular space because they do not freely diffuse across cell membranes. This causes an osmotic gradient that allows water to move from the intracellular to the extracellular space. Two conditions can produce this phenomenon. Hyperglycemia is the most common cause of this disorder. The calculated and measured plasma osmolality will be the same, which is elevated because of hyperglycemia. IV mannitol therapy also demonstrates an elevated plasma osmolality, but the calculated level is lower than the measured value. In either situation, these are not true hypoosmolar states.

Second, **pseudohyponatremia** may occur, also called **factitious hyponatremia.** These terms describe a low serum sodium concentration secondary to volume-displacing effects that can occur with hyperproteinemia and hyperlipidemia. Large macromolecules (e.g., proteins, lipids) are present and fictitiously lower plasma sodium levels, as measured in the clinical laboratory. However, measured plasma osmolality is normal.

These interesting situations must be evaluated in the presence of hyponatremia. Diagnostic work-up for any patient with hyponatremia requires determination of the existence of a hypoosmolar state.

Clinical Features

The clinical syndrome resulting from inappropriate secretion of ADH has the following features:
- Hyponatremia (serum sodium less than normal level of 135 to 147 mEq/L)
- Decreased osmolality of serum and extracellular fluid (less than normal level of 280 to 300 mOsm/kg)
- Excessive water retention (water intoxication)
- Urine osmolality greater than appropriate for plasma osmolality (above 500 mmol/kg), producing less than maximally dilute urine (abnormally high urine specific gravity)
- Continued urinary excretion of sodium (sodium in urine above 20 mEq/L) (washing of sodium in urine)
- Absence of fluid volume depletion (normal skin turgor and blood pressure)
- Suppression of plasma renin
- Normal renal, adrenal, and thyroid function
- BUN possibly low because of volume expansion

- Hypouricemia and hypophosphatemia may be present because of decreased proximal tubular resorption.

The symptomatology experienced by the patient with SIADH depends on the severity, rapidity, and duration of the hyponatremia and decreased plasma osmolality (Box 24-12).[65] Excessive water retention continues despite a decrease in the osmolality of serum and extracellular fluid. Urine is concentrated, and the extracellular fluid expands, and this results in hyponatremia. Patients complain of thirst, anorexia, nausea, and vomiting. Weight gain, lethargy, and muscle weakness occurs. Irritability, personality changes, and mental confusion may occur and lead to seizures and coma.

Diagnosis

Asymptomatic SIADH is often found on routine serum chemistry.[53] SIADH is diagnosed from the combination of hyponatremia, decreased plasma osmolality, and increased urine osmality.[67,53,74,97] Associated lab values may include decreased uric acid, albumin, BUN, and creatinine levels, and increased urine specific gravity.[65] It is possible to do radioimmunoassays

---

BOX 24-12   Signs and Symptoms of SIADH

Mild Hyponatremia: Serum Sodium 125-135 mEq/L
May be asymptomatic
Anorexia
Difficulty concentrating
Fatigue
Headache
Inappropriate behavior
Muscle cramps
Oliguria
Peripheral edema
Weakness
Weight gain

Moderate Hyponatremia: Serum Sodium 115-125 mEq/L
Confusion
Decreased deep tendon reflexes
Hallucinations
Impaired taste
Incontinence
Lethargy
Nausea, vomiting, diarrhea
Oliguria
Personality changes
Thirst
Tremors
Weight gain

Severe Hyponatremia: Serum Sodium <115 mEq/L
Coma
Seizures
Inability to protect airway and mobilize secretions

SIADH, Syndrome of inappropriate antidiuretic hormone secretion.
Data from Keenan AMM: Syndrome of inappropriate secretion of antidiuretic hormone in malignancy, *Semin Oncol Nurs* 15:160, 1999; and Shivnan J, Shelton BK, Onners BK: Bone marrow transplantation: Issues for critical care nurses, *AACN Clin Issues* 7:95, 1996.

of the urine and serum for elevated ADH levels. This is not commonly done because of cost and inconvenience. A water-loading test can also be performed. A calculated amount of water is administered, followed by monitoring intake, output, and specific gravity. This can only be done safely if the serum sodium is greater than 124 mEq/L and the patient is asymptomatic.[7]

Treatment Modalities

The primary treatment of choice for SIADH is to treat or eliminate the underlying cause; however, the sodium level and patient's neurologic status must be stabilized.[53] Treatment decisions are based on the severity of the hyponatremia and symptoms of water intoxication.

Mild hyponatremia is typically treated with fluid restriction (500 to 1000 ml/day). This promotes a negative water balance and will usually correct plasma sodium levels in 3 to 5 days.[53] Mild to moderate hyponatremia that is chronic may be treated with demeclocycline, a derivative of tetracyline (600 to 1200 mg/day orally in divided doses). This drug inhibits the action of ADH on renal tubules so water can be excreted. Fluid restriction is not required with demeclocycline. Side effects and toxicities may include nausea, photosensitivity, reversible diabetes insipidus, and azotemia (more common at higher doses).[97] Dosage must be reduced for patients with decreased renal or hepatic function. Demeclocycline may be used for long-term therapy, but must be used with caution because of nephrotoxicity.[98] Lithium carbonate (900 to 1200 mg/day) and urea (0.5 g/kg/day) are used less frequently.[97] Any drugs that can cause hyponatremia are discontinued (with the possible exception of certain chemotherapeutic agents).

Severe hyponatremia typically develops rapidly, over 1 to 2 days, and is a medical emergency. Untreated, it will progress from seizures and coma to brain herniation and death. Increased intracellular fluid in brain cells (due to extracellular hypoosmolality) increases ICP and decreases cerebral blood flow.[97] Severe cases are treated with hypertonic saline infusions (3%) and Lasix diuresis.[51,99] However, care must be taken not to correct the hyponatremia too quickly, because this can lead to neurologic damage. Osmotic demyelination syndrome can occur within 2 to 6 days of too rapid correction of hyponatremia, particularly in patients with hypokalemia. Symptoms include rapidly progressive lower extremity weakness, dysarthria, and dysphagia. It is recommended to correct serum potassium levels before, or in conjunction with, initiating therapy for hyponatremia. One recommendation for hyponatremia is to begin sodium level correction at a rate not to exceed 0.5 to 1.0 mEq/L per hour.[97] Once mild hyponatremic levels are reached, therapy is changed to fluid restriction or pharmacologic agents such as demeclocycline.[97]

Using chemotherapy to treat the underlying malignancy in a patient with SIADH provides its own set of challenges. One drug used to treat SCLC is cisplatin, which requires the patient to be well hydrated to protect renal tissue from toxicity. Cisplatin can cause SIADH, as well as exacerbate existing SIADH.[65] Administration of cyclophosphamide, used to treat many solid tumors, also requires hydration. Vigorous hydration may exacerbate SIADH.[65] Patients with mild hyponatremia may be gently hydrated with normal saline before chemotherapy and then put on fluid restriction. Moderate SIADH may require saline hydration, electrolyte replacement, and diuresis before chemotherapy. Patients with severe hyponatremia will need to be neurologically stabilized before the initiation of chemotherapy.[7]

Currently, no drugs are available that directly suppress the synthesis or release of ADH from malignant tissue; however, clinical trials are investigating agents that can block the action of ADH at the collecting duct system. These agents are called nonpeptide vasopressin V_2-receptor antagonists.[97]

Nursing Considerations

The primary nursing intervention for a patient diagnosed with the syndrome of inappropriate secretion of antidiuretic hormone (SIADH) is patient education and emotional support to facilitate patient compliance.

Assess for signs or symptoms of alteration in fluid volume (*excess:* rales shortness of breath, neck vein distention, weight gain, and edema of sacrum and/or lower extremities; *deficit:* dry mucous membranes, poor skin turgor, weight loss, rapid and thready pulse, orthostatic hypotension, and restlessness). Auscultate lungs for breath sounds. Monitor cardiac function and tissue perfusion. Monitor intake and output closely. Restrict fluids as ordered (500 to 1000 ml/24 hr). Obtain daily weight. Monitor laboratory values (serum electrolytes, BUN, creatinine, calcium, magnesium) with special attention to the following:

- *Serum plasma osmolality:* As SIADH progresses, plasma osmolality decreases, which causes the brain to swell and level of consciousness (LOC) to decrease. Therefore serum osmolality can predict LOC.
- *Serum sodium:* Hypernatremia may result from overcorrection of low serum levels. Accompanying signs and symptoms of hypernatremia include thirst, dry mucous membranes, irritability, lethargy, and seizures.

Obtain urine osmolality and specific gravity. Determine LOC and note any changes in sensorium. Check muscles and tendon reflexes for twitching. Monitor for seizure activity if serum sodium level is less than 120 mEq/L, and implement seizure precautions (e.g., padded tongue blade and airway at bedside, no oral thermometers). Monitor skin integrity, and provide appropriate skin care. Thoroughly assess the oral cavity, and provide oral care as needed. Use mouthwashes without alcohol content.

Many patients with extreme hyponatremia cannot recollect much of their experience during the SIADH event. This points out the need to provide measures to ensure safety and to reduce anxiety.

Prognosis

The syndrome can be successfully treated, as evidenced by a return to normal levels of serum and extracellular osmolality, serum sodium and urine osmolality, and specific gravity. The rapidity and duration of response depend greatly on the underlying cause. Neurologic impairment from water intoxication is usually reversible.

Usually, SIADH resolves with tumor regression, but it can persist despite control of the tumor. It may recur, suggesting tumor progression, but recurrence is sometimes seen with stable disease during the maintenance phase of therapy. If the underlying cause is not eliminated, the SIADH may be a chronic problem and necessitate ongoing intermittent management.

TUMOR LYSIS SYNDROME

Definition

Tumor lysis syndrome (TLS) is an oncologic emergency that occurs with rapid lysis of malignant cells. The resultant metabolic imbalance can quickly lead to fatal renal, cardiac, and neurologic complications.

Etiology and Risk Factors

Tumor lysis syndrome may occur spontaneously in patients with inordinately high tumor burdens. However, it most commonly results from treatment-related malignant cell death. TLS has been reported to occur with surgery, biotherapy, hyperthermia, hormonal therapy, and radiation therapy, but it is most frequently associated with chemotherapy.[100] Both rituximab and interferon-α as monotherapy have been associated with TLS.[101] TLS may occur anywhere from 24 hours to 7 days after antineoplastic therapy is initiated.[102] The incidence in high-grade non-Hodgkin's lymphomas is estimated as high as 42%, although only 6% are clinically significant.[66] Patients most at risk are those who have large tumor cell burdens with high proliferative fractions (high-grade lymphomas), markedly elevated WBC counts (acute leukemias), elevated LDH (associated with bulky tumors) or uric acid levels, or preexisting renal dysfunction, splenomegaly, or lymphadenopathy.[66] TLS is also seen in CLL in blast crisis, SCLC, metastatic breast cancer, and metastatic medulloblastoma.

Pathophysiology

As malignant cells are lysed, intracellular contents are rapidly released into the bloodstream. This results in high levels of potassium (hyperkalemia), phosphate (hyperphosphatemia), and uric acid (hyperuricemia). Because there is an inverse relationship between phosphate and calcium, a decrease in serum calcium (hypocalcemia) occurs. This metabolic imbalance may be even more pronounced in patients with certain types of cancers. Patients with lymphoblastic leukemia may have 4 times more intracellular phosphate.[101] Leukemic cells are also rich in purine nucleic acids that are metabolized into uric acid by the liver.[100] If the kidneys are unable to sufficiently excrete the by-products of malignant cell death, the clinical situation can rapidly become life-threatening. Hyperkalemia (K >5.5 mEq/L) leads to bradycardia, heart block, ventricular fibrillation, and asystole. Hyperkalemia may be the first metabolic abnormality to manifest, typically within 6 to 72 hours of chemotherapy initiation.[103] Levels greater than 6.5 mEq/L can cause ascending paralysis and respiratory failure. Hypocalcemia can also cause dysrhythmias and cardiac dysfunction. Hyperkalemia, hyperphosphatemia, and hyperuricemia all lead to renal failure. Uric acid is insoluble in acidic urine and can precipitate in the kidneys. Elevated potassium and phosphate both cause renal insufficiency that can progress to renal failure. Hyperuricemia, hyperphosphatemia, and the subsequent hypocalcemia typically develop within 24 to 48 hours.[103] TLS can also stimulate the coagulation cascade that leads to DIC.

Clinical Features

The clinical features of TLS are outlined in Table 24-12. Patients exhibit the signs and symptoms associated with each metabolic abnormality. Early signs may include nausea, vomiting, anorexia and diarrhea, and may be accompanied by muscle weakness and cramping. Later signs may progress to tetany, paresthesias, convulsions, anuria, and cardiac arrest.

Diagnosis

Tumor lysis syndrome is diagnosed by observation of the signs and symptoms outlined in Table 24-21 and by confirmation of abnormal laboratory values. Serum potassium, phosphate, calcium, and uric acid levels are diagnostic. Other important values include serum creatinine, BUN, and urine pH.

Treatment Modalities

The best way to treat TLS is to *prevent* it by recognizing the patient population who is at risk and initiating prophylactic measures before initiation of antineoplastic therapy.[66,104] This includes pretreatment **hydration** to maintain a urinary output of 100 ml/hr. Hydration should begin 24 to 48 hours before treatment and continue for at least 72 hours after treatment.[100] **Diuretics** may be used to promote the excretion of phosphate and uric acid.[102] **Allopurinol** is a xanthine oxidase inhibitor that prevents uric acid formation. It is begun 24 hours to a few days before treatment and should be continued for 3 to 5 days after treatment is completed. Dosage recommendations range from 300 mg/day to a loading dose of 600 to 900 mg followed by 300 to 450 mg/day.[7] Intravenous allopurinol is used for patients who are unable to take an oral formulation.[66,104] Dosages range from 200 to 400 mg/m²/day. Because of the expense, a transition to the oral formulation is implemented as soon as clinically feasible.[66] Side effects of allopurinol may include a rash, eosinophilia, fever, hypersensitivity reaction, and exfoliative dermatitis.[100] **Rasburicase,** a recombinant urate oxidase, is now available for use in the treatment and prevention of chemotherapy-induced hyperuricemia. Unlike allopurinol, rasburicase lowers preexisting uric acid. It has a rapid onset of action and degrades uric acid as opposed to preventing uric acid synthesis. Like intravenous allopurinol, the high cost of therapy is a concern.[66,105] **Sodium bicarbonate** is used to maintain an alkaline urine (pH >7) to prevent uric acid crystallization (50 to 100 mEq/L fluid or 50 mEq by IV bolus).[102] Some controversy exists over whether alkalinization should be continued once treatment is started because of the risk of exacerbating hyperphosphatemia and hypocalcemia.[66] Most references recommend continuing it until uric acid levels stabilize. Acetazolamide, a diuretic, may be used to decrease bicarbonate resorption in the kidney so that it is excreted in the urine where it enhances alkalinization.[104]

Electrolytes, urine pH, and accurate intake and output must be assessed at least every 4 to 8 hours during treatment and for the following 3 to 5 days.[7] If TLS occurs, diuretics are used to prevent volume overload and promote the excretion of potassium in the urine. **Cation-exchange resins,** such as kaexylate, are used to bind with potassium so it can be excreted through the bowel (15 to 30 g with 50 ml 20% sorbitol orally 2 to 4 times a day; or 50 in 200 ml or 20% sorbitol as a retention enema for 30 to 60 minutes).[7] Sodium polystyrene sulfonate may be given orally or by retention enema to treat mild hyperkalemia (<6.5 mEq/L).[104,106] **Insulin-glucose therapy** may be added to enhance the shift of potassium back into the intracellular compartment. (1 unit regular insulin is given for each 4 g glucose, or 50 ml dextrose 50% (D50) and 10 units insulin over 1 hour.) **Calcium gluconate** is used to correct hypocalcemia (10 to 30 ml of 10% calcium gluconate IV push over 1 to 5 minutes with cardiac monitoring).[104,106] Phosphate-binding gels, such as aluminum hydroxide, are given to form an insoluble complex that is excreted by the bowel.[106]

Medications containing phosphate should be discontinued (e.g., clindamycin, sodium-potassium phosphate). Phosphate-containing foods, such as milk, cheese, and carbonated beverages,

TABLE 24-12	Signs and Symptoms of Tumor Lysis Syndrome			
	GI	**RENAL**	**CARDIAC**	**NEUROMUSCULAR**
Hyperkalemia	Nausea Vomiting Diarrhea Anorexia		BP/P changes ECG changes Dysrhythmias Heart block Asystole	Twitching Cramping Weakness Paresthesias Ascending flaccid paralysis
Hyperuricemia	Nausea Vomiting Diarrhea Anorexia	Edema Flank pain Hematuria Oliguria Cloudy, sediment in urine Anuria Azotemia Crystalluria		Lethargy Goutlike symptoms
Hyperphosphatemia		Oliguria Anuria Azotemia Renal insufficiency		
Hypocalcemia			Hypotension Heart block Cardiac arrest	Twitching Cramping Tetany Chvostek's sign* Trousseau's sign* Laryngospasm Paresthesias Seizures Confusion

*See Box 24-3 for definitions.

BP, Blood pressure; *ECG*, electrocardiogram; *P*, pulse.

Data from Arkel TS: Thrombosis and cancer, *Semin Oncol* 27:362, 2000; Gell PHG, Coombs RRA: *Clinical aspects of immunology*, Oxford, 1995, Blackwell Scientific; and Stucky LA: Acute tumor lysis syndrome: assessment and nursing implications, *Oncol Nurs Forum* 20:49, 1993.

may be restricted.[106] Other medications that can further elevate serum phosphate, and thus lower serum calcium, include furosemide, mithramycin, gallium nitrate, and anticonvulsants.[100] Thiazide diuretics, aspirin, and probenecid can elevate uric acid levels.[104] Indomethacin and potassium-sparing diuretics (spironolactone [Aldactone], triamterene [Dyrenium], amiloride HCL [Midamor]) are not recommended.[7,102] Any nephrotoxic medications should be avoided, as should radiographic contrast dyes.

When these measures are not successful, renal dialysis may be necessary.[66,104] Critical laboratory values indicating a need for dialysis include potassium greater than 6 mEq/L, phosphate greater than 10 mg/dl, and uric acid greater than 10 mg/dl.[100]

Nursing Considerations

Oncology nurses should be aware of patients who are at high risk for tumor lysis syndrome (TLS). Nurses take an active role in the prevention of TLS by administering allopurinol and hydration before the initiation of treatment. Careful monitoring of lab values and observing the patient for early, subtle changes allows prompt intervention and the prevention of cardiac abnormalities and renal failure.

Assess medications for those that contain phosphate or spare potassium, and discuss discontinuation with physician. Monitor potassium, phosphorus, calcium, and uric acid levels.

Assess patient for signs and symptoms of TLS (see Table 24-21):
- *Hyperkalemia*—cardiac, GI, neuromuscular
- *Hyperphosphatemia*—renal
- *Hypocalcemia*—cardiac, neuromuscular
- *Hyperuricemia*—GI, renal

Administer diuretics, sodium bicarbonate, cation-exchange resins, insulin-glucose therapy, and phosphate-binding gels as appropriate. Monitor intake and output and notify physician if urinary output is less than 100 ml/hr. Monitor urine pH and maintain above 7.0 with sodium bicarbonate. Prepare the patient and family for dialysis if other measures are not effective. Obtain ECG for potassium greater than 6.0 mEq/L and calcium less than 8.0 mg/dl. Report ECG changes (e.g., peaked and narrow T waves, shortened QT interval, widened QRS complex with decreased amplitude, loss of P wave, ventricular tachycardia, ventricular fibrillation, blending of QRS into T wave). Monitor blood pressure, pulse, and central venous pressure. Be prepared to transfer the patient to the ICU for hemodynamic monitoring.

Assess the patient for jugular venous distention and peripheral edema. Auscultate lung sounds for signs of volume overload, and assess rate and depth of respirations. Keep accurate intake and output. Weigh the patient daily. Monitor blood pressure and pulse. Administer diuretics as ordered.

Prognosis

Successful treatment of TLS depends on preventing renal failure. TLS typically resolves within 7 days, once appropriate treatment is initiated.[88]

Conclusion

Successful management of patients with oncologic complications requires expertise from all members of the health care team. It requires in-depth knowledge in oncology but also in many related areas, such as immunology, pharmacology, cardiopulmonary care, and critical care. The nurse is in a pivotal role as coordinator of the care and as patient advocate to help the patient and family deal with the impact of the illness on their lives.

REVIEW QUESTIONS

✓ Case Study

Fern Williams is a 67-year-old female with a history of adenocarcinoma of the left breast. Her initial diagnosis was made 4 years ago. At the time, she was ER+/PR+, HER2–, and had 3/10 positive lymph nodes. Staging was T2, N1, M0. She is status postchemotherapy with 6 cycles of FAC (5-FU, doxorubicin, and cyclophosphamide) and is currently receiving her third year of tamoxifen therapy. She is widowed and lives alone. However, she is close to her daughter, with whom she has regular contact.

Ms. Williams comes to the clinic accompanied by her daughter, who noticed that her mother was confused and lethargic. Ms. Williams denies pain; however, she does complain of nausea. She can't remember whether she has had difficulty with constipation, but her abdomen is slightly distended.

Physical exam indicates dehydration as exhibited by poor skin turgor. The results of her blood work are as follows:

	ACTUAL VALUES	NORMAL RANGE
Calcium	10.5 mg/dl	9.0-11.0 mg/dl
Phosphorus	2.5 mEq/dl	2.5-4.5 mEq/dl
Alkaline phosphatase	140 units/L	20-125 units/L
Blood urea nitrogen	27 mg/dl	7-25 mg/dl
Creatinine	1.7 mg/dl	0.7-1.4 mg/dl
Potassium	3.9 mEq/L	3.5-5.5 mEq/L
Sodium	150 mEq/L	135-146 mEq/L
Albumin	1.8 g/dl	3.2-5.0 g/dl

Ms. Williams is admitted to the hospital. Hydration is started with normal saline at 200 cc/hr for 24 hours, to be followed by 125 cc/hr. The serum creatinine and sodium are within normal limits within 24 hours. Zoledronic acid is then ordered at 4 mg over 15 minutes. Ms. Williams's calcium begins to drop within 12 hours. It reaches the upper limit of normal within 72 hours. At that time, skeletal survey shows areas of metastatic disease in left iliac crest and L5. The decision is made to discontinue the tamoxifen and initiate therapy with daily letrozole and repeating doses of Zometa every 4 weeks. As her lab values normalize, Ms. Williams no longer complains of nausea and becomes more alert. Physical therapy is ordered to assist her in increasing her weight-bearing activity during the hospitalization. As her hydration improves and activity increases, it is noted that she has a daily bowel movement and is no longer distended. Referral is made to the hospital dietitian to assess Ms. Williams's dietary intake and institute a program to increase her protein intake. Patient and family education includes information on the signs and symptoms of hypercalcemia as well as spinal cord compression (SCC). Ms. Williams is dismissed from the hospital and scheduled to return to clinic within 1 week to recheck her lab results and reinforce patient education.

Ms. Williams has now been diagnosed with recurrent metastatic breast cancer. She has two areas of bony lesions, including her left hip and lumbar spine. Zoledronic acid is instituted to correct her hypercalcemia. It will be continued to reduce the risk of skeletal-related events such as recurrent hypercalcemia, pathologic fracture, and SCC. Her hormonal therapy has been changed to an aromatase inhibitor since she had recurrence of her breast cancer during tamoxifen administration. A key nursing role in this case study is to educate Ms. Williams and her daughter to recognize the signs and symptoms of hypercalcemia. It is important to include family in the education since the lethargy and confusion that may accompany elevated calcium can preclude recognition by the patient. Since Ms. Williams now has progression of disease with bony metastases, she is at risk for SCC. It is critical that she report any signs of back pain immediately. Early recognition and diagnosis of back pain increases the chances of maintaining sensory and motor function.

QUESTIONS

1. Hypercalcemia occurs most commonly in which of the following types of cancer?
   a. Solid tumors
   b. Leukemias
   c. Rhabdomyosarcomas
   d. Preleukemia syndromes and myelodysplasia
2. Why is it important to hydrate the patient before initiation of bisphosphonate therapy?
   a. Bisphosphonates are associated with renal toxicity.
   b. Premature administration causes hyperglycemia.
   c. Dehydration is associated with increased incidence of confusion.
   d. Hydration serves to control further loss of bone strength and durability.
3. For what other oncologic emergency would this patient be most at risk?
   a. Superior vena cava syndrome
   b. Spinal cord compression
   c. Hypersensitivity reaction
   d. Increased intracranial pressure

4. Patient and family education for Ms. Williams should include which of the following?
   a. Report any sign of back pain immediately.
   b. Maintain complete bed rest.
   c. Restrict dietary calcium.
   d. Observe for euphoria.
5. Ms. Williams's serum calcium was within normal limits. Why was she treated for hypercalcemia?
   a. The symptoms of nausea, confusion, and dehydration were diagnostic.
   b. Her low serum albumin masked the elevated serum calcium level.
   c. Patients who received FAC chemotherapy are at high risk for hypercalcemia.
   d. Once a patient is discovered to have any bone metastasis, they are treated for hypercalemia.
6. Additional signs and symptoms of hypercalcemia include which of the following?
   a. Incontinence, sensory loss, and confusion
   b. Diarrhea, rectal bleeding, and fever
   c. Headache, shortness of breath, and blurred vision
   d. Weakness, fatigue, and ECG changes
7. Which of the following can be included among sequelae from hypercalcemia?
   a. Hypertension, motor loss, and collateral circulation
   b. Hypotension, hallucination, and dental caries
   c. Renal failure, cardiac arrest, and ileus
   d. Easy bruising, petechiae, and intracranial bleed
8. As the patient is being hydrated, what lab values should be monitored?
   a. Blood glucose
   b. Tumor necrosis factor-alpha
   c. Serum sodium, serum creatinine, and BUN
   d. Hemoglobin and hematocrit
9. Ms. Williams responded well to therapy. If she had not, what other interventions would be appropriate?
   a. Immobilization
   b. Dietary restriction of calcium
   c. Corticosteroids
   d. Fluid restriction
10. Taking into account the patient's albumin level, what was the value for her corrected serum calcium?
    a. 10.66 mg/dl
    b. 12.26 mg/dl
    c. 13.0 mg/dl
    d. 50.0 mg/dl

ANSWERS

1. **A.** *Rationale:* Solid tumors, particularly lung and breast cancer, make up 80% of malignancy-related hypercalcemia.
2. **A.** *Rationale:* Bisphosphonate administration has been associated with renal toxicity. There has been no association with hyperglycemia. Dehydration may be associated with confusion; however, this is not a relevant point in relation to when bisphosphonates should be initiated. Hydration has no impact on bone strength or durability.
3. **B.** *Rationale:* Ms. Williams is most at risk for SCC because of her recent diagnosis of bony metastases. Breast cancer is not typically associated with superior vena cava syndrome. Hormonal therapy and bisphosphonates are not known to have a high incidence of hypersensitivity reactions. Ms. Williams does not have brain metastases, and so is unlikely to develop increased intracranial pressure.
4. **A.** *Rationale:* Ms. Williams should report any sign of back pain immediately since this is the most common presenting sign of SCC. Bed rest is not in her best interest since non–weight-bearing states can exacerbate bone resorption and high levels of calcium in the serum. Restriction of dietary calcium has not been shown to be effective in correcting hypercalcemia. Mood changes most likely seen with hypercalcemia include lethargy and confusion, not euphoria.
5. **B.** *Rationale:* Low levels of serum albumin may mask calcium levels in the serum. For every 1 g/dl drop in serum albumin, serum calcium must be corrected by 0.8 mg/dl. Nausea, confusion, and dehydration are all symptoms of hypercalcemia, but in themselves are not diagnostic. The type of chemotherapy regimen that is administered is not linked to a patient's risk for hypercalcemia. Treatment of hypercalcemia is not at this point regimented to initiate bisphosphonate therapy; in some cases, the condition may not be treated at all.
6. **D.** *Rationale:* Weakness, fatigue, and ECG changes most accurately reflect additional signs and symptoms of hypercalcemia. Hypercalcemia is not typically associated with blurred vision, shortness of breath, headache, or incontinence. Patients with hypercalcemia are more likely to exhibit constipation, not diarrhea, rectal bleeding, and fever.
7. **C.** *Rationale:* Renal failure, cardiac arrest, and ileus are all sequelae of hypercalcemia. Changes in blood pressure, dental caries, and changes in collateral circulation are not. Easy bruising, petechiae, and intracranial bleeding are associated with DIC.
8. **C.** *Rationale:* It is important to monitor serum sodium, magnesium, and potassium levels during hydration for hypercalcemia. Serum sodium is typically elevated because of dehydration. Serum creatinine and BUN are indicators of renal function. Normal baseline renal function is preferred before the initiation of bisphosphonates. Hemoglobin and hematocrit are indices of anemia and blood loss and are not associated with hypercalcemia.
9. **C.** *Rationale:* Corticosteroids may be employed for hypercalcemia associated with breast cancer owing to their ability to block bone resorption, increase calcium excretion, and decrease GI absorption. However, they are not recommended for chronic administration. Immobilization is contraindicated in this case because of its association with enhanced bone resorption. Dietary restriction has not been shown to be effective. Fluid restriction is also contraindicated since the patient is dehydrated.
10. **B.** *Rationale:* Using the formula to correct serum calcium in patients with low levels of serum albumin: $4.0 - 1.8 \times 0.8 + 10.5 = 12.26$ mg/dl.

REFERENCES

1. Woodard WL III, Hogan DK: Oncologic emergencies: implications for nurses, *Core curriculum for oncology nursing,* ed 4, St. Louis, 2005, Saunders.
2. Oncology Nursing Society, Itano J, Taoka K, editors: *Core curriculum for oncology nursing,* ed 4, St. Louis, 2005, Saunders.
3. Glover DJ, Glick JH: Oncologic emergencies. In Holleb AI, Fink DJ, Murphy GP, editors: *American Cancer Society textbook of clinical oncology,* Atlanta, 1991, American Cancer Society.
4. Flounders JA: Cardiovascular emergencies: pericardial effusion and cardiac tamponade, *Oncol Nurs Forum Vol* 30, No. 2: 2003; retrieved March 13, 2005, from http://www.ons.org/publications/journals/ONF/Volume30/Issue2/300224.asp.
5. Forauer AR, Dasika NL, Femmete JJ et al: Pericardial tamponade complicating central venous interventions, *J Vasc Interv Radiol* 14(2):255, 2003.
6. Hunter JC: Structural emergencies. In Itano JK, Taoka KN, editors: *Core curriculum for oncology nursing,* ed 4, St. Louis, 2005, Saunders.
7. Dietz KA, Flaherty AM: Oncologic emergencies. In Groenwald SL, Frogge MH, Goodman M et al, editors: *Cancer nursing: principles and practice,* ed 3, Boston, 1993, Jones & Bartlett.
8. Jeha S: Tumor lysis syndrome, *Semin Hematol* 38(4):4-8, 2001.
9. Knoop T, Willenberg K: Cardiac tamponade, *Semin Oncol Nurs* 15(3): 168-173, 1999.
10. Joyce M, Cunningham RS: Metastases that interfere with circulation, *Semin Oncol Nurs* 14 (3):230-239, 1998.
11. O'Brien JF: The oncologic crisis, part 2: cardiorespiratory and neurologic emergencies, *Emerg Med* 28:21-44, 1996.
12. Pass HI: Treatment of metastatic cancer. In DeVita VT Jr, Hellman S, Rosenberg SA, editors: *Cancer: principles and practice of oncology,* ed 5, Philadelphia, 1997, Lippincott-Raven.
13. Beauchamp KA: Pericardial tamponade: an oncologic emergency, *Clin J Oncol Nurs* 2:3-98, 1998.
14. Miaskowski C: Oncologic emergencies. In Miaskowski CM, Buchsel P, editors: *Oncology nursing assessment and clinical care,* St. Louis, 1999, Mosby.
15. Krantz JM, Lee JK, Spodick DH: Repetitive yawning associated with cardiac tamponade, *Am J Cardiol* 94(5):701-702, 2004.
16. Fristoe B: Long-term cardiac and pulmonary complications in cancer care, *Nurse Pract Forum* 9(3):177-184, 1998.
17. Guidelines on the diagnosis and management of pericardial diseases, executive summary: the task force on the diagnosis and management of pericardial diseases of the European Society of Cardiology, *Eur Heart J* 25:587, 2004.
18. Shivnan J, Shelton BK, Onners BK: Bone marrow transplantation: issues for critical care nurses, *AACN Clin Issues* 7(1):95-108, 1996.
19. Mangan CM: Malignant pericardial effusions: pathophysiology and clinical correlates, *Oncol Nurs Forum* 19(8): 1215-1221, 1991.
20. Keefe, D: CV emergencies in the CA PT, *Semin Oncol* 27(3):244-255, 2000.
21. Nguyen DM, Schrump DS: Treatment of metastatic cancer, malignant pleural and pericardial effusions. In DeVita VT, Hellman S, Rosenberg SA, editors: *Cancer: principles and practice of oncology,* ed 7, Philadelphia, 2005, Lippincott, Williams & Wilkins.
22. Braunwald E: Pericardial disease. In Braunwald E and others, editors: *Harrison's principles of internal medicine,* ed 11, New York, 1987, McGraw-Hill.
23. Weitzman LB, Tinker WP, Kronzon I: The incidence and natural history of pericardial effusion after cardiac surgery—an echocardiographic study, *Circulation* 69(3):506-511, 1984.
24. Imazio M, DeMichelis B, Parrini I et al: Relation of acute pericardial disease to malignancy, *Am J Cardiol* 95(11):1393, 2005
25. Scott RC III: Evaluation and management of acute pericardial tamponade, *Top Emerg Med* 20(3):95-101, 1998.
26. Spain RC, Wittlesey D: Respiratory emergencies in patients with cancer, *Semin Oncol* 16(6):471-489, 1989.
27. Joiner GA, Kolodychuk GR: Neoplastic cardiac tamponade, *Crit Care Nurse* 11(2):50-55, 1991.
28. Gobel BH: Metabolic emergencies. In Itano JK, Taoka KN, editors: *Core curriculum for oncology nursing,* ed 4, St. Louis, 2005, Saunders.
29. Barbiere CC: Are you listening? Cardiac tamponade: diagnosis and emergency intervention, *Crit Care Nurse* 10(4):20-22, 1990.
30. Baehring JM: Oncologic emergencies, spinal cord compression. In DeVita VT, Hellman S, Rosenberg SA, editors: *Cancer: principles and*

31. Sitton E: Central nervous system metastases, *Semin Oncol Nurs* 1(3)4: 210-219, 1998.
32. Belford K: Central nervous system cancers. In Groenwald SL, Frogge MH, Goodman M et al, editors: *Cancer nursing: principles and practice,* ed 4, Boston, 1997, Jones & Bartlett.
33. Lassman AB, DeAngelis LM. Brain metastases, *Neurol Clin* 21:1-23, 2003.
34. Bucholtz JD: Central nervous system metastases, *Semin Oncol Nurs* 14(1):61-72, 1998.
35. Quinn JA, DeAngelis LM: Neurologic emergencies in the cancer patient, *Semin Oncol* 27(3):311-321, 2000.
36. El Kamar FD, Posner JB: Brain metastases, *Semin Neurol* 24(4): 347-362, 2004.
37. Larson DA, Rubenstein JL, McDermott MW: Treatment of metastatic cancer, metastatic brain cancer. In DeVita VT, Hellman S, Rosenberg SA, editors: *Cancer: principles and practice of oncology,* ed 7, Philadelphia, 2005, Lippincott, Williams & Wilkins.
38. Flounders JA: Spinal cord compression, *Oncol Nur Forum* 30(1):E17-23, 2003.
39. Fuller BG, Heiss J, Oldfield EH: Spinal cord compression. In DeVita VT Jr, Hellman S, Rosenberg SA, editors: *Cancer: principles and practice of oncology,* ed 5, 1997, Philadelphia, Lippincott-Raven.
40. Baehring JM: Oncologic emergencies, increased intracranial pressure. In DeVita VT, Hellman S, Rosenberg SA, editors: *Cancer: principles and practice of oncology,* ed 7, Philadelphia, 2005, Lippincott, Williams & Wilkins.
41. Maher DeLeon ME, Schnell S, Rozental JM: Tumors of the spine and spinal cord, *Semin Oncol Nurs* 14(1, February):43-52, 1998.
42. Gabriel K, Schiff D: Metastatic spinal cord compression by solid tumors, *Semin Neurol* 24(4):375-383, 2004.
43. Schiff D: Spinal cord compression, *Neurol Clin North Am* 21:67-86, 2003.
44. Coleman RE. Metastatic bone disease: clinical features, pathophysiology and treatment strategies, *Cancer Treat Rev* 27:165-176, 2001.
45. Ryu S, Yin FF, Rock J et al: Image-guided and intensity-modulated radiosurgery for patients with spinal metastasis, *Cancer* 97:2013-2018, 2003.
46. Bilsky MH, Boland P, Lis E et al: Single stage, posterolateral transpedicle approach (PTA) for spondylectomy, epidural decompression, and circumferential fusion of spinal metastases, *Spine,* 25(17):2240-2249, 2000.
47. Healey JH, Brown HK. Complications of bone metastases: surgical management, *Cancer* 88(12) (suppl 12):2940-2951, 2000.
48. Shanholtz C: Acute life-threatening toxicity of cancer treatment, *Crit Care Clin* 17(3):483-502, 2001
49. Saad F, Gleason DM, Murray R, et al: Long term efficacy of zoledronic acid for the prevention of skeletal complications in patients with metastatic hormone refractory prostate cancer, *J Natl Cancer Inst* 96(11): 879-882, 2004.
50. Flounders JA: Superior vena cava syndrome, *Oncol Nurs Forum* 30(4):E84-90, 2003
51. Yahalom J: Oncologic emergencies, superior vena cava syndrome. In DeVita VT, Hellman S, Rosenberg SA, editors: *Cancer: principles and practice of oncology,* ed 7, Philadelphia, 2005, Lippincott, Williams & Wilkins.
52. Gowda RM, Khan IA, Metha NJ et al: Cardiac tamponade and superior vena cava syndrome in lung cancer- a case report, *Angiology* 55(6): 691-695, 2004.
53. Haapoja IS, Blendowski C: Superior vena cava syndrome, *Semin Oncol Nurs* 15(3):183-189, 1999.
54. Stewart AF: Hypercalcemia associated with cancer, *New Engl J Med* 352(4):373-379, 2005.
55. Bick RL: Disseminated intravascular coagulation current concepts of etiology, pathophysiology, diagnosis, and treatment, *Hematol Oncol Clin North Am* 17:149-176, 2003.
56. DeSancho MT, Rand JH. Bleeding and thrombotic complications in critically ill patients with cancer, *Crit Care Clin* 17(3, July):599-622, 2001.
57. Gobel BH: Disseminated intravascular coagulation in cancer: providing quality care, *Top Adv Pract Nurs eJournal* 2:2002, retrieved March 13, 2005, from http://www.medscape.com/viewarticle/442737.
58. Arnold SM, Leberman FS, Foon KA: Paraneoplastic syndromes. In DeVita VT, Hellman S, Rosenberg SA, editors: *Cancer: principles and practice of oncology,* ed 7, Philadelphia, 2005, Lippincott, Williams & Wilkins.

59. Shelton BK, Baker L, Stecker S: Critical care of the patient with hematologic malignancy, *AACN Clin Issues: Adv Pract Acute Crit Care* 7(1):65-78, 1996.

60. Gobel BH: Disseminated intravascular coagulation, *Semin Oncol Nurs* 15(3, August):174-182, 1999.

61. Smalley RV, Guaspari A, Haase-Statz S et al: Allopurinol: intravenous use for prevention and treatment of hyperuricemia in patients with leukemia or lymphoma, *J Clin Oncol* 18(8):1758-1763, 2000.

62. Yu M, Nardella A, Pechet L: Screening tests of disseminated intravascular coagulation: guidelines for rapid and specific diagnosis, *Crit Care Med* 28(6):1777-1780, 2000.

63. Arkel TS: Thrombosis and cancer, *Semin Oncol* 27(3, June):362-374, 2000.

64. Barnett ML: Hypercalcemia, *Semin Oncol Nurs* 15(3, August):190-201, 1999.

65. Flombaum CD: Metabolic emergencies in the cancer patient, *Semin Oncol* 27(3):322-334, 2000.

66. Fojo AT: Oncologic emergencies, metabolic emergencies. In DeVita VT, Hellman S, Rosenberg SA, editors: *Cancer: principles and practice of oncology*, ed 7, Philadelphia, 2005, Lippincott, Williams & Wilkins.

67. Heatley S, Coleman R: Product focus. The use of bisphosphonates in the palliative care setting, *Int J Palliat Nurs* 5(2):74-79, 1999.

68. Spratto GR, Woods AL, editors: PDR nurse's drug handbook, Clifton Park NY, 2004, Delmar Learning.

69. Major P, Lortholary J, Hon E et al: Zoledronic acid is superior to pamidronate in the treatment of hypercalcemia of malignancy: a pooled analysis of two randomized, controlled clinical trials, *J Clin Oncol* 19(2, January):558-567, 2001

70. Mann B, Sexton PA: Beta-lactam antibiotics, College of Health and Life Sciences, Fort Hays State University, retrieved July 10, 2005, from http://www.fhsu.edu/nursing/otitis/b-lactam.html.

71. Rosen LS, Gordon D, Kaminski M et al: Treatment of skeletal complications in patients with advanced multiple myeloma or breast cancer, *Cancer* 98(3):1736-1744, 2003.

72. Kovacs CS et al: Hypercalcemia of malignancy in the palliative care patient: a treatment strategy, *J Pain Symptom Manage* 10(3):224-232, 1995.

73. Mundy GR, Guise TA: Hypercalcemia of malignancy, *Am J Med* 103(2):134-145, 1997.

74. Labovich TM: Acute hypersensitivity reactions to chemotherapy, *Semin Oncol Nurs* 15(3):222-231, 1999.

75. Albanell J, Baselga J: Systemic therapy emergencies, *Semin Oncol* 27(3):347-361, 2000.

76. Truini Pittman L, Rossetto C: Pediatric considerations in tumor lysis syndrome, *Semin Oncol Nurs* 18(3 suppl 3):17-22, 2002.

77. Weiss RB: Adverse effects of treatment: miscellaneous toxicities. In DeVita VT, Hellman S, Rosenberg SA, editors: *Cancer: Principles and practice of oncology*, ed 7, Philadelphia, 2005, Lippincott, Williams & Wilkins.

78. Bonosky K, Miller R: Hypersensitivity reactions to oxaliplatin: what nurses need to know, *Clin J Oncol Nur* 9(3):325-330, 2005.

79. Feldweg AM, Lee C-W, Matulonis UA et al: Rapid desensitization for hypersensitivity reactions to paclitaxel and docetaxel: a new standard protocol used in 77 successful treatments, *Gynecol Oncol* 96:824-829, 2004.

80. Markman M: Managing taxane toxicities, *Support Care Cancer* 11:144-147, 2003

81. Quock J, Dea G, Tanaka M: Premedication strategy for weekly paclitaxel, *Cancer Invest* 20:666-672, 2002.

82. Ibrahim NK, Desai N, Legha S et al: Phase I pharmacokinetic study of ABI-007, a cremaphor-free, protein-stabilized, nanoparticle formulation of paclitaxel, *Clin Cancer Res* 8(May):1028-1044, 2002.

83. Abraxane package insert, version 7, 2005, retrieved July 10, 2005, from www.fda.gov/cder/fol/label/2005/021660lbl.pdf.

84. Lieberman P, Kemmp SF, Oppenheimer J et al: The diagnosis and management of anaphylaxis: an updated practice parameter, *J Allergy Clin Immunol* 115(3 Pt 2):S483-S523, 2005.

85. Compton J: Drug update: Use of glucagon in intractable allergic reactions and as an alternative to epinephrine: an interesting case review, *J Emerg Nurs* 23:45, 1997.

86. Bone RC et al: Definitions for sepsis and organ failure and guidelines for the use of innovative therapies in sepsis, *Chest* 101(6):1644-1655, 1992.

87. Talan DA: Sepsis and septic shock, *Emerg Med* 29(March):54-79, 1997.

88. Shelton BK: Sepsis, *Semin Oncol Nurs* 15(3, August):209-221, 1999.

89. Safdar A, Armstrong D: Infectious morbidity in critically ill patients with cancer, *Crit Care Clin* 17(3):531-570, 2001.

90. Astiz ME, Rackow EC: Seminar. Septic shock, *Lancet* 351(9114):1501-1505, 1998.

91. Mutnick AH, Bergquist SC, Beltz E: Bacteremia and sepsis. In Herfindal ET, Gourley DR, editors: *Textbook of therapeutics: drug and disease management*, Baltimore, 1996, Williams & Wilkins.

92. Reigle BS, Dienger MJ: Sepsis and treatment-induced immunosuppression in the patient with cancer, *Crit Care Nurs Clin North Am* 15(1):109-118, 2003.

93. Quadri TL, Brown AE: Infectious complications in the critically ill patient with cancer, *Semin Oncol* 27(3, June):335-346, 2000.

94. Segal BH, Walsh TJ, Gea-Banacloshe JC et al: Infections in the cancer patient. In DeVita VT, Hellman S, Rosenberg SA, editors: *Cancer: principles and practice of oncology*, ed 7, Philadelphia, 2005, Lippincott, Williams & Wilkins.

95. Wheeler AP, Bernard GR: Treating patients with severe sepsis, *N Engl J Med* 349(3):207-214, 1999.

96. Annane D, Sebille V, Charpentier C et al: Effect of treatment with low doses of hydrocortisone and fludrocortisone on mortality in patients with septic shock, *JAMA* 288(7):262-271, 2002.

97. Keenan AMM: Syndrome of inappropriate secretion of antidiuretic hormone in malignancy, *Semin Oncol Nurs* 15:160, 1999.

98. Kapoor M, Chan GZ: Fluid and electrolyte abnormalities, *Crit Care Clin* 17(3):503-529, 2001.

99. Taylor DS: Oncologic emergencies. In Gross S, Wind ML, Bergstrom SK et al: *eMedicine*, retrieved February 6, 2005, from http://www.emedicine.com/ped/topic2590.htm.

100. Ezzone SA: Tumor lysis syndrome, *Semin Oncol Nurs* 15(3, August):202-208, 1999.

101. Altman A: Acute tumor lysis syndrome, *Semin Oncol* 28 (2 Suppl 5):3-8, 2001.

102. Stucky LA: Acute tumor lysis syndrome: assessment and nursing implications, *Oncol Nurs Forum* 20(1):49-57, 1993.

103. Kaplow R: Pathophysiology, signs and symptoms of acute tumor lysis syndrome, *Semin Oncol Nurs* 18(3):6-11, 2002.

104. Gobel BH: Management of tumor lysis syndrome: prevention and treatment, *Semin Oncol Nurs* 18(3):12-16, 2002.

105. Yim BT, Sims-McCallum RP, Cong PH: Rasburicase for the treatment and prevention of hyperuricemia, *Ann Pharmacother* 37(July/August):1047-1053, 2003.

106. Sallan S: Management of acute tumor lysis syndrome, *Semin Oncol* 28(2)(suppl 5):9-12, 2001.

CHAPTER 25

Cancer Clinical Trials

Judith K. Payne

Clinical trials have led the transformation of cancer treatment and symptom management over the last 50 years. Oncology nurses continue to maintain a strong presence and critical force in many aspects of clinical trials focusing on oncology. The roles that oncology nurses are involved in are numerous and range from clinical trial study coordinators, educators, data managers, and as independent investigators. There are numerous controversial and challenging issues related to clinical trials in general, as well as specifically related to stem cell and gene therapy trials, regulatory processes, the relationship between clinical trials and evidence-based practice, federal regulations, protection of human subjects, and the growing awareness of ethical concerns in view of advancing medical technology and treatment.

Historical Perspective

The United States government founded the National Institutes of Health (NIH) in 1887. The purpose of the NIH is to support research into the causes, diagnosis, prevention, and cure of human disease. Many of the early clinical trials in the United States focused on the prophylaxis and the treatment of infectious diseases. By the 1930s, cancer was identified as a major health problem requiring a large-scale national plan of action. In 1937, Congress passed the National Cancer Institute Act, which appropriated $700,000 to establish the National Cancer Institute (NCI), which is the largest of the 12 NIH institutes. The goal of the NCI was to establish a new paradigm in cancer research by conducting its own research agenda, promoting research in other institutions, and coordinating cancer-related activities throughout the United States.[1]

Combined efforts of a wide-scale public and private campaign ultimately resulted in the signing of the National Cancer Act in 1971. This legislation created a national cancer program and was a landmark event in the history of cancer treatment and research.

The Cancer Centers Program of the NCI supports major academic and research institutions throughout the United States to sustain broad-based, coordinated, interdisciplinary programs in cancer research. The NCI and its Cancer Centers Program are dedicated to the advancement of cancer research to ultimately make an impact on the reduction of cancer incidence, morbidity, and mortality. Institutions for cancer center support are subjected to a competitive peer review process that evaluates and ranks applications according to scientific merit. Successful applicants are awarded a P30 Cancer Center Support Grant (CCSG) to fund the scientific infrastructure of the cancer center, including such elements as scientific leadership and administration, research resources that provide ready access to the state-of-the art technologies, and flexible funds that help the center pursue its planned objectives and take advantage of new research opportunities. Those institutions receiving CCSG awards are recognized as NCI-designated under one of two types of designations. **Cancer centers** have a

scientific agenda that is primarily focused on basic or population sciences or clinical research, or any two of the three components. **Comprehensive cancer centers** integrate research activities across three major areas: laboratory, clinical, and population-based research. The goal of all NCI-designated cancer centers is to make significant contributions to advances in cancer research that are key to understanding, preventing, and treating this disease[1]

A summary of NCI cancer programs is described in Table 25-1. These programs include oncology training programs, comprehensive cancer centers, cooperative research groups, community-based research programs, and non–NCI-sponsored research.

Drug Development

The process of drug development is costly and complex and takes years from the point of a conceptual idea to actual commercial use. New drugs for cancer care are developed by the NCI through the Investigational Drug Branch (IDB), a division of the Cancer Drug Therapy and Evaluation Program (CDTEP), and by pharmaceutical companies. A successful pharmaceutical clinical trial requires careful planning and resolution of several key issues before implementation. The primary and secondary objectives of the trial should be carefully determined, with an estimated number of subjects and time required to achieve these goals. It is also necessary to plan for how long it will take to complete the accrual of patients into the trial and follow-up, and increasingly important, to establish how the study will be funded. Following the planning phase, a protocol is written, including a statement of the primary and secondary end points.

CLINICAL TRIALS

Purpose. A clinical trial (also called clinical research) is a research study conducted with human volunteers to answer specific health questions such as whether new treatments are safe and effective, or to find better ways to prevent, screen for, or diagnose disease. There are several types of clinical trials. **Prevention trials** examine ways to reduce the risk, or chance, of developing cancer. **Screening trials** study ways to detect cancer. **Diagnostic trials** study focus on procedures that could be used to identify cancer or other diseases accurately and at an earlier stage. **Treatment trials** are conducted with people who have cancer, and are designed to answer specific questions about, and evaluate the effectiveness of, a new treatment or procedure. **Supportive care trials** explore ways to improve the quality of life of cancer patients and cancer survivors and may include ways to relieve nausea, vomiting, pain, sleep disorders, depression, or other symptoms. **Genetics studies** focus on how genetic makeup can affect diagnosis, detection, treatment, and symptom management, as well as how genetic disorders affect quality of life.

TABLE 25-1	Programs Initiated by National Cancer Institute (NCI) Since 1971
NCI PROGRAMS	**PURPOSE**
Oncology training programs	To provide funding for fellowship programs in medical oncology and radiotherapy. The first certifying examinations for medical oncologists were in 1974.
Comprehensive cancer centers	The NCI developed a network of specialized and comprehensive cancer centers to serve as a national resource for research, as well as a community resource through outreach programs and cancer control, using a multidisciplinary treatment approach. Designation as a comprehensive cancer center requires meeting specific and rigorous criteria established by the NCI. Since its establishment in 1971, when there were only three, the numbers of NCI-designated comprehensive cancer centers have grown to 39.
Cooperative research groups	Cooperative research groups are NCI-supported national networks of researchers, cancer centers, and community physicians who conduct high-quality clinical trials across the United States. Cooperative group clinical trials are funded by the NCI through cooperative agreements. The original purpose of the groups was to test new chemotherapeutic agents developed at the NCI. However, the scope of the program has broadened through the years, and current areas of research include evaluation of multimodality therapies, basic science, supportive care, quality of life, and chemoprevention trials.
Community-based research programs	The NCI *Cooperative Group Outreach Program (CGOP)*, implemented in 1976, was the first comprehensive effort to extend participation in clinical trials to community-based physicians. The *Community Clinical Oncology Program (CCOP)* was initiated by the NCI in 1983 to disseminate state-of-the-art cancer research to patients in community settings. CCOP institutions are groups of community-based physicians who are linked to cooperative groups and cancer centers. *Minority-based CCOPs* are an extension of the CCOP model, which was expanded in 1993 when the NCI funded 13 minority-based CCOPs.
Non–NCI-sponsored research	Although the NCI supports a large network of cancer centers, cooperative research groups, and community programs, most cancer clinical trials are not sponsored by NCI. Comprehensive cancer hospitals enroll patients to NCI studies, but centers and universities also conduct their own cancer research activities. Individual researchers within their own institution frequently develop research studies. Pharmaceutical companies often contract with institutions or individual investigators to evaluate new agents, largely driven by a marked expansion in the field of biotherapy.

PHASES OF CLINICAL TRIALS

Clinical trials involving a new drug or an innovative therapy are often designed in a series of phases.

Phase I clinical trials are the first attempt at evaluating a new drug or new drug combinations in human beings. The primary objective is to determine the maximum tolerated dose, or strength of the therapy, and safety. Investigators conducting phase I trials are determining acceptable toxicity of new agents. The secondary objectives are to study clinical pharmacology and to describe any tumor responses noted in the study.[2] The phase typically uses preexperimental designs (before and after, without a control group). The focus is on developing the best possible and safest treatment, not on efficacy.[3]

Phase II of clinical trials seeks preliminary evidence of the effectiveness of the treatment, typically using preexperimental or quasi-experimental designs. The objective of phase II trials is to establish the value of new treatment in comparison with standard treatment. During this phase, researchers determine the feasibility of conducting a more rigorous test, seek evidence that the treatment holds promise, and look for signs of possible side effects.[3] The trials should have pertinent and objective end points such as symptom control or disease-free interval. According to Collichio, Griggs, and Resenblatt, response rates should not be the only measure of benefit, because they may not **correlate** with patient survival.[2]

The goal of most phase II cancer trials is to determine if the drug has antitumor activity against the tumor type in question.

Phase II trials generally consist of trials of single agents or trials of combinations of agents. Both limit eligibility to patients with a specific diagnosis, and there is no internal control group. This objective is typically measured by response rate.

Tumor response rate is recorded as follows:

1. **Complete response:** The disappearance of all measurable tumor
2. **Partial response:** 50% or greater regression of one or more evaluatable lesions with no progression of any lesion
3. **Stable disease:** Less than 50% reduction in tumor volume or the lack of progression
4. **Progressive disease:** The occurrence of any new lesion during treatment or an increase in size by 25% of one or more lesions. A decline in functional performance status is occasionally classified as progressive disease.[2]

Phase III trials are a complete experimental test of the treatment or intervention with the objective of determining whether it is more effective than the standard treatment. Randomization is critically important for producing reliable results, and therefore most phase III clinical trials employ randomization. These phase III trials often involve the use of a large, heterogeneous sample of subjects, frequently selected from multiple geographic areas (1) to ensure that findings are not unique to a specific single setting and are thus more generalized, and (2) to increase the sample size and therefore the power of the statistical tests.[3] Pharmaceutical companies, private industry, and the NCI have established consortia in order to increase accrual rates. The NCI cooperative groups are called Eastern Cooperative Oncology Group, Cancer and

Leukemia Group B, Gynecologic Oncology Group, Pediatric Oncology Group, National Surgical Adjuvant Breast Project, and the Community Clinical Oncology Program.[1,2] These comparative groups involve hundreds of sites and allow for careful evaluation of treatment feasibility and efficacy in community as well as academic settings. Once a new program or product has shown improvement over previous treatment for a given disease or stage of disease, it becomes the standard of care.[2]

Phase IV clinical trials occur after the decision to adopt an innovative treatment has been made. In this phase, researchers focus primarily on long-term consequences of the intervention or agent, including both benefits and side effects. This phase might use a nonexperimental, preexperimental, or quasi-experimental design.[3]

RESEARCH DATA MANAGEMENT

Research data management is the discipline that involves data collection, storage, retrieval, and quality control of the data required for evaluating the scientific objective of the study.[2] It is a critical part of the research study and determines the success or failure of the study. There are four main components:

- Protocol development
- Data collection
- Computing
- Quality control

Data managers should have an adequate knowledge of tumor biology, medical terminology, and the medical record to allow adequate data collection for subsequent interpretation.[2] A data collection plan outlines how the study will be implemented and includes elements that address the procedures to be used to collect data, the time and costs of data collection, collection forms that facilitate data entry, and development of the codebook. The codebook should contain and define each variable in the study, a descriptive variable label, and the range of possible numerical values of every variable entered in a computer file.[3] Managing data can be a large and complicated process; hence this part of the research process requires organization, adequately trained personnel, space, and a rigorous quality assurance plan that facilitates careful checking of data before data entry.

INSTITUTIONAL REVIEW BOARDS

Institutional review boards (IRBs) are boards that review research projects to ensure that ethical standards are met in relation to the protection of the rights of human subjects.[4] Most hospitals, universities, and other institutions where research is conducted have established formal committees and protocols for reviewing proposed research plans before implementation. These committees are sometimes called human subjects committees, ethical advisory boards, or research ethics committees. If the institution receives funding from the United States government to help support the costs of research, the committee is likely to be called an institutional review board.[3]

The National Research Act of 1974 requires IRBs to be composed of at least five members with professional competence, experience, and qualifications. Membership must include one member whose concerns are primarily nonscientific (such as lawyer, clergy member, or ethicist) and at least one member from outside the institution.[4] Members of IRBs are required to complete annual mandatory training in scientific integrity and prevention of scientific misconduct, as is the principal investigator and research team of a research study.

ETHICAL CONCERNS

The conduct of research mandates not only expertise but honesty and integrity. Right to privacy is a basic and pivotal element underlying all aspects of a clinical trial. This concept assures that all individuals have the right to determine whether private information will be shared with or withheld from others.

The risk/benefit ratio of research is determined on the risks and benefits of a clinical trial. If the risks outweigh the benefits, the study should be revised or a new study developed.[3]

Vulnerable Subjects and Inclusion of Women and Minorities. While adherence to ethical standards is often straightforward, the rights of special vulnerable groups may need to be protected through additional procedures and heightened sensitivity. Vulnerable subjects (the term used in U.S. federal guidelines) may not be capable of giving fully informed consent or may be at high risk of unintended side effects because of their circumstances.[3] Researchers interested in studying high-risk groups need to become familiar with guidelines governing informed consent, risk/benefit assessments, and acceptable procedures for these groups.[4]

Groups that nurse researchers should consider as being vulnerable include the following: children; mentally or emotionally disabled people; institutionalized people; severely ill or physically disabled people; pregnant women; minority groups that may have poor language skills, values, and ethnicity in conflict with research goals; and older adults who may need more assistance with their health care needs than younger adults. Individuals within these groups may experience trust issues with healthcare providers, transportation concerns, and language difficulties.

Certificates of Confidence. Certificates of confidentiality are issued by the NIH to protect the privacy of research subjects by protecting investigators and institutions from being forced to release information that could be used to identify subjects with a research project. Certificates of confidentiality are issued to institutions or universities where the research is being conducted. They allow the investigator and others who have access to research records to refuse to disclose identifying information in any civil, criminal, administrative, legislative, or other proceeding, whether at the federal, state, or local levels. Statutory authority is provided by Section 301(d) of the Public Health Service Act (42 USC 241[d]) to the Secretary of Health and Human Services to authorize persons engaged in biomedical, behavioral, clinical, or other research to protect the privacy of individuals who are the subjects of that research. This authority has been delegated to the NIH. Persons authorized by the NIH to protect the privacy of research subjects may not be compelled in any federal, state, or local proceedings, whether civil, criminal, administrative legislative, or some other type, to identify them by name or other identifying characteristic.

Certificates can be used for biomedical, biobehavioral, clinical, or other types of research that is sensitive. Examples of sensitive research activities include but are not limited to the following: collecting genetic information, psychologic well-being, subjects' sexual preferences or practices, and substance abuse or other illegal risky behaviors. Not eligible for a certificate are projects that are not research, do not collect personally identifiable information, are not reviewed and approved by the IRB, or that collect information that if disclosed would not significantly harm or damage the participant. In general, certificates are issued for single, well-defined research projects rather than groups of classes of projects. In some instances, they can be issued for cooperative multisite projects.

Federal Assurance. Under the Department of Health and Human Services (DHHS) human subjects protection regulations, every institution engaged in human subjects research that is funded or conducted by DHHS must obtain an "Assurance of Compliance" approved by the Office for Human Research Protection (OHRP). The Assurance of Compliance, when granted, is called a Federalwide Assurance (FWA). Both the awarded institution (awardee) and all sites at collaborating institutions (performance sites) must file Assurances. The awardee institution is responsible for ensuring that all collaborating performance sites engaged in the research hold an OHRP Federalwide Assurance prior to their initiation of the research project. An institution becomes "engaged" in human subjects research when its employees or agents intervene or interact with living individuals for research purposes or obtain individually identifiable private information for research purposes. An institution is automatically considered to be "engaged" in human subjects research whenever it receives a direct DHHS award to support such research. In such cases, the awardee institution has the ultimate responsibility for protecting human subjects under the award.

Informed Consent. The concept of informed consent, which acknowledges the rights of patients to participate voluntarily in health care, applies both to clinical practice and clinical research.[5] Informed consent is one of the primary requirements underlying research conducted with humans. Informed consent seeks to ensure that prospective subjects have adequate information regarding the research, are capable of comprehending the information, and can knowledgeably and voluntarily decide whether or not to participate. Information must be provided in a language understandable to the subject and at an appropriate literacy level, usually at an eighth-grade level. Patients are encouraged to ask questions, and the physician or nurse should question the patient to determine his or her level of understanding. The required elements of informed consent include the following:

- Statement of research, purpose of research, expected duration of participation, and description of procedures (including any experimental procedures)
- Description of risks and benefits of the study
- Disclosure of alternative procedures or treatments
- Description of confidentiality; FDA inspection
- Whether compensation and medical treatments are available
- Whom to contact about research, patient's rights, and research-related injury
- Explanation that participation is voluntary and care will not be terminated if participant decides to leave the study

Informed consent in clinical research is recognized as being more stringent than informed consent outside the context of clinical trials. This heightened consent standard exists for a least two reasons. First, from an ethical perspective, a patient who is considering clinical trial participation is always viewed as potentially vulnerable. As a result, the patient may have difficulty in appreciating the differences between the therapeutic and research aspects of a given alternative care or treatment. Without this distinction, patients cannot make uncoerced and autonomous health care decisions.[6] Thus the informed consent process and the ethics of clinical research mandate that a clear distinction be made. Second, physician-investigators are seen as having an intrinsic conflict of interest in their roles as both a provider for an individual patient and a scientific investigator attempting to develop improved medical care and treatment. Within the context of a therapeutic relationship, the physician places the patient's interest above all else.[6] However, within the context of clinical research, researchers may have additional interests that may not be related to their patients' interests. In an attempt to reconcile the importance of these different perspectives, most ethical regulations that govern clinical research have focused on the informed consent process as a means of protecting potentially vulnerable subjects.[6]

BARRIERS TO ENROLLING SUBJECTS IN CLINICAL TRIALS

According to Jemal, more than 1,300,000 new cases of cancer were diagnosed and more than 563,500 cancer deaths occurred in 2005.[7] An estimated 3% to 10% of patients eligible for all NIH-sponsored clinical trials will be enrolled. However, less than 3% of patients receiving cancer therapy are treated through clinical trials. Various reasons are cited for poor patient accrual. Critical barriers to recruitment, enrollment, and retention of patients for clinical trials include fear, distrust of the health care system, misunderstanding of the clinical trial process, the perception that appropriate trials are not available, and the inconvenience of protocol requirements including extra clinic visits for data collection.[8,9] Potential barriers can be viewed from three main perspectives: system-related (including clinical trail design), physician-related, and patient-related.

Physician-related barriers include, in general, a reluctance to offer clinical trials because of the additional time and staff resources required and the randomization process; and some hesitate to create change in their usual practice. Physicians have expressed the following specific concerns: the possible effects on the physician-patient relationship by a randomized clinical trial, difficulty with the informed consent process, general dislike of an open discussion involving uncertainty, perceived conflict between the roles of scientist and clinician, and feelings of personal responsibility if the treatments were found to be unequal.[9] Additional physicians concerns regard the presence of comorbidities in their patients and possible additional side effects or complications.

Patient-related barriers include factors such as financial costs (transportation, lodging, meals, loss of income), concerns of privacy and confidentiality, lack of understanding, fear of research, family influences, anticipated treatment toxicities, and presence of comorbidities that may limit their energy or functional status. An additional primary concern expressed by patients is that they want their physician to choose their treatment rather than be randomized by a computer. An important factor is whether or not the trial offers active treatment in all arms of the study.[10]

System-related barriers include poorly designed clinical trials that may require numerous trips to the clinic or physician office, lack of commitment from administration, limited resources such as inadequate staffing and space, poor staff attitudes, and lack of education.[9] In general, perceived system-related barriers have become increasingly problematic over the past decade. Although appropriately instituted for safety reasons, increased monitoring by both private pharmaceutical companies and federal agencies has added to the complexity of conducting clinical trials. Other system-related barriers include features of poorly designed studies such as frequent trips to physician office or clinic, or complicated studies, narrow eligibility criteria, presence of a no-treatment arm, or large differences between treatment arms.[9]

STRATEGIES TO IMPROVE PATIENT ACCRUAL

Recruitment and enrollment to clinical trials is an arduous job. Limited research exists on which to base clinical trial recruitment strategies; hence most strategies to increase patient accrual are based on trial and error. Research is hard work, and adherence to protocols is critical. Individuals, health care providers, and organizations all have limited time and resources. Caregivers of patients with cancer are often willing, but face time and financial constraints in addition to the sometimes exhausting work involved with being a caregiver. However, there are a few strategies that have been identified as vital to the success of recruitment and enrollment to clinical trials.

Changing the mind-set about research involves developing a new and positive organizational culture or attitude.[9] Health care providers and researchers need to emphasize the fact that patients in clinical trials often receive better care than those not in clinical trials, and that the research environment is a special place. Research usually affords the newest and most innovative treatment, better treatment adherence and follow-up, close monitoring of treatment response and side effects, and surveillance of disease status. Several of the most important ways to make a difference in attitudes are the following: 1) change the mind set within your organization and community about research to one of trust; 2) develop effective communication skills within your office, clinic, and organization; 3) build trust internally, within your office and clinic, and externally, to your community; 4) provide community-based education efforts to inform potential patients on the types of clinical trial available, contact personnel, and how and why clinical research works; and 5) promote a team approach, both internally and to the external community.[9] Communication, effective education, planning, and team work are critical elements that provide the foundation for community awareness, build an organization that supports research, and in the end, provide quality patient care based on evidence and best practice.

Evidence-Based Practice

An important outcome resulting from clinical trials is improved patient care. Evidence-based practice (EBP) involves making clinical decisions on the basis of the best possible evidence.[11] There is general consensus that when enough research evidence is available, it is recommended that the evidence base for practice be based on the research. As more research is done in a specific area, the research evidence can be used to update and refine the guideline.[4] Typically, the best evidence comes from rigorous research such as randomized clinical trials. There is general agreement that findings from rigorous studies are paramount; however, there is no consensus among professional organizations or across health care disciplines about what constitutes rigorous research.[3,4] In an effort to help determine how to rank evidence, several EBP rating systems have been developed. LoBiondo-Wood and Haber provide an overview and summary of EBP rating systems.[4] Two examples of these rating systems include Stetler, Brunell, Giuliano, Morsi, and Prince[12] and the Gerontological Nursing Interventions Research Center (GNIRC),[13] which ranks levels of evidence from strongest to weakest. Summaries of these examples are listed below.
Stetler, Brunell, Giuliano, Morsi, and Price Systems[12]:
  Strength of Evidence
  ▪ Metaanalysis of multiple controlled studies
  ▪ Individual experimental study
  ▪ Quasi-experimental study or match case-control studies
  ▪ Nonexperimental study, such as correlational, descriptive

▪ Case report or systematically obtained, verifiable quality, or program evaluation data
▪ Opinions of respected authorities or the opinions of an expert committee
GNIRC Systems[13]
  Strength and Consistency of Grading the Evidence
  ▪ Evidence from well-designed metaanalysis
  ▪ Evidence from well-designed controlled trials, both randomized and nonrandomized, with results that consistently support a specific action
  ▪ Evidence from observational studies such as correlational, descriptive
  ▪ Evidence from expert opinion or multiple case reports[4]

NURSING'S ROLE AND INFLUENCE

Nurses provide critical influence in all aspects of clinical trials. Roles that nurses have typically managed and excelled at include communicator, collaborator, patient and staff educator, patient advocate, monitor of compliance and adherence and, in general, manager of every phase of clinical trials research. The role of nurses involved with research is one calling for a high level of theoretical expertise and critical thinking skills; the nurse is typically a coordinator who is involved with protocol development and implementation, recruitment, enrollment, data collection and management, and audits conducted by funding agencies and federal compliance regulators.

Greater numbers of nurses than ever are actively involved in clinical trials because of the emphasis on evidence-based practice and the extension of these trials into the community. Nurses practicing in institutions that do not routinely conduct clinical trials still need a working knowledge of research studies because they may have patients who are requesting information about specific trials. In this era of managed care, patients who have elected not to participate in a clinical trial may be referred back to the community setting for treatment and follow-up. The education and support that an informed and knowledgeable oncology nurse can bring to this stressful situation are invaluable.

Considerations for Older Adults

Older adults are still underrepresented in most research clinical trials, especially pharmaceutical trials. Although studies investigating symptom management and individual responses to various treatments have included older adult patients, studies specific to older adults are limited. Many barriers exist that prevent potential older adults from participating in research trials, including fear, distrust, or misunderstanding of the research trial process, lack of awareness of what trials may be available, and subjects' desire to be included in the treatment arm, which researchers cannot guarantee because of randomization.[9,14] Table 25-2 shows a more complete, literature-based list of barriers reported by older adults to participation in clinical research trials.

To increase older adults' enrollment in research trials, health care providers need to create a new approach to recruitment efforts, including specific educational and communication strategies such as education communities; this may help overcome fears, suspicion, and misconceptions surrounding research trials.[9] Clinicians need to take extra time to explain the purpose of the research, the meaning of randomization, and the benefits that derive from research, such as access to new and innovative treatment and frequent follow-up.[9] Excellent communication can help to build trust and should be tailored to accommodate older adults, some of whom who may have poor vision or be hard of hearing. Education strategies for the older adult must focus on repetition and make limited use of printed materials (as well as larger print for those that are used). These efforts must allow for extra time to explain the study and the informed consent process, and address any fears or misconceptions that older adults may have.

Conclusion

We are on the threshold of a new and innovative paradigm in the prevention, detection, treatment, and surveillance of cancer. Exciting new frontiers exist in the areas of novel targeted therapies, stem cell research, and gene therapy. These new areas will present challenging issues that must be approached with careful deliberation of ethical concerns, protocol design, and anticipated outcomes.

A new structure for research is emerging in health care. This movement is called outcomes research, and places its focus on the end results of patient care.[3] Outcomes research is derived from evaluation research. The main elements of this type of research are health, subjects of care (patients), and providers of care. Although most research developed for outcomes studies has been of individual patients, more organizations are now studying the quality of systems of care. The ultimate goal of clinical research is to improve the quality of care delivered to individuals. Clinical trials have been the mainstay of determining best practice and will continue to play a vital role in the emergence of outcomes research.

TABLE 25-2 Barriers to Older Adult Participation in Clinical Research Trials		
BARRIER	PATIENT	PHYSICIAN
Physicians reluctance to enroll older adults		X
Older adults want treatment arm, but researchers cannot guarantee it because of randomization	X	
Physicians are reluctant to enroll older adults because of comorbidities		X
Studies are poorly designed and not tailored to older adults		X
Distrust and fear of health care and research	X	
Additional time required by physician or nurse to explain study and obtain informed consent		X
Research is considered not cost-effective for the private practice physician		X
Transportation costs and additional travel expenses	X	
Caregivers not always available	X	X
High caregiver burden	X	
Physicians lack awareness of available research trials		X
Community and individual resistance to research	X	
Physicians, staff, and office personnel may not be willing to support research because of perceived additional work		X

Data from Payne J: Enrolling elderly cancer patients in clinical trials: changing the mind set. Abstract, Geriatric Oncology Society Program, Geriatric Oncology Society, Sept 18-20, 2003 and Muthty V, Krumholz H, Gross, C: Participation in cancer clinical trials. *JAMA* 291(22): 2720-2726, 2004.

REVIEW QUESTIONS

✓ Case Study

Heather, an oncology APN and adjunct faculty member at a nearby university, and the team of medical oncologists that she works with have been notified by their institutional review board that their new NCI-sponsored chemotherapy trial has been approved for implementation.

The purpose of this phase III study is to determine if the new treatment protocol is more effective than standard care in treating breast cancer patients. Heather knows that these patients will likely experience multiple side effects concurrently, and their follow-up care will be managed in an outpatient clinic. Since Heather will need to coordinate most of their symptom management, she understands that she will need to know the side effects of the chemotherapy drugs being used. Heather and her team of medical oncologists decide they would like to better understand whether the new chemotherapy drug treatment study adversely influences a cluster of symptoms occurring at the same time.

She decides to team up with a nurse researcher and statistician to discuss development and implementation of a companion research study to the phase III study that addresses symptom management at the same time that subjects are completing the chemotherapy treatment trial.

Heather receives advice from the nurse researcher on ways to identify the research problem and which factors to consider in deciding on the best research design to use. The nurse researcher explains that a descriptive design could be used to examine factors that contribute to symptoms occurring concurrently following chemotherapy treatment. Heather and her team decide to study the effects of the new chemotherapy protocol on fatigue, sleep disturbances, depressive symptoms, and hot flashes experienced by women with breast cancer, and begins preparing the final proposal for initiation of the study.

QUESTIONS

1. Which phase of a human investigation trial determines the maximum tolerated dose, or the strength of the therapy and safety?
   a. Phase I
   b. Phase II
   c. Phase III
   d. Phase IV

Continued

REVIEW QUESTIONS—CONT'D

2. What committee assures the rights of human subjects and that informed consent is obtained before they participate in a research study?
   a. Hospital infection control committee
   b. Nursing and medical credentialing committee
   c. Medical review board
   d. Institutional review board

3. The Cancer Centers Program of the NCI was enacted in 1971 to support academic and research institutions throughout the United States with what goal in mind?
   a. To support pharmaceutical companies
   b. To maintain broad-based, coordinated interdisciplinary programs in cancer research
   c. To protect human subjects by focusing on informed consent process
   d. To specifically conduct gene therapy trials

4. The National Research Act (1974) requires that institutional review boards (IRBs) are minimally composed of which of the following:
   a. Five members with professional expertise and qualifications
   b. At least one member whose concerns are related to women's health
   c. Several members from outside the institution
   d. At least one representative from a minority group

5. Which of the following are the best ways to identify a research problem?
   a. Discussing the problem with other experienced health care providers
   b. Reading the literature and identifying gaps in knowledge and noting any discrepancies
   c. Direct observation from clinical practice
   d. Seek input from experts in the topic or clinical area you are interested in studying
      i. c only
      ii. a, b, & c
      iii. c & d
      iv. a, b, c, & d

6. What type of research study design would be best in the case study situation described above?
   a. Experimental
   b. Descriptive
   c. Qualitative
   d. Quasi-experimental

7. Which of the following are considered components of informed consent?
   a. Disclosure of study information to the subject
   b. Comprehension of the information by the subject
   c. Competency of the individual to give consent
   d. Voluntary consent by the individual to participate in research
      i. d only
      ii. a & d
      iii. a, b, & d
      iv. a, b, c, & d

8. Historically, there has been underrepresentation of minorities in clinical trials. Which of the following best explains why minorities are less likely to participate in clinical trials?
   a. Unwillingness of researchers to pay for the participant's time
   b. General distrust of researchers and outsiders doing research in their communities
   c. Lack of individuals' ability to pay for tests involved in study
   d. Religious teachings that discourage research involvement for any reason

9. What factors should you consider when planning research clinical trial information for an audience of older adults?
   a. Older adults often have misperceptions and fear of cancer.
   b. Printed education materials are not always suitable for use by older adults.
   c. The older adult may require more repetition and reinforcement of teaching.
   d. Older adults are often too fatigued to learn new information.
      i. a & b
      ii. b & c
      iii. a, b, & c
      iv. a, b, c, & d

10. Dr. Hennessey has been involved in the institutional review board at Community General Hospital for almost 20 years. Physicians in her group have been hesitent to enroll older adults in clinical trials on several occasions, even though they have has an interest in research and the agent could potentially benefit their patient population. What is(are) the most likely reason(s) for the physicians' hesitancy?
    a. Travel costs, uncertainty, and randomization
    b. Lack of understanding of the benefits of research
    c. Not enough time to adhere to research trial requirements
    d. Office space, staffing, and time constraints

ANSWERS

1. **A.** *Rationale:* Phase I trials are designed to determine maximum tolerated dose, strength, and safety. Phase II trials are used to determine the effectiveness of treatment, and phase III trials are designed to determine whether the new treatment is more effective than the standard treatment. Phase IV trials focus on long-term consequences of the treatment or intervention, including benefits and side effects.

2. **D.** *Rationale:* Institutional review boards are designed to protect the rights of human subjects involved in research studies and ensure that informed consent process is obtained before participation in a study. Infection control committees, credentialing committees and medical review boards **do not** monitor the rights of human subjects and informed consent in research trials. The purpose of hospital infection control committees is to develop and maintain current evidence-based patient-care policies and procedures regarding infection

control, whereas the nursing and medical credentialing committees ensures that physicians and nurses are appropriately licensed and safe to work within their scope of practice. Medical review boards typically review patient cases and determine whether appropriate medical care was provided.

3. **B.** *Rationale:* The purpose and focus of the Cancer Centers Program of the NCI was to sustain broad, coordinated, and interdisciplinary programs in cancer research. The Cancer Center Program was enacted neither to support pharmaceutical companies, nor specifically to protect human subjects or informed consent process. It was also not enacted to specifically conduct gene therapy.

4. **A.** *Rationale:* A requirement mandated by the National Research Act of 1974 that must be strictly adhered to by IRBs states that membership must include five members with professional expertise and qualifications. Violation of this rule by an institution's IRB would violate the National Research Act and cause reprimand and most likely the temporary closure of IRB activities at that institution.

5. **D.** *Rationale:* Research questions stem from problems identified in clinical practice. Therefore the clinical setting of health care providers provides a rich environment for research problems to be identified. The literature also may reveal best practice treatment or interventions and determine the level of evidence to support current practice. Direct observation is another way to identify problems in health care delivery systems and in patient care. Experts can provide one level of evidence and can provide a wealth of clinical or administration information on the topics in which they are experts.

6. **B.** *Rationale:* Descriptive designs are used when researchers want to gain a better understanding of what is happening and search for accurate information about the characteristics of subjects or phenomenon to be studied. Descriptive designs often use surveys to collect data that describes existing variables. Experimental and quasi-experimental designs introduce a treatment or intervention; experimental designs include three explicit criteria (randomization, control, and manipulation), which is the design used in the NCI-sponsored phase III clinical trial in the case study. Qualitative designs describe life experiences and meaning.

7. **D.** *Rationale:* All statements are true. Subjects must understand and comprehend the purpose and significance of the study, and be competent. Competency of a patient is usually determined by the subject's physician. All subjects must voluntarily consent to participate in the study, with no evidence of coercion by the principal investigator or designated research team member.

8. **B.** *Rationale:* Minority groups do not trust researchers in general, and especially those from outside their communities. In the past, members of minorities and vulnerable subjects have been coerced to participate in research without being informed. Examples are prisoners and institutionalized people.

9. **C.** *Rationale:* Older adults often have misconceptions and fears about cancer. Printed materials are not always written at the recommended sixth- to eighth-grade reading level or in larger print, and the older adult may require more repetition of learning. All but choice d are correct; there is no evidence to support that older adults are too fatigued to learn new information.

10. **D.** *Rationale:* Although any of these answers could affect a physician's decision to offer clinical trails, the most likely factors have been found to be office space, uncertainty, and randomization.

REFERENCES

1. National Cancer Institute: National Cancer Institute website. Retrieved April 17, 2006, from http://www.cancer.gov.
2. Collichio F, Griggs J, Rosenblatt J: Basic concepts in drug development and clinical trials. In Rubin P, editor: *Clinical oncology: a multidisciplinary approach for physicians and students*, ed 8, Philadelphia, 2001, WB Saunders.
3. Polit D, Beck C: *Nursing research: principles and practice*, Philadelphia, 2004, Lippincott Williams & Wilkins.
4. LoBiondo-Wood L, Haber J: *Nursing research: methods and critical appraisal for evidence-based practice*, Philadelphia, 2006, Mosby.
5. Applebaum PS, Lindz CN, Meisel A: *Informed consent: legal theory and clinical practice*. New York, 1987, Oxford University Press.
6. Daugherty C: Impact of therapeutic research on informed consent and the ethics of clinical trials: a medical oncology perspective, *J Clin Oncol* 17(5):1601-1617, 1999.
7. Jemal A, Murray T, Ward E et al: Cancer Statistics, 2005, *CA Cancer J Clin* 55(1):10-30, 2005.
8. Connolly N, Schneider D, Hill A: Improving enrollment in cancer clinical trials, *Oncol Nurs Forum* 31(3):610-614, 2004.
9. Payne J: Enrolling elderly cancer patients in clinical trials: changing the mind set. Abstract, Geriatric Oncology Society Program, Geriatric Oncology Society, Sept 18-20, 2003.
10. Jenkins V, Fallowfield L: Reasons for accepting or declining to participate in randomized clinical trials for cancer therapy, *Br J Cancer* 82(11):1783-1788, 2000.
11. Titler M, Mentes J, Rakel B et al: From book to bedside: putting evidence to use in the care of the elderly, *Joint Commission J Qual Improv* 25:545-556, 1999.
12. Stetler C, Brunell M, Giuliano K et al: Evidence-based practice and the role of nursing leadership, *J Nurs Admin* 28(7/8):45-53, 1998.
13. The University of Iowa College of Nursing: Gerontological Nursing Interventions Research Center (GNIRC), retrieved April 2006, from http://www.nursing.uiowa.edu/centers/gnirc/.
14. Munty V, Krumholz H, Gross, C: Participation in cancer clinical trials. *JAMA* 291(22): 2720-2726, 2004.

UNIT FOUR

Cancer Care Supportive Therapies

CHAPTER 26

Nutrition

Lisa Schulmeister

Cancer and its treatment may affect the nutritional status of patients in a variety of ways. Besides being subject to metabolic effects, patients are emotionally stressed when nutritional intake is impaired. Because eating is a basic body function and often a social activity, inability to eat or difficulty in eating may have a profound physical and psychologic impact on patients with cancer and their families.

Undernutrition and malnutrition are major sources of morbidity and mortality among patients with cancer.[1] Nutritional deterioration is associated with decreased survival and quality of life and is the eventual cause of death in approximately 30% of all patients with cancer.[1-3] Early and ongoing assessment of nutritional status and dietary counseling are essential to help prevent nutritional deterioration.

Nutrition also plays a role in the etiology of cancer and its prevention. Cancer is largely a preventable illness, and worldwide evidence indicates that 30% to 40% of all cancers are linked to dietary intake.[4] Diets high in fruits and vegetables and low in saturated fats reduce the risk of developing at least 10 different cancers.[5-8]

Effects of Cancer on Nutritional Status
NUTRITIONAL COMPONENTS AND THEIR FUNCTIONS

Cancer may affect the metabolism of the nutritional components necessary to sustain life: carbohydrates, proteins, fatty acids, vitamins, minerals, and electrolytes. An alteration in the metabolism of these components affects the nutritional status of an individual, that is, the degree to which an individual's need for nutrition is met by intake.

Carbohydrates are the sugars that provide energy for immediate use. They are converted to glycogen or fat for long-term storage or are converted to other molecules in the body. Carbohydrates can be divided into three classes: monosaccharides, disaccharides, and polysaccharides. **Monosaccharides** are simple one-molecule sugars; examples are fructose and dextrose (glucose). **Disaccharides** are two-molecule sugars; an example is sucrose (table sugar). **Polysaccharides** are complex sugars characterized by many molecules; examples are starch and dextran.[9]

Glucose is the fuel for most of the cells of the body. It is metabolized rapidly in the presence or absence of oxygen. Each gram of glucose provides 3.4 kilocalories (kcal). Carbohydrates are also a long-term source of energy. When glucose intake exceeds demand, it is converted into glycogen or fat. Both sources of energy are stored in the body and used when a glucose shortage occurs. When metabolized by certain processes, the glucose molecule can be used as the basis for other molecules, including amino acids and fatty acids.[9]

Amino acids are the building blocks of the body. Proteins are many amino acids joined into one molecule. Amino acids are divided into two categories: essential and nonessential. **Essential** amino acids must be supplied from the diet because the body is unable to synthesize them from glucose or other amino acids. **Nonessential** amino acids need not be supplied from the diet because the body is able to synthesize them.[9]

Functions of amino acids include maintenance and growth. When tissue breakdown exceeds synthesis or when glucose for energy is lacking, the result is wasting of protein from muscles and loss of mass. Amino acids assist in the regulation of body processes and make up many enzymes found throughout the body. Enzymes are the chemical regulators of many of the synthetic processes in the body. During starvation the body uses proteins as a source of energy. Each gram provides 4 kcal.[9]

Lipids and fatty acids serve many roles in the body. **Fatty acids** are basic molecules, and **lipids** are long chains of fatty acids. Lipids may be saturated or unsaturated, depending on the number of double-bonded carbons in their structure. Lipids are an excellent source of energy, supplying 9 kcal/g. They are also the long-term storage form of glucose. Fat-soluble vitamins are transported by lipids. Many fat-soluble vitamins (A, D, E, and K) are transported throughout the body bound to fatty acids. The fat content of food is responsible for the taste of many foods and the feeling of fullness that results from eating. Lipids also provide insulation and padding. The fatty acids are precursors to many hormones, including testosterone and estrogen. They are also the basis for cholesterol.[9]

Vitamins are compounds used in a number of enzymatic steps that regulate many processes. Normal amounts of the adult daily requirements (ADRs) of vitamins are obtained by consuming a balanced diet. Vitamins can be divided into two groups: fat-soluble and water-soluble. **Fat-soluble vitamins** are stored by the body in fat. Deficiencies take a long time to develop because these vitamins are stored. Vitamin A is important in maintaining vision and in tooth and skeletal development, and it acts as a precursor to cholesterol. Vitamin D acts to regulate protein and calcium metabolism. Vitamin E is an antioxidant; that is, it prevents or lessens damage to body tissue caused by atmospheric oxygen. Vitamin K helps maintain the clotting ability of blood.[9]

Water-soluble vitamins are not stored in the body and are readily eliminated in the urine. Deficiencies may develop quickly if inadequate quantities are consumed. Vitamin C is used in the formation of collagen, enhances iron absorption, and serves as an antioxidant. B-complex vitamins are cofactors in many enzymatic reactions.[9]

Macro elements, or **electrolytes,** maintain osmotic pressure and water balance, facilitate nerve conduction and muscle contraction, and perform other functions. The macro elements are sodium, potassium, chloride, calcium, magnesium, phosphorus, and sulfur.[9]

Trace elements are so named because they are needed by the body in small quantities. Deficiencies can develop quickly, but clinical signs of deficiency may not be apparent for a long time. Trace elements include zinc, manganese, copper, chromium, selenium, iron, and cobalt, among others.[9]

SYSTEMIC EFFECTS OF CANCER

The **anorexia-cachexia syndrome** of advanced cancer is characterized by progressive wasting and extensive loss of adipose tissue and skeletal muscle.[10] The syndrome results from a multifactorial process that involves many mediators, including hormones such as leptin, neuropeptides (e.g., melanocortin, orexin, neuropeptide Y, and melanin-concentrating hormone), and cytokines (e.g., interleukin 1, interleukin 6, tumor necrosis factor, and alpha and gamma interferon). These mediators affect the hypothalamus, the area of the brain that controls hunger and thirst, and cause anorexia that ultimately results in cachexia.[11,12] In addition, systemic inflammation is associated with many cancers and has been correlated with hypermetabolism, weight loss, anorexia, and a poor prognosis. A key marker of systemic inflammation is an acute phase protein response induced by proinflammatory cytokines.[13]

Simply increasing nutrient intake does not reverse cachexia.[14] Alterations in the normal metabolism of carbohydrates, proteins, and fats result in increased energy expenditures. A normal body's response is to increase appetite and therefore intake, but the person with cancer experiencing anorexia has further decline in the ability to meet nutritional demands. The process can be exacerbated by psychologic responses: anxiety about cancer and its possible progression, depression, anticipatory phenomena, and learned food aversions.

Vitamin deficiencies observed in patients with cancer include a deficiencies of vitamins A, D, and B_6.[15,16] Vitamin C deficiency also been reported in patients with advanced cancer, and patients with low plasma concentrations of vitamin C have shorter survival times.[17] Iron deficiency may result from the unavailability of iron in the diet, malabsorption, or chronic bleeding.[18]

Fluid and electrolyte imbalances may result from direct and indirect effects of cancer. Parathyroid, lung, kidney, and colon cancers sometimes produce an ectopic parathyroid-like hormone that deposits calcium in the renal tubules and causes renal failure.[19] Hypercalcemia may also cause a concentrating effect that leads to polyuria and water depletion.[20] Leukemia and lymphomas may induce hyperuricemia, hyperphosphatemia, and hyperkalemia as a result of electrolytes released by cellular breakdown.[21] A common presentation of bronchiogenic carcinomas, such as small cell cancer, is the **syndrome of inappropriate antidiuretic hormone secretion (SIADH).** This syndrome is characterized by urinary loss of sodium and excessive retention of water by the renal tubules.[22] Renal cancers may secrete renin and in turn cause increased secretion of aldosterone, resulting in hypokalemia.[23] Treatment with platinum-based chemotherapeutic agents may deplete magnesium and potassium.[24]

EFFECTS OF CANCER

Several local effects of cancer may alter the nutritional intake of the affected individual. Impaired ingestion may be caused by mechanical and anatomic alterations. Patients with cancer of the head and neck area, esophageal cancers, and brain tumors may have difficulty opening the mouth, chewing, and swallowing, and may be at risk for aspiration when they eat and drink.

Obstruction of the esophagus can inhibit the passage of food. Gastric cancers often cause pain and distention. Cancers along the alimentary tract may cause obstructions, and they often inhibit the absorption of nutrients. Pancreatic cancer can cause endocrine and exocrine hormonal insufficiencies that affect nutrient consumption and absorption. Cancer of the small intestine affects the digestion and absorption of food. A fistula of the bowel may develop as a result of tissue necrosis from a gastrointestinal (GI) tract tumor and induce electrolyte imbalance and malabsorption.[25-27]

EFFECTS OF AGING

The older adult has special nutritional needs and requirements that differ from those of other stages of life. Physiologic changes of decreased ingestion and digestion and decreased metabolic rate and excretion can adversely affect nutritional intake, and the presence of impaired mobility or visual impairment can affect the older adult's ability to obtain, prepare, and consume food. Chronic illnesses such as cancer, medication use, and economic factors can further affect the nutritional status of the older adult.[28]

Weight loss and cachexia in elderly patients may have profound consequences. Weight loss and wasting in the elderly diminish self-reliance in activities of daily living and often lead to hospitalization and the need for skilled care. Cachexia has been associated with infections, decubitus ulcer formation, and even death in the elderly.[29]

Nutritional Consequences of Cancer Treatment, Assessment, and Interventions

EFFECTS OF VARIOUS MODES OF TREATMENT

Surgical alterations in any area of the alimentary tract from the mouth to the anus may cause temporary or, occasionally, permanent alterations in nutritional intake or absorptive capabilities. Surgical procedures that alter the patient's ability to chew or swallow may prompt the need for soft or blenderized foods, and tube feedings may be required. Partial or total gastrectomy can cause severe nutritional problems. When the greater portion of the stomach is removed, the intrinsic factor is not produced in quantities sufficient for the absorption of vitamin B_{12}, and pernicious anemia develops. With surgical resection of the stomach, the quantity of food that can be consumed at one time is limited, and frequent, small feedings are necessary. **Dumping syndrome** may also occur after gastrectomy; a few minutes after ingestion, food is dumped into the jejunum, and nausea, cramping, and diarrhea follow. Malabsorption of fat occurs in patients who have undergone a gastrojejunostomy. The duodenum is bypassed, and pancreatic insufficiency results. Malabsorption of fat impairs absorption of fat-soluble vitamins and calcium. Iron absorption is also decreased, and anemia occurs.[30,31]

Radiation therapy may affect the normal tissues surrounding the treatment areas. Patients with cancer of the head and neck have both acute and chronic symptoms. Specifically, the normal tissues of the salivary gland, the oral mucosa, muscle, and occasionally bone may be affected. In the acute phase, inflammation and swelling of tissues with resulting discomfort may affect nutritional intake. Oral mucositis can be complicated with candidiasis. Taste changes, such as a diminished sense of taste or metallic taste when eating red meats, may cause aversion to food and decreased intake. Diminished production of saliva and xerostomia, the perception of dry mouth, are long-term side effects of radiation therapy. Pain and difficulty swallowing often occur. Saliva substitutes and topical anesthetics for oral use may be helpful, and eating moist foods is recommended. Dental caries may occur as a late effect of head and neck radiation. Radiation therapy to the mediastinum for lung or esophageal cancer can cause esophagitis. Dysphagia usually begins within 2 weeks of treatment and can continue for several months afterward. Interventions include topical anesthetics, nonsteroidal antiinflammatory drugs (NSAIDs), systemic analgesics, and histamine blockers to reduce stomach acid reflux. Dietary modifications, such as soft, bland food and liquid supplements, may help maintain intake. Enteral feeding is sometimes necessary during the acute phase if symptoms are severe. Long-term strictures of the esophagus may require periodic dilation.[32,33]

Irradiation of the stomach and the small intestine produces vomiting, anorexia, diarrhea, and gastric distention. Antiemetics taken 30 minutes before treatment, a low-residue and lactose-free diet, and adequate hydration may alleviate or minimize these side effects. Antidiarrheal medications may be necessary to minimize fluid loss and permit oral intake. Generally, these acute effects resolve with the completion of therapy. Long-term side effects of radiation to the intestines that affect nutrition may be chronic obstruction, malabsorption, and fistula formation.[34]

Chemotherapy may produce side effects that impair the patient's nutritional status. Chemotherapy causes nutritional deficiencies by promoting anorexia, mucositis, taste alterations, and nausea and vomiting. Deficiencies of vitamins B_1, B_2, and K and of niacin, folic acid, and thiamine may also result from chemotherapy. Some chemotherapeutic regimens, such as induction therapy for acute leukemia, can cause significant weight loss and hypoalbuminemia. Taste alterations, such as an aversion to red meat and a metallic food taste, are common when platinum-based chemotherapy is administered. Cool foods with little aroma and bland foods are often tolerated well. Topical application of analgesics often minimizes the discomfort of oral mucositis.[35]

The severity of nausea and vomiting and their effect on nutritional status varies from patient to patient and is largely dependent on the emetogenic potential of the chemotherapy agents administered and use of prophylactic antiemetics. Prophylactic antiemetic therapy with $5-HT_3$–receptor antagonists has significantly reduced the acute effects of nausea and vomiting; however, some patients continue to experience nausea several days after chemotherapy. Nausea and vomiting may have a psychogenic component; anticipatory nausea and vomiting before a chemotherapy treatment may occur. Odor, sight, and even the thought of food may produce emesis in some patients. Relaxation and diversion therapy is sometimes indicated. Aversions to specific foods may occur as a result of the association of those foods with nausea and vomiting.[35]

Although chemotherapy is most often associated with effects that contribute to impaired nutritional intake and weight loss, weight gain has been reported to occur in women with breast cancer who receive adjuvant chemotherapy. Exercise has been shown to be a successful intervention to prevent or minimize weight gain.[36]

The side effects of **biotherapy** are generally less severe than those of chemotherapy. Anorexia is a common complaint, and nausea and vomiting occur occasionally. Diarrhea may occur, depending on the agent used. Long-term low-dose treatment may result in fatigue that is intense enough to preclude fixing meals and eating. Interventions may include meal planning for quick, small meals and shopping assistance.

NUTRITIONAL ASSESSMENT

A nutritional assessment can easily be integrated in clinical practice to screen for potential or existing problems in nutritional status, provide a database for individuals at high risk, and determine response to treatment or dietary interventions. Assessment of the patient's eating patterns, nutrient intake, and supplement use and influences on eating habits should be completed before initiation of cancer treatment.[37]

Several methods can be used to estimate or quantify the patient's nutritional status (Box 26-1). A simple method is clinical observation. A thorough nursing history identifies concurrent health problems that may affect nutrition, such as diabetes, hypertension, and malabsorption. Note any psychosocial factors, including the home environment, food preparation methods, and the patient's body image, that may affect nutritional intake. Ability to purchase food and supplements also should be addressed. Physical assessment reflects the patient's overall nutritional status. Examine the hair, teeth, gums, and general muscle tone, since they may be early indicators of nutritional deficiencies. Dentures that fit poorly after weight loss may impair ability to chew. A functional assessment assists in determining patients' ability to prepare meals and feed themselves. Uncontrolled pain can significantly impair appetite and nutritional intake and must be addressed. Fatigue should be assessed for its impact on the ability to obtain food and eat.

Dietary evaluation is a simple and effective tool for assessing nutritional intake. A 24-hour food diary, a complete dietary history with notations of food allergies and preferences, and direct observation of intake coupled with evaluation of nutrient composition are methods for dietary evaluation. Much of this information can be collected from the patient; however, the patient may not report accurately. Direct observation of the patient's intake by a consistent nurse or dietitian is more precise but has limitations for patients who are not hospitalized. Family members can be enlisted to help keep a record at home.

Biochemical measurements include laboratory values such as serum albumin, which is used to estimate visceral protein levels; serum transferrin, which reflects the body's ability to make serum proteins; and total lymphocyte count, which tests immunocompetence. Skin testing can reveal T-cell–mediated immunocompetence, and urine urea nitrogen may be measured to estimate skeletal muscle mass. Serum prealbumin level is a sensitive indicator of changes in nutritional status. Albumin levels take longer to respond to increased intake.[38,39]

Anthropometric measurements are the patient's midarm muscle circumference (MAMC), triceps skinfold thickness (TSF), subscapular skinfold thickness (SST), and weight for height as compared with reference standards. The measurements estimate subcutaneous fat stores, energy reserves, and skeletal muscle protein mass. Moreover, measuring weight and comparing it with the patient's ideal body weight and monitoring changes in weight over time assists in identifying any downward trend in nutritional status. Weight changes also must be assessed in context with the patient's fluid balance, since edema can cause weight gain and dehydration can cause weight loss. Weighing the patient weekly can help assess changes. Daily weights are more appropriate to assess changes in fluid status.[40]

| BOX 26-1 | **Components of Nutritional Assessment** |

Nursing History
Date diagnosed
Type of cancer
Type and duration of therapy
Concurrent medications
Concomitant medical conditions
Surgical procedures
Side effects of therapy
Allergies

Psychosocial Assessment
Home environment
Family support
Coping abilities
Self-image
Perceptions of role of nutrition
Cultural/religious considerations

Physical Assessment
General overall appearance
Hair texture
Skin turgor and integrity
Condition of mouth and gums
Performance status
Alterations in elimination, comfort, gas exchange, or cognition

Dietary Evaluation
24-hour recall of intake
Food preferences
Food allergies
Use of vitamin supplements
Changes in diet or eating on lifestyle patterns
Observation of intake
Evaluation of nutrient composition

Biochemical Measurements
Serum albumin
Serum prealbumin
Hemoglobin, hematocrit
Serum transferrin
Total lymphocyte count
Creatinine
Urine urea nitrogen
Creatinine-height index
Skin testing

Anthropometric Data
Height
Weight
Weight change over time (actual weight compared with ideal body weight)
Triceps skinfold (TSF) thickness
Midarm muscle circumference (MAMC)
Subscapular skinfold thickness (SST)

Since 1982, 71 nutritional screening and assessment tools for use by nurses have been developed. The tools vary in complexity, and many focus on a specific population such as the elderly. Most tools incorporate measurement of food intake, weight, weight change over time, ideal body weight, and sociocultural factors that affect nutritional intake. Some tools include anthropometric and biochemical measures. Although many of these tools are routinely used in clinical practice, few published tools include reports of reliability or validity testing.[41]

NUTRITIONAL INTERVENTION

The extent of nutritional intervention depends on the cause of the nutritional impairment and may be palliative or intensive. Enteral feedings are considered when a mechanical defect precludes ingestion of food. Total parenteral nutrition (TPN) is indicated only when the gut cannot digest, absorb, and excrete nutrients.

The enteral route of nutritional support has been found to be as good as or preferable to parenteral nutrition in terms of maintenance of nutritional status and immune function, prevention of bacterial translocation, and maintenance of normal gut flora; therefore it is always preferable in terms of physiologic response, quality of life, and cost, and should be the method of choice for the nutritional support of patients with cancer.[42] Enteral or parenteral nutrition should be considered only for patients who demonstrate most of the following conditions: (1) inability to eat for a long period of time, (2) weight loss from inability to eat rather than tumor-induced metabolic changes, (3) availability of professional support to reduce complications of therapy, and (4) cancer that can be expected to respond to treatment.[43,44] For example, enteral nutrition support for patients undergoing major abdominal surgery and patients with esophageal cancer being treated with concurrent chemotherapy and radiation therapy has been shown to prevent further nutritional deterioration and is well tolerated.[45,46]

Nutritional Support
ORAL NUTRITION

After the need for nutritional support has been established, the next step is to determine the method of delivery. The degree of intervention is based on the severity and etiology of the nutritional deficiency. Individuals with mild anorexia often respond to dietary counseling. In randomized controlled trials, dietary counseling improved patients' nutritional status, decreased morbidity, and improved quality of life.[47,48] In settings that do not have dietitians available for consultation and counseling, case managers or nurses providing direct care may need to provide nutrition education and counseling.

Patients experiencing mild anorexia may benefit from frequent, small meals and snacks. Foods high in protein, such as cheese, fish, and poultry, and foods high in calories are recommended. Family members and caregivers should offer a variety of foods, since foods not appealing at one time may be favorites at another. Milkshakes, peanut butter on crackers, and prepackaged puddings are snacks that are not only nutritious, but also easy to prepare. Adding dry milk powder to creamed soups or milk increases its calorie and protein content. Providing lists of recommended foods or prepared booklets can give caregivers concrete ideas to implement at home. High-calorie, high-protein supplements such as Sustacal (Mead Johnson), Ensure (Ross), or Citrotein (Sandoz) may be indicated and are most palatable when served cold. Patients need to be monitored for alterations in elimination when using lactose-based products; some patients experience diarrhea and do not tolerate these formulas.

Individuals who have a mild weight loss because of alterations of the oral mucosa or taste alterations may benefit from a high-calorie, bland diet. Avoid seasoning and experimentation with alternative flavorings such as vanilla. Use a topical analgesic to help manage pain and discomfort associated with oral mucositis. Substitute baking soda or use a toothpaste specifically for sensitive mouths if indicated. Patients should avoid commercial mouthwashes, because they contain alcohol, additives, and flavorings that are often painful in situations involving altered oral mucosal integrity. Cold foods, particularly popsicles, ice cream, and frozen yogurt, often have a numbing effect and may be well tolerated. Liquids that are known to have high acidity, such as orange and lemon juices, should be avoided. Patients experiencing xerostomia may encounter difficulties maintaining adequate nutritional intake. The addition of liquids, particularly sauces and gravies, may be helpful.

Psychosocial support is indicated in addition to dietary interventions. Ineffective individual and family coping often occurs when the patient begins to lose weight. Efforts by family members to encourage a better intake are sometimes met with resistance. Frustration for both patient and family results as the patient perceives the relatives to be unsympathetic and lacking in understanding. Family members often perceive a lack of effort by the patient and become frustrated at their inability to do more. Nurses should listen to problems with nutrition and provide guidance and instruction when indicated. It may be helpful to teach families about biologic causes of anorexia to increase understanding of why the patient finds eating so difficult.

Nondietary interventions for patients with a mild weight loss include varying surroundings, eating at the table with family and friends, and arriving at the table immediately before meals to minimize the effect of food odor on appetite. Using small plates and eating more often may be helpful. Relaxation techniques may be useful for some patients.

Medications may be necessary to control the side effects of the disease or treatment that may be affecting intake. Serotonin (5-HT$_3$) blockers have demonstrated effectiveness as prophylactic antiemetic therapy.[49] Antiemetics given 30 minutes before meals and use of artificial saliva to control the symptoms of xerostomia are other examples of pharmacologic interventions. In 30 controlled studies, megestrol acetate (dose range of 320 to 1600 mg/day) improved appetite and prevented or decreased weight loss in patients with advanced cancer and in those undergoing various treatment modalities, such as radiotherapy and chemotherapy.[50] Megestrol acetate has glucocorticoid-like activity and has been linked to the development of Cushing syndrome, new-onset diabetes, and adrenal insufficiency. These secondary conditions can be life-threatening if not recognized.

Dronabinol, δ-9-tetrahydrocannabinol (THC), the active ingredient in marijuana, has also been found to be an effective appetite stimulant in selected patients with advanced cancer and human immunodeficiency virus (HIV) infection. It has been used as an antiemetic for chemotherapy-associated nausea and vomiting.[51]

A variety of **gut-protective nutrients,** such as the amino acid glutamine, are currently being studied to assess their role in stimulating mucosal growth, promoting gut health, and preventing dose-limiting gastrointestinal symptoms during chemotherapy treatment. Omega-3 fatty acids, antioxidants, and L-arginine also are being studied to ascertain their immunonutrient effectiveness.[52]

ENTERAL NUTRITION

Although oral nutrition is preferred, adequate intake may not be possible for patients who have a mechanical impairment in their gastrointestinal tracts. For these patients, it may be necessary to use a feeding tube (enteral nutrition). Using the gut for feeding maintains the GI tract's digestive and absorptive capabilities and assists in maintaining GI motility. Metabolic comparisons show a more nearly normal use of some nutrients with the enteral route than with the parenteral route. A thorough assessment is essential for determining which patients are candidates for enteral nutrition. Mechanical obstruction is the only absolute contraindication to enteral nutrition. Generally, patients with functioning GI tracts who are unable to ingest adequate nutrients to meet their metabolic demands are likely to benefit from tube feedings. They should have a reasonable expectation for improvement through increasing delivery of nutrients, a good support system to help with feedings at home, and reasonable life expectancy.[53]

Tube feedings can be administered by the nasogastric, nasoduodenal, nasojejunal, esophagostomy, gastrostomy, and jejunostomy routes (Fig. 26-1). Passage of the feeding tube through the nose into the stomach or intestine is indicated for short-term feeding. It is best tolerated when a small, flexible feeding tube is used. Larger, stiffer tubes may damage the mucosa of the GI tract and irritate the nose. A feeding ostomy is

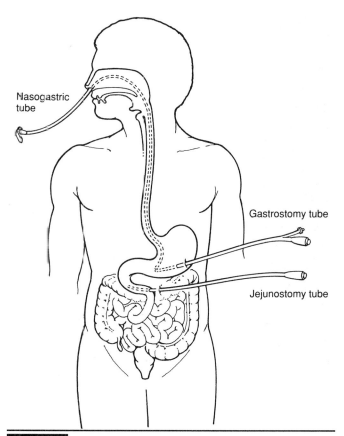

FIG. 26-1 Three routes for tube feeding.

indicated for long-term therapy, whenever obstruction makes insertion through the nose impossible, or after GI surgery. Ostomy tubes eliminate nasal irritation and are more cosmetically acceptable to the patient. Possible complications include infection or skin irritation around the feeding tube site; however, this risk is lessened with appropriate skin care. Percutaneous endoscopic gastrostomy (PEG) or jejunostomy (PEJ) tubes are inserted by GI endoscopy and require a patent esophagus. It is a relatively simple procedure, with the tube being threaded through the abdominal and stomach or jejunal wall over a guidewire. The tube can be used soon after placement. Recovery time is short. It may be possible to place a button gastrostomy into a mature gastrocutaneous fistula and thereby eliminate the need for a protruding tube. If GI endoscopy is not possible, placement is more complicated, requiring laparotomy and a longer recovery time.[54]

Nasogastric, esophagostomy, and gastrostomy feedings allow the digestive process to begin in the stomach. Aspiration may occur more easily with gastric feedings than with intestinal feedings because only the gastroesophageal sphincter is functioning to prevent gastric reflux. Alteration of the gastroesophageal sphincter by tumor or surgery may increase the risk of aspiration. Nasoduodenal, nasojejunal, and jejunostomy feedings, which are delivered directly into the small intestine, may be preferred in these selected patients because they then have the pyloric sphincter to prevent reflux. Tube selection is based on several factors, including the duration of therapy, history of abdominal procedures, GI function, level of debilitation, and the discharge plan. Adequate digestion and absorption occur in the small intestine; however, when feedings are improperly selected or administered, nausea, diarrhea, and cramps can result.[55]

ADMINISTRATION OF TUBE FEEDING

The size of the tube selected for enteral feedings should be the smallest through which the food will flow. A variety of tubes are available. Most are made of soft, flexible material such as polyurethane or silicone rubber. These tubes do not stiffen when exposed to gastric juices and are more comfortable for the patient than are stiff tubes. The tubes are available in different French sizes and lengths, and most are radiopaque.

The volume and concentration of nutriment delivered by tube feeding should meet the individual's specific needs. A patient who has been without adequate food intake before tube feeding requires a period of adaptation before full volume and strength can be tolerated. Isotonic formulas are more easily tolerated than hypertonic formulas and do not require dilution. The duodenum and jejunum are more sensitive than the stomach to both volume and osmolality. Therefore, duodenal or jejunal feeding should be low in osmolality and delivered by continuous drip or pump.

Consultation with the dietary department is usually done to determine the caloric needs and most suitable formula. Water requirements are also calculated. Generally, patients need at least 1 ml fluid per calorie. Formulas range from 75% to 85% water (check exact amount on the product label or product literature). It is usually adequate to presume about 80% for most formulas. Additional water must be given to meet demands. For instance, a patient with 1800 calories delivered by formula needs at least 1800 ml water, 1440 of which will be delivered in the formula (80% of 1800). The remainder must be given as flushes or extra boluses of water. Dehydration is known to occur with tube-fed patients.

Additional fluid may be needed to replace fluid losses from diarrhea, sweating, or wound drainage. Patients who cannot swallow their own saliva because of obstruction may also require extra fluid replacement.

Feedings into the stomach can be done by bolus, gravity, or pump methods. Bolus feedings of enteral formulas are usually administered at 250 to 400 ml over a few minutes, 5 to 8 times daily. Patients who are intolerant of bolus feedings may have nausea, diarrhea, aspiration, abdominal distention, and cramps. Generally, only relatively healthy individuals can tolerate bolus feedings.

Gravity feedings may be intermittent or continuous. Gravity flow rates may be inconsistent and thus must be assessed frequently. Even if checks are made as frequently as every half hour, accidental bolus delivery is possible. Ideally, the tube position should be checked 2 to 3 times daily, and gastric residual should be checked every 2 to 4 hours.

Continuous feedings may be given during the night over 10 to 12 hours or around the clock. Feedings to the distal duodenum or jejunum should be given by continuous pump infusion to prevent dumping syndrome. Start the feeding at 50 ml or less, and advance the amount only if the patient shows no diarrhea, cramping, or other signs of intolerance. When the desired rate has been reached, the strength can be increased as tolerated. Generally, an isotonic or nearly isotonic formula can be started at full strength; hypertonic or concentrated formulas are usually started at half strength (half formula, half water) or at half speed. Adding water or other liquids such as dye can contaminate feedings and should be done as carefully as possible.

Various feeding sets, containers, and pumps are available for tube feeding. Selection of equipment and supplies is based on the formula to be given, rate and frequency of feedings, tube site, and other considerations, including the caregiver's preference. Most feeding bags and administration sets are large enough to accommodate 500 to 1000 ml of formula. To prevent bacterial contamination when a large container is used, the amount of formula in the bag should approximate that which can be given over 8 hours. In warm environments, a feeding bag with a pouch for an ice bag is desirable to prevent curdling of the formula and bacterial growth. New formula should not be added to formula that has already been hanging for 8 hours at room temperature. The container and tubing should be rinsed well before adding formula. With very careful cleaning, a feeding bag may be used for 2 days; however, discarding the bag after 24 hours is recommended. Ready-to-hang enteral feedings can be used for patients who are on stable regimens. They can provide approximately 1000 to 1500 ml of formula in a container that is stable for 24 hours and are as cost-effective as using a bag and multiple cans of formula. Ready-to-hang products decrease the chance for bacterial contamination and are available in screw-top or spikable prefilled bottles or bags.

Several enteral pumps can provide a controlled rate of administration. Most have internal batteries to allow limited mobility and have alarm systems that indicate problems or completion of feeding. Most pumps have occlusion and low-battery alarms and are simply designed to allow easy troubleshooting. An enteral pump is usually indicated if the patient is being fed by the small intestine, if the feedings are given continually around the clock, or if the desired rate is less than 200 ml/hr.

Psychologic Impact of Tube Feeding. Recognition of the psychologic and social needs of the patient receiving tube feedings is an important component of nursing care. Patients facing long-term feedings must adapt to the loss of control over food selection and consumption. Because eating is a social, cultural, and sometimes religious activity, adaptation may be difficult. In addition, alterations of body image related to the presence of a nasogastric or percutaneously inserted feeding tube may cause distress.

Thirst, taste deprivation, and inability to satisfy the appetite are common complaints of tube-fed patients. Patients may feel self-conscious surrounded by the equipment and supplies needed for formula administration and may find mobility limited by the feeding pump and pole. Limiting tube feedings to night hours or using gravity administration may enhance adaptation.

An assessment of the patient's lifestyle, home environment, body image, and motivation for tube feeding is critical before implementing therapy. Exploration of the patient's perceptions of the importance of food and eating will assist in identifying areas of concern and is a good starting point for teaching. Involvement of the patient and family in the tube feedings is helpful. The rationale for all procedures should be described, and the patient and family should be encouraged to assist in the feeding.

Occasionally, patients are allowed some oral intake, usually fluids and soft, bland foods. Patients receiving all their nutrition from tube feedings may be permitted to chew gum or suck on hard candies, thus satisfying their sense of taste and their desire to chew. Some patients may satisfy a craving for a particular food by chewing and then spitting it out if they cannot swallow.

Patients requiring long-term enteral therapy may benefit from meeting with other tube-fed patients. The support and role models provided often ease the transition to tube feeding.

Monitoring the Patient. The patient's weight is a simple test for assessing whether caloric and fluid needs are met. Weighing the patient every 2 or 3 days to start will alert the caregiver to a deviance from the anticipated weight gain or maintenance. If the patient loses weight during tube feeding, adjustments in the rate, the formula, or the calorie content may be made quickly.

Serum proteins may also be monitored, usually every 7 to 10 days to start. In the presence of malnutrition, decreased albumin synthesis occurs. With optimal enterally provided nutritional support, serum prealbumin and protein levels may increase as the patient receives adequate calories and protein; however, abnormal metabolism of nutrients in patients with advanced cancer may preclude significant gains.

When giving intermittent feedings via a nasogastric tube, instill air, then aspirate before checking for residuals before feeding. If fluid can be aspirated, check for indicators of gastric placement. The pH of the aspirated fluid should be less than or equal to 5, and a gastric color, such as grassy green, clear and colorless, or cloudy white, and residual formula from previous feedings should be observable. If fluid cannot be aspirated or pH is 6 or greater, the nasogastric feeding tube may have dislodged. The risk of tube dislodgment is increased by patients' retching, vomiting, severe bouts of coughing, and frequent nasotracheal suctioning. If the risk is low and the tube has remained taped in its original position, the next feeding can be started. If the risk is high and the tube has moved, consider the need for an x-ray study to verify placement.[56]

When giving continuous feedings, if the patient is tolerating the feedings without incident, the mark on the tube's exit site is in its original position, and the most recent x-ray results indicate the placement is correct, the feedings can be continued. If the risk of

displacement is high and the tube has moved, x-ray verification of placement may be needed. The pH measurement is not useful during continuous feedings because the formula raises the pH.[56]

Complications of Tube Feeding. Many of the complications of tube feedings are preventable through appropriate selection of formula and tubes, proper administration, and frequent monitoring. Complications may be mechanical or metabolic and may affect the GI and respiratory systems (Table 26-1).[55]

A common complication is tube clogging that results from inadequate flushing or improper administration of medication. As a rule, tubes should be flushed with 30 to 60 ml water at these times: before and after intermittent feedings, every 4 hours during continuous feedings, before and after medication administration, after checking tube placement, and after checking gastric residual and returning contents. Patency of clogged tubes can often be restored by irrigating the tube with carbonated beverages, such as colas and ginger ale.[54]

Diarrhea is a common problem in tube-fed patients, especially when first begun. If the patient has not been eating, the gut may be intolerant of feeding, and feeding should be started slowly. Isotonic formulas (near 290 mOsm) begun at half rate and slowly increased may be well tolerated. The use of fiber-containing formulas can help provide more normal intestinal function. Infection may occur from contaminated feeding or *Clostridium difficile* infection if the patient has been taking antibiotics. Stool culture can help rule out infectious causes of diarrhea.[54]

PARENTERAL NUTRITION

Parenteral nutrition therapy supplies all of the essential nutrients by means of the intravenous (IV) route. Parenteral therapy may be called hyperalimentation and may be partial or total. Many patients receive partial parenteral nutrition in the form of dextrose solutions as part of their usual care. TPN supplies all the daily requirements for protein and calories directly into the bloodstream. Parenteral nutrition is indicated for patients who have totally nonfunctioning GI tracts, require bowel rest, or are intolerant of enteral therapy. Cancers of the GI tract and related obstructions are often indications for TPN. Because absorption of nutrients is impaired in such patients, TPN is often the only option available.[43]

Components. The three main components of TPN are glucose, amino acids, and fats. The glucose content of TPN, usually in the form of dextrose 50%, provides both immediate and long-term energy. Amino acids or proteins are provided with or without electrolytes and are usually ordered in concentrations of 5.5% or 8.5%. The lower concentration is indicated for patients with hepatic or renal dysfunction or failure. Administration of fats with TPN is required because the TPN solution stimulates the production of insulin, which in turn prevents fat from being metabolized. A fatty acid deficiency may result. Fat is provided through lipid emulsions formulated from safflower and soybean oils emulsified with egg phospholipid. Therefore, lipids are not administered to patients with a history of allergy to eggs. Lipid emulsions usually come in a concentration of 10% or 20% and may be "piggybacked" or added to the TPN solution. Exact formulations are specific to the patient and depend on individual requirements, tolerances, body chemistry, and disease processes. Computer programs have been devised that calculate body composition values and TPN prescriptions.[57]

Administration. TPN solutions may be given continuously or by cycling the infusion over 12 to 20 hours per day. Cycling is

TABLE 26-1 Common Complications of Enteral Nutrition	
COMPLICATION	ETIOLOGY
Mechanical	
Local skin irritation and erosion	Use of rigid, large-bore tubes
Esophagitis, pharyngitis	Use of rigid, large-bore tubes
Tube dislocation	Coughing or pulling on tube, tube migration
Tube occlusion	Kinked tube, inadequate irrigation, formula incompletely crushed, incompatible medications
Gastrointestinal	
Abdominal distention	Rapid infusion rate, delayed gastric emptying, formula intolerance
Nausea, vomiting	Rapid infusion rate, delayed emptying, formula intolerance, malabsorption, electrolyte imbalance, contaminated formula
Diarrhea	Rapid infusion rate, formula intolerance, malabsorption, contaminated formula
Constipation	Long-term use of low-residue solutions, inadequate fluid intake
Respiratory	
Aspiration pneumonia	Gastric reflux of aspiration (especially with large-bore tubes), improper tube placement, large gastric residuals, patient's head elevated less than 30 degrees
Metabolic	
Hyperglycemia	Underlying diabetes, sepsis, stress, intolerance to infusion rate
Hypokalemia	Concurrent diuretic, insulin, or antibiotic therapy
Hyperkalemia	Metabolic acidosis, renal insufficiency, excessive potassium in formula
Hypernatremia, dehydration	Insufficient water (especially if hyperosmolar, high-protein formulas used)

From McClave SA, Chang WK: Complications of enteral access, *Gastrointest Endosc* 58:739, 2003.

most often used for patients receiving TPN at home during the night because it allows them to be mobile during the day. The disadvantage of cycling TPN is that patients must be able to tolerate a high-volume load. Cyclic TPN may be increased slowly at the start and then tapered at the end of the cycle. Programmable pumps are widely used to prevent or minimize hyperglycemia and hypoglycemia as blood sugar levels rise and fall. Compact, portable TPN pumps are also available with programmable functions. The portable pump, worn in a backpack-type carrying bag, is best suited for the ambulatory patient.

Patients requiring long-term parenteral nutrition face different challenges than those needing TPN for only a short time. Long-term therapy is most often accomplished in the home with the patient or designated caregiver performing many of the procedures. Patients must be motivated to receive TPN at home, must be able to provide competent self-care, and have a home with essential resources, such as a telephone, running water, and electricity. Consideration must also be given to the geographic location of the patient's home; patients on home TPN ideally should be able to easily access emergency medical services. Another geographic consideration involves the transportation time between the home and the TPN provider; long driving times may adversely affect the stability of TPN.[58]

Monitoring the Patient and Complications of Therapy. Patients beginning TPN must be monitored frequently to assess side effects and complications of the treatment. Daily monitoring of vital signs, weight, and laboratory values may indicate metabolic changes requiring the adjustment of TPN formula or its rate of administration. The metabolic and technical problems sometimes associated with TPN are numerous. Some are related to the insertion of the central venous access device. Other problems include electrolyte imbalance, infection, and volume overload (Table 26-2).[59]

Hypersensitivity reactions to lipid emulsion containing long-chain fatty acids have been reported. Symptoms of hypersensitivity include flushing, dyspnea, tachycardia, hypotension, and back pain. In patients with cancer, hypersensitivity to lipid emulsion can be mistaken for chemotherapy toxicity. **Refeeding syndrome,** characterized by a rapid drop in levels of potassium, magnesium, and phosphorus, may be precipitated by the introduction of TPN in the severely malnourished patient. Excess amino acid intake can cause elevations in blood urea nitrogen (BUN) and creatinine levels. With frequent monitoring by an experienced staff member or well-educated patient performing self-care, the risk of complications is greatly reduced.

Complementary and Alternative Nutritional Therapies

Dietary supplements and herbs are the most commonly used complementary therapies reported by patients with cancer.[60] The wide use of these therapies has been attributed to, among other things, the passage in 1994 of legislation allowing herbal medicines and other food supplements to be sold over the counter without review by the Food and Drug Administration (FDA).

More than 500 different herbs and nutritional supplements are currently on the market in the United States, and patients often obtain herbs from other countries via the Internet or other means. Patients who use herbal and related remedies do so because of belief in their efficacy, perceived safely, and reasonable cost. However, not all herbs, dietary supplements, and related nutritional therapies are safe and effective. Herbal products with toxic effects include chapparal tea (liver failure); feverfew, ginko, and

TABLE 26-2	Common Complications of Parenteral Nutrition	
COMPLICATION	**ETIOLOGY**	

COMPLICATION	ETIOLOGY
Nonmetabolic	
Allergy or sensitivity	Sensitivity to either amino acid solution or lipid emulsion
Infection	Catheter-related sepsis
Volume overload	Improper pump rate
Catheter placement	Puncture of or injury to nearby organs or vessels
Pneumothorax	
Arterial puncture	
Hematoma	
Thoracic duct puncture	
Brachial plexus injury	
Pulmonary embolism	
Metabolic	
Hyperglycemia/hyperosmo-larity	Inability to metabolize high glucose concentration of formula
Hypoglycemia	When TPN is abruptly discontinued, high insulin levels cause rebound drop in blood sugar
Vitamin or mineral deficiencies	Administration of formulas lacking sufficient vitamins or micronutrients
Fatty acid deficiencies or overload	Insufficient or excessive administration of lipids
Hyponatremia	Formulas without sufficient sodium content
Hypokalemia, hyperkalemia	Insufficient or excessive potassium content
Hypocalcemia, hypercalcemia	Insufficient or excessive calcium content
Hypomagnesemia	Insufficient magnesium or increased metabolism of magnesium

TPN, Total parenteral nutrition.
From Ghabril MS, Aranda-Michel J, Scolapio JS: Metabolic and catheter complications of parenteral nutrition, *Curr Gastroenterol Rep* 6:327, 2004.

ginger (anticoagulation); ma huang or ephedra (central nervous system stimulation); and lobella (coma and death at high doses).[61]

The potential for herb-drug interaction is sufficiently problematic that patients on chemotherapy should be cautioned to discontinue using herbal remedies during treatment. Similar advisories are necessary for patients receiving radiation therapy because some herbs photosensitize the skin and cause severe reactions. The risk of herb-drug interactions appears to be greatest for patients with kidney or liver impairment.[61]

Other related nutritional therapies include megavitamin therapy. However, there is no scientific evidence that megavitamin therapy is effective in treating any disorder. The macrobiotic diet, rooted in ancient Chinese medicine, has been used by patients with cancer and is perceived by some to be a way of life as opposed to a diet. The basic macrobiotic diet consists of 40% to 60% whole cereal grains, 24% to 30% vegetables, 10% to 15% beans and sea vegetables, 5% to 10% fish, and 5% soup. Concerns about this diet include inadequate caloric intake for patients with cancer, and the potential for protein and calcium deficiencies.[62]

Ethical Considerations

As patients with cancer enter the end stage of disease, poor appetite becomes a distressing problem for both patients and families. Poor or absent appetite affects not only physical symptoms but also affects functional, social, and psychologic aspects of patients' quality of life. A number of approaches can be used when appetite declines in the end stage of disease, including education, dietary changes, and appetite stimulants. However, these approaches often are met with minimal or no success and caregivers may voice concern that the patient will "starve to death."

When dying patients are unable to take food or drink, health care providers and caregivers must help the patient decide whether to receive nutrition or hydration by artificial means. Providing this support is an area of ongoing controversy because of the difficulties associated with determining life expectancy, the current emphasis on symptom management, and emerging data that suggest that end-of-life cessation of fluid intake decreases secretions and level of consciousness and thereby improves comfort levels.[63] Decisions about providing nutritional support must be based on the needs, wishes, and expectations of both patients and their families. These decisions also must consider the legal and ethical dilemmas of care provision and the need to ensure that the care provided is based on a true examination of the risks, benefits, and burden to the patient.[64]

Nursing interventions for patients with end-stage disease should be directed at structural or functional deficits such as oral mucositis, nausea, and vomiting, and managing concurrent symptoms such as pain, fatigue, and dyspnea. The use of IV hydration may be helpful in loosening pulmonary secretions, decreasing gastric secretions, and correcting fluid and electrolyte imbalances in select patients who are not imminently near death. However, the potential benefits of IV hydration must be carefully weighed against the potential risk of infection, the effect of the therapy on the patient's quality of life, and the cost of IV therapy. In patients with end-stage disease, dehydration decreases pulmonary secretions and level of consciousness, acting as a natural anesthetic. Maintaining moisture of oral tissues with ice chips and lubricants reduces the most distressing side effect of dehydration.[63-65]

Termination of nutritional support should occur when the patient, the family, the physician, and the nurse judge that the patient no longer benefits from the nutritional support. The decision must be made in accordance with accepted community standards of care and in compliance with applicable law.

Conclusion

Cancer and its treatment affect nutritional status to varying degrees. Patients with local and systemic effects require ongoing assessment and prompt intervention. Nutritional support ranges in complexity depending on needs, and those needs change over time. Oral supplementation, the simplest type of support, is most effective when the patient is highly motivated, has manageable or temporary side effects, and can ingest and digest nutrients. Enteral and parenteral nutrition may be required for individuals with more severe symptoms and for those with demonstrated physical impairments of the GI tract. Despite their complexity, enteral nutrition and parenteral nutrition are often administered in the home, with family members as caregivers. Advances in home therapies and nutritional support have enabled individuals with cancer and nutritional deficiencies to remain at home and have promoted an improved quality of life.

CONSIDERATIONS FOR OLDER ADULTS

- Good nutrition in the later years of life can help lessen the effects of diseases prevalent among older adults, such as cancer, heart disease, diabetes, osteoporosis, and other conditions. Poor nutrition, on the other hand, can prolong recovery from illnesses, increase the costs and incidence of hospitalization, and lead to a poorer quality of life.
- The nutritional status of older adults may be affected by physical limitations or impairment may affect the ability to obtain and prepare food, chew food, swallow, or digest food.
- Older adults may overly restrict nutritious foods because of gastrointestinal disturbances, such as constipation, diarrhea, and heartburn.
- Adverse medication reactions can cause older people to avoid certain foods. Some medications, including several chemotherapy agents, alter the sense of taste, which can adversely affect appetite by adding to the problem of naturally diminishing senses of taste and smell, common as people age.
- Many older adults may require special diets because of comorbid conditions such as diabetes and heart disease.
- Social isolation can also affect nutrition. Older people who find themselves single after many years of living with another person may find it difficult to be alone, especially at mealtimes. They may lose interest in preparing or eating regular meals, or they may eat only sparingly. Older men who live alone may not know how to cook and prepare meals.
- Lack of financial resources may lead older people to choose cheaper, processed foods, which are usually less nutritious than lean meats, fish, and fresh fruits and vegetables.
- Financial problems also contribute to delayed medical and dental treatments that could correct problems that interfere with good nutrition.
- Many older adults receive assistance through the Older Americans Act, which provides nutrition and other services that target older people who are in greatest social and economic need. The program focuses particular attention on low-income minorities and rural populations. Home-delivered meals and congregate nutrition services are the primary nutrition programs funded by this act. The congregate meal program allows seniors to gather at a local site, often the local senior citizen center, a school, another public building, or a restaurant for a meal, plus health screenings, exercise, or recreational activities. The meals provide not only good nutrition, but they also give older people a chance to socialize—a key factor in preventing the adverse nutritional effects of social isolation and a way of keeping people actively and socially engaged.

REVIEW QUESTIONS

✓ Case Study

Mrs. Robinson was recently diagnosed with advanced head and neck cancer. She is 5 feet 6 inches tall and weighs 118 pounds. She states that she weighed 152 pounds 6 months ago and attributes her weight loss to anorexia and recent difficulty with swallowing. A food diary reveals that she consumed 640 calories in the past 24-hour period. The oncologist prescribes megestrol acetate for Mrs. Robinson and schedules her to begin radiation therapy and chemotherapy next week.

QUESTIONS

1. What is an indicator of Mrs. Robinson's anorexia-cachexia syndrome?
   a. Impaired swallowing
   b. Extensive loss of adipose tissue
   c. Inadequate daily calorie intake
   d. Weight loss of 34 pounds over a 6-month period of time

2. Mrs. Robinson asks what can be done to reverse the anorexia-cachexia. What is an appropriate response by the nurse?
   a. "Increase your nutrient intake.'
   b. "Start taking a multivitamin."
   c. "A feeding tube may be indicated."
   d. "Your appetite will improve when you begin cancer treatment."

3. What is Mrs. Robinson at risk for when she eats?
   a. Aspiration
   b. Malabsorption
   c. Gastric distention
   d. Bowel fistula development

4. The nurse informs Mrs. Robinson of an acute side effect of radiation therapy to the head and neck area that she can expect to experience in the first few days of treatment:
   a. Oral mucositis
   b. Xerostomia

c. Dental caries
d. Esophageal stricture

5. Mrs. Robinson states that worries that she will be nause-ated after her first chemotherapy treatment. In addition to instructing her to take an antiemetic, the nurse should advise Mrs. Robinson about what to eat:
a. Liquids only
b. Hot, spicy foods
c. Foods with strong aromas
d. Cool, bland foods with little aroma

6. Which of the following history and assessment findings has the greatest potential to negatively affect Mrs. Robinson's nutritional status?
a. Lives alone
b. Hypertension controlled by an antihypertensive
c. Pain reported to range between 1-3 on a 0-10 scale
d. Fatigue reported to range between 1-3 on a 0-10 scale

7. Which of the following is the most sensitive indicator of changes in nutritional status?
a. Serum albumin
b. Serum prealbumin
c. Serum transferrin
d. Total lymphocyte count

8. Enteral feedings are considered for patients who are unable to do which of the following?
a. Swallow
b. Digest nutrients
c. Absorb nutrients
d. Excrete nutrients

9. A risk associated with use of megestrol acetate as an appetite stimulant is the development of which of the following?
a. Adrenal insufficiency
b. Hyperparathyroidism
c. Addison's disease
d. Syndrome of inappropriate antidiuretic hormone secretion (SIADH)

10. Which of the following types of enteral feedings is delivered into the small intestine?
a. Nasogastric
b. Gastrostomy
c. Jejunostomy
d. Esophagostomy

ANSWERS

1. **B.** *Rationale:* One of the indicators of anorexia-cachexia syndrome is extensive loss of adipose tissue. Impaired swallowing (a) may be a cause of anorexia-cachexia syndrome but is not an indicator of this syndrome. Inadequate daily calorie intake (c) contributes to, but is not an indicator of, anorexia-cachexia syndrome. Weight loss of 34 pounds over a 6-month period (d) is incorrect because anorexia-cachexia syndrome is characterized by progressive wasting, not simply weight loss.

2. **C.** *Rationale:* Mrs. Robinson has impaired swallowing. "Increase your nutrient intake" (a) is incorrect because simply increasing nutrient intake does not reverse cachexia. Cachexia alters the normal metabolism of carbohydrates, proteins, and fats and increases energy expenditures. "Start taking a multivitamin" (b) is incorrect because vitamin supplementation will not reverse and correct anorexia-cachexia syndrome. "Your appetite will improve when you begin cancer treatment"

(d) is incorrect because it is highly unlikely that there will be improvement in appetite and intake when Mrs. Robinson begins radiation therapy and chemotherapy.

3. **A.** *Rationale:* Mrs. Robinson's head and neck cancer has caused impaired swallowing, so her risk of aspiration is high when she eats. Gastrointestinal tract cancers may cause malabsorption (b), but head and neck cancers do not. Gastric cancers, not head and neck cancers, may cause pain and distention (c). Bowel fistula development (d) is associated with cancers of the gastrointestinal tract, not with head and neck cancers.

4. **A.** *Rationale:* Oral mucositis is an acute side effect of radiation therapy to the head and neck area that Mrs. Robinson can expect to experience in the first few days of treatment. Xerostomia (b), dental caries (c), esophageal stricture (d) and are late side effects associated with radiotherapy to the head and neck area.

5. **D.** *Rationale:* These foods are usually tolerated well by patients experiencing nausea. Restricting intake to liquids (a) provides insufficient nutrients. Hot, spicy foods (b) and foods with strong aromas (c) are known to cause or worsen nausea, so these foods should be avoided.

6. **A.** *Rationale:* Living alone is the assessment finding that has the greatest potential to negatively affect Mrs. Robinson's nutritional status, since she has been obtaining and preparing foods for herself and will likely need assistance in these areas once she begins cancer treatment. Hypertension controlled by an antihypertensive (b) will not likely affect Mrs. Robinson's nutritional status, and her hypertension may be better controlled because of her recent weight loss. Pain reported to range between 1-3 on a 0-10 scale (c) is considered to be mild pain; moderate to severe pain can negatively affect nutritional intake. Fatigue reported to range between 1-3 on a 0-10 scale (d) is considered to be mild fatigue; moderate to severe fatigue can negatively affect nutritional intake, since it makes patients lack the energy needed to obtain and prepare food.

7. **B.** *Rationale:* Serum prealbumin is the most sensitive indicator change in nutritional status. Serum albumin levels (a) take longer to respond to increased intake. Serum transferrin (c) and total lymphocyte count (d) are indirect biochemical measurements of nutritional status and are not as sensitive as serum prealbumin levels as indicators of change in nutritional status.

8. **A.** *Rationale:* Enteral feedings are considered when patients have mechanical defects that preclude ingestion of nutrients. Nutrient digestion (b), absorption (c), and excretion (d) are considerations for total parenteral nutrition rather than enteral nutrition.

9. **A.** *Rationale:* Megestrol acetate has glucocorticoid-like activity and has been linked to the development of Cushing syndrome, so Addison's disease (c) is incorrect. Hyperparathyroidism (b) and syndrome of inappropriate antidiuretic hormone secretion (d) are incorrect, because megestrol does not alter parathyroid hormones or cause SIADH.

10. **C.** *Rationale:* Jejunostomy feedings are delivered into the jejunum of the small intestine. Nasogastric (a) gastrostomy (b), and esophagostomy (d) feedings are enteral feedings and allow the digestive process to begin in the stomach, not the small intestine.

REFERENCES

1. Ravasco P, Monteiro-Grillo I, Vidal PM et al: Nutritional deterioration in cancer: the role of disease and diet, *Clin Oncol* 15:443, 2003.
2. Ravasco P, Monteiro-Grillo I, Vidal PM et al: Cancer: disease and nutrition care key determinants of patients' quality of life, *Support Care Cancer* 12:246, 2004.
3. Illman J, Corringham R, Robinson D et al: Are inflammatory cytokines the common link between cancer-associated cachexia and depression? *J Support Oncol* 3:37, 2005.
4. American Institute for Cancer Research: Food, nutrition and the prevention of cancer: a global perspective, retrieved May 21, 2005, from http://www.aicr.org/research/report.lasso.
5. Chao A, Thun MJ, Connell CJ et al: Meat consumption and risk of colorectal cancer, *JAMA* 293:172, 2005.
6. Key TJ, Schatzkin A, Willett WC et al: Diet, nutrition and the prevention of cancer, *Public Health Nutr* 7:187, 2004.
7. van Gils CH, Peeters PH, Bueno-de-Mesquita HB et al: Consumption of vegetables and fruits and risk of breast cancer, *JAMA* 293:183, 2005.
8. Willett WC: Diet and cancer: an evolving picture, *JAMA* 293:233, 2005.
9. Sizer FS, Whitney EN: *Nutrition: concepts and controversies*, ed 9, Pacific Grove, CA, 2003, Brooks Cole.
10. Tisdale MJ: Pathogenesis of cancer cachexia, *J Support Oncol* 1:159, 2003.
11. Ramos EJ, Suzuki S, Marks D et al: Cancer anorexia-cachexia syndrome: cytokines and neuropeptides, *Curr Opin Clin Nutr Metab Care* 7:427, 2004.
12. Argiles JM, Busquets S, Lopez-Soriano FJ: The pivotal role of cytokines in muscle wasting during cancer, *Int J Biochem Cell Biol* 37:1609, 2005.
13. Deans C, Wigmore SJ: Systemic inflammation, cachexia and prognosis in patients with cancer, *Curr Opin Clin Nutr Metab Care* 8:265, 2005.
14. Tijerina AJ: The biochemical basis of metabolism in cancer cachexia, *Dimens Crit Care Nurs* 23:237, 2004.
15. Tangpricha V, Colon NA, Kaul H et al: Prevalence of vitamin D deficiency in patients attending an outpatient cancer care clinic in Boston, *Endocr Pract* 10:292, 2004.
16. Wei EK, Giovannucci E, Selhub J et al: Plasma vitamin B_6 and the risk of colorectal cancer and adenoma in women, *J Natl Cancer Inst* 97:684, 2005.
17. Mayland CR, Bennett MI, Allan K: Vitamin C deficiency in cancer patients, *Palliat Med* 19:17, 2005.
18. Thomas C, Thomas L: Anemia of chronic disease: pathophysiology and laboratory diagnosis, *Lab Hematol* 11:14, 2005.
19. Rabbani SA: Molecular mechanism of action of parathyroid hormone related peptide in hypercalcemia of malignancy: therapeutic strategies, *Int J Oncol* 16:197, 2000.
20. Stewart AF: Clinical practice. Hypercalcemia associated with cancer, *N Engl J Med* 352:373, 2005.
21. Locatelli F, Rossi F: Incidence and pathogenesis of tumor lysis syndrome, *Contrib Nephrol* 147:61, 2005.
22. Langfeldt LA, Cooley ME: Syndrome of inappropriate antidiuretic hormone secretion in malignancy: review and implications for nursing management, *Clin J Oncol Nurs* 7:425, 2003.
23. Karumanchi SA, Merchan J, Sukhatme VP: Renal cancer: molecular mechanisms and newer therapeutic options, *Curr Opin Nephrol Hypertens* 11:37, 2002.
24. Lajer H, Kristensen M, Hansen HH et al: Magnesium and potassium homeostasis during cisplatin treatment, *Cancer Chemother Pharmacol* 55:231, 2005.
25. Campbell BH, Spinelli K, Marbella AM et al: Aspiration, weight loss, and quality of life in head and neck cancer survivors, *Arch Otolaryngol Head Neck Surg* 130:1100, 2004.
26. Levy MJ, Wiersema MJ: Pancreatic neoplasms, *Gastrointest Endosc Clin N Am* 15:117, 2005.
27. Schally AV, Szepeshazi K, Nagy A et al: New approaches to therapy of cancers of the stomach, colon and pancreas based on peptide analogs, *Cell Mol Life Sci* 61:1042, 2004.
28. Visvanathan R, Newbury JW, Chapman I: Malnutrition in older people—screening and management strategies, *Aust Fam Physician* 33:799, 2004.
29. Guigoz Y, Lauque S, Vellas BJ: Identifying the elderly at risk for malnutrition. The Mini Nutritional Assessment, *Clin Geriatr Med* 18:737, 2002.
30. Hyltander A, Bosaeus I, Svedlund J et al: Supportive nutrition on recovery of metabolism, nutritional state, health-related quality of life, and

31. exercise capacity after major surgery: A randomized study, *Clin Gastroenterol Hepatol* 3:466, 2005.
31. Scholmerich J: Postgastrectomy syndromes—diagnosis and treatment, *Best Pract Res Clin Gastroenterol* 18:917, 2004.
32. Barker, BF, Barker GJ: Oral management of the patient with cancer in the head and neck region, *J Calif Dent Assoc* 29:619, 2001.
33. Bruce SD: Radiation-induced xerostomia: how dry is your patient? *Clin J Oncol Nurs* 8:61, 2004.
34. O'Brien BE, Kaklamani VG, Benson AB: The assessment and management of cancer treatment-related diarrhea, *Clin Colorectal Cancer* 4:375, 2005.
35. Sharma R, Tobin P, Clarke SJ: Management of chemotherapy-induced nausea, vomiting, oral mucositis, and diarrhoea, *Lancet Oncol* 6:93, 2005.
36. Schwartz AL: Exercise and weight gain in breast cancer patients receiving chemotherapy, *Cancer Pract* 8:231, 2000.
37. Huhmann MB, Cunningham RS: Importance of nutritional screening in treatment of cancer-related weight loss, *Lancet Oncol* 6:334, 2005.
38. Brugler L, Stankovic AK, Schlefer M et al: A simplified nutrition screen for hospitalized patients using readily available laboratory and patient information, *Nutrition* 21:650, 2005.
39. Robinson MK, Trujillo EB, Mogensen KM et al: Improving nutritional screening of hospitalized patients: the role of prealbumin, *J Parenter Enteral Nutr* 27:389, 2003.
40. Sarhill N, Mahmoud FA, Christie R et al: Assessment of nutritional status and fluid deficits in advanced cancer, *Am J Hosp Palliat Care* 20:465, 2003.
41. Green SM, Watson R: Nutritional screening and assessment tools for use by nurses: literature review, *J Adv Nurs* 50:69, 2005.
42. Schattner M: Enteral nutritional support of the patient with cancer: route and role, *J Clin Gastroenterol* 36:297, 2003.
43. Rivadeneira DE, Evoy D, Fahey TJ et al: Nutritional support of the cancer patient, *CA Cancer J Clin* 48:69, 1998.
44. Wong PW, Enriquez A, Barrera R: Nutritional support in critically ill patients with cancer, *Crit Care Clin* 17:743, 2001.
45. Bozzetti F: Nutrition and gastrointestinal cancer, *Curr Opin Clin Nutr Metab Care* 4:541, 2001.
46. Grobbelaar EJ, Owen S, Torrance AD et al: Nutritional challenges in head and neck cancer, *Clin Otolaryngol Allied Sci* 29:307, 2004.
47. Ravasco P, Monteiro-Grillo I, Vidal PM et al: Dietary counseling improves patient outcomes: a prospective, randomized, controlled trial in colorectal cancer patients undergoing radiotherapy, *J Clin Oncol* 23:1431, 2005.
48. Ravasco P, Monteiro-Grillo I, Vidal PM et al: Impact of nutrition on outcome: a prospective randomized controlled trial in patients with head and neck cancer undergoing radiotherapy, *Head Neck* May 26 [Epub ahead of print]:2005.
49. National Comprehensive Cancer Network: Clinical practice guidelines in oncology. Antiemesis (v. 1.2005), retrieved June 3, 2005, from http://www.nccn.org/professionals/physician_gls/PDF/antiemesis.pdf, 2005.
50. Berenstein E, Ortiz Z: Megestrol acetate for the treatment of anorexia-cachexia syndrome, *Cochrane Database Syst Rev* April 18:CD004310, 2005.
51. Martin BR, Wiley JL: Mechanism of action of cannabinoids: how it may lead to treatment of cachexia, emesis, and pain, *J Support Oncol* 2:305, 2004.
52. Grimble RF: Immunonutrition, *Curr Opin Gastroenterol* 21:216, 2005.
53. Delegge MH: Home enteral nutrition, *J Parenter Enteral Nutr* 26:S4, 2002.
54. Arbogast D: Enteral feedings with comfort and safety, *Clin J Oncol Nurs* 6:275, 2002.
55. McClave SA, Chang WK: Complications of enteral access, *Gastrointest Endosc* 58:739, 2003.
56. Metheny NA, Titler MG: Assessing placement of feeding tubes, *Am J Nurs* 101(5):36, 2001.
57. Schloerb PR: Electronic parenteral and enteral nutrition, *J Parenter Enteral Nutr* 24:23, 2000.
58. Hoda D, Jatoi A, Burnes J et al: Should patients with advanced, incurable cancers ever be sent home with total parenteral nutrition? A single institution's 20-year experience, *Cancer* 103:863, 2005.
59. Ghabril MS, Aranda-Michel J, Scolapio JS: Metabolic and catheter complications of parenteral nutrition, *Curr Gastroenterol Rep* 6:327, 2004.

60. Bernstein BJ, Grasso T: Prevalence of complementary and alternative medicine use in cancer patients, *Oncology* 15:1267, 2001.

61. Sparreboom A, Cox MC, Acharya MR et al: Herbal remedies in the United States: potential adverse interactions with anticancer agents, *J Clin Oncol* 22:2489, 2004.

62. Kushi LH, Cunningham JE, Hebert JR et al: The macrobiotic diet in cancer, *J Nutr* 131:3056S, 2001.

63. van Leeuwen AF, Voogt E, Visser A et al: Considerations of healthcare professionals in medical decision-making about treatment for clinical end-stage cancer patients, *J Pain Symptom Manage* 28:351, 2004.

64. Visser A, van Leeuwen AF, Voogt E et al: Clinical decision-making at the end of life: the role of the patient's wish, *Patient Educ Couns* 50:263, 2003.

65. Schwarte A: Ethical decisions regarding nutrition and the terminally ill, *Gastroenterol Nurs* 24:29, 2001.

CHAPTER 27

Skin Integrity

Kathleen D. Wright

Overview and Introduction

The skin is the largest organ of the body, covering approximately 3000 square inches in the average adult.[1] In its protective function, the skin facilitates the body's homeostatic environment, preventing excessive fluid and electrolyte loss. While serving as a barrier against aqueous, chemical, and mechanical injuries and bacterial and viral infection, the skin also synthesizes vitamin D in the presence of sunlight. The thermoregulatory functions of the skin are mediated through sweating and the circulatory mechanisms of vasoconstriction or dilation. Nerve receptors in the skin provide sensation for pain, touch, temperature, and pressure.[1,2]

Alterations in skin integrity are a significant problem, affecting approximately 10% to 25% of nursing home residents.[3,4] As physiologic changes in the skin render the elderly population at high risk for skin breakdown, end-of-life care often includes wound management. Studies of hospice patients report skin failure prevalence rates of 27% 35%.[5,6] Nursing care for the oncology patient, therefore, must include skills related to skin risk assessment, along with wound assessment and treatment, with recognition that the overall goals for quality of life may not be consistent with wound healing.[7-9]

Definitions

Dry desquamation: Dryness and peeling of the epidermis accompanied by itching, which may be manifested after week 4 of radiation therapy.[1,10,11]

Kennedy terminal ulcer: Sudden onset of yellow, black, or red ulceration, typically located on the coccyx or the sacrum, appearing when death is imminent (within approximately 14 to 21 days).[12]

Moist desquamation: Exposed dermis with erythema, oozing of serous exudates, and localized pain, which may appear after 4 to 6 weeks of radiation therapy.[1,10,12]

Pressure ulcer: Tissue injury or destruction may result from prolonged pressure. Cellular metabolism is compromised by impaired perfusion to the area; cells are denied nutrients for viability and growth, and waste products accumulate, resulting in localized tissue injury or death.[1,10,12,13] The term *decubitus ulcer*, derived from the Latin *decumbere* (to lie down or recline) and used to describe this alteration in skin integrity, would erroneously suggest bed rest as the sole etiology (hence the commonly known lay term, bedsore). Pressure ulcers also may occur as a result of prolonged sitting intervals, or from other external forces such as casts, braces, or splints.[1,14-16]

Pressure ulcer stages as defined by the National Pressure Ulcer Advisory Panel can be recognized by the following descriptors[17,18]:

Stage I: An observable pressure-related alteration of intact skin whose indicators, as compared to an adjacent or opposite area on the body, may include changes in one or more of the following: skin temperature (e.g., warmth or coolness), tissue consistency (e.g., firmness or bogginess), and/or sensation (e.g., pain or itching). The ulcer appears as a defined area of persistent redness in lightly pigmented skin, whereas in darker skin tones, the ulcer may appear with persistent red, blue, or purple hues.

Stage II: Partial-thickness skin loss involving the epidermis and dermis. The ulcer is superficial and appears as a shallow crater or blister.

Stage III: Full-thickness tissue loss involving damage or necrosis of the subcutaneous tissue. The ulcer appears as a deep crater, with or without undermining of adjacent tissues.

Stage IV: Full-thickness tissue loss with extensive destruction, tissue necrosis, or damage to muscle, bone, or supporting structures. Undermining and sinus tracts and/or tunnels may be noted.

Reactive hyperemia (blanchable erythema): Appears as an ill-defined erythematous area at the point of pressure on intact skin, varying in color from pale pink to bright red. Digital compression produces total blanching, and erythema may reappear promptly when fingers are lifted.[1,12,14]

Etiology and Risk Factors

A validated skin risk assessment tool should be used as part of the initial patient evaluation and at regular intervals throughout the treatment of course.[1,10,17,18] See Table 27-1 for the Braden Scale, a frequently used tool for the measurement of skin risk. The minimum data set (MDS) Resident Assessment Instrument, used in the long-term care setting, also includes the intrinsic and extrinsic factors that contribute to pressure ulcer development, including the following[19]:

- Diminished sensory perception or ability to respond meaningfully to sustained pressure and related discomfort
- Prolonged skin exposure to moisture, such as urine, perspiration, or wound drainage
- Diminished physical activity or mobility
- Inadequate fluid and nutritional intake
- Friction and shear

Another significant factor that contributes to skin failure is advanced age. Cellular and structural changes of the skin associated with aging include the following: flattening of the dermal-epidermal junction (resulting in reduced shearing and blistering thresholds and diminished microcirculation to the epidermis); reduction in sebaceous gland secretion and intercellular lipid layers (leading to decreased skin hydration and pruritus); and diminished keratinocyte proliferation and epidermal turnover (causing diminished capacity for wound healing). Chronic health problems, particularly those conditions affecting tissue perfusion (e.g., diabetes, peripheral vascular disease, renal failure, or chronic

TABLE 27-1   **Braden Scale**

Patient's Name _____   Evaluator's Name _____

Date of Assessment _____

	1. COMPLETELY LIMITED	2. VERY LIMITED	3. SLIGHTLY LIMITED	4. NO IMPAIRMENT
Sensory Perception Ability to respond meaningfully to pressure-related discomfort	Unresponsive to painful stimuli (does not moan, flinch, or gasp), because of diminished level of consciousness or sedation. OR Limited ability to feel pain over most of body.	Responds only to painful stimuli. Cannot communicate discomfort except by moaning or restlessness. OR Has a sensory impairment that limits the ability to feel pain or discomfort over $\frac{1}{2}$ of body.	Responds to verbal commands, but cannot always communicate discomfort or the need to be turned. OR Has some sensory impairment which limits ability to feel pain or discomfort in one or two extremities.	Responds to verbal commands. Has no sensory deficit that would limit ability to feel or voice pain or discomfort.
	1. CONSTANTLY MOIST	**2. VERY MOIST**	**3. OCCASIONALLY MOIST**	**4. RARELY MOIST**
Moisture Degree to which skin is exposed to moisture	Skin is kept moist almost constantly by perspiration, urine, etc. Dampness is detected every time patient is moved or turned.	Skin is often, but not always, moist. Linen must be changed at least once a shift.	Skin is occasionally moist, requiring an extra linen change approximately once a day.	Skin is usually dry; linen only requires changing at routine intervals.
	1. BEDFAST	**2. CHAIRFAST**	**3. WALKS OCCASIONALLY**	**4. WALKS FREQUENTLY**
Activity Degree of physical Activity	Confined to bed.	Ability to walk severely limited or nonexistent. Cannot bear own weight and/or must be assisted into chair or wheelchair.	Walks occasionally during day, but for very short distances, with or without assistance. Spends majority of each shift in bed or chair.	Walks outside room at least twice a day and inside room at least once every 2 hours during waking hours.
	1. COMPLETELY IMMOBILE	**2. VERY LIMITED**	**3. SLIGHTLY LIMITED**	**4. NO LIMITATION**
Mobility Ability to change and control body position	Does not make even slight changes in body or extremity position without assistance.	Makes occasional slight changes in body or extremity position but unable to make frequent or significant changes independently.	Makes frequent though slight changes in body or extremity position independently.	Makes major and frequent changes in position without assistance.

Continued

TABLE 27-1   Braden Scale—cont'd

	1. VERY POOR	2. PROBABLY INADEQUATE	3. ADEQUATE	4. EXCELLENT
Nutrition Usual food intake pattern	Never eats a complete meal. Rarely eats more than ½ of any food offered. Eats 2 servings or less of protein (meat or dairy products) per day. Takes fluids poorly. Does not drink a liquid dietary supplement. *OR* Is NPO and/or maintained on clear liquids or IVs for more than 5 days.	Rarely eats a complete meal and generally eats only about ½ of any food offered. Protein intake includes only 3 servings of meat or dairy products per day. Occasionally will take a dietary supplement. *OR* Receives less than optimum amount of liquid diet or tube feeding.	Eats over half of most meals. Eats a total of 4 servings of protein (meat, dairy products) per day. Occasionally will refuse a meal, but will usually take a supplement when offered. *OR* Is on a tube feeding or TPN regimen, which probably meets most of nutritional needs.	Eats most of every meal. Never refuses a meal. Usually eats a total of 4 or more servings of meat and dairy products. Occasionally eats between meals. Does not require supplementation.

	1. PROBLEM	2. POTENTIAL PROBLEM	3. NO APPARENT PROBLEM	
Friction and Shear	Requires moderate to maximum assistance in moving. Complete lifting without sliding against sheets is impossible. Frequently slides down in bed or chair, requiring frequent repositioning with maximum assistance. Spasticity, contractures, or agitation leads to almost constant friction.	Moves feebly or requires minimum assistance. During a move, skin probably slides to some extent against sheets, chair, restraints, or other devices. Maintains relatively good position in chair or bed most of the time, but occasionally slides down.	Moves in bed and in chair independently and has sufficient muscle strength to lift up completely during move. Maintains good position in bed.	**Total Score**

IV, Intravenous (feedings); *NPO*, nothing-by-mouth status; *TPN*, total parenteral nutrition.
Copyright Barbara Braden and Nancy Bergstrom, 1988. Reprinted with permission from the authors.
From Braden B, Bergstrom N: Braden scale for predicting pressure sore risk, retrieved from http://www.bradenscale.com

obstructive pulmonary disease) also place the patient at increased risk for skin failure.[1,10,17,20-22]

Anatomic sites at risk for pressure ulcer development when the patient is in the supine position include the heels, the sacrum, the coccyx, the ischial tuberosities, the elbows, the scapulae, the C7 prominence, the occipital area, and the ears. In the lateral position, the lateral malleoli, the medial malleoli, the greater trochanters, the ears, and the lateral aspects of head sustain increased pressure. In the prone position, the toes, the patellae, the iliac crests, the elbows, the sternum, and the ribs are at greatest risk for pressure ulcer development. The plantar surfaces and heels of the feet, the ischial tuberosities, the sacrum, the coccyx, and the elbows may be compromised by prolonged intervals in the sitting position. External devices such as casts, braces, and splints, as well as catheters and drains or oxygen masks and cannulas, may create pressure-related damage to soft tissues.[1,10,17,23]

Consequences of Cancer and Cancer Treatment

The integumentary system of the oncology patient may be compromised when the appetite wanes as a result of either the cancer or its treatment. Adequate protein stores, vitamin C, and zinc are vital to collagen synthesis.[1,17,24] See Chapter 26 for further discussion on this topic. Chemotherapeutic agents slow the growth of new cells and will further impede wound healing.[1,10,25]

Cellular alterations at an intravenous site or along the vein may result from localized reactions to chemotherapy, such as transient erythema or urticaria. Extravasation of vesicant agents into subcutaneous tissues can create severe skin and tissue damage. Resultant tissue necrosis may require surgical debridement and skin grafting. Cautious and skilled chemotherapy administration is warranted to prevent these painful sequelae.[1,10,25] Refer to Chapter 21 for further information.

Wounds falling within the field of radiation therapy will be more challenging to heal secondary to possible localized damage to the microvasculature and surrounding tissues. Acute epidermal and dermal effects of radiation result from dilatation of the capillaries and increased vascular permeability. Associated skin manifestations during the fourth or fifth weeks of therapy include dry desquamation (pruritus, flaking, or peeling); a brown pigmentation may appear in the affected area as a result of an increase in melanin. With high radiation doses (40 Gy or greater), moist desquamation with unroofing bullae may occur. Irradiated skin may remain chronically thin, dry, and semitranslucent, with the absence of hair follicles, and sweat and sebaceous glands. Other localized late effects of radiation therapy include fibrosis, telangiectasis, and carcinogenesis.[1,10,11] Skin and wound treatments should be selected in collaboration with the radiation oncologist, based on product indications as described in Table 27-2. Concurrent chemotherapy can augment the severity of skin reactions. Affected skin must be protected from chemical, mechanical, and thermal irritants or injuries. Refer to Chapter 20 for further information.

TABLE 27-2   Skin and Wound Care Products

PRODUCT CATEGORY	MANUFACTURERS AND BRAND NAMES
Incontinent Cleansers *Indications:* - Should be used for perineal cleansing on all incontinent clients *Contraindications:* - Known sensitivity to any product ingredients	- *Convatec*, Aloe Vesta Perineal Cleanser - *Carrington*, Carrafoam - *Healthpoint*, Proshield Spray Foam - *Hollister*, Restore Clean N' Moist
Moisture Barriers *Indications:* - Should be applied to the perineum after every incontinent episode *Contraindications:* - Known sensitivity to any product ingredients	- *Convatec*, Aloe Vesta Ointment - *Carrington*, Moisture Barrier - *Healthpoint*, Proshield Plus - *Hollister*, Restore Barrier Cream - *3M*, Cavilon Barrier Cream
Skin Sealants *Indications:* - May be used to provide protection to periwound, peritubular, or peristomal skin - No-sting products provide incontinence protection for those patients for whom routine incontinence products are inadequate *Contraindications:* - Skin sealants containing alcohol should not be used on open areas	- *Convatec*, AllKare - *Smith & Nephew*, Skin Prep - *3M*, No-Sting Barrier Film
Antifungals *Indications:* - For BID application on areas affected with fungal rash - Should be used for 10–14 days minimum for effective treatment *Contraindications:* - Product should not be used PRN	- *Convatec*, Antifungal ointment
Transparent Films *Indications:* - Semipermeable, moisture retentive, and nonabsorptive - Waterproof cover dressing - Primary dressing for shallow wounds with minimal exudate or for protection of high-friction areas *Contraindications:* - Not recommended as primary dressing for moderately or heavily exudating wounds - May cause skin stripping on fragile skin	- *Smith & Nephew*, OpSite - *3M*, Tegaderm
Alginates *Indications:* - Absorption of moderate to heavy exudate - Hydrophilic cleansing action with reduction of surface bacteria	- *Bard*, Algiderm - *Smith & Nephew*, Algisite - *Coloplast*, SeaSorb

Continued

TABLE 27-2　Skin and Wound Care Products—cont'd

PRODUCT CATEGORY	MANUFACTURERS AND BRAND NAMES
Contraindications: - May dehydrate or dessicate wounds with minimal exudate	
Composite Dressing *Indications:* - Primary or secondary dressing with adhesive border *Contraindications:* - Requires intact periwound skin for anchoring adhesive border	- *Smith & Nephew,* Op-site Plus - *3M,* Tegaderm Plus
Foams *Indications:* - Absorption of moderate to heavy exudate - Padding of tracheostomy and other high risk sites *Contraindications:* - May dehydrate/desiccate wounds with minimal exudate - Not for use in sinus tracts	- *Smith & Nephew,* Allevyn - *Beiersdorf,* Cutinova - *Convatec,* Lyofoam
Hydrocolloids *Indications:* - Moisture-retentive and highly occlusive for sites with minimal to moderate exudates - Autolytic debridement - Protection from friction injury and external contaminants *Contraindications:* - Not for use in heavily exudating wounds - May promote hypergranulation	- *Coloplast,* Comfeel - *Convatec,* Duoderm - *Smith & Nephew,* Replicare - *Hollister,* Restore - *3M,* Tegasorb
Hydrogels (Amorphous) *Indications:* - Wound hydrator for sites with minimal to moderate exudate - Autolytic debridement *Contraindications:* - Not for use in heavily exudating wounds - May cause periwound maceration	- *Convatec,* SafGel - *Hollister,* Restore - *Smith & Nephew,* Solosite - *3M,* Tegagel

Assessment

A comprehensive wound assessment should be documented on initiation of care and repeated at regular intervals to determine the effectiveness of the selected treatment modality.[26,27] Wound assessment parameters to be recorded include the following:

- Anatomic location (consider use of anatomic figures for clarity)
- Size in cm (include length × width × depth)
- Presence of undermining or tunneling (indicate direction using clock referents)
- Color of the wound (list percentage of pink, black, yellow tissue)
- Stage (use only for pressure ulcers)
- Drainage (describe volume, color, odor)
- Periwound skin status (note as intact, inflamed, indurated, macerated, denuded)

Although the staging parameter of wound assessment is used for pressure ulcers, the depth of tissue injury or death cannot be accurately determined in wounds with a necrotic base. For necrotic pressure ulcers, document the other wound assessment parameters and indicate that the wound could not be staged because of the presence of eschar or slough.[1,10,17]

The cellular structure of granulation tissue is different than intact subcutaneous and dermal layers; therefore pressure ulcers should not be "reverse staged" during the healing process. Studies have shown that fully remodeled scar tissue only attains approximately 75% of the tensile strength of intact integumentary structures.[1] Note and be attentive to identified areas of scar tissue, since these sites are at greater risk for recurrence of skin breakdown.

Diagnostic work-up may include laboratory studies to assess nutritional status and/or presence of clinical infection. Serum transferrin and prealbumin are measures of visceral protein stores. Evaluating serum creatinine is a method of estimating skeletal muscle mass. A complete blood count can offer additional insights since depressed hemoglobin and hematocrit levels can indicate anemia, and total lymphocyte count indicates both visceral protein status and cellular immune function. An elevated white blood cell count can assist in detection of wound infection.[23,24,28,29]

Punch biopsy is the gold standard for identifying infection in the wound.

In the neutropenic patient, the benefits of a wound biopsy must outweigh the associated risks. It must be noted that swab cultures often reflect surface contaminants despite cleansing and/or irrigation before culture, and that chronic pressure ulcers may be colonized with bacteria that do not impede wound healing. A wound biopsy will facilitate differential diagnosis, should concerns about alternative etiologies exist.[17,30]

Simple x-ray studies and magnetic resonance imaging do not permit definitive diagnosis of osteomyelitis, since the presence of inflammation visualized is nonspecific.[1] A triple-phase bone scan in the presence of an elevated white blood cell count may support associated findings of osteomyelitis.

Interventions

PREVENTIVE SKIN CARE

The identification of patients at high risk for altered skin integrity facilitates implementation of prevention strategies tailored to align with overall management strategies.[1,10,14,17,18] Use a pressure-reducing or pressure-relieving mattress or overlay to reduce pressure on the skin and bony prominences. Avoid use of sheepskin, which can cause heat and maceration. Dense foam overlays must be 3 to 4 inches thick to adequately reduce pressure. Maximizing activity levels will help maintain skin integrity, while preventing stasis-related complications of the circulatory, urinary, and respiratory systems.

Bed-bound patients should be turned and repositioned at least every 2 hours. Pillow or foam wedges will facilitate postural alignment and cushion bony prominences. In the side-lying position, avoid positioning directly on the trochanter. Pressure-relieving and suspension devices should be considered for heel protection. The head of the bed should be maintained at less than 30 degrees of elevation, and lift devices should be used for transfers and repositioning rather than dragging the patient against the bed linens. Chair-bound patients should be instructed to shift weight every 15 minutes, if able, and/or repositioned at least every hour. A pressure-reducing seat cushion should be used, avoiding foam or air "donuts," which actually cause increased pressure at the device-skin contact points.[23,27,29]

Provide skin hygiene, using tepid water and a pH-balanced skin cleanser for bathing and moisturizers to promote skin hydration. Maintain environmental air humidification at or above 40%. Incontinence care should include assessment and treatment of urinary and fecal incontinence. If continence cannot be attained, use absorptive underpads that wick moisture away from the skin. Use briefs only when the patient is out of bed and/or ambulatory, to limit associated heat and maceration. Cleanse the affected area with incontinence cleanser and tepid water at the time of soiling, and regularly apply a topical skin barrier.

Maintain adequate hydration and intake of protein, calories, and essential nutrients. Consider nutritional supplements (e.g., high protein, calorie dense drinks) and additional vitamins and minerals (e.g., vitamin C and zinc, which are essential for wound healing).[17,23,24] Consider aggressive interventions such as enteral or parenteral feedings and/or appetite stimulants if consistent with overall treatment goals (see Chapter 26).

WOUND MANAGEMENT

Wound cleansing should be performed at every dressing change for the removal of surface debris and contaminants, using normal saline (0.9%) or another nontoxic wound cleanser. Commercial antiseptics (e.g., povidone-iodine, hydrogen peroxide, and hypochlorite solutions) are cytotoxic and should not be used to clean open wounds. Heavily contaminated or necrotic wounds require thorough irrigation; use a 19-gauge needle and a 35-ml syringe to create optimal force while minimizing tissue trauma.[1,10,17,23,27,31]

Debridement should be considered for removal of necrotic tissue to promote granulation and reepithelialization. Surgical debridement uses a scalpel, scissors, or laser to remove macroscopically identified necrotic tissue from the wound bed. Mechanical debridement involves the use of whirlpool or pulsatile lavage to remove dead tissue; wet-to-moist dressings also assist in mechanical debridement, since necrotic tissue adheres to the gauze and is lifted away when the dressing is removed. Papain-urea (e.g., Gladase ointment, Smith & Nephew; Accuzyme, Healthpoint) is the active ingredient for selective enzymatic debridement. The body's own enzymes function as autolytic debriders with the use of occlusive dressings.[1,10,17,23,27]

The primary purpose of wound dressings is to maintain a wound environment supportive of moist wound healing and to contain exudate. See Table 27-2 for a summary of skin and wound product selections. Topical antibiotic therapy (e.g., silver sulfadiazine cream or triple antibiotic ointment) may be initiated on clean pressure ulcers that are not healing or that continue to produce exudates after 2 to 4 weeks of consistently attentive wound care. Topical antimicrobials should be used with caution since allergic sensitization and/or resistant organism growth may occur. Discontinue use in 2 weeks if there is no improvement or the ulcer worsens. Wounds resulting in soft tissue infections and/or osteomyelitis require systemic antibiotics for control of the bioburden.[1,10,17,23,27,32,33]

TREATMENT FOR RADIATION-INDUCED SKIN CHANGES

Intact skin within the radiation field should be considered at high risk and protected from trauma. Patient and/or caregiver education should include protection of the irradiated skin from possible injury by avoidance of restrictive clothing, adhesives, heat, or sunlight. Minor skin reactions resulting in dry desquamation necessitate these same precautions, along with keeping the affected skin clean and well hydrated. A topical hydrogel or steroid cream may relieve pruritus or burning.

RadiaCream (Medline) is one skin conditioner that may be used both before and after radiation therapy, preventively and for the treatment of dry desquamation. Moist desquamation should be treated following the principles of wound management listed, using a nonadherent or foam dressing based on the volume of wound exudate. Xenaderm (Healthpoint) or Biafine (Medix) are emulsive ointments that may be selected for the treatment of moist desquamation to promote comfort and granulation in a moist wound healing environment.[1,10,25]

PAIN MANAGEMENT DURING WOUND CARE

Even patients who are cognitively impaired, have an altered mental status, or are otherwise unable to communicate about their pain should be assessed for pain using behavioral observation skills. Appropriate analgesic agents should be provided before wound treatments for maximal effectiveness. Nonpharmacologic measures should also be considered. Allowing the patient or a trusted caregiver to perform dressing changes can decrease anxiety levels and increase the perception of comfort during the dressing changes. A sense of control can be established if patients are permitted to designate the time of day for the dressing change, or offered a "time out" signal to indicate when the caregiver might need to pause and allow the patient to "regroup" before proceeding. Deep breathing, diversion, or imagery techniques have also been found to be effective in promoting patient comfort.

Wound etiology and existing comorbidities should be considered in the selection of wound dressings to promote patient comfort, for example, the need to limit the frequency of dressing changes, protect exposed nerve endings along with periwound skin, and allow removal with the minimum of local trauma to the wound site. The plan for pain management during wound care should be communicated with the patient, caregivers and significant others, and all members of the health care team to ensure a consistent and effective approach to managing the pain of a patient with a wound.[1,10,17,34-36]

CARE OF FUNGATING TUMORS

When malignant tumor cells infiltrate and erode the barrier properties of the skin, a malodorous wound may result. Many of these wounds have proliferative growth that has been likened to a fungus or cauliflower in appearance, hence the term "fungating."[37-39] For the patient with cancer, the presence of this necrotic, exudating lesion can be a constant reminder of the progressive, incurable disease. Approximately 5% to 10% of patients with metastatic cancer will develop a fungating wound, with 62% occurring on the breast.[40,41] The effectiveness of odor-absorbing dressings containing activated charcoal (e.g., Convatec's Carboflex; Johnson & Johnson's Actisorb Plus) is linked with the ability to absorb wound exudate and seal onto the intact periwound skin. A well-documented treatment option for the control of wound odor is topical metronidazole, most often applied in a commercially available gel preparation (e.g., Metrogel, 0.75%, Galderma). Although the use of metronidazole for this indication is not approved by the U.S. Food and Drug Administration, crushed tablets dissolved in normal saline solution and applied with gauze to the wound bed once or twice daily will also suppress odor.[40-50]

MARJOLIN'S ULCERS

A histologic manifestation of carcinoma is often found in various types of chronic, nonhealing wounds. These wounds or lesions, named Marjolin's ulcers after the physician who first documented the problem, most commonly are noted in pressure ulcers, venous ulcers, or burn sites. Although the most commonly observed Marjolin's ulcer is squamous cell carcinoma, basal cell carcinoma and, more rarely, malignant melanoma have also been noted.[51-53]

The mechanism of transformation from a chronic wound to malignant tissue is unknown. It is postulated that repetitive trauma, chronic inflammation, immunosuppression, and a prolonged healing phase create a predisposition.[52] Although the conversion of a chronic wound to a Marjolin's ulcer is relatively rare, a biopsy of a nonhealing wound is necessary to rule out possible malignancy. With a positive biopsy of squamous or basal cell carcinoma, successful outcomes have been reported with wide excision and skin grafting.[51-53]

Outcomes and Ethical Considerations

Wound management for patients receiving palliative care may require recognition that treatment goals are not curative. The group For Recognition of the Adult Immobilized Life (FRAIL) describes a compassionate care model that advocates accepting that complete wound closure and, in some cases, prevention of skin breakdown may not occur.[34] Maintaining patient comfort becomes the primary goal. More specifically, the desired nursing outcomes for wound care include relief of pain, elimination of odor, prevention of infection, and maintenance of function.[5,6] Wound care often is an inevitable part of end-of-life care; palliative treatment protocols should promote compassionate care and patient dignity to maintain and enhance the quality of life for patients with cancer and their significant others.[7,3,21,22,28,36,54-57]

CONSIDERATIONS FOR OLDER ADULTS

- Aging skin is thinner and drier, and produces new cells at a slower pace, which contributes to slower wound healing.
- The epidermal–dermal junction flattens and becomes detached with subtle trauma, resulting in more frequent bruising and skin tears.
- Sebaceous gland secretion and intercellular lipid layers are diminished, leading to decreased skin hydration and pruritus.
- Chronic health problems associated with aging, particularly those conditions affecting tissue perfusion (e.g., diabetes, peripheral vascular disease, renal failure, chronic obstructive pulmonary disease), place the geriatric patient at increased risk for skin failure and extended time frames required for wound healing.

Data from Bryant RA, Nix D: *Acute and chronic wounds: current management concepts,* ed 3, St Louis, 2006, Mosby; Brown DL: *Long term care Resident Assessment Instrument (RAI) user's manual v. 2.0,* Baltimore, MD, 1995, Health Care Financing Administration; Baumgarten M, Margolis D, Gruber-Baldini AL et al: Pressure ulcers and the transition to long-term care, *Adv Skin Wound Care* 16(6):299-304, 2003; Rice KN, Coleman EA, Fish R et al: Factors influencing model of end-of-life care in nursing homes: results of a survey of nursing home administrators, *J Palliat Med* 7(5):668-675, 2004.

REVIEW QUESTIONS

✓ Case Study

Mrs. W. is a 72-year-old woman with infiltrating breast cancer and metastasis to her liver and spine. She has chosen not to receive chemotherapy or radiation therapy. She currently lives with her 45-year-old daughter, who has taken a leave of absence from her employer to care for her mother; another daughter and two sons live in the same town and are willing to assist in their mother's care as needed. Mrs. W. has experienced a loss of appetite resulting in a weight loss of 30 pounds over the last few months. She is experiencing back pain associated with movement that is related to bone metastasis, which has resulted in increasing periods of bed rest. She has also experienced increasingly frequent episodes of both urinary and fecal incontinence. A partial-thickness 1-cm crater exposing the dermis has developed over the coccyx, which is draining a small volume of serous exudate; the wound base is moist and pink, with some periwound skin stripping from tape use. Mrs. W. received radiation therapy to the pelvis for bladder cancer 5 years ago. In addition, the breast cancer has resulted in a malodorous fungating tumor to the left chest wall, which is producing significant volumes of exudate. Hospice services have been arranged to assist the patient and her family in managing her end-of-life care.

QUESTIONS

1. Nutrition to support wound healing should include which of the following combinations?
   a. High-protein diet, vitamin C, and zinc
   b. High-carbohydrate diet and vitamins D and E
   c. High-fat diet, vitamin B, and zinc
   d. Low carbohydrate diet, vitamins D and E

2. What is a laboratory study to evaluate visceral protein stores?
   a. White blood cell count
   b. Serum glucose
   c. Prealbumin
   d. Hemoglobin

3. When considering options for pressure reduction, what is an optimal choice?
   a. Sheepskin mattress overlay
   b. Air ring (donut)
   c. Dense foam mattress overlay, 4 inches thick
   d. Dense foam mattress overlay, 2 inches thick (eggcrate)

4. Based on the case study's descriptors of the partial-thickness wound on the coccyx, how would the site be staged?
   a. Stage I
   b. Stage II
   c. Stage III
   d. Stage IV

5. What should be used to accomplish wound cleansing or irrigation?
   a. Normal saline
   b. Hydrogen peroxide
   c. Povidine-iodine
   d. Acetic acid

6. What would be an appropriate dressing selection for the clean Stage II coccygeal pressure ulcer with scant exudate?
   a. An alginate rope
   b. A hydrocolloid dressing
   c. A transparent dressing
   d. An enzymatic debriding agent

7. Important considerations for management of incontinence include which of the following?
   a. Cleansing the perineum with bar soap and warm water after every incontinence episode
   b. Cleansing the perineum with incontinence cleanser and tepid water followed by application of barrier ointment after each incontinence episode
   c. Application of clean disposable brief after every incontinent episode
   d. Cleansing the perineum with a disposable washcloth and applying a moisturizing lotion

8. Caregiver education related to preventive skin care should include instruction on which of the following?
   a. Regular turning and repositioning, using pillows or foam wedges to maintain body alignment and heel suspension
   b. Keeping the head of the bed elevated more than 40 degrees
   c. Lateral repositioning on trochanters at 90-degree angle
   d. Maximizing time spent out of bed in chair

9. What would be included among appropriate treatment choices for the fungating breast wound?
   a. Hydrocolloid dressings
   b. Metrogel with a charcoal cover dressing
   c. Hydrogel with a composite cover dressing
   d. Saline-moistened gauze dressing

10. Over a very short time, Mrs. W.'s condition deteriorates and the coccygeal pressure ulcer is noted to be covered by a thick layer of black slough. What terminology may be used to describe this wound?
    a. Kennedy terminal ulcer
    b. Stage III pressure ulcer
    c. Osteomyelitis
    d. Friction/shear injury to epidermis

ANSWERS

1. **A.** *Rationale:* Protein, vitamin C, and zinc are vital to collagen synthesis. Collagen forms the framework for cellular migration. Other dietary components (b, c and d) are not as crucial to wound healing.

2. **C.** *Rationale:* Serum prealbumin reflects protein stores and thus nutritional intake over the past few weeks. A shift in white blood cells (a) is measured as an indicator of infection, serum glucose (b) is indicative of the body's ability to metabolize glucose intake, and hemoglobin (d) count is indicative of the oxygen-carrying capacity of the blood.

3. **C.** *Rationale:* A dense foam overlay will provide reduced pressure to this patient's bony prominences. Air rings and donuts (b) and sheepskins (a) are contraindicated and can contribute to skin breakdown; 2-inch foam overlays (eggcrates; d) provide insufficient pressure reduction.

4. **B.** *Rationale:* The wound would be correctly described as a stage II pressure ulcer. A stage I (a) site has no visible opening in the epidermis but presents as an area of redness or altered pigmentation that does not resolve when pressure has been relieved for 30 minutes. In a stage III pressure ulcer (c), tissue injury extends down into the subcutaneous tissue; Stage IV (d) extends into tendon, muscle, or bone.

5. **A.** *Rationale:* Normal saline will effectively remove surface debris and contaminants. Hydrogen peroxide (b) and povidine-iodine (c) have demonstrated cytotoxicity and damage new tissues and prolong wound healing. The use of acetic acid (d) is only indicated for Pseudomonas infection.

6. **B.** *Rationale:* The hydrocolloid dressing will support moist wound healing, while protecting the wound site from contamination related to incontinence. Alginates (a) are designed for use in wounds with large volumes of exudate, whereas transparent dressings (c) have no absorptive capacity. In addition, the transparent dressing may further contribute to periwound skin stripping from adhesives. Enzymatic debridement (d) is not needed as the wound has no necrotic tissue.

7. **B.** *Rationale:* Incontinence cleansers are pH-balanced and contain surfactants, which facilitate cleansing without friction to the perineum. Warm or hot water (a) can cause drying of the skin. Disposable briefs (c) can cause skin rashes related to containment of heat and moisture, and should be

Continued

REVIEW QUESTIONS—CONT'D

reserved for use on patients who are out of bed or ambulatory. Option d does not mention use of an appropriate cleanser or barrier product.

8. **A.** *Rationale:* The patient should be assisted to turn and reposition regularly if consistent with overall management goals. Answer (b) is incorrect; the head of the bed should be kept as low as tolerated to prevent friction and shear injuries related to sliding down in bed. Lateral repositioning need not be at 90 degrees (c), since this may cause significant pressure on the small body surface area of the trochanters; lateral positioning at 40 to 45 degrees is adequate to offload the sacrum. Prolonged sitting (d) can cause pressure ulcer development on the ischial tuberosities.

9. **B.** *Rationale:* Metrogel and charcoal dressings are formulated to control malodorous wounds. Hydrocolloids (a) will

not contain large volumes of wound exudate. Hydrogels (c) are designed to provide moist wound healing, rather than serve in an absorptive function. Saline-moistened gauze (d) will provide neither odor-control nor absorption.

10. **A.** *Rationale:* The Kennedy terminal ulcer (a) is correct, since this phenomenon is demonstrated by rapid deterioration of a wound site, typically occurring over the coccyx or the sacrum, when death is imminent. Answer (b) is incorrect, since the wound cannot be accurately staged when the depth of tissue injury is unknown; the presence of necrotic tissue prevents visualization and measurement of wound depth. The presence of osteomyelitis (c) cannot be accurately diagnosed without bone biopsy or a triple-phase bone scan. Epidermal friction and shear injury (d) is not initially seen as necrotic tissue.

REFERENCES

1. Bryant RA, Nix D: *Acute and chronic wounds: current management concepts,* ed 3, St Louis, 2006, Mosby.
2. Fore-Pfliger J: The epidermal skin barrier: implications for the wound care practitioner, Part I. *Adv Skin Wound Care* 17(8):417-423, 2004.
3. Rhoades JA, Krauss NA: *Medical Expenditure Panel survey, chartbook#3: nursing home trends,* Rockville, Md, 2004, Agency for Healthcare Research and Quality, retrieved May 15, 2005, from http://www.meps.ahrq.gov/papers/cb3_99-0032/cb3.htm.
4. Cuddigan J, Ayello EA, Sussman C et al: *Pressure ulcers in America: prevalence, incidence, and implications for the future,* Reston, Va, 2001, National Pressure Ulcer Advisory Panel.
5. Reifsnyder J, Magee H: Development of pressure ulcers in patients receiving home hospice care, *Wounds Compendium Clin Res Pract* 17(4):74-79, 2005.
6. Tippett, A: Wounds at the end of life, *Wounds Compendium Clin Res Pract* 17(4):91-98, 2005.
7. Markle-Reid M, Browne G: Conceptualizations of frailty in relation to older adults, *J Adv Nurs* 44(1):58-68, 2003.
8. Wenger NS, Shekelle PG: Assessing care of vulnerable elders: a COVE project overview, *Ann Intern Med* 135(8):642-646, 2001.
9. Meehan M: Prevalence of wounds among the frail elderly: a look at its value, *Wounds Compendium Clin Res Pract* 17(4):80-83, 2005.
10. Milne C, Corbett L, Dubuc D: *Wound ostomy and continence nursing secrets,* Philadelphia, 2003, Hanley and Belfus.
11. Bruner D, Haas M, editors: *Manual for radiation oncology nursing practice & education,* Pittsburgh, 2004, Oncology Nurses Society.
12. Kennedy, KL: Kennedy terminal ulcer, retrieved May 14, 2005, from www.kennedyterminalulcer.com.
13. Zeleznik J, Agard-Henriques B, Schnebel B: Terminology used by different health care providers to document skin ulcers: the blind men and the elephant, *J WOCN* 30(6):324-333, 2003.
14. Maklebust J, Sieggreen M: *Pressure ulcers: guidelines for prevention and management,* ed 3, Springhouse, Pa, 2001, Springhouse.
15. Sibbald RG, Campbell K, Coutts P et al: Intact skin—an integrity not to be lost, *Ostomy Wound Manage* 49(6):27-41, 2003.
16. Gunningberg L, Ehrenberg A: Accuracy and quality in the nursing documentation of pressure ulcers, *J WOCN* 31(6):328-335, 2004.
17. Hess KT: *Clinical guide: Wound care,* ed 5, Springhouse, Pa, 2005, Springhouse.
18. Ayello EA, Braden B: How and why to do pressure ulcer risk assessment, *Adv Wound Care,* 15(3):125-131, 2002.
19. Brown DL: *Long term care Resident Assessment Instrument (RAI) user's manual v. 2.0,* Baltimore, Md, 1995, Health Care Financing Administration.
20. Baumgarten M, Margolis D, Gruber-Baldini AL et al: Pressure ulcers and the transition to long-term care, *Adv Skin Wound Care* 16(6):299-304, 2003.
21. Rice KN, Coleman EA, Fish R et al: Factors influencing model of end-of-life care in nursing homes: results of a survey of nursing home administrators, *J Palliat Med* 7(5):668-675, 2004.

22. Covinsky KE, Eng C, Lui LY et al: The last two years of life: functional trajectories of frail older people, *J Am Geriatr Soc* 51(4):492-498, 2003.
23. Ratliff C, Bryant D: *Guidelines for the prevention and management of pressure ulcers,* Glenview, Ill, 2004,Wound, Ostomy and Continence Nurses Society.
24. Harris C, Fraser C: Malnutrition in the institutionalized elderly: the effects on wound healing, *Ostomy Wound Manage* 50(10):55-63, 2004.
25. Polovich M, White J, Kelleher L: *Chemotherapy and biotherapy guidelines & recommendations for practice,* Pittsburgh, Pa, 2005, Oncology Nurses Society.
26. Pierce B: Wound assessment and palliative care, *Extended Care Product News* 100(4):16-17, 2005.
27. Ratliff C: WOCN's evidence-based pressure ulcer guideline, *Adv Skin Wound Care* 18(4):204-208, 2005.
28. Brown P, Maloy J: *Quick reference to wound care,* Sudbury, Mass, 2005, Jones & Bartlett.
29. Bolton L, McNees P, Van Rijswijk L et al: Wound-healing outcomes using standardized assessment and care in clinical practice, *J WOCN* 31(2):65-71, 2004.
30. Bill TJ, Ratliff C, Donovan A et al: Quantitative swab culture vs. tissue biopsy: a comparison in chronic wounds, *Ostomy Wound Manage* 47(1): 34-37, 2001.
31. Rodeheaver G: Wound cleansing, wound irrigation, wound disinfection. In Krasner DL, Rodeheaver GT, Sibbald RG, editors: *Chronic wound care: a clinical source book for healthcare professionals,* ed 3, Wayne, Pa, 2001, HMP Communications.
32. Siem C, Wipke-Tevis D, Rantz M: Skin assessment and pressure ulcer care in hospital-based skilled nursing facilities, *Ostomy Wound Manage* 49(6):42-57, 2003.
33. Norton L, Sibbald RG: Is bed rest an effective treatment modality for pressure ulcers? *Ostomy Wound Manage* 50(10):41-53, 2004.
34. Wright K, Shirey J: A pain management protocol for wound care, *Ostomy Wound Manage* 49(5):18-20, 2003.
35. Kazanowski M, Laccetti M: *Pain,* Thorofare, NJ, 2002, Slack.
36. Fleck C: Ethical wound management for the palliative patient, *Extended Care Product News* 100(4):38-46, 2005.
37. Grocott P: The palliative management of fungating malignant wounds, *J Wound Care* 9(1):4-9, 2000.
38. Laverty D: Fungating wounds, informing practice through knowledge and theory, *Br J Nurs* 12(15):S29-S40, 2003.
39. Schiech L: Malignant cutaneous wounds, *Clin J Oncol Nurs* 6(5): 41-44, 2002.
40. Dowsett C: Malignant fungating wounds: assessment and management, *Br J Community Nurs* 7(8):394-400, 2002.
41. Naylor W: Assessment and management of pain in fungating wounds, *Br J Nurs* 10(6):S24-S30, 2001.
42. Wilkes L, White K, Beale B: Malignant wound management: what dressings do nurses use? *J Wound Care* 10(3):65-69, 2001.

43. Kalinski C, Schnepf M, Laboy D et al: Effectiveness of a topical formulation containing metronidazole for wound odor and exudate control, *Wounds* 17(4):84-90, 2005.

44. Boon H, Brophy J, Lee J: The community care of a patient with a fungating wound, *Br J Nurs* 9(6):S35-S38, 2000.

45. Moore K, Schmais L.: *Living well with cancer,* New York, 2001, Berkley.

46. Kelly, N: Malodorous fungating wounds: a review of current literature, *Prof Nurse* 17(5):323-326, 2002.

47. Bird C: Managing malignant fungating wounds, *Prof Nurse* 15(4): 253-256, 2000.

48. Naylor W: Malignant wounds: etiology and principles of management, *Nurs Standard* 16(52):45-53, 2002.

49. Piggin C: Malodorous fungating wounds: uncertain concepts underlying the management of social isolation, *Int J Palliat Nurs* 9(5):216-221, 2003.

50. Lisle J: Managing malignant fungating lesions, *Nurs Times* 97(2):36-37, 2001.

51. Snyder R, Stillman R, Weiss S: Epidermoid cancers that masquerade as venous ulcer disease, *Ostomy Wound Manage* 49(4):63-66, 2003.

52. Malheiro E, Pinto A, Choupina M et al: Marjolin's ulcer of the scalp, *Ann Burns Fire Disasters* 14(1):39-43, 2001.

53. Bello Y, Rohrer T, Phillips T: Diagnostic dilemmas, *Wounds,* 12(5): 350-355, 2000.

54. Shugarman L, Lorenz K, Lynn J: End-of-life care: an agenda for policy improvement, *Clin Geriatr Med* 21(1):255-272, 2005.

55. Fleck C: Dawn of advanced skin care, *Extended Care Product News* 95(5):34-39, 2004.

56. Langemo D, Bates-Jensen B, Hanson D: Pressure ulcers in individuals at the end of life. In Cuddigan J, Ayello E, Sussman C, Editors: *Pressure ulcers in America: prevalence, incidence and implications for the future,* Reston, Va, 2001, National Pressure Ulcer Advisory Panel.

57. Chaplin J: Wound management in palliative care, *Nurs Standard* 15(19):39-42, 2004.

CHAPTER 28

Bone Marrow Suppression

Barbara Holmes Gobel
and Colleen O'Leary

Overview and Introduction

Myelosuppression is the most common dose-limiting side effect related to chemotherapy administration, and it is potentially the most life-threatening side effect of chemotherapy. Chemotherapy, as well as certain biotherapies and radiation therapy, can destroy the proliferating progenitor blood cells (granulocytes, megakaryocytes, and the erythrocytes) of the bone marrow. Not only do these therapies affect the progenitor blood cells of the bone marrow, but they affect the mature circulating cells and lead to the cell count nadir that occurs with these therapies. The destruction of the progenitor blood cells and the circulating blood cells can result in treatment-related neutropenia, thrombocytopenia, and anemia.

Risk factors related to the various cytopenias include patient-related risk factors, treatment-related risk factors, and disease-related risk factors. Patients suffering from protein-calorie malnutrition and cancer cachexia have an increased risk of infection. Another patient-related risk factor in the development of myelosuppression is the age of the patient.[1] Younger patients have been found to be less likely to experience severe cytopenias from chemotherapy because their marrow is more cellular and less fatty. Prior treatments with chemotherapy and radiation therapy are a risk factor in the duration and degree of treatment-associated myelosuppression. The majority of chemotherapy drugs cause some degree of myelosuppression. The duration and degree of the myelosuppression related to chemotherapy drugs is associated with the mechanism of action of the drugs; for example, cell cycle–specific drugs can produce rapid cytopenias. Also, dose intensification and combinations of chemotherapies can produce severe and prolonged neutropenia. Myelosuppression is often more severe in patients whose disease has originated in the bone marrow or that spreads to the bone marrow, since tumor cells in the marrow will physically crowd out progenitor blood cells.

Definition

Myelosuppression is a condition in which there is a marked decrease in the circulating neutrophils, the megakaryocytes, and the erythrocytes of the bone marrow. Myelosuppression is caused by disease and, in many patients, it is caused by the treatment of the disease. Myelosuppression can be caused by chemotherapy, biotherapy, surgery, and radiation therapy. The resulting clinical conditions associated with myelosuppression include neutropenia, thrombocytopenia, and anemia. Each of these clinical conditions poses significant problems and can prove to be life-threatening for the patient with cancer. The care of the patient who experiences myelosuppression is complex, and requires well thought-out plans of care and critical decision making skills of the nurse.

Neutropenia
Overview

Neutropenia is a condition in which there is a marked decrease in circulating neutrophils. It has significant negative clinical outcomes for patients; for example, it is one of the greatest predictors of life-threatening infection in patients with cancer. Neutrophils are the first line of defense against bacterial infection and account for 50% to 60% of the total number of white blood cells (WBCs). Chemotherapy-induced neutropenia (CIN) is the major dose-limiting toxicity of systemic cancer chemotherapy, and is associated with significant morbidity, mortality, and cost.[2] Neutropenia is frequently managed by reducing or delaying the chemotherapy doses, which can result in lower overall survival.[3]

Definition

The Infectious Disease Society of America (IDSA) defines neutropenia as an absolute neutrophil count (ANC) less than 500/mm³, or an ANC of 500 to1000/mm³ in patients in whom further decline is anticipated.[4] The ANC is calculated by multiplying the WBC by the percentage of bands and segmented neutrophils (Box 28-1). The ANC is a benchmark to determine persons at risk for developing infection. The risk of infection is significant when the ANC is lower than 500/mm³, and it is considered to be high when the ANC lower than 100/mm³.

The degree and duration of neutropenia can help to determine the risk of infection. Short-term neutropenia is defined as lasting less than 10 days, and is associated with less risk of infection, whereas long-term neutropenia exceeds 10 to 14 days.[5] Each chemotherapy agent has a relatively predictable period of neutropenia following administration. The nadir, which is the point of lowest WBC level following treatment, usually occurs 7 to 10 days after therapy. Cell cycle–specific drugs produce rapid nadirs in 7 to 14 days, whereas cell cycle–nonspecific drugs cause nadirs in 10 to 14 days.[6] There are also some cell cycle–nonspecific drugs such as the nitrosoureas that produce a delayed and prolonged neutropenia. For adults, the nadir associated with nitrosoureas can occur at 26 to 63 days, whereas in children the nadir occurs at 21 to 35 days.[6] This places the patient at a great risk for infection and other complications associated with neutropenia.

Etiology

The earliest identifiable cell of the neutrophil lineage is the myeloblast. Differentiation from the myeloblast to the segmented neutrophil takes 7 to 14 days. A large number of both mature and immature neutrophils are located in the bone marrow of healthy adults. Circulating neutrophils have a half-life of only 6 to 9 hours. Since the life span of the neutrophil is so short, the bone marrow must constantly produce neutrophils. When chemotherapy is given, the bone marrow is suppressed and stem cells may be damaged.

BOX 28-1	**Absolute Neutrophil Count Calculation**

The absolute neutrophil count (ANC) is calculated as follows:

$$ANC = \frac{Segmented\ neutrophils + bands}{100} \times white\ blood\ cell\ (WBC)\ count$$

The example shows how to calculate the ANC of a patient with the following counts:

Segmented neutrophils = 40, bands = 6, WBC = 2500

$$ANC = (40 + 6) = \frac{46}{100} = .46$$

$$.46 \times 2500 = 1150$$

$$ANC = 1500$$

The neutrophil count is lowered as the mature cells die and are not replaced.

Approximately 70% to 75% of the deaths from acute leukemia and 50% of the deaths in patients with solid tumors are related to infection secondary to neutropenia.[7] At least half of the neutropenic patients who become febrile have an established or occult infection, and at least 20% of the patients with neutrophil counts below 100/mm[3] have a documented bacteremia.[4]

Risk Factors

All patients who are treated with chemotherapy are at risk for the development of neutropenia and complications associated with neutropenia. Identified risk factors for neutropenia can be classified as patient-specific, disease-specific, or treatment-specific (Table 28-1). Patient-specific risk factors include age, gender, performance status, nutritional status, comorbid conditions, and pretreatment health.

PATIENT-SPECIFIC RISK FACTORS

According to a review of 18 published risk models developed to assess neutropenia, advanced age and performance status were validated in at least two of the models.[3] Furthermore, another review of 10 studies found higher age to be a general risk factor for the development of severe neutropenia.[2] Older patients are often treated with lower chemotherapy doses to minimize the occurrence of neutropenic complications. However, older patients with cancer can obtain the same benefit from aggressive chemotherapy as younger patients[8]; therefore, effective management of the risk of neutropenia is crucial so full-dose chemotherapy can be administered to this population of patients. Three additional studies also show that poor performance status is a significant risk for neutropenia.[2] These studies also supported that in older adults, physiologic age or frailty may be a more accurate predictor of risk than chronologic age.

There is an increased risk for neutropenia in patients who also have comorbid conditions. Renal and heart disease increase the risk for febrile neutropenia in patients with non-Hodgkin's lymphoma, as well as in patients with breast cancer.[2] Comorbidities such as sepsis, pneumonia, hypertension, prior fungal infections, and chronic obstructive pulmonary disease have been shown to increase

TABLE 28-1	**Risk Factors for Neutropenia and Neutropenia-Related Events**

Patient-Specific Factors	Age >65 years
	Poor performance status
	Comorbid conditions
	• With non-Hodgkin's lymphoma
	  Renal disease
	  Cardiovascular disease
	• With breast cancer
	  Liver disease
	  Renal disease
	  Cardiovascular disease
	• Sepsis
	• Pneumonia
	• Hypertension
	• Fungal infections
	  Immune deficit and/or decreased WBCs
	Hemoglobin <12 g/dl
	Albumin <35 g/l
	Female
	Open wounds

Disease-Specific Factors	Hematologic malignancies Lung cancer Advanced cancer Uncontrolled cancer Bone marrow involvement Elevated LDH in lymphoma
Treatment-Specific Factors	Chemotherapy regimen High-dose cyclophosphamide Etoposide High-dose anthracycline Intensity of regimen Current or prior radiation therapy Extensive prior chemotherapy Absence of CSF therapy

CSF, Colony-stimulating factor; *LDH*, lactate dehydrogenase; *WBC*, white blood cell.

the risk for serious neutropenic complications, including prolonged hospitalizations for febrile neutropenia and death.[2]

Pretreatment health, as established by laboratory values, has been shown to be predictive of neutropenia as well. Decreased WBC levels, hemoglobin levels below 12g/dl and serum albumin concentrations of 3.5 g/L or less show greater risk for severe neutropenia.[2] The National Comprehensive Cancer Network (NCCN) also indicate female gender, poor nutritional status and low albumin, open wounds, and tissue infection as patient-related risk factors (see Table 28-1).[9]

DISEASE-SPECIFIC RISK FACTORS

Patients with hematologic malignancies are at a greater risk than patients with solid tumors for the development of neutropenia. This is probably because of the underlying disease process as well as the intensity of treatment required for hematologic malignancies. Both advanced disease and uncontrolled cancer have been identified as significant predictors of hospitalization for neutropenia and serious neutropenic complications, including death.[2] In addition to these risk factors, the NCCN also identifies patients with lung cancer, marrow involvement, and elevated lactate dehydrogenase (LDH) (as seen in patients with lymphoma) at a higher risk for neutropenia.[9]

TREATMENT-SPECIFIC RISK FACTORS

Treatment-specific risk factors can also be a determinant in the risk for neutropenia. Some chemotherapy regimens are more myelo-suppressive than others, which puts the patient at a higher risk for neutropenia. High-dose cyclophosphamide, the use of etoposide, and high doses of anthracyclines have all been identified as significant predictors of severe neutropenia.[2] Other treatment-related predictors identified by the NCCN include intensity of the regimen, concurrent or prior radiation therapy, extensive prior chemotherapy, and the absence of colony-stimulating factor (CSF) therapy.[9]

Assessment

HISTORY

A thorough history of patients is important in assessing for the presence or risk of neutropenia. The history should include a review of previous cancer therapies including chemotherapy, biotherapy, radiation therapy, or multimodal therapies. A review of current antibiotic regimens may reveal the use of agents such as trimethoprim-sulfamethoxazole (Bactrim) or amphotericin B, which can decrease the neutrophil count.[10] A review of comorbid conditions as well as current medication use, including hematopoietic growth factors, should be included. Common medications that may cause neutropenia include phenytoin (Dilantin), procainamide (Pornestyl), amoxicillin (Amoxil), cimetidine (Tagamet), captopril (Capoten), enalapril (Vasotec), ibuprofen (Motrin), and ranitidine (Zantac).[1]

PHYSICAL EXAMINATION

Assessment of signs of infection is an important focus of the physical examination of the neutropenic patient. The usual objective signs of infection such as redness, swelling, and pus formation may not be apparent with a decreased neutrophil count. Fever is the most common and important sign of infection and may be the only response to infection in neutropenic patients. Therefore, antipyretic use in the neutropenic patient should be carefully considered. Fever in the patient with neutropenia is defined by three oral temperatures above 100.4° F or 38° C in a 24-hour period, or one temperature above 101.3° F or 38.5° C.[4] Fever is significant in patients with an ANC less than 500/mm³.

The most commonly infected sites in a patient with neutropenia include the anus, the perineum, the skin and mucous membranes, the respiratory tract, the gastrointestinal (GI) tract, and the genitourinary (GU) tract. The respiratory tract is assessed for cough, abnormal breath sounds, and characteristics of expectorants (e.g., color, amount, and viscosity). The GI tract is assessed for abdominal tenderness, stiffness, guarding, and diarrhea. The skin, the anus, and the perineum are assessed for any breaks in integrity and for subtle signs of infection. All catheter exit sites are assessed for edema, drainage, erythema, and tenderness. Tenderness and erythema along the subcutaneous tunnel of an indwelling catheter may indicate a tunnel tract infection. The mucous membranes should be inspected for redness, tenderness, and ulceration. In addition, the oral cavity should be inspected

for thrush and plaque (Table 28-2). Because mucositis can easily progress to secondary infection, oral cultures for fungus and viruses should be obtained.[5] Camp-Sorrell[11] also recommends including assessments of changes in mental status and nutritional status. Protein-calorie malnutrition causes lymphopenia, diminished levels of the complement system, and a decrease of immunoglobulins (Ig) IgA, IgE, IgG, and IgM.[12]

A complete blood count (CBC) with a differential and the ANC are important indicators for neutropenia. However, the diagnosis of bloodstream infections requires blood cultures taken before the administration of antibiotics. Blood cultures are obtained at the first fever and may continue daily as long as the patient remains febrile, until the source of infection is identified or the neutrophil count returns to normal. The current standard requires a minimum of 20 ml/culture set and two sets per episode of fever.[5] There are controversies over the optimal way to obtain blood cultures. Some of these controversies regard whether to obtain cultures from both peripheral and central line sites, and what the adequate volume of blood is for a culture.

Chest radiographs (CXRs) may reveal diffuse infiltrates. Serial CXRs have been useful in illustrating subtle changes in patients with prolonged neutropenia. Computed tomography (CT) has demonstrated pneumonia in up to 60% of cases of neutropenic patients with fevers of unknown origin lasting 48 hours, notwithstanding a normal CXR.[5] Invasive bronchoscopic procedures are used to determine lower respiratory tract infections.

If diarrhea is present the patient should be tested for the presence of *Clostridium difficile*. This bacteria causes toxin release and is treated with an antifungal medication. Patients with prolonged neutropenia are also at risk for an inflammation of the small intestine or colon, called typhlitis, which can progress to bowel perforation.

The most commonly used scale for grading the severity of the neutropenia associated with cancer chemotherapy is the common terminology criteria (CTC) of the National Cancer Institute (NCI). This scale categorizes neutropenia into five grades: grade 0 is a normal WBC and grade 5 is death.[13] However, the

TABLE 28-2	Assessment for Signs of Infection
SYSTEM	**ASSESS FOR**
Respiratory tract	Abnormal breath sounds
	Cough
	Characteristics of expectorants (e.g., color, amount, and viscosity)
Gastrointestinal (GI) tract	Abdominal tenderness
	Stiffness
	Guarding
Genitourinary (GU) tract (perineum and/or anus)	Breaks in integrity
	Subtle signs of infection
Skin (catheter sites)	Edema
	Drainage
	Erythema
	Tenderness
Mucous membranes	Redness
	Tenderness
	Ulceration

grade of neutropenia toxicity related to chemotherapy does not always correlate directly with the incidence of infection.

Interventions

A discussion of interventions should include both interventions found to be effective in the prevention of neutropenia as well as those used for the treatment of confirmed neutropenia. These interventions can be categorized further to include nonpharmacologic as well as pharmacologic interventions.

NONPHARMACOLOGIC INTERVENTIONS

Although neutropenia itself may not be entirely preventable in patients with cancer receiving chemotherapy, biotherapy, or radiation therapy, there are many interventions that have been shown to be effective in the prevention of infections. There are many nonpharmacologic interventions for the prevention of infection. Handwashing remains the single most important intervention to prevent infection. The use of antimicrobial soap and water or alcohol-based hand rubs, when hands are not visibly soiled, is recommended.[14] Other hygiene-related prevention strategies identified include avoidance of urinary catheterization, frequent oral care, and care of malignant cutaneous wounds. Limiting visits to immunosuppressed patients by persons who have symptoms of respiratory infection is also a recommendation that is well supported in the literature.[15]

The use of neutropenic precautions is well established. However, these precautions can vary from institution to institution, and many are based on tradition rather than scientific evidence. It has long been the practice to limit the intake of fresh fruits and vegetables in neutropenic patients. However, very little evidence supports dietary restrictions for neutropenic patients as long as principles of safe food handling are adhered to, including thorough washing of fruits and vegetables before consumption.[7] Other preventive measures that have been found to be effective in the management of neutropenic patients include daily bathing, with attention to meticulous personal hygiene and perineal care; giving meticulous care to all catheters; changing water in pitchers, denture cups, and nebulizers daily; administering nothing per rectum including suppositories, thermometers, and enemas; initiating bowel regimens to avoid constipation; and taking vital signs every 4 hours with complete assessments every 12 hours for hospitalized patients.[11]

PHARMACOLOGIC INTERVENTIONS

Prophylactic treatment of infection with oral antibiotics in neutropenic patients is often used. The fluoroquinolones (e.g., ciprofloxacin [Cipro], levofloxacin [Levaquin], and moxifloxacin [Avelox]) have potent activity against gram-negative aerobes and little effect on aerobes. The prophylactic use of these drugs has been shown to decrease febrile episodes and reduce overall mortality in neutropenic patients.[16]

Hematopoietic growth factors (HGFs) are used to reduce the period of neutropenia, which is the highest period of risk for infection. These glycoproteins activate the production and maturation of specific cell lines. Granulocyte colony-stimulating factor (G-CSF) prompts neutrophil growth, whereas granulocyte-macrophage colony-stimulating factor (GM-CSF) stimulates both neutrophils and macrophages. The NCCN has established practice guidelines for the use of CSFs to assist in their appropriate prophylactic use.[9]

The initial evaluation for the use of CSFs is to identify the risk of chemotherapy-induced neutropenia and febrile neutropenia. The risk is based on patient, treatment, and disease risk factors, as previously discussed. Those with a risk of less than 10% are considered at low risk, of 10% to 20% at intermediate risk, and of more than 20% at high risk.[9] Other factors taken into consideration for the use of CSFs include the treatment intent and overall quality of life.

The use of growth factors as a method to prevent infection has been well established. In a cumulative study of 1544 control patients and 1547 patients receiving G-CSF, the relative risk of febrile neutropenia was significantly decreased by the addition of G-CSF in all disease types.[17] Until 2003, filgrastim (Neupogen) was the G-CSF that was primarily used for the prevention of chemotherapy-induced neutropenia. In 2003 there was release of a pegylated, longer-acting formulation of G-CSF, pegfilgrastim (Neulasta). Campos, Folbe, Mezaand, and others found that there was a significant decrease in febrile neutropenia, hospitalizations associated with neutropenia, and antiinfectives use for patients who received pegfilgrastim as compared to filgrastim (Table 28-3).[18]

The NCCN has also developed practice guidelines for the administration of both filgrastim and pegfilgrastim (Box 28-2).[9] The once-per-cycle pegfilgrastim may allow for better adherence to the recommended dosing schedule as compared to filgrastim, which requires daily dosing. In the study mentioned above, greater than 80% of patients received pegfilgrastim at the recommended times versus less than 50% of patients who received filgrastim.[18]

Once a neutropenic infection has been established, it is imperative to begin antimicrobial treatment as soon as possible. The practice of empiric therapy, which is antibiotic therapy that is started before the specific organism is identified, was begun when it was shown that between 48% and 60% of febrile neutropenic patients eventually had proven sites of infection.[19] This practice began in the early 1970s, when mortality was up to 95% in febrile neutropenic patients. Since the initiation of empiric therapy, the mortality rate is less than 5% to 10%.[20] The IDSA updated evidence based guidelines in 2002 for the use of antimicrobial agents to treat neutropenic patients (Table 28-4). The choice of antibiotic is based on host factors, the risk of neutropenia, clinical presentation, and duration of neutropenia and fever.

Aminoglycosides interfere with cell wall synthesis to destroy bacteria and are effective against gram-negative organisms.

TABLE 28-3   Comparison of Pegfilgrastim and Filgrastim[18]

CSF USED	ANTIMICROBIAL USE NEEDED	EPISODES OF FEBRILE NEUTROPENIA (FN)	HOSPITALIZATION FOR FN
Pegfilgrastim	24.5%	6.3%	3.6%
Filgrastim	32.4%	10.7%	6.6%.

BOX 28-2   **Summary of Practice Guidelines for Administration and Maintenance of Colony-Stimulating Factors (CSF)[9]**

Filgrastim:

- Start 1–3 days after completion of chemotherapy and treat through postnadir recovery
- Give daily dose of 5 mcg/kg (rounded to the nearest vial size) until ANC is normal or near normal

Pegfilgrastim:

- Use with chemotherapy regimens given every 3 weeks
- Some efficacy in chemotherapy regimens given every 2 weeks
- Start 1–3 days after completion of chemotherapy and treat through postnadir recovery
- One dose of 6 mg per cycle of treatment

Close monitoring of drug levels is essential, since they have a narrow therapeutic and toxicity margin. Renal function is assessed daily through laboratory values as well as monitoring of fluid intake and output. The cephalosporins also interfere with cell wall synthesis. The third-generation cephalosporins, such as ceftazidime (Tazadime), are very effective against gram-negative organisms as well as limited types of gram-positive organisms. Fourth-generation cephalosporins, such as cefapime (Moxapime), are effective against both gram-negative and gram-positive organisms. The penicillins are effective against gram-negative organisms. Aztreonam (Azactam) can be used for patients who are allergic to penicillins. Fluoroquinolones are synthetic antibiotics that are effective against gram-negative organisms. vancomycin (Vancocin) is effective for treating gram-positive organisms. Vancomycin is frequently used empirically in patients with indwelling catheters undergoing myelosuppressive therapy.[4]

Despite a lack of evidence to support their use, antifungal medications are often used when a patient remains febrile 5 to 7 days after empiric antibiotic therapy is begun. The drug of choice to treat fungal infections remains amphotericin B, despite its severe toxicities. Side effects related to amphotericin B

TABLE 28-4   **2002 IDSA Guidelines for Use of Antimicrobial Agents in Neutropenic Patients with Cancer**

Initial Evaluation	Determine whether the patient is at low risk for complications; determine whether vancomycin is needed.
Initial Antibiotic Therapy	*Oral Route*—For low risk adults only; use ciprofloxacin plus amoxicillin-clavulanate
	Monotherapy, with vancomycin not indicated—Choose therapy with one of following agents: cefapime or ceftazidime, or imipenem or meropenem.
	Two drugs without vancomycin—Choose aminoglycosides plus penicillin, cephalosporin (cefapime or ceftazidime), or carbapenem.
	Vancomycin plus one or two antibiotics, if criteria for use of vancomycin are met—Choose cefipime or ceftazidime plus vancomycin, with or without an aminoglycoside; carbapenem plus vancomycin with or without aminoglycoside; or penicillin plus aminoglycoside and vancomycin.
Modification of Therapy during the First Week of Treatment	*Patient becomes afebrile in 3-5 days*—If etiologic agent is identified, adjust therapy to appropriate drug. If no etiologic agent identified and patient is low-risk initially, and oral antibiotic was initiated, continue use of same drug. If patient was low-risk and therapy was intravenous, change to oral ciprofloxacin after 48 hours plus amoxicillin-clavulanate for adults or cefixime for children. If patient was high-risk and intravenous therapy was started, continue use of same drug.
	Persistent fever throughout first 3-5 days—Reassess therapy on day 3. If no clinical worsening, continue same antibiotic. Stop vancomycin if cultures do not yield organism. If disease progresses, change antibiotic. If febrile after 5 days, consider adding antifungal with or without change in antibiotic.
Duration of Antibiotic Therapy	*Patient is afebrile by day 3*—If ANC is >500/mm³ for 2 consecutive days, there is no definite site of infection, and cultures do not yield positive results, stop antibiotic therapy when patient is afebrile for >48 hours. If ANC <500/mm³ by day 7, the patient was low-risk, and there are no subsequent complications, stop therapy when the patient is afebrile for 5-7 days. If patient initially high-risk and there are no subsequent complications, continue antibiotic therapy.
	Persistent fever on day 3—If ANC is >500/mm³, stop antibiotic therapy 4-5 days after the ANC is >500/mm³. If ANC <500/mm³, reassess and continue antibiotic therapy for 2 weeks; reassess and consider stopping therapy if no disease site is found.
Use of Antiviral Drugs Granulocyte Transfusions	Antiviral drugs are not recommended for routine use unless clinical or laboratory evidence of viral infection is evident.
	Granulocyte transfusions are not recommended for routine use.

ANC, Absolute neutrophil count.
Used with permission from Hughes WT, Armstrong D, Bodey GP et al: 2002 Guidelines for the use of antimicrobial agents in neutropenic patients with cancer, *Clin Infec Dis* 34(6):730-751, 2002.

include nephrotoxicity (90%); fever, chills, and rigors (80% to 90%); anorexia (50%); headache (45%); vomiting; and anemia.[21] New lipid formulations of amphotericin B (Ambisome) with less nephrotoxicity are now available.

Imidazoles are antifungals that block the synthesis of fungal cell walls. Other antifungals, the triazoles, have good oral absorption and penetrate into the cerebrospinal fluid. Two large studies have shown these agents to be effective in preventing candidal infections.[22] Triazoles have greater efficacy and less toxicity than the imidazoles.[23]

If neutropenia continues and antimicrobial coverage is not adequate, sepsis can quickly develop. Mortality rates from sepsis range from 30% to 80%.[24] Most of the organisms that cause sepsis are gram-negative. If sepsis develops, the patient will have insufficient cardiovascular function, microvascular perfusion, and oxygenation of tissues. The early symptoms of sepsis include fever, rigors, tachypnea, tachycardia, and mental status changes. Increasing sepsis can lead to multiorgan failure and death. Careful assessment and early interventions may hinder the development and progression of sepsis in the neutropenic patient.

Thrombocytopenia

Overview and Definition

Thrombocytopenia, a decrease in the circulating platelet count below 100,000/mm[3], is the most common platelet abnormality associated with cancer. The platelet count is considered to be the single most significant factor for predicting bleeding in the patient with cancer.

Platelets, also known as thrombocytes, are developed from megakaryocytes in the bone marrow. Control of bleeding requires adequate numbers of circulating platelets, as well as their functional capacity to assist in hemostasis or clotting of the blood. Hemostasis is initiated by vascular or tissue injury and culminates in the formation of a firm mechanical barrier: a clot that is made up of platelets and fibrin. The initial events after vessel injury, which provide a temporary cessation of bleeding, include local constriction of the damaged vessel; platelet adherence to the structures within the damaged vessel wall; secretion of multiple components, including nucleotide adenosine diphosphate (ADP),[25] which causes platelets to become "sticky" and thereby increases their adherence to other platelets; and the development of a large platelet aggregate or hemostatic plug, followed by the initiation of the coagulation mechanism, which results in a firm mechanical clot.

Etiology

INCIDENCE

Thrombocytopenia is a common complication related to cancer and cancer treatment. Bleeding, as a manifestation of thrombocytopenia, occurs more frequently in hematologic cancers compared with solid tumors. Hematologic cancers affect the bone marrow, resulting in thrombocytopenia or platelets with altered function. The bone marrow is also a target of chemotherapy and radiation therapy in these cancers, which worsens the thrombocytopenia. Bleeding that results from thrombocytopenia is a cause of morbidity and mortality in patients with acute leukemia. Life-threatening hemorrhage has

been associated with a variety of clinical conditions, including acute myeloid leukemia and in acute promyelocytic leukemia.[26]

The bleeding that occurs as a result of thrombocytopenia can be occult and difficult to detect, or it can present as frank bleeding. The manifestations of bleeding can range from pinpoint petechiae to life-threatening hemorrhage. The most common manifestations of bleeding related to thrombocytopenia include multiple petechiae, purpura, ecchymoses, menorrhagia, epistaxis, and oozing from mucous membranes and localized injuries (e.g., venipuncture or injection sites), as well as frank bleeding from organ sites (e.g., intracranial or gastrointestinal bleeding).

RISK FACTORS

Disease-Related Risk Factors

Platelet production. Cancers involving the bone marrow, such as leukemia, lymphoma, and multiple myeloma, alter platelet production. A low platelet count is directly proportional to the degree of bone marrow infiltration by tumor cells. When tumor invades the bone marrow, the resulting thrombocytopenia is generally part of the pancytopenia that occurs with tumor invasion.[27]

Platelet distribution. Hypersplenism may occur in cancer, particularly in the hematologic cancers. Hypersplenism may also occur as a result of metastasis to the spleen, which is seen in lung, breast, stomach, and prostate cancers. Splenic vein obstruction, seen with pancreatic cancer, can lead to thrombocytopenia caused by congestive splenomegaly.[28] An enlarged spleen may sequester up to 90% of circulating platelets. The bone marrow responds to this lack of circulating platelets by increasing platelet production, but these cells are also sequestered, leading to a worsening of the splenomegaly.[29]

Platelet destruction. Idiopathic thrombocytopenia purpura (ITP) and thrombotic thrombocytopenia purpura (TTP) are both associated with accelerated destruction of platelets. ITP is an autoimmune-mediated thrombocytopenia in which antibodies are formed against the individual's own platelets. The bone marrow continues to produce normal to increased numbers of platelets with ITP, but the alloantibodies destroy the platelets in the general circulation, leading to mild to severe bleeding.[30] ITP is seen most frequently in persons with chronic lymphocytic leukemia, acute lymphocytic leukemia, Hodgkin's disease, and non-Hodgkin's lymphoma.[31] TTP is a severe microvascular disorder of platelet clumping. Although it is an immune-mediated disorder, it is generally thought to be precipitated by medications or bacterial endotoxins related to infection. Both disorders can lead to thrombocytopenia and bleeding.

Treatment-Related Risk Factors

Chemotherapy and biotherapy. Chemotherapy is the most common treatment-related risk factor associated with the development of thrombocytopenia. Chemotherapy temporarily destroys the proliferating cells of the platelet line in the bone marrow, resulting in a decrease in the production of platelet precursors. At the same time, the mature platelets in the general circulation are being cleared at the end of their life span: the average life span of platelet is 7 to 10 days. Chemotherapy-induced thrombocytopenia generally occurs within 7 to 14 days after the administration of chemotherapy, and recovery is seen within 2 to 6 weeks. The severity of chemotherapy-induced thrombocytopenia is associated with the types of chemotherapy drugs used, the dosages of the drugs, the intervals between treatments, previous cancer treatments, and concomitant therapies. Thrombocytopenia associated with biotherapy is not as common as with chemotherapy.

Radiation therapy. The occurrence and extent of thrombocytopenia induced by radiation therapy is associated with the amount of bone marrow in the radiation field. Sites of bone marrow production, including the sternum, the ilia, and the metaphyses of the long bones, that receive 20 Gy or more are at risk for the development of thrombocytopenia.[11] Platelet precursors, or megakaryocytes, are affected 1 to 2 weeks after exposure to radiation, and recovery of platelets takes about 2 to 6 weeks. Because of the localized nature of radiation therapy in most cases, the untreated marrow is able to compensate for the damage to the treated marrow. Radiolabeled monoclonal antibodies deliver radiation directly to tumor cells, resulting in less radiation damage to surrounding cells. However, they may cause temporary thrombocytopenia.[32]

Medication-related risk factors. Multiple drugs are known to cause platelet destruction and dysfunction. Drug-induced thrombocytopenia may be caused by a decreased production of platelets, a nonimmune direct effect on circulating platelets, or by an immune-mediated suppression or destruction of platelets. Some agents that may cause a decreased production of platelets include estrogens, alcohol, thiazine diuretics (as well as furosemide), phenothiazines, antimetabolites, antimitotic chemotherapy drugs, benzene and benzene derivatives, ionizing radiation, nitrogen mustard, and tricyclic antidepressants.[27]

Heparin is the most common drug to cause a nonimmune direct effect on circulating platelets. Heparin may cause a direct aggregating effect on platelets, leading to reversible platelet clumping and resulting in minor bleeding or other complications, or it may lead to the more serious problem of heparin-induced thrombocytopenia (HIT) that may result in serious bleeding. Low-molecular-weight heparins are associated with a lower risk of HIT.[33]

Other drugs that may affect platelet aggregation include aspirin and the nonsteroidal antiinflammatory drugs (NSAIDs). However, aspirin is the only drug that has been shown to cause a significant increase in bleeding. Aspirin places patients are at risk for bleeding because it inactivates platelet cyclooxygenase, thereby preventing the release of vasoactive substances and prolonging the bleeding time. Alterations in platelet aggregation may last up to 4 days after the ingestion of aspirin. The NSAIDs affect platelet aggregation in a similar manner, but their effect lasts only as long as the active drug remains in the circulation. The COX-2 inhibitors have minimal effect on platelets and are an important option for patients with cancer, but should be used with the same caution, (i.e., contraindication is a history of heart disease).[34]

Two drugs that are known to produce drug-induced immune thrombocytopenia include quinine and quinidine.[35] The platelet count may drop rapidly upon sensitization to these drugs. Bleeding may occur as soon as hours after they are ingested. (See Table 28-5 for a list of medications that may alter the platelet count or function.)

Assessment for Thrombocytopenia and Bleeding

HISTORY

The patient history can elicit information about the potential for thrombocytopenia as well as the potential and actual problem of bleeding in the patient with cancer. Key aspects of the patient history include the following:

- Previous cancer treatment, including treatment with chemotherapy, biotherapy, radiation treatment, or a combination of treatments

TABLE 28-5　Medications Known to Affect Platelet Count and Function

MECHANISM OF ACTION	MEDICATION OR OTHER AGENT
Decreased production of platelets	Alcohol
	Estrogens
	Furosemide
	Nitrogen mustard
	Thiazine diuretics
	Ionizing radiation
	Tricyclic antidepressants
	Antimitotic chemotherapy
	Benzene and benzene derivatives
Nonimmune effect on platelets	Heparin
	Aspirin
	Nonsteroidal antiinflammatory drugs (NSAIDs)
Immune-mediated suppression or destruction of platelets	Quinine
	Quinidine

- Review of all medications that the patient is taking, including over-the-counter and herbal medications, with a focus on medications that may alter platelet production or function
- Signs and symptoms of bleeding including headaches, epistaxis, petechiae, easy bruising, gingival bleeding, change in color of stools or urine, and painful joints
- Acute infections (bacterial and viral) that may increase the risk of disseminated intravascular coagulation (DIC)
- Concomitant disorders, such as ITP, that may increase the risk of bleeding
- Transfusion history, including recent transfusions, history of reactions, and response to transfusions

PHYSICAL EXAMINATION

The individual at risk for bleeding related to thrombocytopenia requires routine assessment of all body systems. A thorough physical assessment can detect early signs of bleeding. Bleeding can occur from any part of the body, but common sites of hemorrhage include the brain, the nose, the bladder, the gingiva, and the GI tract. See Box 28-3 for the physical examination of the patient with actual or potential bleeding.

LABORATORY DATA

Laboratory screening tests are done to determine the risk of bleeding related to thrombocytopenia, to measure platelet loss, and to determine the pathophysiology of thrombocytopenia. The screening tests that are done include measuring the platelet count and bleeding time and examining bone marrow aspirate. In addition to screening tests, a number of diagnostic tests may be done to determine and evaluate internal bleeding. These diagnostic tests may include ultrasound, angiography, plain film radiographs, CT scans, and magnetic resonance imaging (MRI).

Platelet Count. The platelet count is the most significant indicator of the potential for bleeding related to thrombocytopenia.

BOX 28-3   **Physical Examination of the Patient with Actual or Potential Bleeding**

Eyes and Ears
Visual disturbances (e.g., diplopia, blurred vision), increased scleral injection, periorbital edema, eye or ear pain

Nasopharynx and/or Oropharynx
Epistaxis; bleeding, ulcerations, or petechiae on the nasal or oral mucosa

Central Nervous System
Mental status changes (may indicate intracranial hemorrhage) including restlessness, confusion, lethargy, dizziness, obtundation, seizure and coma; neurologic changes (may indicate intracranial hemorrhage) including paralysis, change in speech, widening pulse pressure, change in pupil size and reactivity, change in motor strength, and complaint of headache

Integumentary
Bleeding from anywhere on entire skin surface, including skin folds; bruising, purpura, petechiae, ecchymoses; pallor and jaundice; oozing from venipuncture sites, sites of invasive procedures, or indwelling tubes or catheters

Cardiopulmonary
Changes in vital signs including hypotension and tachycardia, tachypnea; peripheral pulses; color and temperature of all extremities; crackles, wheezes, stridor, complaints of dyspnea; hemoptysis, cyanosis

Gastrointestinal
Hematemesis, rectal or abdominal pain, rectal bleeding, blood in stools, bleeding hemorrhoids

Genitourinary
Intake and output, hematuria, character and amount of menses

Musculoskeletal
Warm, tender, swollen joints; diminished mobility of joints

The platelet count measures the number of platelets in the circulating blood. A normal platelet count is considered to be between 150,000 mm³ and 400,000 mm³. A platelet count below 100,000 mm³ is considered to be indicative of thrombocytopenia, and the potential for bleeding is increased. A platelet count below 10,000 mm³ is considered to be indicative of severe thrombocytopenia and can be life-threatening because of intracranial or gastrointestinal bleeding.

Bleeding Time. The bleeding time measures the time that it takes for a small skin incision to stop bleeding. A normal bleeding time is between 1 and 9 minutes. The results depend on the platelet number and function, and the ability of the capillary wall to vasoconstrict. Prolonged bleeding times may be associated with thrombocytopenia and with drugs that affect platelet function.

Bone Marrow Aspiration. Examination of the bone marrow aspirate helps to determine the etiology of the thrombocytopenia. Reduced megakaryocytes in the bone marrow demonstrates an underproduction of platelet precursors, which generally occurs either from the disease crowding marrow elements out of the marrow or from damage to the marrow from treatment. Adequate to increased numbers of platelets in the marrow demonstrates that the platelets are being destroyed in the peripheral blood by the immune system or that the platelets are being sequestered in the spleen.

Therapeutic Interventions and Nursing Care
PREVENTION OF BLEEDING

General Nursing Measures. Prevention of bleeding in a patient who is thrombocytopenic is critical to the safety of the patient. Patients whose platelet counts are 50,000/mm³ or below are generally placed on bleeding precautions (Table 28-6). Although these precautions may be managed by the nurse when the patient is in the hospital, the patient and family need to be aware of the bleeding precautions so that they can minimize the potential for bleeding at home and can help to ensure the safety of the patient.

Environmental safety concerns are valid whether the patient is at home or in the hospital. All objects that the patient may slip on or fall over, such as clutter or throw rugs, should be minimized. Patients who are severely thrombocytopenic should be taught to seek assistance with walking, especially if they feel dizzy or are sedated.

All unnecessary procedures are avoided in the patient who is at risk for bleeding. These procedures include intramuscular and subcutaneous injections, rectal temperatures or suppositories, and any indwelling catheters. The smallest gauge needle is used if the patient requires an injection. The injection site requires firm pressure for 3 to 5 minutes, followed by the application of a pressure dressing to avoid a hematoma. (A hematoma may become more readily infected in a patient who is also granulocytopenic.) Cold compresses or application of a topical thrombin may also be needed to control the bleeding. Pressure dressings are also necessary after a bone marrow biopsy in a patient who is thrombocytopenic. The patient is instructed to lie on the site after the marrow for at least 10 minutes. The physician should be notified if the bleeding does not stop within 10 minutes.

Personal hygiene is critical for maintaining good skin integrity. Along with stressing the importance of daily showering, the skin should be kept moist with the use of an emollient cream or lotion. No studies to date demonstrate that the use of an antibacterial soap protects the integrity of the skin more than a bar or a liquid, nonantibacterial soap. Care should be taken to minimize skin breaks by promoting practices such as the use of paper tape only. Patients should be taught to use only electric razors.

It is imperative to avoid any activities in the patient who is at risk for bleeding that increase intracranial pressure. These activities include retching and vomiting, forceful nose blowing, frequent and forceful coughing, and bearing down using the Valsalva maneuver with bowel strain. Close monitoring and management of nausea, vomiting and retching are required. The use of H_2 blockers or proton pump inhibitors may decrease the risk of upper GI bleeding in patients who are on corticosteroids.[27] Patients should be taught not to pick their noses or blow forcefully when they are thrombocytopenic, since both practices may precipitate bleeding. The nares can be cleaned and moistened by the application of saline or a water-soluble lubricant, using cotton tipped applicators. Humidified oxygen helps to decrease

TABLE 28-6   Bleeding Precautions for Thrombocytopenic Patients

PROBLEM	DESIRED OUTCOME	NURSING INTERVENTIONS
Environmental safety precautions	The patient will be protected from bumps or falls. The patient will experience no bleeding to minimal bleeding. The patient and family will verbalize understanding regarding environmental safety precautions.	1. Clear clutter in patient's hospital room, or teach family to keep clutter clear at home. 2. Remove any throw rugs that the patient may trip over. 3. Teach patients to ask for assistance with walking when weak or dizzy.
Unnecessary procedures and care for necessary procedures	The patient will experience no bleeding to minimal bleeding. The patient and family will verbalize understanding regarding the need to avoid all unnecessary procedures.	1. Avoid all unnecessary procedures including intramuscular and subcutaneous injections, rectal temperatures, suppositories, and indwelling catheters. 2. Apply pressure to injection sites for at least 5 minutes. 3. Apply cold compresses and topical thrombin to injection sites for continued bleeding. 4. Apply pressure dressings to bone marrow sites.
Personal hygiene and maintenance of skin integrity	The patient will experience no bleeding to minimal bleeding. The patient and family will verbalize understanding of the needs for personal hygiene and to maintain skin integrity.	1. Encourage daily showering or bathing. 2. Use an emollient lotion on patient's skin. 3. Use paper tape only. 4. Use electric razor only.
Activities that increase intracranial pressure	The patient will experience no bleeding to minimal bleeding. The patient and family will verbalize understanding of the need to avoid activities that increase intracranial pressure.	1. Teach patient not to pick nose or blow forcefully. 2. Teach patient to clean nares with saline-moistened cotton applicators. 3. Medicate patient to minimize nausea, vomiting, retching, and coughing. 4. Administer stool softeners and laxatives to keep bowel movements soft. 5. Provide for humidified oxygen when oxygen is required. 6. Instruct patients on the need for a high-fiber diet with adequate fluid intake.
Oral hygiene	The patient will experience no bleeding to minimal bleeding. The patient and family will verbalize the need for good oral hygiene.	1. Use a lip lubricant and mouth moisturizer regularly. 2. Keep lips, gums, teeth, and mucous membranes clean through regular cleansing and use of mouth rinses. 3. Use soft-bristled toothbrush or moistened swabs for cleansing. 4. Use only alcohol-free mouth rinse. 5. Avoid use of dental floss and toothpicks if platelet count is <50,000 mm^3 or the patient is bleeding. 6. Avoid use of dental prosthetics, including dentures, if the mouth is sore or irritated.
General considerations	The patient will experience no bleeding to minimal bleeding.	1. Monitor platelet count and other lab data related to the potential for bleeding, and report abnormal values. 2. Assess vital signs q4hr or more often as indicated. 3. Assess each organ system for signs and symptoms of bleeding. 4. Review medication list for any medications that may cause or exacerbate the patient's bleeding. 5. Administer recombinant thrombopoietin as indicated. 6. Administer platelet transfusions as indicated.

the drying of the nares. Cough medication, especially those medications containing codeine or hydrocodone, can help to minimize the cough and potential bleeding. Bowel strain can be avoided by attention to the frequency and character of patients' bowel movements and the administration of laxatives and stool softeners. While instructions on the need for a high-fiber diet and proper fluid intake are appropriate for most patients, any patient who is taking opioids should also be taking laxatives because of the constipating effect of these medications.

Good oral hygiene and systematic assessment of the mouth can help to minimize bleeding and infection in the patient who is thrombocytopenic. A good lip lubricant and mouth moisturizer can help to prevent cracks in the lips, gums, tongue, and the mucous membranes. A soft-bristled toothbrush is needed for any patient whose platelet count is 50,000/mm³ or above. If the platelet count is less than 50,000/mm³ or the patient is bleeding from the gums or oral membranes, soft Toothettes or mouth swabs are used to avoid trauma. Flossing of the gums is avoided when the platelet count drops below 50,000/mm³ or if the patient is bleeding. An alcohol-free mouth rinse is recommended, since mouth rinses containing alcohol can be drying and irritating to the mucous membranes. Likewise, lemon and glycerine swabs are also contraindicated because of their drying character. Any kind of dental prosthetic, including dentures, should not be placed in the mouth if it is sore or irritated.

Hematopoietic Growth Factors. Several hematopoietic growth factors have been studied to evaluate their effect on the growth and proliferation of megakaryocytes.[36,37] The only platelet growth factor that has demonstrated significant clinical efficacy, and that is approved by the U.S. Food and Drug Administration (FDA) for the treatment of severe chemotherapy-induced thrombocytopenia, is recombinant human interleukin-11, or oprelvekin (Neumega).[38] Oprelvekin has demonstrated in randomized placebo-controlled trials that its use can decrease the need for platelet transfusions, and that it can shorten the duration of thrombocytopenia.[39] Platelet counts should be monitored during the time of the expected nadir and until adequate recovery has occurred (i.e., platelet counts have reached 50,000/mm³).

Platelet Transfusions. National guidelines on the treatment of chemotherapy-induced thrombocytopenia were recently published by the American Society of Clinical Oncology (ASCO).[40] These guidelines are evidence-based recommendations based on well-designed nonexperimental trials. The current recommendations include the use of prophylactic platelet transfusions when the platelet count is 10,000/mm³ or less, when the platelet count is less than 20,000/mm³ with necrotic tumors (e.g., bladder or colorectal cancers), or when the performance status is significantly decreased. Transfusions of platelets even when the platelet count is over 10,000/mm³ may be needed in patients with evidence of bleeding or with hyperleukocytosis, in the presence of high fevers, and in patients undergoing invasive procedures.[40] Platelet transfusions are generally ineffective and considered to be unnecessary in patients with ITP unless the patient is bleeding, and are contraindicated in patients with TTP.[27]

Patients may receive either random-donor platelets, single-donor platelets, or human leukocyte antigen (HLA)–matched platelets. Random-donor platelets are pooled from 4 to 8 donor units of whole blood and have a volume of approximately 200 ml. Random-donor platelets expose patients to multiple tissue antigens, which may lead to refractoriness (or lack of response) to platelets.

There is an increased risk of hepatitis with the use of random-donor platelets because of the use of multiple donors. Single-donor platelets are removed by apheresis from a single donor; the number of platelets in a single-donor unit equals approximately the number of platelets in 5 random donor units. Single-donor platelets are often used when patients become refractory to random donor platelets. The risk of viral infection is reduced with the use of single-donor platelets. HLA-matched platelets are platelets that are matched at the HLA complex on the leukocyte. HLA-matched platelets are often used when the patient becomes refractory to single-donor or multiple-donor platelets. Platelets can be stored up to 5 days at room temperature with gentle agitation.

Leukoreduced platelets, from which the WBCs are mostly filtered out, should be used in patients who are severely immunocompromised or who are candidates for stem cell transplantation. Leukoreduction of platelets is done to prevent the development of alloimmunization from antibodies carried by the leukocytes in blood products. Prestorage leukoreduction of platelets is preferred, since most febrile, nonhemolytic transfusion reactions are due to cytokines that are released from leukocytes into the plasma during storage.[40,41] Bedside leukocyte reduction filters can be used if prestorage leukoreduced platelets are not available. Leukoreduction of platelets also helps to decrease febrile reactions to platelets, to decrease the transmission of cytomegalovirus, and to decrease the chance of immunocompromised patients developing graft-versus-host disease.[42]

Irradiation of platelets with ultraviolet B (UVB) light may be indicated in patients with severe immunodeficiency or in patients who are candidates for stem cell transplantation. The process of irradiation kills the lymphocytes in the platelet pack, but it spares the platelets. This process helps to prevent alloimmunization to platelets and graft-versus-host disease in immunocompromised patients.[43] Platelet cross-matching can also be done to attempt to decrease the risk of alloimmunization to platelets. The cross-matching process can detect antibodies in the patient's serum that will react with platelets in potential donor units.[44]

INTERVENTIONS

One of the most important interventions related to bleeding is patient and family education. The patient and family need to be taught to recognize signs and symptoms of bleeding and to report them to their health care provider immediately. Patients and families need to understand the importance of bleeding precautions because of the potentially-life threatening nature of bleeding related to thrombocytopenia.

Direct measures to stop bleeding are instituted immediately with any bleeding related to thrombocytopenia. Direct pressure can be applied to the bleeding site. Invasive pressure management may be needed if the bleeding is from an internal organ. For example, if the patient is experiencing a GI bleed, a balloon tamponade may be required to stop the bleeding. If the patient is experiencing epistaxis, place the patient in a high Fowler's position and apply steady firm pressure to the area of the nostrils below the bridge of the nose. If the bleeding does not stop with pressure alone, an ice bag can be applied to the area, or topical thrombin or topical epinephrine can be applied to the nares. The nares may require packing if these measures do not stop the bleeding within 5 minutes.

Bleeding from oral lesions can be minimized by frequent, but gentle, mouth care. Rinsing the mouth with cool water or saline may help to minimize the bleeding by promoting vasoconstriction. The mouth may require suctioning with a flexible suction catheter. Topical thrombin may be applied to oral lesions to control bleeding.[45]

Platelet therapy is required for active bleeding related to thrombocytopenia. One unit of platelets should increase the recipient's platelet count by 10,000/mm[3]. Several factors affect the patient's response to platelets, including infection, hypersplenism, the presence of fevers, DIC, and the presence of serum antibodies that may increase refractoriness to platelets. Platelets can be obtained by apheresis up to every other day from a particular donor to whom a patient experiences a good response. The administration of acetaminophen, antihistamines, and steroids are often used to premedicate a patient before platelet transfusions to minimize the chance of a febrile nonhemolytic transfusion reaction, although there is no evidence in the literature to support this practice.

Anemia

Overview

Treatment-induced anemia occurs less frequently than neutropenia or thrombocytopenia. The life span of the red blood cell (RBC) (120 days) helps to account for the less frequent occurrence of treatment-induced anemia, in that the bone marrow begins to recover from the therapy before the number of circulating RBCs decreases significantly. Treatment-induced anemia is less life-threatening than either neutropenia or thrombocytopenia, but it can negatively affect a patient's quality of life (QOL).[46] Anemia also has the potential to delay critical drug therapy. Anemia is often manifested by pallor, fatigue, headaches, irritability, feeling cold, and dyspnea on exertion. The degree and severity of the anemia depend on the intensity and frequency of treatment. The decrease in oxygen related to anemia may progress slowly or rapidly depending on the underlying mechanism. To compensate for hypoxia, the body increases cardiac output, dilates peripheral blood vessels, and redirects oxygen to vital organs. This compensation can result in murmurs, dyspnea, tachycardia, palpitations, and pedal edema.

Definition

Anemia is defined as a reduction in the normal concentration of hemoglobin (Hgb) or RBCs in the blood. A decrease in the hematocrit (Hct) or the number of RBCs may also be used to define anemia. The hemoglobin level is used most often because of its accuracy and reproducibility and because it is the value most often related to the physiologic consequences of anemia.[47] Anemia is defined as an Hgb level below 12 g/dl. Mild anemia is defined as an Hgb level of 8 to 12 g/dl in adults and 7 to 10 g/dl in children. Severe anemia is defined as an Hgb level below 8 g/dl.

Etiology and Risk Factors

Treatment-induced anemia can occur in the context of chemotherapy administration, biotherapy, radiation therapy (if the radiated sites are areas of active marrow development), or surgery (related to blood loss), and stem cell transplantation. The most common drugs to cause chemotherapy-induced anemia are those drugs that are nephrotoxic, such as cisplatin (Platinol), ifosfamide (Ifex), interferon, and interleukin-2.[48] The kidney is primarily responsible for the development of endogenous erythropoietin,

which is necessary for erythropoiesis. Thus nephrotoxic drugs can blunt the body's ability to perform erythropoiesis.

The anemia associated with cancer treatment can be exacerbated by other risk factors. These risk factors include blood loss from the GI or the GU tract, inadequate diet with insufficient intake of folate, multiple drug therapies (e.g., alcohol, aspirin, and the NSAIDs), infection, renal insufficiency, and bone marrow infiltration; patients with chronic disease and those with a preexisting anemia (e.g., thalassemia or iron deficiency anemia) are also at risk.

Assessment

HISTORY

Early recognition and treatment of anemia is essential for the patient with cancer. Conducting a thorough history and physical assessment can help nurses monitor patients who are at risk for the development of anemia. The history should include cancer diagnosis, staging and areas of metastases, renal disease, current medications, treatment course and response (including past side effects), dietary patterns for the prior 3 months, acute or chronic blood loss during the prior 6 months, chronic infection or inflammatory disease, reports of any new symptoms within the prior 3 to 6 months, and reports of fatigue-related lifestyle changes during the prior 3 to 6 months.[49] Symptoms of anemia develop when the RBC mass or the hemoglobin supply decreases, because fewer cells are available to transport oxygen throughout the body which results in hypoxia. These symptoms depend on such things as the rate at which the anemia develops, age of the individual, and individual compensatory mechanisms and activity level.[49]

PHYSICAL EXAMINATION

A history that suggests risk or evidence of anemia should be followed by a physical examination (Table 28-7). The patient's general appearance may include pallor and lethargy; however, if anemia is mild, there may be no overt signs. In moderate to severe anemia, the pulse and respirations may be increased. Postural hypotension may also be present with severe anemia. The integument may reveal pallor and dryness of the skin and mucous membranes; brittle, ridged, concave, flattened, or spoon-shaped nails; and brittle, fine hair. Exam of the head, eyes, ears, nose and throat (HEENT) may show atrophy of the papillae of the tongue; a smooth, shiny, beefy-red appearance of the tongue, glossitis or cheilitis (fissuring of the angles of the mouth); and pale conjunctiva or sclera. Cardiovascular symptoms include tachycardia, mild cardiac enlargement and, in severe anemia, functional systolic murmurs. Hepatomegaly or splenomegaly in severe anemia may be revealed with assessment of the abdomen. Although confusion may be present with severe anemia (due to a lack of circulating oxygen), generally there are no unusual neurologic findings.

It is equally important for the nurse to review all diagnostic tests and findings. A routine CBC will show decreased hemoglobin, decreased hematocrit, and decreased reticulocyte count. Other values that are important to monitor include folate, ferritin, vitamin B_{12}, bilirubin, iron, and the total iron-binding capacity.

Fatigue may be the first and most common indication of anemia: 80% to 90% of patients who receive chemotherapy report being fatigued.[50] Patients with cancer have rated fatigue as the leading complaint, outweighing nausea and vomiting.[51] The closer the hemoglobin levels are to normal, the greater improvement in

TABLE 28-7	Clinical Signs of Anemia	
SIGN OR SYMPTOM	**MILD ANEMIA**	**SEVERE ANEMIA**
Hemoglobin level	Adults: 8-12 g/dl Children: 7-10 g/dl	Adults: <8 g/dl Children: <7 g/dl
Hematocrit	Adults: 31%-37% Children: 34%	Adults: <25% Children: <20%
Associated symptoms	Pallor Fatigue Palpitations Slight dyspnea Sweating on exertion	Angina Headache Dizziness Irritability Tachypnea Compensatory tachycardia Dyspnea on exertion and at rest
Skin	Pallor	Pallor Sensitivity to cold
General	Fatigue	Fatigue Exercise intolerance
Pulmonary	Dyspnea with exertion	Dyspnea at rest
Cardiovascular	Tachycardia Palpitations with exertion	Tachycardia Palpitations at rest Systolic ejection murmur
Gastrointestinal	None	Anorexia Indigestion
Genitourinary	None	Menstrual problems Male impotence
Central nervous system	Dizziness Headaches Irritability	Difficulty sleeping Difficulty concentrating

functional status and QOL. Fatigue is described as the sensation of tiredness. Like pain, fatigue is a self-perceived, self-reported sensation. There is evidence to show that fatigue as experienced by cancer patients is different than fatigue experienced by healthy individuals.[52] There are a variety of psychometric tests available to measure fatigue. One of the most commonly used tests to measure fatigue is the Brief Fatigue Inventory (BFI) numeric scale, using a Likert scale of 0 to 10 to grade the fatigue (0 = no tiredness or fatigue, 10 = worst possible fatigue).[53] The BFI is both reliable and valid. Since fatigue is a self-perceived symptom, it is appropriate for the patient to grade his or her own fatigue.

Interventions

To treat anemia effectively, the underlying cause of the anemia must first be identified. If the anemia is related to iron deficiency, supplemental iron may be administered. In general, serum ferritin levels less than 100 ng/ml or transferrin saturation levels less than 20% are taken as evidence of functional iron deficiency, and oral or intravenous supplementation may be warranted.[54] Oral iron, administered with vitamin C, can only

increase the iron stores by 1 mg/day, whereas intravenous iron can increase the iron stores by 800 to 900 mg/day.

Attending to symptoms related to hypoxia is important. Improved hemoglobin has been shown to have a positive impact on both chemotherapy and radiation therapy. Anoxic tumor cells are 2 to 3 times more resistant to radiation therapy than normally oxygenated cells.[55] The use of supplemental oxygen is appropriate if saturation is less than 90%. Teaching patients to rest and conserve energy is also beneficial.

In patients with cancer, fatigue is not necessarily linked to exertion or activity; it is not completely relieved by sleep or rest and is described as unremitting and severe. There has been recent progress in evaluating and treating cancer-related fatigue. Interventions that have shown to be effective include mild to moderate aerobic exercise, conservation of energy, managing other symptoms, providing for adequate nutrition, and supplemental oxygen if the patient is hypoxic.

Consistently across studies, aerobic exercise has shown to be the most effective measure to decrease fatigue in cancer patients.[56-58] Aerobic exercise in these studies has included walking, cycling, and swimming. There has been little study to determine the impact of strength training on fatigue or the combination of strength and aerobic training. Safety precautions relative to individual patients and disease processes must be taken into consideration with any exercise program.

RBC transfusion and erythropoietic therapy have been the primary modes of treating anemia associated with cancer. Current NCCN guidelines recommend transfusion and/or erythropoietic therapy for symptomatic patients.[54] If the patient's hemoglobin level is between 10 and 11 g/dl, the panel recommends the consideration of erythropoietic therapy with or without transfusion.[54] If the patient's hemoglobin level is lower than 10g/dl, the panel strongly recommends erythropoietic therapy.[54]

If hematocrit drops below 25%, the hemoglobin drops below 8 g/dl, or cardiopulmonary symptoms develop, transfusion of 1 to 2 units of packed RBCs over 2 to 3 hours is warranted. RBC transfusions provide a short-term solution, but have significant risks such as the potential transmission of infectious agents as well as transfusion reactions. RBCs should be leukocyte depleted, or a bedside leukocyte reduction filter is used in patients who are immunosuppressed. If the patient is severely immunocompromised, irradiated packed RBCs are administered. One unit of packed RBCs can raise the hematocrit by 3% and hemoglobin by 1 g/dl. The patient should be monitored according to institutional guidelines.

Recombinant human erythropoietin, epoetin alfa, is currently used to treat chemotherapy-induced anemia. Several studies[54,59-61] have shown that both the short-acting agents (epoetin alfa) and the long-acting agents (darbepoetin alfa) are well tolerated and effective in alleviating anemia and its symptoms in patients with cancer. Erythropoietic therapy is effective in increasing hemoglobin levels, decreasing RBC transfusion requirements, and improving the patients' QOL. The agents differ in their biochemical structure and serum half-life, which allows for alternative dosing and scheduling. Table 28-8 lists the current recommended dosing for these agents.[59] Response to treatment should be monitored and adjusted according to results in the individual patient. The NCCN[54] recommends that in patients who respond to therapy, which is measured by a hemoglobin increase by 1 g/dl, the erythropoietin therapy should be continued to maintain optimal

TABLE 28-8	Treatments for Anemia
DARBEPOETIN ALFA	**EPOETIN ALFA**
• Indicated dose is 2.5 mcg/kg weekly. • 200 mcg every 2 weeks is the common clinical dose. • Higher starting doses followed by less frequent maintenance doses are being explored.[51] • Studies showed correlation between rise in hemoglobin and decrease in fatigue.[51]	• Indicated dose is 150 units/kg 3 times weekly. • 40,000 units weekly are clinically effective and are most commonly prescribed. • Higher starting doses followed by less frequent maintenance doses are being explored.[51]

hemoglobin. Assessment of patients with no response to therapy should be performed at 4 weeks for epoetin alfa and 6 weeks for darbepoetin alfa.[54] Doses should be titrated to maintain an optimal hemoglobin level of 12 g/dl. Erythropoietic therapy should be discontinued and transfusion initiated if there is no hemoglobin response at 8 to 12 weeks of therapy.

Follow-up therapy is indicated for all patients who have received erythropoietic therapy. Symptoms should be evaluated with each visit. If hemoglobin levels increase by more than 1 g/dl in a 2-week period, the dose should be reduced by 25%.[54] If the hemoglobin level exceeds 12 g/dl, therapy should be discontinued, and if the patient's hemoglobin then falls below 12 g/dl, therapy should be resumed at 25% less than the prior dose.[54]

Outcomes

PATIENT OUTCOMES

Most patients undergoing treatment for cancer will develop myelosuppression, or one or more of its manifestations (neutropenia, thrombocytopenia, and anemia), at some point in the course of their treatment. Patients and families play a critical role in the prevention and management of many of the complications related to myelosuppression. Nurses are in a key position to educate patients and families about side effects of treatment and how to prevent and manage these side effects.

Outcomes Related to Neutropenia. The primary outcome desired with regard to neutropenia is that the patient will be free of infection. After appropriate teaching, the patient and family will be able to do the following: identify risk factors that have the potential to cause infection; regularly assess for signs and symptoms of infections and report any positive signs and symptoms of infection to the appropriate health care team members; and identify and use appropriate interventions to prevent or manage infection.

Outcomes Related to Thrombocytopenia. The primary outcome desired pertaining to thrombocytopenia is that the patient will experience no life-threatening bleeding. Patient and family education is critical to preventing bleeding related to thrombocytopenia. After appropriate teaching, the patient and family will be able to do the following: identify risk factors with the potential to cause bleeding; assess for the presence of bleeding; use appropriate interventions to prevent or manage bleeding; identify safety measures to prevent falls or accidents when the

platelet count is low; and report any signs or symptoms of bleeding to the appropriate health care team members.

Outcomes Related to Anemia. The primary outcome desired in relation to anemia is that the patient will not experience significant fatigue or dyspnea. After appropriate teaching, the patient and family will be able to do the following: identify the signs and symptoms of anemia; identify risk factors with the potential to cause anemia; identify safety measures to prevent incidents related to fatigue, syncope, or dizziness; use appropriate interventions (including adequate nutrition) to prevent and manage anemia; and report any signs or symptoms of anemia to the appropriate health care team members.

NURSING-SENSITIVE PATIENT OUTCOMES

Nursing sensitive patient outcomes are patient outcomes that are amenable to nursing intervention. Nursing-sensitive patient outcomes represent the impact of nursing interventions on areas such as a patient's symptom management, functional status, QOL, psychologic distress, cost, and utilization of healthcare resources.[62] Measurement of nursing-sensitive outcomes is important for the patient (to ensure patients' ability to receive care that enables them to achieve the best outcomes), nursing (to demonstrate the impact of nursing on patient care and outcomes related to care), and policy makers (to secure appropriate funding for nursing and for reimbursement purposes).[62]

The prevention and management of myelosuppression offers a number of opportunities to demonstrate nursing-sensitive patient outcomes. Prevention of infection related to neutropenia is within the scope of nursing. Not only do nurses teach patients and families about methods to decrease infection, but the daily practices of nursing such as handwashing and close attention to assessment of the patient can help to prevent infection. Early detection of infection provides the patient the best opportunity for a positive outcome. Thorough nursing assessment of the patient and close monitoring of lab values can assist in early identification of infection. Becoming familiar with the standards and guidelines for administration of growth factors as well as empiric antimicrobial therapy will allow the nurse to advocate best practice for the patient. Once the patient demonstrates signs and symptoms of infection, it is imperative for the nurse to proceed quickly. Fever in a neutropenic patient makes blood cultures necessary, and close attention must be paid to quick administration of antibiotics after the blood cultures have been obtained.

Preventing and managing bleeding are key nursing actions in managing the patient with thrombocytopenia. Safety of the patient with a low platelet count is critical. By attending to the safety of the patient, poor outcomes such as an intracranial bleed may be prevented. Early detection of bleeding can help to prevent life-threatening complications in the thrombocytopenic patient. A thorough head-to-toe examination of the patient who is at risk or is experiencing bleeding is done frequently. Rapid response to bleeding is critical in the thrombocytopenic patient, and this includes administration of platelets. Knowledge of the different types of platelet products and the problem of refractoriness and alloimmunization allows the nurse to advocate for the appropriate platelet product for the patient.

Early detection of anemia can help to decrease the negative impact of this symptom on patients. Early detection is done through close attention to lab values, but also by listening to patients and their subjective complaints. Although patients often compensate for decreasing hemoglobin, their subjective complaints of fatigue or dyspnea can be an early symptom of low hemoglobin. Educating patients and families on the signs and symptoms of anemia is key in helping to maintain patients' QOL. When patients do experience the effects of anemia, the nurse can help to identify ways to maximize activity tolerance and describe strategies to conserve energy. Nurses can help to establish sleep and rest patterns to achieve optimal performance of activities. Monitoring of lab values related to erythropoietic therapy (platelet transfusions or CSF therapy), especially monitoring the impact of CSFs on the hemoglobin level, helps to optimize patients' well-being.

Ethical Considerations

Myelosuppression from disease or treatment places the patient with cancer at risk for significant morbidity and mortality. The neutropenia, the thrombocytopenia, and the anemia related to myelosuppression can all be potentially life-threatening in the patient with cancer. Side effects from cancer treatment, including pain, fatigue, and nausea and vomiting, may also affect the patient who is treated for cancer. It is critical that patients undergoing cancer treatment understand the risks and benefits of the treatment.

The patient's QOL is important to evaluate throughout treatment. Poor QOL during chemotherapy can negatively influence a patient's willingness to continue treatment.[63] Padilla and Ropka cite several studies that indicate that the QOL in patients with neutropenia is reduced.[63]

The management of neutropenia may include chemotherapy dose reductions or delays. It is not clear from current research what the impact of dose reductions or dose delays is on patient survival. Every attempt should be made to keep the patient on the intended schedule of therapy. One method to decrease the duration and severity of neutropenia is the use of CSFs. Since current data indicate that the pegylated form of G-CSF is comparable in efficacy to the short-acting form, patient lifestyle and QOL are valid criteria for choosing the type of CSF to use.

The management of thrombocytopenia and anemia include the use of blood products. All blood products have inherent risk associated with their use, and the patient must be aware of these risks. Knowing the religious or cultural beliefs of the patient is crucial. If a patient is opposed to blood component therapy because of religious or cultural beliefs, other options must be considered and discussed with the patient.

The use of thrombopoietic and erythropoietic therapy must be clearly explained to patients. It is important that patients understand the time that these products take to be effective. There have been studies that indicate negative side effects related to the use of erythropoietic therapy.[54] Seizures, hypertension, thrombosis, and pure red cell aplasia are among the adverse effects of erythropoietic therapy. In addition, the NCCN reports two studies that have reported decreased survival in patients with cancer who have received erythropoietic therapy.[54] Further study is necessary to investigate the long-term and survival issues related to patients with cancer and cancer treatment.

CONSIDERATIONS FOR OLDER ADULTS

- Advanced age increases risk for developing severe neutropenia.[2]
- Effective management of neutropenia is crucial to be able to administer full-dose chemotherapy to older adult patients with cancer.[2]
- Comorbidities such as renal and heart disease increase the risk for febrile neutropenia.[2]
- Ability to self-administer colony-stimulating factors must include assessment of visual acuity, as well as fine motor skills, of older adults.
- A complete medication history is vital since multiple drugs are known to cause platelet destruction and dysfunction.[27]
- Encourage moisturizing dry skin with emollient cream or lotion to maintain good skin integrity.
- Encourage mild to moderate aerobic exercise such as swimming or walking to help alleviate cancer-related fatigue.
- Pluripotent hemopoietic stem cell reserves are decreased in persons aged 65 and older, causing increased risk of myelosuppression.[64]
- The use of colony-stimulating factors and erythropoietin may reduce the mortality and morbidity of myelosuppression in older patients who receive chemotherapy.[65]

REVIEW QUESTIONS

✓ Case Study

DM is a 54-year-old female who was recently diagnosed with acute promyelocytic leukemia (APML). Her admission labs included a WBC count of 87,000/mm³, an Hgb level of 7 g/dl, and platelets of 9,000/mm³. She was initially treated with hydroxycarbamide (Hydrea) to rapidly decrease her WBC count, 2 units of packed RBCs, and 1 unit of platelets obtained by apheresis. Upon the results of her bone marrow biopsy and insertion of a central-line catheter, DM was started on chemotherapy (cytosine arabinoside, or cytarabine [Cytosar-U, Ara-C], and daunorubicin) and all-trans retinoic acid (ATRA) therapy. DM was also started on prophylactic ciprofloxacin (Cipro). The Hydrea therapy was discontinued after the cytarabine and daunorubicin were initiated.

On day 9 of her chemotherapy regimen DM's counts were as follows: WBC count of 2500/mm³, Hgb of 7.6 g/dl, and platelets of 8,000/mm³. At 10 AM on day 9, the patient's temperature was 102.7° F, and she had a blood pressure of 100/70, respirations of 22, and pulse of 110. Blood cultures were immediately obtained, and the patient was started on a broad-spectrum antibiotic within 1 hour of the temperature reading. Vancocin was also started at this time. She also received 2 units of packed RBCs and 1 unit of platelets obtained by apheresis. Later that day, DM began to have an uncontrolled nose bleed, and it was noted that she had frank blood in her urine. Her posttreatment platelet count from the morning revealed a platelet count of 7,000/mm³. DM also complains of dizziness and significant fatigue.

QUESTIONS

1. The RN would expect to see neutropenia in DM for what reasons?
   a. Her admission WBC and her Hgb
   b. History of extensive prior chemotherapy

Continued

REVIEW QUESTIONS—CONT'D

c. DM is unwilling to get out of bed and exercise

d. Marrow involvement of her disease and her Hgb

2. What is this patient's absolute neutrophil count on the day of her first febrile episode? (polysegmented neutrophils (segs) = 40, bands = 6)

   a. 1000

   b. 1150

   c. 2500

   d. 3500

3. What is the rationale for the initiation of the Vancocin on day 9?

   a. Vancocin is good antifungal coverage.

   b. Vancocin is good for gram-positive bacteria, which is often seen with central-line catheters.

   c. Vancocin is good for gram-negative bacteria, which is often seen with central-line catheters.

   d. Vancocin is a broad-spectrum antibiotic, which is necessary until the specific bacteria have time to grow.

4. What is the primary reason that hematopoietic growth factors (HGFs) are used for neutropenia?

   a. To prevent the occurrence of neutropenia

   b. To promote the growth of neutrophils and lymphocytes

   c. The HGFs provide symptom relief to patients: patients state that they feel better on HGFs.

   d. The HGFs have been found to reduce the period of neutropenia, which is the highest period of risk for infection.

5. Why is DM at high risk for bleeding?

   a. Platelets may be sequestered in an enlarged spleen.

   b. Leukemia invades the bone marrow, resulting in thrombocytopenia.

   c. DM is suffering from heparin-induced thrombocytopenia (HIT).

   d. Her age puts her at great risk for bleeding when she receives the chemotherapy.

6. Appropriate nursing measures to help stop DM's nosebleed include which of the following?

   a. Cold compresses to the bridge of the nose, topical thrombin applied to the nares, and administration of platelets

   b. Packing the nose with gauze that has been soaked in topical thrombin and administration of platelets

   c. Holding all platelet products since DM is not responding to platelet administration

   d. Administer a sedative to the patient for her anxiety and hold all blood products, since she is not responding to RBCs or platelets.

7. On day 9, it is identified that DM's platelets decreased after she received a unit of platelets. It is suspected that DM is refractory to the platelets that she is receiving. What steps can be done for patients who are refractory to platelets?

   a. Use only random-donor platelets.

   b. Use random-donor platelets that have been irradiated.

   c. Hold platelets, since patients who are refractory to them will not benefit from their administration.

   d. Use single-donor platelets, cross-matched platelets, or HLA-matched platelets, all of which are leukoreduced.

8. The anemia that DM demonstrates on admission is due to what risk factor?

   a. Bone marrow infiltration of her leukemia

   b. Unknown cause of anemia upon diagnosis of leukemia

   c. Poor nutrition—her husband states that she has not eaten well over the past 2 weeks

   d. The patient is experiencing nephrotoxicity from her chemotherapy agents, which contributes to the anemia.

9. What is the most appropriate response when DM complains of fatigue?

   a. "The fatigue will be taken care of by erythropoietin agents."

   b. "You must walk at least 3 miles a day to gain benefit from aerobic exercise for your fatigue."

   c. "Fatigue is common with the cancer experience and there is not much that you can do about it."

   d. "Your hemoglobin levels must be treated with a blood transfusion, and you may feel better after the blood; and moderate aerobic exercise has been found to be beneficial with treatment-related disease."

10. What is the rationale for using red blood cell transfusions to treat DM rather than starting her on recombinant human erythropoietin?

   a. DM is symptomatic because of her anemia.

   b. Red blood cell transfusions are effective in providing a better quality of life.

   c. Red blood cell transfusions have no risks.

   d. DM has asked for red blood cell transfusions rather than recombinant human erythropoietin because it works faster.

ANSWERS

1. **D.** *Rationale:* Pretreatment health as established by laboratory values has been shown to be predictive of neutropenia, including hemoglobin levels lower than 12 g/dl. Another significant risk factor in the development of neutropenia includes the marrow involvement seen with hematologic malignancies such as leukemia. No information was given about any previous chemotherapy that this patient may have received. The patient's unwillingness to get out of bed and exercise has no impact on her neutrophil count.

2. **B.** *Rationale:* ANC = % neutrophils, segs (40%) + bands (6%) ÷ 100 × WBC = 1150

3. **B.** *Rationale:* Vancocin provides good coverage for the gram-positive cocci often found in central-line catheter infections.

4. **D.** *Rationale:* Hematopoietic growth factors for neutropenia reduce the period of neutropenia, which is the highest period of risk for infection. Growth factors do not prevent neutropenia altogether. Filgrastim and pegfilgrastim are single-lineage growth factors and promote the growth of neutrophils, not lymphocytes. Filgrastim and pegfilgrastim have not been shown in studies to directly provide any specific symptom relief to patients.

5. **B.** *Rationale:* One of the primary risk factors for bleeding in the patient with cancer is disease (leukemia) that invades the bone marrow. The disease can push out the normal elements of the marrow such as platelets and leave the patient at risk for

bleeding. An enlarged spleen can sequester platelets, but there is no evidence of this in DM. The existence of HIT can also decrease platelet counts, but again there is no evidence of this in DM. DM's age is not a risk factor in the development of a decreased platelet count.

6. A. *Rationale:* Appropriate nursing measures to help stop the nosebleed include cold compresses to the bridge of the nose (to cause vasoconstriction of the vessels of the nose), application of topical thrombin to the nares, and administration of platelets. Packing the nose with gauze soaked in thrombin is generally not within the scope of practice of a staff nurse. The patient may benefit from some antianxiety medication, since bleeding is anxiety provoking, but holding platelets is not appropriate in bleeding patients.

7. D. *Rationale:* When patients begin to demonstrate refractoriness to platelets, the most appropriate nursing actions are to continue to transfuse with single-donor platelets, cross-match the patients' platelets per order (to detect antibodies in the patient's serum that will react with platelets in potential donor units), provide HLA-matched platelets, and administer only leukoreduced platelets (can prevent the development of alloimmunization or refractoriness to platelets). Irradiation of platelet products can also help to prevent alloimmunization to platelets.

8. A. *Rationale:* DM's primary risk for anemia with her diagnosis of leukemia is her disease. Bone marrow infiltration from the leukemia decreases the space allowed for the bone marrow to produce normally functioning red blood cells. Since red blood cells have a life span of approximately 120 days, it is unlikely that her poor nutrition over the past 2 weeks can account for the anemia. Nephrotoxicity can contribute to anemia by decreasing the production of hemoglobin, but there is no evidence in the case to support this finding.

9. D. *Rationale:* Appropriate teaching regarding the patient's complaint of fatigue include the need to treat her anemia with transfusion therapy, and when she feels better (e.g., lack of dizziness) that moderate aerobic exercise has been found to provide benefit in managing treatment-related fatigue. Chemotherapy-induced anemia is expected with treatment of APL and is most appropriately treated acutely with red blood cell transfusions. There is no evidence to support that a certain type of aerobic exercise, or a certain distance walked, will provide the most benefit for relief of fatigue.

10. A. *Rationale:* Symptomatic anemia is generally treated with red blood cell transfusions, even though red cell transfusions have risks such as transfusion of bacteria or communicable diseases. Both transfusion therapy and administration of erythropoietic agents have been shown to increase the quality of life. It is always important for the nurse to know the rationale for treatment to be able to explain it to the patient and family.

REFERENCES

1. Godwin JE, Shin PD: Neutropenia, retrieved November 4, 2005, from www.eMedicine.com, 2005.
2. Lyman GH, Lyman CH, Agboola O: Risk models for predicting chemotherapy-induced neutropenia, *Oncologist* 10(6):427-437, 2005.
3. White N, Maxwell C, Michelson J, Bedell C: Protocols for managing chemotherapy-induced neutropenia in clinical oncology practices, *Cancer Nurs* 28(1):62-69, 2005.
4. Hughes WT, Armstrong D, Bodey GP et al: 2002 Guidelines for the use of antimicrobial agents in neutropenic patients with cancer, *Clin Infec Dis* 34(6):730-751, 2002.
5. Wujcik D: Infection. In Yarbro CH, Frogge MH, Goodman M, editors: *Cancer symptom management,* Sudbury, Mass, 2004, Jones & Bartlett.
6. Barton-Burke M., Wilkes GM, Ingwersen, KC: *Cancer chemotherapy: a nursing process approach,* ed 3, Sudbury, Mass 2001, Jones & Bartlett.
7. Larson E, Nirenberg A: Evidence-based nursing practice to prevent infection in hospitalized neutropenic patients with cancer, *Oncol Nurs Forum* 31(4):717-723, 2004.
8. Balducci L, Repetto L: Increased risk of myelotoxicity in elderly patients with non-Hodgkin's lymphoma, *Cancer* 100(1):6-11, 2004.
9. National Comprehensive Cancer Network: *Clinical practice guidelines in oncology: myeloid growth factors in cancer treatment* (v. 2.2005), 2005, August. Retrieved October 28, 2005, from http://www.nccn.org/professionals/physician_gls/PDF/anemia.pdf
10. Barber FD: Management of fever in neutropenic patients with cancer, *Nurs Clin North Am* 36(4):631-644, 2001.
11. Camp-Sorrell D: Myelosuppression. In Itano JK, Taoka KN, editors: *Core curriculum for oncology nursing,* St. Louis, 2005, Saunders.
12. Rust DM, Simpson JK, Lister J: Nutritional issues in patients with severe neutropenia, *Semin Oncol Nurs* 16(2):152-162, 2000.
13. Crawford J, Dale DC, Lyman GH: Chemotherapy-induced neutropenia, *Cancer* 100(2):228-237, 2003.
14. Sehulster LM, Chinn RYW, Arduino MJ, et al: Guidelines for environmental infection control in health-care facilities. Recommendations from CDC and the Healthcare Infection Control Practices Advisory Committee (HICPAC). Chicago IL; American Society for Healthcare Engineering/American Hospital Association; 2004. Retrieved October 28, 2005, from www.cdc.gov/ncidod/hip/enviro/guide.htm
15. Friese CR: Measuring oncology nursing-sensitive patient outcomes: evidence based summary, retrieved October 25, 2005, from http://onsopcontent.ons.org/toolkits/evidence/Clinical/pdf/PreventionSummary.pdf, 2004.
16. Gafter-Gvili A, Fraser A, Paul M et al: Meta-analysis: antibiotic prophylaxis reduces mortality in neutropenic patients, *Ann Intern Med* 142(2):979-995, 2005.
17. Kuderer NM, Crawford J, Dale DC et al: Meta-analysis of prophylactic granulocyte colony stimulating factor in cancer patients receiving chemotherapy, *J Clin Oncol* 23(16S suppl 1):8117, 2005 (abstract).
18. Campos LT, Folbe M, Meza L et al: Frequency of neutropenia-related events during chemotherapy and the use of pegfilgrastim and filgrastim in community practice: results of the ACCEPT study, *J Clin Oncol* 23(16S suppl 1):8115, 2005 (abstract).
19. DeMichele A, Glick JH: Overview of diagnosis and management of oncologic emergencies. In Lenhard RE, Osteen RT, Gansler T, editors: *The American Cancer Society's clinical oncology,* Atlanta, 2001, American Cancer Society.
20. Feld R: Multinational cooperation in trials and guidelines dealing with febrile neutropenia, *Int J Antimicrob Agents,* 16(2):185-187, 2000.
21. Aoun M: Standard antifungal therapy in neutropenic patients, *Int J Antimicrob Agents* 16(2):143-145, 2000.
22. Slavin MA, Osborne B, Adams R et al: Efficacy and safety of fluconazone prophylaxis for fungal infections after marrow transplantation: a prospective, randomized double-blind study, *J Infec Dis* 171(6): 1545-1552, 1995.
23. dePauw BE, Meis JFGM: Progress in fighting systemic fungal infections in haematological neoplasia, *Supp Care Cancer* 6(1):31-38, 1998.
24. Klastersky J: Empirical treatment of sepsis in neutropenic patients, *Int J Antimicrob Agents* 16(2):131-133, 2000.
25. Packham MA: Role of platelets in thrombosis and hemostasis, *Cancer J Physiol Pharm* 72(3):278-284, 1994.
26. Tallman MS: Bleeding in acute leukemia, *Pathophysiol Haemostasis Thromb* 33(suppl 1):48-49, 2003.

27. Gobel BH: Bleeding. In Yarbro CH, Frogge MH, Goodman M, editors: *Cancer nursing principles and practice*, Sudbury, Mass, 2005, Jones & Bartlett.

28. Yamakado K, Nakatsuka A, Tanaka N et al: Malignant pleural venous obstructions treated by stent placement: significant factors affecting patency, *J Vasc Interv Radiol* 12(12):1407-1415, 2001.

29. CancerSourceRN.com: Bleeding in cancer, retrieved October 10, 2005, from www.cancersourcern.com/Nursing/CE/CECourse.cfm?courseid=62&contentid=20166, 2000.

30. Pamuk GE, Pamuk ON, Baslarz Z et al: Overview of 321 patients with ITP. Retrospective analysis of the clinical features and response to therapy, *Ann Hematol* 81(8):36-440, 2002.

31. Silverman MA: Idiopathic thrombocytopenic purpura, retrieved October 1, 2005, from www.emedicine.com/emerg/topic282.htm, 2004.

32. Tunistra N: Outpatient administration of radiolabeled monoclonal antibodies, *Clin J Oncol Nurs* 7(1):106-108, 2003.

33. Hirsh J, Heddle N, Kelton JG: Treatment of heparin-induced thrombocytopenia: a critical review, *Arch Int Med* 164(4):361-369, 2004.

34. Verburg KM, Maziasz TJ, Weiner E et al: COX-2-specific inhibitors: definition of a new therapeutic concept, *Am J Therap* 8(1):49-64, 2001.

35. Reddy JC, Shuman MA, Aster RH: Quinine and quinidine-induced thrombocytopenia: a great imitator, *Arch Int Med* 164(2):218-220, 2004.

36. Demetri GD: Pharmacologic treatment options in patients with thrombocytopenia, *Semin Hematol* 37 (2 suppl 4):11-18, 2000.

37. Reid TJ, Rentas FJ, Ketchum LH: Platelet substitutes in the management of thrombocytopenia, *Curr Hematol Rep* 2(2):165-170, 2003.

38. Weich NS, Wang A, Fitzgerald M et al: Recombinant human interleukin-11 directly promotes megakaryocytopoiesis in vitro, *Blood* 90(10):3893-3902, 1997.

39. Isaacs C, Robert FA, Bailey FA et al: Randomized placebo-controlled study of recombinant human interleukin-11 to prevent chemotherapy-induced thrombocytopenia in patients with breast cancer receiving dose-intensive cyclophosphamide and doxorubicin, *J Clin Oncol* 15:3368-3377, 1997.

40. Schiffer KC, Anderson CL, Bennett S, Bernstein LS: Platelet transfusions for patients with cancer: clinical practice guidelines of the American Society of Clinical Oncology, *J Clin Oncol* 19:1519-1538, 2000.

41. Da Ponte A, Bidoli E, Talamini R et al: Pre-storage leucocyte depletion and transfusion reaction rates in cancer patients, *Transfus Med* 15(1):1365-1374, 2005.

42. Perrotta PL, Snyder EL: Transfusion therapy. In DeVita, VT, Hellman S, Rosenberg SA, editors: *Cancer principles and practice of oncology*, Philadelphia, 2001, Lippincott, Williams & Wilkins.

43. Dzik WH, Anderson JK, O'Neill EM et al: A prospective, randomized clinical trial of universal WBC reduction, *Transfusion* 42(9):1537-1545, 2002.

44. Sloan SR, Silberstein LE: Transfusion medicine. In Furie B, Cassileth PA, Atkins MB et al, editors: *Clinical hematology and oncology: clinical presentation, diagnosis, and treatment*, Philadelphia, 2003, Churchill Livingstone.

45. Friend PH, Pruett J: Bleeding and thrombotic complications. In Yarbro CH, Frogge MH, Goodman, M, editors: *Cancer symptom management*, Sudbury, Mass, 2004, Jones & Bartlett.

46. Ross SD, Fahrbach K, Frame D, et al: The effect of anemia treatment on selected health-related quality-of-life domains: a systematic review, *Clin Ther* 25(6):1786-1805, 2003.

47. Demetri GD, Anderson KC: Disorders of blood cell production in clinical oncology. In Abeloff MD, Armita, editors: *Clinical oncology*, Philadelphia, 2004, Churchill Livingstone.

48. Polovich M, White JM, Kelleher LO, editors: *Chemotherapy and biotherapy guidelines and recommendations for practice*, Pittsburgh, 2005, Oncology Nursing Society.

49. Matthews LV: Alterations in ventilation. In Itano JK, Taoka KN, editors: *Core curriculum for oncology nursing*, St. Louis, 2005, Saunders.

50. Kuhn JG: Chemotherapy-associated hematopoietic toxicity, *Am J Health-Syst Pharm* 59(suppl 4):S4-S7, 2002.

51. Teeple CL: Myelosuppression: anemia and thrombocytopenia. In Polovich MP, White JM, Kelleher LO, editors: *chemotherapy and biotherapy guidelines and recommendations for practice*, Pittsburgh, 2005, Oncology Nursing Society.

52. Barsevick AM, Whitmer K, Walker L: In their own words: using the common sense model to analyze patient descriptions of cancer-related fatigue, *Oncol Nurs Forum* 28(9):1363-1369, 2001.

53. Oncology Nursing Society: Clinical practice/evidence based summaries (n.d.), *Measuring oncology-nursing-sensitive patient outcomes: evidence based summaries*, retrieved October 28, 2005, from http://www.ons.org, 2004.

54. National Comprehensive Cancer Network: *Clinical practice guidelines in oncology: cancer and treatment related anemia* (v. 2.2005), 2005, August. Retrieved November 6, 2005, from http://www.nccn.org/ professionals/physician_gls/PDF/myeloid_growth.pdf

55. Weiss MJ: New insights into erythropoietin and epoetin alfa: mechanisms of action, target tissues, and clinical applications, *Oncologist* 8(suppl 3):18-29, 2003.

56. Mock V, Pickett M, Ropka ME et al: Fatigue and quality of life outcomes of exercise during cancer treatment, *Cancer Pract* 9(3):119-127, 2001.

57. Nail LM: Fatigue in patients with cancer, *Oncol Nurs Forum* 29(3):537-544, 2002.

58. Schwartz AL, Thompson JA, Masood N: Interferon-induced fatigue in patients with melanoma: a pilot study of exercise and methylphenidate, *Oncol Nurs Forum* 29(7):E85-90, 2002.

59. Henry DH, Handy CM: Optimizing patient care: minimizing the impact of chemotherapy-induced toxicities, *Spotlight on Symposia from ONS 29th Annual Congress in Anaheim, CA*, retrieved October 25, 2005, from http://www.ons.org, 2005.

60. Herrington JD, Davidson SL, Tomita DK et al: Utilization of darbepoetin alfa and epoetin alfa for chemotherapy-induced anemia, *Am J Health-Syst Pharm* 62(1):54-62, 2005.

61. Mughal TI: Current and future use of hematopoietic growth factors in cancer medicine, *Hematol Oncol* 22(3):121-134, 2004.

62. Given BA, Sherwood PR: Oncology Nursing Society report on nursing-sensitive patient outcomes-A white paper, *Oncol Nurs Forum* 32(4):773-784, 2005.

63. Ropka ME, Padilla G, Gillespie TW: Risk modeling: applying evidence-based risk assessment in oncology nursing practice, *Oncol Nurs Forum* 32(1):49-56, 2005.

64. Baraldi-Junkins, CA, Beck AC, Rothstein G: Hematopoiesis and cytokines. Relevance to cancer and aging, *Hematol Oncol Clin North Am* 14(4):45-61, 2000.

65. Balducci L, Hardy C, Lyman GH: Hemopoietic reserve in the older cancer patient: clinical and economic considerations, *Cancer Causes Control* 7(6):539-547, 2000.

CHAPTER 29

Oral Mucositis

Janet S. Fulton and Michelle L. Treon

Overview and Introduction

Oral mucositis is a major complication of cytotoxic chemotherapy and radiation therapy. It involves a complex interaction including host factors, treatment factors, oral microflora, and epithelial regeneration and is associated with significant pain, dysphagia, and dysguesia. Oral mucositis represents a significant risk factor for systemic infections, particularly in patients with neutropenia. Mucositis is experienced by about 40% of chemotherapy patients and up to 80% of bone marrow transplant patients.[1,2] In addition, bone marrow transplant patients rated oral mucositis as the single most debilitating side effect of treatment, over nausea and vomiting, diarrhea, and fatigue.[1] Oral mucositis can be a dose-limiting toxicity, ultimately affecting rate of survival.[3] In addition, oral mucositis can increase length of hospital stay and increase cancer-related treatment costs.[4,5] At present, no treatment exists to completely prevent the development of oral mucositis; however, good oral hygiene and attention to management of mucositis-related symptoms such as pain can reduce complications and improve quality of life.

Definitions

Mucositis, the inflammation of the mucosal tissue, can occur anywhere in the gastrointestinal (GI) tract.[6] Oral mucositis specifically designates the condition of tissue breakdown in the oral and oropharyngeal mucosal lining. The term **oral mucositis** was first used in the 1980s to distinguish it from mucositis in other parts of the GI tract.[7] Oral mucositis is associated with erythema, inflammation, and ulceration that results in pain and dysguesia (taste changes) that can lead to impaired hydration and nutrition. It is also a significant risk factor for systemic infection.[8] The severity and duration of oral mucositis is known to significantly influence quality of life.[9,10]

Prevalence

The incidence of oral mucositis varies and is highly influenced by the type of cancer treatment; however, an estimated 400,000 people develop oral complications from cancer each year.[11] The incidence of oral mucositis among patients receiving adjunctive chemotherapy has been estimated to be around 10%; the incidence rate increases to 40% for patients receiving primary chemotherapy. For patients undergoing hematopoietic stem cell transplant with myeloablative conditioning regimens, the incidence of oral mucositis is around 80%; and with radiation therapy for head and neck cancer to fields involving the oral cavity, the incidence is 100%.[8]

Complications associated with oral mucositis include pain, infection, salivary gland dysfunction, taste dysfunction, dysguesia, and malnutrition. Oral mucositis and associated complications can be detrimental to a patient's clinical outcome, especially when the management of mucositis requires reducing the dose of treatment, which occurs in approximately 50% of chemotherapy patients.[8] The incidence of mucositis and associated complications varies depending on the number and severity of risk factors.

Risk Factors

The risk for developing oral mucositis includes several predisposing factors that are either patient- or treatment-related. Patient factors include age, gender, oral hygiene, salivary secretion rate, genetic factors, body mass index (BMI), smoking practices (past and present), and previous cancer treatments.[12]

AGE

Patients 20 years of age and younger are considered at increased risk because of increased epithelial mitotic rates and increased epidermal growth factor receptors in epithelial tissue. Younger patients also have a higher incidence of hematologic malignancies, which are associated with greater immunosuppression.[13] Older patients are at risk as a result of declining kidney function with lower creatinine clearance rates, which alters chemotherapy excretion and allows drugs to circulate longer and cause greater cell damage.[14,15] Also, older adults are at increased risk for oral mucositis when 5-fluorouracil (5-FU) is included in the chemotherapy regime.[16]

GENDER

Limited research has suggested that gender may be a predisposing risk factor; however, the evidence is not clear.[17-19] Gender has emerged as a risk factor for patients taking fluorouracil chemotherapy. Among patients taking 5-FU in a study by Sloan and Loprinzi, women reported oral mucositis more often and as having greater severity compared to men, and the incidence of severe or very severe mucositis was higher for women compared to men.[17] Additional studies demonstrated a similar trend of higher and more severe occurrence of oral mucositis among women taking 5-FU compared to men; however, the physiologic mechanism responsible for this difference is not evident.[17,18]

Differences across gender were present for patients receiving placebo and for those receiving mucositis interventions, suggesting that the differences are not easily explained by arguing for a different response by women to particular mucositis interventions. Additional studies have explored differences in nonhematologic responses to cancer treatment, including oral mucositis; findings suggest that there are differences by gender.[20,21]

ORAL HYGIENE

Preexisting oral health influences both the development and the severity of treatment-related mucositis.[22] Oral health status can increase risk of mucositis if preexisting dental problems are not resolved before treatment begins. Preexisting oral disease can predispose oral tissue to insult.[8,23] Specific risk factors include mucosal lesions, dental caries and endodontic disease, as well as periodontal disease, poorly fitting dentures, orthodontic appliances, temporomandibular joint dysfunction, and salivary abnormalities. Resolving dental problems can take time, so the patient should be evaluated by the dental team at least 1 month before beginning therapy, whenever possible.[8]

SALIVARY SECRETION

Saliva protects the oral mucosa from infection. Decreased salivary secretion leads to an increase in debris, plaque deposits, and growth of infectious microbes that can lead to opportunistic microorganisms entering gum tissues and an increased incidence of local and systemic infections.[24] Factors that contribute to oral tissue drying are also risk factors for development of oral mucositis, including dehydration, oxygen therapy, mouth breathing, and tachypnea. In addition, some medications can be drying on oral tissue such as anticholinergics, antidepressants, antihistamines, antihypertensives, diuretics, opiates, phenothiazines, and sedatives.[2] Local tissue irritation or infection caused by *Candida* species or oral herpes simplex can further predispose dry tissue to damage or prolong healing.[2]

TOBACCO USE AND SMOKING

Tobacco use (smoking and smokeless tobacco) initiates cellular changes to the tissues of the oral mucosa, particularly the surface epithelial cells, causing increased pigmentation and epithelial thickening. Smoking tobacco reduces available oxygen, which impairs tissue healing and increases the risk for overgrowth of anaerobic organisms. Neutropenic patients may be at additional risk, since smoking tobacco is known to reduce neutrophil function.[25] Smokeless tobacco can result in changes in keratin production, gingival tissue damage, and long-term risk of malignant oral lesions. In addition, many long-term smokers and tobacco users are predisposed to periodontal disease and delayed tissue healing.[25] A history of recent smoking has been linked to higher grades of oral mucositis among patients undergoing bone marrow transplant.[9]

GENETICS

Emerging research evidence suggests that mucositis risk may be genetically influenced. Persons with genetically determined deficiencies in enzymes necessary for metabolism of chemotherapy drugs may be an increased risk for toxicities including mucositis. Genetics may also influence any risk related to gender and ethnicity, though additional research is needed to identify the influence of genetics on physiology.[6]

NUTRITIONAL STATUS AND BODY MASS INDEX

Nutritional status can be a risk factor at the beginning or during the course of therapy. Patients who begin therapy with less than ideal body weight, or are deficient in essential nutrients, may experience more severe side effects than those with no nutritional concerns.[9] Patients with caloric and protein malnutrition are at risk for decreased wound healing that may lead to prolonged recovery from treatment-induced damage to the oral epithelium.

Weight and BMI have been linked to increased severity of mucositis. Overweight patients with a BMI of 25 or more, and obese patients with a BMI equal to or greater than 30, experienced increased severity of mucositis compared to patients of normal weight. The difference was attributed to a higher absolute dose of chemotherapy drug received in bone marrow transplant conditioning regimes (including cyclophosphamide, busulfan, and total body irradiation), and differences in drug distribution through tissues compared to leaner individuals.[9] Other research has not supported this finding and has suggested that BMI is not a risk factor.[26]

OTHER RISK FACTORS

The risk of developing oral mucositis is also dependent upon treatment factors including type of treatment (e.g., chemotherapy, biotherapy, or radiation therapy), delivery and dosing sequencing, and concurrent therapies. Generally, higher doses of chemotherapy, fractionated radiation, or combining chemotherapy and radiation will place the patient into the highest risk category.[12] Box 29-1 lists antineoplastic chemotherapeutic agents with high potential to cause oral mucositis, though it is important to note that lists of chemotherapy agents with high potential for mucosal damage are inconsistent.[27] Also, the relationship between risk and dose of chemotherapy, and risk and chemotherapy combinations, is poorly understood.[28]

Specific patient populations are more likely to develop oral mucositis based upon standard treatment regimens for some types of cancers. The head and neck cancer patients experience oral mucositis at exceedingly high rates, since localized radiotherapy targets tumors near or involving the oral cavity, and the oral tissues are more likely to receive direct insult from radiation.[29,30] In addition, the type of radiation is an important factor: altered fractionation radiation therapy will lead to a 100% rate of oral mucositis development, whereas conventional radiation has a slightly lower incidence.[31] Box 29-2 lists risk factors for oral mucositis during radiation therapy.

Patients undergoing stem cell transplant typically receive a preparatory regime involving high-dose myeloablative chemotherapy with or without simultaneous total body irradiation. These treatments result in an incidence rate of oral mucositis that ranges from 50% to 100% of patients, with a higher risk associated with allogeneic transplants than with autologous

---

BOX 29-1	**Mucosatoxic Chemotherapeutic Agents***

6-Mercaptopurine	Docetaxel	Mechlorethamine
6-Thioguanine	Doxorubicin	Methotrexate
Actinomycin D	Epirubicin	Mitomycin
Bleomycin	Etoposide	Mitoxantrone
Busulfan	5-Fluorouracil	Melphalan
Capecitabine	Fludarabine	Paclitaxel
Carboplatin	Gemcitabine	Procarbazine
Cisplatin	Hydroxyurea	Teniposide
Cyclophosphamide	Idarubicin	Thiotepa
Cytarabine	Ifosfamide	Topotecan
Daunorubicin	Irinotecan	

*Listed in alphabetical order.
Adapted from Hsu K, Toljanic JA, Bedard JF et al: Oral toxicity associated with chemotherapy. *Up-to-Date*. Retrieved September 11, 2006 from http://www.utdol.com/utd/store/index.do.

BOX 29-2   Risk Factors for Oral Mucositis during Radiation Therapy

Treatment-Related Risk Factors

Higher cumulative dose of radiation therapy (5000-6000 cGy)

Hyperfractionation schedule

Concurrent use of chemotherapy

Treatment of tongue, soft palate, and floor of mouth

Treatment field includes salivary glands or sites near dental fillings with metallic restorations

Patient-Related Risk Factors

Preexisting dental problems

Use of irritating substances (e.g., smoking)

Younger age

From Shih A, Miaskowski C et al: Mechanisms for radiation-induced oral mucositis and the consequences, *Cancer Nurs* 26(3):222-229, 2003.

transplants.[31] Some of the antineoplastic agents used in these treatments have a high mucotoxic nature, including methotrexate, melphalan, irinotecan, and cyclophosphamide.[32]

A commonly used antineoplastic chemotherapy agent associated with an increased risk for oral mucositis is 5-FU. 5-FU alone contributes to the development of oral mucositis in 10% to 15% of patients who are treated with the agent, but incidence increases to around 40% when combined with platinum-based antineoplastic agents, plus radiation or taxane agents.[18,32] Furthermore, when these three treatments are combined (i.e., taxane, platinum, and radiation), the rate of oral mucositis increases to over 60%.[6]

Etiology

NORMAL ORAL ANATOMY AND PHYSIOLOGY

Under normal conditions, oral tissue is pink, moist to observation, and without breaks or irregularity in integrity. Nonkeratinized stratified squamous epithelial cells, originating from the stratum basale, are progressively flattened as they transform to outer-layer oral tissue. Thus they become elastic and flexible, putting these cells at risk for damage. The hard palate and tongue contain both keratinized and nonkeratinized cells. Cells containing keratin are strengthened by this protein. Keratin functions as a buffer for the cell structure against stress by protecting cell shape and viability; and on the surfaces of cells, the protein functions as special glue holding epithelial cells together. Keratin-containing cells still proliferate at a fast rate, but slower than nonkeratinized cells. The fastest areas of proliferation are found on the floor of the mouth and underside of the tongue.[33] The floor of the mouth has an average epithelial turnover rate of 20 days, the hard plate of 24 days.[33] The oral cavity also contains normal balanced flora.

PATHOPHYSIOLOGY

The pathobiologic response of oral tissue to cancer therapy (i.e., radiation and chemotherapy) is not fully understood. Until recently, oral mucositis was thought to be the result of damage to the epithelium and degradation of mucosal stem cells in the basal

layer.[34-37] Atrophy, thinning, and ulceration of the mucosa were thought to be the consequence of the inability of the mucosal epithelium to renew itself. Mucosal epithelial damage was viewed as caused directly by radiation and indirectly by antineoplastic chemotherapeutic agents, because these therapies do not differentiate between highly replicating cancer cells and highly replicating normal cells. The pathobiologic basis of support for this view was the belief that normal, highly replicating cells of the mucosal epithelium were indiscriminately damaged.

The inability to find suitable interventions to prevent or manage oral mucositis suggested that the rationale for therapy was based more on assumptions than on a clear understanding of the pathobiology leading to mucositis development. Recently, a more complex perspective has been emerging, supported by considerable effort to develop an animal model for the study of human oral mucositis. Hamsters are now the preferred animal for studying mucositis, because they have large cheek pouches that provide sufficient tissue for evaluation, their oral bacterial flora is similar to that of humans, their oral mucosa and bone marrow respond to myeloablative chemotherapy (conditioning regimes for hematologic stem cell transplant) in much the same way as that of humans, they develop mucositis in response to radiation therapy similarly to humans, and they have blood cells that are comparable to humans' and therefore can be studied using existing laboratory instruments and procedures.[38] Mice are also being used in some situations to investigate very specific types of research questions.[39-41] Thus laboratory animal models are replacing older techniques of clinical observation and histologic examination of tissue from autopsy and are providing more precise understanding of the pathobiologic mechanisms involved in mucositis. New understandings are creating new opportunities for interventions that will reduce both incidence and severity of cancer treatment–related oral mucositis.

The idea that only the epithelium was involved in the development of mucositis was challenged by early hamster studies, where it was discovered that, following mucosal irradiation, damage occurred in the endothelium of blood vessels walls and connective tissue of the submucosa. This endothelial blood vessel damage preceded observable mucosal epithelial damage by about a week, suggesting that damage to the endothelium of blood vessels was related to radiation-induced mucositis. It was then discovered that proinflammatory cytokines were increased in the blood of patients who received myeloablative chemotherapy and experienced nonhematologic toxicity such as mucositis. This pattern of response was also demonstrated in hamsters: cytokines increased in the submucosa as mucositis developed in response to chemotherapy. When these cytokines were attenuated by pharmacologic manipulation, the occurrence of mucositis was reduced in hamsters.[39-41] Further, it was noted that patients with systemic diseases that predisposed cells to apoptosis (a form of cell death necessary to make way for new cells and to remove cells whose DNA has been damaged) were more likely to develop mucositis compared to patients who had higher resistance to cell death.[39-41] Increased levels of cytokine platelet-activating factor have been detected after radiation, and increased apoptosis of submucosal fibroblasts has occurred in response to chemotherapy and radiation. Macrophages have been noted to accumulate in the submucosa after radiation treatment. These responses suggested that radiation and chemotherapy do not cause mucositis by damaging the basal layer of the epithelium, but rather by activating injury-producing pathways.[38,42]

These pathways in turn activate transcription factors that lead to the up-regulation of genes that modulate the damage response. By mapping gene expression, researchers have seen that transcription factors act as master switches that control an individual patient's mucosal response to radiation and chemotherapy.[39-41] The transcription factor called nuclear factor-κB (NF-KB) has emerged as significant, since it appears to control around 200 genes associated with mucositis.[43] Thus it is a complex, interdependent sequence of events that eventually damages and destroys epithelial stem cells. It has further been demonstrated that mucositis develops across time and involves five loosely divided stages including initiation, message generation, signaling and amplification, ulcer formation, and healing.[39-41]

PATHOBIOLOGIC MODEL

Sonis created a five-phase model to explain the developmental process of oral mucositis.[39-41] These phases are not exact and vary depending on the cancer treatment-related insult. For example, the commonly used fractionated radiation dosing regimens produce phases that can overlap, because the insult occurs with small doses applied over time. However, a short but intense chemotherapeutic insult, such as occurs with conditioning regimens for hematologic stem cell transplant, will produce distinct phases.

Phase I: Initiation. Initiation phase begins with the delivery of a chemotherapeutic or a radiation treatment. The injury-initiating event affects the basal epithelium, connective tissue, and blood vessels. Damage results from the activation of free radicals known as reactive oxygen species (ROS) that target the DNA. Direct damage to the DNA of epithelial basal cells leads to cell death. By damaging the basal cell DNA, the once balanced process of proliferation and desquamation becomes so severely disrupted that cellular erosion eventually occurs. However, ROS also set in motion a cascade of biochemical events that lead to additional tissue injury.[39-41]

Phase II: Up-Regulation and Message Generation. Once the injury has been initiated, an up-regulation and message generation begins. The up-regulation of genes results in the production of proinflammatory cytokines including tumor necrosis factor-alpha (TNF-α), and the interleukins IL-1β and IL-6. Cytokines are chemical messengers that initiate biologic actions. Increased levels of these cytokines stimulate early damage to connective tissue and endothelium and initiate signaling that reduces epithelial oxygenation, resulting in basal cell injury and death. In addition, chemotherapy and radiation cause direct damage to tissue through other non-DNA–related chemical actions.[39-41]

Phase III: Amplification and Signaling. After the tissue is injured, chemical changes continue in the mucosal tissue, intensifying the processes begun during phase II. TNF-α activates a pathway of reactions that eventually result in cell death. The actions of the pathway involve both the epithelium and elements of the submucosa. During this phase of intense biochemical actions in the tissue, there are few clinical indicators of tissue damage. Tissue integrity is maintained, and patients have few symptoms.[39-41]

Phase IV: Ulceration. The loss of mucosal integrity makes itself evident as ulceration that is severely painful and distressing for patients. The oral nerve endings are freely exposed to the chemical stimulators of pain and inflammation of nearby tissue. If microorganisms (bacteria, viruses, or fungi) colonize the ulcerated area, it can lead to bacteremia or septicemia, a potentially life-threatening condition in the presence of neutropenia. In addition, cell wall products from bacteria likely penetrate the submucosa and activate the release of additional proinflammatory cytokines, leading to further tissue injury and intense pain.[39-41]

Phase V: Healing. Healing results after new chemical messengers released from the extracellular matrix direct the epithelium along the margins of the ulcer to divide, migrate, and differentiate into new, healthy tissue. Once the surface of the ulcer is covered with epithelium, the tissue begins to form layers, normal tissue configuration occurs, and the ulcer heals. Once the ulcer heals, symptoms resolve (see Figure 29-1).[39-41]

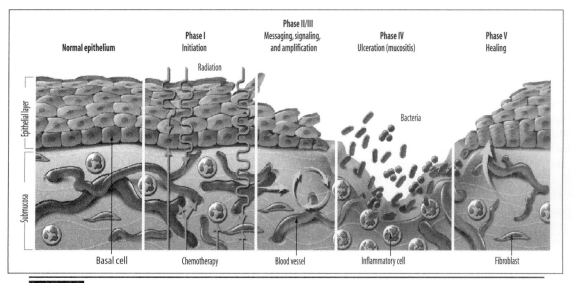

FIG. 29-1 Phases of development of oral mucositis. (From Peterson DE: New strategies for management of oral mucositis in cancer patients, *Support Oncol* 4(2 Suppl 1):11, 2006.

Consequences

PAIN

A widely accepted definition of pain is "an unpleasant sensory and emotional experience associated with actual or potential tissue damage, or described in terms of such damage."[44] Pain from oral mucositis is the result of tissue damage.

Pain is perceived through chemical nociception.[45] Nociception occurs through two specific types of pain fibers, fast, myelinated A-δ fibers and unmyelinated C fibers. These fibers transmit noxious stimuli from the primary afferent nociceptors (PAN) to the dorsal horn and to the spinal cord after cellular injury or after the initiation of the inflammatory response. In the oral tissue, the nerve endings exist as free nerve endings in the PAN microenvironment. When tissue is damaged, chemicals are released including dopamine, norepinephrine, bradykinin, histamine, phospholipase, arachidonic acid, cyclooxygenase, and prostaglandin. These chemicals activate nociception by causing the nerves to fire an action potential. Prostaglandin is especially important because it additionally causes sensitization of the nerve endings, meaning it lowers the threshold for an action potential to fire. Further, prostaglandin also attracts leukocytes and increases cellular permeability, starting the process of inflammation. Another important chemical in nociception is substance P (SP). SP is located in the dorsal root ganglia and in the PAN microenvironment itself, causing additional vasodilatation and additional bradykinin and histamine release, and facilitating C fiber action potential transmission.[45]

While tissue damage occurs, the inflammatory process also begins; phagocytes rush to the injured site, and vasodilatation occurs from histamine release, ultimately resulting in more vasodilatation and increased cellular permeability. Increasing a cell's permeability allows protein exudates, cellular debris, and excess fluid to gather. As the protein content rises interstitially, osmosis attracts tissue fluid from surrounding blood vessels, causing edema. The increased cellular pressure leads to irritation of the PAN nerve endings via pressure on the mechanoreceptors. Furthermore, the buildup of this cellular debris barricades the lymphatic system, preventing lymphatic fluid return and venous blood flow, leading to edema at the site of injury. If the inflammatory process escalates, it can ultimately result in cellular hemorrhage and bleeding. This occurs when the accumulation of vasodilator chemicals exceeds the interstitial pressure, resulting in cellular rupture.[45]

Bone marrow transplant patients reported mouth sores as the single most debilitating side effect, stating that mouth sores made it difficult or impossible to eat, swallow, drink, and talk; and among these patients almost 70% received opioid analgesics, most frequently morphine, to relieve oral pain.[1] Additional studies have similarly found that from the patient's perspective, pain is the most distressing symptom of oral mucositis.[46,47]

INFECTION

An intact oral mucosa and normal salivary flow provide a barrier that reduces the risk of microorganisms invading the epithelium. Loss of the oral epithelium as a protective barrier provides a portal of entry for microorganisms into the systemic circulation. Once mucosal integrity is altered, local and systemic infections can be caused by indigenous oral flora, as well as nosocomial and opportunistic organisms, predisposing the patient to bacteremia, septicemia, and fungemia.[48,49] Both indigenous oral flora and hospital-acquired pathogens have been associated with bacteremia and septicemia.[8] In addition, some microorganisms may be involved in up-regulating proinflammatory cytokines via bacterial metabolic products. As the absolute neutrophil count falls 1500/mcL, and the duration of neutropenia is prolonged, the incidence and severity of infection rises.[8,39-41] Decreased or altered salivary flow can also increase the risk for infection of oral origin.[8]

Bacterial infections may be primary or secondary. Gram-positive organisms including α-hemolytic streptococci and Enterococcus species are associated with systemic infections originating from mucositis.[8] Streptococcus oralis and S. mitis are among the most common bacteria isolated from blood. S. mitis is associated with adult respiratory distress syndrome (ARDS) especially among patients receiving high-dose cytarabine.[49] Gram-negative organisms include Pseudomonas aeruginosa, Neisseria species, and Escherichia coli. Secondary infections can result from acute episodes of underlying periodontal disease exacerbated by chemotherapy-induced myelosuppression.[8,50] Extensive ulceration associated with periodontal disease may not be directly observable, especially during myelosuppression, when signs of inflammation may be masked. However, periodontal disease can be a source for disseminating oral microorganisms, especially during neutropenic periods.[3]

The majority of fungal oral infections are caused by Candida species. C. albicans accounts for the majority of fungal infections; however, other Candida species may also infect cancer patients including C. krusei, C. tropicalis, C. parapsilosis, and C. glabrata.[49] Herpes group viral infections caused by oral lesions can range from mild to serious in patients receiving cancer treatment. The severity of and the distressing symptoms associated with herpes viral infections is related to immunocompetence: the more compromised the patient's immunity, the greater the severity of the infection. Herpes simplex, varicella zoster, and Epstein-Barr viruses occur as reactivation of a latent virus. Cytomegalovirus can result from either reactivation of a latent virus or a newly acquired virus. These viruses cause oral lesions and pain, but they can also be fatal depending on the degree of immunosuppression.[8] Epstein-Barr virus is associated with increased risk for lymphomas of the head and neck region in hematopoietic stem cell transplant patients who are immunocompromised for prolonged periods. After cancer treatment, anti-Epstein Barr titers often decrease, and they can increase with disease recurrence.[8] Viral cultures are needed for accurate diagnosis.

BLEEDING

Bleeding, usually involving the gums, can occur during chemotherapy-induced thrombocytopenia and/or coagulopathy. Oral bleeding may be minimal, with petechiae located on the lips, the soft palate, or the floor of the mouth, or it may be severe, with oral hemorrhage, especially in the gingival crevices. Bleeding may occur spontaneously from sites of underlying periodontal disease or may be trauma induced, underscoring the need for pretreatment of any existing periodontal disease. Ulcers caused by the herpes simplex virus may bleed continuously during periods of thrombocytopenia. Spontaneous gingival oozing may occur when platelet counts diminish to less than 30,000/mm³, and the risk of bleeding is higher for patients receiving high-dose chemotherapy or undergoing hematopoietic stem cell transplant.[8]

XEROSTOMIA

Saliva is necessary for the normal execution of oral functions such as taste, swallowing, and speech. Xerostomia, the sensation of dry mouth, is often thought to be a relatively minor treatment-related symptom with few deleterious effects; however, many patients find xerostomia a significant source of distress.[29,51] Caused by a marked reduction in salivary gland secretion, clinical symptoms and signs of xerostomia include dryness, a sore or burning sensation, especially involving the tongue, cracked lips, slits or fissures at the corners of the mouth, changes in the tongue surface, difficulty wearing dentures, and increased frequency and/or volume of fluid intake. Both chemotherapy and radiation therapy can result in xerostomia. Patients receiving radiation therapy for head and neck cancer all experience some degree of xerostomia.[8]

Saliva contains proteins, electrolytes, antimicrobial elements (bactericidal substances, proteolytic enzymes, and antibodies), enzymes that act on starch, and mucus, a lubricant. Saliva inhibits dental caries and protects the mouth from infection. Xerostomia alters the mouth's normal physiology and reduces its buffering capacity and mechanical cleansing ability, contributing to dental caries and the progression of periodontal disease.[51] In a healthy mouth, approximately 1.5 liters of saliva is produced every day, with increased flow in response to stimulation (e.g., chewing). Unstimulated whole salivary flow rates of less than 0.1 ml/min are considered indicative of xerostomia; normal salivary flow rate is 0.3 to 0.5 ml/min.[51]

ECONOMIC IMPACT

Mucositis is not only associated with increased morbidity and symptom distress; it is also associated with increased cost of care resulting from changes in therapy, additional therapy, and increased hospitalization.[4,5] A review of the clinical consequences of oral mucositis among patients treated for head and neck cancers found that approximately 33% of patients who developed severe oral mucositis were hospitalized, compared to 16% of patients with moderate mucositis, 21% of patients with mild mucositis, and 11% of patients with no oral mucositis.[52] Among all autologous bone marrow transplant patients, patients with oral ulcerations had a hospital length of stay of 34 days compared to 29 days for patients without ulcerations. Patients with oral ulcerations complicated by streptococcal infection stayed in the hospital 6 days longer than patients with oral ulcerations without septic complications (40 days compared to 34 days). The researchers estimated a cost savings in excess of $1 million in length of stay for 100 patients if mucositis could be completely prevented.[4] In a separate study looking at outcomes of hematopoietic stem cell transplant, each 1-point increase in severity of mucositis on the 5-point Oral Mucositis Assessment Scale (OMAS) was associated with a more than twofold increase in infection, 2.7 additional days of total parenteral nutrition, 2.6 additional days in the hospital, and more than $25,400 in additional hospital charges. Most importantly, an increase in severity of mucositis is highly correlated with an increase in mortality at 100 days after transplant.[5]

Assessment and Measurement

Multiple measurement instruments and scales are available for assessing the oral cavity, varying in complexity, focus, reliability,

and validity (See Appendix B).[53-55] Scales and grading guidelines often include a mix of objective, subjective, and functional parameters that vary in wording, format, reliability, and ease of use. Measurement scales developed for research and involving specific populations have been used in or adapted for other populations with or without validation or reliability testing. Achieving good patient outcomes is highly dependent on having valid and reliable measurement instruments to assess mucositis and evaluate outcomes of care that are selected to match the purpose of the measurement.

CANCER-FOCUSED ASSESSMENT INSTRUMENTS

In an early study of the outcomes of oral care for older adults, DeWalt demonstrated that oral care interventions by nurses can produce significant changes for the better.[56] To conduct the research, an oral rating scale was developed that included salivation, tongue moisture, tongue color, palate, gingival tissue, membranes, lip texture, lip moisture, and soft tooth debris. Although not specifically a cancer-focused assessment, the DeWalt instrument influenced development of the Beck Oral Exam Guide (OEG) and Beck Oral Perception Guide (OPG).[57] The OEG and OPG were developed for a study that explored the effectiveness of oral care protocols for patients receiving cancer treatments and were among the first scales to assess oral mucositis in cancer patients receiving cancer treatments. OEG included eight subscales: lips, tongue, mucous membranes of the palate, the uvula, and the tonsilar fossa, gingiva, teeth, saliva, voice, and ability to swallow. Each subscale included one to three items: for example, the category lips included texture, color, and moisture—all rated from 1 (normal) to 4 (severe level of alteration). Across the subscales, the instrument measured a total of 15 mostly objective signs, the exception being pain (subjective measure) in the descriptors of swallowing (functional measure). The companion instrument was the OPG, designed to measure the patient's perception of his or her mouth. Using the same eight subscales, the OPG asked patients to rate a perception. Perception is not well defined; however, the instrument seems to be measuring a perception of comfort rated along a 1-to-4 continuum. The amount of detail makes these instruments difficult to use in clinical practice.

A survey of cancer nurses in Canada, conducted by the Western Consortium for Cancer Nursing Research (WCCNR) in the 1980s, identified chemotherapy-related mucositis as a research priority. The consortium developed and later revised a mucositis staging system to support its research in the area of mucositis management.[58] Similar to the World Health Organization (WHO) grading scale, the descriptors for the WCCNR scale are more specific clinical indicators of mucositis severity (see Appendix B, Table B-1). Eight anatomic and functional descriptors are listed in the first version: mucosal color, lesions, bleeding, moisture, edema, infection, ability to eat and/or drink, and discomfort were grouped to reflect four distinct stages, from 0 (normal) to 3 (severe alterations) based on results of discriminate analysis.[58]

The Oral Assessment Guide (OAG) was developed by Eilers and colleagues to meet the need for a clinically reliable assessment instrument (see Appendix B, Table B-2).[59] It includes the eight subscales and uses a 3-point scale that ranges from 1 (normal) to 3 (severe alteration). The eight subscale scores are added to obtain an overall score between 8 (normal) and 24 (severe alterations). The subscale scores can also be used independently. The items are objectively rated and focus on physiology and function. In addition, the assessment guide identifies clinical tools needed for assessment of each parameter—such as tongue blade for assessing gingiva, and the method for measuring (e.g., *gently press tissue with tip of blade*). The inclusion of specific instructions increases the guide's clinical usefulness. Reliability and validity measures were established for this instrument.[59]

Several oral assessment guides and grading scales have been developed that focus on mucositis associated with high-dose chemotherapy and hematopoietic stem cell transplant. The Oral Mucositis Rating Scale (OMRS) was created in 1988 by Kolbinson and colleagues as part of a study that assessed oral changes following bone marrow transplant.[60] In this study, multiple changes were observed in the mucosa, the tongue, and the gingival, along with patient complaints of dryness and pain. A 91-item assessment scale was created that included the anatomic locations of lips (upper and lower), labial mucosa (upper and lower), buccal mucosa (upper and lower), palate (hard and soft), floor of mouth, gingiva, and tongue (dorsal, lateral, and ventral). The OMRS assesses each location for atrophy, pseudomembrane, erythema, hyperkeratosis, lichenoid keratosis, ulceration, and edema and/or cellulitis. Separate visual analogue scales measure the patient's perception of pain and dryness. The OMRS is a comprehensive tool for measuring a broad range of oral tissue changes associated with cancer therapy. The OMRS was used to develop an index for assessing acute oral mucositis after bone marrow transplant, the Oral Mucositis Index (OMI). The OMI excluded items that did not change markedly in the posttransplant period—measures of the hard palate and gingival areas—and retained items that were most problematic—ulceration and pseudomembranous changes.[61] The OMI consists of 34 pathophysiologic items—atrophy, pseudomembrane, erythema, and edema in eight anatomic areas: lips (upper and lower), labial mucosa (upper and lower), buccal mucosa (right and left), tongue (dorsal, lateral and ventral), floor of the mouth, and soft palate. Changes are rated from 0 (normal) to 3 (severe). Subjective measures of pain and dryness were eliminated. The researchers concluded that the OMI, which relies on objective assessment, adequately measures oral mucositis associated with bone marrow transplant and can be used for studies examining change over time, testing oral care protocols, and examining relationships between oral mucositis and other treatment-related complications. Reliability and validity measures have been established for both the OMRS and the OMI.[61]

The Oral Mucositis Index-20 (OMI-20) is a shortened version of the OMI developed by McGuire and colleagues in consultation with the developers of the OMI to test the effects of a psychoeducational nursing intervention (see Appendix B, Table B-3).[62] OMI-20 measures four types of mucosal changes—atrophy, edema, erythema and ulceration—in nine anatomic areas: dorsal and lateral tongue, upper and lower labial mucosa, right and left buccal mucosa, floor of mouth, soft palate, and dorsal, lateral, and ventral tongue. Ratings are summed across mucosal changes and anatomic areas, yielding a score ranging from 0 to 60, with higher scores representing greater mucositis. In addition, the nine items measuring erythema and ulceration can each be summed to obtain an erythema subscale score and an ulceration subscale score. OMI-20 captures changes associated with the pathophysiologic phases of developing and resolving mucositis and is a stable measure of mucositis over time.[62] Compared to the 34 item OMI, the OMI-20

provides consistent, reproducible scores when used by non–dental health professionals to measure oral mucositis.[62]

The Oral Mucositis Assessment Scale (OMAS) was developed by Sonis and colleagues as an easy and reproducible scoring system for mucositis to support multicenter clinical trials and measure changes over time (see Appendix B, Table B-4).[63] OMAS includes both objective and subjective indicators of mucositis. It focuses on mucous membranes and does not include other changes occurring in the oral cavity. The objective measures include ulceration, pseudomembranes, and erythema. Patient-reported measures include pain and perceived ability to swallow, as well as a functional measure of ability to swallow (degree to which food intake is limited). OMAS demonstrated good reliability and validitity; however, it should be noted that the individuals who participated in the instrument's development were highly experienced at evaluation of the oral cavity.

Assessment scales have been developed specifically for patients receiving radiation therapy. Spijkervet and colleagues developed a scoring system for mucositis related to radiation therapy of the head and neck.[64] It is based on two indicators: local signs of mucositis (i.e., white discoloration, erythema, pseudomembranes, and ulceration) scored between 0 (normal) and 4 (more severe), and the physical size of the sign (in cm) in each of the anatomic areas. The nine anatomic areas are left and right buccal mucosa, soft and hard palate, left and right dorsum and borders of the tongue, and floor of the mouth. The scoring system is considered complex, with overlapping areas.[54]

The MacDibbs Mouth Assessment also was developed specifically to measure oral mucositis in patients receiving head and neck radiation therapy.[65] The instrument has 14 items grouped into four major sections: patient information, examination, potassium hydroxide smear for fungus, and herpes simplex virus culture. The patient information section includes seven subjective measures: pain, dryness, eating, talking, swallowing, tasting, and saliva production—measured on a 0 (no problem) to 3 (severe problem) rating scale. The examination section includes five objective measures: size of the largest ulcer, the presence or absence of vesicles (+ or −), red areas (+ or −), or white patches (+ or −). Ulcers are measured using a Hu-Friedy probe, a color-coded probe using alternating silver and black bands that mark 3, 6, and 12 mm. Content validity and interrater reliability was excellent for 13 items on the tool (100%). Reliability and validity data are available. It was noted that larger ulcers were more difficult to measure, because the maximum size that could be directly measured with the periodontal probe was 12 mm. The MacDibbs instrument has been recommended for both clinical practice and research.[65]

Several additional grading scales have been developed that focus on cancer and cancer treatment–related mucositis. In reviewing and selecting an instrument for use, the most important criterion is the purpose of the assessment. Each available scale is different and yields different data.

CLINICAL TOXICITY ASSESSMENT SCALES

Clinical toxicity assessment scales are commonly used for measuring toxic side effects of cancer-related treatments. The WHO index is a simple grading scale along a 5-point continuum that measures objective signs (e.g., erythema and ulcers), subjective symptoms (e.g., soreness), and functional performance (e.g., ability to eat) (see Appendix B, Table B-5).[66] The descriptors are somewhat ambiguous, and reliability and validity are not established for this instrument; nonetheless, it is used as a general measurement scale and for comparison to other instruments.[54]

The National Cancer Institute (NCI) Common Toxicity Criteria measures anatomic and functional components of mucositis similar to the WHO index (see Appendix B, Table B-6). The NCI *Common Terminology Criteria for Adverse Events* is a descriptive terminology that can be used for reporting treatment-related adverse events related to clinical trials.[67] An adverse event is defined as any unfavorable and unintended sign, symptom, or disease temporally associated with the use of a medical treatment procedure that may or may not be considered related to the medical treatment or procedure. Within the criteria, adverse event terminology is specific and standardized, thus allowing for comparison of events as related to treatments and populations. The criteria include a specific grading scale for oral mucositis and one for xerostomia. Although these grading scales take into consideration both objective and subjective measures and have been helpful for comparison research looking across national and international clinical trials, these instruments are limited in scope.[28] The WHO scale and the NCI Common Toxicity Criteria are most frequently used to measure toxicity in clinical trials. The Radiation Therapy Oncology Group (RTOG) has a similar scale to measure radiation-related toxicity, which can be found online at *www.rtog.org*.

SELECTING AN INSTRUMENT

Instruments have been developed for specific purposes, including research to test nursing care protocols and for comparison across multicenter clinical trials.[57,62,63] Patient outcomes improve when an assessment instrument is routinely used, as Graham demonstrated in evaluating outcomes of a quality improvement program.[68] However, in clinical practice, oral assessment instruments and grading scales are not routinely used.[69] Before selecting an assessment instrument, consider the purpose of the assessment.

Instruments may be used to examine change over time, test interventions, or explore the relationships between oral mucositis and other complications. Eilers and Epstein outline several purposes for oral assessments.[28] One purpose is to measure differences between patients at a point in time. Instruments used for this purpose (i.e., discriminative instruments) should be able to identify change when it is present and should not find change when it is not present. A second purpose is predictive, to make a classification into a set of predetermined categories, such as determining a level-of-risk category. A third purpose involves detecting change across time (i.e., longitudinal change) for individuals or groups. Instruments used for measuring longitudinal change are referred to as evaluative instruments.[28]

Once the purpose is determined, decide on the endpoint. Different instruments measure different dimensions of mucositis. Some instruments focus entirely on objective physical parameters, and others include subjective patient perception. Where patient participation is required, as in reporting intensity of pain, the target patient group must be able to participate. Some instruments are designed for specific populations, such as patients receiving bone marrow transplant or patients receiving radiation therapy for head and neck cancer. Reliability and validity will have to be reestablished if an instrument designed and tested for one population is used for another population. Reliability and validity also will have to be reestablished if items are added to or deleted from an instrument.

Consider the level of training necessary for raters to be proficient in use of the assessment instrument, availability of training materials, and cost of training and equipment such as dental mirrors or special lighting. Also consider patient burden. Frequent or probative assessment may not be well tolerated by patients experiencing severe mucositis-associated pain, bleeding or other distressing symptoms.

Research has not established the timing for measurement. DeWalt coordinated assessment times with the delivery of routine oral care for older adults in the presence of interventions such as continuous nasal oxygen, mechanical suctioning, and keeping the patient on nothing-by-mouth (NPO) status.[56] Assessment scores may vary based on the window of time between activities such as oral care or eating and assessment.[28] Assessment scores may also vary depending on cancer treatments. If the purpose is to monitor longitudinal change, consider an instrument that can be used in different settings (e.g., inpatient, outpatient, home care) so as to capture patterns of change across time.

Interventions

The incidence of oral mucositis and related complications can be reduced significantly when an aggressive approach to oral care is initiated; however, to date no interventions are available that will completely prevent the development of mucositis. Current efforts to better understand the pathophysiology of oral mucositis is providing opportunity for targeted pharmacologic interventions, and preliminary studies are demonstrating promising new approaches to prevent or reduce the severity of oral mucositis.[30,70,71] Good oral hygiene and palliative symptom control remain among the best strategies to date.

PRETREATMENT ASSESSMENT

Pretreatment oral care strategies to minimize oral mucositis and related complications include establishing a baseline assessment with which all subsequent examinations can be compared and risk factors identified for the development of oral complications. A complete evaluation by a dentist should include information about number of teeth, dental caries, teeth requiring restoration, endodontic disease, teeth with pulpal infection, teeth requiring endodontic treatment, periodontal disease status, teeth requiring extraction, and any other urgent conditions. Ideally, this examination is performed 2 to 4 weeks before treatment.[67] Early evaluation gives time for healing, should dental procedures be indicated. Specific interventions are needed to address any of the following: mucosal lesions, dental caries and endodontic disease, ill-fitting dentures, orthodontic appliances, temporomandibular joint dysfunction, and salivary abnormalities.[67] Prophylactic antibiotic therapy and/or platelet transfusion may be indicated.

Soft-bristle toothbrushes are recommended, though electric or ultrasound toothbrushes may be used if the patient is skilled at using the appliance and will not traumatize oral tissues. Soft tooth-cleaning sponges do not thoroughly cleanse the teeth, although they are good for cleaning the maxillary and mandibular alveolar ridges of edentulous areas, the palate, and the tongue.[67]

ROUTINE ORAL CARE

All patients should receive routine oral care, either self-performed or provided by nurses. Routine oral hygiene helps reduce the incidence and severity of mucositis by reducing plaque build-up and clearing debris, which, in the presence of decreased saliva, can lead to increased inflammation of oral tissues. Inflammation of tissues weakens the mucosal lining, allowing for entry of bacteria into surrounding tissues. Toothbrushing and oral rinses 2 to 3 times a day and daily flossing remove plaque mechanically. Specific care routines may vary depending on personal preference and individual care needs. Routine oral care for cancer patients has not been extensively researched; however, the value of basic oral care is assumed for maintaining oral health and reducing oral complications.[72] Risk factors should guide interventions. Targeting high-risk patient groups for intensive or specialized interventions should not take preference over providing basic care for all patients receiving cancer treatments.[27]

Products selected for oral care such as toothpaste and mouth rinses should contain fluoride while avoiding strong flavors that can irritate. Mouthwashes containing alcohol should be avoided. Instead, use bland saline or sodium bicarbonate rinses. Dentures should be cleaned twice a day and rinsed well. In addition, dentures should be soaked daily in antimicrobial solution and clean water. Patients with removable dental appliances should take care to remove and clean the appliance. Ill-fitting dentures should be avoided and appropriate adjustment made to ensure a nonirritating fit. Orthodontic appliances with brackets and wires should be used with caution and only when conditioning has occurred.[6,67] Table 29-1 outlines routine oral hygiene practices.

PROTOCOLS

Protocols, also called standardized care plans or standing plans of care, are systematic approaches used by clinicians to promote and carry out basic oral care.[72] Protocols can guide clinicians in assessment, prevention, and treatment of mucositis and resulting secondary complications. Oral-care protocols generally include the following key points: First, oral care should begin before cancer treatment is initiated. Second, adequate hydration is essential to keep the oral tissues moist. Third, a grading scale must be used before and during treatment to adequately assess the patient's response to cancer-related treatment side effects. Fourth, research is needed to determine the most appropriate assessment parameters, interventions, and agents for managing mucositis.

Evidence supports the use of standardized oral care protocols for the prevention and management of oral mucositis.[57,73-75] Beck demonstrated significant improvement in oral status in patients receiving chemotherapy when an oral care protocol was used.[57] Kenny found that adding patient education into the intervention contributed more to reducing complications than the actual procedures and agents used in oral-care protocols.[73] Using collaborative, process-oriented criteria, Yeager and colleagues demonstrated that although implementing oral-care protocols in routine hospital nursing practice is a complex and challenging process, it can have a positive impact on patient outcomes.[74]

Used consistently, protocols can decrease the incidence and severity of mucositis, compared to the variations and gaps in care that can result from individual clinicians making independent decisions about care. Developing an oral-care protocol is an interdisciplinary responsibility that should include nurses, dentists, dental hygienists, pharmacists, and physicians. Protocols should be based on scientific evidence, national and international standards, and best practices. Different protocols may be needed for different

TABLE 29-1   Routine Oral Hygiene Care

Toothbrushing
Electric or ultrasound toothbrushes (only if used without causing trauma)
Soft nylon-bristled brush (2-3 rows) with frequent rinses
Foam toothbrushes
- Use only when a regular toothbrush is not feasible
- Use with antimicrobial rinses when possible
- Brush teeth and mucosal surfaces 2-3 times a day
- Rinse frequently

Dentifrice
Toothpaste with neutral taste; flavoring agents can be irritating
Fluoride recommended

Flossing
Once daily
Atraumatic technique

Rinses
Rinse after brushing with water or a bland rinse for 30 seconds
- 0.9% saline
- Sodium bicarbonate solution
- 0.9% saline plus sodium bicarbonate solution
Avoid mouthwashes containing alcohol and strong flavors

Fluoride
Apply a fluoride solution daily
- 1.1% neutral sodium fluoride gel
- 0.4% stannous fluoride gel
Brush on gel for 2-3 minutes
Expectorate and rinse mouth gently

Denture Care
Clean twice a day and rinse well
Soak daily in an antimicrobial solution and clean water
Avoid ill-fitting dentures

Data from Eilers J: Nursing interventions and supportive care for the prevention and treatment of oral mucositis associated with cancer treatment, *Oncol Nurs Forum* 31(4 Suppl):13-23, 2004; Eilers J, Epstein JB: Assessment and measurement of oral mucositis, *Semin Oncol Nurs* 20(1):22-29, 2004; Rubenstein EB, Peterson DE Schubert M et al: Clinical practice guidelines for the prevention and treatment of cancer therapy-induced oral and gastrointestinal mucositis, *Cancer* 100(9 Suppl): 2026-2046, 2004; Sonis ST, Elting LS et al: Perspectives on cancer therapy-induced mucosal injury: pathogenesis, measurement, epidemiology, and consequences for patients, *Cancer* 100(9S Suppl):1995-2025, 2004; National Cancer Institute: *Oral complications of chemotherapy and head/neck radiation, (PDQ) health professional version,* 2006, Author.

populations depending on both patient- and treatment-related risk factors. Many of the products and agents that have been used to manage oral mucositis lack adequate scientific support of effectiveness; however, emerging evidence, along with a clearer understanding of the pathophysiology of oral mucositis, is providing better scientific support for selected product use.[32,57,76]

Include patient education as an intervention in all oral-care protocols; international guidelines for oral care recommend patient education to help reduce the severity of oral mucositis. Patients are expected to self-manage oral care, yet not all patients have good oral care practices. In addition, most patients will be unaware of any modifications in self-care practices that may be necessary because of cancer treatment–related side effects.

Family members should also be included in educational programs: individuals learn basic hygiene practices such as oral care from family members. Proper oral care practices should be addressed with both the patient and the family. Protocols should include guidelines for initial assessment of patient learning needs and strategies for evaluating teaching and learning.[77]

Staff education is also important and should be included in strategies to initiate oral-care protocols. Little information about oral care is available in basic nursing education textbooks, especially oral care for high-risk and specialty patient groups, and evidence suggests that nurses are not always aware of or use guidelines published by professional organizations.[72,78] Oral care often reflects individual nurse preferences and relies on tradition, which leads to wide variations in practice.[79] Staff education is necessary to address gaps in knowledge, support consistent and reliable oral assessment, eliminate ineffective practices, and reinforce a standard of care.

PREVENTION AND MANAGEMENT OF MUCOSITIS

Routine oral care using scientifically sound principles and evidence-based practices will help prevent or minimize oral complications related to cancer treatments. Patients are advised to maintain adequate hydration, avoid mechanically or chemically irritating foods, and avoid alcohol and tobacco.[27] In addition, a number of products, agents, and procedures have been included in interventions to prevent or minimize mucositis.

Toothbrushes. Brushing natural teeth is always preferred when possible. An electric toothbrush may be used without causing trauma to gums and surrounding tissue. A soft-bristle toothbrush is recommended for high-risk patients. Any toothbrush should be replaced on a regular basis.[77]

If a toothbrush cannot be used, remove plaque and debris with a dry gauze pad. Lemon and glycerin swabs are not recommended for oral care. The oily character of the swabs makes them inadequate to remove debris. Glycerin is drying and hydroscopic; it takes up and retains moisture, and overall has tissue-drying effects. Acid contained in the lemon may decalcify teeth and cause pain when mucositis is present.[80,81]

Bland Rinses. Bland rinses are used to loosen and remove debris and maintain moisture.[24] Commonly used bland rinses include sterile water, normal saline, salt and soda (0.5 teaspoon each of table salt and sodium bicarbonate in 8 ounces of warm water), and sodium bicarbonate (1 teaspoon in 8 ounces of water). Sterile water and normal saline solutions are considered the least damaging. Sodium bicarbonate is considered effective at removing debris without harming underlying tissue. Few studies have systematically examined the use and effectiveness of bland rinses; the Multinational Association of Supportive Care in Cancer/International Society for Oral Oncology (MASCC/ISOO) was not able to recommend guidelines for bland rinses because of insufficient evidence.[72]

Commercial mouthwashes can cause irritation, ulceration, and sloughing related to the addition of oils, astringents, and antiseptic agents. Commercial products may contain as much as 25% alcohol and should be avoided because of the drying effects to the mucous membranes.[82] Furthermore, commercial mouthwashes have the potential to cause irritation and aggravate erythema, ulceration, and epithelial sloughing.[24]

Moisturizing Agents. Lip moisturizers include mineral oil, petroleum jelly, and water-based lubricating jelly. Mineral oil

and petroleum jelly form a protective coating on the lips and help reduce moisture evaporation. Water-based lubricating jelly forms a film on the lips that prevents moisture evaporation. Topical application of lanolin and aloe vera has been recommended.[73] Some lubricating jellies and other products for lip care contain glycerin and other ingredients that can be drying in high concentrations or with prolonged use.

Antiseptic Agents. Antiseptic agents for mouth care include chlorhexidine, hydrogen peroxide, and povidone-iodine. Chlorhexidine is a broad-spectrum antimicrobial with ability to bind to oral surfaces with minimal GI absorption, thereby limiting adverse systemic effects.[83] Commonly used to treat dental conditions in noncancer patients, chlorhexidine has been used as both a mouthwash and gargle in an attempt to prevent and treat oral mucositis in high-risk cancer patients.[84] However, clinical trials in cancer patients have failed to demonstrate therapeutic effects of chlorhexidine for the prevention and treatment of oral mucositis, and it might even be detrimental.[85-87] Gram-negative infections have been reported when chlorhexidine mouthwashes are used.[7] Currently, chlorhexidine is *not* recommended to prevent oral mucositis in patients with solid tumors of the head and neck who are undergoing radiotherapy or to treat established mucositis in patients receiving chemotherapy.[77]

Hydrogen peroxide may be useful in removing crusty debris. Oxygen, liberated from the peroxide by the peroxidase enzyme in the saliva, will froth and bubble, thereby loosening degenerated tissue and debris.[88] Long-term use of hydrogen peroxide as an antiseptic is discouraged.[27] Hydrogen peroxide at full strength may break down newly granulating tissue and disrupt normal flora and may exacerbate dryness, which leads to burning, stinging, and pain when applied to fragile oral tissue.[24,89]

Povidone-iodine has broad-spectrum antimicrobial activity against bacteria, fungus, yeast, and some viruses and has been used to prevent and treat chemotherapy-induced and radiation-induced oral mucositis.[7] It has been reported as well tolerated when used as a dilute (1:8) oral rinse, although it can be irritating.[90] Povidone-iodine swabs available in most clinical settings contain a 10% concentration and should not be used for oral care.[27] Studies to date have included povidone-iodine as one of several agents in an oral care intervention; thus no data are available to demonstrate the effectiveness of povidone-iodine as a single-agent intervention.[90,91] Swallowing povidone-iodine solution is absolutely contraindicated.[90] The overall usefulness of povidone-iodine in prevention and management of oral mucositis lacks adequate scientific evidence, and its use can lead to unintended consequences; further research is needed.

Antibiotic lozenges containing polymyxin E, tobramycin, and amphotericin B, either alone or in combination, have shown ability to eliminate microbial flora; however, selective decontamination has not been shown to reduce the incidence or severity of mucositis.[7] Antimicrobial lozenges are *not* recommended for prevention of radiation-induced oral mucositis.[77]

Cryotherapy. Oral cryotherapy is recommended before bolus infusions of 5-FU infusions. Ice chips are placed in the mouth for 5 minutes before the bolus infusion and continued for 25 minutes after administration.[92] By producing vasoconstriction in oral tissues, less of the drug circulates through the tissue, resulting in decreased blood flow to the oral mucous membranes during the period of peak drug concentration: 5-FU has a short half-life (about 10 minutes). The principle behind this intervention is consistent with the current pathophysiologic model of mucositis. With less drug circulating through the tissue, proliferating layers of the mucosa are protected, which in turn prevents future damage.[3,77,93] Patients treated with bolus doses of edatrexate should undergo 20 to 30 minutes of oral cryotherapy to minimize mucositis.[77] Cryotherapy is also recommended to prevent oral mucositis in patients receiving high-dose melphalan.[77] In addition to being nontoxic and inexpensive, this intervention has been demonstrated to be effective in several studies.[7,93-95]

Mucosal Protectants. Mucosal protectants contain binding or coating agents such as milk of magnesia, kaolin with pectin suspension, and mixtures of aluminum and/or hydroxide suspensions (e.g., many antacids) and have been used primarily for treatment of peptic ulcer disease. Such mixtures are believed to protect the mucosa and prevent ulceration. Mucosal protectants include sucralfate suspension, amifostine, prostaglandin E_2, and commercial products with hydroxypropyl cellulose (Zilactin), and polyvinylpyrolidone/sodium hyalurondate (Gelclair). Sucralfate, a basic aluminum salt, forms an ionic bond to proteins, and it forms a pastelike coat upon contact with mucosa, where it is thought to protect against prostaglandin release from local tissue. Clinical trials have not shown consistent results in modifying mucositis severity and associated symptoms.[96-100] Sucralfate is *not* recommended for prevention of radiation-induced oral mucositis.[77]

Amifostine is an antioxidant that acts as a free-radical scavenger that selectively protects normal cells from radiation.[92] Evidence suggests that it is beneficial in reducing the risk and severity of radiation-induced oral mucositis.[101] The optimal dose has not been determined, and research to date involves primarily head and neck patients receiving radiation therapy.[27,92] It can be administered either intravenously or subcutaneously.

Prostaglandin E_2 also has been suggested as a protective agent; however, study findings are mixed, demonstrating both significant reduction in pain severity and no difference.[102-104] It has been associated with higher incidence of herpes simplex virus and treatment-associated adverse events including vomiting, diarrhea, and fever.[27] Further research is needed.

Zilactin is a biofilm that forms a barrier over denuded and painful areas of the mouth. It stays in place, is flexible, and can remain in place for extended periods of time, up to 6 hours. Gelclair is a concentrated gel that forms a thin adhesive layer over the oral mucosa when it is rinsed within the mouth. Both Zilactin and Gelclair form a barrier that shields exposed or sensitized nerve endings from overstimulation; thus they both facilitate eating, drinking, and talking. Gelclair is considered a class 1 medical device.[27] Further research is needed on both products.

Multiagent rinses, also known as *magic mouthwash* and *mucositis cocktails,* are combinations of ingredients. Such mixtures often lack evidence of clinical effectiveness but continue to be used based on preferences of individual care providers and established hospital routines.[7] When used, the ingredients in these rinses should be identified. Alcohol should be eliminated.

Antiinflammatory Agents. Antiinflammatory agents that have been used to reduce mucositis-related inflammation and pain include steroids, indomethacin, allopurinol, prostaglandin E_1, and benzydamine.[105] Clinical evidence suggests that these agents may be helpful in minimizing mucositis; however,

evidence from controlled clinical trials is not available. Only benzydamine is recommended for prevention of radiation-induced mucositis in patients with head and neck cancer receiving moderate-dose radiation therapy.[77]

Kamillosan liquidum rinse and chamomile have also been suggested specifically for oral inflammation. Kamillosan liquidum showed unfavorable results in clinical trials.[27] Chamomile did not demonstrate significant reduction in 5-FU–induced mucositis; however, it was perceived by patients as soothing.[106] Chamomile contains ingredients that are antiinflammatory, antispasmodic, and antibacterial. It is inexpensive, well-tolerated, and frequently used despite the absence of data-based evidence.[7]

Growth Factors. The growth factors granulocyte colony-stimulating factor (G-CSF) and granulocytemacrophage colony-stimulating factor (GM-CSF) have been administered to prevent or minimize oral mucositis-related breakdown of the epithelium and enhance defense mechanisms. Both agents can be administered topically or by mouthwash. Clinical trials involving G-CSF and GM-CSF have demonstrated mixed results, and their use is considered investigational.[7,27,92] Some evidence suggests that these agents, particularly GM-CSF, may be more efficacious when used prophylactically.[27,101] The systemic use of GM-CSF is associated with significant side effects including local skin reaction, fever, bone pain, and nausea.[92]

There are promising study results that indicate that recombinant human keratinocyte growth factor-1, Palifermin, can prevent and/or minimize oral mucositis. Palifermin is a man-made version of a naturally occurring human protein called keratinocyte growth factor (KGF). KGF stimulates the growth of cells in the skin and on the surface layer of the mouth, the stomach, and the colon. Like the natural KGF, Palifermin also stimulates cells on the surface layer of the mouth to grow, leading to faster replacement of these cells. Palifermin was approved for use in the United States in 2004. MASCC/ISOO mucositis guidelines recommend that patients with hematologic malignancies receiving high-dose chemotherapy and total body irradiation with autologous stem cell transplant also receive Palifermin at a dosage of before the conditioning regimen and for 3 days posttransplant.[77]

Management of Complications

PAIN

The principles of oral pain management are the same as for other cancer-related pain: pain history, physical assessment, and direct treatment aimed at the cause of the pain; pain relief; and monitoring the effectiveness of interventions. Systemic approaches to the management of acute and persistent mucositis pain includes scheduled around-the-clock analgesics. The route of administration should be selected carefully, because swallowing pills may be difficult and may increase pain. For moderate mucositis, combinations of opioid and nonopioid drugs are recommended. When pain is unrelieved or mucositis is severe, sustained-release oral doses or continuous intravenous infusions of morphine may be required until healing occurs.

Patient-controlled analgesia (PCA) offers patients more control over pain relief. An advantage of the PCA system is that it often allows a set-up of baseline pain management through a continuous drip mode, and additionally allows the patient to administer boluses of pain medication for break-through pain. Other modes of delivery can be beneficial to manage pain, such as oral, transmucosal, and transdermal routes.[32]

Local agents, such as dyclonine hydrochloride, 0.5% to 1%, Xylocaine Viscous 2%, and diphendyramine hydrochloride (Benadryl elixir), may be effective in controlling pain, especially mild pain associated with only a few ulcerations. Topical anesthetic agents can be sprayed on, applied directly to painful areas, or swished and swallowed or expectorated. The numbness that results decreases taste and thermal perception. Mucosal protectants hydroxypropyl cellulose and polyvinylpyrolidone/sodium hyalurondate also provide local pain control. Topical capsaicin preparations are reported to be effective in controlling oral mucositis pain.[7] Capsaicin, the active (hot) ingredient in peppers that produces burning pain, stimulates polymodal nociceptors—pain receptors found in skin and mucous membranes that are sensitive to noxious heat, mechanical, and chemical stimuli. Capsaicin's potential derives from its ability to elevate the pain threshold in areas to which it is applied. Using an extemporaneous formulation of cayenne pepper in candy taffy, patients reported some relief from mucositis pain.[107] Commercial oral capsaicin formulations are investigational, and topical lotions and creams containing capsaicin are available without a prescription for external use only.

Topical anesthetics may minimize pain temporarily, but are frequently formulated with additives that can intensify and prolong oral mucositis. Systemic analgesics, including opioids, are indicated to alleviate discomfort.

INFECTION

Antibiotics used during prolonged neutropenia alter oral flora, creating a favorable environment for fungal overgrowth that may be exacerbated by concurrent steroid therapy. Early detection and treatment of local fungal infections is imperative, because systemic fungal infections are associated with high mortality rates.[8] Prophylaxis against fungal superinfection is generally recommended and includes using topical antifungal agents such as nystatin or clotrimazole as "swish and swallow" mouthwashes or in troche (dissolvable pastille) form. Evidence suggests that agents that are absorbed or partially absorbed from the GI tract prevent oral candidiasis in patients receiving treatment for cancer.[108] In addition, prophylactic treatment with antifungal agents, either absorbed or partially absorbed, should be used when the risk for infection is high based on the type of cancer or cancer treatment.[109] Topical antifungal prophylaxis and treatment can clear superficial oropharyngeal infections; however, these topical agents are not well absorbed and may be ineffective against more deeply invasive infections. To treat deep infections, systemic agents such as ketaconazole and fluconazole may be needed. In addition to *Candida* species, other fungi (e.g., *Aspergillus* and *Rhizopus* species) are also known to known cause oral infections among cancer patients.[8] Microbiologic determination of the causative organism is important, and systemic therapy should be used for severely immunocompromised patients.[8]

To prevent or minimize herpes simplex infections, acyclovir or valacyclovir is the treatment of choice.[8,110] It should be initiated prophylactically for patients who are seropositive, when severe immunosuppression is anticipated. Acyclovir decreases viral shedding, thus reducing healing time. For patient not receiving prophylactic treatment, outbreaks of herpes simplex tend to occur during the white blood cell nadir initiated by chemotherapy or radiation therapy.[8]

Varicella zoster distributes along dermatomes and tends to appear several weeks after chemotherapy treatments are completed. Acyclovir, valacyclovir, and famciclovir are the treatments of choice. Acyclovir should not be routinely used to prevent mucositis in patients receiving chemotherapy.[77] Cytomegaloviral infections are characterized by multiple mild to moderate ulcerations with irregular margins; these include nonspecific pseudomembranous fibrin exudate-covered ulcerations with granulomatous-appearing bases. Ganciclovir is the treatment of choice.[8,111]

BLEEDING

Bleeding may occur during treatment-induced thrombocytopenia and/or coagulopathy. Spontaneous gingival oozing may occur when platelet counts fall below $30,000/mm^3$. Sites of underlying periodontal disease may bleed spontaneously or may be trauma induced. Oral bleeding may be minimal, with petechiae located on the lips, the soft palate, or the floor of the mouth; or it may be severe, with oral hemorrhage especially in the gingival crevices or from herpes simplex virus ulcers.[8]

Using toothbrushes and dental floss when platelet counts are low is controversial because of the potential to induce bleeding; however, oral care should be modified and not eliminated during periods of severe thrombocytopenia. Oral care should be gentle. Use a very soft toothbrush, sponge, or gauze pad, and a technique that is adequate to remove plaque and debris. Ice chips and ice water irrigations may provide comfort and control bleeding. Vasoconstrictors such as epinephrine can be used topically to reduce blood flow through local vessels. Topical thrombin or a fibrinolysis inhibitor such as aminocaproic acid can be used for patients with minor oral hemorrhage secondary to thrombocytopenia.[8] The clots that form are friable and easily dislodged. Use extreme care when cleaning teeth around newly formed clots. In the presence of thrombocytopenia with continued bleeding, platelet transfusion may be indicated.

XEROSTOMIA

Daily use of fluoride toothpaste and/or topical fluoride is necessary to minimize caries formation during incidences of xerostomia. In addition, management of xerostomia involves two primary types of treatment: salivary stimulation and salivary substitutes.

Salivary flow is controlled largely by the parasympathetic nervous system and can be stimulated by taste, touch, and pressure. Interventions that stimulate receptors within the mouth will act directly on the parasympathetic nerves, namely, the efferent pathways. Patients should consume foods that require chewing. Reduced mastication will contribute to atrophy of salivary glands.[51] Although sugary, sweet foods promote salivation, patients should avoid sugar because it can promote demineralization of dental enamel and potentate caries formation. Patients can use sugar-free candy or sugar-free chewing gum to stimulate saliva.[112]

Sialogogues contain the cholinergic drug pilocarpine. These agents pharmacologically stimulate salivary flow from intact and responsive salivary glandular tissues, thus restoring salivary flow.[51,113] Sialogogues are particularly helpful for treatment of dry mouth from salivary gland hypofunction caused by radiotherapy for cancer of the head and neck. Pilocarpine is the only drug approved for use as a sialogogue. Given orally 3 times a day, pilocarpine typically increases salivary flow within 30 minutes after ingestion; however, maximal response may be achieved only after continual use is established.[113]

Synthetic saliva is recommended in situations involving excessive dryness. Saliva substitutes are palliative agents that relieve the discomfort of xerostomia by temporarily wetting the oral mucosa and replacing some missing constituents of saliva. Natural saliva contains mucous and serous secretions with many and complex functions; it is difficult to replace.[24] Commercially available artificial saliva products contain mucins, sorbitol or xylitol, mineral salts, and fluorides. Used in spray form, the effects of these agents last 1 to 2 hours.[51] When artificial saliva was compared to low-tack, sugar-free chewing gum for management of xerostomia in patients with advanced cancer, both products were effective, and the chewing gum was rated more acceptable to patients.[114]

Outcomes

Outcomes should focus on how cancer and cancer treatment–induced oral mucositis is affected by nursing interventions; these are called nursing-sensitive outcomes. Nursing-sensitive outcomes are those patient outcomes arrived at, or significantly affected, by nursing interventions or interventions delivered by nurses in collaboration with other health care providers. The interventions must be within the legal scope of

---

BOX 29-3   **Summary of Evidence-Based Clinical Practice Guidelines for Care of Patients with Oral Mucositis**

Foundations of Care

Patient Education: Patient education should address knowledge and skill-learning needs for self-care to reduce severity of oral mucositis from chemotherapy or radiation therapy. Educational outcomes should be evaluated.

Staff Education: Staff education should address knowledge and skill-learning needs related to reducing severity of oral mucositis from chemotherapy or radiation therapy. Educational outcomes should be evaluated.

Oral Care Protocols: Oral care protocols are systematic approaches used by clinicians to direct basic oral care independent of agents and products used. Protocol development should be multidisciplinary. Clinical outcomes of oral care protocols should be evaluated.

Products: A soft toothbrush should be used that is replaced on a regular basis.

Pain Control: Patient-controlled analgesia with morphine is the treatment of choice for oral mucositis pain in patients undergoing hematopoietic stem cell transplantation (HSCT).

Radiation Therapy–Prevention

- Midline radiation blocks and three-dimensional radiation treatment are recommended to reduce mucosal injury.
- Benzydamine is recommended for prevention of radiation-induced mucositis in patients with head and neck cancer receiving moderate-dose radiation therapy.
- Sucralfate is *not* recommended for prevention of radiation-induced oral mucositis.
- Antimicrobial lozenges are *not* recommended for prevention of radiation-induced oral mucositis.
- Chlorhexidine is *not* recommended to prevent oral mucositis in patients with solid tumors of the head and neck who are undergoing radiotherapy.

Standard-Dose Chemotherapy–Prevention

- Patients receiving bolus 5-fluorouracil (5-FU) chemotherapy should undergo 30 minutes of oral cryotherapy to prevent oral mucositis.
- Patients treated with bolus doses of edatrexate should undergo 20 to 30 minutes of oral cryotherapy to minimize mucositis.
- Acyclovir and its analogues are *not* recommended for routine use to prevent mucositis.

Standard-Dose Chemotherapy–Treatment

- Chlorhexidine is *not* recommended to treat established oral mucositis.

High-Dose Chemotherapy with or without Total Body Irradiation Plus Hematopoietic Cell Transplantation (HSCT)–Prevention

- Patients with hematologic malignancies receiving high-dose chemotherapy and total body irradiation with autologous stem cell transplant should receive keratinocyte growth factor-1 (Palifermin) at a dosage of 60 mcg/kg/day for 3 days before conditioning treatment and for 3 days after transplant for the prevention of oral mucositis.
- Cryotherapy is recommended to prevent oral mucositis in patients receiving high-dose melphalan.
- Pentoxifylline is *not* recommended to prevent mucositis in patients undergoing HSCT.
- Low-level laser therapy (LLLT) requires expensive equipment and specialized training. Because of interoperator variability, clinical trials are difficult to conduct, and their results are difficult to compare; nevertheless, the panel is encouraged by the accumulating evidence in support of LLLT. The panel suggests that, for centers able to support the necessary technology and training, LLLT be used to attempt to reduce the incidence of oral mucositis and its associated pain in patients receiving high-dose chemotherapy or chemoradiotherapy before HSCT.

From Multinational Association of Supportive Care in Cancer/International Society for Oral Oncology (MASCC/ISOO): Summary of evidence-based clinical practice guidelines for care of patients with oral and gastrointestinal mucositis (update), Metairie, LA, 2005, Author; retrieved from http://www.mascc.org/media/Resource_centers/Guidelines_table_12_Oct_05.pdf.

nursing practice and central to the delivery of nursing care. For example, selecting a type of toothbrush is a nursing judgment based on a nursing assessment of the degree of mucositis. The toothbrush is used to deliver a nursing intervention, oral care, and the intervention can be directly linked to the patient's outcome. Good assessment supports good judgment in selecting equipment which, in turn, supports delivery of a nursing intervention—all of which leads to good patient outcomes. The logical link between nursing actions and patient outcomes makes the outcome nursing-sensitive.

In collaborative care, nursing-sensitive outcomes may be apparent when nursing care is absent. For example, an interdisciplinary oral care protocol for bone marrow transplant patients is nursing-sensitive because nursing is integral to actualizing the protocol—nurses implement the protocol and use independent judgments during the delivery of the care. Without nursing, and nursing judgment, the protocol would not lead to improved patient outcomes. Likewise, without multidisciplinary collaboration, oral care outcomes would be compromised. Therefore, collaborative care is interdependent care, and discipline-sensitive outcomes become apparent in the absence of a particular discipline.

Evaluation of quality of care and effectiveness of nursing interventions for patients with cancer and their families is measured in outcomes. When delivering interventions to prevent or manage oral mucositis, nurses are accountable for the results of their care: the patient outcomes. The selection of outcome(s) to measure depends on multiple considerations such as setting, patient population, type of intervention, level of expertise of the provider and so forth. Evaluation should be longitudinal and consider short- and long-term outcomes. For example, a short-term goal for oral care may be to reduce or maintain reduced levels of plaque and debris. A long-term goal may be prevention of dental caries at specified time intervals after cancer treatment–induced mucositis. The time of measurement becomes important when interventions are evaluated. Measurement must take place at the time(s) consistent with the expected effects of the intervention (outcome). For example, the amount of plaque may be determined after oral care interventions, where the prevention of caries can only be determined at longer time intervals of months to years. Measurement of outcomes should occur in a timely manner so as to control for other confounding factors and more accurately ensure that the outcomes are attributed to nursing interventions. For more information on measuring oncology nursing–sensitive patient outcomes, visit the Oncology Nursing Society Evidence-based Practice web site at *http://www.ons.org/outcomes/measures/symptomexperience/mucositisummary.shtml.*

Ethical Considerations

Currently, no oral care intervention has been shown to be uniformly efficacious across multiple cancer population or treatment groups. No evidence-based therapy standard has been developed. However, knowledgeable experts in the field and clinical observations clearly signal that nurses should routinely provide oral care that includes regular cleansing of the teeth and mucosal tissues using nontraumatizing products and agents. Further, experts agree on the need for nurses to be guided by oral care protocols. Protocols standardize care practices, removing the variability of individual provider preference and leading to more consistent care.

Ethical dilemmas arise in situations where conflict exists between personal values and professional values, personal values and a patient's values, and among professional values. The American Nurses Association *Code of Ethics for Nurses* has five core values: respectful care, quality of life, competence, collegiality, and fairness.[115] These core values should be the guiding principles for delivery of care. For example, the multidisciplinary process of creating oral care protocols should be framed in collegiality and fairness since expertise is needed from the disciplines of nursing, dentistry, pharmacy, and medicine. The multidisciplinary team should work collaboratively to design care protocols that emphasize respect for patients in the context of cancer, when the disease and its related treatments cause multiple challenges. Care protocols should also promote quality of life. In some situations, it may be appropriate to include quality of life measures in ongoing evaluation of care.

Care protocols should reflect thoughtfully considered scientific and clinical evidence. Evidence-based protocols will help ensure that the care to be delivered is competent and that patients will achieve the best possible outcomes. Delivering competent care also means that staff who are expected to deliver oral care have access to education about scientific and clinical evidence and the care protocol. Staff should receive regular feedback about patient outcomes and have opportunity for input into modifications in care protocols or system-related issues that affect care delivery. As with all cancer nursing care, it is important to develop mechanisms for addressing values conflicts.

CONSIDERATIONS FOR OLDER ADULTS

Age-Related Changes That Affect Drug Absorption and Secretion
- Age-related decreases in liver blood flow may lead to decreased clearance of drugs, increased circulating drug, and increased drug related mucosal toxicity.
- Age-related decreases in glomerular filtration rate may lead to decreased drug excretion, increased circulating drug, and increased drug–related mucosal toxicity.
- Age-related changes in body composition with increased fat tissue and decreased total body water may lead to increased plasma concentration of drug and increased drug-related mucosal toxicity.
- Age-related decreased hematopoietic reserve may prolong periods of myelosuppression and contribute to risk and severity of mucositis.
- Age-related changes in the oral mucosa include decreased salivary flow, and diminished keratinization of the mucosa may contribute to increased risk of mucositis.

Age-Related Care Considerations
- The risk of mucositis increases with age.
- Older adults experience greater severity of oral mucositis when 5-fluorouracil is included in the chemotherapy regimen.
- Dentures and dental appliances can increase the risk for irritation and ulceration during treatments.
- Education programs for older adults should address beliefs and self-care practices about oral care.
- Drugs used to manage comorbidities may cause xerostomia.
- A pretreatment dental exam should be performed.

Incorporating nursing's core values into the process of care delivery is an important consideration for building an atmosphere of ethical care. Ethical conflicts should be identified and addressed. The standards for oral care for cancer patients is rapidly developing and as such are vulnerable to conflict as care providers struggle to deliver the best possible care in the face of changing evidence.

Conclusion

Oral mucositis develops in the context of cancer and cancer-related treatments. Preventing and managing mucositis requires a collaborative multidisciplinary effort. Many oral care interventions lack good scientific evidence and have become part of practice in the absence of more evidence-based options. New and emerging interventions, along with older interventions that are undergoing rigorous scientific evaluation, are providing new insights into better care options for mucositis. No single care standard exists; however, evidence suggests that care protocols do lead to better patient outcomes. Patient outcomes of mucositis care are nursing-sensitive, and nursing is responsible for ensuring that cancer patients across multiple settings of care receive evidence-based care.

REVIEW QUESTIONS

✓ Case Study

JT—a 21-year-old, 6-foot, 195-pound, male college student—was diagnosed with acute lymphoblastic leukemia (ALL). Since diagnosis he completed induction chemotherapy with cyclophosphamide, vincristine, doxorubicin, and dexamethasone; during the therapy, he eventually developed oral mucositis that was scored as grade 2 according to the National Cancer Institute (NCI) Common Toxicity Criteria. He experienced a 15-pound weight loss and complained of overwhelming fatigue that resulted in dropping classes. JT then completed consolidation chemotherapy with an additional five cycles, each with intrathecal methotrexate. He reported oral tenderness and taste alterations with each cycle and lost another 8 pounds over the time of consolidation therapy. JT achieved a complete remission of ALL and was placed on maintenance chemotherapy of 6-mercaptopurine and methotrexate. Fourteen months later, JT had gained back the weight he lost and had returned to school full-time; however, his follow-up blood tests revealed increasing white cell counts with high levels of circulating blasts. JT completed salvage and reinduction chemotherapy that included vincristine, daunorubicin, and asparaginase. After achieving a second complete remission, plans are being made for an autologous bone marrow transplant that includes a conditioning regime of high-dose cyclophosphamide, high-dose etoposide, and total body irradiation. A pretransplant dental evaluation found two new cavities.

QUESTIONS

1. Early in the course of induction chemotherapy, JT did not experience mucositis, and chlorhexidine solution was included in oral care. Based on the action of chlorhexidine, which of the following are the best instructions for its use by patients undergoing induction chemotherapy?
   a. Use chlorhexidine mouthwash before each meal and at bedtime.
   b. Use chlorhexidine with a swish-and-spit technique after meals and at bedtime.
   c. Apply chlorhexidine mouthwash with a soft-bristle toothbrush after meals and at bedtime.
   d. Use chlorhexidine as needed for pain management.

2. As induction therapy proceeded, JT began experiencing pain associated with grade 2 oral mucositis and was medically managed with low-dose intravenous morphine. In addition to physician-prescribed narcotics, which of the following nonpharmacologic interventions could the nurse implement?
   a. A bland rinse with sterile water and sodium bicarbonate
   b. A full-strength hydrogen peroxide mouthwash
   c. Xylocaine Viscous 2% mouthwash
   d. G-CSF mouthwash

3. JT's grade 2 mucositis made eating normal foods difficult. In making dietary modifications when mucositis is present, which of the following is the best option?
   a. The patient's favorite food—spicy taco
   b. Large chocolate milkshake
   c. Room-temperature applesauce
   d. Protein shake

4. After completing induction chemotherapy, JT's oral mucositis continued to worsen, and he lost 15 pounds. According to the NCI Common Toxicity Criteria for oral mucositis, weight loss is indicative of which grade of mucositis?
   a. Grade 1
   b. Grade 2
   c. Grade 3
   d. Grade 4

5. When JT began a course of consolidation chemotherapy treatments, which of the following were considered risk factors for development of oral mucositis?
   a. Younger age
   b. Previous chemotherapy treatment
   c. A history of weight loss while on treatment
   d. Dental caries

6. During an outpatient visit for consolidation chemotherapy treatment, JT is assessed as experiencing grade 1 mucositis according to the NCI Common Toxicity Criteria. Which of the following oral care recommendations should the nurse make?
   a. Rinse mouth with mint-flavored fluoride containing commercial mouthwash twice a day.
   b. Brush with a soft-bristle toothbrush with fluoride toothpaste after each meal and before bed.

Continued

REVIEW QUESTIONS—CONT'D

c. Brush with a regular toothbrush with a flavored fluoride toothpaste and floss 3 times a day.

d. Clean teeth with lemon-flavored foam swabs every 4 hours.

7. After JT's third cycle of consolidation chemotherapy, he complains of oral tenderness, and upon visual assessment, a red area approximately 1 cm × 1 cm in size is visualized directly behind the upper teeth. When documenting the assessment findings, which anatomic region is included?

a. *Palatine velum* (lower soft palate)

b. *Palatum molle* (soft palate)

c. *Lingua* (tongue)

d. *Palatum durum* (hard palate)

8. JT comes to the outpatient infusion area for his fifth and final cycle of consolidation chemotherapy treatment and tells the staff that he and his friend smoked cigars in celebration of the arrival of his best friend's first child. What should the nurse remind JT?

a. Smoking cigars can cause canker sores.

b. Smoking cigars can prevent bacteria from replicating in the mouth.

c. Smoking brings extra oxygen to the mouth.

d. Smoking impairs oral tissue healing.

9. As plans for JT's bone marrow transplant are made, he tells the nurse that one problem he is not looking forward to experiencing again is oral mucositis because it was so painful. What is the standard of care for bone marrow transplant patients experiencing mucositis-related pain?

a. Patient-controlled analgesia with morphine

b. Morphine as needed (PRN), with acetaminophen for breakthrough pain

c. Topical pain relief such as xylocaine, capsaicin, or chamomile

d. Round-the-clock use of mucosal protectants, also known as oral bandages

10. After bone marrow transplant, the Oral Assessment Guide (OAG) is used to assess for mucositis; why?

a. The OAG is a good subjective measure of all aspects of mucous membranes and teeth.

b. The OAG is routinely used by dentists for oral assessment

c. The OAG has been proven to be the best instrument to use for patients undergoing bone marrow transplant.

d. The OAG relies on objective measures and includes oral structures in addition to mucous membranes.

ANSWERS

1. **C.** *Rationale:* A chlorhexidine mouthwash acts as a broad-spectrum antiseptic, antiplaque, and antifungal intervention that is best utilized after meals and at bedtime to reduce bacteria in the oral cavity. Using the mouthwash in conjunction with brushing further reduces the bacterial content on surfaces. Using chlorhexidine before eating does not reduce the bacterial load after meals. Swishing and spitting does not provide enough friction to remove bacteria from surfaces, although this technique may be used as a last resort with more advanced oral mucositis when brushing causes too much pain. Chlorhexidine has antiplaque and antimicrobial action and is effective in reducing gram-positive and gram-negative bacteria, but does not contain analgesic components.

2. **A.** *Rationale:* Bland rinses are nonpharmacologic interventions. Sterile water is gentle on oral tissue, and sodium bicarbonate is effective for removing debris without harming underlying tissue. Full-strength hydrogen peroxide as a mouthwash is currently not an evidence-based intervention and is potentially harmful to delicate oral tissue. Xylocaine Viscous requires a physician prescription and is not an independent nursing intervention. Growth-factor mouthwashes are investigational and are not independent nursing interventions.

3. **D.** *Rationale:* A protein shake will provide the most calories and protein to promote tissue healing and with the least amount of sugar, which helps prevent bacterial growth in the oral cavity. Although patient preferences should be considered, hot and spicy foods can irritate damaged oral tissue, and hard, crunchy foods can cause further damage to delicate oral tissue. Milkshakes will provide calories and are easy to swallow; however, they typically have a high sugar content that promotes bacterial growth on oral surfaces. Although applesauce is easy to swallow and has low sugar content, it does not provide enough calories or protein for tissue healing.

4. **C.** *Rationale:* Difficulty with maintaining sufficient caloric intake that results in a 15-pound weight loss is a consequence of inadequate oral alimentation. At grade 1, normal dietary intake is still achievable. At grade 2, the patient can still swallow a modified diet without difficulty. Although the patient's 15-pound weight loss is significant, it is not life-threatening (grade 4).

5. **B.** *Rationale:* Previous chemotherapy is a known risk factor for development of oral mucositis with subsequent chemotherapy treatment. Although younger age is a risk factor from a growth and development perspective, JT is an adult. Weight loss is not a risk factor by itself; however, it is likely that oral mucositis contributed to the weight loss and therefore the patient could be at risk for nutritional compromise. Likewise, the presence of dental caries is not a risk factor by itself; however, it may signal the need for improved dental hygiene and increased oral self-care practices.

6. **B.** *Rationale:* Utilizing a soft-bristle toothbrush for performing oral care is recommended for plaque removal without causing mucosal damage. Fluoride toothpaste helps prevent dental caries. Commercial mouthwashes can contain high concentrations of alcohol and thus cause further mucosal dryness. Although fluoride-containing products are recommended, strongly flavored products can be irritating to already compromised oral tissue. Lemon swabs are acidic and can cause additional pain.

7. **D.** *Rationale:* The palatum durum is the region behind the teeth where the alveolar arches meet the gums. The palatine velum is the lower portion of the soft palate. *Palatum molle* is the term for *soft palate*, and *lingua* is the anatomic term for the *tongue*.

8. **D.** *Rationale:* Smoking either cigars or cigarettes causes cellular changes that prevent oral tissue from healing quickly, which delays healing after mucositis. Smoking cigars does

not cause canker sores, though it can be irritating to local tissue. Smoking actually increases the risk for overgrowth of anaerobic organisms; furthermore, it reduces oxygen available to oral tissue to aid in the repair.

9. A. *Rationale:* Systemic approaches to the management of acute and persistent mucositis pain include patient-controlled around-the-clock analgesics. Intravenous route should be selected when swallowing pills that are difficult and that cause pain. PRN dosing will not provide adequate baseline coverage. Patients with severe mucositis often have difficulty swallowing pills, including acetaminophen, which is also not the best option for pain management in a neutropenic population because it can mask a fever. Although topical anesthetics may minimize pain temporarily, they are frequently formulated with additives that can intensify and prolong mucositis. Mucosal protectants, although they provide local relief, are inadequate to manage pain associated with severe mucositis.

10. D. *Rationale:* The OAG relies on objective (observable), rather than subjective, measures and measures a comprehensive list of parameters: voice, swallow, lips, tongue, saliva, mucous membranes, gingiva, and teeth (dentures). It is not an instrument routinely used by dentists for oral assessment; it was developed for assessment of mucositis in cancer patients. Research has not established that OAG is the best instrument for assessing oral mucositis among patients undergoing bone marrow transplant. Other instruments such as the Oral Mucositis Index (OMI) and Oral Mucositis Assessment Scale (OMAS) have also been used to assess mucositis among bone marrow transplant patients along with NCI Common Toxicity Criteria for patients undergoing investigational protocol treatments.

REFERENCES

1. Bellm LA, Epstein B, Rose-Ped A et al: Patient reports of complications of bone marrow transplantation, *Support Care Cancer* 8(1):33-39, 2000.
2. Gerpen RV: Stomatitis, *Clin J Oncol Nurs* 7(4):471-474, 2003.
3. Sonis ST, Fey GE: Oral complications of cancer therapy, *Oncology* (Williston Park) 16(5):680-686, discussion 686, 691-692, 695, 2002.
4. Ruescher T, Sodeifi A, Scrivani SJ et al: The impact of mucositis on alpha-hemolytic streptococcal infection in patients undergoing autologous bone marrow transplantation for hematologic malignancies, *Cancer* 82(11):2275-2281, 1998.
5. Sonis ST, Oster G, Fuchs H et al: Oral mucositis and the clinical and economic outcomes of hematopoietic stem-cell transplantation, *J Clin Oncol* 19(8):2201-2205, 2001.
6. Sonis ST, Elting LS, Keefe D et al: Perspectives on cancer therapy-induced mucosal injury: pathogenesis, measurement, epidemiology, and consequences for patients, *Cancer* 100(9 Suppl):1995-2025, 2004.
7. Kostler WJ, Hejna M, Wenzel C et al: Oral mucositis complicating chemotherapy and/or radiotherapy: options for prevention and treatment, *CA Cancer J Clin* 51(5):290-315, 2001.
8. National Cancer Institute: Oral complications of chemotherapy and head/neck radiation, (PDQ) Health professional version, 2006, retrieved October 11, 2006, from www.cancer.gov/cancertopics/pdq/supportivecare/oralcomplications.
9. Robien K, Schubert MM, Bruemmer B et al: Predictors of oral mucositis in patients receiving hematopoietic cell transplants for chronic myelogenous leukaemia, *J Clin Oncol* 22(7):1268-1275, 2004.
10. Bruce SD: Pain management issues and strategies in oral mucositis, *Oncol Support Care Q* 3(2):18-27, 2005.
11. Brown CG, Wingard J: Clinical consequences of oral mucositis, *Semin Oncol Nurs* 20(1):16-21, 2004.
12. Avritscher EB, Cooksley CD, Etling LS: Scope and epidemiology of cancer therapy-induced oral and gastrointestinal mucositis, *Semin Oncol Nurs* 20(1):3-10, 2004.
13. Cheng KK, Molassiotis A, Chang AM et al: Evaluation of an oral care protocol intervention in the prevention of chemotherapy-induced oral mucositis in paediatric cancer patients, *Eur J Cancer* 37(16):2056-2063, 2001.
14. Pico L, Avila-Garavito A, Naccache P: Mucositis: its occurrence, consequences, and treatment in the oncology setting, *Oncologist* 3(6):446-451, 1998.
15. Raber-Durlacher E, Weijl NI, Abu Saris M et al: Oral mucositis in patients treated with chemotherapy for solid tumors: a retrospective analysis of 150 cases, *Support Care Cancer* 8(5):366-371, 2000.
16. Bond SM: Symptom management of mucositis. An evidence-based approach to the treatment and care of the older adult with cancer. In Cope DG, Reb AM, editors: *An evidence-based approach to treatment and care of older adults with cancer,* Pittsburgh, 2006, Oncology Nursing Society.
17. Sloan JA, Loprinzi CL, Novotny PJ et al: Sex differences in fluorouracil-induced stomatitis, *J Clin Oncol* 18(2):412-420, 2000.
18. Chansky K, Benedetti J, Macdonald JS: Differences in toxicity between men and women treated with 5-fluorouracil therapy for colorectal carcinoma, *Cancer* 103(6):1165-1171, 2005.
19. Vokurka S, Bystricka E, Koza V et al: Higher incidence of chemotherapy induced oral mucositis in females: a supplement of multivariate analysis to a randomized multicentre study, *Support Care Cancer* 14(9):974-976, 2006.
20. Dibble SL, Padilla GV, Dodd MJ et al: Gender differences in the dimensions of quality of life, *Oncol Nurs Forum* 25(3):577-583, 1998.
21. Gremel ER, Padilla GV, Grant MM: Gender differences in outcomes among patients with cancer, *Psychooncology* 7(3):197-206, 1998.
22. Raber-Durlacher JE: Current practices for management of oral mucositis in cancer patients, *Support Care Cancer* 7(2):71-74, 1999.
23. Woo SB, Sonis ST, Monopoli MM et al: A longitudinal study of oral ulcerative mucositis in bone marrow transplant recipients, *Cancer* 72(5):1612-1617, 1993.
24. Miller M, Kearney N: Oral care for patients with cancer: a review of the literature, *Cancer Nurs* 24(4):241-254, 2001.
25. Taybos G: Oral changes associated with tobacco use, *Am J Med Sci* 326(4):179-182, 2003.
26. Vokurka S, Bystricka E, Koza V et al: The comparative effects of povidone-iodine and normal saline mouthwashes on oral mucositis in patients after high-dose chemotherapy and APBSCT—results of a randomized multicentre study, *Support Care Cancer* 13(7):554-558, 2005.
27. Eilers J: Nursing interventions and supportive care for the prevention and treatment of oral mucositis associated with cancer treatment, *Oncol Nurs Forum* 31(4 Suppl):13-23, 2004.
28. Eilers J, Epstein JB: Assessment and measurement of oral mucositis, *Semin Oncol Nurs* 20(1):22-29, 2004.
29. Rose-Ped AM, Bellm LA, Epstein JB et al: Complications of radiation therapy for head and neck cancers. The patient's perspective, *Cancer Nurs* 25(6):461-467, quiz 468-469, 2002.
30. Hwang D, Popat R, Bragdon C et al: Effects of ceramide inhibition on experimental radiation-induced oral mucositis, *Oral Surg Oral Med Oral Pathol Oral Radiol Endod* 100(3):321-329, 2005.
31. Sonis ST: Oral mucositis in cancer therapy, *J Support Oncol* 2(6 Suppl 3):3-8, 2004.
32. Rubenstein EB, Peterson DE, Schubert M et al: Clinical practice guidelines for the prevention and treatment of cancer therapy-induced oral and gastrointestinal mucositis, *Cancer* 100(9 Suppl):2026-2046, 2004.
33. McGuire DB: Mucosal tissue injury in cancer therapy. More than mucositis and mouthwash, *Cancer Pract* 10(4):179-191, 2002.
34. Daeffler R: Oral hygiene measures for patients with cancer. II, *Cancer Nurs* 3(6):427-432, 1980.
35. Ducjak LA: Mouth care for mucositis due to radiation therapy, *Cancer Nurs* 10(3):131-140, 1987.
36. Coleman S: An overview of the oral complications of adult patients with malignant haematological conditions who have undergone radiotherapy or chemotherapy, *J Adv Nurs* 22(6):1085-1091, 1995.

37. Shih A, Miaskowski C, Dodd MJ et al: Mechanisms for radiation-induced oral mucositis and the consequences, *Cancer Nurs* 26(3):222-229, 2003.

38. Sonis S, Edwards L, Lucey C: The biological basis for the attenuation of mucositis: the example of interleukin-11, *Leukemia* 13(6):831-834, 1999.

39. Sonis ST: A biological approach to mucositis, *J Support Oncol* 2(1): 21-32, discussion 35-36, 2004.

40. Sonis ST: The pathobiology of mucositis, *Nat Rev Cancer* 4(4):277-284, 2004.

41. Sonis ST: Pathobiology of mucositis, *Semin Oncol Nurs* 20(1):11-15, 2004.

42. Sonis ST, O'Donnell KE, Popat R et al: The relationship between mucosal cyclooxygenase-2 (COX-2) expression and experimental radiation-induced mucositis, *Oral Oncol* 40(2):170-176, 2004.

43. Sonis ST: The biologic role for nuclear factor-kappaB in disease and its potential involvement in mucosal injury associated with anti-neoplastic therapy, *Crit Rev Oral Biol Med* 13(5):380-389, 2002.

44. Puntillo KA, Miaskowski C, Summer G: Pain. In Carrieri-Kohlman V, Lindsey A, West C, editors: *Pathophysiological phenomena in nursing: human response to illness*, ed 3, St. Louis, 2003, Saunders.

45. Miaskowski C: Biology of mucosal pain, *J Natl Cancer Inst Monogr* (29):37-40, 2001.

46. McGuire DB, Yeager KA, Dudley WN et al: Acute oral pain and mucositis in bone marrow transplant and leukemia patients: data from a pilot study, *Cancer Nurs* 21(6):385-393, 1998.

47. Bellm LA, Cunningham G, Durnell L et al: Defining clinically meaningful outcomes in the evaluation of new treatments for oral mucositis: oral mucositis patient provider advisory board, *Cancer Invest* 20(5-6): 793-800, 2002.

48. Rapoport AP, Miller Watelet LF, Linder T et al: Analysis of factors that correlate with mucositis in recipients of autologous and allogeneic stem-cell transplants, *J Clin Oncol* 17(8):2446-2453, 1999.

49. Scully C, Sonis S, Diz PD: Oral mucositis, *Oral Dis* 12(3):229-241, 2006.

50. Raber-Durlacher JE, Epstein JB, Raber J et al: Periodontal infection in cancer patients treated with high-dose chemotherapy, *Support Care Cancer* 10(6):466-473, 2002.

51. Holmes S: Xerostomia: Aetiology and management in cancer patients, *Support Care Cancer* 6(4):348-355, 1998.

52. Vera-Llonch M, Oster G, Hagiwara M et al: Oral mucositis in patients undergoing radiation treatment for head and neck carcinoma, *Cancer* 106(2):329-336, 2006.

53. Dodd MJ: The pathogenesis and characterization of oral mucositis associated with cancer therapy, *Oncol Nurs Forum* 31(4):5-11, 2004.

54. Hyland SA: Assessing the oral cavity. Instruments for clinical health-care research. In Frank-Stromborg M, Olsen SJ, editors: *Instruments for clinical health-care research*, Boston, 2004, Jones & Bartlett.

55. Gerpen RV: An overview of oral mucositis, *Oncol Support Care Q* 3(2):4-10, 2005.

56. DeWalt EM: Effect of timed hygienic measures on oral mucosa in a group of elderly subjects, *Nurs Res* 24(2):104-108, 1975.

57. Beck S: Impact of a systematic oral care protocol on stomatitis after chemotherapy, *Cancer Nurs* 2(3):185-199, 1979.

58. Western Consortium for Cancer Nursing Research (WCCNR): Assessing stomatitis: refinement of the WCCNR stomatitis staging system, *Can Oncol Nurs J* 8(3):1605, 1998.

59. Eilers J, Berger AM, Peterson MC: Development, testing, and application of the oral assessment guide, *Oncol Nurs Forum* 15(3):325-330, 1988.

60. Kolbinson DA, Schubert MM, Flournoy N et al: Early oral changes following bone marrow transplantation, *Oral Surg Oral Med Oral Pathol* 66(1):130-138, 1988.

61. Schubert MM, Williams BE, Lloid ME et al: Clinical assessment scale for the rating of oral mucosal changes associated with bone marrow transplantation. Development of an oral mucositis index, *Cancer* 69(10):2469-2477, 1992.

62. McGuire DB, Peterson DE, Muller S et al: The 20 item oral mucositis index: reliability and validity in bone marrow and stem cell transplant patients, *Cancer Invest* 20(7-8):893-903, 2002.

63. Sonis ST, Eilers JP, Epstein JB et al: Validation of a new scoring system for the assessment of clinical trial research of oral mucositis induced by radiation or chemotherapy. Mucositis Study Group, *Cancer* 85(10): 2103-2013, 1999.

64. Spijkervet FK, van Saene HK, Panders AK et al: Scoring irradiation mucositis in head and neck cancer patients, *J Oral Pathol Med* 18(3):167-171, 1989.

65. Dibble SL, Shiba G, MacPhail L et al: MacDibbs mouth assessment. A new tool to evaluate mucositis in the radiation therapy patient, *Cancer Pract* 4(3):135-140, 1996.

66. World Health Organization: *Handbook for reporting results of cancer treatment*, Geneva, 1979, Author.

67. National Cancer Institute: Common terminology criteria for adverse events, v.3.0, 2006, retrieved October 11, 2006, from http://ctep.cancer.gov/forms/CTC.

68. Graham KM, Pecoraro DA, Ventura M et al: Reducing the incidence of stomatitis using a quality assessment and improvement approach, *Cancer Nurs* 16(2):117-122, 1993.

69. Fulton JS, Middleton GJ, McPhail JT: Management of oral complications, *Semin Oncol Nurs* 18(1):28-35, 2002.

70. Barasch A, Peterson DE: Risk factors for ulcerative oral mucositis in cancer patients: unanswered questions, *Oral Oncol* 39(2):91-100, 2003.

71. Peterson DE: New strategies for management of oral mucositis in cancer patients, *J Support Oncol* 4(2 Suppl):9-13, 2006.

72. McGuire DB, Johnson J, Migliorati C: Promulgation of guidelines for mucositis management: educating health care professionals and patients, *Support Care Cancer* 14(6):548-557, 2006.

73. Kenny SA: Effect of two oral care protocols on the incidence of stomatitis in hematology patients, *Cancer Nurs* 13(6):345-353, 1990.

74. Yeager KA, Webster J, Crain M et al: Implementation of an oral care standard for leukemia and transplantation patients, *Cancer Nurs* 23(1):40-47; quiz 47-48, 2000.

75. Sadler GR, Stoudt A, Fullerton JT et al: Managing the oral sequelae of cancer therapy, *Medsurg Nurs* 12(1):28-36, 2003.

76. Sadler GR, Oberle-Edwards L, Farooqi A et al: Oral sequelae of chemotherapy: an important teaching opportunity for oncology health care providers and their patients, *Support Care Cancer* 8(3):209-214, 2000.

77. Multinational Association for Supportive Care in Cancer/International Society for Oral Oncology (MASCC/ISOO): (2005). Summary of evidence-based clinical practice guidelines for care of patients with oral and gastrointestinal mucositis (update), Metairie, LA, 2005, Author.

78. Hudson J. Personal communication, October 3, 2006.

79. McGuire DB: Barriers and strategies in implementation of oral care standards for cancer patients, *Support Care Cancer* 11(7):435-441, 2003.

80. Sonis S, Kunz A: Impact of improved dental services on the frequency of oral complications of cancer therapy for patients with non-head-and-neck malignancies, *Oral Surg Oral Med Oral Pathol* 65(1):19-22, 1988.

81. Mueller BA, Millheim ET: Pharmaceutical aspects of mucositis mouth-wash mixtures, *Am J Health Syst Pharm* 52(22):2596-2597, 1995.

82. Beck SL, Yasko JM: Guidelines for oral care, Crystal Lake, IL, 1993, Sage Products.

83. Rutkauskas JS, Davis JW: Effects of chlorhexidine during immunosuppressive chemotherapy. A preliminary report, *Oral Surg Oral Med Oral Pathol* 76(4):441-448, 1993.

84. Ferretti GA, Raybould TP, Brown AT et al: Chlorhexidine prophylaxis for chemotherapy and radiotherapy-induced stomatitis: a randomized double-blind trial, *Oral Surg Oral Med Oral Pathol* 69(3):331-338, 1990.

85. Spijkervet FK, van Saene HK, Panders AK et al: Effect of chlorhexidine rinsing on the oropharyngeal ecology in patients with head and neck cancer who have irradiation mucositis, *Oral Surg Oral Med Oral Pathol* 67(2):154-161, 1989.

86. Dodd MJ, Larson PJ, Dibble SL et al: Randomized clinical trial of chlorhexidine versus placebo for prevention of oral mucositis in patients receiving chemotherapy, *Oncol Nurs Forum* 23(6):921-927, 1996.

87. Foote RL, Loprinzi CL, Frank AR et al: Randomized trial of a chlorhexidine mouthwash for alleviation of radiation-induced mucositis, *J Clin Oncol* 12(12):2630-2633, 1994.

88. Beck S: Prevention and management of oral complications in cancer patients. In Hubbard PGS, Knopf T: *Current issues in cancer nursing practice*, Philadelphia, 1990, Lippincott.

89. Shih A, Miaskowski C, Dodd MJ et al: A research review of the current treatments for radiation-induced oral mucositis in patients with head and neck cancer, *Oncol Nurs Forum* 29(7):1063-1080, 2002.

90. Adamietz IA, Rahn R, Bottcher HD et al: Prophylaxis with povidone-iodine against induction of oral mucositis by radiochemotherapy, *Support Care Cancer* 6(4):373-377, 1998.

91. Rahn R, Adamietz JA, Boettcher HD et al: Povidone-iodine to prevent mucositis in patients during antineoplastic radiochemotherapy, *Dermatology* 195(Suppl 2):57-61, 1997.

92. Peterson DE, Beck SL, Keefe DM: Novel therapies, *Semin Oncol Nurs* 20(1):53-58, 2004.

93. Rocke LK, Loprinzi CL, Lee JK et al: A randomized clinical trial of two different durations of oral cryotherapy for prevention of 5-fluorouracil-related stomatitis, *Cancer* 72(7):2234-2238, 1993.

94. Mahood DJ, Dose AM, Loprinzi CL et al: Inhibition of fluorouracil-induced stomatitis by oral cryotherapy, *J Clin Oncol* 9(3):449-452, 1991.

95. Cascinu S, Fedeli A, Fedeli SL et al: Oral cooling (cryotherapy), an effective treatment for the prevention of 5-fluorouracil-induced stomatitis, *Eur J Cancer B Oral Oncol* 30B(4):234-236, 1994.

96. Epstein JB, Wong FL: The efficacy of sucralfate suspension in the prevention of oral mucositis due to radiation therapy, *Int J Radiat Oncol Biol Phys* 28(3):693-698, 1994.

97. Allison RR, Vongtama V, Vaughan J et al: Symptomatic acute mucositis can be minimized or prophylaxed by the combination of sucralfate and fluconazole, *Cancer Invest* 13(1):16-22, 1995.

98. Loprinzi CL, Ghosh C, Camoriano J et al: Phase III controlled evaluation of sucralfate to alleviate stomatitis in patients receiving fluorouracil-based chemotherapy, *J Clin Oncol* 15(3):1235-1238, 1997.

99. Carter DL, Hebert ME, Smink K et al: Double blind randomized trial of sucralfate vs placebo during radical radiotherapy for head and neck cancers, *Head Neck* 21(8):760-766, 1999.

100. Dodd MJ, Miaskowski C, Greenspan D et al: Radiation-induced mucositis: a randomized clinical trial of micronized sucralfate versus salt & soda mouthwashes, *Cancer Invest* 21(1):21-33, 2003.

101. Clarkson JE, Worthington HV, Eden OB: Interventions for preventing oral mucositis for patients with cancer receiving treatment, *Cochrane Database Syst Rev* (3): CD000978, 2003.

102. Porteder H, Rausch E, Kment G et al: Local prostaglandin E$_2$ in patients with oral malignancies undergoing chemo- and radiotherapy, *J Craniomaxillofac Surg* 16(8):371-374, 1988.

103. Matejka M, Nell A, Kment G et al: Local benefit of prostaglandin E$_2$ in radiochemotherapy-induced oral mucositis, *Br J Oral Maxillofac Surg* 28(2):89-91, 1990.

104. Labar B, Mrsic M, Pavletic Z et al: Prostaglandin E$_2$ for prophylaxis of oral mucositis following BMT, *Bone Marrow Transplant* 11(5):379-382, 1993.

105. Lalla RV, Schubert MM, Bensadoun RJ et al: Anti-inflammatory agents in the management of alimentary mucositis, *Support Care Cancer* 14(6):558-565, 2006.

106. Fidler P, Loprinzi CL, O'Fallon JR et al: Prospective evaluation of a chamomile mouthwash for prevention of 5-FU-induced oral mucositis, *Cancer* 77(3):522-525, 1996.

107. Berger A, Henderson M, Nadoolman W et al: Oral capsaicin provides temporary relief for oral mucositis pain secondary to chemotherapy/radiation therapy, *J Pain Symptom Manage* 10(3):243-248, 1995.

108. Worthington HV, Clarkson JE, Eden OB: Interventions for preventing oral mucositis for patients with cancer receiving treatment. Cochrane Database Syst Rev (2): CD001972, 2006.

109. Clarkson JE, Worthington HV, Eden OB et al: Interventions for treating oral candidiasis for patients with cancer receiving treatment. Cochrane Database Syst Rev (1): CD001972, 2004.

110. Leflore S, Anderson PL, Fletcher CV: A risk-benefit evaluation of acyclovir for the treatment and prophylaxis of herpes simplex virus infections, *Drug Saf* 23(2):131-142, 2000

111. Zaia JA: Prevention of cytomegalovirus disease in hematopoietic stem cell transplantation, *Clin Infect* Dis 35(8):999-1004, 2002

112. Bruce SD: Radiation-induced xerostomia: how dry is your patient? *Clin J Oncol Nurs* 8(1):61-67, 2004.

113. Bruce S: Pilocarpine hydrochloride, *Clin J Oncol Nurs* 7(2):240-241, 2003.

114. Davies AN: A comparison of artificial saliva and chewing gum in the management of xerostomia in patients with advanced cancer, *Palliat Med* 14(3):197-203, 2000.

115. American Nurses Association: *Code of ethics for nurses*, Washington, DC, 2001, Author.

CHAPTER 30

Psychosocial Care

Judith A. Shell

I wanted a perfect ending so I sat down to write the book with the ending in place before there even was an ending. Now I've learned the hard way that some poems don't rhyme, and some stories do not have a clear beginning, middle, and end. Like my life, this book has ambiguity. Like my life, this book is about not knowing, having to change, taking the moment and making the best of it without knowing what is going to happen next.

– Gilda Radner[1]

Introduction

All cancer patients and families face challenges during their life cycle; some are sudden and untimely (unexpected death or disaster), whereas others are expected (divorce and remarriage or retirement). The cancer illness in one member of a family will alter the emotional balance, finances, division of responsibility, and social activities of the spouse or partner, as well as the rest of the family.[2] How patients and families become organized, and how they communicate and solve problems together to cope with the threat often foretells their ability to recover. A support network of extended family, friends, neighbors, spiritual counselors, employers, and available community resources will also contribute to the recovery process.

Many patients, even today, consider a cancer diagnosis as a sentence of impending and painful death, with the result that it has great psychologic impact on their functioning and that of their family. Initially, a psychologic crisis is created, which causes many emotions ranging from the anxiety, anger, fear, and depression caused by the often emotionally paralyzing diagnosis and treatment options, to despair and hopelessness.[3] Following this immediate crisis response, Weisman and Worden's landmark study described the "existential plight" of the individual during the first 100 days after diagnosis.[4] The patient attempts to address the meaning of the illness, and the possible changes in life patterns and the life-altering decisions that must be made; the possibility of dying is also included. This "plight" must not be underestimated, because there are a wide range of responses encountered as patients search for and try to make sense of the meaning of cancer. Patients must be cautioned not to consider their responses abnormal or maladaptive, because there is nothing "normal" about getting a cancer diagnosis.

Along with these genuine emotional responses, patients experience the sense of a total loss of control. One of the greatest fears that cancer patients often express is that of the loss of control. Patients are burdened with the need to comply with tests (often on different days at various facilities) or several different doctor appointments (often to receive chemotherapy or radiation therapy), and these obligations cause other losses such as ability to work or care for the family. Schedules and plans are a thing of the past, and patients often focus primarily on the demands of the illness and getting well. As one patient explained, "I just couldn't do anything. I couldn't think. I couldn't read. I couldn't work. And it went on for weeks."[5] Indeck and Bunney report that as patients begin to create meaning in relation to the illness, they experience a sense of victory over the many life-changing events, which leads to an increased sense of some control.[3] As an increased sense of control emerges, patients can think more efficiently and act constructively; they can become active rather than passive in their plan of care.

This chapter will identify psychosocial factors of adjustment for patients and families during the many phases of the cancer trajectory including diagnosis and treatment, after treatment, progressive disease, and completion of life, as well as long-term survival. Intervention strategies will be offered for all phases of psychosocial circumstances. Cancer patients and families can have a more positive and empowering experience, and an increased survival rate if good psychosocial management is integrated into their plan of care.[6,7] There may also be a reduction in problem-oriented physical distresses such as discomfort and side effects and affairs of daily living such as relationship and vocational issues, and a significant reduction in emotional distress such as depression, hopelessness, confusion, anxiety, and avoidance; quality of life will likewise be enhanced.[8-10] Psychosocial suffering must be recognized and awareness heightened of those patients at increased risk for distress, such as those with a history of emotional problems, a lack of resources, and/or advanced disease.[11]

Patient/Family Response along the Cancer Continuum

PATIENTS' EMOTIONAL RESPONSE AND ABILITY TO COPE

On learning of a cancer diagnosis, patients experience new and multiple kinds of distress that they must learn to cope with. Denial, the "it can't be true" phenomenon, is often initially used and is a very adaptive temporary response. In immediate succession come anger (why me?), fear (doesn't cancer mean death?), general anxiety (fear of the unknown), "test" anxiety (waiting for results), and mourning their many losses. They must also be prepared to learn the foreign language of medicine, make choices that are life-changing decisions, and all the while wonder if they are "going crazy—am I losing my mind?" These are all examples of the kinds of distress that patients must now handle as a conglomerate, whereas previously they may have encountered them only on an individual basis.[12,13]

One important factor affecting how patients respond to the diagnosis of cancer is how they are told the news. Although initially, it is usually the responsibility of the primary physician or surgeon to deliver "sad and bad" news to the patient and family, oncology nurses usually participate in this endeavor as well, either by accompanying the physician or by reinforcing what has been said. Recent literature has provided some general principles through which a recommended process was developed (Table 30-1). Fallowfield noted that "professional detachment" can offend the recipient of bad news; therefore, we must develop the skills to deliver information, in a truthful yet gentle manner, that can maintain hope and a sense of reassurance.[14] Other elements (principles) that influence response include developmental tasks and goals according to age, prior levels of psychologic and social adjustment to illness, religious and cultural attitudes, the level of social support, the potential for rehabilitation, and the patient's own personality.[12,15]

Although patients may be informed of the diagnosis in an empathic and appropriate manner, they may still feel overwhelmed, with a sense of lost equilibrium that precipitates a crisis. However, adjustment to a chronic illness like cancer can occur more rapidly in those who exhibit more resiliency factors such as problem-solving communications, equality, spirituality, flexibility, truthfulness, hope, family hardiness, family time and routines, social support, and health.[16] Whether or not the newly diagnosed patient adjusts gradually or more rapidly, numerous coping tasks must be managed (Table 30-2).

ROLE ADJUSTMENT AND ALTERED RELATIONSHIPS

Once the patient is projected into the cancer domain, various factors will alter established roles and relationships. The ability to fulfill usual roles and responsibilities will change, new roles will be added, and role relationships with others will operate in a modified manner. The usual functions associated with being a spouse or partner and lover, parent, sibling, child, friend, employer, employee, or any other group will shift dramatically. Changed relationships may manifest themselves by a new separateness, increased concern and kindness, or by distancing and avoidance.[17] The nature of the new roles and relationships can create feelings of incompetence and discomfort. These people who have become cancer patients are now labeled as "different."

Because the perception may now exist that this person is different somehow, it might be necessary for that person to set the tone for maintaining relationships. This can create a feeling of overwhelming frustration, because the patient is also trying to recover and heal. There will often be a new sense of awareness about such issues as who helps with household chores, who takes time to be attentive and visit, and who listens when the patient feels like talking about illness. However, troubled thoughts of abandonment may intermittently surface if anticipated support is felt to be lacking.[15]

The desire for privacy can actually cause problems, because the patient may not want to share much information regarding the illness with many people other than immediate family, at least initially. Consequently, when information is kept private, isolation results. Social isolation can be due not only to privacy factors, but also to the stigma of cancer, to the anger of family and friends because the patient developed the disease, and to the fact that disability has arisen and prevents participation in many social activities. Family and friends want to help, but often it is by voicing cheery encouragement, rather than allowing the patient to ask for what he or she needs and or feels would be helpful. Occasionally, friendships that were cultivated before the illness do not remain intact for various reasons and may have to be discontinued.

Sexual health and the sexual relationship are important aspects of the patient's very being; however, focus is usually centered on the physical well-being of the patient, especially during diagnosis. As the patient traverses the treatment process and beyond, sexual functioning can be threatened via numerous influences including fear of contagion, disfiguring surgery, fertility issues, chemotherapy side effects like fatigue and malaise, nausea and vomiting, and pain.

TABLE 30-1	**Recommended Steps for Breaking Bad News**
STEPS	**PROCESS**
1. Privacy and adequate time	Provide quiet space. Provide enough time for thought and questions. Ideally, family member(s) should be present.
2. Assess understanding	Is patient aware of situation and prognosis? Ask patients how much information they want. Be aware of culture, race, religion, and social background.
3. Simple, honest information	Speak simply, and avoid medical jargon. Use the word "cancer." Consider writing information down.
4. Advocate expression of feelings	Normalize feelings of numbness, disbelief, and anger. Respond with empathy and warmth.
5. Promote a broad time frame	Avoid definite time scale; be realistic. Reassure and provide support to promote comfort.
6. Arrange a review	Plan a discussion to review the situation soon after the initial consult.
7. Discuss treatment options	Clearly relate treatment options, and encourage patient and family to participate in final decisions.
8. Offer assistance to tell others	Support communication of diagnosis between family and friends. Promote use of family therapist to help with children.
9. Provide resource information	Offer referral to various support services and personnel, e.g., groups, funds, therapists for families.
10. Document information given	Document concisely all information given and people involved in consultation sessions.

From Girgis A, Sanson-Fisher RW: Breaking bad news: consensus guidelines for medical practitioners, *J Clin Oncol* 13(9):2449, 1995.

TABLE 30-2	Typology of Coping Tasks of Chronically Ill Adults
BROAD TASK CATEGORY	**SUBCONCEPTS IN THE CATEGORY**
1. Maintaining a sense of normalcy	Hiding, minimizing illness and/or responding to curious inquiries of others
2. Modifying daily routine; adjusting lifestyle	Living as normally as possible despite daily therapy and obvious symptoms Providing for safety
3. Obtaining knowledge and skill for continuing self-care	Having internal awareness Monitoring effects of therapy
4. Maintaining a positive self-concept	Integrating illness into self-concept Maintaining or enhancing self-esteem
5. Adjusting to altered social relationships	Experiencing loneliness or social isolation Undergoing patient or other initiated disengagement Preserving relationships with friends and family who satisfy dependency needs Maintaining family solidarity
6. Grieving over losses concomitant with chronic illness	Losing physical abilities, function Losing status Losing income and social relationships Losing roles and dignity Dealing with financial losses
7. Dealing with role change	Losing roles—social, work, family Gaining roles—dependent help seeker, self-care agent, chronically ill patient
8. Handling physical discomfort	Handling illness-induced discomfort Handling pain caused by therapy
9. Complying with prescribed regimen	
10. Confronting the inevitability of one's own death	
11. Dealing with social stigma of illness or disability	
12. Maintaining a feeling of being in control	Exerting cognitive control Exerting behavioral control Exerting decisional control
13. Maintaining hope despite uncertain or downward course of health	Experiencing effects of hope Finding meaning in physical changes

From Miller JF: Analysis of coping with illness. In Miller JF, editor: *Coping with chronic illness: overcoming powerlessness*, Philadelphia, 1992, Davis. Used with permission

PSYCHOLOGIC DISORDERS: ANXIETY AND DEPRESSION

Two of the most frequent and common psychologic disorders in cancer patients are anxiety and depression. These feelings are normal, since cancer is an obvious threat to the person's very well-being. However, many myths and assumptions exist which suggest that "all" cancer patients must be depressed and require psychiatric intervention. In reality, Massie and others report that several psychosocial studies indicate cancer patients do experience illness-related emotional distress; however, they are for the most part psychologically healthy.[18]

Anxiety. Normally, anxiety occurs at different points throughout the course of illness and treatment. Technically, anxiety disorders are classified in the *Diagnostic and Statistical Manual of Mental Disorders* (*DSM-IV-TR*).[19] Although the most common anxiety response in cancer patients is classified in the *DSM-IV* as adjustment disorder with anxious mood (with or without depression), the other types include generalized anxiety disorder, panic disorder, phobias, posttraumatic stress disorder, and anxiety due to medical illness.[19]

Adjustment disorder with anxious mood is commonly referred to as reactive or situational anxiety and is caused by the normal or expected fears that occur after diagnosis and during treatment. Patients often experience tension, nervousness, feeling upset, and

an inability to sleep.[20] This acute form of anxiety can occur during various phases of the illness:

- When awaiting procedures and tests
- When awaiting test results and diagnosis
- When anticipating major treatment (surgery, chemotherapy and/or biotherapy, radiation)
- At completion of treatment
- Upon learning of relapse
- When anticipating more (and often more severe) treatment
- During advanced illness
- On anniversary dates of diagnosis, treatments, or other related events[15,18]

Symptoms of acute anxiety may also surface as a result of pain, uncontrolled or conditioned nausea and vomiting, hypoxia, treatment withdrawal, and various medications.

Chronic anxiety, which precedes a cancer diagnosis, may exacerbate the generalized anxiety disorders, phobias, and panic states. This creates greater risk for the individual because she or he may perceive an increased threat from cancer and be overwhelmed with symptoms of fatigue, restlessness and inability to concentrate, irritability and tension, rapid heart rate, losing control, and feelings of "going crazy."[20] McDaniel and co-workers remind us that, "because of the level of anxiety and concern exhibited in most families with sick members, it is especially important to respond to their story with empathy, respect, and a lack of blame and to emphasize the strengths exhibited by the family in their response to this crisis."[21]

Depression. Although sadness and a sense of hopelessness may be considered normal reactions to the cancer diagnosis, other factors can contribute to a depressed mood. Disease-related tests, treatments, side effects, and medications such as chemotherapy, biotherapy, and steroids can contribute to depressed mood; so can a biologic depression not necessarily related to the present event. Other risk factors include the severity of the disease, particular disease sites (pancreatic or head and neck), lack of social support, fear of uncontrolled pain, and other stressful life events.[18,22] Depression, as with anxiety, is diagnosed according to the DSM-IV.[19] The criteria stipulate that the patient must experience symptoms of depression for at least 2 weeks, and at least four of several conditions must be present, such as anorexia, fatigue, weight loss, and insomnia. Consequently, a diagnosis of depression can be difficult to make because of the fact that these particular symptoms of depression mimic the side effects of cancer and its treatment.

Although it is considered common during the first 7 to 14 days to observe a depressive mood if a preexisting depressive disorder was present (e.g., a bipolar mood disorder), it can be difficult to determine the actual cause of the depression.[18,23] As well, many times depression is undertreated or ignored because it is not recognized, and because it is considered to be customary for cancer patients to be depressed.[24] Whether the etiology is from the stressful cancer event, biologic in nature, or from medications, the patient deserves to be treated just as aggressively for the depression as for the cancer or other treatment-related side effects.

FAMILY EMOTIONAL RESPONSE AND ABILITY TO COPE

A cancer diagnosis is perhaps one of the most profound stressors an individual can experience. The physical disease process affects only its host, but the experience of illness and the inherent potential for stress is shared by the entire family. How patients and their families cope with the cancer experience has a profound effect on the perceived level of suffering. Cancer demands new ways of coping for both the patient and the family as they face changes in the way they define themselves personally and as a family unit. A family's ability to cope with the emotional, physical, and relational challenges that the diagnosis and treatment of cancer can impose will be influenced by a variety of factors, some of which may be the cancer prognosis, the level of support available to the family, family illness beliefs, the family's sense of agency, their degree of hope, and the family's level of communication around their feelings, needs, and wants.[25]

Support. It is common for patients with serious illness and their families to feel isolated even from close friends and family members. McDaniel and colleagues note the importance of the emotional bonds, the sense of support and being cared for, and being loved by a community of family, friends, and professionals, and suggest that this may be the most powerful psychosocial factor in health and illness.[21] Additional extended support networks may include volunteer organizations, church groups, or other community groups and can be instrumental in providing emotional support for the entire family.

Illness Beliefs. Susan Sontag reminded us that "everyone who is born holds dual citizenship, in the kingdom of the well and in the kingdom of the sick," and although some citizens escape personal illness for much of their lives, most will be affected at least indirectly by the illness beliefs of a loved family member.[26] We cannot escape the broad brush of the illness experience and its meaning as it paints confusion, fear, disability, and sometimes death on family and friends. Often, little attention is paid to the impact a prior illness experience has on the manner in which patients and their families deal with a diagnosis of cancer. Current attitudes, understandings, fears, hopes, ability to cope and so forth are all crafted, in part, by past experiences with serious illness. Each family, with its own unique illness story and meaning, will be challenged to cope with the plethora of emotional themes that emerge in the face of a cancer diagnosis and its treatment.

Agency. For those families experiencing cancer who walk the illness journey with their loved one, cancer may be the most "out of control" experience they have ever participated in. Loving family members who once were competent protectors, caretakers, and providers can feel helpless in the company of cancer and a health care system that may seemingly wedge themselves between patient and loved ones, and alter the ways in which they are accustomed to experiencing one another. Our health care system is organized, in large part, for the convenience of health care providers and the efficacy of their work; it powerfully invites a passive "good patient and family" role and a sense of helplessness and loss of agency. An increase in the sense of agency may be provided for families by helping them accept what they cannot change and to work to change what they can.[10]

Hope. Some patients have likened the experience of cancer to a roller coaster ride with the unpredictable highs and lows of hope and despair. Beliefs have a significant influence on the way in which people can hold hope during an illness experience. Hope is not the same as desires and expectations and is not exclusive to the wish for a cure; thus, patients and their families can explore the possibility of holding hope for a broad range of physical, emotional, and relational outcomes. The dominant medical system may not address the idea of hope and optimism in the illness experience, yet an understanding of the existence of hope can be ascertained by asking family members their beliefs about the future with the illness. McDaniel and colleagues suggest that patients and their families generally feel discouraged during the early phases of an illness and find it difficult to hold hope.[10] Still, they also look eagerly for positive stories from those who have had a similar condition. After the illness seems more stabilized, patients and families are often reassured and become more hopeful.[10]

Communication. Most people have not been raised in an atmosphere that fosters awareness of the importance of talking about illness, its challenges, and the feelings that accompany it. Patients and families may experience less anxiety when they are able to communicate honestly with one another; and yet, there is a great tendency to try to say the right thing, to cheer one another up too quickly, or to try to protect one another from the real emotions that each is experiencing. A failure to communicate with one another leads to unnecessary tension, misunderstanding, and suffering that will adversely affect the family's ability to cope with the illness experience. An honest and open atmosphere of communication can convey a sense of trust and respect for each family member's ability to cope with the truth and manage the challenges that lie ahead.[27] Patients and family members also benefit most from honest and direct communication from the medical and nursing team about prognosis, treatment options, and possible outcomes. Physicians, nurses, and other health care providers vary in what they tell patients and families; this may be in part because they are uncertain about the course the illness may take. The family's sense of agency and connectedness to one another and to the health care team during the time of illness can be strengthened by frequent and honest conversation with the entire health care team.[27]

ROLE ADJUSTMENT, ALTERED RELATIONSHIPS, AND FAMILY ORGANIZATION

Family adaptability is a quality required for well-functioning families but is particularly necessary for families facing serious illness. Illness and its challenges have been said to arrive like an unwanted, demanding, and unsettling guest that requires the entire household to shift and reorganize the ways in which it has been experiencing family routine and relationships with one another. According to Rolland, the ability of a family to adapt to changing circumstances or life cycle developmental tasks is balanced by a family's need for enduring values, traditions, and predictable, consistent rules for behavior.[28]

A serious illness can derail a family from its natural life cycle momentum as the family struggles to maintain a challenging balancing act. They must adjust physical, emotional, relational, and financial demands so that they can respond to the needs of their sick member and help implement the treatment plan, while at the same time continue their own lives in a normal fashion. Families may not be prepared for the role shifts and relationship skews that may occur within the domain of serious illness. Changes in family organization will be needed as disorder continues to intrude on normal family and individual members' life cycle development.[28]

Stay-at-home moms, who enjoy their role and experience as primary caregivers to their young children, may be required to get a job outside the home when the father becomes too ill to continue to work. Fathers who take pride in their ability to be providers and protectors of the family can experience emotional as well as physical suffering when cancer treatment and its side effects render them unable to be productive in their professions. If a married adult daughter decides to take care of her ill mother, not only must she cope with the stresses of an additional household member who is ill, but she must also continue to accommodate the needs of her own family. In the family with adolescents or young dependent adults, the serious illness of a parent can impede the completion of the major life cycle task of weaning children from parents. Not only does the parental illness interfere with the adolescents' achievement of independence through the usual rebellion and focus outside of the family, but the adolescent may be called on to act as parental surrogate with siblings, which holds him or her tightly to the family.[29] Brown noted that those deaths or serious illnesses whose victims are in the prime of life are the most disruptive to the family function; this may be, in part, because it is during this life phase that an individual has the greatest responsibilities.[29] Illness can also test the role and organizational flexibility of the extended family when, for instance, a grandmother becomes sick and can no longer take care of herself.

Will the adult children be able to take care of their mother, and will the mother be able to shift her role from caregiver to care receiver?

Within the context of illness, flexibility and adaptability can help a family better manage the myriad changes that have the potential to disrupt family organization, values, traditions, rules, and particularly the manner in which family members relate to one another and the roles that each person plays. Family strength requires clear, yet flexible, boundaries and subsystems to mobilize alternative coping patterns when stressed by the challenges of illness and disability.[28]

FACING CANCER WITH A SPOUSE

For many couples, there are no family stories about how to cope with life-threatening or terminal illness, and they may be unprepared for the strains of living with serious illness. This illness can have a devastating effect on a couple's relationship if their joint dreams have not considered what life together with illness would involve. Serious illness or disability can offer opportunity for growth and understanding in a relationship, but it can also confuse, frustrate, and distance a couple from one another, and can powerfully challenge the relationship rules, boundaries, and family organization of the couple.

The dimension of time is a central organizing principle for most couples and families dealing with a long-term condition.[30] Family members adapt best when they understand the strengths and vulnerabilities connected to their past experiences and, at the same time, are able to integrate these prior experiences with the current illness in a useful way. Whatever a couple's history together, illness will challenge them with a balancing act that juggles maintaining normalcy within the relationship, while at the same time caring for a partner with an uncertain cancer diagnosis.

The spouse has been identified as the most pivotal person within the patient's social support network, and a spouse often uses words to describe his or her own suffering in language similar to that of the ill person; tension, anxiety, depression, loss, grief, isolation, and fear of death or recurrence. In a study of women with breast cancer, marital support was conceptualized as the perceived degree of satisfaction with a spouse's response to emotional and interactional needs during the diagnostic, postsurgical, adjuvant therapy, and ongoing recovery phases.[31] When a spouse learns that his loved one has cancer, myriad emotions flood his being, perhaps the most profound being fear and shock. A spouse may wonder what his ill partner needs from him during the time of crisis and how, or if, he will be able to help. The emotional support that a spouse is able to offer will play a major role in how well a patient is able to cope with the disease, and how the disease will draw a couple closer to, or distance them from, one another.

The ill spouse will need both emotional and concrete support in many ways. How well a partner can accomplish this support will depend on the strengths of the relationship, the resources available, the ability of the well spouse to understand what is happening to his partner, and each partner's response to the illness experience. What can a spouse do to help?

- *Listening* is reportedly one of the most supportive ways to help a partner with a serious illness.[10] Illness can be an isolating experience, especially when there isn't a safe person to share feelings with. Listening promotes safety and connection, both for the patient and the spouse.

- *Staying emotionally responsive* even when the patient turns inward and takes time to process is important. It can take a great deal of energy to be ill, and many patients "recharge" their batteries by becoming introspective at times, but this is not a cue to withdraw from the patient.
- *Offering physical closeness*, while at the same time showing acceptance of the full range of feelings, supports the ill spouse's need for assurance that she is still loved and understood. It can be difficult to maintain optimism while at the same time avoiding the temptation to deny the ill spouse's painful illness experience. This conduct is needed and appreciated and is a way of validating the experience of the ill spouse.
- *Respect the need of the ill spouse to remain in control of her life.* Depending on the stage of the illness, much of what a patient called "normal" may be taken away. A partner can support the patient by understanding her great sense of security and accomplishment in retaining as much of what was "normal" as possible in a very abnormal experience. Concrete ways in which the spouse can support the ill partner are to help handle daily household and child-rearing tasks and, most importantly, to be able to handle shifts in family roles and activities. Most families can find methods to adapt to changes when open discussion is offered to ease the tensions and fears.

Psychosocial Adjustment and Quality of Life

INITIAL DIAGNOSIS AND TREATMENT

Individuals diagnosed with cancer often face uncertainties about their mortality, the future course of their illness, their ability to care for themselves and their families, their physical capabilities, the effects of symptoms, and threatened relationships. The emotional repertoire ranges from denial, anger, and fear, to anxiety, depression, guilt, loss, and loneliness, and is shared and experienced by family members as well as the patient. The initial diagnosis can be one of the most emotionally stressful periods of the cancer time frame, and the patient's need to learn how to go on living in a purposeful way despite the uncertainty, fear, and worry can seem an impossible task.

The primary concern of a newly diagnosed person is life versus death, and it is not uncommon for family members to worry for the patient and for themselves as they grapple with the uncertainty that a cancer diagnosis can bring.[18] Fear during this period can be crippling and is often rooted in uncertainty. During the diagnostic period, the individual, the family, and friends can be overwhelmed and unable to comprehend all of the information provided by a nurse or physician. This information often seems vague, expansive, and detached to many patients and families. Many individuals feel numb or shocked and particularly vulnerable in instances when they are told the diagnosis while alone; even greater distress is reported by those told of their diagnosis while in a recovery room or over the telephone.

Patients with cancer can be supported in their efforts to adjust to the stress that accompanies the initial diagnosis by thoughtful and respectful communication practices. If suspicions of cancer are confirmed, it should be the physician who tells the patient, with family present. The physician should explain the disease and available medical treatments. This experience helps give the patient an increased sense of confidence that the truth is being told and that no one is withholding information. This practice also provides opportunity for patient and family members to ask questions and share in the interpretation and understanding of the diagnosis. Some patients have reported a need to have their sense of personal tragedy acknowledged, but without familiar and caring support around them they are often unable to speak honestly about their emotions.[32] However, each individual is unique, and some patients prefer to have privacy while being told the diagnosis.

According to the National Cancer Institute (NCI), the stress of a cancer diagnosis can cause a wide range of physical symptoms such as increased heart rate and blood pressure, headaches, muscle pains, dizziness, loss of appetite, nausea, diarrhea, trembling, weakness, tightness in throat and chest, and sleep disturbances.[33] Some believe that stress can affect the body's immune system and its role in fighting disease. Oncology nurses care not only for physical needs, but they also are an important source of emotional support at this phase of the illness by attentive and patient listening to the patient's hopes and concerns, and by expressing empathy with what they are going through. Furthermore, education at appropriate moments and helping patients discover and express their needs to other health care providers, family, and friends can help sustain emotional stability.

THE CRISIS AND DISRUPTION OF TREATMENT

The rigorous schedule and the side effects of surgery, chemotherapy, and radiation treatment often require the combined efforts of many family members to provide the best physical and emotional support to the patient. Enormous blocks of time are spent traveling to and from clinics, undergoing laboratory tests, waiting in doctors' offices, and lying in hospital beds. The treatments for cancer can interfere significantly with diet, sexuality, lifestyle, relationships, recreation, and other taken-for-granted activities of daily living. Treatment is exhausting and can create frustration, irritability, fear, and hopelessness.

According to Rolland, the complexity, frequency, and efficacy of a treatment regimen and the amount of home as opposed to hospital-based care required by an illness can vary widely across disorders and will have important implications for individual and family adaptation.[28] To understand more clearly the impact of cancer treatment on the patient and family, one must consider the fit between the demands of the illness and the family pattern of functioning. For instance, a family accustomed to and comfortable with working together toward a goal will probably have less trouble adapting to illness disorders that involve regular teamwork as part of the treatment regimen.

Cancer therapies can place demands on the patients' spirit as well as the body. During treatment, it is common for individuals to grieve the loss of feeling that life is open-ended, that health is a given, and that one is in control of one's body. Other feelings that may arise are anger, depression (caused by anger turned inward), anxiety, a sense of being helpless or out of control, and an intense feeling of vulnerability that can be accompanied by feelings of betrayal and unfairness. Help and encouragement for patients to gather wanted information, to take an active part in the treatment process when possible, and to find the support they need to deal with their feelings will all contribute to a sense of well-being during the treatment phase. As patients learn how illness and treatment can affect their bodies and are able to stay informed about their progress, they may naturally become more engaged in the entire course of therapy. Encouraging a patient to ask questions of the physician, nurse, and other members of the team will empower them and decrease their feelings of vulnerability. Patients can be further encouraged to keep their health care team informed of their physical and emotional responses to the treatment regimen. Often patients are reluctant to report signs and symptoms of illness or side effects because they do not consider them important enough or do not want to "bother" anyone. Education regarding the value in providing this information can be instrumental in creating a collaborative atmosphere that cares for both emotional and physical aspects of the patient.

The manner in which a partner responds to the ill spouse is often correlated with how well patients cope, and can be important to their psychologic well-being. One report suggested that a couple's adjustment to changes after diagnosis and treatment of cancer depended on two things.[34] The first was the degree of a spouse's involvement in treatment planning; this suggested that spouses who remain outside this process and offer no help at this stage may have greater difficulty after treatment completion. Second, when the patient was hospitalized for treatment, the extent of the partner's contact with the patient, how often visits occurred, and telephone calls made was an indicator of how easily they were able to become integrated into the new circumstances related to the illness.[34]

Family physicians, nurses, and family therapists are beginning to recognize that the impact of physical illness reaches beyond biologic processes, and that behavioral and social factors play a role in disease etiology and health maintenance.[35] The recognition of this relationship has led to changes in the way spouses, partners, and other family members are included in decisions around treatment issues. Because of the close relationship with the patient and family, the nurse is often in a position to decide when conversation around illness is appropriate or necessary, and how best to include illness issues into conversations with family members. These decisions can best be made through an understanding of how family members interact with one another, both in the present and in the past.

POSTTREATMENT PHASE

Treatment Followed by Cure. Most patients and families will attest to the fact that nearly all control within their lives is lost during diagnosis and treatment for cancer. However, they now may feel an even greater loss of control when treatment ends because of the fact that they are no longer doing anything active to battle cancer. Some feel that this has truly been the battle of their lives. Many patients report that throughout this struggle, the medical procedures and side effects they endured were just as traumatic as the cancer diagnosis itself.[36] They feel just as triumphant that they have been able to survive the treatment for cancer and consider this an independent victory in itself.

Although the patient's success is now a realistic concept, it is also met with uncertainty and ambivalence. Health has been restored; however, there are many emotional feelings and physical side effects (intermediate and long term) to process. The troublesome and possibly serious physical side effects may include chronic fatigue, lymphedema, psychoneurologic difficulties, disfigurement due to loss of limb or other surgeries, stunted growth, problems with fertility, secondary tumors, and damage to major organ systems.[37] As patients begin to deal with the physical impact of treatment, they begin to understand that a new person has evolved with new physiologic responses and uncertainties. How are these dilemmas resolved? As these intermittent anxieties are encountered, the patient may begin to assign meaning to the experience and incorporate a notion of self as important, significant, and worthy of love and appreciation. Adult survivors confess that to recognize and accept the "new" self, they must grieve the loss of the "old" self as they once knew it.[38] If they fail to successfully overcome the anxiety, discomfort, and disabling physical conditions, healthy psychologic growth may be hindered.[11] A review by the physician and reinforced by the nurse of the information originally (at diagnosis) given to the patient and family regarding the possible long-term consequences of cancer treatment can help patients prepare and offset emotional pain caused by not understanding physical responses. Because the focus at the time of diagnosis is the elimination of the malignancy, this information should again be reinforced during routine follow-up examination at the end of medical treatment.

Survival is usually the goal of successful cancer treatment for the patient and the family. The ultimate goal, however, may encompass a "quality" survival that allows the patient to transcend the terror of diagnosis and treatment, create a new life style congruous with a chronic illness, and renew the practice of accomplishing life goals. This may, in part, be attained through normalization and recognition of patient and family resiliency (strengths) and the hard work it took to triumph over adversity (Table 30-3).[39]

Remission Followed by Recurrence. Once again, the sense of personal control surfaces as we speak about the fear of recurrence. Herold and Roetzheim describe five possible scenarios for living that can play into the fear of recurrence and negative stress.[40] They include living without recurrence for many years, living an extended period with no cancer and then surrendering to a quick death from a recurrence or second malignancy, living with alternating intervals of cancer recurrence, living beyond projected death, or dying from unrelated disease or other reasons unrelated to cancer.[40] Once recurrence is identified, patients' feelings range from complete surprise, disappointment, and hopelessness, to relief from the uncertainty of when it would happen.[35] Although the breadth of feelings and fears is wide, discussions, decisions, and preparation must be made to face this adversary again: discussions of the significance of the feelings and fears, decisions regarding treatment options, preparations for treatment, and potential for success or failure.[12]

As the impact begins to affect the patient and family, issues and questions will arise related to how they feel about incorporating cancer treatment again into their lives, and adjustments will again have to be made to the caretaker roles. There may be greater feelings of loss, greater fears, increased hopelessness, and an increased danger of dying. When treatment for the recurrence nears its end, the patient and family will once again need to deal with the results of treatment (test results, and success or failure) and decide what their next step will be.[12,15] Emphasizing personal and family strengths and normalizing the innumerable feelings that surround the significance of recurrence and the termination of treatment for the second time may again assist in restructuring family roles, and in the expression of special needs and concerns of the patient and caregivers. Now that it is certain never to leave conscious awareness, patient and family must learn how to *live* with cancer rather than harboring a focus on *dying*. Even though

TABLE 30-3	Indicators of Family Strengths
CATEGORY	INDICATORS
Values	Commitment to the family as a group
	Respect for and trust in each other
	Investment in improving relationships
	Willingness to seek help for problems
	Value for family rituals and traditions
	Strong sense of spirituality
	Belief in service to others[60-62]
Competencies	Assorted list of problem-solving and coping strategies
	Flexibility and adaptability in roles, especially in times of crisis
	Knowledge and skills used to recognize concerns, identify needs, and specify desired outcomes
	Planning ability to meet goals
	Ability to identify, obtain, and manage resources for meeting the family's needs
	Ability to see positive aspects of life
	Ability to initiate and maintain social support[60-62]
Interactional patterns	Expression of appreciation, warmth, support, and nurturance
	Engage in proactive problem solving
	Positive communication patterns—good listening—sharing ideas—conveying negative emotions creatively and constructively
	Seek opportunity to spend time together
	Engage in leisure time together
	Sense of plan and humor
	Relaxed home environment[60-62]

cancer recurrence is not an unusual event, there is little in the research literature to afford us knowledge regarding how cancer patients express their fears or cope with recurrence of their illness, according to Mahon and Casperson.[41] Lavery and Clarke, however, assert that those patients who engage in problem-focused coping strategies, like changing eating habits and seeking more information about cancer, actually report fewer feelings of helplessness and rated their adjustment to living with cancer as excellent.[42]

PROGRESSIVE DISEASE AND COMPLETION OF LIFE

Daily Living with Illness, Progressive Deterioration, and Providing Comfort. In all phases of cancer, it is important for life to go on as usual, or at least as usual as possible. In the diagnostic stage, the patient and family are usually immobilized by shock, fear and, often, denial. In the crisis phase of cancer, a patient and the family may be united in their mission to devote all efforts to fight the disease, but progression to the advanced phase of illness can be particularly difficult. This now means that for most patients who accepted the diagnosis, any lingering hope for a cure is relinquished. The attention of terminally ill patients may be focused zealously on the specifics of their bodily condition that could indicate the signs of worsening

disease. However, even in the advanced stages of cancer, there may be spells of improvement, which can cause confusion for patients and families who have already accepted and resigned themselves to the inevitability of death.

As the symptoms of progressive disease begin, the sufferer loses faith in the dependability and adaptability of basic bodily processes that the rest of us rely on as part of our general sense of well-being. This loss of confidence can lead to demoralization and hopelessness. Some patients, at this point, will blame themselves for the advanced disease, because they feel that if their will power or desire to live and ability to fight had been stronger, they could have overcome the cancer. Rolland noted that it is important to hold a flexible belief that defines success in terms of active participation rather than in terms of a purely biologic outcome.[30] Those terminally ill patients who have only one acceptable outcome, a cure, and who feel that they have "lost" the battle with cancer will be further burdened with feelings of guilt if they believe that they could have "willed" the cancer away.

Progressive disease may demand even more intense psychosocial adjustment that will best be supported by close family and friends, with additional support coming from nurses and other health care staff, counselors, therapists, and support groups. Fawzy and others have shown a significant reduction in such psychologic symptoms as anxiety and depression in patients who participated in group interventions.[43] With group participation, the patient may not be able to change the status of the illness, but may be able to improve how he or she deals with the illness and its challenges. Being among supportive people who have a similar condition can promote honest communication about the illness experience and can promote emotional healing, lessen feelings of isolation, and encourage patients to begin to reorder their lives and pay attention to what is valued most.

A diagnosis of progressive or advanced disease is an opportunity to gain a greater level of appreciation for those aspects of life that can still be enjoyed, and a chance to redirect one's life in new and productive ways. Many cancer patients say that until they were faced with their own mortality, they never realized how important family is, how much they are loved, how deep their faith is, how emotionally strong they can be, and how blessed they have been in life. Although patients with end-stage illness may no longer be able to hope for a cure, support can be provided to find other ways to hope that give meaning to their lives. Individuals dying of cancer have learned to hope for acceptance of the illness, dying in the presence of their loved ones, finishing old business before they say goodbye, taking one last trip to see loved ones, or finishing a simple project.

Human contact and relationships are domains of existence that are valued by all people, healthy and ill alike, and these seem to be of particular importance for those people who have had their relationships threatened by severe illness. Maintaining a meaningful relationship for the seriously ill patient requires continued presence and availability, often in the midst of considerable pain, fear, sorrow, anger, and grief. Additional comfort can be provided and patient self-esteem enhanced by empathic listening and helping the patient maintain as much independence and personal control as possible. Patients can be encouraged to make decisions regarding their own care, establish daily routine and set realistic personal goals, make plans for their future, the moment of death, and who they want in attendance, and to participate in their own funeral arrangements. One patient expressed a real feeling of control over her death as she worked with her daughter to plan her own funeral and wake.

LONG-TERM SURVIVAL

Optimally, cancer survivorship would indicate a renewed enthusiasm for and enjoyment of life. Realistically, the cancer survivor experiences concerns related to physical sequelae (second malignancies, organ dysfunction, residual fatigue, disability, and disfigurement) and continuing emotional distress (hypervigilance, chronic anxiety, and depression). Gorman discussed three phases of survivorship: acute survival, extended survival, and permanent survival.[12] Acute survival relates to the cancer diagnosis and a goal to survive aggressive medical treatment. Extended survival begins as treatment for cancer ends (remission) and the potential for recurrence is confronted. Permanent survival is related to a "cure," and the likelihood of recurrence is minimal. Long-term survival is not an isolated experience, but rather, one that falls within the continuum of experiences and earlier phases of life.[44]

A new group of survivors has emerged, and these individuals have come together through various forums to search, explore, and learn together. They attend meetings, share newsletters, and write books. They exchange "war" stories and work together to achieve quality time. They have found meaning and usefulness in the concept of survival rather than cure. The organization called the National Coalition for Cancer Survivorship (NCCS) was thus formed, and it defines survivorship as a dynamic process of living with, through, and beyond cancer.[45]

An estimated 8 million Americans with a history of cancer share survivorship concerns. In an attempt to call public attention to the survivor's needs, the American Cancer Society (ACS) put forth "The Cancer Survivor's Bill of Rights." These rights address medical care, personal life adjustment, job opportunities, and insurance coverage. The aim is to have society foster a truly normal life span for cancer survivors.

Despite progress in treatment, cancer continues to be associated with negative outcomes. With such a prevailing attitude, often too little thought is given to aggressive rehabilitation. The growing survivorship movement has refocused concern on life after treatment and the rehabilitation needs of cancer patients. The continued struggle of living with residual disease or treatment effects defines rehabilitation needs. The rehabilitation philosophy has become a component of survivorship and focuses on self-care and maximizing potential for wellness.[46]

Interpersonal Difficulties. Effective survivorship skills may influence the patient's management of the inner turmoil of being a cancer survivor as he or she relates to others on a long-term basis. Working to find spiritual meaning may help to put cancer in its place and to understand other people's discomfort and biases related to the cancer experience.[47] Telling one's cancer story about victory over the illness can reduce the fears and misconceptions that others often carry; this empowers the patient and transforms him or her from victim to victor.[48] Storytelling that gives meaning to the illness may also help with survivor "guilt." This very real feeling arises when other family or friends with cancer do not do as well or die from the disease, whereas the patient has survived.

A sensitive interpersonal difficulty for survivors involves intimacy, marriage, and reproduction. Mann reported that for most married couples, cancer is not related to a decrease in the goodness and worth of the marital relationship. However, "if one partner becomes distressed, it is more likely that the other partner will also become distressed. Recent studies have shown that negative aspects of the marital relationship may have a much stronger association with the patient's emotional functioning than the supportive aspects of the relationship."[49] Possible changes in reproduction are explained by Herold and Roetzheim as being due to decreased fertility, and they report that fertility rates in cancer survivors range from 40% to 85% of expected rates."[40] These patients will most likely benefit from being informed early (before treatment begins) about possible sterility effects, so they can plan for procedures such as sperm banking or embryo preservation.

Workplace Challenges and Discrimination. Approximately 25% of Americans in the workplace or seeking to enter it experience some form of job discrimination, including demotions, firings, unwanted transfers, social isolation and animosity, and required medical examinations unrelated to job efficiency.[50] Discrimination still abounds because of many myths: cancer is a terminal disease, cancer is contagious, or cancer survivors are more of an economic burden than they are productive employees.[50]

Employment often means more than a source of income. A job or career may confer feelings of identity and self-worth. Most successfully treated cancer patients are able to resume previous occupations with minor or no alteration in circumstances. Those who do face problems when returning to work cite the attitudes of employers and co-workers as a major concern, and nurses should prepare patients for the possibility of such reactions.[46] Some patients recognize their own attitudes as the obstacle, along with fear of recurrence and fatalism about the disease. Some cancer survivors are hesitant to change positions because of specific concerns about obtaining insurance benefits, and feel locked into their present position. Actual discrimination may be difficult to prove because it can be subtle. The Americans with Disabilities Act (ADA) of 1990 requires equal opportunity in selection, testing, and hiring of qualified applicants with disabilities.[51] Under the act, anyone who has had cancer is considered disabled. This law prohibits discrimination against workers with disabilities and is similar to the Civil Rights Act of 1964 and Title V of the Rehabilitation Act of 1973.

The ADA covers discrimination that may occur in hiring, promotion, pay, job training, benefits, and firing. Since 1994, the law applies to any private employer with 15 or more employees, state and local government agencies, labor organizations, religious bodies that are employers, and Congress. A different law covers federal government employees. Individuals who are familiar with these laws can protect themselves from discrimination through preventive strategies. Unless the effects of disease or treatment directly affect the individual's ability to perform the essential functions of a job, there is no obligation to disclose information. It is important not to lie, but it is also unnecessary to volunteer information. The employee should be prepared to educate the employer and to stress specific job qualifications and abilities. The emphasis must be on present ability to perform the job, not on disability or medical history. The Equal Employment Opportunity Commission (EEOC) bears the federal government's responsibility of enforcing the standard. Local government offices can assist in investigations or claims.

Any person with a history of cancer who meets specified job qualifications and can perform the essential functions of the employment position is protected under the ADA. The employer is required to provide reasonable accommodations, which includes retraining, special devices, or a change in part of the job such as flexible scheduling. In effect, such accommodations make the disabled enabled.

When residual effects of disease or treatment alter the individual's ability to continue in the pre-illness job, vocational rehabilitation intervention may be necessary. Retraining, partial disability, or full disability may be the only alternatives. In these situations, a rehabilitation team with programs and services in place is needed to smooth transition from the encounters with acute care and ambulatory care settings to self-care in the home setting.

Finances, Insurance, and the Law. An individual's insurance coverage and financial resources greatly influence access to and quality of care. The uninsured and underinsured are limited to indigent care providers or state and federal programs with limited resources. Limited coverage and services can place individuals in the compromised position of underreporting health problems. This situation fosters delayed diagnosis and treatment, increased acuity, and spiraling of health care costs.

The cost of care adds to the individual's and family's burden of living with cancer. They may be faced with the dilemma of forced choices: limited job mobility, paying medical bills versus living expenses, not reporting symptoms, seeking financial assistance, changing relationships, and coping with insurance limitations. All are a subtle form of discrimination.

Insurance companies can decide the type of insurance contract they will sell and to whom. Contracts are negotiated with employers and with individuals, and the cost is determined by coverage limits. The individual with evidence of persistent or recurrent disease may be considered a high risk to the insurance industry. The concept of excess mortality (observed death rates as opposed to standard expected rates) is used in calculating premiums. Private insurance companies can establish waiting periods, deny coverage, and cancel policies based on the provision of each policy.

Currently, no federal law guarantees a right to adequate health insurance. Cancer survivors do have the opportunity of keeping the health insurance obtained through their employer even after they are no longer employed. This opportunity is provided through the Comprehensive Omnibus Budget Reconciliation Act (COBRA) and the Employee Retirement and Income Security Act (ERISA). The COBRA plan can provide short-term coverage while the individual is seeking new employment or a new group plan. ERISA entitles the individual to file a claim when benefits are denied through discrimination. ERISA is enforced by the Pension and Welfare Benefits Administration of the United States Department of Labor. Support is afforded the individual with financial concerns by assessing their situation and educating them about rights and resources.

Making Choices and Regaining Control. Long-term survival has created unique challenges for cancer survivors, but it has also permitted them to return to their families and perform a wide variety of social roles. There are several opportunities for this population to make positive choices, to regain control, and achieve a heightened quality of life. These opportunities take shape through varied approaches, which may include the following:

- Engaging in positive affirmations to enhance self-esteem
- Rearranging schedules or activities to adjust to residual deficits
- Using makeup, hairstyles, or clothing to disguise scars or defects
- Putting cancer in its place and into the past rather than choosing to be preoccupied with recurrence
- Most importantly, NEVER postponing a pleasure[52]

Many feel an increased sense of control as they reprioritize their lives and activities to include volunteering to help others with cancer or to accomplish a long time goal in a more immediate fashion.[44] Gorman noted that "others may make difficult decisions more easily (e.g., leaving a destructive relationship, completing work towards a longed-for degree) because of a sense of urgency created by having a potentially fatal illness."[12]

As the social climate continues to improve, and more well-known people like athletes and celebrities share and publicize early detection and their positive cancer experiences, fears and misconceptions will be dispelled. There will be less stigma associated with cancer and more open communication, and people surviving cancer will experience less shame and have less difficulty in relationships, which will promote less isolation from family, friends, employers, and others.

Assessment

PROMOTING A HEALTHY RESPONSE TO ANXIETY AND DEPRESSION

Anxiety. Assessment is necessary to determine the cause of the anxiety in any given individual; reasons for anxiety during the cancer experience have been previously identified. To construct an appropriate plan of care and intervention, it is helpful to know where the patient is in the course of illness. Commonly, there are two types of intervention, nonpharmacologic and pharmacologic, and either or both will be beneficial at various points along the cancer continuum.[20]

Many assessment techniques are helpful within the nonpharmacologic class of interventions. Initially, it is important to demonstrate interest by using open-ended questions, and McDaniel and co-workers suggest several questions to elicit the patient's and family members' illness perceptions.[21] Some examples:

- What do you think caused your problem?
- What do you think your sickness does to you? How does it work?
- What do you fear most about your sickness?
- What might make healing now a struggle for you?[21]

Anxiety questionnaires such as the trait scale of the State-Trait Anxiety Inventory and the Hospital Anxiety and Depressions scale may also be employed to assess for anxiety. However, Stark and others studied 178 subjects and concluded that these questionnaires may be able to assess for anxiety symptoms adequately, but do not adequately discriminate abnormal anxiety.[53] Once a cause for the anxiety is identified, validation of the patient's feelings and information that anxiety is quite normal in relation to cancer will provide reassurance. A reframing (creating a different story) for the patient's perception of the potential threat may also reduce stress and anxiety.[11] Other strategies, both cognitive and behavioral, will teach coping skills and help the patient maintain control when anxiety arises.

Depression. Depression is one of the most underrecognized symptoms, especially in advanced cancer. Lloyd-Williams reported that as much as 80% of psychologic morbidity in the cancer population goes unrecognized and/or untreated.[54] Factors that contribute to a depressed and hopeless state have been previously identified. Barriers to a diagnosis of depression in the cancer patient may include the inability to distinguish the physical manifestations of a depressive disorder from the cancer or treatment related side effects. As well, there are no biologic markers for depression, nor are there any effective diagnostic tests.[54] Bowers and Boyle discuss various screening tools that may be employed to ascertain whether or not depression may exist (e.g., the DSM, a single-item screening question, a screening questionnaire, and a diagnostic interviews). [22] Patients should be screened routinely for depression via questions and/or screening instruments, because they often will not volunteer this information if left on their own, and consequently their depression fails to be detected or an intervention made.[55,56] (See Box 30-1 for sample assessment questions.)

If patients are severely depressed or suicidal, they should be evaluated for potential to do immediate harm to themselves (e.g., do they have a plan?). If a strong potential for self-harm is evident, assistance may be needed to hospitalize them where psychiatric help is readily available.[18] However, many cancer patients suffer from a "situational" depression, which lasts about 2 weeks and can be managed briefly by the oncology nurse, and more consistently by a medical family therapist or a psychiatric clinical nurse specialist or nurse practitioner.[9] Often, the most helpful type of therapy is with the entire family, in which unresolved issues can be identified and discussed. Family as well as the patient may share in the depressed mood due to stress from the illness, and all may have a sense of guilt, shame, and resentment because of these occult feelings.

The National Comprehensive Cancer Network (NCCN) has established guidelines for distress management and recommend a self-report "distress thermometer" and a checklist to determine the distress level in cancer patients. Their definition of distress in cancer is "a multifactorial unpleasant emotional experience of a psychological (cognitive, behavioral, emotional), social, and/or spiritual nature that may interfere with the ability to cope effectively with cancer, its physical symptoms and its treatment. Distress extends along a continuum, ranging from common normal feelings of vulnerability, sadness, and fears to problems that can become disabling, such as depression, anxiety, panic, social isolation, and existential and spiritual crisis."[57] The distress thermometer instructs patients to "circle the number (0-10) that best describes how much distress you have been experiencing in the past week including today."[57] A score of 5 and above requires further evaluation. The patient is also instructed to complete a multiple-category (family, emotional, physical, practical, and spiritual) problem checklist for noting problems over the past week. The patient simply checks a "yes" or a "no" to indicate the problem. If there is an indication of moderate to severe distress, the patient is referred to a mental health or social work provider, and if the distress is deemed mild, the primary oncology team continues to care for the patient, and no other referral is given at the time.

Interventions

ANXIETY

Although cognitive-behavioral therapy is used by psychotherapists as part of a brief therapy model, nurses can also practice some of these techniques. A cognitive intervention may be used in an attempt to prevent anxiety or when anxious moments occur. Patients can be helped to reduce negative self-talk, reframe obstacles as challenges, and expand possibilities. A patient with colon cancer can be taught to identify a self-defeating belief (e.g., "No one will ever find me attractive now that I have an ostomy") and to substitute it with a self-enhancing belief (e.g., "My sexuality is more than just the appearance of my abdomen").[20] One of the authors' patients was encouraged to experience the pain she was having from thoracic surgery as what was necessary to help cure her of her lung cancer, rather than as a fear that her cancer had returned. This reframing of an obsessive recurrence "phobia" helped to prevent the severe anxiety she felt when she experienced sharp shooting pain within her chest.

Behavioral techniques can offer stress reduction and teach patients coping skills if they are exposed to an anxiety-producing thought or event. Relaxation or distraction using music and techniques such as breathing exercises and yoga, guided imagery, biofeedback, and meditation make up several behavioral components of nondrug therapy.[58,59] A psychotherapy consult may be appropriate to learn hypnosis and self-hypnosis, and in cases of severe phobias or panic attacks, eye movement desensitization and reprocessing (EMDR) procedures might be considered.

Support groups such as I Can Cope and educational services like those provided by the ACS and NCI offer emotional and educational information and help reduce anxiety while the patient learns cognitive and behavioral techniques.[3] Many patients and families continue to use these kinds of services even after cancer treatment has subsided. However, individual and/or family psychotherapy is often a more desirable option in that it provides a safe and professional setting in which to process emotional and private issues inappropriate to support groups or doctor visits.

For cancer patients and families who would benefit from individual or family counseling, a psychotherapeutic model of crisis intervention or brief therapy is advocated by Barbara Andersen.[60] Brief cognitive-behavioral therapy uses the following:
• Expeditious diagnosis and assessment
• A focus on the present time and current issues

BOX 30-1 **Sample Assessment Questions**

1. Do you feel like you're moving or thinking in slow motion?
2. Have you found you're having to push yourself to do the things you liked to do?
3. Has your spouse expressed concern about how you're doing? Has your family noted changes in you? In what way?
4. What keeps you going? From whom do you derive support?
5. Where is hope for you, or on what do you have hope?
6. Have you been so fidgety or restless that you haven't been able to sit still?
7. Were you feeling like this before you became ill, or is this a recent change for you?

- A limited number of therapeutic goals
- Specific suggestions and guidance from the therapist
- Confrontation and change in perceptions, interpretation, assumptions, and attributions
- Behavioral and practical therapeutic techniques and interventions

Greer and co-workers reported that patients who receive health education, brief, problem-focused cognitive-behavioral psychotherapy, and support services had significantly reduced emotional and physical distress; fewer episodes of anxiety, depression, and other psychologic symptoms; a better outlook on life; and more cooperative and realistic involvement with their medical treatment.[61]

Pharmacologic intervention for anxiety is usually accomplished with drugs from the benzodiazepine family; however, stronger antipsychotic medications like phenothiazine can be used if a patient is severely anxious. There are several commonly prescribed benzodiazepines for anxiety in cancer patients. They include the short-acting drugs such as lorazepam (Ativan) and oxazepam (Serax); an intermediate-acting drug, alprazolam (Xanax); and several long-acting drugs such as chlordiazepoxide (Librium), diazepam (Valium), and clorazepate (Tranxene).[18] Because the benzodiazepines can cause respiratory depression, antihistamines can be used for patients with serious breathing impairment. Other drugs can be used such as the tricyclic antidepressants; however, they are usually used to treat depression and anxiety together and will be discussed at a later time. Cancer patients often have underlying medical problems that can create agitation and restlessness. Careful assessment helps ensure that the correct medication is being used to treat the appropriate symptom, and that the underlying pathologic condition is being addressed.[20]

DEPRESSION

During initial conversation with the patient, a validation of feelings is important, albeit avoiding premature reassurance. Body language can also be significant as a communication tool; effective eye contact, active listening, and a caring touch demonstrate interest and sensibility. Although reflective interaction can help patients admit and accept feelings, it can also frustrate patients if this type of response is not used skillfully. If a patient simply hears her statement repeated back to her, she may feel as if the interviewer possesses little if any understanding. Open-ended questions encourage patients to express thoughts and feelings. Cloutier and Ferrall caution care providers to remember that depressed individuals often sense others' reluctance or discomfort when initiating conversation about their depressed mood.[15] Because depression often accompanies anxiety, relaxation or diversion methods (e.g., music, relaxation therapy, guided imagery) are most useful.

When considering the use of medication for depression, it is important to ascertain whether the depression is severe, recurrent, or accompanied by psychotic symptoms. If any are the case, medication is begun immediately with psychotherapy to follow. There are many antidepressant drug families on the market that include the tricyclic antidepressants, the selective serotonin reuptake inhibitors (SSRIs), and the monoamine oxidase inhibitors (MAOIs). The most popular tricyclic antidepressants are amitriptyline (Elavil), doxepin (Sinequan), and imipramine (Tofranil); the SSRIs include fluoxetine (Prozac), paroxetine (Paxil), sertraline (Zoloft), escitalopram oxalate (Lexapro), and duloxetine (Cymbalta); the MAOIs include phenelzine (Nardil) and tranylcypromine (Parnate). For an in-depth discussion of the pros and cons of each medication, refer to Diamond in *Instant Psychopharmacology*.[62] Because the side effects of cancer treatment can mimic depressive symptoms, attention to the signs of depression is imperative to ensure proper treatment for this devastating sense of hopelessness.

MOBILIZING SOCIAL SUPPORT SYSTEMS

During the time of illness, there are a multitude of social support systems for the patient to draw on, and family and friends are customarily the first to offer their assistance. Family members, along with others in the social system, can play a significant role in how the patient copes and adjusts to this illness.[63,64] In addition, other systems can become involved, especially if family and friends are scarce or can't be mobilized; awareness of available support services in the community and how to activate them may be necessary for patient welfare.

Another notable task is to convince the patient, who already feels like a burden, that these systems are there to help and will affect recovery in a positive manner. The most common systems to be recognized, along with family and friends, include neighbors, co-workers, and fellow members of spiritual communities; health care professionals like nurses, physical therapists, and community and home care agencies; psychosocial professionals like social workers, clergy, counselors, and therapists.[49]

To activate these systems, it is helpful to include family members and friends, and to encourage participation in treatment planning conferences or when discussion centers around changes in the patient's condition. Families, friends, and even co-workers feel much more like partners when inspired to participate in support group activities or programs like the "We Can Weekend" sponsored by the ACS. Groups such as these help to normalize the cancer experience and validate individual meanings of illness. Fellow group members may be able to model effective coping strategies and help the patient and family to concentrate on realistic goals.[45]

When patients require specialized care to attend to physical or psychosocial needs after discharge from the hospital or while being treated as an outpatient, more structured services may be needed to support families in the form of home care nurses or therapists. Other assistance in the form of a homemaker service may also be needed to carry out household responsibilities. A referral list of the various support professionals who specialize in cancer care may be needed to maintain the patient and family system and is a helpful addition for all patients and families seeking support.

In addition to these positive outcomes, negative consequences are reported in the literature as well. Cloutier and Ferral noted that invasion of privacy, unkept promises, unwelcome advice, forced dependency, and encouraged noncompliance with treatment are examples of negative consequences of interactions with outside individuals, groups, and systems.[15] Awareness and monitoring for these possibilities will enable the patient and family to use appropriate support systems and benefit from their services.

MAINTAINING COMMUNICATION

How does one best talk with someone who has cancer? Families generally do not talk with one another about their illness concerns, yet when family members are able to discuss their needs and desires they generally do better in managing the illness experience.[27,49] The key to coping with cancer is communication and, because cancer is a chronic as well as an acute illness, the diagnosis signifies a great threat that can only be managed by patient and family members if there is conversation about it.

Commonly, the manner in which family members have communicated with one another before cancer will be similar to the way they will communicate in the midst of illness. If family members have been open with their feelings and emotions, it is likely that they will react in a similar fashion, although this is not always the case. The fear of the unknown often leaves a patient and family unsure of how to speak about what they are feeling. Open communication is enhanced by asking open-ended questions such as, "What are you feeling?" rather than just "How are you feeling?" Open-ended questions have the potential to invite an honest sharing of feelings, to strengthen a family's sense of connectedness, and to provide emotional support.

Although there may be just one illness, there is never just one illness story in a family. Each member will have his own unique view about the meaning of the symptoms and the impact of the illness on the family.[10] Within families there is often a desire to protect one another from additional emotional stress, and so communication can break down as individuals keep feelings, wants, and needs to themselves. Family members can be helped to realize that different perceptions, meanings, and emotions are to be expected, and they can be encouraged to hear and appreciate one another's experiences. Respectful listening to one another and an open acceptance of the experiences of others can promote empathy within the family. Dakof and Liddle, in their research with cancer patients, found no one particular communication style that was most adaptive for all individuals and couples facing illness.[65] The findings showed that the couples in which both members wanted to talk about the illness did well, and couples where both agreed that they did not want to talk about the illness also did well, suggesting that family members can be supportive of one another without communicating about the illness.

Nurses not only have an opportunity to promote communication within the family, they have a responsibility to maintain an ongoing conversation with the patient regarding prognosis, disease course, and treatment plans. Honest communication provides patients with the critical information needed to decide how to respond to the illness and may allow them a greater sense of competency and confidence in their ability to manage the illness experience.[21] Openness, honesty, respect, clarity, responsibility, accountability, and a willingness to listen and learn are qualities that will promote and maintain effective communication between the patient and family members, as well as between the patient, the family, and health care providers.

PROMOTING THE SENSE OF AGENCY

The empowerment of the patient and all members of a family is essential to their coping with the crisis of illness. When patients are able to mobilize all of their physical, emotional, spiritual, and relational resources toward the goal of health and wellness, life is experienced more fully; the patient and loved ones are able to take back some control that cancer and its treatment took from them. Some 30 or 40 years ago, patients did not know they had options. They were passive, and their role was to follow the physicians' instructions and interventions and to pray, if the patient was so inclined. Today, patients can choose to be an active part of the team working toward their recovery, or they can still choose to be somewhat passive, handing over most of the responsibility for their recovery to the health care team.[18] The choice to enhance the sense of agency has never been more available than it is today. Although there is a choice, there is no right or wrong, no good or bad choice. The patient's choice must be honored, because no one knows more about what is good and right than the patient herself.

All individuals are unique and will have coping strategies that work especially well for them and their families. There is no one way to navigate the emotional seas of cancer, but there are some attitudes and strategies that seem to be empowering and promote a renewed sense of agency for many patients. According to Spiegel and Diamond, patients can help in the fight for recovery by making plans for the future as a way of unconsciously not giving up, fighting unwanted aloneness by communicating to friends and family what is wanted and expected of them, and doing whatever possible to keep relationships and intimacy alive.[66] Patients can use methods to evoke the relaxation response, regain and maintain as much control of life as is reasonable, become partners with the physician and nurse in the recovery effort, be with other people who have cancer as a way of being validated and understood, and do what is possible to keep hope alive. These ideas are not easy to accomplish, nor is each useful for every patient, but experience has shown that some patients gain a sense of agency and an improved quality of life when they are able to intentionally incorporate these ideas into their illness experience.

When families are better able to cope with the crisis of an illness, they begin to feel more competent and in control of the illness experience. With a greater sense of control, families will feel less trapped by illness and have greater enthusiasm for constructing more enriched lives.[21] Quality of care is enhanced when patients and families have opportunities to learn more about the disease and discover new and useful coping strategies. Information can be shared about how others are coping, and this can encourage patients and families to read more and ask questions. Additional possibilities for future change and a renewed sense of agency may be made available as past illness experiences are explored, and a discussion ensues that examines which illness beliefs constrain and which facilitate the management of illness.[67] An important developmental challenge is to create a meaning for the illness experience that can promote a sense of competency and mastery: an empowering narrative. Rather than viewing competency and mastery in a rigid way that focuses only on biologic outcomes as the sole determinant of success, facilitators can suggest that agency and mastery be defined in a more "holistic" sense. A "holistic" view will consider involvement and participation in the overall process as a viable and more realistic criteria of competence and agency.[68]

INFORMATIONAL SUPPORT TO MAINTAIN INDEPENDENCE

It is said that *knowledge is power;* and for the patient and family with cancer, knowledge can promote the feeling of increased control and independence, especially for the patient. Before illness progresses and treatment begins, patient roles are essentially the same as before. However, as disease progresses, role responsibilities change dramatically; still, when the patient is kept well informed, roles may be able to be maintained to some degree.

Patients and families find it most helpful if there are professionals to answer their questions regarding medical issues surrounding the diagnosis, treatment and its options, and side effects, as well as to help them clarify their concerns and articulate their fears and needs.[18] When patients can develop specific questions and role play creatively, they can more effectively respond to closed, uninformative conversation or reports from medical personnel.

There may be various logistics behind patients' failure to keep follow-up appointments: they may require more information, and the importance of maintaining appropriate health care may have to be stressed. If the patient lacks transportation, has lost medical insurance, has problems with day care, or is hindered by a language barrier, referrals can be made to social service agencies. Many other resources are available and range from audiotapes and videotapes for the illiterate, to teleconference programs, the computer and the Internet, community workshops, and the national programs listed at the end of this chapter. Preserving patients' independence by way of knowledge throughout the cancer experience can improve self-esteem and provide the necessary encouragement, patience, and stamina to continue their courageous fight.

ASSISTING THE PATIENT AND FAMILY WITH GOAL SETTING

At varying stages of the illness experience, patients may begin to prioritize their lives in a way that honors life with illness, gives clarity to what they really value about living, and encourages them to choose intentionally how they will engage each day they live. Often, patients will realize how much of life they have been "accumulating" that has not been particularly significant, and will decide to set new goals for themselves that better incorporate more of the meaningful aspects of life that have been neglected. Patients facing a life-threatening illness may at some time begin to realize that "the ultimate value of illness is that it teaches us the value of being alive."[69]

Patients may need help to simplify goals and to notice and appreciate the small achievements that come along.[10] Cancer is stressful, and although some stress can be helpful as a means of pushing us to take action, too much stress can harm our health and make us feel like we are losing control.

It is important to consider goals that will support the whole patient: the patient's emotional, spiritual, physical, and relational well-being. Goals should be empowering and appropriate for the patient's stage of cancer, support healthy self-esteem, be measurable and realistically achievable, give joy, and help the patient experience illness not as a tragedy but rather as a different way of living. Because the illness experience is shared in varying degrees by the entire family, the patient may want members of the family to participate in setting goals, and may also want the nurse to monitor their progress and assess the usefulness of established goals. Goals will naturally change over the course of the illness.

ASSISTING THE PATIENT AND FAMILY TO REVEAL ILLNESS HISTORY AND ITS MEANING

One of the most important roles that a health care provider can play in the lives of patients and families challenged by a chronic or terminal illness is to be a witness to the stories of their experience and the meaning they attach to their experience of illness.[70] These stories cannot be told unless someone listens, and although being an audience to the story is not a cure for the illness, it is often a critical source of comfort and healing. A simple question, "Has anyone else in your family had cancer?" can open a conversation that may inform a listener about the patient's understanding of the illness and possible myths they may be holding onto that are not supportive of hope and control.

Beliefs about what is normal and abnormal, and the importance a family places on conformity and excellence in relation to the average family, will significantly affect the family's ability to adapt to illness.[68] Families desperately want to know that they are doing the best they can under the circumstances. The establishment of a community of families with shared experiences reduces their sense of isolation and helps them realize that their reactions, feelings, and struggles are "normal" for the illness experience.[71] Groups offer the advantage of publicly sharing stories of illness history and meanings with people in similar situations.

Bruner emphasizes meaning-making as a key feature of human experience and suggests that it is by participation in culture that meaning is rendered public and shared.[72] People with cancer and other chronic illness do not often have the opportunity to share the meanings they have made of their situation and therefore are vulnerable to isolation. A patient's and family's capacity to find meaning in their dilemma can greatly affect their ability to cope. Questions can be entertained that open discussion around the meanings made of the illness. These are some suitable questions:

- "How often does your family talk about the illness and its impact on everyone's life?"
- "Do you think there is a reason the illness occurred?"
- "How do you approach the future?"
- "Can your illness bring your family closer?"
- "How could it separate you?"

Perhaps some of the most pivotal challenges for individuals with cancer are how to make sense of senselessness, how to find a reason to live in the face of a chronic illness, and how to really live well with illness. Individuals may be called on to realize that they may not always be cured of illness, but that maybe they can strive to be emotionally and spiritually healed and embrace all of their experiences, even illness. As nurses listen to the sometimes agonizing stories of their patients, they can be comforted in the knowledge that it is not only in the physical "doing" that they care for their patients, but that their best intervention may be just "being" who they are in that precious moment when a patient shares her story and knows that she is heard and understood.

ADDRESSING THE NEEDS OF FAMILY CAREGIVERS

Family members, not professionals, are the primary health care providers for most patients.[27,73] Caregivers have a demanding and exhausting job and may find it difficult to care for themselves in light of their partner or family member's illness. Few people seem to recognize the danger and the losses to the caregiver. Society lacks adequate terms to express the experience of caring, so the experience of caregiving goes mainly unrecognized.[27] Because the obvious focus of concern is on the person who is ill, few recognize the overwhelming sense of anxiety, fear, guilt, depression, grief, and isolation that the caregiver experiences. In a study of mastectomy, testicular, and colon cancer patients, it was found that spouses reported as many psychologic problems as the patients, and similar ones.[74] Nurses can support the caregivers in the family by inquiring about the resources the family has available to them and by informing them of community support systems and counseling services available. Participation in support groups is shown to be very helpful in the support of family caregivers. Studies reveal that caregiving partners with sufficient social support and self-care exhibited significantly better coping skills that can have a direct effect on promoting the highest quality of life for partners and patients.[75,76]

The Family Life History model, which was designed to be broadly applicable to situations where families are having to cope with physical illness, suggests that a process unfolds in many families with chronic illness in which family life is increasingly organized around illness-generated needs and demands.[77] As the illness is allowed to dictate the parameters of family life, family caregivers as well as other family members' priorities inevitably and increasingly emphasize an illness-centered family organization.

Support can be provided to family caregivers by helping them make decisions about the role that the illness should be allowed to have in the family. Families can be advised to take a closer look at current resources available and to consider reallocation of resources in a way that meets the needs of the patient but also the needs of the caregivers and other family members.

Critical to meeting the demands of caregiving is the family's ability to renegotiate rigid role definitions, acknowledge the caregiver's expression of personal limits, and engage in discussions around issues of balance, flexibility, and shared participation of responsibilities.[30] The National Family Caregivers Association has suggested that some basic principles of empowerment can help caregivers find a sense of direction. Caregiver tips are noted in Box 30-2.

PROMOTING HOPE

Of all the ingredients in the will to live, hope is the most vital: the emotional and mental state that motivates us to keep on living, to accomplish things and succeed. Hope is a component of a positive attitude and acceptance of our fate in life. Hope influences survival, is a source of energy, enables healthy coping, and saves individuals from the pain of an agonizing state.[78] In addition, hope is a prerequisite for effective coping and a significant factor in physical and emotional well-being.[79] When patients are robbed of hope, they feel cheated of the promise of a future and will succumb to depression. When people fall to that low emotional state, their will to live is threatened and their bodies may shut down. The tumultuous illness journey is marked with periods of high hopes and deep despair, neither of which may make sense at the time they present themselves. Although patients can at times feel at the mercy of the highs and lows of emotions, they can often learn to anticipate and cope with them and discover ways to keep the flames of hope burning.

Most individuals, when asked to explain how they have managed to transcend their problems, will report that they have gone through a similar process of emotional recovery in the past. Further conversation can explore the ways in which the patient and family have managed to keep hope alive in the past, and what the inherent strengths were that the family had drawn on to do so.

BOX 30-2   10 Tips for Family Caregivers

1. Caregiving is a job and respite is your earned right. **Reward yourself** with respite breaks often.
2. **Watch out** for signs of depression, and don't delay in getting professional help when you need it.
3. When people offer to help, **accept the offer** and suggest specific things that they can do.
4. **Educate yourself** about your loved one's condition and how to communicate effectively with doctors.
5. There's a difference between caring and doing. **Be open to technologies and ideas** that promote your loved one's independence.
6. **Trust your instincts.** Most of the time they'll lead you in the right direction.
7. Grieve for your losses, and then allow yourself to **dream new dreams.**
8. **Stand up for your rights** as a caregiver and a citizen.
9. **Seek support from other caregivers.** There is great strength in knowing you are not alone.
10. Caregivers often do a lot of heavy lifting, pushing, and pulling. **Be good to your back.**

Reprinted with permission of the National Family Caregivers Association, Kensington, MD, the only organization for all family caregivers. 1-800-896-3650; www.nfcacares.org.

Being able to find something important yet realistic to hope for is important for patients and their families. Some families experiencing cancer realize that they are able to shift their hope for a cure to the hope of being able to use their remaining time together to the utmost, hope that their loved one does not suffer, or even for a peaceful transition from life to death. In one qualitative study with 30 cancer patients, hope was identified and equated with a person's search for meaning and value in one's life.[80]

Hope-inspiring interventions used by nurses caring for cancer patients and their families included prayer and faith in God, support from family and friends, and positive relationships with the health care team. These interventions promoted confidence in the treatment plan, spousal devotion for the patient, optimistic attitude, physical presence of loved ones at the patient's bedside, and talking to others.[81] Nurses often influence the spouse and patient's hopes through the information they provide, and they must be mindful of the professional power they wield in dispensing information to patients and families.

Outcomes

Because the literature reminds us that we are in the earliest stages of learning in regard to the needs of the cancer population, there is potential to contribute to this literature by recording our work, creating research studies that will reveal and assess strategies, and providing data on successful interventions. In addition, more work must be done in relation to healthy members of the patient's family and increased study of the psychosocial needs and adjustment of cancer survivors. Our challenge is to cultivate patient and family strengths and resources, and to improve psychologic functioning and adjustment to illness through the provision of strategies at the most appropriate point in time during the illness trajectory, the mobilization of support, and the inspiration of hope.

Psychosocial services and psychotherapeutic interventions should be available to cancer patients and families, and directly involved in their care in conjunction with oncologic medical treatment. Nurses serving the oncology population in all settings have the capability to face unique challenges and the opportunity to affect not only physical deficits, but also to provide understanding and empathy to all those they minister to.

REVIEW QUESTIONS

✓ Case Study

Mr. J. was a 42-year-old Caucasian male who was married and had two teenage children. He was diagnosed with osteogenic sarcoma of his left femur, and had several courses of chemotherapy locally before he had limb-salvage surgery at a large university hospital in a city about 100 miles away. He was then scheduled for three courses of chemotherapy after the surgical area had healed.

Mr. J. was an equine (horse) veterinarian, a second career for him. Initially, when he heard his diagnosis, he became very distraught. He thought he might lose his leg to the cancer, and then he would no longer be able to practice veterinary medicine with horses. His surgeon had told him, in fact, that whether or not he was able to save the leg, Mr. J. should consider another career because if a horse kicked his operated leg, he would definitely lose it altogether. Another concern Mr. J had was whether the clinic would hold his job open for him even though it would be several months before he could return to work full time. There would also be much less money coming into the household, and although his wife worked full-time in an office, he worried about getting behind with bill payment with only one salary coming in. He had two teenagers to support (one was to go to college the next year), and he was also helping his elderly parents financially. During the surgery, Mrs. J. had to stay in a motel and eat all of her meals in a restaurant, which was another added expense.

About 6 months before he was diagnosed and had to begin chemotherapy, he had had a hair transplant because he had begun to develop male pattern balding. When he found out that he would lose his hair, he was extremely upset. Although he was able to discuss his feelings about his changing body image with his wife, he began to feel very overwhelmed, anxious, and depressed. He was not only worried about his present diagnosis and treatment, but also about how he would look after the surgery, if his hair would grow back, if he would still have a job, and most importantly, whether or not he would be cured of his cancer or if he would suffer a recurrence.

ASSESSMENT AND INTERVENTION

The clinical nurse specialist (CNS) addressed psychosocial issues during the entire treatment trajectory to ensure that Mr. and Mrs. J. felt well supported. Mrs. J. was always included in conversations with Mr. J., when she was able to be present at clinic visits, to ascertain how she was coping with the added responsibilities of activities of daily living along with caring for Mr. J. The children also had several sessions with the CNS to ensure that they understood what was going on with their father's treatment and to address all questions. The CNS did an assessment using the Beck Depression Inventory and a structured interview with open-ended questions for anxiety and depression.[82] The following interventions were provided:

1. Provide empathic communication regarding cancer diagnosis and acknowledge crisis this information causes for patient and family.
2. Assist to verbalize fears related to the disease process and survival potential.
3. Acknowledge fear of inability for Mr. J. to do his job and concern about job security. Inform him of his legal rights regarding the Americans with Disabilities Act.
4. Acknowledge patient's sense of responsibility for his family and his extended family. Discuss fears regarding financial status and provide social service referral to discuss financial concerns.
5. Acknowledge and assist to verbalize distress over hair loss and negative body image.
6. Allow patient to tell his story and explore the meaning of his illness.
7. Acknowledge and normalize negative moods and behaviors such as difficulty sleeping, loss of appetite, and difficulty in concentrating and with short-term memory, and provide suggestions for antidepressant and/or antianxiety medication.
8. Encourage continued conversation with Mrs. J. regarding patient's thoughts and feelings of inadequacy as a provider, low self-esteem, fears of how the surgery would affect his body image and his career, and fears regarding the possibility of recurrence and the loss of life.
9. Normalize Mrs. J.'s fears and encourage her to take time out for herself.

OUTCOMES

1. Patient verbalized satisfaction with information given regarding his diagnosis and the understanding shown by the surgeon and CNS. Crisis interventions decreased feelings of being overwhelmed with the changes that had to take place within the family.
2. Mr. J. felt comfortable expressing his fears and actively learned about his disease process and prognosis.
3. Mr. J. talked at length to the surgeon about his future ability to function as an equine veterinarian and contacted a lawyer about his legal rights.
4. Mr. J. was able to discern what his present responsibilities were for his family and communicated with social services to stabilize his financial status.
5. Distress over hair loss and negative body image was discussed, and other remaining attractive attributes were accentuated.
6. Mr. J. told several stories of previous experiences in his family with cancer and how each person tapped into strengths and resources that were provided by extended family.

Continued

REVIEW QUESTIONS—CONT'D

7. Suggestions for antidepressant and antianxiety medications were accepted, and Mr. J.'s physician prescribed a medication that was effective for him.
8. Mr. And Mrs. J. remained close all during the treatment process and were able to communicate their fears, needs, and desires appropriately.
9. Mrs. J. reported that she took a half day a week off to pamper herself, and this helped her cope with the treatment process.

QUESTIONS

1. Cancer patients' rehabilitation needs are legally best addressed by which of the following?
   a. Americans with Disabilities Act (1990)
   b. Title V Rehabilitation Act (1973)
   c. Civil Rights Act (1964)
   d. Patient Self-Determination Act (1991)
2. Initially, when a person learns he has cancer, what is the first psychologic circumstance that happens?
   a. The patient attempts to address the meaning of the illness.
   b. There is a psychologic crisis.
   c. The patient falls into an "existential plight."
   d. Nothing. The patient is completely numb.
3. Cancer patients and families can have a more positive experience if which of the following occurs?
   a. Problem-solving techniques are taught immediately after the physician tells the patient of the diagnosis.
   b. The physician and nurse first tell the patient the "bad news" about the cancer diagnosis and treatment, and then tell the family.
   c. The patient is told nothing of the illness, especially if he has a history of emotional problems and a lack of resources.
   d. Good psychosocial management is integrated into the patient's entire plan of care.
4. Breaking the news that the patient has cancer should include which of the following?
   a. A message delivered with professional detachment
   b. Simple, honest information and a discussion of treatment options
   c. Discouraging the expression of feelings
   d. Assume the patient understands, if he or she poses no questions, and move on
5. When the nurse is assessing the patient for acute anxiety, which of the following should she do?
   a. Assess for symptoms of chronic anxiety, which creates greater risk that the patient will experience acute anxiety.
   b. Assess for panic disorder.
   c. Blame the patient for being ridiculous, because the cancer just isn't that bad.
   d. Disregard the patient's story because that has nothing to do with the symptoms of rapid heart rate, fatigue, and restlessness.
6. Why is it believed that serious illness is the most disruptive to family function in families who are in the prime of life (in their late thirties to forties)?
   a. These families most always have teenagers who are in trouble.

   b. These families have no sense of "personal boundaries."
   c. They have rarely experienced illness before.
   d. They are in the phase of life that has the greatest responsibilities.
7. Long-term survival for cancer patients entails which of the following?
   a. Little worry about recurrence
   b. Renewed intimacy and anticipation of having children
   c. Concerns about physical sequelae and continued emotional distress
   d. Returning to their job with no fears of discrimination
8. Nurses can best assist patients and families with open communication by doing what?
   a. Asking open-ended questions, which invites the sharing of feelings
   b. Encouraging patients to keep most illness concerns to themselves so they do not worry family members needlessly
   c. Reminding patients that their story is really not unique, because they have cancer just like all of the other patients
   d. Withholding most information, because details will just confuse patients and families anyway
9. What makes being a witness to the patient's story important?
   a. This can help cure the illness because it promotes comfort and healing.
   b. It helps inform the nurse about the patient's understanding of the illness.
   c. It really isn't important to listen to these stories, because there are usually more important duties to accomplish.
   d. The nurse should know everything about the patient so she can make the treatment decisions for the patient.
10. Family members who are caregivers should be encouraged and reminded to do which of the following?
    a. Make sure the loved one's illness or disability always takes "center stage."
    b. Try not to accept help from those who offer because illness is a private matter.
    c. Remember to value and be good to yourself, because your job is difficult.
    d. Try to do the most you can for a loved one, because independence is not important at such a critical time.

ANSWERS

1. **A.** *Rationale:* Although other acts are similar, the Americans with Disabilities Act says that anyone who has had cancer is considered disabled and requires equal opportunity in selection, testing, and hiring of qualified applicants. The ADA covers discrimination that may occur in hiring, promotion, pay, job training, benefits, and firing. Since 1994, the law applies to any private employer with 15 or more employees, state and local government agencies, labor organizations, religious bodies that are employers, and Congress. The other three do not.
2. **B.** *Rationale:* A cancer diagnosis causes many emotions ranging from the anxiety, anger, fear, and depression of the often emotionally paralyzing diagnosis and treatment

options, to despair and hopelessness, which initially causes a psychologic crisis. (a), (c), and (d) may occur at a later time; however, once the realization of the diagnosis is understood, the *first* psychologic event is "crisis," and the brain doesn't know what to do yet.

3. **D.** *Rationale:* Good psychologic management throughout the treatment trajectory will empower patients and reduce problem-oriented physical distress such as discomfort and side effects and will reduce emotional distress such as depression and hopelessness. Problem-solving techniques should not be taught when the patient is in crisis; patient and family should be told together so they are all receiving the same information and can process it together; and patients must always be given appropriate information so they can be a partner in their care. Resources are almost always available (see Box 30-3).

4. **B.** *Rationale:* Information should be related truthfully yet gently to maintain hope and a sense of reassurance. It should be simply stated using the word "cancer," and written information reinforces what has been said. When "professional detachment" is used, it can offend the recipient of bad news; if the client is discouraged from expressing feelings, the nurse or physician cannot normalize the feelings of numbness, disbelief and anger; assumptions are inappropriate, since this leads to mind-reading, which is not good communication.

5. **A.** *Rationale:* Chronic anxiety that precedes the cancer diagnosis may exacerbate the generalized anxiety disorders, phobias, and panic states. This creates greater risk for the individual because he or she may perceive an increased threat from cancer and be overwhelmed with symptoms of fatigue, restlessness, and so on. The most common anxiety response in cancer patients is classified in the *DSM-IV* as adjustment disorder with anxious mood (with or without depression). There are several other subtypes that can be part of the adjustment disorder with anxious mood including panic disorder, phobias, and posttraumatic stress disorder. A patient's report of symptoms should never be disregarded.

6. **D.** *Rationale:* These families usually have the responsibility of careers, children in the home, and elderly parents who often become their responsibility at this time in their life (the "sandwich generation"). The other answers are not inclusive enough and only touch on one aspect rather than the particular phase of life the family is experiencing.

7. **C.** *Rationale:* Successful treatment is often met with uncertainty and ambivalence. Health has been restored; however, there are many emotional feelings and physical side effects (intermediate and long-term) to process. Serious physical side effects may include chronic fatigue, psychoneurologic difficulties, disfigurement due to loss of body part, problems with fertility, and secondary tumors, to name a few. Cancer patients are almost *always* worried about a recurrence. The patient may not have a partner or may be older and not within childbearing age. Even with new laws, there is often discrimination if an employer learns a person has had cancer.

8. **A.** *Rationale:* Open-ended questions have the potential to invite an honest sharing of feelings, to strengthen a family's sense of connectedness, and provide emotional support. Honest communication provides patients with the critical information needed to decide how to respond to the illness and may allow them a greater sense of competency and confidence in their ability to manage the illness experience. Openness, honesty, respect, clarity, responsibility, accountability, and a willingness to listen and learn are qualities that will promote and maintain effective communication between the patient and family members, as well as between the patient, the family, and health care providers.

9. **B.** *Rationale:* When the nurse has information relative to patients' understanding of their illness, they can dispel possible myths patients may be holding onto that are not supportive of hope and control. Being an audience to the story is not a cure for the illness but is often a critical source of comfort and healing, and when nurses listen to their patients' stories, they can be comforted in the knowledge that it is not only in the physical "doing" that they care for their patients, but that their best intervention may be just "being" who they are when a patient shares her story and knows that she is heard and understood. Today, patients can choose to be an active part of the team working toward their recovery, or they can still choose to be somewhat passive, handing over most of the responsibility for their recovery to the health care team.

10. **C.** *Rationale:* Studies reveal that caregiving partners with sufficient social support and self-care exhibited significantly better coping skills that can have a direct effect on promoting the highest quality of life for partners and patients. The National Family Caregivers Association encourages caregivers to choose to take charge of their life, and not to let their loved one's illness or disability always take center stage. When people offer to help, caregivers are advised to accept the offer and suggest specific things that they can do. Patients should be encouraged to maintain their independence since this enhances their feeling of control and significance.

BOX 30-3 **Psychosocial Resources**

Associations and Advocacy Groups

Alliance for Lung Cancer Advocacy, Support and Education (ALCASE): Dedicated to helping people living with lung cancer. Programs include education, early detection, psychosocial support and advocacy issues. 1601 Lincoln Avenue, Vancouver, WA 98660. 800-298-2436. Website: http://www.alcase.org.

American Association of Retired Persons (AARP): Services provided include information and supplemental insurance. Fees vary based on policy chosen. 202-434-2277.

American Brain Tumor Association: Services offered include free publications on brain tumors, social service consultation by telephone, a mentorship program, support group lists, a resource list of physicians, and a pen pal program. 2720 River Road, Suite 146, Des Plaines, IL 60018. 800-886-2282. Website: http://www.abta.org.

American Cancer Society (ACS): Programs offered include children's camps, Hope Lodge, I Can Cope, Look Good ... Feel Better, Man to Man, Reach to Recovery, Road to Recovery, and TLC for breast cancer patients. Services offered include education, free publications, support groups lists, and many others depending on the particular state or community. 1599 Clifton Road NE, Atlanta, GA 30329. 800-ACS-2345. Website: http://www.cancer.org.

Blood and Marrow Transplant Information Network: Services include a quarterly newsletter for bone marrow, peripheral stem cell, and cord blood transplant patients, a book describing bone marrow transplants (BMTs) and peripheral blood stem cell transplants (PBSCTs), an attorney list to help resolve insurance problems, a patient-to-survivor telephone link, and a directory of transplant centers. 2900 Skokie Valley Road, Highland Park, IL 60035. 847-433-3313. Website: http://www.bmtnews.org.

Cancer Care, Inc: Services include free professional counseling, support groups, education and information, and referrals for patients and families to assist with psychological and social issues. 275 Seventh Avenue, New York, NY 10001. 800-813-HOPE. Website: http://www.cancercare.org.

Choice in Dying: Advocates recognition and protection of individual rights at the end of life. Services include counseling regarding preparation and use of living wills and durable powers of attorney for healthcare. 1035 30th Street NW, Washington, DC 20007. 800-989-WILL. Website: http:// www.choices.org.

CONVERSATIONS: The International Ovarian Cancer Connection: Services provided include a free monthly newsletter (CONVERSATIONS! The International Newsletter for Those Fighting Ovarian Cancer) and a survivor-to-fighter matching service. P.O. Box 7948, Amarillo, TX 79114. 806-355-2565. Website: http://www.ovarian-news.org.

Corporate Angel Network, Inc (CAN): Provides free plane transportation for cancer patients going to and from cancer treatment centers. There are no financial requirements or limits on number of trips. One Loop Road, Westchester County Airport, White Plains, NY 10604. 914-328-1313. Website: http://www.corpangelnetwork.org.

Dave Dravecky's Outreach of Hope: Offers encouragement and hope through the love of Jesus Christ to those suffering from cancer or amputation. Services offered include prayer support, correspondence, resource referral, and encouraging literature. 13840 Gleneagle Drive, Colorado Springs, CO 80921. 719-481-3528. Website: http://www. outreachofhope.org.

International Association of Laryngectomees (IAL): Services offered include preoperative and postoperative visits to laryngeal cancer patients, support education for laryngectomees and families, educational materials, and an annual meeting and Voice Restoration Institute at a rotating location each year. 7822 Ivymount Terrace, Potomac, MD 20854. 301-983-9323.

International Myeloma Foundation: Services provided include a quarterly newsletter, "Myeloma Today," education about myeloma, and patient and family seminars. 2129 Stanley Hills Drive, Los Angeles, CA 90046. 800-452-CURE. Website: http://www.myeloma.org.

Kidney Cancer Association: Services provided include providing information to patients and families and acts as advocate. 1234 Sherman Avenue, Suite 203, Evanston, IL 60202. 800-850-9132. Website: http://www.nkca.org.

Leukemia Society of America: Services provided include free educational materials, patient aid, peer support, family support groups, and education regarding leukemia, lymphoma, Hodgkin's disease, and myeloma. 600 Third Avenue, New York, NY 10016. 800-955-4LSA. Website: http://www. leukemia.org.

Mathews Foundation for Prostate Cancer Research: Services provided include customized information packages and individual answers to questions about the disease and its symptoms and treatment therapies. 11242 NE 58th Street, Kirkland, WA 98033. 800-234-6284. Website: http://www. mathews.org.

Mautner Project for Lesbians with Cancer: Services provided include support, education, information, and advocacy for health issues relating to lesbians and families with cancer. 1707 L Street NW, Suite 500, Washington, DC 20036. 202-332-0662. Website: http:// www.mautnerproject.org.

National Alliance of Breast Cancer Organizations (NABCO): Services provided include information, assistance, and referral, education for the public, and links underserved women to medical services. 9 East 37th Street, 10th Floor, New York, NY 10016. 888-80-NABCO. Website: http://www.nabco.org.

National Cancer Institute (NCI): Services provided include a nationwide telephone service that answers questions and free information booklets about cancer. 800-4-CANCER. Website: www.nci.nih.gov.

Patient Advocate Foundation (PAF): Services provided include education relative to managed care terminology and policy issues, legal intervention services, and counseling to resolve job and insurance problems. 780 Pilot House Drive, Suite 100C, Newport News, VA 23606. 800-532-5274. Website: http://www.patientadvocate.org.

Southwest Airlines: Provides air transportation for medical need with written request and physician letter. 214-904-4103.

BOX 30-3   **Psychosocial Resources—cont'd**

Support for People with Oral and Head and Neck Cancer, Inc. (SPOHNC): Services provided include support and information addressing the emotional, psychological, and humanistic needs of oral and head and neck cancer patients/families. PO Box 53, Locust Valley, NY 11560. 561-759-5333. Website: http://www.spohnc.org.

United Ostomy Association, Inc: Services provided include educational materials (some free of charge) and rehabilitation of all ostomates. 19772 Macarthur Boulevard, Suite 200, Irvine, CA 92612. 800-826-0826. Website: http:// www.uoa.org.

Well Spouse Foundation: Services provided include support groups and newsletters for partners and caregivers of the chronically ill. 800-838-0879 or 212-724-7209.

Y-ME: National Breast Cancer Organization: Services provided include hotline counseling, educational programs, open door meetings for breast cancer patients, families, and friends, and a Y-ME Men's Support Line. 212 West Van Buren Avenue, Chicago, IL 60607. 800-221-2141 (24 hour), 800-986-9505. Website: http://www.y-me.org.

Financial Resources

Social Security Administration

Supplemental Security Income (SSI): A federally funded income maintenance program for the aged, blind, or disabled. There are restrictions on amount of income and assets a recipient may have.

Social Security Disability (SSD): A federally funded program for the disabled and for survivors of a decreased wage earner.

For the above programs, contact the local Social Security Office, or call 800-772-1213.

Community for Agriculture: Services provided include publication of a state-by-state analysis of health insurance programs for high-risk individuals, including plan information and cost. 800-850-3276.

National Insurance Consumer Organization: Services provided include assistance with insurance problems. 703-549-8050.

Energy Assistance: Services provided include financial assistance offered by many states to low-income households to help pay energy costs. Contact the local Department of Social Services, local infoline, or local fuel bank.

U.S. Department of Veterans Affairs: Services provided include benefit information to veterans regarding educational assistance, disability compensation, medical care, life insurance, burial benefits, and dependent benefits.

Survivor Services

Cancervive: Assists cancer survivors to face and overcome the challenges of having cancer. 310-203-9232.

Coping Magazine: Bimonthly publication dedicated to patients, families, and friends involved with cancer. 615-790-2400.

National Coalition for Cancer Survivorship: Provides peer support and information to patients and families regarding issues of survivorship. 301-650-8868.

The Wellness Community: Services provided include professionally led support groups, education, stress management, and social networking with a focus on health and well-being for individuals recovering from cancer. 35 East 7th Street, Suite 412, Cincinnati, OH 45202. 888-793-WELL. Website: http://www.wellness-community.org.

Websites

American Cancer Society—www.cancer.org
CancerCare—www.cancercare.org
Cancer and Careers—www.cancerandcareers.org
Gilda's Club—www.gildasclub.org
Susan G. Komen Foundation—www.komen.org
People Living with Cancer—www.plwc.org
Sharsheret—www.sharsheret.org
Susan Love's Web site—www.susanlovemd.org
The Wellness Community—www.thewellnesscommunity.org
Young Survival Coalition—www.youngsurvival.org

REFERENCES

1. Radner G: *It's always something*, New York, 1989, Simon & Schuster.
2. Kaye J, Gracely E: Psychological distress in cancer patients and their spouses, *J Cancer Educ* 8(1):47, 1993.
3. Indeck BA, Smith PM: Community resources. In Devita VT, Hellman S, Rosenberg S, editors: *Cancer: principles and practice of oncology*, ed 6, Philadelphia, 2001, Lippincott-Raven.
4. Weisman J, Worden W: The existential plight in cancer: significance of the first 100 days, *Int J Psychiatry Med* 7(1):1, 1976.
5. Hagopian GA: Cognitive strategies used in adapting to a cancer diagnosis, *Oncol Nurs Forum* 20(5):759, 1993.
6. Fawzy FI, Fawzy NW, Hyun HC et al: Malignant melanoma: effects of early structured psychotic intervention, coping, and affective state on recurrence and survival 6 years later, *Arch Gen Psychiatry* 50(9):681, 1993.
7. Fawzy FI, Fawzy NW, Arndt LA et al: Critical review of psychosocial interventions in cancer care, *Arch Gen Psychiatry* 52(2):100, 1995.
8. Edgar L, Rosgerger Z, Nowlis D: Coping with cancer during the first year after diagnosis: assessment and intervention, *Cancer* 69(3):817, 1992.
9. Fuller S, Swensen C: Marital quality and quality of life among cancer patients and their spouses, *J Psychosoc Oncol* 10(3):41, 1992.
10. Tope D, Ahles T, Silberfarb P: Psycho-oncology: psychological well-being as one component of quality of life, *Psychother Psychosom* 60(3-4):129, 1993.

11. Holland J: *Psycho-oncology*, New York, 1998, Oxford University Press.
12. Gorman LM: The psychosocial impact of cancer on the individual, family, and society. In Carroll-Johnson RM, Gorman LM, Bush NJ, editors: *Psychosocial nursing care: along the cancer continuum*, Pittsburgh, 1998, Oncology Nursing Press.
13. Holland J, Rowland J, editors: Psychological care of the patient. In Holland J, editor: *Handbook of Psycho-oncology*, New York, 1989, Oxford Press.
14. Fallowfield L: Giving sad and bad news, *Lancet* 341(8843):476, 1993.
15. Cloutier A, Ferrall S: Psychosocial aspects of complex responses to cancer. In Barry P, editor: *Psychosocial nursing: care of physically ill patients and their families*, ed 3, Philadelphia, 1996, Lippincott.
16. McCubbin HI, McCubbin M, Thompson E et al: Families under stress: what makes them resilient? *J Fam Consumer Sci* 2:55, 1997.
17. Cole-Kelly, K: Two families, two stories: courage and chronic illness. In McDaniel S, Hepworth J, Doherty W, editors: *The shared experience of illness: stories of patients, families, and their therapists*, New York, 1997, Basic Books.
18. Massie MT, Chertkov L, Roth AJ: Psychologic issues. In Devita V, Hellman S, Rosenberg S, editors: *Cancer: principles and practice of oncology*, ed 5, Philadelphia, 1997, Lippincott-Raven.
19. American Psychiatric Association: Diagnostic and statistical manual of mental disorders, ed 4, Text revision, Washington DC, 2000, Author.
20. Bush NJ: Anxiety and the cancer experience. In Carroll-Johnson RM, Gorman LM, Bush NJ, editors: *Psychosocial nursing care: along the cancer continuum*, Pittsburgh, 1998, Oncology Nursing Press.
21. McDaniel SH, Hepworth J, Doherty WJ: *Medical family therapy: a biopsychosocial approach to families with health problems*, New York, 1992, Basic Books.
22. Bowers L, Boyle DA: Depression in patients with advanced cancer, *Clin J Onc Nurs* 7(3):281, 2003.
23. Holland J: *Depression in cancer patients is underrecognized, undertreated*, Psychiatric Update Memorial Sloan Kettering Cancer Center, *Oncol News Int* 1996.
24. Albright AV, Valente SM: Depression and suicide. In Carroll-Johnson RM, Gorman LM, Bush NJ, editors: *Psychosocial nursing care: along the cancer continuum*, Pittsburgh, 1998, Oncology Nursing Press.
25. Zabalegui A: Coping strategies and psychological distress in patients with advanced cancer, *Onc Nurs For* 26(9):1511, 1999.
26. Sontag S: *Illness as metaphor*, New York, 1978, Farrar, Straus & Giroux.
27. Given BA, Given CW, Kozachik S: Family support in advanced cancer, *CA Cancer J Clin* 51(4):213, 2001.
28. Rolland JS: *Families, illness, & disability*, New York, 1994, Basic Books.
29. Brown FH: The impact of death and serious illness on the family life cycle. In Carter B, Goldrick M, editors: *The changing family life cycle: a framework for family therapy*, Boston, 1989, Allyn & Bacon.
30. Rolland JS: A journey with hope, fear, and loss: young couples and cancer. In McDaniel SH, Hepworth J, Doherty WH, editors: *A shared experience of illness: stories of patients, families, and their therapists*, New York, 1997, Basic Books.
31. Hoskins CN, Baker S, Sherman D et al: Social support and patterns of adjustment to breast cancer, *Sch Inq Nurs Pract* 10(2):99, 1996.
32. Lind S: Telling the diagnosis of cancer, *J Clin Oncol* 7(5):583, 1989.
33. National Cancer Institute: *Taking time: support for people with cancer and the people who care for them*, In the National Institutes of Health booklet, 1999, National Institute of Health.
34. Ayers L: *The answer is within you*, New York, 1994, Crossroads Publishing.
35. Young D, Rosenthal D: Couples' experience of illness: the daily lives of patients and spouses, *Families Systems Health* 17:64, 1999.
36. Carter SE: End of treatment: laugh or cry? *Community Oncology* 1(3):179, 2004.
37. Shell JA, Bell K, Dougherty M: Gonadal toxicities. In Liebman M, and Camp-Sorrell D, editors: *Multimodal therapy in oncology nursing*, St. Louis, 1996, Mosby.
38. Nessims S, Ellis J: *Cancervive*, Boston, 1992, Houghton Mifflin.
39. Buckley MR, Thorngren JM, Kleist DM: Family resiliency: a neglected family construct, *Fam J* 5:241, 1998.
40. Herold AH, Roetzheim RG: Cancer survivors, *Cancer Diagn Treat* 19: 779, 1992.
41. Mahon SM, Casperson DS: Psychosocial concerns associated with recurrent cancer, *Cancer Pract* 3(6):372, 1995.
42. Lavery JF, Clarke VA: Causal attributions, coping strategies, and adjustment to breast cancer, *Cancer Nurs* 19(1):20, 1996.
43. Fawzy FI, Fawzy NW, Arndt LA et al: Critical review of psychosocial interventions in cancer care, *Arch Gen Psychiatry* 52(3):100, 1995.
44. Pelusi J: The lived experience of surviving breast cancer, *Oncol Nurs Forum* 24(8):1343, 1997.
45. Herbst S: Survivorship: redefining the cancer experience, *Oncol Nurs Forum* 2:527, 1995.
46. Henderson PA: Psychosocial adjustment of adult cancer survivors: their needs and counselor interventions, *J Counsel Develop* 75:188, 1997.
47. Abdallah-Baran R: Nurturing spirit through complementary cancer care, *Clin J Onc Nurs* 7(4):468, 2003.
48. Leigh S: Cancer survivorship: a consumer movement, *Semin Oncol* 10(8):783, 1994.
49. Mann S: Cancer in the marital context: a review of the literature, *Cancer Investigation* 16(3):188, 1998.
50. Hoffman B: Employment discrimination: another hurdle for cancer survivors, *Cancer Invest* 9(5):589, 1991.
51. Americans with Disabilities Act of 1990, 42 U.S.C.A. 12101 et seq. (West 1993).
52. Carnevali DL, Reiner AC: *The cancer experience: nursing diagnosis and management*, Philadelphia, 1990, Lippincott.
53. Stark D, Kiely M, Smith A et al: Anxiety disorders in cancer patients: their nature, associations, and relation to quality of life, *J Clin Onc* 20(14):3137, 2002.
54. Lloyd-Williams M: Difficulties in diagnosing and treating depression in the terminally ill cancer patient, *Postgrad Med* 76:555, 2000.
55. Hotopf M, Chidgey J, Addington-Hall J et al: Depression in advanced disease: a systematic review. Part 1. Prevalence and case finding, *Palliat Med* 16(1):81, 2002.
56. McDonald MV, Passik SD, Dugan W et al: Nurses' recognition of depression in their patients with cancer, *Oncol Nurs Forum* 26(3):593, 1999.
57. National Comprehensive Cancer Network: Clinical practice guidelines in oncology: distress management v. 1.2005, retrieved December 13, 2005, from http://www.nccn.org/professionals/physician_gls/PDF/distress.pdf.
58. Danton WG, Altrocchi J, Antonuccio D, Basta R: Nondrug treatment of anxiety, *Am Fam Phys* 49(1):161, 1994.
59. Massie MJ, Shakin EF: Management of depression and anxiety in cancer patients. In Breadboard W, Holland JC, editors: Washington, DC, 1993, American Psychiatric Press.
60. Andersen B: Psychosocial interventions for cancer patients to enhance the quality of life, *J Consult Clin Psychol* 60(4):552, 1992.
61. Greer S, Moorey S, Baruch JDR et al: Adjuvant psychological therapy for patients with cancer: a prospective randomized trial, *BMJ* 304(6828):675, 1992.
62. Diamond RJ: *Instant Psychopharmacology*, ed 2, New York, 2002, W.W. Norton.
63. Manne S, Taylor K, Dougherty J, Kemeny N: Supportive and negative responses in the partner relationship: their association with psychological adjustment among individuals with cancer, *J Behav Med* 20:101, 1997.
64. Pistrang N, Barker C: The partner relationship in psychological response to breast cancer, *Soc Sci Med* 40:789, 1995.
65. Dakof G, Liddle H: *Communication between cancer patients and their spouses: is it an essential aspect of adjustment?* Paper given at the American Psychological Association Annual Meeting, Boston, August 12, 1990.
66. Spiegel D, Diamond S: *Psychosocial interventions*. In Educational Booklet, 1998, American Society of Clinical Oncology, Philadelphia, 1998, WB Saunders.
67. Wright LM, Watson WL, Bell JM: *Beliefs: the heart of healing in families and illness*, New York, 1996, Basic Books.
68. Rolland JS: Beliefs and collaboration in illness: evolution over time, *Family Systems Health* 16:7, 1998.
69. Frank A: *At the will of the body: reflections on illness*, Boston/New York, 1991, Houghton Mifflin.
70. Seaburn D: A mother's death: family stories of illness, loss and healing, *Families Systems Health* 14:3, 1996.
71. Steinglass P: Multiple family discussion groups for patients with chronic medical illness, *Family Systems Health* 16:55, 1998.
72. Bruner J: *Acts of meaning*, Cambridge, 1990, Harvard University Press.

73. McDaniel SH, Campbell TL: Family caregiving and coping with chronic illness, *Families Systems Health* 16; 1998.
74. Baider L, Kaplan De-Nour A: Adjustment to cancer: who is the patient— the husband or the wife? *Isr J Med Sci* 24:631, 1998.
75. Lutzky SM, Knight BG: Explaining gender differences in caregiver distress: the roles of emotional attentiveness and coping styles, *Psychol Aging* 9:13, 1994.
76. Morse SR, Fife B: Coping with a partner's cancer: adjustment at four states of illness trajectory, *Oncol Nurs Forum* 25(4):751, 1998.
77. Steinglass P, Bennett LA, Wolin SJ: *The alcoholic family*, New York, 1993, Basic Books.
78. Miller JF: Developing and maintaining hope in families of the critically ill, *ACCN Clin Issues Crit Care Nurs* 2:307, 1992.
79. Herth K: The relationship between level of hope and level of coping responses and other variables in patients with cancer, *Oncol Nurs Forum* 16(1):67, 1989.
80. O'Connor A, Wicker C, Germino B: Understanding the cancer patient's search for meaning, *Cancer Nurs* 13(3):167, 1990.
81. Patel CTC: Hope-inspiring strategies of spouses of critically ill adults, *J Holistic Nurs* 14(1):44, 1996.
82. Beck AT, Shaw BF, Emery G: Cognitive therapy of depression, New York, 1975, Guilford.

CHAPTER 31

Sexuality

Judith A. Shell

The diagnosis of a chronic illness like cancer can be a significant crisis in the lives of individuals and families.[1,2] Crises can undermine the client's self-esteem and self-efficacy, and it is not unusual for them to lose skills they have already developed for dealing with difficult situations. Generally, patients are unprepared for the physical changes, alternating periods of stability and change, and the uncertainty of future functioning. Because of multiple losses, chronic illness demands new ways of coping, changes in patient and family self-definitions, and various periods of adaptation.[1,3]

Even though the mirror may not reflect immediate outward alterations in physical appearance, the image presented can no longer be trusted: the body has betrayed its keeper. Various treatments (surgery, chemotherapy, and radiation therapy) can be devastating, and the effects of treatment can cause changes in body image even when no outward change in appearance may be obvious. The sense of being feminine or masculine may be hindered simply because of the fact that helpful drugs like narcotics and antinausea medication, along with the general feelings of fatigue, may influence the sexual response cycle. Patients and partners need to be made aware that many means of communication and sexual expression can provide satisfaction and pleasure throughout the cancer experience, both physically and emotionally. Rolland reminds us, "Often the diagnosis of a serious condition can heighten feelings associated with loss in such a terrifying way that couples react either by pulling away from one another or clinging to each other in a fused way. Being a caregiver, receiving caregiving, or seeing the visible signs of illness or emotional strain can become implosive reminders of loss. Couples adapt best when they learn to deal with these facts of life and use that consciousness in an empowering manner to live more fully rather than constrain their relationship.[3]

The routine discussion of sexuality and sexual function with the oncology survivor will normalize this aspect of potential patient concern and promote beneficial quality of life. Regardless of age, marital status, or sexual orientation, sexual health can be advanced by promoting prevention through assessment, education, and intervention, and by providing information when the patient has a question or problem throughout treatment and beyond. Emphasis should always be placed on characteristics that will remain intact after treatment, since patients often tend to focus on what they will lose. Today, nurses tend to be more liberal and aware of the importance of human sexual function; however, Brunner and Boyd have admonished us for continuing to not communicating sufficient information regarding sexuality issues to the cancer population.[4] As a result, changes in practice are needed to reduce (1) personal feelings of anxiety regarding sexual topics, (2) embarrassment about obtaining a sexual history, and (3) negative societal stereotypes about sexuality and chronic illness or disability (see Table 31-1).

Definitions

Although sexuality remains a sensitive topic, sexual rehabilitation has taken on new significance and substance in the past decade owing to better education concerning human sexuality and a change in attitude; there is an increased demand for candid discussion of the sexuality issues related to cancer treatment.[1] The standard of physical attractiveness is also beginning to change from one of only slim and slender youth to include that of the 50- to 60-year-old who may be somewhat overweight. At present, thanks to new legislation, active patient advocacy groups, and more sensitive media attention and portrayal, people with physical impairments are more active and visible, and the concept of "normal" is expanding.

Sexuality is a term that can mean different things to different people. The definition Weiss offers best details male and female humanness:

Sexuality isn't really about the things we've been taught to think it is. It isn't about pleasing others, nor is it about owning or controlling others. It isn't about intercourse or having babies. It isn't about competition and beauty contests or proving ourselves more beautiful or sexy than others. It isn't about giving others pleasure so we can feel loved by them, nor is it about trading our bodies for financial, material, or emotional security and comfort. It isn't even only about having orgasms and other pleasurable physical sensations. Sexuality is about connecting our head with our gut through our heart. It's about genuinely caring for ourselves, finding ecstasy in simply being alive, and giving creative voice to our ideas and feelings. It's about bridging physical pleasures with spiritual awareness and serenity. It's about opening ourselves to the sensations of the body and to the joys of the imagination and the heart. It's about sharing and enjoying our sexual selves with partners we feel affectionate and safe with, and it's about loving ourselves and others.[5]

Etiology and Risk Factors

Four decades ago, Masters and Johnson stated that almost half of all couples who are physically and psychologically "healthy" have had sexual problems at some time during their relationship.[6] In the 1990s they continued to educate the public about how health problems and chronic illness can affect sexual relationships.[7] It is reasonable to assume, then, that many individuals with cancer, and particularly those who must undergo treatment, will have some type of sexual concerns, given the added pressures of their disease. These concerns, in turn, can affect a relationship if the patient has a spouse or partner.

A person's sexual expression varies throughout the life cycle. Although personal beliefs and values are influential, interference with the psychosexual stages of development by an event such as disease may affect sexual function. Shell noted, "If the patient is young and just beginning to embark upon relationship and career,

TABLE 31-1	Necessary Information to Promote Communication
SUBJECT	**KNOWLEDGE**
Cancer diagnosis	Extent of sexual problems generated by cancer
Nurse comfort discussing sexuality with patients and partners	Practice in the development of skills to consult and talk with patients and partners
Awareness of the normal sexual concerns related to cancer and its treatment	General and specific information to be shared with patient and partner in relation to expressed sexuality concerns to augment quality of life
Increase the ability to either initiate conversation, or facilitate the patient's initiation of the conversation.	Knowledge of resources and referrals that are available for support

their focus will probably be one of courtship, marriage and procreation. Their sexuality interests will be much different from those of a middle age or older group of patients who now envision their sexuality and intimate sexual relationship to be one of physical nearness, intimate communication, pleasure seeking and companionship."[8] For the cancer patient, passage from one stage to the next may be precluded by the disease and its treatment or prognosis.

In addition to these stages, various other factors of importance should be considered. The patient's personal reaction to the illness and previous experience with the disease should be explored. If the patient has a spouse or partner, consideration should be given to the couple's prior strengths and the stability of the relationship. What were their feelings toward sexuality before the disease? If the partners were supportive before diagnosis, they tend to be supportive after diagnosis.[2]

Sexual orientation is another factor that may be missed or ignored because appropriate questions were not asked because of lack of experience or misperceptions. Since all individuals are not in heterosexual relationships (and may not be in a relationship at all), it is imperative to appreciate that the patient may be gay, lesbian, or bisexual. Exclusion of the partner from participation during and in the treatment process may precipitate anxious decision making for the patient and preclude any outward signs of affection between the couple during hospitalization, office, or home visits.[9]

Consequences of Cancer and Cancer Treatment

Once patients are assured of survival beyond the initial diagnosis, the quality of their lives becomes a concern. Will they be able to function as "normal" people do? Taken-for-granted activities like work, recreation, travel, parenting, and sex take on a new importance. While undergoing treatment or in the recovery period, patients will experience fluctuating degrees of fatigue, anorexia and nausea, and discomfort and debilitation. These will affect their level of sexual interest and ability and their sense of

adequacy and self-esteem. Depending on the type of cancer and therapy used, specific physiologic and psychologic changes can interrupt normal sexual functioning and feelings of femininity or masculinity.[1,10]

SENSE OF ADEQUACY

Femaleness and maleness is not only expressed in the bedroom. Sexuality is a part of all of the activities in which a person engages from work to political discussions, decorating one's home, eating a meal, and watching a movie, to arguments, child-rearing, and expressions of affection. For some people, the mere process of being ill may cast doubt on their sexual identity and response, which in turn will reflect on their sense of adequacy. Because of the seriousness of their illness, cancer patients are often too embarrassed to raise questions about their sexual concerns. They may feel that worrying about such a relatively unimportant matter as sex is unjustified. However, it must be emphasized that a sexual relationship is a physical and emotional source of satisfaction and great pleasure and also the most intimate way we share ourselves with others.

Male and female sexual response is normally integrated into the sexual response cycle (excitement, plateau, orgasm, and resolution). The **male sexual response** (desire, subjective arousal, erection, emission, orgasm, and ejaculation has separate mechanisms of control and can therefore be affected independently.[11] Although cancer therapy may destroy the capability for an erection, the pleasure of sexual arousal and orgasm often remain intact. Long, Burnett, and Thomas provide a thorough description of the physical changes during the sexual response cycle, along with a conceptual model of sexual desire.[11] Detailed photographs of the internal and external changes of the penis, the vagina, and the breast during sexual intercourse are provided by Masters and others.[7] Schover and colleagues present an in-depth explanation of male and female sexual response during the cancer experience.[12]

Female sexual response (desire, subjective arousal, vaginal expansion and lubrication, and orgasm) is less well understood. Women with cancer may lose sexual desire during debilitating treatment, especially if the therapy affects the structure or innervation of the clitoris or the vagina. These effects, along with painful intercourse, are factors that tend to interfere with orgasm. In addition, emphasis is placed on perceived damage resulting from therapy, which women feel may lead to rejection from their partner.[13]

Because the capability of relating sexually is extremely important in our culture, some patients may declare a lost interest in sex just to protect themselves from the embarrassment of lost orgasmic function or erectile failure. Moreover, added sexual inadequacy that is the result of a potentially fatal disease often leads to a threatened self-image. Syrjala and others inform the reader that, even though newer techniques and therapies are being used, between 10% and 90% of cancer survivors report sexual problems depending on gender, diagnosis, and type of treatment.[14] In addition, sexual dysfunction apart from a cancer diagnosis may also be present as a result of premorbid factors. Chronic illnesses such as diabetes, heart disease or hypertension, increased age, emotional difficulties such as anxiety and depression, and/or substance abuse with alcohol or drugs may all contribute to sexual dysfunction in this population.[14]

SENSE OF SELF-ESTEEM

Even when there is no organic illness, feelings of unworthiness and incompetence can lead to a negative body image.[11] Cancer patients are at greater risk of having a negative body image because of mutilating surgery and other devastating side effects (e.g., weight loss or gain, hair loss, decreased saliva production). Cancer and its treatment can produce considerable loss of economic independence, alter role behavior, change significant relationships, and reduce sexual responsiveness. What follows is fear of abandonment, withdrawal, and probable sexual dysfunction. To enhance sexual self-esteem, preservation or resumption of the ability to function sexually and/or to see oneself as a sexual being becomes of paramount importance. Many times patients feel sexual desires but take it for granted that their partner does not desire them. The partner, in turn, worries that the patient may be too sick to want sexual activity and feels guilty about having a sexual interest in someone who is sick and under treatment. Unfortunately, if these misconceptions persist, patients and their partners are likely to avoid the intimate and/or sexual contact that may provide much needed comfort and solace.

Alternatives to stereotypical sexual behavior must be ascertained, and each patient's unique sexual identity acknolwedged.[7] This promotes the ability to be free of fixed ideas and to continue to discuss sexual concerns at all stages of cancer and its treatment, regardless of the patient's circumstances, age, or sexual orientation. It must never be assumed that the patient who has raised no questions has no concerns. Concentrated attention must be given to the issue of sexuality just as it is given to other aspects of cancer care.

Assessment and Common Problems, Issues, and Concerns

Assessment and common problems will be covered in site-specific sections. Most discussions in the literature related to sexual problems of cancer patients are relegated to malignancies of the genital organs or the breast, because cancer in these areas is most likely to directly cause sexual dysfunction. Consequently, head and neck cancers, sarcomas that result in amputation, hematologic malignancies, and lung cancers are frequently overlooked or barely mentioned. Therefore, a nursing approach to these concerns will be addressed first.

HEAD AND NECK CANCER

Physical and Psychosocial Parameters. Although the social significance of youth and facial beauty continues to be profound and is exemplified through movies, television, and magazines, it is beginning to be somewhat less dramatic. However, when patients are portrayed on television, they often continue to be perfectly made up (unless a patient on *ER*), and the few older people represented in the mass media are also fairly attractive.

The impact of head and neck cancer can be particularly devastating because the defects can be immediately recognizable, or a voice can be raspy and difficult to understand. The patient feels grossly unattractive and frequently has difficulty with life's most basic needs, such as talking, eating, and even breathing. Given these fundamental problems, it is not surprising that little or no attention is given to the need for closeness, touching, and genital sexual pleasures.

Sexual relationships may be influenced by the patient's age, smoking and drinking habits, and the general emotional impact of treatment. Many patients are more than 60 years of age at the time of diagnosis and may be entering a period of adjustment to a decrease in frequency of sexual intercourse, although desire can remain about the same.[15] The patient may also be an alcoholic, which will influence treatment and the rehabilitation process. Intimacy, trust, and open communication are frequently nonexistent in alcoholic relationships because intimacy is too threatening to the alcoholic individual.[16]

Patients with head and neck cancer often require rehabilitation, if extensive surgery was required; this may begin to be accomplished with reconstructive surgery or prostheses or both. It is important to remember that the expectations of how patients think they will look may differ from actual rehabilitative results. Consequently, patients may suffer one or more disappointments, as illustrated by the following anecdote.

A woman had an oral prosthesis made. The match and the appearance were excellent, and she regained confidence and employment and she delighted in sociability. Her praise and gratitude were profuse. However, once when we had lunch together she said, "I have so much to be thankful for and yet …" and she turned away and she touched the prosthesis. "When I laugh, this never laughs, and when I take it off I sometimes wonder if I can go on."[17]

Patients with head and neck cancer will necessarily face lingering cosmetic and functional impairments, which will affect their body image and sexuality. If a tracheostomy must be placed, esophageal speech or the use of an electronic device to speak may be embarrassing, especially if the patient is female. The tracheostomy may also produce hissing sounds, and a partner may fear suffocating the patient during intercourse. Several patients have expressed problems with a diminished quality of life amid feelings of anger, frustration, and a lack of self-esteem after experiencing side effects such as xerostomia, lack of the ability to taste, fatigue, and skin changes.[18] Poor body image, along with a decrease in libido, will most likely be the result of dysphagia, pain, and disfigurement and will compromise confidence in sexual expression.

SARCOMAS OF BONE AND SOFT TISSUE AND LIMB AMPUTATION

Physical and Psychosocial Parameters. There continues to be a dearth of information regarding the sexual adjustment of those with upper or lower extremity amputation. Commonly, concentration is placed on the patient's functional problems during and after prosthetic rehabilitation, and reference to sexuality is often omitted.[19]

If major limb amputation is necessary, it can create emotional hurdles for the patient's self-perception, as well as for acceptance by the patient's partner (Fig. 31-1). A decrease in self-esteem and a negative body image are common because of the presence of a gross defect that is obvious even when covered with clothes. Limb amputation creates several potential sexual problems, which include the simple mechanics of body positioning during intercourse, immobility because of physical isolation, amputee fetishism, and phantom pain sensations.[20]

Amputees are understandably apprehensive about their physical capabilities, but this fear often subsides once they begin prosthetic training, ambulation, or articulation. As patients become

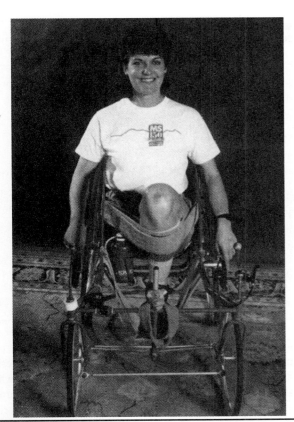

FIG. 31-1 Lou Keyes, hemipelvectomy patient, in her racing wheelchair. Lou also used a prosthetic device proficiently, and crutches when she was in a hurry.

more independent, confidence in their sexuality usually returns.[19] Some patients with lower extremity amputation fail to gain satisfaction from a prosthesis. Those patients then resort to using crutches rather than be restricted by the somewhat awkward movement of artificial limbs, and this may directly affect their sense of self image. They forfeit a better cosmetic appearance, however. The range of problems an amputation causes often depends on its extensiveness. For example, a woman with a shoulder disarticulation may find that simple tasks like styling hair and getting clothing to look good are difficult. Less dramatic upper extremity amputations allow for easier manipulation of a conventional hand prosthesis, a hook prosthesis, or a myoelectric-powered hand (Fig. 31-2).

The most prevalent worries for patients with hip disarticulations and hemipelvectomies are socket discomfort, mobility, and energy expenditure.[20] With an exoskeletal device for disarticulation or hemipelvectomy, the socket area envelops the entire pelvis and adds to hip and waist measurements (Fig. 31-3). One woman stated that she couldn't tuck her blouses in and thought her clothes looked too big. Women often have difficulty wearing sanitary pads during menses and may wish to use double tampons. All amputees must deal with undesirable noises produced by prosthetic joints, and even buying a pair of shoes can be disconcerting.

For patients without partners, there may be a support group or sporting activities to become involved in, such as wheelchair racing. The more the patient gets out and regains self-confidence, the easier it will be to meet and interact with other people. (For more information, contact Lower Extremity Amputees Providing Support [LEAPS] at 816-361-3206.)

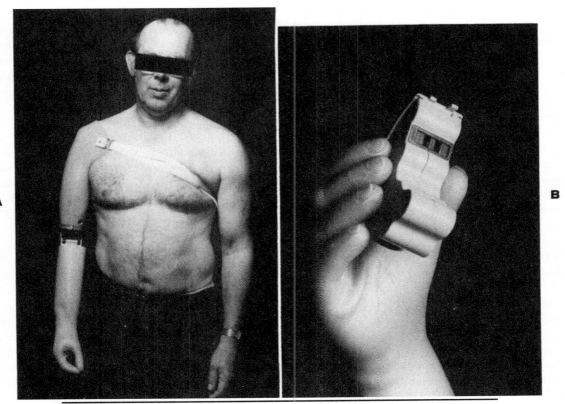

FIG. 31-2 **A,** Above the elbow, myoelectric prosthesis. **B,** Myoelectric hand grasping object.

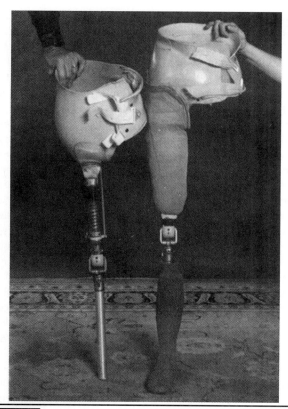

FIG. 31-3 Prosthesis on left is a hip flexion bias system without a rotator knee and no flexibility in the socket. Prosthesis on the right is a hip flexion bias system with a rotator knee and partially flexible socket.

HEMATOLOGIC MALIGNANCIES

Physical and Psychosocial Parameters. Although the diagnosis of lymphoma or leukemia or multiple myeloma can be terrifying, treatment does not comprise surgery or amputation, which can cause disfigurement. What the individual may not realize, however, is that chemotherapy and radiation therapy can be just as devastating to sexuality. Most men and women experience reduced desire for sexual intercourse during chemotherapy treatments, particularly during the first few days after receiving the drugs. This is usually the result of increased weakness, fatigue, and intermittent nausea and vomiting. Also, whether the patient is young or old, male or female, defacement caused by hair loss can destroy self-confidence. Another problem for patients with acute myelocytic leukemia is the prolonged hospitalization during chemotherapy with consequent lack of privacy.

Lack of sexual eagerness can also be induced by an effect on the testes or ovaries caused by chemotherapy. Ovarian dysfunction is progressive, and women may experience symptoms such as amenorrhea or irregular menses, hot flashes, decreased libido, and vaginal dryness.[21] Testicular dysfunction occurs more abruptly and results in oligospermia (decreased sperm) or azoospermia (absent sperm), as well as difficulty with erections caused by peripheral neuropathies.[22] Fortunately, these problems are often temporary, and hormone levels and sexual desire return to normal after chemotherapy or radiation therapy ends.

Myelosuppression and its consequences can cause fatigue and shortness of breath, which decrease sexual desire. Concern about bleeding and infection will be present because of low platelet and white blood cell (WBC) and absolute neutrophil counts. A perfect environment for a vaginal yeast infection may be created, which inflames the lining of the vagina and causes itching and burning during intercourse. The male patient's ability to have an erection may also be affected.

A discussion will most likely be needed to assess the feelings of the spouse or significant other, particularly if a bone marrow transplant (BMT) has been required. These patients may experience sexuality issues for years after BMT treatment, in particular with a negative impact on the human sexual response and the ability to have children.[23] It is helpful to identify ways family and friends can support the patient's feelings of self-worth and masculinity or femininity during and after the treatment trajectory. Tierney explains, "Social factors may contribute to sexual dissatisfaction in transplant recipients. In the context of sexuality, the most important social relationship is that of the intimate partner. Variables influencing this relationship include partner uncertainty and anxiety, difficult communicating, and role shifting within the couple during treatment and recovery."[23]

One of the most stressful events for any patient is alopecia.[24] Some patients may feel that hair loss is even worse than amputation, and because of its effect on body image, sexual inadequacy can ensue. Sensitivity should be used when explaining this side effect to any patient, male or female, and patients should be provided with the information presented in Box 31-1.

BREAST CANCER

Physical and Psychosocial Parameters. Physiologically, removal of a breast should not decrease sexual desire or activity, but in reality studies have demonstrated high levels of stress in regard to sexual functioning among mastectomy patients.[25] Mastectomy creates an obvious change in the body's contour, which can lead to fears about loss of identity as a woman and as a desirable sexual being. The partner's perceived importance of a breast can also affect the woman's perspective, should she choose mastectomy, even though reconstruction today is more prevalent and has better results.[26]

| BOX 31-1 | Suggestions for Patients Who Experience Alopecia |

Use a mild, protein-based shampoo, cream rinse, and conditioner.
Rinse the hair well and pat dry, *not* vigorously.
Shampoo every 4 to 7 days.
Avoid excessive brushing and use a wide-toothed comb or brush.
Avoid hair spray and hair dye.
Permanents are okay, but if hair loss is expected, it is best to wait for regrowth to perm the hair.
Avoid electric hair dryers and curling irons, clips, bobby pins, barrettes, and pony tails.
Many types of hats and caps are available.
Purchase some kind of head wrap or turban, whether it is winter or summer, because the hair helps to keep the head warm. Even in warm weather, the head can get very cold if left uncovered in an air-conditioned environment.
Use sunscreen on scalp when outside.

The patient who is treated with breast-conserving surgery and radiation therapy has concerns about her sexuality as well. Although this patient's breast is preserved, she may experience a skin reaction and increased fatigue while receiving radiation treatment. This can last for several weeks and also lead to decreased desire for sexual activity. Long-term depression and maladjustment are not as likely in this population, but it is just as important to assist these patients with their doubts and anxieties.[26]

A woman's response to treatment for breast cancer and its corresponding threat to sexuality will depend on several conditions[27]:

- Her feelings about her femininity
- The value she bestows on her missing breast
- Her physical discomfort
- The response of her spouse or partner
- The reinforcement she receives regarding her sexual identity
- Her sense of self-worth

The status of the patient's preoperative sexual relationship and her interpretation of sexual satisfaction must also be ascertained. Cultural and religious attitudes will also influence "acceptable" sexual practices.

Couples may not be sure how to begin to experience the loss of a breast or the reaction of the breast to radiation therapy together. One behavior seen on television is where the woman disrobes in front of her spouse to show him her changed body and the scar. A more reasonable and less threatening activity may be for both members of a couple to stand nude together in front of a mirror and express the thoughts and feelings this elicits. In this circumstance, the patient is likely to feel less vulnerable, because she and her partner are both nude. Of course, not all couples will be able to accept or handle this type of exercise, and they should be encouraged to use their own coping strategies. Because coping mechanisms will vary from person to person and couple to couple, numerous behaviors will be exhibited. These will range from allowing the partner to participate in care and view the mastectomy scar or radiation area immediately, to not allowing anyone but the nurse or physician to see the wound.

Rehabilitation may consist of reconstructive surgery, which may be done immediately or several months after treatment is complete. Occasionally, surgical repair must be done before good reconstruction can be accomplished. Although the reconstructed breast will never look like the original breast, some women exercise this option because they think it looks and feels more natural. One factor that women are often not prepared for with either mastectomy and reconstruction or breast-conserving treatment is the lack of sensation or numbness in the reconstructed breast or that of the breast area. This is disconcerting and uncomfortable, and can hinder sexual arousal, particularly during foreplay.[26]

Unmarried patients with breast cancer may have increased insecurities related to meeting new partners and dating, and when and how to tell them about their diagnosis and physical condition.[28] An excellent resource for this population, as well as for married women, is the Reach to Recovery program. This American Cancer Society (ACS) program tries to pair the patient with a volunteer mastectomy patient of the same race, side of mastectomy, social status (single, married, widowed, divorced) and, in some areas, sexual orientation. The volunteer explains exercises for the affected side's arm, tells where to get prostheses and clothing, and gives emotional support.

FEMALE PELVIC AND GENITAL CANCER

Physical and Psychosocial Parameters. As in breast cancer, the surgery needed to cure women of cancers of the genital organs can considerably inhibit a woman's sexuality.[13]

A threat to a woman's capability of being physically sexual can lead to a lost sense of femininity and consequent fluctuations in self-esteem and body image.[29] The female sexual response cycle will most likely be affected if treatment affects the structure and innervation of the clitoris or the vagina. Surgical resection or radiation therapy for cancer of the cervix, the uterus, the ovary, the vulva, the vagina, and the bladder can be either simple or extensive. Women faced with this type of treatment have many apprehensions:

- Threat to life
- Feelings of lost femininity
- Concern about what the external area will look like
- Questions about the ability to have intercourse and, if they do, fears that it will be painful
- Fear that along with the loss of fertility will come loss of vitality and orgasmic potential
- Fear of physical aging, diminished libido, loss of vaginal lubrication, and dyspareunia
- To prevent extensive morbidity and sexual dysfunction from the concerns just mentioned, early intervention with counseling is imperative for the gynecologic cancer patient.

Radical Hysterectomy. The surgical procedure of radical hysterectomy shortens the vaginal canal (up to one half), but this consequence is not believed to be sexually appreciable in all cases. Penile thrusting may be uncomfortable, because the trigone of the bladder and sigmoid colon may be closely associated with the new vaginal apex. Delayed resumption of bladder function introduces an embarrassing problem. If a long-term indwelling catheter is present, vaginal sexual relations can be impeded. To prevent dislodgment, the catheter can be placed up over the lower abdomen and taped into place. Vaginal dryness, atrophy, and pain can be caused by radical hysterectomy and often, women are advised to use oral estrogen replacement therapy or estrogen creams, tablets, or the product Estring (estradiol vaginal ring) (see interventions section later in chapter). Most of these products can raise the blood levels of estrogen, and this is often considered dangerous if a woman has an estrogen-sensitive tumor.[30] The Estring may be a safer alternative, because changes in blood levels of estradiol are very small and temporary.[30] However, it has not been tested in breast cancer survivors as yet and cannot be recommended without caution.

Women who have undergone radical hysterectomy may also realize a decrease in sensation in the nipples and the clitoris, decreased libido, and a decrease in the intensity of orgasms.[13] This decreased sensation may be due simply to a deficiency in testosterone. Testosterone levels are usually obtained during the middle third of the menstrual cycle; however, "the free testosterone index (total testosterone divided by sex hormone-binding globulin [SHBG]) correlates with bioavailable testosterone [and] may be a substitute evaluation" since this cancer population has had hysterectomy.[31] Although there are no approved methods of replacing testosterone in women in this country, androgens have been used off-label for replacement. Testosterone injections usually provide above-normal levels for women, and the patch may also supply a dose that is too high.[31] Phase III studies are underway using a testosterone patch, but the U.S. Food and Drug Administration (FDA) has required more safety data before allowing it onto the commercial market. Dr. Patricia Ganz, professor and director of The Division of Cancer Prevention and Control at Jonsson Comprehensive Cancer Center in Los Angeles, CA, offers her patients a compounded cream of testosterone propionate 2% in petrolatum after careful assessment. She uses a pea-size amount to the skin twice a week or as needed (email communication, June 3, 2003).

Pelvic Exenteration. The adjustment to this particular surgery may comprise several factors.[12] These can include adaptation to a urinary conduit, bowel conduit, or both, and this can cause worry about appearance and appliance fit, possible leakage, and odor. The vulva will be extensively denervated, which results in a decrease in erotic sensation. Creation of a neovagina may also be necessary. Clitoral swelling and pain may occur, requiring a clitoridectomy for relief. It is understandable that many patients report decreased frequency of sexual activity and satisfaction and a loss of sexual self-confidence.

To ensure the most beneficial adjustment psychologically and sexually for the patient and her partner, it is necessary to provide specific alternatives and realistic information *before* surgery. Many women complain of the inability to voluntarily constrict the vaginal introitus, and for those women with a neovagina, some allege that it is too short or too large or associate it with an increased chronic discharge.[12] Some women retain the ability to have an orgasm, but others lose it or achieve orgasm only with extra effort. Also, after reconstruction, vaginal sensation is usually decreased. To promote total healing and the ability to detect early recurrence, a waiting period of 6 weeks to 2 months is advised before resumption of sexual intercourse.[13]

Radical Vulvectomy and Cystectomy. Cancer of the vulva usually occurs in women who are well past menopause, and these older women are often reluctant to seek treatment until the disease has progressed. As a result, the therapy can have a particularly frightful impact on body image and sexual identity.[32]

For early-stage disease, patients are usually treated with skinning vulvectomy (a partial vulvectomy of the superficial skin), laser treatment, or wide local excision rather than simple vulvectomy. With a skinning vulvectomy, a split-thickness graft from the inner thigh is often applied to cover the denuded area.[33] This procedure gives an optimal cosmetic and functional result. Laser treatment involves destruction of the lesion by vaporizing the tissue. Healing is excellent with this procedure, but a thorough pathologic review cannot be done of the diseased specimen.[33] Patients have few complaints of dyspareunia or decreased sexual responsiveness with laser therapy. In radical vulvectomy, the fine sensory perception experienced during foreplay is destroyed and must be compensated for by excitement of other erogenous zones such as the earlobes, the breasts, the fingers, the toes, and the inner thighs.[32] Patients comment that adequate information is rarely given to help them begin to alter their sexual expectations, and others state that the treatment is embarrassing and creates a feeling of isolation.[32]

Little is mentioned in the literature concerning women undergoing cystectomy and the sexual problems that arise from excision of the bladder and more than one third of the vagina.

Problems identified are vaginal tightness and dryness and self-conscious anxiety because of the ostomy.[34] Either a continent urinary reservoir, which has to be catheterized frequently, or a urostomy stoma will be placed. Problems with body image and sexual desire may be negatively affected, which is similar to those who have had stoma placement from colon cancer. Scarring can develop, as well as numbness and lost sensation, because of impaired innervation of the perineum. Gallo-Silver explained that women can still have a positive sexual experience with their partners even after radical cystectomy with stoma placement: "Although Helen did not want to experiment with vaginal penetration, she and Max enjoyed physical intimacy by using a side by side position in which Max approached her lubricated inner thighs from behind her. This position also protected and avoided the ostomy site."[35]

Radiation Therapy. Both external therapy and internal radiation insertion (brachytherapy) can cause irritating side effects to the perineal area, which are disruptive to sexual activity. Diarrhea, skin reaction of the external genitalia, and especially vaginal irritation, stenosis, and dryness are the most troublesome.[36] To prevent a diminished sense of femininity, a discussion with pertinent facts and preventive interventions should precede radiation therapy. The vagina will react to radiation by becoming shorter and narrower and will have adhesions and problems with lubrication.

MALE PELVIC CANCER

Physiologic and Body Image Alterations. Societal expectations of men have changed little since the 1980s. They are supposed to be heroes and good providers, to hide their emotions and be strong, not to touch each other unless engaging in sports, not be dependent on another, and periodically to relate on an emotional level. Masculinity is also equated with activity and productivity; a man must never admit to possible physical problems and should always be in control.[10,37] Consequently, when the male patient experiences a malignancy in the pelvis or genital area, his entire self-image may be threatened. According to Alfonso and others, sexual dysfunction was more common in males (82%) than in females (61%) in both experimental and control groups in their cohort of 107 cancer patients.[10] When the malignancy involves the prostate, the testicle, or the penis, there can be a temporary or permanent disturbance in relation to erection, emission, and/or ejaculation. Orgasm is not as frequently affected and can actually be achieved even when genital function is lost.[38]

Prostate. Surgery for prostate cancer has a definite impact on male sexual potency, depending on how extensive it is. When transurethral resection (TUR) is used in early-stage disease, approximately 79% of these patients experience scanty or absent ejaculation and have problems with incontinence and erectile dysfunction (ED).[39] With nerve-sparing surgical techniques, men can achieve erections with better success; however, return of erectile function may take up to 6 months.[39] A metaanalysis of 40 articles found that treatment for prostate cancer with radiotherapy produced a lower rate of treatment-related ED compared to surgery. Pretreatment erectile function was considered, and the surgical procedures included radical prostatectomy or a nerve-sparing procedure (unilateral or bilateral).[40] However, problems can occur when radiation is used in lieu of surgery because of probable fibrosis of the pelvic arteries. Erectile impotence can vary from 40% to 46% after treatment with external radiation, and the dose to the bulb of the penis is of consequence as reported by Fisch and others: "Increasing doses of radiation therapy to the bulb of the penis decreases the number of nitric oxide-producing cells. Nitric oxide is essential to obtain and maintain an erection... as such, the efficacy of sildenafil citrate in brachytherapy-induced ED may be related to its ability to enhance the effect of nitric oxide."[41] Interstitial treatment may be used if tumor burden is small, and the incidence of impotence is reported between 2% and 51%; however, when ED is reported in the area of 50%, brachytherapy had been combined with external beam radiotherapy.[42] Other sexuality disorders may include a reduction or absence of ejaculate volume, painful ejaculation and hemospermia, a decreased frequency and rigidity of erections, and a decreased libido.[37]

Endocrine treatment (castration, estrogen, and/or a luteinizing hormone/regulatory hormone [LH/RH] antagonist [Lupron]) commonly causes difficult and embarrassing problems such as gynecomastia, phallic atrophy, loss of libido, and erectile impotence.[43] Many men experience physical debilitation, depression, anxiety, and pain, all of which may decrease sexual desire.

One important aspect of care may be to help the patient and his partner develop a change in attitude toward sexual intercourse if erection is no longer possible or if it is impaired. The goal of an intimate interlude may no longer be penile vaginal or anal intercourse, but rather one of caressing and fondling each other with the desire to achieve pleasant stimulation with possible orgasm. Even if frequency drops, the potential for sexual arousal remains with the correct stimulus.

Testicle. Not surprisingly, men with cancer of the testicle not only have problems with fertility, but also with their intimate relationships.[44] This population is generally young (15 to 34 years old) and in a crucial stage in life, and cancer treatment produces organic problems and sexual anxieties leading to dysfunction. However, testicular cancer, generally the seminomatous type, may also be diagnosed during midlife (ages 40 to 50 years). When more treatment than unilateral orchiectomy is necessary, sexual dysfunction increases. Extensive surgery (retroperitoneal lymph node dissection [RLND]), radiation, and chemotherapy may cause erectile and orgasmic dysfunction.[44] With RNLD, sympathetic ganglia are often damaged and can result in "dry orgasms" caused by retrograde ejaculation. However, fertility may be preserved with nerve-sparing surgery.[44] It must be stressed that normal sexual desire and pleasurable sensations, erection, and orgasm will probably continue after treatment. If sexual desire is lost, serum testosterone should be checked; replacement therapy may be needed.

Penis. Penile cancer, although very rare, results in the greatest risk of sexual dysfunction. Partial or total penectomy is usually needed to control the cancer. If partial penectomy is done, the penile stump usually can become erect with stimulation and remain so long enough for intercourse with antegrade ejaculation. If the entire glans penis is removed, a perineal urethrostomy is created behind the scrotum.[45] When it is stimulated to orgasm, ejaculation takes place through the perineal urethrostomy. Counseling for this man and his partner must include reassurance that both can be satisfied in several different ways.

Cystectomy. Radical cystectomy is similar to radical prostatectomy except that with cystectomy, urethrectomy may be included, which further damages penile innervation or blood flow.

The other major difference is that a urinary diversion must be done, which can result in the need for an ostomy appliance. Many patients choose to have a continent internal urinary reservoir or ileocolonic neobladder, and those men are reported to remain more sexually active than men with appliances.[34] Problems with sexual function are similar to those with radical prostatectomy since the prostate is removed; no ejaculate is present, and the sensation of orgasm may be diminished.[34]

COLORECTAL CANCER

Physical and Psychosocial Parameters. Surgery for colorectal cancer often has a profound effect on body image and sexual responsiveness. Because of the societal taboos centered around eliminative functions, many men and women feel disgusted that their feces are now eliminated through an opening on their abdomen.[46] Women undergo feelings of having been violated, whereas men experience the surgery as castration or mutilation.[46] Some patients report embarrassment because they equate the cleaning of their stomas with masturbation. Others are distressed because they have no "vacation" from stoma maintenance. They must always make sure that there are adequate facilities for cleaning themselves in private; consequently, leisure activities may be compromised.[46]

Regardless of the type of surgical diversion performed (colostomy, ileostomy, or urinary diversion), patients express many common reactions, which may include (1) greater-than-expected fatigue and weakness; (2) feelings of fragility and vulnerability to harm; (3) despair at the initial viewing of the stoma; (4) feelings of invalidism and depression; (5) fear of accidents, odor, leakage, and staining; (6) excessive emotional investment in the stoma; and (7) feelings of lost personal control.[47] Problems for both spouses and partners relative to acceptance of the ostomy may be realized in suffering sexual inadequacy, a lack of feeling desirable, and being lovable. (Desensitization may be enhanced if the partner views the stoma at an early stage.) Lesbians and gays will have the same concerns; furthermore, Turnball reports, "If anal sex has been a part of an individual's sexual repertoire—whether gay or straight—removal of the rectum and closure of the anus presents a sexual impairment. A stoma should never be used as a substitute for the anus, as this activity can cause trauma to the stomal tissue and necessitate further surgery."[47]

LUNG CANCER

Physical and Psychosocial Parameters. Unlike many other malignancies discussed in this chapter, lung cancer has a less optimistic prognosis unless it is diagnosed in the early stages and surgery is performed. However, even if disease is outside the lung, treatment with chemotherapy and radiation therapy is producing longer intervals of controlled disease.[48] There is a lack of information in the literature relative to psychosocial issues, particularly sexuality concerns, with regard to the person with lung cancer. Some researchers are including sexuality issues within their studies (e.g., loss of libido), and one study has focused only on sexuality in lung cancer patients.[49] A reason for this may be that these patients are often diagnosed with advanced disease that progresses rapidly, and their performance status is often very poor. Because treatment for these people is often palliative rather than curative, it is important to consider their feelings of masculinity, femininity, and self-esteem, along with the basic aspects of care such as pain control. The patient and partner must make significant decisions and adjustments, which often affects the patient's sense of self-esteem and worthiness: (1) if the patient has been a smoker, he or she will probably have tremendous feelings of guilt to cope with or overcome; (2) if the patient's performance status is poor and remains so as a result of fatigue and weakness, he or she will be unable to continue as a productive member of the family; (3) if the patient or the partner decide to take treatment (chemotherapy, radiation therapy), energy must be expended to decrease or manage the side effects; and (4) if the patient or the partner decide not to take treatment, there will be issues to resolve such as coping with an early death and caregiving. All of these factors will have an effect on the relationship the patient has with a spouse or partner, and it is no wonder that there may be little time, energy, or desire for intimacy. Patients and partners need encouragement to experience sexual closeness that does not necessarily lead to intercourse, because intercourse can exacerbate fatigue and dyspnea.

Considerations for Older Adults

Even though much of society finds it difficult to believe that their parents and their elderly grandparents are engaging in sexual activity, the American Association for Retired Persons (AARP) reported, in a study with 1384 adults with partners 45 years of age and older, that they engaged about once a week in kissing and hugging (average 85%), sexual touching or caressing (average 75%), and sexual intercourse (average 53%) during a 6-month period of time.[50] Older adults often face a double bias about their sexuality. It is assumed that "old" people are (1) too ill to be thinking sexually and (2) incapable of sexual activity. If attitudes such as these prevail, chances are few that sexual issues will be considered in these patients' general health care.[37,51]

Personal attitudes related to sexuality and the aging population must be examined and questions asked, such as "How do I feel about my elderly parents or grandparents having sex?" "If I see two elderly people kissing and fondling each other, how do I react?" (Fig. 31-4) Because the "baby boomers" have decided that they are not going to grow old gracefully, information relative to sexual health and behavior in the 40- to 80-year-old age group must be scrutinized. When providing sexual counseling for older adults, keep in mind that all couples will not be interested in improving their sexual activity; consequently, a focus on various aspects of femininity and masculinity can be emphasized. However, it can be ascertained during assessment whether or not abstinence is chosen because that is what the couple feels is expected of them. For those patients who still have the desire for sexual involvement, consult the Considerations for Older Adults Box.

Special Issues Influencing Sexuality

THE GAY OR LESBIAN PATIENT

It must never be assumed that all patients have or wish to have a partner or that all partners are of the opposite sex. Knowledge and sensitivity about any patient with cancer is imperative, as is a nonjudgmental disposition. All patients are entitled to competence and a caring attitude from their caregivers. However, the literature and research that offers information concerning the gay and lesbian cancer population is limited.[9,52] There are several books on counseling gay and lesbian people and couples; however, few are written specifically in relation to cancer care.[53]

The sociocultural structure of gay relationships differs from that of lesbians. Six types of sociosexual relationships have been identified for the male, ranging from one-night stands to stable cohabitation or "marriage."[52,54] Less is known about lesbian relationships, but there is less promiscuity, and more lesbians marry.[52] The gay and lesbian sexual repertoire and erotic positions are similar to those of heterosexuals except when limited by identical anatomy. As with heterosexuals, the precancer sexual relationship has an important effect on the stability of the postcancer relationship. If the patient has been diagnosed with cancer and still has to "cruise" (look for a sexual partner), it will be as

---

CONSIDERATIONS FOR OLDER ADULTS

- A weak back or muscles can be helped by exercising those muscles. This will also help the person have more energy and feel more sexually attractive.
- A nutritional diet using the food guide pyramid can help prevent or decrease depression and apathy, which may decrease sexual performance and interest.
- For partners to achieve lubrication and erection, longer precoital stimulation may be needed to compensate for slowed physical response.
- Because of musculoskeletal changes, various positions for intercourse may have to be tried to promote comfort and save energy.[52,53]
- Both partners may not achieve orgasm; however, sexual pleasuring can still be enjoyed. Also the male may have little or no ejaculate.[7]
- During prolonged hospitalization or nursing home confinement, privacy should be provided for couples to hold, touch, fondle, and have intercourse if desired. This holds true for couples of any age.
- Warm baths, gentle massage, caressing and touching, masturbation, and fantasy all provide a sense of satisfaction and reassurance.
- Cleanliness, skin care (including makeup, perfume, and aftershave), hair care, mouth care, and attractive clothing can enhance feelings of masculinity and femininity.

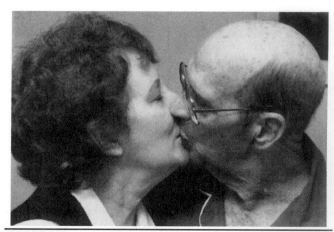

FIG. 31-4   Henry and Margie share a tender moment.

difficult to deal with the new body image as it is for the heterosexual patient. Because staff members may be inexperienced at being sensitive to behavioral cues, they may be unsuccessful in obtaining information about sexual orientation because they do not ask the right questions. Rather than asking about a spouse, husband, or wife, questions can be asked about whether the patient is sexually active or has a significant other.[52] If the partner is treated like a spouse and involved in the patient's treatment process, this will likely promote self-confidence and self-esteem in both members of the couple.[52]

STERILITY, INFERTILITY, AND PREGNANCY

Although cancer affects many young people in their prime reproductive years, it also affects those in midlife and later (women in their 40s and men in their 50s and 60s) who still may wish to have children. The patient's age, gender, and stage of development and the type, dose, and duration of therapy are all integral factors in the damage caused to reproductive tissue. Many concerns are reported in relation to reproductive damage and future capacity: (1) abnormal sexual development, impaired sexual performance, and infertility; (2) potential damage to germ cells, producing chromosomal changes; (3) transmission of the cancer-bearing gene to offspring; (4) problems with childbearing capabilities; and (5) likelihood of marriage.[55,56] Cancer transmission has not been reported except for genetic forms of cancer. Increased spontaneous abortion with combination therapy (radiation and chemotherapy) is known to occur.[55] The young cancer survivor tends to be less likely to marry than the average person.

Generally, male fertility is more susceptible to early damage than female fertility because of the constant mitotic cycles needed for spermatogenesis, as compared with the relative inactivity of the female oocyte. Consequently, many chemotherapy agents alone, and especially in combination, can cause azoospermia, oligospermia, or permanent sterility.[22] Alkylating agents such as nitrogen mustard, cyclophosphamide, and chlorambucil cause sterility in the majority of treated male patients. However, depending on the drugs used, drug dose, and length of treatment, fertility may return, and the time frame can vary from 15 to 49 months after completion of therapy.[56] Successful pregnancy is often limited because of abnormalities of the pretreatment sperm specimen. However, with the advent of assisted reproductive technologies (ART) such as in vitro fertilization (IVF), gamete intrafallopian transfer (GIFT), and zygote intrafallopian transfer (ZIFT), men with lower than normal sperm concentration can take advantage of semen cryopreservation.[22] In vitro fertilization or intracytoplasmic sperm injection (ICSI) is a newer technique whereby the egg is injected with a single, isolated sperm and is cultured until an embryo develops; the embryo is then transferred to the uterus.[22]

Again, age plays a role in a woman's possibility of ovarian dysfunction after treatment with chemotherapy, because there are progressively fewer germ cells in the aging ovary. As with boys, the ovarian function of prepubertal girls seems less susceptible to damage from chemotherapy. One other major concern for women is cancer and pregnancy. It is reported that 1 in 1800 pregnant women will have cancer, and all forms of neoplasms are found during pregnancy, with lymphoma and breast, cervical, ovarian, and colorectal cancers occurring most frequently.[20] In making a decision whether to treat the patient during pregnancy, several factors should be considered: (1) "gestation age of the fetus; (2) maternal and fetal health at the time of diagnosis; (3) mother's prognosis and likelihood of future pregnancies after treatment; and (4) the known teratogenic effects of the drugs to be used."[57] If the administration of chemotherapy is initiated *after* the first trimester, surprisingly few complications are associated with treatment. Also, pregnancy after chemotherapy is not usually discouraged, although some oncologists are concerned about recurrence facilitated by hormonal and immunologic changes. Because little scientific data support these worries, women should consider ultimate prognosis and the desire for children.

Finally, the children of patients treated with chemotherapy must be considered. No known studies are available that show an increase in congenital anomalies or other diseases in these children.[57] If the parent is treated with a combination of chemotherapy and radiation therapy, there appears to be a higher rate of complications of pregnancy. Wives of male patients have more spontaneous abortions, and female patients have more offspring with a variety of problems. Many scientists feel that prolonged observation must be done to better define the possible mutagenic nature of chemotherapy and radiation therapy in these children.

Assessment and Assessment Instruments

NURSING ASSESSMENT TECHNIQUES

When performing a sexual health assessment, several elements can enhance both the nurse's and the patient's comfort during the discussion.[22] Key elements that will promote optimal patient teaching can be found in Box 31-2.

BOX 31-2   Sexual Health Assessment

Privacy is essential when doing the assessment. If the patient is not in a private room, move to another area if possible. An office, conference room, or a vacant patient room is preferable.

Assure the patient of confidentiality. This tends to decrease the level of anxiety markedly. Usually it is good to include the partner, but it may be necessary to meet privately with the patient at first to establish rapport.

Try to obtain a sexual history early in your association with the patient (see the approaches described in text). This implies that sexuality is an important and natural part of good health. Fatigue and how it can affect the patient's sexual activity may be included during an explanation of chemotherapy side effects. In this way, one can introduce the concept, talk about it somewhat, and come back to it without making the patient uncomfortable.

Avoid overreaction in your verbal and nonverbal communication. Wide eyes and an open mouth are not conducive to trust. Also try not to be bored. Listening with genuine interest helps to convey acceptance.

Move from less sensitive to more sensitive issues.

Determine the patient's goals for treatment.

Realize when a problem is too complex to handle or when you do not know enough to be therapeutic, and refer the problem on (e.g., clinical nurse specialist, psychologist, sexual rehabilitation counselor).

There are several different approaches to sexual history taking. Three sets of questions are presented here.

McPhetridge included assessment of the effects of the illness on sexuality as a part of the nursing history. For our purposes, these questions might read as follows:

- Has having cancer (or its treatment) interfered with your being a mother (wife, husband, father, partner)?
- Has your cancer (or its treatment) changed the way you see yourself as a man (woman)?
- Has your cancer (or its treatment) caused any change in your sexual functioning (sex life)?
- Do you expect your sexual functioning (sex life) to be changed in any way after you leave the hospital or after treatment is finished?[58]

The PLISSIT is a model frequently used for sexuality counseling or as a nursing intervention. Each step is taken depending on the nurse's knowledge and comfort level.[59]

P = Permission: Promotes discussion and encourages the couple to continue in their present pattern of sexual activity plus suggests some risk taking

LI = Limited Information: Includes the permission already given plus some new information specific to their sexuality concerns

SS = Specific Suggestions: May include new activities for the couple, which may entail "homework"

IT = Intensive Therapy: When the couple is referred on to a therapist for more intense treatment

Interventions

The interventions that follow will be in the order of presentation in the chapter, and they do not have a strong evidence-based foundation. At present, there are very few randomized controlled intervention trials; however Shell assessed the literature from the past 20 years and reported on an in-depth examination of evidence-based research relative to sexual function in the cancer population.[60]

HEAD AND NECK CANCER

To freshen stale breath caused by a dry mouth (from radiation therapy) sugarless mints and artificial saliva will help.[18] Artificial saliva (Moi-Stir [Kingswood Labs]; Xerolube [Colgate Oral Pharm]) also helps prevent tooth decay. Patients may have a decreased sense of smell, so that perfumes cannot be appreciated; however, candles, scented or not, can provide a relaxed ambience for both patient and partner, though the fragrance will not be appreciated by the patient.

Partners should be made aware that the patient's heavy breathing may sound different. If the larynx is removed, a sexy voice, whispered love talk, and other eroticisms will be eliminated.

Tracheostomies should be cleaned of mucus and covered lightly during sexual activity. (For information on obtaining tracheostomy covers, contact Byram Health Care Center, Greenwich, CT 06380, 800-354-4054.) Various positions may have to be tried for sexual activity, because the partner may be fearful of cutting off the patient's air supply. (See Schover's *Sexuality and Cancer: For the Woman[Man] Who Has Cancer and Her[His] Partner*[61,62]). Patients, especially women, may wish to wear a fancy nightgown with a high neck, or other erotic neckwear. Men may wish to wear a dickey.

LIMB AMPUTATION

After some experimenting, some amputees find that intercourse can be maintained without any modification or adjustment of positions. Although some patients may expend slightly more energy, which may result in mild fatigue, this rarely hampers sexual function. If balance and movement are a problem, pillows or other forms of support may be used to maintain a level pelvis.[20]

Lovemaking does not always have to occur in the bedroom. A sofa or large chair can be used to balance on, or the female lower amputee can lean against a chair while her partner enters her from behind. An upper extremity amputee may wish to use a side-lying position with the existing arm free to balance.

Hemipelvectomy patients may have extra folds of skin used to make their flaps. Because these patients may be uncomfortable exposing themselves to their partner, these skin folds can be held in place by a "compression sock." This sock compresses the folds into a hip-like shape, and the sock can then be modified with an opening in the crotch to allow for intercourse.

HEMATOLOGIC MALIGNANCIES

The patient who is neutropenic (WBC below 1000/mm³; platelets below 20,000/mm³) should be advised against oral, penile or vaginal, and anal sexual manipulation. Remind the patient and partner that gratification may be derived from touching and holding. If the patient's complexion is pale because of decreased erythrocytes, encourage bright-colored clothing and the use of make-up to enhance appearance.

To avoid fatigue, a nap before intercourse may be helpful. The supine position or a side-lying position uses less energy. Also, avoid temperature extremes if possible. Intercourse can be planned for after the administration of antiemetics and pain medications and when the medications will be most effective, and advise patients to avoid the stress of heavy meals and liquor before intercourse. The couple may wish to bathe together. Bubbles, a little candlelight, romantic music, and some wine (in plastic glasses) make for an intimate experience. The couple can share each other's company without performance anxiety, and the warm water may help ease some general aches and pains.

The importance of contraceptive measures during chemotherapy and radiation must be emphasized to all patients. Although chemotherapy will affect sperm count and ovulation, the patient cannot depend on this alone for contraception.[56,57] Teratogenic effects are seen during the first trimester of pregnancy, especially if the woman is under treatment.[57] Encourage sperm banking before initiation of chemotherapy.

BREAST CANCER

Until a woman is ready to disrobe or let her partner touch the wound and/or radiation area, she can wear a fancy camisole or short nightgown. This camouflages the area but is still sexually stimulating for the couple. To minimize a direct view of the woman's missing breast, the partner may assume the superior position (missionary position) or use a rear-entry position. *The New Joy of Sex: A Gourmet Guide to Lovemaking in the Nineties* edited by Dr. Alex Comfort, is an excellent reference for positions a couple may use to increase sexual pleasure.[63] The couple may make love by candlelight to decrease the impact of the change in body contour. Concentration on a certain sexual task (sensate focus) may increase stimulation and reduce appearance concerns. One suggestion is a touching exercise, explained in depth in Schover's book *Sexuality and Cancer: For the Woman Who Has Cancer, and Her Partner*.[62] The focus is initially on massaging the extremities and back and ignoring the genital sexual organs, and the result is relaxation and sensual pleasure.

Because many women derive great pleasure from stroking, sucking, and manipulation of the breast during foreplay, the remaining breast (if mastectomy has occurred) or both breasts can continue to be stimulated if the woman so desires. If reconstruction has taken place, remind the patient that there will most likely be no sensation in the affected breast. Reassure the patient that manipulation will not cause another breast cancer.

FEMALE PELVIC AND GENITAL CANCER

Gynecological Cancers. Sexual intercourse should not be resumed until 6 to 8 weeks after gynecological surgery (hysterectomy, vulvectomy, pelvic exenteration). This waiting time will promote healing, and rehabilitation may be needed if reconstruction of the vagina has been done or a neovagina has been created.

Alternatives to intercourse must be provided and encouraged even if intercourse is possible. These include nudity and cuddling with general pleasuring, autoeroticism and mutual masturbation, oral-genital stimulation, anal love play, and fantasy with DVD or videos. The Kama Sutra created by the Sinclair Intimacy Institute is a good choice; it can be found on the Web at *www.BetterSex.com*.

Kegel exercises (tensing and relaxing the pelvic muscles) will help to relieve tension, increase elasticity, reduce urinary incontinence, and decrease dyspareunia. During sexual activity, the hips may be elevated to improve stimulation. If rear entry is preferred, the thighs may be adducted and lubricated to emulate a deeper vaginal barrel. More control is afforded in the female superior position, but it may not be as comfortable. Vaginal estrogen products which decrease dryness and irritability are an option, and several are on the market such as Ogen Vaginal Cream (estropipate), a vaginal cream; Vagifem tablets (estradiol hemihydrate); and Estring (estradiol vaginal ring). The tablets and Estring are the least absorbed systemically.

If radiation has been administered to the pelvis, the following interventions may be helpful:

- Encourage a woman to continue intercourse during treatment until it becomes uncomfortable and to resume when the vagina is healed. This helps prevent adhesions and shortening of the vagina.
- If she does not have a partner, she should be encouraged to use a dilator (available in sizes from extra small to large) on a daily basis, and one should also be used while the woman cannot tolerate intercourse. Sensitivity must be used when explaining dilator use. A water-soluble lubricant must be used for intercourse or when using a dilator, since the ability of the vagina to lubricate will be damaged from the radiation.
- A lubricant can be applied either privately or as part of foreplay. Lubricants include Astroglide (BioFilm, Inc., Vista, CA), Slippery Stuff, KY jelly products, and others. They are obtained at any local drugstore or supermarket. Replens is another vaginal moisturizer; it can be applied on a daily basis and is especially useful in women who have had total body radiation.[46]

Cystectomy. If the bladder has had to be removed and the vagina is dry and tight, estrogen products may be used for the dryness along with vaginal dilators to decrease dyspareunia.[12] A fabric cover may be worn over the urostomy stoma appliance, and women may wear feminine lingerie during sexual activity. Kegel exercises may help to relieve perineal tension for both men and women and decrease dyspareunia for women. (See also information under Colorectal Cancer).

MALE PELVIC CANCERS

Prostate Cancer. Many men become sexually aroused by reading and/or viewing erotic books, pictures, or movies. Long periods of foreplay, including romantic dinners, showering or bathing together, and using different rooms for lovemaking, may be stimulating. A changed or new environment such as a local motel or house sitting for a friend may bring new excitement.

If a full erection is not possible, mutual masturbation with a partner may allow the patient to reach orgasm and ejaculation. The partner should massage the penis in a downward motion with pressure beginning at the base of the penis. The penis should not be pulled up toward the abdomen, or it can lose blood. A female partner can assist erection by inserting a partially erect penis into the vagina and flexing her perineal muscles, like Kegel exercises.

During ejaculation, semen may be propelled into the bladder, which may threaten the man's sense of masculinity.[37] However, a partner may enjoy oral stimulation more because she or he no longer has to experience the taste of semen. If the patient has problems with urinary incontinence, he should empty his bladder before intercourse and perhaps wear a condom, if this becomes worrisome to his partner. Remind the couple that urine is sterile and will not harm the partner.

To enhance or acquire an erection, intracavernous penile injections, urethral suppositories, and oral medications are pharmacologic options. Both electrical and hand-operated vacuum devices are available, as well as penile implants (see Fig. 31-5). The risks and benefits of penile implants should be explained to the couple. Many urologists recommend waiting 6 months after surgery before installing a prosthesis, and the patient and partner may choose from several different types of prosthesis (see Table 31-2).[12]

Testicular Cancer. Remind the patient that often people feel awkward and anxious when resuming sexual activity, but sexual relations, if physiologically possible, may resume about 6 weeks after pelvic surgery. Stress the fact that normal sexual desire and pleasurable sensations, erection, and orgasm will probably continue. If sexual desire is lost, serum testosterone should be checked; replacement therapy may be needed. α-Adrenergic–stimulating drugs can increase ejaculation and occasionally the intensity of orgasm for some patients who have had RLND.[64] If retrograde ejaculation is a problem because of RLND and cannot be reversed, there is a technique that can be used to harvest sperm after orgasm. Postorgasmic urine is immediately voided into a sterile container, and viable sperm cells are centrifuged out. They are then placed in a nutrient solution that prepares them for use in artificial insemination.[65] Sperm banking may be an option worth exploring, if the number and motility of the sperm are adequate. This is costly, and the success of future artificial insemination is not guaranteed. However, if the patient is interested, sperm banking must be done before chemotherapy begins or between the first and second treatments.

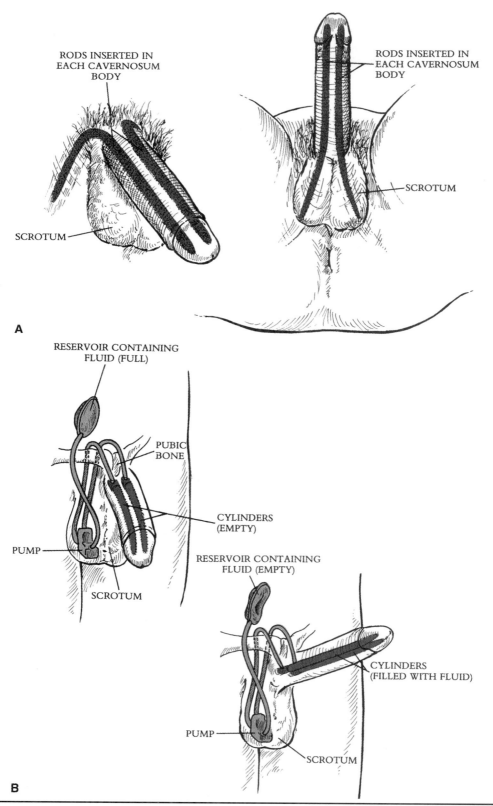

FIG. 31-5 Penile prostheses can be of two types. **A,** In one type, two semirigid silicone rods are implanted into the penis. **B,** In the second type two expandable cylinders are inserted into the penis and are connected by a tubing system to a fluid-filled bulb. (From Denney N, Quadagno D: *Human sexuality*, St. Louis, 1988, Mosby.)

TABLE 31-2	Interventions for Erectile Dysfunction (ED)	
PHARMACOLOGIC INTERVENTIONS		
DRUG	**ACTION**	
Sildenafil (Viagra): oral medication	Dilates blood vessels to enhance inflow to the corpus cavernosum. It does not increase desire. In brachytherapy-induced ED, sildenafil is started at 50 mg 1 hour before intercourse; if not effective in 3 doses, it is increased to 100 mg for 3 doses. If still not effective, drug is discontinued.[63]	
Alprostadil (MUSE: Medicated Urethral System for Erection) urethral suppository from 125 to 1000 mcg, or alprostadil injection into base of penis	Promotes erection within 5 to 7 minutes and lasts up to 1 to 1.5 hours. For injection, use tiny ⅜-inch needle to inject into base of penis.[65] Suppositories are expensive and not covered by insurance ($20 to $25 each).	
Vacuum Erection Devices		
A cylindrical tube is placed over the penis, a vacuum is created, an erection occurs, a soft rubber O-ring is placed on the base of the penis, and the vacuum tube is removed and intercourse is possible.	The O-ring can be left in place for 25 to 30 minutes. The vacuum device works best for patients who are able to achieve a partial erection on their own.	
Penile Prosthesis		
Semirigid implants: paired silicone-covered malleable metal rods are placed in the corpora cavernosa.	This is the simplest of the prostheses to implant and has the least chance of mechanical failure. The penis is always semierect and concealment is a potential problem with some clothing.	
Self-contained inflatable prosthesis: paired silicone cylinders that have a pump at the prosthesis tip and a reservoir within the shaft that transfers fluid so the cylinders become firm.	This surgery is simpler than with the multicomponent inflatable prostheses. It does not increase girth significantly when inflated and is not as soft or concealable when deflated.	
Inflatable penile prostheses: soft paired silicone inner tubes filled with solution that comes from a reservoir placed under the glans penis. When more fluid is pumped into the inner tubes, the erection becomes larger and firmer.	Prosthesis provides a more natural erection with total patient control; the erection lasts indefinitely until the patient transfers the fluid back into the reservoir. The surgical implant is more complicated and has a higher chance of mechanical failure.	

Loss of a testicle can cause embarrassment that may be remedied by a saline implant. Reinforce the fact that the cancer is not contagious through sexual activity, and if radiation therapy is used, the partner will not be contaminated. Encourage both partners to ask directly for the type of caressing and touching they prefer. For those patients with permanent erectile difficulties, see the penile implant suggestions in Table 31-2.

Penile Cancer. If the penis is completely removed, some couples may wish to use a phallic-shaped vibrator as a substitute penis for partner satisfaction. Stimulation of the mons pubis, the perineum, and the scrotum can produce orgasms with pleasurable contractions in the remaining cavernous musculature.[37] If only partial penectomy has occurred, men often report erections and orgasms of normal or near normal intensity with the phallic stump.[37] Finally, female partners must be advised (without instigating avoidance of sexual contact) to have a yearly Papanicolaou (Pap) smear, because they may be at increased risk for cervical cancer from exposure to the human papillomavirus.[28]

Cystectomy. If a stoma is in place, it should be emptied before intercourse, and some patients may wish to secure the stoma bag with a supportive belt. Like women, men may choose to wear a cover over their ostomy bag. Men may also wish to wear provocative underwear (silk boxer shorts) and expose only their genitalia during intercourse. To avoid friction on the stoma and pouch, other positions besides the missionary position may be tried. Some patients like to have their stomas touched during lovemaking, but they must be reminded that the stoma is fragile

and too much rubbing may cause tearing. Objects should not be placed into the stoma.

Colorectal Cancer. If a stoma is in place, the pouch should be prepared before sexual activity by emptying and ensuring the seal. If the ostomy is "dry" or controllable with irrigation, a small cover or patch may be sufficient cover. Attractive camouflage like a cummerbund or a cloth cover for the pouch can also be worn. The pouch can be deodorized (1 or 2 drops of Banish is helpful), and foods that cause gas should be avoided. Comfortable positions have to be tested (e.g., lateral scissors position, rear entry), and to protect from leakage, a rubber sheet may be placed under the sheet with a towel on top of the sheet. If an accident occurs, a shower together may be the best prescription.

For men, underwear with an opening up the center is provocative and also provides a cover. They may experience retrograde ejaculation after colorectal surgery and should be warned of this to prevent thoughts that "things aren't working quite right." Penile implants are an option for men unable to have an erection.

Most important, a good sense of humor is necessary, because accidents will happen. The couple may even consider rehearsing for when that time comes. Encourage them to "save water and shower with a friend."

LUNG CANCER

When experiencing sexual closeness, the significant other should continue to treat the patient as a partner rather than an invalid These are the few moments when the patient can feel "alive" and like a normal person again. It is important that the spouse or partner can be near to the patient when in an office setting or in a hospital bed. Being physically close, hand holding, and sharing an intimate moment will enhance feelings of intimacy, especially when the patient is getting treatment or is hospitalized.

When making love, soft caressing or light massage with oils or creams is sensual and can help reduce pain and discomfort. Decrease environmental irritants, perfumes, colognes, and hairsprays that can trigger bronchospasm. Mutual masturbation while watching adult movies promotes intimacy and conserves energy. During intercourse, take extra pillows and covers off the bed to allow the patient to feel less "closed in."

Making love on a pad on the floor may help remove the fear of sinking into a soft surface and not getting enough air. Instruct patients and partners to avoid long kisses on the mouth, which can create a fear of not getting enough air to breathe, and to avoid positions that put pressure on the chest and restrict breathing. The use of a waterbed should be considered. Movement of the water will move the patient without much effort, and reduce energy exertion during sex.

Outcomes

Today patients survive longer after their treatment for cancer. Survivorship, in turn, speaks to rehabilitation with the intent of helping restore the patient's sexual function, followed closely by the goals of reestablishing self-image and self-esteem. Each patient's sexuality is unique and is reflected in touching, smelling, hearing, tasting, and visual stimulation. These create for the patient and partner their own special intimacy, sense of affection, and physical gratification. Many references have been made and suggestions given in this chapter, but when there are *no* acceptable alternatives within a relationship, this choice should also be normalized and the couple helped to use their own coping strategies and strengths. The values and beliefs of the couple are important to the use and success of various alternatives. What may be an acceptable expression for some may not be for others. Sometimes all they need is to be given permission to try something different. Encourage them to take the risk, and be there to support them.

OUTCOMES EVALUATION MEASURES

Presently, the challenge is to create more intervention-based controlled trials to enhance and improve the sexual function of the person with cancer and their partner. Barton and others present examples of various research assessment instruments in use that can be adapted to the clinical setting.[66] One example is the Derogatis Interview for Sexual Functioning (DISF), which also has a self-report component; it measures the quality of sexual function in five segments (sexual cognition and fantasy, sexual arousal, sexual behavior and experiences, orgasm, and drive and relationship).[67] This instrument parallels the sexual response cycle, it has a female and male version, and it takes less than 15 minutes to complete. Studies regarding the sexual function of patients with head and neck, prostate, and lung cancer have used this brief instrument.[60]

There are several studies available that document that there is a problem relative to sexual function when a person is diagnosed with cancer.[60] There are many questions to be answered with controlled trials, and they may include the following:

1. What kinds or combinations of interventions would be most effective in promoting sexual adjustment after the cancer diagnosis?

2. When should an intervention be performed, and should interventions involve structured medical and/or psychosocial education?

3. Patient adjustment times usually occur at diagnosis, after surgery, during adjuvant treatment, during recovery, and posttreatment. Is it best to provide intervention(s) during all phases of adjustment or at one particular point in time?

4. Do intervention techniques developed for healthy people provide appropriate information to people with cancer and their partners?[60]

Most evidence currently available is of the lowest level, and interventions are provided according to published practice guidelines from the Oncology Nursing Society and the ACS, and from expert authorities, agencies, and committees. "Although practice guidelines and expert opinions should not be ignored, oncology nurses are obligated to patients and their partners to use their expertise and knowledge to participate in research that provides accurate, state-of-the-art interventions."[60]

ETHICAL CONSIDERATIONS

Although there is an entire chapter on ethical issues and legal-ethical dilemmas within oncology care, it is understood that when any subject is discussed with a patient, it must be done with complete confidentiality, and this is now the law. However, when we discuss one of the most sensitive and intimate aspects of who a person is and what their relationships are like, it is even more crucial that a discussion be done with respect, candor, and objective professional interest. This also means that the interviewer should be nonmoralistic, reassuring, and empathic. Any overreaction or underreaction may be offensive and set up a negative climate. Some particularly sensitive issues may be a person's sexual orientation, the inability to conceive children, or a human immunodeficiency virus (HIV) diagnosis. Patients must feel a stalwart trust that the information they offer will be held in strict confidence and not be part of a lunchroom or other friendly discussion. Because of the type of extended and familiar relationship that exists between the oncology professional and the patient and the partner, the information they divulge must be honored and held in strictest confidence.

The ability to intervene appropriately and with correct and complete information is always the nurse's goal. If a patient comes for care with a sexuality problem, either an individual or a couple issue, it should be managed by a practitioner with the most appropriate education, knowledge, and experience to do so. Intercession without these abilities, or incorrect or missing information may result in harm for both patient and partner. It is imperative to know when to make a referral to a psychotherapist or other provider for more intensive treatment.

Summary

As health care professionals continue to struggle to understand and be comfortable with their own sexuality, cancer patients continue to ask for help in dealing with disease and treatment-related sexuality issues. In this situation it is important to extend our efforts beyond the disease and focus on the whole patient. For all of us, receiving sexual pleasure and closeness is linked to a sense of belonging and worthiness. Being accepted is intimately bound to self-esteem. As Cantor put it, "Self-esteem is the sum total of all our feelings about ourselves ... it is the reputation we share of ourselves with ourself."[68]

REVIEW QUESTIONS

✓ Case Study

Mrs. D. was a 38-year-old Hispanic woman who was married and had one 5-year-old child. She was energetic and often went dancing with her husband and sisters. She was diagnosed with breast cancer and had a mastectomy with lymph node dissection; 6 of 15 lymph nodes were positive. Mrs. D. was a homemaker and also worked outside the home. She was attractive, of slim build, of average height with long black hair, and her husband took great pride in her beauty. She had hoped that she could be treated with lumpectomy and radiation therapy; however, her physician told her that her tumor was too large. Consequently, she had a mastectomy, which made her sad because she did not want to loose her breast. She explained that she was already "small breasted," and losing one breast made her feel like she was losing part of her sense of self and femininity. Although her husband seemed very supportive of the treatment, she remained anxious. She required adjuvant treatment with radiation therapy and chemotherapy, and was informed of the risk of immediate reconstruction and complications resulting from postreconstruction radiation; however, Mrs. D. decided to have immediate reconstruction with a transverse rectus abdominus myocutaneous (TRAM) flap anyway. After surgery, she remarked that she thought she looked quite "normal," especially with clothes on, and definitely decided to have nipple reconstruction at a later time. However, she was surprised that her reconstructed breast was completely numb; this upset her because breast manipulation was a favorite foreplay activity, and the breast that had been removed was also the most sensitive. She then worried about her arousal ability and ability to lubricate vaginally during intercourse. Mr. D. experienced reluctance to touch not only Mrs. D.'s reconstructed breast, but her other breast as well; consequently, she began to feel self conscious when naked in front of him. They had always been sexually compatible, and this situation puzzled her, even though she thought it may be because Mr. D. was afraid that he would hurt her.

Mrs. D. went through eight courses of chemotherapy, which caused hair loss and weight gain. She had always been thin, and the weight gain affected her self-image negatively. She also had intermittent problems with nausea, vomiting, and fatigue.

About 10 months after treatment, Mrs. D. had a local recurrence, and it was decided that she should undergo a stem cell transplant. She had started having intermittent periods again, but now she knew that sterility was certain with this treatment. She and Mr. D. were happy with their only child; however, Mrs. D. hoped to avoid a drug-induced menopause. The high-dose chemotherapy again caused hair loss, but this time her eyebrows and eyelashes were also affected, which made her feel even more ravaged by the treatment. Although she participated in the American Cancer Society's "Look Good, Feel Better" program, she still felt uncomfortable with how she looked when she had to pencil-in eyebrows and use fake eyelashes. She purchased a new wig; however, she was concerned about whether her husband would still find her attractive, even though he continued to voice his support. One problem that remained since her mastectomy was that Mr. D. remained reluctant to touch her breasts, even though she repeatedly told him that she was healed and had no pain. She explained that she and Mr. D. had slowly

begun to engage in more intimate lovemaking, and now that she had to experience more devastating treatment, she worried whether their relationship would ever be normal again. Because her body had betrayed her again, she felt angry and vulnerable, with a low sense of self-esteem and femininity; she said she was a changed person and had many body image concerns. Mrs. D. did well with the stem cell transplant process, and her sexuality concerns continued to be discussed at subsequent visits.

ASSESSMENT AND INTERVENTION

The clinical nurse specialist (CNS) addressed sexual function during the entire treatment trajectory to ensure that Mrs. D. knew that all aspects of who she was as a woman were important. Because the issues of self-esteem, self-efficacy, and body image were addressed, Mrs. D. was able to feel validated and to express her concerns. The following interventions were provided:

1. Acknowledge and assist to verbalize losses and fears, and discuss body modifications with both partners. Assist couple to accept changes and accentuate what remains normal.
2. Acknowledge disappointment over numbness of reconstructed breast and fears of inability to become sexually aroused. Advise of other body areas that are erogenous and easily stimulated, and of various vaginal lubricants and moisturizers (Astroglide, Slippery Stuff, Replens). Promote nonperformance closeness and touching.
3. Discuss reluctance to be naked, and encourage use of feminine lingerie during intercourse, possible changes in positions during intercourse, use of candles for light, and accentuating other attractive physical aspects of her body.
4. Acknowledge and assist to verbalize distress over body image side effects during treatment such as hair loss and weight gain. Encourage purchase of wigs, hats, and scarves and services such as "Look Good Feel Better." Offer realistic compliments.
5. Refer to dietician.
6. Acknowledge and assist to verbalize grief over further body betrayal and future fertility issues, and teach about methods to control menopausal symptoms such as hot flashes.
7. During extreme fatigue, advocate for time for fun and companionship, laughter, listening to music, simple communication, and being emotionally available to each other as a couple.
8. Referral of couple to a sex therapist re further issues with Mr. D.'s behaviors, and Mrs. D.'s anger and continued loss of sense of self-esteem and femininity.

OUTCOMES

1. Grief, loss, fears, and body modification issues were verbalized re lost breast, lost sense of self, and fear of hurting the patient. Changes were acknowledged, and "normal" aspects of her body were accentuated by the couple.
2. Disappointment and fears were acknowledged, patient learned about other erogenous areas of her body such as ear lobes, inner thighs. Astroglide and Replens were used to keep the vagina moist and to prevent dyspareunia. They took bubble baths together, which enhanced their closeness.

Continued

REVIEW QUESTIONS—CONT'D

3. Seductive lingerie was used and positions changed during intercourse to the couple's delight. Lighting was subdued, with candles.
4. Distress over body image side effects was acknowledged, and other remaining attractive attributes were accentuated. The "Look Good, Feel Better" class was attended, with pleasing results and compliments accepted.
5. Grief over further body betrayal and future fertility issues was voiced. Information about control of menopausal symptoms acknowledged.

QUESTIONS

1. Once a woman is diagnosed with breast cancer, she may be concerned about several issues related to sexuality, including which of the following?
   a. Denial of cancer disease
   b. Complexity of chemotherapy regimen
   c. Altered body image, self-esteem, impact on femininity, and sexual function
   d. Potential for disease spread or death
2. When a woman is ill, she may begin to doubt her sexual ability. Which of the following may affect this feeling?
   a. Questions about her cancer treatment and its side effects
   b. The effect the illness will have on her ability to respond sexually re arousal, vaginal lubrication, hot flashes, and so on
   c. Whether or not she has a supportive extended family
   d. Disinterest in sex, because it is not important in our society after 30 years of age
3. Some women with breast cancer who have mastectomy may choose to have reconstruction whether or not they have chemotherapy and/or radiation therapy. What is the most important issues to explain to her?
   a. She will most likely experience numbness in the reconstructed breast.
   b. She will always experience unusual sensations after radiation to the breast area.
   c. She will most likely have hot flashes after her chemotherapy.
   d. She will be able to allow her partner to manipulate her breasts even though she has had reconstruction.
4. What are some sexual concerns that potentially arise in connection with side effects from chemotherapy?
   a. Myelosuppression related to fatigue, infection, and bleeding
   b. Loss of the ability to go dancing because of fatigue
   c. Intermittent nausea and vomiting
   d. Complete hair loss, which affects body image and sense of self esteem
5. Patients' sexuality concerns related to reproductive damage include which of the following?
   a. Damage to germ cells, transmission of cancer-bearing genes, childbearing, and finances
   b. Infertility, childbearing, damage to germ cells, and finances
   c. Damage to germ cells, childbearing, infertility, and marriage likelihood
   d. Infertility, damage to germ cells, transmission of cancer-bearing genes, and pain

6. What interventions to promote sexual expression are suggested for women with mastectomy who have had treatment for breast cancer?
   a. Use of fancy lingerie to camouflage surgical area, a change of positions during intercourse to decrease attention to surgical area, and use of candles to subdue light.
   b. Use sugarless mints and artificial saliva help to freshen stale breath.
   c. Sexual intercourse should not be resumed until 6 to 8 weeks after surgery.
   d. Kegel exercises may help to relieve perineal tension and decrease dyspareunia.
7. Issues related to sexuality concerns can be of a physical nature; however, which of the following are questions related to the *inner* sense of femininity?
   a. The nature of or whether there is the threat of death
   b. Communication with partner related to their day, the relationship, their feelings, and emotional availability
   c. Whether or not there is anxiety and/or depression
   d. Whether or not there will be adequate time for activities of daily living
8. Assessment will always include the spouse or partner and whether or not the couple will cope with the diagnosis of breast cancer. What is most important factor that influences the stability of their relationship after the cancer diagnosis?
   a. Whether the couple had a strong relationship before the cancer diagnosis
   b. Whether the patient had any previous experience with a chronic disease
   c. Whether the couple had a good sex life before cancer
   d. Whether the couple had sexual relations before marriage or commitment as a couple
9. Mr. D. continued to have an aversion toward touching Mrs. D.'s reconstructed breast even after several conversations with her regarding her comfort. What would be an appropriate intervention for the CNS to do now that several months have elapsed?
   a. Confront Mr. D. with his behavior and inform him that this is making Mrs. D. uncomfortable.
   b. Ignore this situation, because Mrs. D. has just gone through a stem cell transplant and he has other things to worry about.
   c. Refer Mr. & Mrs. D. to a sex therapist for in-depth therapy.
   d. Refer Mr. D. to a support group for husbands of cancer patients.
10. The CNS was able to address sexuality issues with Mrs. D. without hesitation. This type of assessment should always be included when caring for cancer patients. When is the best time to assess for sexuality concerns?
   a. Concerns really shouldn't be addressed unless the cancer is relative to a sexual aspect of the body such as the breast or gynecologic area.
   b. Sexuality concerns are best addressed when the cancer is first diagnosed so the patient knows what to expect.
   c. Sexuality concerns are really best addressed by the physician and by the nurse only if requested to do so.
   d. Sexuality issues should be addressed at initial diagnosis, intermittently during treatment, and posttreatment.

ANSWERS

1. C. *Rationale:* After issues related to the cancer diagnosis have been discussed, sexuality issues including altered body image, self-esteem, impact on femininity, and sexual function will then be of concern. The remaining choices are related to the cancer diagnosis and will usually be discussed before sexuality.

2. B. *Rationale:* If the cancer involves the breast and the woman has to have chemotherapy, the drugs may affect the sexual response cycle (arousal and vaginal lubrication), and a hormone such as tamoxifen may cause hot flashes that can impede sexual activity. The remaining choices are related to her treatment, her family's involvement, and to a myth.

3. D. *Rationale:* Many women already believe that a bump to the breast or other accident caused the cancer; she and partner must realize that they will not cause another cancer if breasts are manipulated. Other, specific issues need not be explained if the patient does not have that particular treatment. However, no matter what the treatment, she may always worry about manipulating the other breast and causing another cancer.

4. D. *Rationale:* Hair loss affects body image for weeks to months and is readily visible to family and the public. It also distorts how a woman *looks*. The remaining choices are concerns related to physical maladies that are readily (within several days) corrected, are not readily visible, and don't affect body image.

5. C. *Rationale:* This relates directly to reproductive damage (e.g., damage to germ cells, childbearing, infertility, and marriage likelihood). The remaining choices are aspects not directly related to reproductive damage (e.g., transmission of cancer-bearing genes, finances and pain).

6. A. *Rationale:* These interventions all create illusion or diversion from the breast area and may provide an increased sense of relaxation. The remaining choices are specific interventions related to other cancers such as head and neck and gynecologic cancers.

7. B. *Rationale:* The sense of femininity also includes being a partner, wife, and/or lover, and communication with a partner regarding daily activities, the relationship, and emotional availability reaffirms this sense. The remaining choices relate to fears (death and time for activities) and psychologic disorders.

8. A. *Rationale:* Research tells us that the most important aspect of how a couple will handle the cancer illness is how strong the relationship was before the illness.

9. C. *Rationale:* It is important to be able to recognize that a referral should be made to a psychotherapist when a deep-seated psychosocial problem exists and remains over a long period of time. This problem has not been able to be resolved with the interventions of the CNS, and Mr. D. would be benefited more by psychotherapy with a sex therapist than confrontation, ignoring the issue, or sending him to a support group that may or may not talk about sexuality issues.

10. D. *Rationale:* Sexuality concerns should be addressed all along the treatment trajectory so that patients know that all aspects of their personhood are important. If sexuality is only addressed at one particular point in time during treatment, or only if asked about, the patient and the partner may believe that this is the only time they are permitted to speak about it, or they may not feel comfortable addressing it at all.

REFERENCES

1. Jeffry D: Overview: Cancer survivorship and sexual function, *J Sex Ed Ther* 26(3):170, 2001.
2. Manne S: Cancer in the marital literature: a review of the literature, *Cancer Invest* 16(3):188, 1998.
3. Rowland J: In sickness and in health: the impact of illness on couples' relationships, *J Marital Fam Ther* 20(4):327, 1994.
4. Brunner DW, Boyd CP: Assessing women's sexuality after cancer therapy: checking assumptions with the focus group technique, *Cancer Nurs* 22(6):438-447, 1999.
5. Weiss K: *Women's experience of sex and sexuality*, Center City, MN, Hazelden Educational Materials, 1992.
6. Masters W, Johnson V: *Human sexual response*, Boston, 1966, Little, Brown.
7. Masters W, Johnson V, Koloday R: *Heterosexuality*, New York, 1994, Harper Perennial.
8. Shell J: Sexuality and sexual dysfunction. In Hass ML, Hogle WP, Moore-Higgs G, Gosselin-Acomb, editors: *Radiation therapy: a guide to patient care*, Philadelphia, Mosby (in press).
9. Fields B, Scout: Addressing the needs of lesbian patients, *J Sex Ed Ther* 26(3):182, 2001.
10. Alfonso C, Cohen MA, Levin M et al: Sexual dysfunction in cancer patients: a collaborative psychooncology project, *Int J Mental Health* 26(1):90, 1997.
11. Long L, Burnett JA, Thomas RV: *Sexuality counseling: an integrative approach*, New Jersey, 2006, Merrill/Prentice Hall.
12. Schover L, Montague D, Lakin M: Psychologic aspects of patients with cancer: sexual problems of patients with cancer. In DeVita VT, Hellman S, Rosenberg SA, editors: *Cancer: principles and practices of oncology*, ed 5, Philadelphia, 1997, Lippincott-Raven.
13. Lefkowitz GK, McCullough AR: Influence of abdominal, pelvic, and genital surgery on sexual function in women, *J Sex Ed Ther* 25(1):45, 2000.
14. Syrjala K, Schroeder T, Abrams J et al: Sexual function measurement and outcomes in cancer survivors and matched controls, *J Sex Res* 37(3):213, 2000.
15. Sexuality Information and Education Council of the United States: *Fact sheet: sexuality in middle and later life*, Report 30:1, 2001/2002: Author.
16. Minarik P: Psychosocial intervention with ineffective coping responses to physical illness: depression related. In Barry P, editor: *Psychosocial nursing*, ed 3, Philadelphia, 1996, Lippincott.
17. Curtis T, Zlotglow I: Sexuality and head and neck cancer, *Front Radiat Ther Oncol* 14:26, 1979.
18. Nordgren, M, Abendstein H, Jannert M et al: Health-related quality of life five years after diagnosis of laryngeal carcinoma, *Int J Radiat Oncol Biol Phys* 56(5):1333, 2003.
19. Williamson GM, Walters AS: Perceived impact of amputation on sexual activity: a study of adult amputees, *J Sex Res* 33(3):221, 1996.
20. Shell JA, Miller ME: The cancer amputee and sexuality, *Orthopedic Nurs*, September-October:53, 1999.
21. Syrjala KL, Roth-Roemer SL, Abrams JR et al: Prevalence and predictors of sexual dysfunction in long-term survivors of marrow transplantation, *J Clin Oncol* 16(9):3148, 1998.
22. Leonard M, Hammelef K, Smith GD: Fertility considerations, counseling, and semen cryopreservation for males prior to the initiation of cancer therapy, *Clin J Oncol Nurs* 8(2):127, 2004.

23. Tierney DK: Sexuality following hematopoietic cell transplantation, *Clin J Oncol Nurs* 8(1):43, 2004.

24. Williams J, Wood C, Cunningham-Warburton P: A narrative study of chemotherapy-induced alopecia, *Oncol Nurs Forum* 26(9):1463, 1999.

25. Gantz PA, Rowland JH, Desmond K et al: Life after breast cancer: understanding women's health-related quality of life and sexual functioning, *J Clin Oncol* 16 (2):501-514, 1998.

26. Wilmoth MC, Ross JA: Women's perception: breast cancer treatments and sexuality, *Cancer Pract* 5(6):353, 1997.

27. Andersen B, Golden-Kreutz D: Sexual self-concept for the woman with cancer. In Baider L, Cooper CL, Kaplan De-Nour A, editors: *Cancer and the family*, New York, 1996, Wiley.

28. Schover L: *Sexuality and fertility after cancer*, New York, 1997, Wiley.

29. Andersen BL, Woods XA, Copeland LJ: Sexual self-schema and sexual morbidity among gynecologic cancer survivors, *J Consult Clin Psychol* 65(2):221, 1997.

30. Whittelsey FC: The secrets about sex, *Mamm* May:49, 1999.

31. Davis S: Testosterone and sexual desire in women, *J Sex Ed Ther* 25(1):25, 2000.

32. Green MS, Naumann RW, Elliot M et al: Sexual dysfunction following vulvectomy, *Gynecol Oncol* 77(1):73, 2000.

33. Eifel P, Berek J, Thigpen JT: Gynecologic tumors. In DeVita VT, Hellman S, Rosenberg SA, editors: *Cancer: principles and practices of oncology*, ed 6, Philadelphia, 2001, Lippincott-Raven.

34. Ofman US: *Preservation of function in genitourinary cancers: psychosexual and psychosocial issues,* New York, 1995, Marcel Dekker.

35. Gallo-Silver L: The sexual rehabilitation of persons with cancer, *Cancer Pract* 8(1):10, 2000.

36. Lamb MA: Effects of cancer on sexuality and fertility of women, *Semin Oncol Nurs* 11(2):120, 1995.

37. Shell J: Treatment of sexual dysfunction in male cancer survivors. In Kandeel F, Lue T, Swerdloff R et al, editors: *Male sexual dysfunction: pathophysiology and treatment*, New York, Marcel Dekker (in press).

38. Baniel J, Israilov S, Segenreich E et al: Comparative evaluation of treatments for erectile dysfunction in patients with prostate cancer after radical retropubic prostatectomy, *Brit J Urol Internat* 88:58, 2001.

39. Talcott JA, Rieker P, Clark JA et al: Patient-reported impotence and incontinence after nerve-sparing radical prostatectomy, *J Natl Cancer Inst* 89(15):1117, 1997.

40. Robinson JW, Dufour MS, Fung TS: Erectile functioning of men treated for prostate carcinoma, *Cancer* 79(3):538, 1997.

41. Fisch BM, Pickett B, Weinberg V et al: Dose of radiation received by the bulb of the penis correlates with risk of impotence after three-dimensional conformal radio-therapy for prostate cancer, *Urology* 57(5):955, 2001.

42. Beckendorf V, Hay M, Rozen, R: Changes in sexual function after radiotherapy treatment of prostate cancer, *Br J Urol* 77(1):118, 1996.

43. Brunner DW, Hanlon A, Nicolaou N et al: Sexual function after radiotherapy + androgen deprivation for clinically localized prostate cancer in younger men (age 50-65), *Oncol Nurs Forum* 24:327, 1997 (abstract).

44. Jonker-Pool G, van Basten JP, Hoekstra HJ et al: Sexual functioning after treatment for testicular cancer: comparison of treatment modalities, *Cancer* 80(3):454-464, 1997.

45. Smith D, Babian R: The effects of treatment for cancer on male fertility and sexuality, *Cancer Nurs* 15(4):271, 1992.

46. Shell JA: Sexual functioning: body image. In Dow K, editor: *Nursing care of women and cancer*, St. Louis, 2006, Mosby.

47. Turnbull GW: Sexual counseling: the forgotten aspect of ostomy rehabilitation, *J Sex Ed Ther* 26(3):189, 2001.

48. Kris MG: Lung cancer cure, care and cost: let the data be your guide, *J Clin Oncol* 15(9):3027, 1997.

49. Shell JA: *The longitudinal effects of cancer treatment on sexuality in individual with lung cancer*, Unpublished doctoral dissertation, Michigan State University, East Lansing Mi, 2002.

50. American Association of Retired Persons: *Modern maturity sexuality study*, Washington, DC, 1999, Author.

51. Shell, J: Sexuality issues for the older adult with cancer. In Cope D, Reb A, editors: *An evidence-based approach to the treatment and care of the older adult with cancer*, Pittsburgh, 2006, Oncology Nursing Press.

52. Barret B, Logan C: *Counseling gay men and lesbians: a practice primer*, Pacific Grove, CA, 2002, Brooks/Cole.

53. Butler S, Rosenblum B: *Cancer in two voices*, Duluth, MN, 1991, Spinsters.

54. Shernoff M: Monogamy and gay men, *Networker* March/A pril:63, 1999.

55. Schahin MS, Puscheck E: Reproductive sequelae of cancer treatment 2, *Obstet Gynecol Clin North Am* 5:423, 1998.

56. Meistrich M, Vassilopoulou-Sellan R, Lipshultz L: Gonadal dysfunction. In DeVita VT, Hellman S, Rosenberg SA, editors: *Cancer: principles and practices of oncology*, ed. 6, Philadelphia, 2001, Lippincott-Raven.

57. DeLaat CA, Lampkin BC: Long-term survivors of childhood cancer: evaluation and identification of sequelae of treatment, *Cancer J Clin* 42(5):263, 1992.

58. McPhetridge L: Nursing history: one means to personalize care, *Am J Nurs* 68(1):73, 1968.

59. Cooley M, Yeomans A, Cobb S: Sexual and reproductive issues for women with Hodgkin's disease: application of PLISSIT model, *Cancer Nurs* 9(5):248, 1986.

60. Shell JA: Evidence-based practice for symptom management in adults with cancer: sexual dysfunction, *Oncol Nurs Forum* 29(1):53, 2002.

61. Schover L: *Sexuality and cancer: for the man who has cancer, and his partner*, ed 3, Atlanta, 2001, American Cancer Society.

62. Schover L: *Sexuality and cancer: For the woman who has cancer, and her partner*, ed 3, Atlanta, 2001, American Cancer Society.

63. Comfort A: *The New Joy of Sex: a Gourmet Guide to Lovemaking in the Nineties*, New York, 1991, Mitchell Beazley Publishers.

64. Crenshaw JL, Goldberg JP: *Sexual pharmacology*, New York, 1996, Norton.

65. Schover L: *Sexual problems in men with pelvic or genital malignancies: workshop on psychosexual and reproductive issues affecting patients with cancer*, San Antonio, TX, January, 1987, American Cancer Society.

66. Barton D, Wilwerding MB, Carpenter L et al: Libido as part of sexuality in female cancer survivors, *Oncol Nurs Forum* 31(3):599, 2004.

67. Derogatis LR: *The DISF/DISF-SR manual*. Baltimore, 1987, Clinical Psychometric Research.

68. Cantor R: Self-esteem, sexuality and cancer-related stress, *Front Radiat Ther Oncol* 14:51, 1980.

CHAPTER 32

Functional Status in the Patient with Cancer

Sandra A. Mitchell

Overview

Increasingly, there is an emphasis in cancer care on the outcomes of treatment: not just overall survival or time to disease progression, but also on the functional status and quality of life (QOL) of the individuals living through and beyond their treatment. Many cancer patients live with significant morbidity and functional losses caused by the disease and its treatment. Limitations in the ability to perform needed and valued activities independently and to participate in community life are costly to the individual, to the family, and to society. Rehabilitation has been defined as the process by which a person is restored to an optimal physiologic, psychologic, social, and vocational status.[1] Structured rehabilitation programs have the potential to blunt some of the negative side effects of cancer treatment, in particular, reduced functional capacity and health-related quality of life.

Functional status as it results from the care delivered by both staff nurses and advanced practice nurses has been identified as an outcome variable of clinical and conceptual interest to oncology nurses.[2] An Oncology Nursing Society (ONS) initiative to develop nursing-sensitive outcome measures identified "return to usual function" as one of the first of a series of outcomes to receive focused study, along with fatigue, nausea, and the prevention of infection.[3] Functional status is also an important aspect of cancer patients' perceived QOL; most of the prominent QOL measures used in cancer care, including the EORTC-QLQ-C-30, and the Functional Assessment of Cancer Therapy (FACT) scales, include functional status as part of their conceptual and operational definition of the concept of QOL. Functional status is also conceptually linked with the patient's experience of symptoms and is identified as a consequence of symptoms in the theory of unpleasant symptoms (Fig. 32-1), and as an outcome of effective symptom management in the University of California at San Francisco (UCSF) Symptom Management Model (Fig. 32-2).[4,5,6]

However, despite its clinical and conceptual importance as a component of QOL and symptom management, to date functional status has received little directed attention in the oncology literature.[7] There is a large body of conceptual and empirical work elucidating the concept of quality of life, and a smaller body of philosophical work exploring cancer rehabilitation, and yet the subject of function in the patient with cancer has remained largely underdeveloped, both conceptually and empirically.

This chapter will examine the conceptual and operational definition of functional status, discuss the risk factors for functional losses in patients with cancer, review the measures that clinicians and researchers can use to assess functional status in patients with cancer and to measure the outcomes of interventions designed to improve functional status, and outline interventions that may improve functional status and prevent functional decline in patients during and following the experience of cancer and its treatment.

Definitions and Conceptual Models

Functional status may be broadly defined as a systematic evaluation of the level at which a person is functioning in areas such as physical health, self-maintenance, role activities, intellectual status, social activity, attitude toward the world and toward self, and emotional status.[8] Health-related QOL may be defined as the impact of cancer on physical symptoms, affective status, functional status, and social support.[9]

Several conceptual models of functional status have been proposed, although none has achieved predominance within the specialty area of cancer care. Within rehabilitation medicine, the most prominent model of functional status is the International Classification of Functioning, Disability and Health (ICF) of the World Health Organization (WHO).[10] Developed from a synthesis of the Nagi Disablement model and the International Classification of Impairments, Disabilities and Handicaps, this conceptual model, as shown in Fig. 32-3, has three main constructs: (1) body structures and functions, (2) activities, and (3) participation.[11-13] These three spheres of human functioning are depicted as occurring at the level of the body or body part or system, the whole person, and the whole person in a social context. Within this model, disability results from dysfunction at one or more of these same levels, in the form of impairments (i.e., problems, such as significant deviation or loss, in body function or structure), activity limitations (i.e., difficulties an individual may have in executing an activity, task, or action), and participation restrictions (i.e., problems an individual experiences with involvement in life situations and roles). Functioning and disability result from the interaction between health conditions (i.e., diseases, disorders, and injuries) and contextual factors within the environment and the person. The framework is helpful in drawing a distinction between an *impairment* in body structures or body function (e.g., decreased proximal muscle strength) and the *consequence* of that impairment for normal activity and a satisfactory level of participation (e.g., ability to climb stairs and take public transit to appointments). Although there has been criticism of the ICF framework for its emphasis of negative terms such as impairment, disability, and handicap, the ICF framework may be particularly useful as a model of functional status in understanding functional status from a social perspective, and in formulating health policy change and advocating

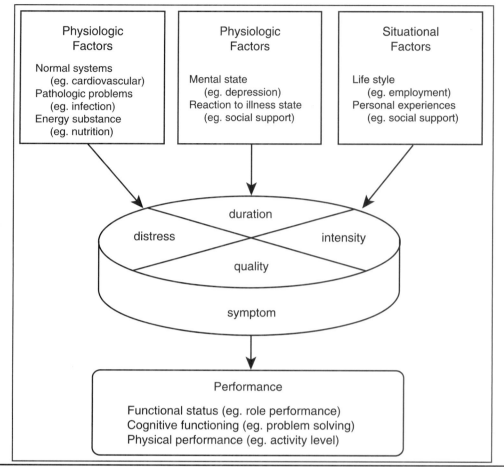

FIG. 32-1 Conceptual model in which functional status is relevant outcome variable: the Middle Range Theory of Unpleasant Symptoms. (From Lenz ER, Pugh LC, Milligan RA et al: The Middle-Range Theory of Unpleasant Symptoms: An update, *ANS Adv Nurs Sci* 17(3):1-13, 1995.)

for societal, community, and systems enhancements that improve accessibility.

Leidy[14] has proposed an alternative model of functional status (see Fig. 32-4); one that is potentially more helpful in directing clinical intervention to improve functional status and limiting functional decline in patients with chronic illness. She defines functional status as a multidimensional overarching conceptual framework through which the performance of necessary and desired human activities and roles may be understood.[14] Within Leidy's model, functional status is composed of four dimensions: capacity, performance, reserve, and capacity utilization.[14] **Functional capacity** is an individual's maximum potential to perform activities, whereas **functional performance** is defined as the physical, psychologic, social, occupational, and spiritual activities that individuals do in the normal course of their lives to meet basic needs, fulfill usual roles, and maintain their health and well-being.[14] Functional capacity reflects the maximum possible level of function, whereas functional performance is what individuals actually do in their day-to-day lives. Individuals choose to function at a level of performance that reflects their greatest physical and psychological comfort. The term **functional reserve** refers to this difference between functional capacity and functional performance. Functional reserve is the latent functional ability that can be called upon in time of perceived need. Finally, **functional capacity utilization** is the extent to which

capacity is called upon to achieve a given level of performance. Functional capacity utilization is what accounts for the common observation that two people with the same apparent functional capacity can display different levels of functional performance.[14] Functional status is also likely to be influenced by health perceptions. For example, a person who most observers would judge to be well, but who views himself as ill, may have a low level of functional performance in relation to his capacity.[14]

Each of these dimensions of functional status is evaluated differently. For example, exercise tolerance testing, the 2-, 6- or 12-minute walk, and other tests such as grip strength and the "timed up-and-go" have been used to quantify a patient's capacity for physical activity and function. On the other hand, functional performance is often captured through self-report measures such as the Functional Performance Inventory or the Sickness Impact Profile.[15,16] The physical function, role physical, emotional role function, and social function subscales of the SF-36 also qualify as functional performance indicators under this framework.

Leidy's framework is useful as a model to guide both practice and research, since the model can integrate functional status with all of the following: disease and treatment-related factors; biologic or physiologic factors; level of premorbid conditioning; symptoms, mood, motivation and self-efficacy; expectations; lifestyle; and environmental support and accommodation.

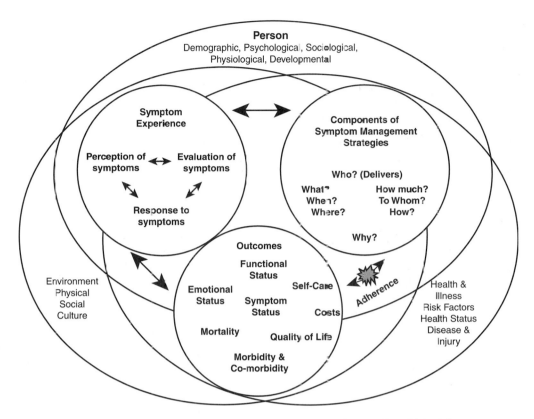

Larson, P.J., Uchinuno, A., Izurni, S., Kawno, A., Takemoto, A., Shigeno, M. et al (1999). An integrated approach to symptom management. *Nursing and Health Sciences, 1*, 203-210.

FIG. 32-2   Conceptual model in which functional status is relevant outcome variable: University of California at San Francisco model for symptom management. (From Larson PJ, Uchinuno A, Izumi S et al: An integrated approach to symptom management. *Nurs Health Sci* 1(4):203-210, 1999.)

The impact on capacity, capacity utilization, and reserve of each of these factors is considered individually and in concert. Similarly, the model can be used to define nursing interventions to elevate functional capacity (e.g., exercise) and improve performance (through home supports or functional accommodations), thereby reducing capacity utilization and expanding functional reserve.

In summary, no model of functional status has been proposed to guide clinical practice or research specifically in oncology, although a model for conceptualizing and measuring physical functioning in cancer survivorship studies has recently been proposed.[17] Attention to the development of conceptual models of functioning in patients with cancer would promote clarity and precision in terminology. Furthermore, it would stimulate an expanded and more sophisticated approach to the measurement of functional status as an outcome and would improve the translation into practice of research findings concerning functioning during and following the diagnosis of cancer.

Risk Factors for Functional Losses During and Following Cancer and Its Treatment

Cancer and its treatment pose several risks for functional loss across the treatment trajectory, and various sociodemographic and treatment-related factors influence an individual patient's risk profile. The relative contributions of the treatments

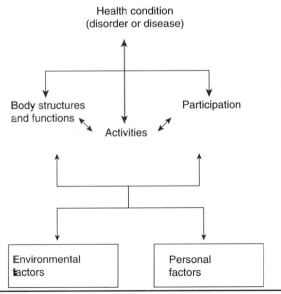

FIG. 32-3   World Health Organization International Classification of Functioning, Disability and Health (ICF). Model of Functioning and Disability. All rights reserved by the World Health Organization.

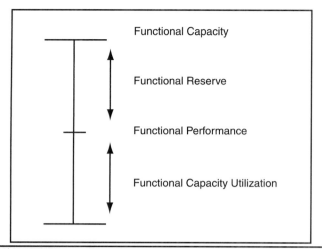

Functional Capacity

Functional Reserve

Functional Performance

Functional Capacity Utilization

FIG. 32-4 Visual representation of Leidy's analytic framework of functional status. (From Leidy NK: Functional status and the forward progress of merry-go-rounds: toward a coherent analytical framework, *Nurs Res* 43: 196-202, 1994.)

themselves (radiation, chemotherapy, biotherapy, molecularly targeted therapies, and hematopoietic stem cell transplantation) is unknown, as are the side effects of disease and treatment including fatigue, peripheral neuropathy, asthenia, and protein-calorie malnutrition, together with inactivity (and the factors that contribute to inactivity such as pain, dyspnea, fatigue, depression). Functional status is also contingent upon motivation, cognition, and sensory capacity, including vision and hearing. Alterations in any of these components as a result of the cancer diagnosis and its treatment can result in functional losses. Additional complications can accrue from functional loss including falls, incontinence, malnutrition, decreased socialization, depression, loss of independence, and increased risk for long-term institutionalization, and each of these can worsen functional status. Some of the factors contributing to functional status losses during and following cancer and its treatment are listed in Box 32-1. Thomas and Dodd have proposed a model of morbidity in patients with cancer that nurses can use to profile patients at greatest risk for functional status decline and to design targeted intervention programs.[18]

Efforts to systematically characterize the impact of cancer and its treatment on functional status have been severely limited by the absence of a clear consistent definition of functioning, a limited conceptual understanding of functional status, and confusion in the way measures of "functioning" have been applied and interpreted. Terms such as functional status, physical functioning, functional limitations, and QOL are sometimes used interchangeably. Measures such as the SF-36 are construed in some studies as a measure of QOL, whereas in another study as a measure of function. Further, most of the studies evaluating functional status in patients with cancer have relied heavily on self-report measures, with limited application of performance-based measures of function.

IMPACT OF DISEASE AND TREATMENT ON FUNCTIONAL STATUS

Studies have explored the impact of cancer and its treatment on functional status in women with breast cancer, in older adults newly diagnosed with breast, colon, lung and prostate cancer,

following hematopoietic stem cell transplantation, in survivors of breast cancer, in survivors of other solid and hematologic malignancies, and in patients at the end of life. Symptom distress from single symptoms such as pain or dyspnea and the distress experienced as a result of symptom clusters has also been shown to affect functional status.

Kroenke and colleagues observed that in women with breast cancer, young women (those less than 40 years old) experienced the greatest relative decline in physical role function compared with women ages 41 to 64 years and those greater than 65 years of age.[19] It was also found that young women experience greater absolute functional losses in physical role function, bodily pain, social function, and mental health, compared with middle-aged or elderly women with breast cancer.[19] These larger declines in young women were not due to more severe disease or more aggressive treatment.[19] Michael and colleagues report that social isolation before the diagnosis of breast cancer was associated with a greater risk of decline in role function and social function following the diagnosis of breast cancer.[20] A substantial portion of newly diagnosed breast cancer patients experience cognitive dysfunction, and during adjuvant chemotherapy, more than 50% of women experience cognitive dysfunction that persists for at least a year after treatment.[21,22] Breast cancer survivors are troubled by upper extremity functional limitations from swelling, numbness, and pain.[23] At the end of life, patients experience significant compromise in functional well-being, including distressing symptoms, a lack of independence, and an inability to participate in usual activities.[24] Ethnicity was associated with impaired physical functioning in cancer survivors, with Hispanic

---

BOX 32-1   Factors Contributing to Functional Decline in Patients with Cancer

- Inactivity
- Bed rest
- Deconditioning
- Physical restraints
- Muscle weakness
- Decreased muscle mass
- Protein-calorie malnutrition
- Anorexia and/or cachexia
- Constipation/diarrhea
- Incontinence
- Fatigue
- Pain
- Dyspnea
- Depression
- Peripheral neuropathy
- Lymphedema
- Diminished range of motion and contractures
- Cognitive dysfunction
- Hemiparesis
- Changes in visual acuity and visual field losses
- Hearing loss secondary to chemotherapy-induced ototoxicity
- Polypharmacy
- Medication side effects and drug-drug interactions

and African American individuals experiencing more problems with physical function.[25,26] Hewitt, Rowland, and Yancik found that cancer survivors are more likely to report functional limitations and difficulties with activities of daily living than age-matched individuals without cancer, and cancer survivors with comorbidities experience even greater functional compromise.[27,28] Compared to women with a history of breast cancer, individuals with a history of lung or respiratory cancer and leukemia or lymphoma reported poorer health status.[27]

PATTERNS OF FUNCTIONAL STATUS CHANGE ACROSS THE CANCER TRAJECTORY

Most studies of functional status in patients with cancer have been cross-sectional in design and offer limited information about patterns of functional decline or recovery across the cancer experience. In one of the few studies that has examined functional loss across a treatment trajectory, it was noted that in sedentary women undergoing radiation for breast cancer, both younger and older participants lost an average of 4% of their initial maximal aerobic capacity across the 7 weeks of radiation treatment.[29] Given and colleagues and Kurtz and colleagues have extensively studied the patterns of physical function in older adult patients undergoing treatment for breast, colon, lung, or prostate cancer.[30-33] In their samples of older adults with cancer, Given and colleagues found that those patients who had surgery followed by adjuvant chemotherapy or radiotherapy had more difficulties with physical function than those who were treated with surgery alone.[31] Watters and others report that although physical and role function was impaired during treatment in women receiving adjuvant therapy for breast cancer, these dimensions had recovered to baseline by 6 months after therapy.[34] In their longitudinal study of patients newly diagnosed with breast, lung, colorectal, or prostate cancer, Given and others found that although all patients had compromised functioning at 6 to 8 weeks after diagnosis, they showed improvements in their functional status when followed across the year after receiving their diagnosis.[30] In a sample of older adult patients with breast, colorectal, lung, or prostate cancer, Hodgson and Given observed that individuals who demonstrated functional recovery had less symptom severity and higher psychologic well-being at baseline compared with those who did not have functional recovery.[35]

FUNCTIONAL STATUS FOLLOWING HEMATOPOIETIC STEM CELL TRANSPLANTATION (HSCT)

Prior research exploring the functional status of patients after HSCT suggests considerable variability. Some patients experience few post-HSCT complications and report a gradual achievement of a functional status comparable, in one or more dimensions, to age-matched healthy individuals and a resumption of school and/or work. However, other patients report a variety of residual difficulties in physical function, cognitive function, and role and occupational functioning.[36-44]

Few studies have explored functional status following HSCT from a longitudinal perspective. Andrykowksy, Henslee, and Farrall found in their small sample of 16 participants that there was little change in functional status across time beyond a mean of 28 months after transplant, suggesting that a ceiling effect in terms of further improvements in functional status may be

achieved approximately 2 years after HSCT.[43] Similarly, Syrjala and colleagues noted that most improvements in physical functioning occurred between 90 days and 2 years after transplant, with recovery complete for about 75% of patients by 2 years, although an additional 10% to 20% of patients made some improvement in functioning between 2 and 4 years after transplant.[45] In contrast, particularly in patients older than 25 years at the time of HSCT, recovery may be nonlinear, with functional status continuing to improve significantly with time, suggesting that recovery may be somewhat delayed in older patients.[46]

Factors associated with reduced physical functioning and incomplete resumption of social function include chronic graft-versus-host disease (GVHD), second malignancy, and neurologic or psychologic problems.[46-48] Although some studies suggest that older age at transplantation may have negative effects on long-term physical functioning, other studies have failed to find a relationship between older age at transplant and impairments in QOL during survivorship following the procedure.[43,47]

Specifically in relationship to sexual function, studies have reported that HSCT survivors experience difficulties with sexual interest activity, pleasure, and ability.[37,49-51] Impotence and/or erectile difficulties are experienced by 25% to 40% of male transplant recipients, and at least 20% of transplant survivors experience alterations in body image.[51-53] Survivors of HSCT also experienced higher psychosexual dysfunction compared with healthy subjects.[52] Factors that have been found to be predictors of difficulties with sexual function following HSCT included younger age, lower serum levels of gonadal hormones, female gender, dissatisfaction with appearance, dissatisfaction with the quality of the relationships with spouse or partner, and the occurrence of chronic GVHD.

SYMPTOM DISTRESS AND FUNCTIONAL STATUS

Although distressing symptoms are prevalent among patients with cancer, symptoms are not consistently linked with compromised functioning across all disease sites and at all time points in the cancer trajectory. Pain, peripheral neuropathy, hot flashes, urinary dysfunction, dyspnea, anorexia-cachexia have been associated with poorer function. Following allogeneic stem cell transplantation, both extensive chronic GVHD and severe fatigue have been shown to negatively affect functional status. In a group of patients with mixed tumor types receiving chemotherapy, the symptom cluster of pain, fatigue, depression, and sleep insufficiency adversely affected functional status.[54] In a cohort of lung cancer patients, the symptom cluster of fatigue, nausea, weakness, appetite loss, weight loss, altered taste, and vomiting was negatively correlated with functional status, and greater symptom severity was associated with more limitations in physical and role function.[55] Particularly among older cancer patients and those with breast or lung cancer, symptom intensity, multiple concurrent symptoms, and higher levels of comorbidity correlate with poorer physical functioning.[30,33,35,56] Following surgery for breast, colorectal, lung, or prostate cancer, in patients with newly diagnosed lung cancer, and in women undergoing radiotherapy for breast cancer, higher levels of symptom severity were associated with diminished functional recovery.[35,57,58] Functional limitations are also associated with greater symptom distress, as well as more overall distress for patients and increased distress and disruption to daily schedules for their family caregivers.[32,33,59,60-63]

In randomized clinical trials, cognitive and behavioral nursing interventions to manage cancer-related symptoms have been shown to be effective in limiting the deleterious effects of symptom distress on functional status.[64]

Assessing Functional Status

Functional status evaluation in the patient with cancer is important for many reasons. In the clinical setting, baseline and longitudinal evaluation of functional status in the patient with cancer offers information with which to benchmark patient's response to treatment, to plan service delivery to meet patient needs across care settings, and to evaluate the quality of care. Functional status is a key clinical indicator, and declining functional status is associated with mortality, extended lengths of hospital stay, the need for institutionalization, and higher health care costs. A focus on functional status also serves to reduce fragmentation and discontinuity. Precise functional assessment conducted at regular intervals serves to detect early deterioration and allow for immediate intervention.

The clinical assessment of function should include two dimensions: **functional ability**, which is defined as the capability to perform the daily activities and tasks normally expected of individuals to care for themselves and fulfill fundamental needs, and **functional performance,** which is defined as an individual's actual performance of activities and tasks associated with life roles.[65] Three levels of functional ability have been described and are shown in Table 32-1: basic activities of daily living (ADLs), instrumental activities of daily living (IADLs), and mobility.[66] In functional assessment instruments that focus on activities of daily living, this classification of ADL, IADL, and mobility has become standard. Individuals may be totally independent, partially independent, or dependent in their ability to perform these activities.

As shown in Table 32-2, a wide variety of approaches to functional evaluation have been described.[67-69] These may be questionnaires, or they may be performance measures in which direct observation is made of what the patient is capable of doing. In addition to providing prognostic and outcomes information, both performance-based measures and self-report can be used to target interventions toward improving overall functional capacity and performance. Examples of two functional status measures, the Katz Index of Activities of Daily Living and the Functional Performance Inventory are given in Boxes 32-2 and 32-3.[15,70]

The Katz Index of Activities of Daily Living is useful in evaluating independent functioning for each activity, or the degree and type of assistance needed for each activity. The Functional Performance Inventory is an example of a multidimensional measure of functional status across a variety of domains. The Functional Performance Inventory evaluates functional status from a broader perspective than that of ADLs. Both measures may be useful clinically in describing baseline functioning, setting goals, and monitoring abilities, and can be used in research as outcomes measures to evaluate the effectiveness of interventions.

FUNCTIONAL STATUS MEASUREMENT IN PATIENTS WITH CANCER

The measures most frequently employed in studies of functional status in patients with cancer are SF-36, the Karnofsky Performance Scale (KPS), and Eastern Cooperative Oncology Group (ECOG) Performance Status.[71] Performance status scales such as KPS and ECOG have utility for specific purposes; however, these instruments offer a limited evaluation of functional status, may be insensitive to subtle changes over time, and may suffer from variable interrater reliability. While the SF-36 has the advantage of allowing comparison with population norms, both the SF-36 and the KPS may be insensitive to changes in functional status, particularly in patients at the lowest and highest levels of function. The confounding of indicators of symptom status and physical function within the SF-36 also makes this instrument problematic for evaluating the impact of symptoms on functional status.

Several measures of functional status are designed to evaluate both cancer symptoms and the degree to which in the past 24 hours those symptoms interfered with seven daily activities including normal work, walking, sleep, mood, relations with other people, enjoyment of life, and general ADLs. This approach is potentially promising, since the examination of symptoms and their functional impact can be partitioned. However, the psychometric properties of this measurement model for evaluating the impact of symptoms on functional status has not been systematically assessed, and little is known about the reliability, validity, and sensitivity to change over time of these measures. Like other measures of functional status that operationalize function in terms of ADLs and IADLs, there may also be ceiling effects that limit sensitivity.

TABLE 32-1 Three Levels of Functional Ability		
ACTIVITIES OF DAILY LIVING (ADLs)	**INSTRUMENTAL ACTIVITIES OF DAILY LIVING (IADLs)**	**MOBILITY**
Bathing	Using the telephone	Walking (balance, gait distance, capacity)
Dressing	Driving	Leaving one's residence
Toileting	Shopping	Moving from one location to another using
Continence	Housekeeping	public transit
Feeding	Cooking	
Transferring	Laundry	
	Managing finances	
	Administering medications	

TABLE 32-2   Measures of Functional Status

MESURE	CONCEPTUAL AND MEASUREMENT MODEL	RELIABILITY, VALIDITY, AND RESPONSIVENESS	BURDEN	CULTURAL AND LANGUAGE ADAPTATIONS	COMMENTS– STRENGTHS AND WEAKNESSES
ADL Measures: Barthel Index; Katz Index of Activities of Daily Living, Physical Self-Maintenance Scale (PSMS); Nagi Functional Difficulty Index, Functional Status Index (Jette), Enforced Social Dependency Scale (McCorkle)	Measure functional independence in domains of personal care, basic ADLs, and mobility	Good internal consistency, test-retest reliability, and concurrent validity	Self-administered in 5 minutes	Japanese	Significant ceiling effects and therefore low levels of disability may not be detected, reflecting its origins as a measure for severely ill individuals
Functional Independence Measure (FIM)	Eighteen items covering independence in self-care, sphincter control, mobility, locomotion, communication, and social cognition. Seven-point ordinal ratings represent gradations of independence and the amount of assistance a patient requires.	Good test-retest and internal consistency reliability. Satisfactory convergent validity with other measures of functional independence in ADLs	Clinician rating scale; takes 30 minutes to complete and score	Japanese, French, German, and Swedish	
Human Activity Profile (HAP)	HAP is a measure of physical activity and consists of a list of 94 activities ranked in ascending order of the level of energy required to perform each activity. The HAP therefore provides a survey of activities performed across a wide range of energy requirements. Subjects are asked to assign each activity	Satisfactory test-retest and internal consistency reliability. Good discriminant and concurrent validity demonstrated in populations including individuals with COPD, osteoarthritis, ESRD, and chronic pain. In COPD studies, there was good correlation with maximum oxygen uptake (VO_2 max),	Self-administered in 5–8 minutes	English, Chinese. German translation in development	Healthy population reference norms have been established. Limited use in patients with cancer, although an abstract reports the use of the HAP as part of rehabilitation assessments of survivors of childhood sarcoma. Inclusion in a larger study as an outcome measure for clinical trials should

Continued

TABLE 32-2   Measures of Functional Status—cont'd

MEASURE	CONCEPTUAL AND MEASUREMENT MODEL	RELIABILITY, VALIDITY, AND RESPONSIVENESS	BURDEN	CULTURAL AND LANGUAGE ADAPTATIONS	COMMENTS– STRENGTHS AND WEAKNESSES
	to one of three categories: "still doing this activity," "have stopped doing this activity," or "never did this activity." The maximum activity score is the number between 1 and 94 identifying the activity with the highest oxygen-consumption requirement that the subject still performs. The adjusted activity score is the difference between the maximum activity score and the number of activities that the subject has stopped performing, which gives a better estimate of the range of activities performed and the presence of impairment.	suggesting that the HAP is a valid measure of physical performance. Questionnaire has also been used to measure physical activity in healthy populations.			probably include a phase where the concurrent validity and reliability of the HAP is assessed in patients with GVHD (a great study would be one that attempts to validate the HAP in this patient population with accelerometry data and SF-36 data). One of the strengths of this tool is its sensitivity to change (evaluated in non–cancer patient populations), and the availability of reference norms.
Health Assessment Questionnaire (HAQ)	Measures difficulty in performing activities of daily living including dressing and grooming, rising, eating, walking, hygiene, reach, grip and outdoor activities. The questionnaire is based on a hierarchical model that considers the effect of a disease in terms of death, disability, discomfort, the side effects of treatment, and medical costs.	Good internal consistent and test-retest reliability. Satisfactory concurrent validity. Modest responsiveness to change demonstrated in the arthritis patient population in which it was developed.	Self administered in 5-8 minutes	Spanish, French, Dutch, and Swedish	Major criticism is that the HAQ, in counting only the highest score in each section, does not use all the information collected. In comparing scores over time, therefore, improvements in less severely affected areas of functioning may be missed. It is a good descriptive instrument, but may be less appropriate as a tool for measuring clinical change in outcomes studies. In addition, there is little psychometric information on its adequacy as a tool in non–arthritic patient populations.
SF-36, SF-12	The SF-36 (and its 1-page 2-minute survey form, the SF-12) is a multipurpose, generic health survey that yields an 8-scale profile of functional health	Reliability estimates extensively established, and usually exceed 0.9. Studies to date have yielded content, concurrent, criterion, construct,	Self-administered in 5-10 minutes	Translated into more than 20 languages and used in more than 50 countries.	Used successfully in more than 600 randomized controlled trials. Proven responsive in more than 40 disease conditions Accepted by the FDA as

Instrument	Description	Reliability/Validity	Time	Languages	Comments
	and well-being, as well as psychometrically based physical and mental health summary measures and a preference-based health utility index. The subscales are physical functioning, role functioning, bodily pain, general health, vitality, social functioning, role-emotional functioning, and mental health. With version 2, a sixfold increase in the range of scores covered was achieved, and floor and ceiling effects were minimized.	and predictive evidence of validity. The content areas not included in the SF-36 are sleep adequacy, cognitive functioning, sexual functioning, health distress, family functioning, self-esteem, eating, recreation and hobbies, communication, and symptoms and problems specific to one condition (SF-36 is intended as a generic measure).			proof of benefit for improved functioning and other patient-reported outcomes. Adopted as the standard of measurement by key government agencies, including the AHRQ and MEPS. Norm-based Scoring algorithms are available. The principal strength of the SF-36 is the availability of considerable information about norms and benchmarks in both "well" and "sick" populations. The authors themselves point out, however, the strengths of using the SF-36 as a generic core, and combining it with other, more precise, general, and condition-specific measures.
Cancer Rehabilitation Evaluation System (CARES)	Cancer-specific QOL instrument. Patients rate cancer-related problems encountered on a daily basis. There are 139 items (88 for all patients, and 51 for patients in specific situations). Items are scored using a 5-point Likert scale. These yield 5 summary scales and 31 subscales for detailed scoring. Categories for broader scoring include physical, psychosocial, marital, medical interaction, and sexual function.	Reliability and validity established in patients with breast cancer and those with lung cancer, patients undergoing HSCT, and cancer survivors.	Average of 20 minutes to complete	Language translations not available	Strength is inclusion of items addressing family functioning, sexual functioning, marital interaction, and interaction with medical care team. Focus on Rehabilitation needs would complement other measures, although CARES-SF has not demonstrated itself to be a sensitive outcomes measure.
Functional Assessment of Cancer Therapy (FACT)	General QOL instrument intended for use with cancer patients. FACT-G is the core instrument, with multiple disease-, treatment-, and condition-specific subscales to complement the FACT-G including one for BMT. Items are measured on a 5-point Likert scale, and yield four domains: physical, social and	Well-established test-retest, internal consistency reliability, and good discriminant validity and responsiveness demonstrated against measures such as the Functional Living Index- Cancer (FLIC), ECOG Performance Status, and POMs.	Average of 5 minutes to complete	Available in more than 15 languages	In lung cancer the FACT-G physical and functional well-being indices have been combined with lung cancer subscales to create a Trial Outcome Index (TOI). This is reported to be an efficient and precise index of physical and functional outcomes of different treatment strategies in lung cancer.

TABLE 32-2 Measures of Functional Status—cont'd

MEASURE	CONCEPTUAL AND MEASUREMENT MODEL	RELIABILITY, VALIDITY, AND RESPONSIVENESS	BURDEN	CULTURAL AND LANGUAGE ADAPTATIONS	COMMENTS- STRENGTHS AND WEAKNESSES
	family, emotional, and functional well-being. Subscale scores are added to obtain a total score.				
EORTC-QLQ-C-30	Core measure of QOL and functional well-being, with cancer-, disease-, and condition-specific modules that can be added. A module of high-dose chemotherapy has been developed and is in final testing phases. The QLQ-C30 consists of 30 items comprising 5 functional scales (physical, role, cognitive, emotional, and social), 3 symptom scales (fatigue, pain, and nausea and vomiting) a global health status and QOL scale, 5 single items, which assess additional symptoms commonly reported by cancer patients (dyspnea, appetite loss, sleep disturbance, constipation, and diarrhea) and financial difficulties resulting from the disease.	Satisfactory reliability extensively demonstrated in cancer population. Convergent, discriminant, and concurrent validity established in many different cancer populations. Limited use in long-term follow-up studies of cancer patients versus those on active treatment. Good responsiveness to change demonstrated.	5-10 minutes	Available in more than 40 languages	No authorized physical or psychosocial summary scores. Norms in large samples of cancer patients available.
Functional Living Index-Cancer (FLIC)	Cancer-specific, functionally oriented QOL instrument. Linear analogue scales are used to produce 5 domains, specifically physical well-being and ability, emotional state, sociability, family situation, and nausea.	Internal consistency reliability is reported to be at least 0.7. Limited exploration of concurrent validity and discriminant validity; some evidence of convergent validity with independent measures of symptoms and anxiety in patients with lung cancer.	Self-Administered in less than 10 minutes	Available in at least 15 languages	More recently, there has been limited use of the FLIC as a HRQOL measure in cancer care, as it has been eclipsed by the FACT and EORTC-QLQ.
Functional Performance Inventory	Self-report measure of functional performance developed from an analytical framework of functional status, and from qualitative studies of COPD patients. Performance is defined as the day-to-day activities patients	Test-retest and internal consistency reliability has been evaluated. Face validity has been established through qualitative studies. Concurrent and discriminant validity demonstrated in patients	Time to complete is not formally reported, but would be estimated to be approximately 5-8 minutes.	English	No reported use to date in patients with cancer. It has been used as an outcomes measure in clinical trials of treatments for COPD.

Instrument	Description	Time to Complete	Language	Reliability/Validity	Comments
	do to meet basic needs, fulfil usual roles, and maintain their health and well-being. Items are scaled on a 4-point scale (from "activity can be performed easily" to "activity is no longer performed for health reasons"). There is a category for nonapplicable. Domains include body care (9 items), household maintenance (21 items), physical exercise (7 items), recreation (11 items), spiritual activities (5 items), and social activities (12 items).			with different levels of perceived illness severity and activity limitation, and in relationship to FEV1 on PFTs in patients with COPD.	
Sickness Impact Profile (SIP)	Generic measure used to evaluate the impact of disease on both physical and emotional functioning. Patients are asked to respond to the items as they are on that day. 136 items yield two overall domains (physical and psychosocial), and 12 categories (sleep and rest, eating, work, home management, recreation and pastimes, ambulation, mobility, body care and movement, social interaction, alertness behavior, emotional behavior, and communication).	Approximately 20 minutes to complete	English	Good test-retest and internal consistency reliability reported. Some evidence of concurrent, convergent, and divergent validity, and sensitivity as an outcomes measure in clinical trials of asthma, and in COPD and cancer	Although the SIP is a widely used general health status measure, there are problems with scoring of SIP*, that lead to inconsistent and illogical scores. Strategies have been developed to address these issues and to modify the tool to limit response burden, but there has been limited subsequent use of the tool to evaluate the revised instrument and scoring system, in terms of reliability and validity.
Edmonton Functional Assessment Tool (EFAT)	Designed as a measure of functional status through a declining course in palliative care, the tool evaluates functional status along several dimensions including communication, mental alertness, pain, sensation, respiratory function, balance, mobility, activity level, wheelchair mobility, and ADLs. The instrument also includes a single	Completed in approximately 10 minutes	English	Satisfactory interrater reliability and concurrent validity. Discriminant validity in distinguishing functional status of patients in inpatient hospice and those in home hospice	The measure confounds symptom evaluation (e.g, pain, respiratory symptoms) and functional status, and confounds the impact of symptoms such as pain on functioning. Significant ceiling effects, since measure is designed to differentiate patients even at the lowest levels of functioning.

Continued

TABLE 32-2	Measures of Functional Status—cont'd			
MEASURE	CONCEPTUAL AND MEASUREMENT MODEL	RELIABILITY, VALIDITY, AND RESPONSIVENESS	BURDEN	CULTURAL AND LANGUAGE ADAPTATIONS	COMMENTS– STRENGTHS AND WEAKNESSES
Enforced Social Dependency Scale	item to summarize performance status. Some established reliability and validity, mostly in cancer and other progressive diseases				Primarily a measure of functional dependence rather than functional status. Most items focus on basic ADLs

*See, for example, Pollard B, Johnston M: Problems with the sickness impact profile: a theoretically based analysis and a proposal for a new method of implementation and scoring, *Soc Sci Med* 52(6):921-934, 2001.
ADLs, Activities of daily living; *AHRQ*, Agency for Healthcare Research and Quality; *BMT*, bone marrow transplant; *COPD*, chronic obstructive pulmonary disease; *cGVHD*, chronic graft-versus-host disease; *ECOG*, Eastern Cooperative Oncology Group; *ESRD*, end-stage renal disease; *FDA*, U.S. Food and Drug Administration; *FEV1*, forced expiratory volume in 1 second; *HRQOL*, health-related quality of life; *HSCT*, human stem cell transplantation; *MEPS*, Medical Expenditure Panel Survey; *PFTs*, pulmonary function tests; *POMs*, profile of mood states; *QOL*, quality of life; *VO₂*, oxygen uptake.

| BOX 32-2 | **Functional Status Measures: Katz Index of Activities of Daily Living (ADLs)** |

1. Bathing (Sponge, Shower, or Tub)

Independent: Receives no assistance (gets in and out of tub if tub is usual means of bathing)

Assistance: Receives assistance in bathing only one part of the body (such as the back or a leg)

Dependent: Receives assistance in bathing more than one part of the body (or not bathed)

2. Dressing

Independent: Gets clothes and gets completely dressed without assistance

Assistance: Gets clothes and gets dressed without assistance except in tying shoes

Dependent: Receives assistance in getting clothes or in getting dressed or stays partly or completely undressed

3. Toileting

Independent: Transfers to the toilet in a bathroom for the elimination process, cleans self, and arranges clothes without assistance (may use object for support such as cane, walker, or wheelchair), and may manage night bedpan or commode, emptying it in the morning

Assistance: Receives assistance in going to the toilet, in cleansing self, in arranging clothes after elimination, or in use of night bedpan or commode

Dependent: Doesn't transfer to the toilet in a bathroom for the elimination process

4. Transfer

Independent: Moves in and out of bed as well as in and out of chair without assistance

Assistance: Moves in and out of bed or chair with assistance

Dependent: Doesn't get out of bed

5. Continence

Independent: Controls urination and bowel movement completely by self

Assistance: Has occasional "accidents"

Dependent: Supervision helps keep urine and bowel control; catheter is used, or is incontinent

6. Feeding

Independent: Feeds self without assistance

Assistance: Feeds self except for getting assistance in cutting meat or buttering bread

Dependent: Receives assistance in feeding or is fed partly or completely by using tubes or intravenous fluids

From Kats S, Ford AB, Moskowitz RW: Studies of illness in the aged: the index of ADL: a standardized measure of biological and psychological function, *JAMA* 185:914-915, 1963.

Although most studies used a questionnaire approach to evaluate functional status, the other method of evaluating functional status entails observing what the patient is capable of doing, often referred to as performance measures. These performance measures either classify the patient based on a gestalt impression using scales, such as KPS or ECOG Performance Status, or characterize the patient's function based on his or her performance on one or more standardized tests or tasks. The Edmonton Functional Assessment Tool and the Thorne-KPS represent efforts to develop a performance scale analogous to the KPS for use in a palliative care population.[72,73] However, like KPS, these instruments offer only a limited evaluation of functional status, may be insensitive to subtle change over time, and may suffer from poor reproducibility when the patient is rated by different clinicians. Few studies have used an objective test battery to evaluate functional performance in patients with cancer, although there is evidence to support the reliability, validity, and feasibility of these tests of functional performance.[74] Typically, these tests of physical functional performance include the time taken to complete various tasks (e.g., picking up coins, tying a belt, reaching up, putting on a sock, standing from sitting, a 50-foot fast walk, a 50-foot walk at preferred speed), the distance walked in 6 minutes (6-minute walk test), and the distance reached forward while standing (standing forward reach). The use of performance-based tests also offers the possibility of quantifying the time and effort burden imposed on patients living with cancer by the daily tasks involved in self-care or mobility. Simmonds noted that the patient group took approximately twice as long as the control group of healthy individuals to complete most tasks and were only able to walk half the distance of the healthy group on the 6-minute walk.[74] The moderate statistical relationships between self-report of function and performance tests in this sample of cancer patients suggest that these methods of measuring function are complementary, and that both have applicability for assessment and for outcomes evaluation in clinical practice and research.[74] Box 32-4 has standardized instructions for performing the walk test.

CONSIDERATIONS IN SELECTING A FUNCTIONAL STATUS MEASURE FOR THE ONCOLOGY PATIENT

The selection of a measure of functional status should be guided by the purpose for measuring functional status and the functional status domains of greatest relevance, and tailored to the needs of the population that will be evaluated. Purposes of evaluating functional status could include (a) screening, (b) assessment, or (c) monitoring.[75] When screening for functional compromise, the measure chosen should be specific (i.e., capable of differentiating individuals with functional compromise from those without), brief, inexpensive, and appropriate for administration by paraprofessional staff. An example of a measure developed for screening for functional dependence in the oncology population has recently been described.[76] The 12 items of the Short Functional Dependence Measure evaluate the extent of dependence in basic and instrumental activities of daily living. An instrument for assessment must be able to detect incremental changes in functional status; it should also have response choices that are not too large or too inclusive, since such measures will be insensitive to small but clinically important changes in functioning. In addition, an instrument for assessment should demonstrate limited floor or ceiling effects in a heterogeneous population. Monitoring of functional status involves rescreening or retesting specific problem areas at specified intervals following an intervention, based on the anticipated trajectory of improvement expected from that intervention.

BOX 32-3   Functional Status Measure: Functional Performance Inventory Short Form

Functional Performance Inventory—Short Form

This questionnaire asks about how your health usually affects your day-to-day activities. Please circle the number that best describes how difficult it is for you, in general, to do the following activities. Circling 1 means you do the activity easily, with no difficulty at all; 2 means you do it with some difficulty; 3 means you have much difficulty; and 4 means you no longer do this activity because of your health. If you have never done, or choose not to do, an activity for reasons other than your health, please circle N/A (not applicable)

Activity	DO with...			DON'T DO because...	
	No Difficulty	Some Difficulty	Much Difficulty	Health Reasons	Choose Not To
Body Care					
Dressing and undressing	1	2	3	4	N/A
Showering or bathing	1	2	3	4	N/A
Caring for your feet	1	2	3	4	N/A
Washing your hair	1	2	3	4	N/A
Shaving or applying makeup	1	2	3	4	N/A
Maintaining the Household					
Groceries and Meals					
Preparing meals/cooking	1	2	3	4	N/A
Grocery shopping	1	2	3	4	N/A
Carrying groceries	1	2	3	4	N/A
Activities Around the House or Apartment					
Vacuuming or sweeping	1	2	3	4	N/A
Moving furniture, changing sheets, or washing windows	1	2	3	4	N/A
Cleaning bathrooms or washing floors	1	2	3	4	N/A
Mowing the lawn, shoveling snow, raking, or heavy gardening	1	2	3	4	N/A
Going to appointments (such as doctors or dentists)	1	2	3	4	N/A
Physical Exercise					
Regular stretching, moving, or lifting light weights	1	2	3	4	N/A
Walking up and down a flight of stairs	1	2	3	4	N/A
Short walks around the neighborhood or mall	1	2	3	4	N/A
Long, fast walks (more than 20 minutes)	1	2	3	4	N/A
Activities such as swimming or bicycling	1	2	3	4	N/A
Recreation – Activities for Personal Pleasure					
Taking vacations	1	2	3	4	N/A
Activities Away from the House or Apartment					
Indoor activities such as shopping or museums	1	2	3	4	N/A
Going to the movies	1	2	3	4	N/A
Activities in and Around the House or Apartment					
Sitting outside	1	2	3	4	N/A
Reading	1	2	3	4	N/A

BOX 32-3 Functional Status Measure: Functional Performance Inventory Short Form—cont'd

Activity	DO with...			DON'T DO because...	
	No Difficulty	Some Difficulty	Much Difficulty	Health Reasons	Choose Not To
Spiritual Activities					
Attending religious services	1	2	3	4	N/A
Going to religious ceremonies	1	2	3	4	N/A
Personal reading, meditation, or prayer	1	2	3	4	N/A
Visits from spiritual friends or teachers	1	2	3	4	N/A
Social Interaction—Family and Friends					
Dinner, cards, bingo, or other activity in your home	1	2	3	4	N/A
Places other than your home	1	2	3	4	N/A
Helping Family or Friends					
Going to the store, giving rides, doing repairs or other favors	1	2	3	4	N/A
Helping in the care of children	1	2	3	4	N/A
Travel					
Distant or overnight travel to visit others	1	2	3	4	N/A

Individual functional status instruments may demonstrate floor or ceiling effects with specific patient populations, and this can contribute to insensitivity of the measure with that population. Floor effects occur when most patients are already at the lowest level of functioning encompassed by a measure. Such a measure will therefore be insensitive to continued worsening of functional status. When a measure demonstrates ceiling effects, it is because most patients are already at the highest level of functioning captured by a measure. A measure with ceiling effects will be unable to detect improvements in functional status. For example, many functional status instruments that focus on activities of daily living will show ceiling effects when used with a high-functioning ambulatory oncology population. Similarly, measures that may be more suitable for an ambulatory oncology population will show floor effects when used with a population at the end of life, since these patients will tend to score at the lowest end of the instrument's range.

Some of the considerations in selecting an instrument to measure functional status in patients with cancer are listed in Table 32-3. Among the most important criteria in selecting a functional status instrument for screening, assessment, or monitoring is the relevance and usefulness of the measure's individual items to the aspect of functional status of greatest interest (e.g., independence in activities of daily living, physical activity, ability to function in valued roles, extent to which symptoms interfere with function). Sometimes the purpose of functional evaluation is to detect impairment in specific organ systems that are important to the maintenance of functional status or that limit capacity. In this case, specific measures of impairment such as walk distance, grip strength, or range of motion may be better than a self-report measure.

Other important factors to consider in evaluating functional performance include literacy level, language spoken, cultural background, and economic resources. Literacy level and the language spoken are important if the assessment requires completion of a questionnaire. Beyond language, cultural expectations and norms may also influence functional performance. Further, economic resources can affect the kinds of functional support resources available to the client including home care supports and coverage for durable medical equipment and rehabilitation services.

COMPREHENSIVE GERIATRIC ASSESSMENT (CGA)

Efforts have been made to test the applicability of a multidimensional approach, termed comprehensive geriatric assessment (CGA), to the functional assessment of the older adult cancer patient.[77,78] CGA is defined as multidisciplinary evaluation in which the multiple problems of older persons are assessed, the service needs, resources, and strengths of the person are identified, and a coordinated comprehensive care plan is developed.[67,79] The elements of CGA include evaluation of functional dependence in ADLs and IADLs, symptom distress, comorbidity, cognition, mood disturbance, nutrition, polypharmacy, living conditions, and social support, as well as an evaluation for the presence of geriatric syndromes such as incontinence, diminished sensory acuity, and risk for falls. This approach has been successfully applied in geriatrics since the early 1970s, and efforts are underway to validate a CGA-based scale for use in older adults with cancer.[80] CGA has been shown to add substantial information on the functional assessment of older cancer patients, including patients with a good performance status.[81] The CGA model

---

BOX 32-4   **Performance-Based Measure of Physical Function: Walk Time**

What's Needed:

- Mechanical lap counter
- Stop watch
- Marker rings for anchoring turn-around points of lap course
- Marker for anchoring partial lap
- 50-foot length of cotton cord to measure lap

Procedure:

1. Establish a lap course of 50 feet; a clinic or office hallway is often a good choice. The lap course should be straight, without obstacles or traffic, and well lit. Use the 50-foot cotton cord included in the tool kit to measure a 50-foot lap. Mark the start and finish points of the lap (turn-around points) with the marker rings.
2. The patient should be wearing appropriate shoes for walking. Assess the patient briefly to confirm that he or she is feeling well, and is without dizziness, lightheadedness, chest pain, or shortness of breath. Bring the patient over to the hallway course you have established.
3. Set the lap counter and stop watch to 0.
4. Explain the test to the patient. "The object of this test is to walk as far as possible for 2 (or 6 or 12) minutes. You will walk back and forth in this hallway. You are permitted to slow down, to stop, and to rest as necessary. You will be walking back and forth between the marker rings. You should pivot briskly around the marker rings and continue back the other way without hesitation. Now I am going to show you. Please watch the way I turn without hesitation."
5. Demonstrate by walking one lap yourself. Pivot briskly at the marker ring.
6. Continue with instructions: "Are you ready to do that? I am going to use this counter to keep track of the number of laps you complete. I will click it each time you turn around at the ring marker. Remember that the object is to walk AS FAR AS POSSIBLE for 2 minutes, but don't run or jog. Are you ready to start?"
7. As soon as the patient starts to walk, start the timer.
8. Do not talk to anyone during the walk. Watch the patient and do not allow yourself to be distracted and lose count of the laps. Each time the participant returns to the starting line, click the lap counter once.
9. When the stopwatch shows that 1 minute has elapsed, tell the patient, "You are doing well; you have 1 minute to go."
10. When the stopwatch shows that there is 15 seconds remaining, say, "In a moment, I am going to tell you to stop. When I do, just stop right where you are, and I will come to you."
11. When the full 2 minutes have elapsed, say, "Stop"; walk over to the patient, and mark the spot where he or she stopped by placing the ring marker on the floor.
12. Measure the distance in feet covered in the final partial lap. Record this distance and the number of laps, and calculate the total distance traveled in 2 minutes.

Total distance walked in 2 minutes: Number of laps _____ (× 50 feet) + final partial lap: _____ feet = _____ feet walked in 2 minutes

---

strikes a balance between patient self-report of functioning, clinician assessment, and performance test measures. For the older adult, CGA may offer an especially valuable methodology for the evaluation of functional status, particularly during times of transition between care settings (for example, hospital to home), when specialty care is fragmented, and in those who have recently developed impairments in functional status.

Nursing Interventions to Promote Functional Recovery or Limit Functional Decline

Functional status evaluation is the basis upon which to direct interventions that promote rehabilitation, optimize role fulfillment, and limit functional decline. The attitudes, personality, previous lifestyle, and coping patterns of individuals have a significant effect on their reactions to functional loss and to rehabilitative efforts. An individual who has felt that life has consistently disappointed his expectations or someone who uses her situation for secondary gains such as attention getting will respond to interventions to promote functioning differently than someone who is optimistic, who has approached problems as challenges to be

overcome, or who has valued personal independence. Similarly, the reaction of the family, caregivers, and the social system can influence responses. Families and caregivers who insist on doing everything for the individual can diminish self-esteem, whereas treating the person as a responsible individual and encouraging self-care and independence can help promote a sense of worth and normality.

To promote functional recovery or limit functional decline, interventions are designed to help individuals improve their functional capacity and functional performance toward maximal independence, well-being, and satisfaction. General rehabilitative principles are given in Box 32-5. Social workers, physical therapists, occupational therapists, speech and language therapists, and vocational counselors may all be good sources of information about local community resources for rehabilitative needs.

COMPREHENSIVE MULTIDISCIPLINARY REHABILITATION PROGRAMS

Relatively few oncology-specific comprehensive multidisciplinary rehabilitation programs are described in the literature; however, those that have been described and evaluated report that

TABLE 32-3   Considerations in Selecting an Instrument to Measure Functional Status

CONSIDERATION	COMMENT
Relevance and usefulness of the individual items to the functional domains of interest	Functional status data must be useful for their intended purpose. Knowledge of activities of daily living may be of limited interest in a high-functioning ambulatory population, or in patients at the end of life for whom effective symptom control and an opportunity to contribute to valued roles and activities may be more relevant.
Established reliability, validity, and sensitivity to change in patient population	In general, functional status instruments have had limited psychometric evaluation in the oncology population. This is an important priority for future research so that an instrument with known reliability and validity can be selected.
Ceiling or floor effects expected to be limited in patient population	Functional status instruments can suffer from ceiling or floor effects in specific populations, rendering the measure insensitive to changes in functional status over time.
Patient acceptability and/or burden	Functional status measures should be pilot-tested with the population before final selection to determine that the measure(s) are seen as relevant by the population, and that the burden associated with completing the measures is acceptable.
Reading levels and/or translations available	Some functional status instruments are available in other languages or have been developed to accommodate low-literacy individuals.
Resources required for administration, scoring, and interpretation	Some measures require professional staff for administration, or complex computer-based scoring algorithms and training to interpret the scores may be required.
Whether initial or follow-up evaluations will be conducted remotely (e.g., by Internet, telephone) or in a clinical setting	Performance-based measures of function are not amenable to administration via telephone or Internet. This may be a limitation, particularly if follow-up and/or monitoring will be done remote to the clinical setting.

BOX 32-5   General Principles of Rehabilitative Care

- Functional status is influenced by physiologic aging changes, acute and chronic illness, and adaptation to the physical environment.
- Evaluate for underlying causes of functional decline when a change in functional status is noted.
- In working with clients, emphasize function rather than dysfunction, and capabilities rather than disabilities.
- Rehabilitation is an individualized process, and it requires a multidisciplinary team for optimal results.
- Demonstrate hope, optimism, interest, determination, patience, and humor; these encourage patients in their rehabilitative efforts.
- Recognize and praise accomplishments.
- Include patient and family in multidisciplinary team conferences whenever possible.
- Institutional routines can promote a tendency for caregivers to do things for patients they could otherwise do for themselves if given time and flexibility. Although doing for clients allows the tasks to be completed efficiently, the therapeutic benefits to the individual client of independence should supersede staff's desires for efficiency or adherence to institutional routines.
- Do not equate functional loss with a loss of maturity, intelligence, or independence; continue to treat the individual as an adult with goals and preferences, and the capacity and desire to solve problems and make decisions.
- Educate clients and families on the value of independent functioning, and causes and consequences of functional decline.
- Identify prevent and treat complications of functional loss such as skin breakdown, muscle weakness, pulmonary compromise, social isolation, and depression.
- Manage pain and other symptoms.
- Balance activity with rest periods.
- Design environments to facilitate access with handrails, wide doorways, raised toilet seats, shower seats, enhanced lighting, and chairs of various types and height.

Data from Bottomley JM, Lewis CB: Principles and practice of geriatric rehabilitation. In Bottomley JM, Lewis CB, editors: *Geriatric rehabilitation: a clinical approach,* ed 2, Upper Saddle River, NJ, 2003, Prentice Hall; Eliopoulos C: *Gerontological nursing,* ed 6, Philadelphia, 2005, Lippincott, Williams & Wilkins.; and Kresevic DM, Mezey M: Assessment of function. In Mezey M, Fulner T, Abraham I et al, editors: *Geriatric nursing protocols for best practice,* ed 2, New York, 2003, Springer.

comprehensive rehabilitation can achieve substantial improvements in functional status. Several recent studies have shown that comprehensive rehabilitation programs are effective in improving (1) functional outcomes in women with breast cancer, (2) functional and peak exercise capacity in patients with lung cancer, (3) reduction in fatigue and improvements in physical functioning, role functioning due to physical problems, psychologic functioning, and physical symptoms distress in cancer survivors, and (4) improvements in functional status in patients with mixed diagnoses, some of whom were malnourished, had advanced cancers, or were elderly.[82-93] Examples of rehabilitative therapies that may be useful for patients during and following cancer treatment are listed in Box 32-6.

ASSISTIVE TECHNOLOGY

Assistive technology can benefit individuals with physical, sensory, or cognitive impairments. Examples of assistive technology include mobility aids (e.g., wheelchair, motorized scooter, walker, cane), grasping aids, back-saving solutions, devices for blindness and low vision, assistive listening devices, electronic aids for daily living, alternative and augmentative communication devices, and memory and/or organizational aids. Transfer aids such as a transfer board, a transfer bench, and a shower chair can assist with safe and efficient transfers. For patients who spend prolonged time sitting in a wheelchair, a proper seating system is often required to limit the development of secondary problems such as a pressure ulcer or musculoskeletal pain. In addition to devices, participation in valued activities and roles is also restored or sustained through modifications to transportation equipment, telecommunication equipment, computers, and home, work, school, and community environments.

Properly used, assistive technologies can optimize independent mobility, enhance functional performance, and limit the development of secondary problems that can result from functional dependence. However, this equipment should be individually selected and fitted for a patient's size, need and capacity. A physical, occupational, or speech and language therapist or an orthotist or prosthetist should be consulted for selection, fitting, and instructions for use of a cane, walker, wheelchair, orthotic device, or other assistive technology.

EXERCISE AND ACTIVITY

Increasing the level of activity and exercise is an essential component of a plan to optimize or preserve functional status. Inactivity and sedentarism by themselves cause rapid deterioration in physical function, and the theoretic rule of thumb for athletes is that 3 days of training for each day lost from training are required to recover prior function.[94] Bed rest and inactivity also cause muscle atrophy, particularly in thigh and calf muscles, which are critical for ambulation and maintenance of functional status.[95] The complications that result from inactivity can affect the neurosensory, cardiovascular, respiratory, gastrointestinal, and musculoskeletal systems.[66]

Exercise training also has the potential to reduce the risk factors for the development of cancer and other chronic diseases. It can improve psychologic health, preserve cognitive function, reduce symptoms including depression and fatigue, and strengthen a sense of well-being, personal control, and self-efficacy.[96,97] Participation in regular exercise has many other benefits including enhanced circulation, promotion of joint motion, improvements in muscle strength and endurance, maintenance or improvement of cardiopulmonary capacity, and prevention of contractures and other complications of inactivity.

Exercise prescription is guided by the purposes of training, current and prior health status, and an exercise evaluation including an assessment of fitness level. Examples of low to moderately intense exercises to improve active or passive range of motion are ambulation, bicycling, and muscle-strengthening resistive exercises. Lower exercise intensities and duration may be required in individuals with anemia or thrombocytopenia. Individuals with compromised skeletal integrity—secondary, for example, to bone metastases or osteopenia and/or osteoporosis—may be able to participate in non–weight-bearing aerobic activities including cycling or rowing. Eliopoulos provides a thorough description of basic range of motion exercises.[98] Although not specifically for patients with cancer, guidelines for exercise prescription are available through the American College of Sports Medicine.[99] Gentle resistive exercise with elastic bands such as Theraband, and repeatedly walking or bicycling for even just a few minutes at a time during several sessions per day can help to build stamina.[100]

BOX 32-6

Therapies to Enhance Function Applicable to Individuals with Cancer

- Gait and/or balance training
- Provision of assistive ambulatory devices (e.g., quad cane, hemiwalker)
- Ambulation on different types of surfaces (e.g., stairs)
- Provision and/or modification of shoe gear and orthotics
- Education and provision of bracing and splinting
- Range of motion, strengthening, coordination exercises
- Sensory integration
- Electrical stimulation for pain management
- Positioning and posturing
- Breathing exercises
- Chest physical therapy
- Relaxation exercises
- Conditioning and endurance exercises
- Strengthening and flexibility exercises
- Modalities to decrease pain and edema
- Alternative interventions—qigong, yoga, aquatics
- Family and patient education for home management
- Training in activities of daily living (e.g., grooming, dressing, cooking)
- Transfer training (e.g., toilet, bathtub, car)
- Energy conservation training
- Endurance for participation in activities of daily living
- Activities to enhance function of upper extremities
- Training to compensate for visual–perceptual problems
- Provision of adaptive devices (e.g., reachers, special eating utensils)
- Interventions to improve and/or normalize language production
- Use of voice amplifiers and/or alternate communication devices
- Reading, writing, and math retraining
- Functional skills such as checkbook balancing, making change
- Therapy for swallowing disorders
- Oral muscular strengthening

Referral for physical therapy can be extremely helpful when commencing an exercise program, particularly in individuals who are severely deconditioned, since physical therapy can offer an appropriately-paced and tailored exercised routine together with close monitoring of responses to exercise. Consideration should also be given to consulting with a physician or nurse practitioner for prescreening of individuals before beginning an exercise program if there are concerns about cardiopulmonary, skeletal, or other contraindications to physical activity.

As with any exercise program, caution must be taken.[101] Some of the signs that indicate a need to stop exercise include a resting heart rate greater than or equal to 100 beats per minute, an exercise heart rate greater than or equal to 35% above the resting heart rate, increase or decrease in systolic blood pressure by 20 mm Hg, pulse oximetry less than 95%, angina, dyspnea, pallor, cyanosis, dizziness, diaphoresis, pain, shortness of breath, muscle cramping, or joint pain. Individuals can be taught to use a rating of perceived exertion (RPE) scale to gauge their exercise intensity. For moderate-intensity exercise, their RPE should be about 11 to 13 on a scale of 6 to 20.[99]

BOWEL AND BLADDER CONTINENCE

Incontinence can have a profound impact on general health and self-esteem. Incontinence of bowel or bladder can lead to infections, skin breakdown, falls, anorexia, depression, and social isolation. There are rehabilitative approaches that successfully promote urinary and fecal continence.[102-104] The specific plan should be tailored to the etiology of the incontinence and to factors such as limited ambulation or diminished mental status that may be contributing to incontinence.

NUTRITION

Ensuring adequate intake of protein, calories, nutrients, and fluids is an important goal in all patients with cancer because of both hypermetabolism and the risks of therapy-related malnutrition. Declining functional status can make shopping for food and meal preparation difficult, and muscle weakness, fatigue, dyspnea, and depression, together with other symptoms such as mucositis that result in functional changes in chewing and swallowing, contribute directly to inadequate intake of food and fluids. This becomes a circular process, since cachexia and protein-calorie malnutrition cause further muscle wasting, weakness, and functional loss.[105] Interventions include referral to a clinical dietician, together with specific measures to meet the additional needs for protein and calories secondary to hypermetabolism, to build lean body mass, and to address the consequences of functional disability (e.g., difficulties with meal preparation, anorexia, cachexia, functional problems with chewing and swallowing) on nutrient intake. The outcomes of nutritional intervention can be monitored through evaluation of body weight, skin fold thickness, lean muscle mass, and daily food diaries.

EMOTIONAL SUPPORT

Many losses and unwanted changes accompany a decline in functional status. These may include changes in role, income status, social networks, independence, self-image, self-esteem, and QOL. Reactions to these losses can include anxiety, anger, frustration, sadness, and denial. Individuals do not experience these reactions to the grieving process or the rehabilitative process

in a stepwise or sequential manner, and may vacillate between hope and a determination to improve, and discouragement and resignation. Denial can lead to unrealistic plans, the search for a healer or strategy that will offer a more optimistic outlook, or nonadherence to the plan of care. Emotional support that offers acceptance and an opportunity to discuss values and personal goals, explore options for problem solving, and discuss the emotional impact of functional changes can be helpful in supporting the grieving process.

CAREGIVER SUPPORT

Patients experiencing functional losses place additional demands on their family caregivers. If these caregivers are older adults or have health problems themselves, the additional burden of caring for a parent, partner, or friend experiencing the functional losses of cancer may exceed available resources or may result in the caregiver neglecting his or her own health care needs. A recent study noted that compared to family caregivers of patients with intact functional status, family caregivers of cancer patients with functional losses experienced increased distress and disruption to daily schedules.[32,61] Assessment of the home environment should include an assessment of the abilities, capacity, and needs of the individual(s) providing care. Adaptive equipment and the provision of home health services, together with caregiver education and access to respite care, are important elements of service delivery to support the caregivers of cancer patients experiencing functional losses.

Outcomes Evaluation

All of the measures previously described for the evaluation of functional status can be used to evaluate the outcomes of interventions designed to improve functional status. Instruments should be chosen with attention to their reliability, validity, measurement properties in the population of interest (e.g., responsiveness and sensitivity to change, anticipated ceiling or floor effects). Thoughtful consideration must also be given to the most appropriate time points at which to measure the achievement of functional status outcomes.

There is also debate in the oncology nursing community about optimal as opposed to acceptable outcomes of interventions to improve functional status. The Oncology Nursing Society's Oncology Nursing Sensitive Outcomes Project team chose "Return to Usual Function" for their outcomes measurement initiative (http://www.ons.org/outcomes). However, this may be a limiting definition, particularly in situations where functional status is expected to continue to decline (e.g., in terminally ill patients), or where return to usual function is not possible but return to optimal function within limits is achievable (e.g., patient with laryngectomy who uses a speech production device). Fawcett, Tulman, and Samarel suggest that the goal of nursing intervention is to help the individual attain the highest possible and most desirable level of function.[106] The definition of the outcome to be achieved through interventions to improve functional status will continue to be a topic of discussion, whether it be a return to usual function or the achievement of optimal function within the limits imposed by the disease and its treatment.

A related issue in the measurement of functional status as an outcome of care is the evaluation of comorbidity, since this is an important variable that can negatively affect functional status in patients with cancer. A variety of indices are available to evaluate the presence of comorbidities including the Kaplan-Feinstein Index, the Charlson index, the Index of Coexistent Disease, and the Functional Comorbidity Index (FCI). Among the advantages of the FCI for use in studies of functional status are the facts that (1) the FCI addresses comorbidities such as visual impairment or osteoarthritis, which affect function but which may not affect mortality, (2) it is simple to administer and to score, and (3) the FCI's explicit outcome of interest is physical function, whereas the other comorbidity indices have a stronger association with mortality outcomes.[107]

Ethical Considerations

In delivering ethically appropriate nursing care to patients with cancer who are at risk for or who have experienced a decline in functional status, nurses apply the ethical principles of respect for persons and autonomy. Respect for persons presumes that all individual human beings are free and responsible persons and should be treated as such in proportion to their ability in the circumstances. Respect for persons also requires that individuals are treated with respect for and with recognition of their human dignity. Individuals with reduced decisional capacity (i.e., ability or competence to make decisions) are entitled to appropriate protection; however, the assessment of decisional capacity is complex and is rarely absolute.[108] Decisional capacity may fluctuate over time, or may be affected by the side effects of medications or treatment. Often, decisional capacity is decision-specific, meaning that different levels of capacity are required depending upon the potential consequences of the decision.

Autonomy is the capacity for self determination and includes the principle of a person's being respected as an autonomous agent. To respect an autonomous agent is to acknowledge that person's right to make choices and take action based on his or her own values and belief system. Respect not only involves refraining from interfering with others' choices, but may also include providing them with the necessary conditions and opportunities for exercising autonomy, although respect for autonomy does not imply that one must cooperate with another's actions. The principle of respect for autonomy implies that one should be free from coercion in deciding to act, and that others are obligated to protect confidentiality, respect privacy, and tell the truth. On the other hand, health care professionals' actions, rules, or policies do not respect patient autonomy when they attempt to dictate what is best for the patient without considering the patient's own beliefs and value system; it is the competent patient's right to determine what is truly in his or her own best interest. However, health care professionals do have expertise that the patient and family may not possess, and this incurs the obligation to act beneficently in recommending treatments and approaches that they believe will truly benefit the patient. Nonetheless, this expertise does not give them the right to make decisions for the patient.

In the area of functional health, interventions promote the principle of autonomy when they help patients set and achieve individually meaningful rehabilitation goals and to become independent in areas important to them. Efforts to improve functional status must begin with a joint identification by the patient and the health care team of areas of limitation. Together they must develop approaches that allow the patient to optimize his or her functioning and QOL within the limits imposed by cancer. Optimal functioning following the diagnosis and treatment of

cancer may involve choices and trade-offs that individual patients can best judge for themselves. For example, consider the patient with severe peripheral neuropathy who holds the goal of returning to parenting responsibilities after treatment. This person's rehabilitative goals may include learning adaptations to be able to perform household tasks safely and effective pain management, whereas vocational counseling to allow this person to return to work may not be of interest. On the other hand, a patient who identifies returning home as his or her goal may decide that the most important priority is to learn how to manage stairs or to safely transfer in and out of the shower, but may be less interested in nutritional status. An assessment of functional performance in the areas of ADLs and role performance can lay the foundation for patients setting incremental, achievable, and realistic goals. Functional assessment can also inform the patient's priorities for self-care, for example, by contributing to an understanding of how compromised nutrition contributes to the loss of lean muscle mass and results in weakness and difficulties with ambulation. Nursing care that is directed toward restoring or supporting functional performance must be based on a fundamental respect for human dignity and a faith in the strength of the human spirit. Patients must also be supported by nurse-patient relationships that are grounded by authenticity, trust, mutuality, and hope.

Conclusions and Directions for Research

Despite the acknowledged importance of functional status in patients with cancer, there has been relatively little systematic exploration of this variable in patients with cancer. Most studies have been cross-sectional, providing a limited exploration of patterns of functional recovery or decline across the cancer experience. Functional status as discussed in current cancer literature is also characterized by the use of a restricted range of measures to operationalize functional status (predominantly KPS and the SF-36), and by the emphasis on self-report measures rather than performance-based measures. There is limited empirical work that identifies methods for valid and reliable measurement of functional status in specific tumor groups, both during and after specific types of cancer treatment, and only sporadic study of the patterns of functional recovery following treatment or of the impact on function of symptom prevalence, intensity, and distress. Likewise scanty are discussions of how self-care and restorative interventions such as exercise, relaxation training, educational interventions, traditional rehabilitation programs, or nurse service delivery models affect functional status as an outcomes variable. Measurement issues include how the concept of function should be operationalized (e.g., objective measures versus self-report), from whose perspective function should be measured (i.e., patient, family, or health care provider), and the optimal time points for detecting changes improvement or decline in function across the cancer trajectory.[109,110] A wider array of clinically sensitive measures of function, with established psychometric properties in patients with cancer, is needed so that researchers and clinicians can tailor the selection of a measure to the specific patient population, as well as to their purpose (screening, longitudinal evaluation, outcome measurement) in evaluating function.

A priority area for further research is greater feasibility, acceptability, and psychometric evaluation of the performance test battery in patients across the disease spectrum, from diagnosis to survivorship or terminal care, and in patients with a wide range of tumor types. However, such performance measures may not truly reflect actual functioning, because the accommodations people make in their homes for decreased function may not be available to support their performance in the clinic environment. In addition, performance test measures do not capture a patient's level of satisfaction with his or her functional status. These measures may be insensitive in distinguishing the impact of symptoms, affect and mood, and motivation on functional performance, and they do not directly indicate specific areas of need for rehabilitation, support services, or assistance.

Although functional status and patterns of functional recovery and decline across the cancer experience have been in explored in patients with breast, lung, colorectal, and prostate cancer, there has been only limited exploration of functional status in patients with primary brain tumors or hematologic malignancies, especially patients with multiple myeloma and non-Hodgkin's lymphoma. In addition, there have been no studies of functional status in adolescent or young adult patients, and few studies of functional status in non-Caucasian patients. The need to study functional status in non-Caucasian samples is underscored by studies that suggest that relative to their Caucasian counterparts, Hispanic and African American cancer survivors may experience more difficulties with ADLs.[25,26] Studies of symptom prevalence and distress and clinical trials of symptom management approaches should incorporate measures of functional status as a correlate or outcome. However, questions remain about the best way to measure this variable, whether by self-report or performance, and about which instruments are best for which purposes.

REVIEW QUESTIONS

✓ Case Study

Mr. Grant is a 66-year-old widowed individual newly diagnosed with Stage IIIA multiple myeloma. He has multiple osteolytic bone lesions involving ribs, vertebrae, and femur. He lives alone; however, his daughter lives close by and visits on weekends and occasionally during the week. The patient is retired but golfs at least weekly; he volunteers at the local school, helping to mentor children in reading. His multiple myeloma was diagnosed when he came for care of a pathologic compound fracture of his right humerus. He is right-handed. His current medications include sustained-release morphine, which provides good pain control. He is admitted to the hospital for open reduction of the fracture and to receive initial treatment with high-dose dexamethasone. He has made a good postoperative recovery, although on functional evaluation he has steroid-induced proximal muscle weakness and has lost some muscle mass as a result of inactivity. In terms of his basic ADLs and instrumental ADLs, because of his humeral fracture, he is somewhat dependent on others for driving, shopping, and meal preparation. Although it takes more time than in the past, the patient is independent in bathing, dressing, and grooming. With the assistance of the nursing staff, he has developed a written schedule for the times his medications are due, and you have asked his nurse practitioner to direct the pharmacy to dispense his discharge medications in nonchildproof containers to make it easier for him to open medication containers using his left hand. Because of proximal muscle weakness, he has some difficulty with climbing stairs and rising from a seated position. His home is on one level, and a raised toilet seat is provided. His daughter has agreed to provide transportation to and from his clinic appointments; arrangements are also made for the patient to receive home delivery of meals. A program of proximal muscle-strengthening exercises is recommended by the physical therapist at the time of discharge, and he is referred for outpatient physical therapy to promote right shoulder range of motion and to assist with recovery of right upper-extremity dexterity.

When you next see the patient he returns to the clinic after two cycles of treatment with vincristine, doxorubicin, and dexamethasone (VAD) chemotherapy. He has made a good postoperative recovery, although proximal muscle weakness is still problematic, particularly in the lower extremities. He has very limited activity, and has been unable to return to previously enjoyable pursuits such as golf, which also provided him with an opportunity for companionship and social support. Owing to therapy with vincristine, the patient has developed peripheral neuropathy, and has some difficulty with fine motor tasks such as buttoning his shirt. He is also reporting significant fatigue, and you note that he is mildly anemic. He indicates that he has not returned to his volunteer role at school, and he has not felt like attending church or other social gatherings to which he is invited. He denies having pain and indicates that although he sleeps well at night, he also naps frequently during the day. Although frustrated and at times discouraged by the absence of the clinical improvement he had expected, the patient denies significant mood disturbances such as anxiety or depression.

Based on this functional assessment, you note that he has fatigue, restrictions in role performance, limited social and vocational role function, and increasing limitation in basic ADLs such as dressing. You suggest that a trial of a slow taper of his sustained-release morphine be considered under close supervision of the team, and that measures such as treatment with epoetin alfa to elevate hemoglobin be considered. You are concerned that some of his fatigue and excessive daytime sleepiness is related to treatment with narcotics, and since he has received several cycles of chemotherapy treatment, his pain may be improving. A slow narcotic taper will allow the patient and the health care team to determine the dose of narcotic that is needed to control pain, without incurring excess sedation or other deleterious side effects. A prescription for breakthrough analgesic is provided, and the patient is instructed not to taper faster than recommended and to contact the team immediately should he develop pain. You also recommend that the patient might benefit from a course of physical therapy, together with an exercise program of walking. A referral for occupational therapy is made for instruction in techniques for managing ADLs for those with neuropathy, and for a review of safety principles to limit falls in those with peripheral neuropathy.

Continued

REVIEW QUESTIONS—CONT'D

When the patient returns to clinic 6 weeks after completing VAD chemotherapy, he is in complete remission, and is making some slow progress in the area of fatigue. He denies having pain, and is taking a lower dose of sustained-release morphine. Although he has not yet resumed his volunteer activities, he reports that he has joined his golfing partners for lunch one afternoon after they had played a round; he enjoyed that opportunity to see friends again and to resume a component of his normal routine, although he acknowledges he will likely not be able to resume golfing for many months to come. However, he has joined a group for mall walking, so that he has an exercise program that he can participate in during the inclement winter months.

QUESTIONS

1. Which of the following is an example of instrumental activity of daily living, or IADL?
   a. Dressing
   b. Moving from one location to another
   c. Using the telephone
   d. Feeding self

2. Of the following, which would be the most important criterion to be considered when selecting a functional status measure for screening in clinical practice?
   a. Measure should be able to detect clinically important changes in functioning.
   b. Measure should differentiate individuals with and without functional compromise, be brief, and be easy to score and interpret.
   c. Measure should be able to detect subtle changes in function.
   d. Measure should be based on a variety of sources of information, including self-report, performance-based measures, and clinician evaluation of functioning.

3. Which of the following is true about the risk factors for functional loss during and following cancer and its treatment?
   a. The treatment modality (i.e., radiation, chemotherapy, surgery, biotherapy, or molecularly targeted agent) and the side effects of treatment are the two most significant risk factors for functional loss.
   b. The relative contributions of polypharmacy, malnutrition, inactivity, and comorbidity to functional loss during and following treatment are unknown.
   c. Motivation, expectations, and mood are significant predictors of those individuals who will develop functional losses.
   d. Age is a significant risk factor for functional loss during and following treatment.

4. Exercise tolerance testing, the 2-, 6- or 12-minute walk, and other tests such as grip strength and the "timed up-and-go" are examples of measures of what?
   a. Functional capacity
   b. IADLs
   c. Functional performance
   d. Participation restrictions

5. Which of the following statements is true about recent studies of function in older adults with cancer?
   a. Cognitive and behavioral nursing interventions to manage cancer-related symptoms have little effect on functional status.
   b. Comprehensive geriatric assessment (CGA) is only useful in evaluating older adults with cancer who have poor performance status.
   c. Symptom intensity and the presence of multiple concurrent symptoms is correlated with poorer physical functioning.
   d. Comprehensive rehabilitation is unlikely to be effective in achieving functional improvements in debilitated older adults with cancer.

6. Which of the following is true of exercise and/or activity and functional status in patients with cancer?
   a. Benefits of regular exercise include improvements in cardiopulmonary capacity and muscle strength and endurance, a reduction in fatigue and depression, and an improved sense of well-being.
   b. Examples of low- to moderate-intensity exercises include brisk walking, slow jogging, and rowing.
   c. To be of benefit in improving functioning, preventing muscle atrophy, and reversing deconditioning, exercise should be performed continuously for 30 to 60 minutes.
   d. Bone metastases or osteopenia and/or osteoporosis are a contraindication to aerobic exercise.

7. An individual who is coping with a decline in functional status is assessed to be setting unrealistic plans, demonstrating nonadherence to recommendations, and at the same time endlessly searching for solutions that offer a more optimistic outlook. These would all be most characteristic of which of the following emotional reactions?
   a. Anger
   b. Resignation
   c. Search for control
   d. Denial and minimization

8. Which of the following best describes the primary purpose of a functional status evaluation?
   a. Plan rehabilitation treatment/care and evaluate progress toward goals.
   b. Assess rehabilitation potential and predict improvements in functional status.
   c. Ensure a comprehensive evaluation of the older adult with cancer.
   d. Systematically assess neurologic status.

9. Let's return to the case discussed above, involving a patient with Stage IIIA multiple myeloma with multiple osteolytic bone lesions who is receiving outpatient chemotherapy. The patient's daughter asks to meet with you. She is concerned because her father is not using his wheeled walker at home. You meet with the patient and his daughter to discuss their respective viewpoints on this situation. The daughter notes that her father is frail and lives alone, and she fears that he is at significant risk to fall and sustain a fracture. After all he has been through with chemotherapy treatment, she feels that a fracture will just set him back further and that it is unnecessary for him to take that risk. However, her father states that he is strong enough to walk without a walker, that he hasn't fallen yet at the hospital or at home, and that using the walker makes him feel more like 'an invalid'. The nurse notes that this patient has made sound and reasonable judgments regarding

other aspects of his care and treatment, and his daughter verifies that he is managing his affairs at home well, and has agreed to other home supports such as visiting nursing and an emergency call system for his home. Resolving this case requires that the nurse primarily consider which of the following ethical constructs?

a. Autonomy
b. Beneficence
c. Surrogate decision making
d. Decision-making competence

10. You are a nurse on an inpatient oncology unit, and you are considering a measure of functional status that you will administer upon admission to your unit and 3 days before discharge to evaluate the outcome of rehabilitative and supportive care interventions delivered on your unit. Your unit cares mostly for patients admitted with febrile neutropenia, those with complications of radiotherapy such as dehydration, and patients with pain, intractable nausea and vomiting or other distressing symptoms at the end of life. Your average length of stay is 5 to 8 days, and patients are primarily discharged to home, although some are transferred to hospice. Which of the following types of functional status measures might be the most appropriate selection to measure this outcome?

a. 6-minute walk time
b. A measure of independence in basic ADLs
c. A measure of independence in basic ADLs and IADLs and performance and/or participation limitations such as ability to fulfill roles as worker, spouse, and parent
d. A checklist of common symptoms

ANSWERS

1. **C.** *Rationale:* Dressing and feeding self are examples of basic ADLs. Moving from one location to another is an example of mobility.

2. **B.** *Rationale:* The purposes of functional status evaluation include screening, assessment, and monitoring for change. Measures for screening should be brief, specific (capable of differentiating individuals with functional compromise from those without), and easy to score and interpret so that they can be administered by professional and paraprofessional staff. On the other hand, measures for assessment should be able to detect incremental changes in functional status, should be sensitive to clinical important changes in functioning, and should not demonstrate significant ceiling or floor effects in the intended population. A measure for screening should emphasize self-report, clinician ratings, or both. Performance-based measures may be optimally applied for assessment and monitoring of changes in functional status over time.

3. **B.** *Rationale:* Treatment-related factors such as treatment modality, its intensity, and its associated side effects may influence an individual patient's risk profile, The relative contributions of the treatment modality itself, together with polypharmacy, protein-calorie malnutrition, inactivity, and comorbidities, are unknown. Motivation, expectations, and mood may also influence functional losses; however, no prior study has identified these as significant

predictors of functional losses. On the other hand, unrelieved symptoms have been shown to predict those individuals who will develop functional limitations. Although older adults with comorbidities may be at greater risk for functional loss during and following treatment, age per se is not a risk factor for functional loss.

4. **A.** *Rationale:* Performance-based measures of function are considered measures of functional capacity (reflecting the maximum possible level of function), whereas functional performance is what individuals actually do in their day-to-day lives. IADLs include tasks such as using the telephone, driving, shopping, managing finances, and administering medications. Participation restrictions reflect problems an individual experiences with involvement in life situations and roles. Participation restrictions are typically gauged by self-report, since performance-based measures reflect the maximum possible level of function, not role performance in daily life.

5. **C.** *Rationale:* Symptom intensity and the presence of multiple concurrent symptoms has been shown to be associated with poorer physical functioning. However, cognitive and behavioral nursing interventions to manage cancer-related symptoms can be effective in limiting the deleterious effects of symptom distress on functional status.[64] Comprehensive geriatric assessment has been shown to add substantial information to the functional assessment of older cancer patients, including patients with a good performance status.[81] Recent studies have shown that comprehensive rehabilitation programs are effective in improving functional status in patients with mixed diagnoses, some of whom were malnourished, had advanced cancers, or were elderly.[87-93]

6. **A.** *Rationale:* The benefits of regular exercise include improvements in cardiopulmonary capacity and muscle strength and endurance, a reduction in fatigue and depression, and an improved sense of well-being, including personal control and self-efficacy. Examples of low- to moderate-intensity exercises include active or passive range of motion, ambulation, bicycling, and muscle-strengthening resistive exercises. Gentle resistive exercise and walking or bicycling performed for even just a few minutes and repeated during several sessions per day can help to build stamina. Before commencing an exercise program, patients with metastatic or osteopenic and/or osteoporotic bone lesions should be carefully screened by a physician or nurse practitioner; however, these morbidities are not a contraindication to aerobic exercise per se, and patients may be able to participate in non–weight-bearing aerobic activities including cycling or rowing.

7. **D.** *Rationale:* Although it is difficult to judge a coping strategy from a brief clinical vignette, individuals who are seeking more control or experiencing anger or resignation may demonstrate nonadherence to recommendations. However, these emotional responses would not be expected to be associated with setting unrealistic plans and seeking solutions that offer a more optimistic outlook. The characteristics of setting unrealistic plans, demonstrating nonadherence to recommendations and at the same time searching for solutions that

Continued

REVIEW QUESTIONS—CONT'D

offer a more optimistic outlook most likely suggest denial or minimization of the functional losses.

8. **A.** *Rationale:* Measures of functional status are primarily helpful in setting goals, planning rehabilitative interventions, and evaluating outcomes. They may also help with continuity of care, particularly as patients move between settings. However, they cannot predict rehabilitative potential, the trajectory of functional recovery, or the likelihood that there will be improvement in functional status, since this is dependent upon a complex interplay of clinical factors, health history, premorbid level of functioning, strength, and aerobic conditioning, together with individual attributes, including motivation.. Functional status evaluations can be applied to any developmental group, not just the older adult. Comprehensive geriatric assessment includes evaluation of functional dependence in ADL and IADLs, together with other dimensions, such as symptom distress, polypharmacy, and social support, that may be problematic for the older adult. Alterations in neurologic status may result in functional status decline; however, neurologic status is best assessed directly and specifically through tests of muscle strength and evaluation of the cranial nerves, cerebellar function, and cognition.

9. **A.** *Rationale:* Although all four ethical principles might bear on this case, the principle of autonomy, or self-determination, is a central tenet. This value is expressed in a strong commitment and respect for the right of the individual to hold views, make decisions, and take voluntary actions based on personal preferences and beliefs. Respect for autonomy assumes primacy even when the health care team hold the opinion that a different course of action will produce the greatest benefit for the patient. Beneficence (doing good) and nonmaleficence (avoiding doing evil) are not specific moral rules and cannot

by themselves tell us which concrete actions constitute doing good and avoiding evil. Surrogate decision making does not have a role at this time, since there is clear evidence that the patient is able to meaningfully participate in decision making, and there is no evidence that decision-making competence is constrained. Respecting that the patient has the final decision about using a walker, the nurse might explain the risks of pathologic fracture, given the patient's osteolytic bony lesions, and might offer encouragement for patient to consider having the walker available in his home to use, perhaps in situations where he is at greatest risk of fall (e.g., walking on uneven surfaces, in inclement weather, when fatigued, when weakened in the first few days following treatment).

10. **C.** *Rationale:* A checklist of symptoms may be helpful in predicting those individuals at greatest risk for functional losses. However, it cannot characterize the nature of functional changes, and it is not useful as a direct measure to evaluate the outcome of interventions to improve functioning. Although it is a sensitive measure of incremental changes in functional capacity, the 6-minute walk time is not an ideal screening measure for functional compromise, since it is not specific to functional performance and may not be ideal in differentiating individuals with functional compromise from those without. It is also not a measure that can be administered by paraprofessional staff. In a patient population with a short average length of stay, and who are admitted during the course of treatment, a measure of independence in basic ADLs such as bathing, dressing, and feeding self may demonstrate ceiling effects and be therefore insensitive to dependencies in IADLs or role performance and/or participation restrictions.

REFERENCES

1. Watson PG: The optimal functioning plan: a key element in cancer rehabilitation, *Cancer Nurs* 15(4):254-263, 1992.
2. Doran DM: Functional status. In Doran DM, editor: *Nursing sensitive outcomes: state of the science*, Boston, 2003, Jones & Bartlett.
3. Gobel BH, Beck SL, O'Leary C: Nursing-sensitive patient outcomes: the development of the Putting Evidence Into Practice Resources for Nursing Practice, *Clin J Oncol Nurs* 10(5):621-624, 2006.
4. Armstrong TS: Symptoms experience: a concept analysis, *Oncol Nurs Forum* 30(4):601-606, 2003.
5. Lenz ER, Pugh LC, Milligan RA et al: The Middle-Range Theory of Unpleasant Symptoms: an update, *Adv Nurs Sci* 19(3):14-27, 1997.
6. Larson PJ, Unchinuno A, Izumi S et al: An integrated approach to symptom management, *Nurs Health Sci* 1(4):203-210, 1999.
7. Bourbonniere M, Sutherland N: *Oncology nursing sensitive outcomes resource guide: return to usual function*, Pittsburg, PA, 2004, Oncology Nursing Society.
8. McCorkle R, Benoliel, Donaldson G et al: A randomized clinical trial of home nursing care for lung cancer patients, *Cancer* 64(6):1375-1382, 1989.
9. Cooley ME: Quality of life in persons with non-small cell lung cancer: a concept analysis, *Cancer Nurs* 21(3):151-161, 1998.
10. Halbertsma J, Heerkens YF, Hirs WM et al: Towards a new ICIDH, *Disabil Rehabil* 22(3):144-156, 2000.
11. World Health Organization: *International classification of impairments, disabilities and handicaps: a manual of classification related to the consequences of disease*, Geneva, 1980, Author.
12. Verbrugge LM, Jette AM: The disablement process, *Social Sci Med* 38(1):1-14, 1994.
13. Nagi SZ: A study in the evaluation of disability and rehabilitation potential: concepts, methods and procedures, *Am J Pub Health* 54(9):1568-1579, 1964.
14. Leidy NK: Functional status and the forward progress of merry-go-rounds: toward a coherent analytical framework, *Nurs Res* 43(4):196-202, 1994.
15. Leidy NK: Psychometric properties of the functional performance inventory in patients with chronic obstructive pulmonary disease, *Nurs Res* 48(1):20-28, 1999.
16. Bergner M, Bobbitt RA, Pollard WE: The sickness impact profile: validation of a health status measure, *Med Care* 14(1):57-67, 1976.
17. Bennett JA, Winters-Stone K, Nail L: Conceptualizing and measuring physical functioning in cancer survivorship studies, *Oncol Nurs Forum* 33(1):41-49, 2006.
18. Thomas ML, Dodd MJ: The development and testing of a nursing model of morbidity in patients with cancer, *Oncol Nurs Forum* 19(9):1385-1395, discussion 1395, 1992.
19. Kroenke CH, Rosner B, Chen WY et al: Functional impact of breast cancer by age at diagnosis, *J Clin Oncol* 22(10):1849-1856, 2004.
20. Michael YL, Kawachi I, Berkman LF et al: The persistent impact of breast carcinoma on functional health status: prospective evidence from the nurses' health study, *Cancer* 89(11):2176-2186, 2000.
21. Cimprich B, Ronis DL: Attention and symptom distress in women with and without breast cancer, *Nurs Res* 50(2):86-94, 2001.
22. Wefel JS, Lenzi R, Theriault RL et al: The cognitive sequelae of standard-dose adjuvant chemotherapy in women with breast carcinoma: results of

a prospective, randomized, longitudinal trial, *Cancer* 100(11): 2292-2299, 2004.

23. Polinsky ML: Functional status of long-term breast cancer survivors: demonstrating chronicity, *Health Soc Work* 19(3):165-173, 1994.

24. McMillan SC, Weitzner M: How problematic are various aspects of quality of life in patients with cancer at the end of life? *Oncol Nurs Forum* 27(5):817-823, 2000.

25. Deimling GT, Schaefer ML, Kahana B et al: Racial differences in the health of older-adult long-term cancer survivors, *J Psychosoc Oncol* 20(4):71-94, 2002

26. Kim Y, Stein K, Baker F et al: The effects of problems in daily living and ethnicity on quality of life of cancer survivors, *Psychooncology* 13(S1):P7-2, 2004.

27. Hewitt M, Rowland JH, Yancik R: Cancer survivors in the United States: age, health, and disability, *J Gerontol A Biol Sci Med Sci* 58(1):82-91, 2003.

28. Garman KS, Pieper CF, Seo P et al: Function in elderly cancer survivors depends on comorbidities, *J Gerontol A Biol Sci Med Sci* 58(12):1119-1124, 2003.

29. Drouin J: Exercise in older individuals with cancer, *Top Geriatr Rehabil* 20(2):81-97, 2004.

30. Given CW, Given B, Azzouz F et al: Comparison of changes in physical functioning of elderly patients with new diagnoses of cancer, *Med Care* 38(5):482-493, 2000.

31. Given B, Given C, Azzouz F et al: Physical functioning of elderly cancer patients prior to diagnosis and following initial treatment, *Nurs Res* 50(4):222-232, 2001.

32. Kurtz ME, Kurtz JC, Given CW et al: Relationship of caregiver reactions and depression to cancer patients' symptoms, functional states and depression—a longitudinal view, *Soc Sci Med* 40(6):837-846, 1995.

33. Kurtz ME, Kurtz JC, Stommel M et al: Physical functioning and depression among older persons with cancer, *Cancer Pract* 9(1):11-18, 2001.

34. Watters JM, Yau JC, O'Rourke K et al: Functional status is well maintained in older women during adjuvant chemotherapy for breast cancer, *Ann Oncol* 14(12):1744-1750, 2003.

35. Hodgson NA, Given CW: Determinants of functional recovery in older adults surgically treated for cancer, *Cancer Nurs* 27(1):10-16, 2004.

36. Bush NE, Haberman M, Donaldson G, et al: Quality of life of 125 adults surviving 6-18 years after bone marrow transplantation, *Soc Sci Med* 40(4):479-490, 1995.

37. Hayden PJ, Keogh F, Ni Conghaile M et al.: A single-centre assessment of long-term quality-of-life status after sibling allogeneic stem cell transplantation for chronic myeloid leukaemia in first chronic phase, *Bone Marrow Transplant* 34(6):545-556, 2004.

38. Kiss TL, Abdolell M, Jamal N et al: Long-term medical outcomes and quality-of-life assessment of patients with chronic myeloid leukemia followed at least 10 years after allogeneic bone marrow transplantation, *J Clin Oncol* 20(9):2334-2343, 2002.

39. Schmidt GM, Niland JC, Forman SJ et al: Extended follow-up in 212 long-term allogeneic bone marrow transplant survivors: issues of quality of life, *Transplantation* 55(3):551-557, 1993.

40. Sutherland HJ, Fyles GM, Adams G et al: Quality of life following bone marrow transplantation: a comparison of patient reports with population norms, *Bone Marrow Transplant* 19(11):1129-1136, 1997.

41. Andrykowski MA, Bishop MM, Hahn EA et al: Long-term health-related quality of life, growth, and spiritual well-being after hematopoietic stem-cell transplantation, *J Clin Oncol* 23(3):599-608, 2005.

42. Andrykowski MA, Altmaier EM, Barnett RL et al: Cognitive dysfunction in adult survivors of allogeneic marrow transplantation: relationship to dose of total body irradiation, *Bone Marrow Transplant* 6(4):269-276, 1990.

43. Andrykowski MA, Henslee PJ, Farrall MG: Physical and psychosocial functioning of adult survivors of allogeneic bone marrow transplantation, *Bone Marrow Transplant* 4(1):75-81, 1989.

44. Molassiotis A, Boughton BJ, Burgoyne T et al: Comparison of the overall quality of life in 50 long-term survivors of autologous and allogeneic bone marrow transplantation, *J Adv Nurs* 22(3):509-516, 1995.

45. Syrjala KL, Chapko MK, Vitaliano PP et al: Recovery after allogeneic marrow transplantation: prospective study of predictors of long-term physical and psychosocial functioning, *Bone Marrow Transplant* 11(4):319-327, 1993.

46. Chiodi S, Spinelli S, Ravera G et al: Quality of life in 244 recipients of allogeneic bone marrow transplantation, *Brit J Haematol* 110(3):614-619, 2000.

47. Duel T, Van Lint MT, Ljungman P et al: Health and functional status of long-term survivors of bone marrow transplantation, *Ann Intern Med* 126(3):184-192, 1997.

48. Worel N, Biener D, Kalhs P et al: Long-term outcome and quality of life of patients who are alive and in complete remission more than two years after allogeneic and syngeneic stem cell transplantation, *Bone Marrow Transplant* 30(9):619-626, 2002.

49. Edman L, Larsen J, Hagglund H et al: Health-related quality of life, symptom distress and sense of coherence in adult survivors of allogeneic stem-cell transplantation, *Eur J Cancer Care* 10(2):124-130, 2001.

50. Marks DI, Gale DJ, Vedhara K et al: A quality of life study in 20 adult long-term survivors of unrelated donor bone marrow transplantation, *Bone Marrow Transplant* 24(2):191-195, 1999.

51. Wingard JR, Curbow B, Baker F et al: Sexual satisfaction in survivors of bone marrow transplantation, *Bone Marrow Transplant* 9(3):185-190, 1992.

52. Molassiotis A, Van den Akker OBA, Milligan DW et al: Gonadal function and psychosexual adjustment in male long-term survivors of bone marrow transplantation, *Bone Marrow Transplant* 16(2):253-259, 1995.

53. Wolcott DL, Wellisch DK, Fawzy FI et al: Adaptation of adult bone marrow transplant recipient long-term survivors, *Transplantation* 41(4):478-484, 1986.

54. Dodd MJ, Miaskowski C, Paul SM: Symptom clusters and their effect on the functional status of patients with cancer, *Oncol Nurs Forum* 28(3):465-470, 2001.

55. Gift AG, Jablonski A, Stommel M et al: Symptom clusters in elderly patients with lung cancer, *Oncol Nurs Forum* 31(2):202-212, 2004.

56. Kurtz ME, Kurtz JC, Stommel M et al: The influence of symptoms, age, comorbidity and cancer site on physical functioning and mental health of geriatric women patients, *Women Health* 29(3):1-12, 1999.

57. Kurtz ME, Kurtz JC, Stommel M et al: Symptomatology and loss of physical functioning among geriatric patients with lung cancer, *J Pain Symptom Manage* 19(4):249-256, 2000.

58. Graydon JE: Women with breast cancer: their quality of life following a course of radiation therapy, *J Adv Nurs* 19(4):617-622, 1994.

59. Pasacreta JV: Depressive phenomena, physical symptom distress, and functional status among women with breast cancer, *Nurs Res* 46(4):214-221, 1997.

60. Sarna L: Effectiveness of structured nursing assessment of symptom distress in advanced lung cancer, *Oncol Nurs Forum* 25(6):1041-1048, 1998.

61. Given CW, Stommel M, Given B et al: The influence of cancer patients' symptoms and functional states on patients' depression and family caregivers' reaction and depression, *Health Psychol* 12(4):277-285, 1993.

62. Lin CC, Lai YL, Ward SE: Effect of cancer pain on performance status, mood states, and level of hope among Taiwanese cancer patients, *J Pain Symptom Manage* 25(1):29-37, 2003.

63. Syrjala KL, Langer SL, Abrams JR et al: Recovery and long-term function after hematopoietic cell transplantation for leukemia or lymphoma, *JAMA* 291(19):2335-2343, 2004.

64. Doorenbos A, Given B, Given C et al: Reducing symptom limitations: a cognitive behavioral intervention randomized trial, *Psychooncology* 14(7):574-584, 2005.

65. Richmond T, Tang S, Tulman L et al: Measuring function. In Frank-Stromborg M, Olsen SJ, editors: *Instruments for clinical health-care research*, ed 3, Boston 2004, Jones & Bartlett.

66. Bottomley JM, Lewis CB: Principles and practice of geriatric rehabilitation. In Bottomley JM, Lewis CB, editors: *Geriatric rehabilitation: A clinical approach*, ed 2, Upper Saddle River, NJ, 2003, Prentice Hall.

67. Chen CCH, Kenefick AL, Tang ST et al: Utilization of comprehensive geriatric assessment in cancer patients, *Crit Rev Oncol Hematol* 49(1):53-67, 2004.

68. Garman KS, Cohen HJ: Functional status and the elderly cancer patient, *Crit Rev Oncol Hematol* 43 (3):191-208, 2002.

69. Goodwin JA, Coleman EA: Exploring measures of functional dependence in the older adult with cancer, *Medsurg Nurs* 12(6):359-366, quiz 367 2003.

70. Katz S, Ford AB, Moskowitz RW et al: Studies of illness in the aged: the index of ADL: a standardized measure of biological and psychosocial survivors, *JAMA* 185:914-919, 1963.

71. Ware Jr JE, Sherbourne CD: The MOS 36-item short-form health survey (SF-36). I. Conceptual framework and item selection, *Med Care* 30(6):473-483, 1992.

72. Kaasa T, Wessel J: The Edmonton functional assessment tool: further development and validation for use in palliative care, *J Palliat Care* 17(1):5-11, 2001.

73. Nikoletti S, Porock D, Kristjanson LJ et al: Performance status assessment in home hospice patients using a modified form of the Karnofsky Performance Status scale, *J Palliat Med* 3(3):301-311, 2000.

74. Simmonds MJ: Physical function in patients with cancer: psychometric characteristics and clinical usefulness of a physical performance test battery, *J Pain Symptom Manage* 24(4):404-414, 2002.

75. Sehy YB, Williams MP: Functional assessment. In Stone JT, Salisbury SA, Wyman JF, editors: *Clinical gerontological nursing: a guide to advanced practice*, ed 2, Philadelphia, 1999, W.B. Saunders.

76. Goodwin JA, Coleman EA, Shaw J: Short Functional Dependence Scale: development and pilot test in older adults with cancer, *Cancer Nurs* 29(1):73-81, 2006.

77. Terret C, Albrand G, Droz JP: Geriatric assessment in elderly patients with prostate cancer, *Clin Prostate Cancer* 2(4):236-240, 2004.

78. Extermann M, Meyer J, McGinnis M et al: A comprehensive geriatric intervention detects multiple problems in older breast cancer patients, *Crit Rev Oncol Hematol* 49(1):69-75, 2004.

79. Reuben DB: Geriatric assessment in oncology, *Cancer* 80(7):1311-1316, 1997.

80. Monfardini S, Ferrucci L, Fratino L et al: Validation of a multidimensional evaluation scale for use in elderly cancer patients, *Cancer* 77(2):395-401, 1996.

81. Repetto L, Fratino L, Audisio RA et al: Comprehensive geriatric assessment adds information to Eastern Cooperative Oncology Group performance status in elderly cancer patients: an Italian Group for Geriatric Oncology study, *J Clin Oncol* 20(2):494-502, 2002.

82. Gordon LG, Scuffham P, Battistutta D et al: A cost-effectiveness analysis of two rehabilitation support services for women with breast cancer, *Breast Cancer Res Treat* 94(2):123-133, 2005.

83. Karki A, Simonen R, Malkia E et al: Efficacy of physical therapy methods and exercise after a breast cancer operation: a systematic review, *Crit Rev Phys Rehabil Med* 13(2-3):159-190, 2001.

84. Strauss-Blasche G, Gnad E, Ekmekcioglu C et al: Combined inpatient rehabilitation and spa therapy for breast cancer patients: Effects on quality of life and CA 15-3, *Cancer Nurs* 28 (5):390-398, 2005.

85. Spruit MA, Janssen PP, Willemsen SCP et al: Exercise capacity before and after an 8-week multidisciplinary inpatient rehabilitation program in lung cancer patients: a pilot study, *Lung Cancer* 52(2):257-260, 2006.

86. Van Weert E, Hoekstra-Weebers J, Otter R et al: Cancer-related fatigue: predictors and effects of rehabilitation, *Oncologist* 11(2):184-196, 2006.

87. Cole RP, Scialla SJ, Bednarz L: Functional recovery in cancer rehabilitation, *Arch Phys Med Rehabil* 81(5):623-627, 2000.

88. Sabers SR, Kokal JE, Girardi JC et al: Evaluation of consultation-based rehabilitation for hospitalized cancer patients with functional impairment, *Mayo Clin Proc* 74(9):855-861, 1999.

89. Guo Y, Palmer JL, Kaur G et al: Nutritional status of cancer patients and its relationship to function in an inpatient rehabilitation setting, *Support Care Cancer* 13(3):169-175, 2005.

90. Marciniak CM, Sliwa JA, Spill G et al: Functional outcome following rehabilitation of the cancer patient, *Arch Phys Med Rehabil* 77(1):54-57, 1996.

91. Scialla S, Cole R, Scialla T et al: Rehabilitation for elderly patients with cancer asthenia: making a transition to palliative care, *Palliat Med* 14(2):121-127, 2000.

92. Garman KS, McConnell ES, Cohen HJ: Inpatient care for elderly cancer patients: the role for geriatric evaluation and management units in fulfilling goals for care, *Crit Rev Oncol Hematol* 51(3):241-247, 2004.

93. Rao AV, Hsieh F, Feussner JR et al: Geriatric evaluation and management units in the care of the frail elderly cancer patient, *J Gerontol A Biol Sci Med Sci* 60(6):798-803, 2005.

94. Coyle EF: Detraining and retention of adaptations induced by endurance training. In ACSM: *Resource manual for guidelines for exercise testing and prescription*, ed 4, Baltimore, 2001, Williams & Wilkins.

95. Michael K: Relationship of skeletal muscle atrophy to functional status: a systematic research review, *Biol Res Nurs* 2(2):117-131, 2000.

96. Galvao DA, Newton RU: Review of exercise intervention studies in cancer patients, *J Clin Oncol* 23(4):899-909, 2005.

97. Stricker CT, Drake D, Hoyer KA et al: Evidence-based practice for fatigue management in adults with cancer: exercise as an intervention, *Oncol Nurs Forum* 31(5):963-976, 2004

98. Eliopoulos C: *Gerontological nursing*, ed 6, Philadelphia, 2005, Lippincott, Williams & Wilkins.

99. American College of Sports Medicine: *ACSM's Guidelines for exercise testing and prescription*, ed 7, Philadelphia, 2005, Lippincott, Williams & Wilkins.

100. Dimeo F, Rumberger BG, Keul J: Aerobic exercise as therapy for cancer fatigue, *Med Sci Sports Exer* 30(4):475-478, 1998.

101. Winningham ML, MacVicar MG, Burke C.: Exercise guidelines for cancer patients: guidelines and precautions, *Phys Sports Med* 14(10):125-134, 1986.

102. Mitchell Beddar SA, Holden-Bennett L, McCormick AM: Development and evaluation of a protocol to manage fecal incontinence in the patient with cancer, *J Palliat Care* 13(2):27-38, 1997.

103. Ostaszkiewicz J, Roe B, Johnston L: Effects of timed voiding for the management of urinary incontinence in adults: systematic review, *J Adv Nurs* 52(4):420-431, 2005.

104. Ouslander JG, Griffiths PC, McConnell E et al: Functional incidental training: a randomized, controlled, crossover trial in Veterans Affairs nursing homes, *J Am Geriatr Soc* 53(7):1091-1100, 2005.

105. Muscaritoli M, Bossola M, Aversa Z et al: Prevention and treatment of cancer cachexia: new insights into an old problem, *Euro J Cancer* 42(1):31-41, 2006.

106. Fawcett J, Tulman L, Samarel N: Enhancing function in life transitions and serious illness, *Adv Pract Nurs Q* 1(3):50-57, 1995.

107. Groll DL, To T, Bombardier C et al: The development of a comorbidity index with physical function as the outcome, *J Clin Epidemiol* 58(6):595-602, 2005.

108. Checkland D, Silberfeld M: Reflections on segregating and assessing areas of competence, *Theor Med* 16(4):375-88, 1995.

109. Hakamies-Blomqvist L, Luoma ML, Sjostrom J et al: Timing of quality of life (QoL) assessments as a source of error in oncological trials, *J Adv Nurs* 35(5):709-716, 2001.

110. Hollen PJ, Gralla RJ, Rittenberg CN: Quality of life as a clinical trial endpoint: determining the appropriate interval for repeated assessments in patients with advanced lung cancer, *Support Care Cancer* 12(11):767-773, 2004.

CHAPTER 33

Patient Education

Patricia Agre and
Ann Marie Shaftic

Introduction

Patient education has never been more important than it is today. Patients are responsible for so many of their care activities that without it treatment may be compromised, complications and side effects may increase, and outcomes may be suboptimal. This is as true for cancer as it is for diabetes, asthma, and other chronic conditions. However, education of patients with cancer has particular challenges and, perhaps, some incentive components. Cancer raises the specter of death in a way that other diseases may not. Thus the educator has anxiety to overcome as a barrier to learning. On the positive side, a diagnosis of cancer can be so frightening that patients are often strongly motivated to learn whatever they need to learn to live. The educator of the patient with cancer has to take both factors into account when working with cancer patients and their families.

The entire health care team is responsible for teaching, but nurses play a crucial role. They are responsible for preparing patients before tests, procedures, and treatment. They care for the patient during hospitalizations and outpatient treatments. They do much of the discharge teaching, whether following surgery, for chemotherapy administration, or for radiation treatments. They are often the first ones contacted when questions or problems arise. And, they frequently spend more time with patients than any other members of the team.

Although patient education is an important part of the professional nurse's responsibilities, except for learning theory, it remains a small part of nursing education. Nurses are almost always taught *what* to teach, but they may not learn or have opportunities practicing *how* to teach. This chapter will review key principles of patient education and will provide some guidance for improving this critical nursing role.

Definitions

Action verbs—Verbs that indicate the doing of something (e.g., *state, describe, demonstrate*)

Adult learning theory—Malcolm Knowles' theory describing the adult learner as independent, self-directed, and problem-centered

Basic literacy skills—Skills that are required for reading simple text

Behavioral learning theory—A theory that covers learning based on observable behaviors

Cloze technique—A reading comprehension assessment technique that has a reader replace the appropriate word in text that has every fifth or sixth word deleted

Cognitive learning theory—Theory describing acquisition of knowledge through mental processes

Culturally competent—Capable of recognizing and respecting cultural differences

Fry—A test of readability that counts words and syllables

Goals—Broad aims of teaching

HIPAA privacy rules—Health Insurance Portability and Accountability Act, rules from the U. S. Department of Health and Human Services (USDHSS) that protect patients' privacy

Informed consent—A discussion and document that informs patients about invasive procedures and clinical trials; the patient must sign consent to indicate permission to proceed

Learning needs assessment—An assessment of what patients know, what they want to know, and how they want to learn

Learning theory—A theory that describes how people learn new information or skills

Limited English proficiency—Describes the person who does not speak English fluently

Literacy—The ability to read, write, and do quantitative tasks

Literacy assessment tools—Tools that assess an individual's reading and, sometimes, numeracy (working with numbers) skills

Motivational learning theory—Theory that describes the role of motivation in learning

Objectives—Aims that describe who will do what by when

Readability—The reading level of a text

REALM-R—Rapid Estimate of Adult Literacy in Medicine—Revised, a word pronunciation test

SIRACT—Stieglitz Informal Reading Assessment of Cancer Text, an informal reading inventory

SMOG—Simple Measure of Gobbledygook, a reading level assessment tool that uses sentences and syllables

Social learning theory—Learning theory that describes observational learning

Teachable moment—An "aha" moment when someone is particularly ready to learn

TOFLA—Test of Functional Literacy of Adults, a reading assessment that uses the cloze technique

Learning Needs Assessment

A learning needs assessment establishes the specifics of what a patient needs to learn about his or her diagnosis, treatment, and self-care. It leads to a nursing diagnosis and plan of care. It also identifies barriers to learning and the patient's preferred learning method. Finally, it tells the nurse what a patient's goals are for learning about his or her diagnosis and treatment.

A learning needs assessment is a first and important step in educating patients. Experienced nurses may know what they must teach and also what they would add for interested patients. However, a needs assessment provides two additional pieces of information. It tells the nurse what the patient already knows or thinks he or she knows and what the patient wants to know. Without this step, next steps may be ineffective or wasted. Misinformation and flawed understanding can only be righted if the nurse is aware of them. As with any learning, cancer patient education begins with building a fundamental knowledge base on the cancer and its treatment. If the basic understanding is wrong, the foundation for learning is faulty. For example, a common misconception is that metastatic breast cancer that has spread to the lung is now lung cancer. Another is that taking pain medication will lead to an addiction to it. This is especially problematic because pain interferes with a return to activity, which slows recovery—and thus, unrelieved pain slows recovery.

The needs assessment should explore understanding in addition to characteristics of the patient as learner. These are some questions to ask during a learning needs assessment:

- Can you tell me what you understand about your cancer and your cancer diagnosis, and its treatment?
- Are you someone who wants to know as much as possible, or would you say you only want to know what you need to know to take care of yourself?
- Do you have any physical limitations?
- Do you have any cultural or religious beliefs that I should know about to help give you the best care possible? For example, if you need to be on a special diet, are there foods you don't eat? Do you have religious beliefs that would prevent you from having transfusions? Do you need to pray at specific times during the day?
- Is there a learning style you prefer? For example, would you rather read about something or watch a video or DVD? Do you like learning in a one-on-one situation or in a class? (If no media exist, or no classes are given, the nurse should think about what it means to ask this question. It sets up an expectation that the nurse can provide it. On the other hand, a quick sketch or drawing can help the visual learner; a tape recorder can help the aural learner; informally gathering a group of patients with similar learning needs may help the person who wants to take part in a shared experience.)

The assessment should also include barriers that might have to be discovered by more subtle means than asking. For example, cognitive impairments may become obvious during a nursing assessment, but asking outright if someone has trouble thinking and understanding could be awkward. On the other hand, most patients will admit, "My memory isn't as good as it once was." Emotional states may or may not be obvious, but it is generally easier to ask a patient about anxiety, fear, depression, and sorrow than about impairments to cognition.

Findings from the learning needs assessment must be documented. This documentation tells other members of the health care team where they should start their teaching. It helps to eliminate duplication and to ensure that topics not covered at one time won't be neglected altogether. Reassessments are equally important. They establish what the patient remembers from an earlier teaching session and even more importantly, what the patient does not remember. The documentation, therefore, should include both topics covered by teaching and outcomes achieved, such as that the patient can state the common side effects of doxorubicin.

The Teaching Plan

GOALS AND OBJECTIVES

The nurse should develop a teaching plan that is based on the needs assessment and the nursing diagnosis. The first step is to identify a goal of the teaching. This can be short-term or long-term, but it is generally broad. For example, "Mr. Smith will learn how to manage his self-care needs" is an admirable (and necessary) goal. It provides the framework for the teaching, but it doesn't identify specifics, and therefore, it does not allow any evaluation. The objectives of teaching do each of those things. They state *who* will do *what*, and *when*. For example: "Before his discharge, Mr. Smith will select foods that are low in salt from a menu." The *who* (Mr. Smith) will do *what* (select foods low in salt) and *when* (before discharge) are spelled out. An objective always includes the *who, what,* and *when*. Only with concrete objectives is it possible to evaluate learning goals. Each goal is likely to have many objectives. Mr. Smith may need to learn about his diet, his activities, his medications, and any other self-care skills he needs during his recovery. These are all part of the broad goal of having him learn how to manage at home.

LEARNING THEORY

Experienced nurses may know intuitively what the theory is behind much of their teaching, but newer nurses should spend time thinking about why one approach might be more effective than another. Whole books are written on multiple and individual learning theories.[1-3] The interested nurse will benefit from reading classic textbooks and research that uses specific theories. However, for this chapter we will summarize five important theories, although there are many more.

The most common theory nurses use is cognitive. **Cognitive learning** theory describes what we cannot see, which in this case is what happens to the information when it enters the patient's mind.[4] Good teachers have techniques for gaining and keeping students' attention. They might tell a story or relate the teaching to something funny or surprising or memorable. They might engage the students' imagination. However they do it, they have a gift that makes learning easier. Exceptional nurse teachers have the same skills, and they also have the added advantage that most patients are motivated to understand their cancer or their cancer treatment or how to manage a side effect. Motivated patients are likely to be attentive patients, even when the teacher is inexperienced.

Cognitive learning starts when the teacher begins telling or showing. If the patient attends to the information, the information goes into the patient's short-term memory. What happens next is crucial. Some of it will be forgotten almost immediately, some will be forgotten within days, and some will, it is hoped, be encoded into long-term memory for retrieval when it is needed. A key to encoding is to provide the patient with a way to retrieve the information. Relating it to an experience the patient has already had, to something the patient already knows, to a mnemonic, or to a story are just some ways to help patients access information newly stored in long-term memory. Encouraging the patient to use the information or apply it helps make it familiar and of practical value. For example, if the teaching session concerns management of chemotherapy-related nausea, the nurse might ask the patient what foods she might avoid or eat to prevent or minimize the symptom. If the teaching is about preoperative preparation, the question might focus on what the patient might take instead of aspirin for pain. If the teaching is about radiation simulation, asking the patient to describe how he will manage when he has to lie still on the table for a long period will focus his thoughts on being prepared.

Behavioral learning is learning that can be observed by observing behaviors. The traditional example is Pavlov's dogs. In cancer care, one of the most common examples of behavioral learning is anticipatory nausea and vomiting that some patients experience on seeing their chemotherapy unit or even in driving to the clinic. Behavioral learning takes place when patients are taught to change dressings, when they use behavior modification to manage anxiety, and when they use distraction techniques to get through painful procedures. Nurses often shine in these situations, and many build a repertoire of tools they can teach patients to use.

Social learning is another important learning theory.[5,6] It posits that we learn by watching. Advertisements are often based on social learning. The famous basketball player wears name brand sneakers, so aspiring basketball players buy them. A glamorous actress eats a certain cereal; a commercial hopes the viewer thinks, "She looks so good; I'll eat the same cereal." For nurses, an application of social learning that is particularly effective is introducing a new patient to a patient who has successfully managed an ostomy or amputation or mastectomy. Reach-to-Recovery is a prime example. It is a powerful learning tool to see someone who is healthy, looks good, and is back at work.

Motivational learning is another important theory that nurses often use.[7] It can be intrinsic or extrinsic. Smokers may be encouraged to quit because they have young children and do not want to risk getting cancer. This motivation comes from within. Extrinsic motivation occurs when something beyond the patient's control exerts an influence. No smoking policies in the workplace may prod people into quitting. Cost hikes in a carton of cigarettes can motivate a smoker to quit. Motivational learning theory has many uses in cancer patient education, especially in encouraging compliance with difficult treatments.

A final theory, **adult learning theory**, describes the learner.[3,8] Adults are self-directed and independent. An eighth-grade teacher can exert pressure on her students to pay attention so they can pass a test and move into ninth grade. The nurse teacher has no such carrot with which to pressure his or her patients to learn what they do not want to learn. Rather, the nurse must somehow convince the patient to want to learn. Adults build on past experiences. Patients who have had a parent or friend die of cancer have that experience as a basis to anticipate their own journey with cancer. Adults are goal-oriented. They want to know what they need to do to realize a specific outcome. Finally, adults are motivated to learn by problem-solving needs.

Teaching Methods

ONE-ON-ONE

The nurse will do most of his or her teaching one-on-one at the point of service. It is practical, convenient, and efficient. Often, it is done informally during a procedure or other nursing activity, such as explaining side effects while hanging IV medications. Other times, it may be more formal, with the nurse concentrating just on teaching. One-on-one teaching has many advantages over other forms of teaching. One important one is the opportunity for eye contact (which is appropriate for Americans, though it may not be in some cultures). When the nurse is looking at a patient, she or he can pick up signs of confusion, boredom, disinterest, or engagement. This facilitates the nurse's ability to customize the teaching to the individual.

A puzzled expression should trigger the nurse to ask, at a minimum, if the patient has any questions. Ideally though, the nurse would explore what the patient might not have understood. For example, the nurse might say, "This is really complicated. Tell me what you understand so far so I can make sure I've been clear." It is always helpful to make the patient feel that it is the nurse's job to teach in a way that facilitates learning, rather than the onus being on the patient to understand. If the patient looks bored or tired, the nurse can respond in other ways. "I know this is difficult to understand, but you need to know how to care for the drain when you go home. Do you think you will be able to concentrate for a few more minutes?" "You look a little tired right now. I'm going to let you rest for a bit and come back later." "I know this has been a long morning for you, but we didn't get through all that you need to learn about the procedure you will have and the things you need to do beforehand. Would it be possible for me to call you tomorrow at home so we can review the rest?" The nurse could also suggest taking a quick break from that topic and talking about how the patient feels or something the patient likes to do (granted—this assumes the luxury of plenty of time, something that few nurses have). If the patient is engaged, asks questions, and tries to apply the learning, the nurse has a wonderful opportunity to provide comprehensive information and to give the patient additional resources for learning. "Do you have Internet access? www.nccn.org (the site of the National Comprehensive Cancer Network, or NCCN) has a really complete description of your cancer and all its treatment options."

Verbal teaching is often accompanied by demonstrations. The nurse uses the patient's drain, catheter, wound, and so on, to demonstrate its care. The patient returns the demonstration, either right away or during a subsequent teaching session. Sometimes, the demonstration uses drawings or models.

Limited English Proficiency and Teaching. An increasingly common dilemma in all of health care is the patient with limited English proficiency (LEP). If the nurse does not speak the patient's language, one-on-one teaching becomes complicated. The ideal solution is having access to a professional translator who is knowledgeable about the patient's culture and is conversant with medical and oncologic terminology. This situation exists in very few institutions. Some institutions have a volunteer translator staff, and many others use telephone services such as the AT&T language hotline. When none of these resources is available, nurses enlist other staff, who may or may not be nurses, or family members accompanying the patient. Whatever the solution, nurses using anything other than the experienced and culturally competent translator should be aware of potential problems. Just as a patient may misunderstand what the nurse explains, so may the translator, especially if that person does not have medical knowledge. The translator may impart his or her own understanding, and prejudices or personal concerns could creep into explanations. For example, a translator who believes that a patient needs rest after surgery may not emphasize the importance of having the patient get out of bed and walk. A translator may feel so sympathetic with a patient's situation that she or he does not accurately translate bad news. It is always in the nurse's and the patient's best interests to confirm the message the translator translates.

GROUP TEACHING

When several patients are scheduled to have the same procedure or begin chemotherapy or radiation therapy, it is very efficient to teach a group. Group teaching requires fewer person hours, and a single nurse can accomplish the goals of many, compared to one-on-one teaching. If members of the group actively participate, group dynamics can make the teaching more interesting, pertinent, and lively. One patient's questions may help another to recognize that she, too, wants to know the answer but would have forgotten to ask. Another patient's personal story may make the instructions more real. For example, a patient might have had a complication from surgery and may emphasize to the group how important coughing is, or getting adequate pain relief, or paying close attention to drainage from a wound.

PRINT MATERIALS

Most nurses have access to print materials to support their teaching. These can be purchased, obtained free from various organizations and the National Cancer Institute (NCI), or produced in-house. They can be as simple as a 1-page fact sheet or as comprehensive as a 50-page booklet. Print materials are especially useful as supplements to verbal instruction. Since patients are unlikely to remember everything a nurse tells them, a booklet or fact card serves as a reference and reminder. These can be even more effective teaching tools if the nurse personalizes them by highlighting or marking important sections or making notations that apply to the individual patient.

Literacy. An issue that has been gaining attention is literacy. Of adult Americans, 43% scored at a basic or below-basic level on prose literacy (which would be the type needed to understand patient education booklets) in the recent National Assessment of Adult Literacy survey.[9] The survey, based on 19,000 adults representing adults ages 16 years and older in the United States, found that 14% had below-basic reading skills (meaning they had very limited skills), and 29% were at the basic level, meaning they could do everyday literary activities such as reading bus schedules or signs. Another 44% were at the intermediate level, and 13% were proficient. These data are essentially unchanged from the 1992 data on the National Adult Literacy Survey.[10] Most studies done to assess patients' reading levels have taken place as part of a research study in hospitals or clinics serving low socioeconomic patients or patients who are on Medicare.[11,12] Results reflect the aims and methods of each study, making them somewhat difficult to interpret. Initially, studies reported words such as "randomly," "systemically," "emesis," and "voided" that the typical patient could not understand.[13,14] Later studies reported what a patient could or could not do, such as following medication instructions after reading a piece of text.[15] The common theme of all studies is that low literacy increases the risk for poor health and poor health outcomes.[16,17]

Literacy assessment tools. A variety of assessment tools can be used to assess a patient's literacy level. Some test pronunciation only, and others, comprehension. The REALM-R is a word recognition test.[17] It correlates well with other assessments, including the TOFLA, but it does not confirm comprehension. A much-used comprehension assessment is the TOFHLA (Test of Functional Health Literacy in Adults).[18-20] It uses a cloze technique, which eliminates every fifth or sixth word and has the reader pick the missing word from a list. A new test, specific for cancer patients, is the SIRACT.[21] This informal reading inventory has one-page texts on cancer topics written at specific grade levels. Each has five questions following the passage, the answers to which are found in the passage. It is currently being used in a clinical trial, and only preliminary data are available.

Some researchers advise testing all patients, and others believe it should only be done in a research setting.[22] Many now agree that a baseline should be established for a clinic or hospital, and that all print materials should be at a particular level based on baseline results. Whether a baseline is established or not, the nurse should understand that it isn't possible to know how well people read by talking to them.[23] Poor readers may say they left their glasses at home or they would prefer to read the material later, but highly literate people may also forget their glasses or prefer to read materials in the privacy of their homes. Although poor readers are more likely to be older, poorer, and less educated, that generalization cannot and should not be applied to any individual. It is simply not possible to tell how well anyone understands print materials except by testing. To be cautious, nurses should assume that patients read four grade levels below the last grade of school completed. However, they should also understand that people who have not finished eighth grade may read at a college level, and those with a college education may read at a basic level only.[22] If the content in the text is important to the patient's understanding of critical concepts, the patient should be asked to describe in his or her own words the key points in print materials that supplement teaching.

Readability. A related issue is the readability of print materials. Only recently have the NCI and the American Cancer Society (ACS) become proactive in creating print materials at sixth-grade levels. Much of what is currently available, whether it is hospital-produced or it comes from a patient advocacy group, is written at or above a ninth-grade level.[24-26] At the very least, nurses should know how well patients have to read to understand the materials they give out. Two methods of assessing readability can be done with pencil and paper. The SMOG is a well-respected, quick, and simple estimation of readability based on the number of polysyllabic (three or more syllables) words in 10-sentence samples drawn from the beginning, the middle, and the end of the booklet.[27] Many sites on the Internet, easily found by searching on the keyword *SMOG readability*, provide formulas and conversion tables to calculate the reading grade level according to SMOG.

The Fry formula is another widely accepted means of measuring readability, which is also easily accessed by searching the Internet (keyword: *Fry readability*).[27] For this method, the average number of sentences and the average number of syllables in three 100-word passages are plotted on a graph.

Although the SMOG, the Fry or some similar assessment tool is necessary for materials not developed within the nurse's institution (or for which a Microsoft Word version is not available), the easiest and fastest solution to determining the readability of a Microsoft Word document is to use the Flesch-Kincaid tool found in the tools menu of Microsoft Word. Under "Options" and then "Spelling and Grammar," select "Check grammar with spelling" and "Show readability statistics." After running a spelling and grammar check of the document, a summary of various statistics will pop up, including the Flesch reading ease score, the Flesch-Kincaid grade level and the percentage of sentences using the passive voice.

One caveat for readability is that it is not exact. Each formula will give slightly (sometimes highly) different results.[28] What is considered an eighth-grade level according to one may come out as a seventh- or ninth-grade level using another. Nevertheless, the formulas provide a much better idea of the reading level than even an expert would predict by merely reading a passage.

However, after a patient has read a booklet, the committed educator should actively engage him or her in a discussion of its key points. Even a well-written booklet with a sixth-grade reading level may be confusing to someone who is unfamiliar with the content.

MEDIA

Video. If video is available, it is an extremely useful and well-received tool in patient education. Most patients love videos. Many manufacturing companies produce videos for their products (e.g., catheters, drains, inhalers), pharmaceutical companies may do videos on drugs such as low-molecular-weight heparin, and advocacy groups do them on support issues. Comprehensive and clinical cancer centers frequently have overview videos for topics such as chemotherapy or radiation therapy. Many are willing to sell them at cost or at a reasonable rate.

It is also possible to produce a video, even for nurses with no personal experience in the field. When a topic is identified, and research confirms that a video on the topic is not available, the nurse would begin by doing an outline on *what* has to be covered. The next step is to determine *how* the topic will be covered. Will it be visually demonstrated—for example, step-by-step dressing change? Will it be a series of "sound bites" from people who have been satisfied with a particular treatment? Will it be a "talking head" describing treatment options? Or, will it be a story of a journey, or an orientation, or perhaps an explanation of how to prepare for ___ (your choice)? The next step is to determine a price range that is within the patient education budget and contact a script writer and a production company. (Some production companies can do both.) Some hospitals have in-house video departments, but most do not. Any independent company should provide demo tapes for review. This makes it easier for nurses to know whether they think the company will produce a video that will meet their patients' needs. When the company has been selected, the nurse then works with them, beginning with the outline and the nurse's idea of the kind of video that is needed. The company can then easily orchestrate all remaining steps. An important piece of advice from experienced producers is to build in money in the budget for professional talent. Nurses may demonstrate techniques or explain concepts (briefly), but nursing skills do not often include acting in front of a camera.

CD-ROM. Many in-house facilities can now produce CD-ROMs, and many programs on cancer are available commercially. Producing a CD-ROM is a bit more complicated than doing a video, but it can be done, even by a novice, as long as help is available. It is still not common for the older cancer patient to be highly computer-literate, which makes navigation the most critical element in the design. It can be as simple as back and forward buttons, or it can have multiple paths to more information. Whatever the depth of content and number of choices a user can make, it is important to make it easy to get back to a central point without having to "go back" 10 screens. If help is not available within a hospital, and a budget will not support a commercial producer, a local college may have a computer programming department whose students may be willing to donate time and effort to have a product for their portfolio.

DVD. DVDs combine techniques used in CD-ROMs and video. They allow the user to go directly to a desired topic (track). They may replace both the video and CD-ROM in the future. A video can be copied or converted to a DVD format with direction from the nurse on titles for specific tracks.

The Internet. The Internet is an amazing source of information for those who know how to search and who understand the pitfalls of trying to find "the right answer."[29] Nurses can help their patients by providing web addresses to reliable sites. These include *www.cancer.gov, www.cancer.org*, and *www.nccn.org*, various well known advocacy sites such as *www.leukemia.org*, and medical organizations such as *www.asco.org*. Patients and their families should be told that much misinformation is on the Web, and they should become grounded in the basics about their cancer before surfing independently. If they begin to use a search engine, they should look at the author (is it someone trying to sell something, or is it a recognized cancer center or university?) and the date the information was posted (it may be out of date). Some sites will have references supporting the information. Patients should be told that any site that provides information that is contrary to that found in other sites should be viewed with suspicion.

Organizing the Teaching

Perhaps the most important thing for nurses to consider when planning their teaching is to look at the topics that "should" be covered at particular times, consider what is realistically possible, and then determine how to cover the rest. Using a prostatectomy as an example, nurses instruct patients on when to stop taking aspirin and nonsteroidal antiinflammatory drugs (NSAIDs), herbal remedies that might interfere with surgery, preadmission testing, what the patient must do to prepare for surgery including bowel preparation, the actual surgical procedure including the possibility that it would not proceed if cancer is found outside the gland, the possibility of permanent impotence and temporary incontinence, control of pain following surgery, expectations for activities after surgery (e.g., coughing and deep breathing and exercise), and psychosocial services that are available. Logically, it would be difficult for even an eager and motivated patient to retain all of this information, especially given that many nurses will have only 30 minutes to do the teaching. What is the solution? There is no single best solution, but trying to cover all of it at one time is likely to fail.

One approach the nurse might take is to think about what the patient needs to know for his safety: stopping aspirin and NSAIDs, eliminating any herbal remedies that can interfere with platelet function or anesthesia, and bowel preparation. She or he might then consider what the patient should know about the surgery and its impact on the patient's physical functioning: normal anatomy, what will be removed, possible impotence, temporary incontinence, and short- and long-term solutions to these side effects. (If these are things about which the patient has no knowledge, they clearly take on the status of need-to-know, not for safety, but for informed decision making.) Finally the nurse should consider all of the nice-to-know information: where the patient's family should wait to speak with the surgeon, how pain will be managed, and what the patient should expect in terms of progress each hospital day and returning to work or usual activities.

The need-to-know topics must, absolutely, be covered, and the nurse should have a plan on how and when she or he will do so. They might come first or last, but should probably not come in the middle of the teaching session. They should be reinforced with print material, and the nurse should highlight their importance. Bowel preparation, especially, should be organized in a logical progression. "Two days before surgery, start...." On the other hand, if the nurse finds that the patient does not use aspirin or NSAIDs and never takes herbal remedies, this teaching is no longer as important. "Since you never take aspirin, I don't need to review all of the medicines that have aspirin, but please remember that if you have a headache, take an acetaminophen product such as Tylenol."

The bulk of the teaching is on the surgery and what will happen afterwards. The surgeon will have explained much of it already, so the nurse's task is primarily review. The needs assessment will establish what the patient already knows and understands. Since patients are likely to be most interested in these topics, it will be easier to hold the patient's attention. Although not all topics will have to be covered in the same detail for each man—for example, options for treating impotence may not be of interest if a man is not sexually active or has no partner—the nurse cannot assume that she or he can independently make a decision about what will be important to the patient. The nurse might present a list of topics and ask the patient to prioritize. Whatever is not covered during the teaching session can then be the subject of assigned reading in the days before the operation. This gives the patient a chance to digest new information slowly and call with questions.

Finally, the nurse can choose which nice-to-know information to explain verbally and point out where to read the rest. The nurse might prioritize the patient's reading list. "It's important for you to know what resources you can call on in the days after surgery. This card describes the services we can offer you." "There are several options for you if you remain impotent even after nerve-sparing surgery. You can read about them in this booklet."

Most nurses begin at the beginning: for example, this is what you have, this is how you'll be treated, and this is what it feels like or what you can expect. Some use brief explanations, and some go more in-depth. Most have their own styles, which they have developed with trial and error. No matter what their style, nurses should keep the learning needs assessment in mind when beginning a teaching session. Teaching should start at a point where the patient has some knowledge. For example, a patient may know only that he has prostate cancer. He may not have a clear understanding of where the prostate is located and thus, may not know to be concerned about or even ask about side effects of treatment. It is simple enough to show the patient a diagram and begin the teaching for surgery by pointing out the nearby anatomy. Another reasonable approach is to begin the teaching by asking what the patient's key questions are. Adults are goal directed and will readily engage in teaching that addresses their concerns. These teachable moments should never be wasted. A question or problem is the perfect opening to a teachable moment.

When the patient's concerns have been addressed, the nurse can then go back and finish teaching the remaining information by reestablishing the framework and filling in the missing pieces. "We've talked about the things that most concern you, so now let's go back and talk about how you do the bowel preparation and the things you will need to do after the operation is over to reduce the chance of complications."

Whether the teaching flows from an answer to a question or from an overview of a treatment, it should be organized in a way that makes it easy for the patient to remember. Teaching that skips around will not allow the patient to set up a storing mechanism in long-term memory that serves to retrieve the information later.

A patient may have all the letters for a word, but if she or he doesn't know how to arrange the letters, they are meaningless. Just as we need a telephone book to access many phone numbers, patients need some mechanism that lets them "look up" new information. This is often based on logic, one building block after another. Without an organizing structure, new information is likely to be lost to long-term memory. For example, in preparing a patient for a procedure, the nurse might briefly review the purpose of the procedure and how it will help in the patient's care. She or he might then say, "Let me describe what you might feel during the procedure so you will know what to expect." This anchors the teaching with something the patient is likely to want to know.

Evaluation

Any teaching that involves critical decision making, patient safety, and important quality of life issues should be evaluated to make sure the patient understood the information. Most people require practice and reinforcement before new information becomes learned information. Students read textbooks, take notes in class, and use, write about, memorize, or discuss before they are tested. Patients, on the other hand, may have only a 30-minute session with the nurse, who must cover simulation for radiation therapy, a description of what it will be like to have the radiation, the schedule for status checks, side effects and their management, and so on. Logically, the patient is not going to remember everything. It is therefore the nurse's responsibility to ensure that the patient has retained the critical pieces or has supplemental material to which to refer. There are many ways to do this, but the *least* effective may be the most common, namely, the "Do you have any questions?" approach. This is not evaluation.

The nurse should devise a strategy to ensure that the patient does, in fact, understand. One technique is to ask the patient to explain in his or her own words what the nurse has reviewed. This may be uncomfortable at first, but if it's done with some kind of explanation that makes it clear the nurse is just making absolutely sure the patient has the information, most patients will not be offended. For example, the nurse might say, "I've given you a lot of information and sometimes I forget something and I may not be as clear as I think I am. Can you tell me in your own words what I've just told you? That way I can pick up anything I've left out."

Practice and return demonstrations are very important when the patient is learning a skill. As a patient goes through the process of self-injecting or changing a dressing, the nurse can provide helpful hints that might make it easier for the patient to remember specific steps later. For example, the nurse might say, "Bubbles are fine in champagne or carbonated water, but not in a syringe. Always remember to check for air before you inject the medicine." Food choices can be used to see if a patient understands the concept of low-salt foods or clear liquids. Patients can be asked to select a food from a list or describe what foods they would or would not purchase in a grocery store or restaurant.

Engaging the patient in discussion can also alert the nurse to misunderstandings. For example, the nurse might ask if the patient has ever had a similar procedure or has ever had to make a difficult choice and then use that to engage in a pros and cons discussion.

Documentation

All nurses know that if it isn't recorded, it wasn't done. However, that is a risk management issue. A patient educator is also interested in what has been covered in prior teaching sessions, what knowledge the patient has already demonstrated, and what the patient has had trouble understanding. Documentation refreshes a nurse's memory when seeing a patient days or weeks later, and it informs another nurse of what has been covered and what the patient can state, demonstrate, explain, describe, identify, and so on. Documentation of patient education should be succinct and should describe what the patient is able to do after the teaching session. Action verbs are important if the patient has demonstrated learning. If not, it is equally important to document what the patient cannot do. Finally, problem areas should be identified, such as "Mrs. Smith forgets to maintain sterile technique when drawing up her medication." Documentation is the basis for ongoing evaluation of learning. Table 33-1 has examples of some objectives of teaching and examples of documentation of some possible outcomes.

Family Education

Patients' families may have similar and overlapping learning needs, but they may also have very different needs. Family members may want more information, may need more direction if they will add a care-taking role to their other roles, or may

simply have different concerns. Often, a patient's family sits in during consultations with the doctor or nurse. In this case, the nurse may assume the patient approves of the family member having information. On occasion, a family member may call and ask the nurse about the patient or some part of the patient's care. In this case, HIPAA privacy rules must be enforced, and the nurse may not provide any information without the patient's knowledge and permission. More information is available on the USDHSS Web page under HIPAA, at *www.hhs.gov/ocr/hipaa*. It is wise to confirm with the patient the names and relationships of people who can ask for and be given information. It might also be wise to confirm with the patient any limitations on the type of information that can be given to family members.

After HIPAA concerns are addressed, the nurse can address the family's educational needs. Given that time is finite and the nurse's primary responsibility is the *patient's* learning, the nurse need not do a formal needs assessment for family members. Rather, she or he should answer their questions and make eye contact from time to time during a teaching session aimed at the patient to be sure that they are following along. If the family member will be doing any part of the home care, the nurse should

TABLE 33-1	Learning Objectives and Possible Outcomes	
LEARNING OBJECTIVE	**POSSIBLE OUTCOMES**
The patient and/or care partner is able to	
1. Describe the purpose of the prescribed treatment.	a. Ms. Smith states that her treatment might slow the progression of the cancer. b. Ms. Smith states that the treatment is designed to cure the cancer. c. Ms. Smith cannot describe the purpose of the treatment. She states, "I'm not sure; it's what the doctor wants me to do." The doctor has been informed of this.
2. List the drugs she will receive.	a. Ms. Smith identifies her chemotherapy drugs including which she will get by intravenous route in clinic and which she will take by mouth at home. b. Ms. Smith is not able to name her chemotherapy drugs, but states that she will get three different ones by vein. The nurse reinforced the names and highlighted them on the fact cards.
3. List the most common side effects of treatment.	a. Ms. Smith can recall four side effects: nausea and vomiting, low white blood cell count, mouth sores, and redness of the skin. She cannot name any other side effects. She was given fact cards with all side effects and asked to keep them in a place where she could review them if she developed any symptoms that she did not expect. b. Ms. Smith cannot describe any side effects, but states that she knows they are listed on the fact cards, which she will keep in her medical file.
4. List the supportive care medications to manage side effects while undergoing treatment.	a. Ms. Smith correctly described how to take Imodium if she has diarrhea beginning the day after treatment. b. Ms. Smith relates that she knows to take her antiemetic medicine before she comes in for her chemotherapy. c. Ms. Smith correctly demonstrates how to inject herself with granulocyte colony-stimulating factor.
5. State the reasons for contacting the physician or the nurse.	a. Ms. Smith lists the five reasons to call the doctor or nurse: fever ≥100.5° F; diarrhea; black stools or any sign of bleeding; pain, redness, swelling, or blistering near the injection site; and mouth sores. b. Ms. Smith cannot identify the reasons to call the doctor. Nurse gave her the fact cards and highlighted the reasons to call the doctor section. Nurse will reinforce these with her at her next visit. c. Ms. Smith cannot identify the reasons to call the doctor. Nurse reviewed them with her daughter who was with her during the teaching session. The daughter stated that she would make sure to watch for any of these side effects.

teach and document just as she or he does with the patient. Informed caregivers are an important part of the team.

Ethical Considerations

On occasion, nurses must deal with ethical issues having to do with patient education. Some examples involve informed consent for clinical trials, noncompliance with instructions, cultural conflicts, and family disagreements. Most pediatric cancer patients and some adult cancer patients go on clinical trials. All are given an informed consent to read in addition to having discussions with their doctor or the trial's principal investigator. The consent may be written at a very high reading level, the amount of information it contains may be overwhelming, and the concepts described may be medically sophisticated. Following an informed consent consultation, it may be the nurse who reviews what will happen. During the discussion, the nurse may realize that the patient really does not understand the protocol, even though she or he signed the consent. What is the nurse's responsibility? She or he must alert the physician and ideally, have the patient reeducated and consent regiven, if only verbally. This is easy to advise, but may be difficult to do for a variety of reasons. Patients may not understand what they do not understand; they may need to believe that drugs on a phase I trial will cure them; and they may simply say, "I'll do whatever the doctor advises, so I don't need more information." This makes it awkward for the nurse to know how to proceed. However, clarifying misunderstanding and alerting the physician about the misunderstanding is the only ethical response possible.

Another dilemma is how to respond with the noncompliant patient. Here, nurses must first examine their teaching and the patient's understanding of the teaching. Is the problem that the patient does not understand how a treatment works and why compliance is important? Here is a prime example of the need for a reassessment of learning needs. If noncompliance is based on a lack of understanding of the "why" something is needed or "how" it works, reeducation may solve the problem. If the noncompliance is for reasons other than lack of understanding, then motivation may be the culprit. Are the side effects intolerable? Is there a way to help the patient manage, physically and cognitively? If the nurse determines that the patient has the knowledge needed to understand why compliance is important, but still is not compliant, the nurse must then explain what noncompliance will mean to the success of the test or treatment, report it to the patient's physician, document what the patient knows and the stated reasons for noncompliance, and finally, respect the patient's autonomy.

Some nurses will face cultural conflicts with patients from different ethnic backgrounds or with unfamiliar religious beliefs and practices. Madeleine M. Leininger's huge body of work on transcultural nursing is the ideal starting place to learn about these issues.[30,31] Accommodating some cultural beliefs and behaviors is easy, such as making sure Orthodox Jews and Muslims do not have pork on their dinner plate; whereas others are more difficult, such as allowing gypsies to place a sprinkling of dirt on bed linens. Some cultures reward those who boldly advocate for themselves or family members; others reward those who are quiet and reserved. The demanding patient or family member may be from a culture that expects the family to push aggressively for services, whereas members of another culture might not speak up even when it is important to do so, such as for pain management. Culturally competent care takes many forms: from physical care,

to respect for a patient's religious needs, to involvement in decisions. In some cultures, decisions are made by the patient; in others they may be made by the entire family, the elders in the family, or the older dominant male. The nurse should understand, respect, and work with the patient's cultural beliefs even though she or he may not share them. Nurses should ask patients about specific beliefs, practices, and customs that may be relevant and important during nursing care and hospitalization.

Unfortunately, it may be impossible to go through a cancer nursing career without experiencing a family controversy. Conflict may arise even in healthy and loving families, but cancer issues can definitely exacerbate strained relationships. The nurse must be a sensitive, diplomatic, and respectful advocate for his or her patient. Family quarrels may impede teaching, and they can imperil a patient's recovery, mood, energy, and quality of life. At the first sign of problems that interfere with a nurse's effort to provide instructions for the patient's well-being, the nurse would do well to garner support from peers, managers, and the patient advocate's office. At times, the nurse may be in a position to broker a resolution by pointing out the negative impact quarreling can have on the patient. On occasion, however, a hospital's ethics committee may have to be consulted.

Considerations for Older Adults

Cancer is a disease primarily of the older adult, and it is the leading cause of death in those aged 60 years and older.[32] The U.S. Census Bureau projects that 1 out of 5 Americans in 2030 will be age 65 or older.[33] Seniors are more likely than middle-aged adults to have physical and cognitive limitations, have comorbidities, be frail or have frail caregivers, and have financial needs. These can all be a challenge for the nurse who provides instructions, explanations, and skill-building sessions. However, it is important to remember that the old (65 years old and above) are a heterogeneous group. There is a wide variance in their abilities and independence. The fortunate nurse will find a geriatric assessment on the patient's medical chart, and this should serve as a basis on which to do a learning needs assessment. For example, comorbidities may increase the risk of adverse outcomes from surgery or chemotherapy. Functional dependence should alert the nurse to assess the patient's ability to get help when needed, to take medications properly, or to understand when to call the doctor. It is also important to assess financial and insurance status. Fixed income and lack of insurance can make it more difficult for patients to take advantage of costly treatments that may prolong life and improve quality of life. Finally, social support may be critical to the success of the teaching sessions; an older patient may need help to successfully complete a treatment regimen.

Normal aging reduces visual acuity, but aging is also associated with macular degeneration, glaucoma, and cataracts. Even people who stay current with ophthalmic care and have good glasses may need reading material to be printed in larger font sizes as they age. However, few patient education materials come in large font sizes. Hearing loss may or may not be recognized. The hard of hearing who use hearing devices may be able to hear easily in one-on-one conversations, but less well when background noise intrudes. Some elders do not recognize or acknowledge any difficulty with hearing. This can result in lots of repetition for the nurse, or in the patient pretending to hear while simply tuning out. Arthritis and frailty can interfere with physical skills that may be important for self-care. An additional problem is the high risk for a decline in activities of daily living with hospitalized older patients.[34] These and additional physical limitations, perhaps caused by a cancer treatment or a comorbidity, necessitate creativity, skill, and patience on the nurse's part.

The first step is a thorough assessment of physical and cognitive abilities. Does the patient have physical limitations that will make self-care difficult? Is she forgetful? Does he have impaired decision-making skills? Is she motivated to understand her treatment plan? Based on this assessment, the nurse must individualize a teaching plan that encompasses strategies to minimize barriers to teaching and learning and maximize the patient's abilities and skills. The second step is to make sure the patient understands and agrees with the goal of teaching.[34] Although this is true for teaching any age, the goals may be implicit with younger patients. However, they must be addressed directly with the older patient.

Perhaps the first teaching session for a senior who is hospitalized, and even for an older ambulatory patient who is living and functioning independently, is to make sure the patient understands the relationship between mobility and functional decline. Older patients may be less inclined than younger ones to walk or exercise, especially if they experience side effects such as pain or nausea and vomiting. In this group, good antiemetic and pain management is essential to keep them active. Patients who have low mobility levels are at high risk of adverse outcomes and a decline in activities of daily living, and nurses should include it as part of their cancer care teaching.[35]

Older patients have a wealth of life experiences on which a nurse can build. The nurse should explore a patient's past experiences that may be pertinent to learning new information related to the cancer. The nurse should try to make them relevant and use them as stepping stones to reach a specific objective. For example, many older patients will have had side effects from medications. A discussion of those outcomes can be used to help the patient understand the importance of reporting new symptoms. The patient might be a cook or have other hobbies that can be used as a bridge to understanding. "Do you ever use cornstarch to thicken sauces? You know that you can't put it directly into a hot liquid. It just clumps and doesn't thicken the liquid. If you take this pill with food, it won't work either. In order for it to work properly, you must take it on an empty stomach."

Teaching sessions may have to be broken down into multiple parts, with more repetition. It is important to provide quiet and private space for teaching seniors. Distractions may be even more of a problem for this age group than for younger patients. Confirm that the patient can read the print in any booklets or fact sheets. Use reminder aids, such as compartmental weekly medicine containers, refrigerator checklist magnets, telephone calls from family or friends, log sheets, and patient journals. Have the patient repeat instructions and practice skills over and over. Try to incorporate instructions into a patient's daily routines, since it may be difficult to convince an elder to change behaviors or establish new routines. Involve significant others if necessary.

REVIEW QUESTIONS

✓ Case Study

Mr. Mendez is a 72-year-old male diagnosed with colorectal cancer in June 2005. He completed 6 cycles of chemotherapy and then underwent a restaging CT scan. It indicated that he had metastatic disease. In hearing this news the patient became angry and asked how this could happen to him. The physician gently reminded him that there was always the chance that the treatment would not work, but that a new treatment could be effective. The nurse then met with him to review the side effects and treatment schedule.

The patient exhibited signs of high anxiety. He continually asked why this was happening to him. The nurse let him talk, and then reinforced the doctor's explanation that the new treatment has been effective in some patients and acknowledged the importance of hope. She then said his new chemotherapy would be different from the first one and would have different side effects that he needed to know about. She asked if he had specific questions about the new treatment he would be starting, and if they could talk about what he should expect and look for. She also asked if he knew anything about the new chemotherapy, or if he remembered what the doctor had told him. Mr. Mendez could not remember what the doctor had told him about the new chemotherapy, and the nurse realized after telling him about the new drugs that he did not remember anything she had said. She pointed out that she was sure it would be hard for him to remember the side effects because he was thinking about the bad news and was not able to concentrate. She gave him a side effects sheet as a reference for use at home

and highlighted the important information on it. She then asked what he understood about the diarrhea he was likely to experience. The patient replied "All I need is some Imodium to control the diarrhea, and if it should happen, I can skip my next treatment." The nurse then recognized that he did not understand the importance of taking Imodium, and might, therefore, be noncompliant with her instructions. She elected not to reinforce her instructions, because Mr. Mendez was not receptive at that time. Instead, she asked if she could call him on the day after his treatment to see how he was doing and discuss what he should do if he was experiencing side effects.

Mr. Mendez had come alone to his appointment. He did not want his family involved immediately. He felt it was his problem, and they did not need to know anything more. He said he would discuss it with his family when he felt ready. The nurse offered several reasons for him to involve the family, such as support with side effects management, their need to feel that they can help, and their need to feel included. Mr. Mendez repeated his intent to inform them only when he felt ready.

The nurse phoned Mr. Mendez the day after treatment and asked about diarrhea. Mr. Mendez said he had had several loose and watery stools, but it was no big deal. He said he did not want to take "another pill." The nurse asked if he was feeling light-headed, dizzy, or weak. He denied having any of these symptoms. The nurse then suggested that if he had any further episodes of diarrhea, he should call her, so she could make sure it would be safe for him not to take the Imodium. He agreed that he would call her.

Continued

REVIEW QUESTIONS—CONT'D

QUESTIONS

1. In assessing Mr. Mendez's readiness to learn, what should the nurse ask?
   a. About side effects associated with his previous chemotherapy
   b. What coping skills he used previously in adapting to treatment
   c. How willing he is to undergo a new chemotherapy regimen
   d. What he wants to know about the new chemotherapy

2. What should the nurse have done when she realized Mr. Mendez did not remember anything she said?
   a. Repeat her teaching.
   b. Talk louder.
   c. Give him print materials, highlight important sections, and arrange to continue the teaching on the phone in 24 hours.
   d. Ask Mr. Mendez if she could give the instructions to a family member.

3. If a patient does not want to learn, what is the first thing a nurse should do?
   a. Explain why the topic is important.
   b. Report it to the doctor.
   c. Enlist the aid of the family.
   d. Respect the patient's right not to learn.

4. A nurse might use behavioral learning theory to accomplish which of the following?
   a. Explain the side effects of a drug.
   b. Discuss various smoking cessation aids.
   c. Help prepare a patient for a painful procedure.
   d. Counter a patient's fear of having an ostomy.

5. Which of the following describes likely characteristics of adult learners?
   a. Need a lot of repetition
   b. Are dependent on the nurse
   c. Need extra time to learn new skills compared to young adults
   d. Are self-directed and problem oriented

6. Which of the following is used in the best approach to teaching patients with limited English proficiency?
   a. Family members who speak English because they know the patient
   b. A culturally competent professional translator who understands oncologic terminology
   c. The AT&T language hotline, because the operators can quickly identify the patient's language or dialect
   d. A nursing peer because she or he understands cancer-related information

7. A person with basic literacy skills can read which of the following?
   a. Only things like signs or a train schedule
   b. Simple prose text
   c. An eighth-grade textbook, unless it is on science
   d. Most novels that are 200 pages long or less

8. Which of the following is true of patients who do not read well?
   a. They may be embarrassed, but will always tell the nurse.
   b. They often say they have left their glasses at home.
   c. They always bring a relative or friend who can read.
   d. They will have difficulty learning even when the teaching is verbal.

9. What should the nurse always do when beginning a teaching session?
   a. Begin at a basic level.
   b. Assume the patient has some knowledge.
   c. Ask if the patient has questions.
   d. First review the learning needs assessment.

10. When teaching older adults, what should the nurse do?
   a. Assume the patient will have comorbidities that will make learning difficult.
   b. Make sure the patient understands the goals of teaching.
   c. Assume the patient will be compliant.
   d. Speak loudly and slowly.

ANSWERS

1. **D.** *Rationale:* Ascertaining what the patient wants to know about the new chemotherapy is one of the steps in a learning needs assessment. Having side effects is not in and of itself a patient education issue; it's how to manage them that is an educational issue. Coping skills used previously in adapting to treatment and how willing he is to undergo a new chemotherapy regimen could be related to education, but (d) is the better answer.

2. **C.** *Rationale:* It's better to allow the patient time to read over print materials and come back to the teaching at another session. Repeating the teaching to a resistant patient is likely to be a waste of time. Talking louder does not address nonlearning, except if the patient is hard of hearing. Mr. Mendez clearly did not want to involve his family.

3. **A.** *Rationale:* Explaining why the topic is important might help the patient recognize what is at stake. It may be necessary to report it to the doctor later, but not as a first step. Respecting the patient's right not to learn would be the last step, and enlisting the aid of the family might be a HIPAA infringement if the patient did not want the family involved.

4. **C.** *Rationale:* Helping to prepare a patient for a painful procedure is an area where behavioral learning theory comes into play, because patients actually do something to cope with the discomfort. Cognitive learning theory would be better to explain the side effects of a drug; whereas to discuss various smoking cessation aids, motivational theory is likely a better approach; and to counter a patient's fear of having an ostomy, social learning theory is a better approach.

5. **D.** *Rationale:* Being self-directed and problem oriented describes one of the attributes of adult learners. The need for repetition, dependence on the nurse, and the need for extra time to learn new skills compared to young adults may apply to an individual, but not to a group.

6. **B.** *Rationale:* A culturally competent professional translator who understands oncologic terminology is the best resource in teaching patients with limited English proficiency. The other choices are all secondary and inferior solutions. Using family members who speak English is the least acceptable solution, because the nurse cannot know what the family member is actually telling the patient.

7. **B.** *Rationale:* A person with basic literacy skills can read simple prose text, according to the National Assessment of Adult Literacy descriptions of the skills of below-basic, basic, and intermediate readers. The ability to read only things like signs or a train schedule describes a person with below-basic skills, and eighth-grade textbooks and 200-page novels fall within the range of intermediate-level readers.

8. **B.** *Rationale:* Patients who do not read well often say they have left their glasses at home. Patients will rarely admit they cannot read. Some will, and some will not, bring someone with them (but that person may not know the patient cannot read); and poor reading skills may have nothing to do with learning ability or intelligence.

9. **D.** *Rationale:* It is best to first review the learning needs assessment, because it will tell the nurse what the patient already knows and what the patient wants to learn. It is invalid to assume that the patient has either some knowledge (b) or no knowledge (a). It might be good to begin the actual teaching by asking if the patient has questions, *after* first reviewing the learning needs assessment.

10. **B.** *Rationale:* Making sure the patient understands the goals of teaching is a key in getting someone to focus on the teaching. The other answers imply assumptions that may or may not be valid.

REFERENCES

1. Bigge ML, Shermis SS: *Learning theories for teachers,* ed 6, Upper Saddle River, NJ, 2004, Allyn & Bacon.
2. Hergenhan BR, Olson MH: *Introduction to the theories of learning,* ed 7, Upper Saddle River, NJ, 2005, Prentice Hall.
3. Merriam SB: *The new update on adult learning theory: new directions for adult and continuing education,* San Francisco, 2001, Jossey-Bass.
4. Flannery DD: *Applying cognitive learning theory to adult learning: new directions for adult and continuing education,* San Francisco, 1993, Jossey-Bass.
5. Bandura A: Social cognitive theory: An agentic perspective, *Ann Rev Psychol* 52:1-26, 2001.
6. Bahn D: Social learning theory: its application in the context of nursing education, *Nurse Ed Today* 21:110-117, 2001.
7. Volet S, Jarvela S: *Motivation in learning contexts: theoretical advances and methodological implications,* Elmsford, NY, 2001, Pergamon Press.
8. Knowles MS: *The modern practice of adult education: andragogy vs. pedagogy,* New York, 1970, Association Press.
9. US Department of Education: *National assessment of educational progress,* Washington, DC, 2005, National Center for Education Statistics.
10. Kirsch IS, Jungeblut A, Jenkins L et al: *Adult literacy in America: a first look at the results of the National Adult Literacy Survey,* Washington, DC, 1993, National Center for Education Statistics.
11. Williams MV, Parker RM, Baker DW et al: Inadequate functional health literacy among patients at two public hospitals, *JAMA* 274(21): 1677-1682, 1995.
12. Davis T, Michielutte R, Askov EN et al: Practical assessment of adult literacy in health care, *Health Ed Behav* 25(5):613-624 1998.
13. Spees CM: Knowledge of medical terminology among clients and families, *IMAGE J Nurs Scholar* 23(4):225-229, 1991.
14. Waggoner WC, Mayo DM: Who understands? A survey of 25 words or phrases commonly used in proposed clinical research consent forms, *IRB* 17(1):6-9, 1995.
15. Moon RY, Cheng TL, Patel KM et al: Parental literacy level and understanding of medical information, *Pediatrics* 102(2):e25, 1998.
16. Mayer G, Villaire M: Low health literacy and its effects on patient care, *J Nurs Admin* 34(10):440-442, 2004.
17. Bass PF, Wilson JF, Griffith CH: A shortened instrument for literacy screening, *J Gen Intern Med* 18:1036-1038, 2003.
18. Parker RM, Baker DW, Williams MV et al: The Test of Functional Health Literacy in Adults: a new instrument for measuring patients' literacy skills, *J Gen Intern Med* 10:537-541, 1995.
19. Aguirre AC, Ebrahim N, Shea JA: Performance of the English and Spanish S-TOFHLA among publicly insured Medicaid and Medicare patients, *Patient Ed Couns* 56:332-339, 2005.
20. Nurss JR, Parker RM, Williams MV et al: *TOFHLA: Test of Functional Health Literacy in Adults,* Snow Camp, NC, 1995, Peppercorn Brooks & Press.
21. Agre P, Steiglitz E, Milstein G: The case for development of a new test of health literacy. *Oncol Nurs Forum* 33(2):283-290, 2006.
22. Davis TC, Kennen EM, Gazmararian JA et al: Literacy testing in health care research. In Schwartzberg JG, VanGeest JB, Wang CC, editors: *Understanding health literacy,* Chicago, 2005, American Medical Association Press.
23. Lindau ST, Tomori C, Lyons T et al: The association of health literacy with cervical cancer prevention knowledge and health behaviors in a multiethnic cohort of women, *Am J Obstet Gynecol* 186:938-943, 2002.
24. Albright J, de Guzman C, Acebo P et al: Readability of patient education materials: implications for clinical practice, *Appl Nurs Res* 9(3):139-143, 1996.
25. Cooley ME, Moriarty H, Berger MS et al: Patient literacy and the readability of written cancer educational materials, *Oncol Nurs Forum* 22(9):1345-1351, 1995.
26. French KS, Larrabee J: Relationships among educational material readability, client literacy, perceived beneficence, and perceived quality, *J Nurs Care Qual* 13(6):68-82, 1999.
27. Quirk PA: Screening for literacy and readability: implications for the advanced practice nurse, *Clin Nurse Specialist* 14(1):26-32, 2000.
28. Meade CD, Smith CF: Readability formulas: cautions and criteria, *Patient Ed Couns* 17:153-158, 1991.
29. Biermann JS, Golladay GJ, Greenfield MLVH et al: Evaluation of cancer information on the Internet, *Cancer* 86(3):381-90, 1999.
30. Leininger MM, McFarland MR: *Transcultural nursing: concepts, theories, research and practice,* ed 3, New York, 2002, McGraw-Hill Medical.
31. Leininger MM, McFarland MR, editors: *Culture care diversity and universality: a worldwide nursing theory,* ed 2, Sudbury, Mass, Jones & Bartlett.
32. Jemal A, Siegel R, Ward E et al: Cancer statistics, 2006, *CA Cancer J Clin* 56(2):106-130, 2006.
33. He W, Sengupta M, Velkoff VA et al: *65+ in the United States: 2005,* Washington, DC, 2006, National Institute on Aging and U.S. Census Bureau.
34. Graf C: Functional decline in hospitalized older adults, *Am J Nurs* 106(1):58-67, 2006.
35. Brown CJ, Friedkin RJ, Inouye SK: Prevalence and outcomes of low mobility in hospitalized older patients, *J Am Geriatr Soc* 52:1263-70, 2004.

CHAPTER 34

Palliative Care

Debra E. Heidrich

Approximately 564,830 Americans will die of cancer in 2006.[1] Health care professionals are generally not as comfortable dealing with issues related to death and dying as they are with supporting the patient through curative treatment. Knowledge and skill in providing physical and emotional comfort to dying patients and their families is essential to providing optimum care to persons with advanced, progressive diseases.

Until recently, the focus of the health care system, as well as of nursing and medical education, was on cure and the prolongation of life. Issues related to death and dying were often avoided. A 1999 analysis of the textbooks most often used in nursing education showed that only 2% of overall content and 1.4% of chapters in these texts were related to end-of-life care.[2] This study has had an impact, as have those that illustrate that the care of persons with advanced illnesses is deficient, such as the Study to Understand Prognoses and Preferences for Outcomes and Risks of Treatments (SUPPORT) (discussed below).[3] More and more health care facilities are starting palliative care programs, nursing and medical texts and journals have more content related to end-of-life care, and some schools of nursing and medicine are integrating end-of-life care into their curricula.[4]

This chapter reviews the palliative care concept, the identification of patients and families for whom palliative care is appropriate, and management of symptoms commonly experienced by persons with advanced diseases.

The History and Evolution of Hospice and Palliative Care

Palliative care is a relatively new specialty that focuses on promoting, through optimal management of physical, psychosocial, emotional, and spiritual symptoms, the best possible quality of life for patients facing serious, life-threatening illness. This specialty grew out of the hospice movement and is continuing to evolve as more palliative care teams are integrated into health care systems, more palliative care content is taught in schools of medicine and nursing, and more research is conducted to support an evidence base for palliative interventions. A review of hospice provides a background to understand the broader concept of palliative care.

HOSPICE

The modern hospice movement began in England in 1967 when Dame Cicely Saunders, frustrated with the care given in the traditional health care system to dying patients, founded St. Christopher's Hospice. Her vision was patient-centered care provided by an interdisciplinary team that used the best medical and nursing science to address physical, psychosocial, emotional, and spiritual comfort. The principles of patient-centered, holistic care provided by an interdisciplinary team are the foundation of hospice care provided throughout the world today. The combination of lessons learned at St. Christopher's and publications on death, dying, and grief (such as the landmark works by Kübler-Ross and Worden) heightened the awareness that the care of persons in the last stages of life should and could improve.[5,6]

In the United States, the hospice movement began when Florence Wald, dean of the Graduate School of Nursing at Yale University, inspired by a lecture given by Cecily Saunders, resigned her position as dean to study at St. Christopher's Hospice. In 1974, Wald founded the New Haven Connecticut Hospice. Unlike St. Christopher's, the New Haven Hospice was a home care–based program.

Many other hospices opened across the United States during the 1970s. However, the growth of hospice programs was hampered by inadequate payment for services by third party payers. In 1982, Congress authorized the hospice Medicare benefit. (See Table 34-1 for more information on the Medicare hospice benefit.[7]) With a source of funding available, the number of hospice programs grew, as did as the number of patients receiving hospice care. There are now approximately 3,300 hospice programs in the United States, serving an estimated 950,000 patients annually. Cancer diagnoses account for 49% of hospice program admissions.[8]

Despite the increase in the number of patients receiving hospice services over the 3 decades since passage of the hospice Medicare benefit legislation, most Americans still die in hospitals or nursing homes. Some patients who die in hospitals or nursing homes are receiving hospice care, but those numbers are relatively few.[8,9] And, although patients are eligible for hospice care with a prognosis of 6 months, the median length of stay in hospice programs in 2003 was only 22 days.[8] Barriers that interfere with initial and timely referrals to hospice programs include (1) discomfort in discussing end-of-life care issues by patients, family members, and health care professionals; (2) difficulty in determining a prognosis of 6 months or less; (3) lack of information or misinformation about hospice care by patients, family members, and health care providers; and (4) real or perceived requirement to discontinue life-prolonging therapies in order to receive hospice services.[10] Organizations like the National Hospice and Palliative Care Organization (NHPCO), the Hospice and Palliative Nurses Association, and the American Academy of Hospice and Palliative Medicine are working to address the barriers that interfere with hospice care. (See Chapter 35 for further discussion of hospice and, particularly, how it is delivered in the home setting.)

PALLIATIVE CARE

Since the majority of deaths in the United States do not occur in the hospice setting, it is important to look at the type of care provided at the end of life in other settings. The SUPPORT study was conducted in five major medical centers over several years in

TABLE 34-1	The Hospice Medicare Benefit

Eligibility Criteria	The patient must
	    Be eligible for Medicare Part A
	    Be certified as having a terminal diagnosis with a prognosis of
	    6 months or less by a physician
	    Agree to waive traditional Medicare coverage for the terminal illness
	    Enroll in a Medicare-approved hospice program

Services Covered	All services for the terminal illness:
	    Physician care
	    Nursing care
	    Medical equipment
	    Medical supplies
	    Medications for symptom control and pain relief (there may be a small copayment)
	    Home health aide and homemaker services
	    Physical and occupational therapy
	    Speech therapy
	    Social work services
	    Dietary counseling
	    Grief and loss counseling for the patient and family
	    Short-term inpatient care
	    Short-term respite care
	    Volunteer services

Services Not Covered	Treatment intended to cure the terminal illness Prescription medications to cure the terminal illness rather than for symptom control Care from any provider or in any facility that isn't arranged by the hospice team Room and board
Benefit Periods	There are two 90-day periods followed by an unlimited number of 60-day periods. At the start of each period of care, the hospice medical director must recertify that the patient is terminally ill

Payment for Services	Hospice programs are paid a per diem rate to provide all of the services
	The per diem rate is based on the level of care:
	    Routine home care
	        Must account for at least 80% of all care provided by a hospice program
	        Includes private home, assisted living facility, boarding home, or long-term care facility
	    Respite care—short-term inpatient care to relive caregivers
	    General inpatient care for management of uncontrolled physical or psychosocial problems
	    Continuous home care for management of uncontrolled physical or
	        psychosocial problems in the home

Centers for Medicare and Medicaid Services: *The hospice benefit*, CMS Publication No. 02154. Baltimore MD, 2005, Author.

the early 1990s. This study showed that many hospitalized patients die prolonged and painful deaths, receiving unwanted, expensive, and invasive care.[3] This type of death is in stark contrast with what patients say they want at end of life (see Box 34-1).[11] Clearly, there is a gap between what people want and what they are receiving.

Similarly, the Institute of Medicine issued a report in 1997 calling for systems changes to assure the public of "reliably excellent and respectful" care at the end of life.[12] Palliative care is one response to the inadequacies in the prevention and relief of symptoms and distress in persons approaching death.

The basic philosophy of palliative care is essentially the same as hospice care. Indeed, hospice care is viewed as part of the palliative care continuum. The National Consensus Project for Quality Palliative Care (NCPQPC) defines palliative care as "medical care provided by an interdisciplinary team... focused on the relief of suffering and support for the best possible quality

of life for patients facing serious life-threatening illness, and their families. It aims to identify and address the physical, psychological, spiritual, and practical burdens of illness."[13] The interdisciplinary approach, the focus on psychosocial, emotional, and spiritual symptoms as well as physical symptoms, and inclusion of the family in the unit of care are key features that distinguish palliative care from routine symptom management. See Box 34-2 for a summary of the practice guidelines outlined by the NCPQPC.

Palliative care can and should be initiated at the diagnosis of a serious, life-threatening illness and continued throughout the course of the illness across all care settings. As illustrated in Figure 34-1, palliative care is started along with life-prolonging therapies at initial diagnosis. As the disease progresses, there is a greater and greater emphasis on palliative interventions as opposed to life-prolonging interventions. Hospice care is the part of the palliative care continuum when the emphasis is no longer

---

BOX 34-1   **Conditions and Attributes Important to Patients at End of Life***

Be kept clean
Name a decision maker
Be mentally aware
Have a nurse with whom one feels comfortable
Know what to expect about one's physical condition
Have someone who will listen
Maintain one's dignity
Trust one's physician
Have financial affairs in order
Be free of pain
Maintain a sense of humor
Say goodbye to important people
Be free of shortness of breath
Be free of anxiety
Have physicians with whom one can discuss fears
Be at peace with God
Not be a burden to family
Be able to help others
Have a physician who knows one as a whole person
Resolve unfinished business with family or friends
Have physical touch
Know that one's physician is comfortable talking about death and dying
Share time with close friends
Believe family is prepared for one's death
Pray
Feel prepared to die
Have funeral arrangements planned
Presence of family
Treatment preferences in writing
Not be a burden to society
Feel one's life is complete
Not die alone
Remember personal accomplishments
Receive care from personal physician

*More than 70% of study participants rated these items as important; presented in rank order.
Adapted from Steinhauser, KE, Christakis, NA, Clipp, EC et al: Factors considered important at the end of life by patients, family, physicians, and other care providers, *JAMA* 284(19):2476-2482, 2000.

on prolongation of life, but primarily on comfort. In the United States, this is often defined as the last 6 months of life, based on the eligibility requirements for the hospice Medicare benefit.

Comprehensive palliative care requires the expertise of medicine, nursing, social work, chaplaincy, counseling, nutrition, rehabilitation, pharmacy, therapists, and other health team professionals to meet the multidimensional needs of patients and their families who are facing serious, life-threatening illnesses. To be successful, palliative care must be integrated into the care provided in all health care settings, including inpatient units, intensive care units, emergency departments, ambulatory care clinics, nursing homes, home care, assisted living facilities, and nontraditional settings. There are many different models for providing palliative care, including consultant service teams,

dedicated inpatient units, clinic- or outpatient-based services, palliative care in the home care setting, or hospice-based palliative care in the home, and various combinations of two or more of these.

At the time of diagnosis, all patients, no matter what their diagnosis and prognosis, should receive optimal management of their physical, psychosocial, emotional, and spiritual symptoms. It is the role of all health care professionals to integrate the principles of palliative care into their work.[14] The role of the palliative care team at this time may include addressing any difficult-to-control symptoms, advance care planning, and psychosocial support. As the disease progresses, the need for palliative interventions increases. Whereas the palliative care team might provide care on an "as needed" basis early in the diagnosis, its expertise is needed on an ongoing basis as the disease progresses. Because the majority of palliative care is provided in the last year of life, this chapter focuses on the care of patients and their families with a prognosis of 12 months or less.

Who Will Die from Cancer?

Advances in cancer prevention, detection, and treatment have increased the 5-year relative survival rate for all cancers from 50% in mid-1970s to 64% in the late 1990s.[1] Despite these improvements, 36% of persons diagnosed with cancer will die from their cancer. The question becomes this: How can we identify who will be in this 36% and provide them with the appropriate palliative care?

The type of cancer provides one clue as to which patients are more likely to die from their disease. Cancers of the lung, the colon and rectum, the breast, the pancreas, and the prostate, as well as leukemia, are associated with the highest mortality rates, accounting for approximately 60% of all cancer deaths in both males and females.[1] Among these cancers there is wide variability on survival based on tumor size, histologic grade, and number of metastatic sites. In general, larger, poorly differentiated tumors and the presence of distant metastasis are poor prognostic indicators. A referral to a palliative care team is appropriate for patients with stage IV disease. And, those persons whose disease progresses while on treatment or with short progression-free intervals after completing a course of treatment have a worse prognosis.

Figure 34-2 shows the typical dying trajectory for cancer patients. This model is based on monitoring dependence in activities of daily living (ADLs) over the last 12 months of the lives of 897 persons with cancer and supports the idea that functional or performance status is an indicator of length of life for cancer patients—the poorer the functional status, the shorter the survival.[15] Multiple studies of patients enrolled in palliative care programs report that a Karnofsky performance status score of 50% suggests a life expectancy of less than 8 weeks.[16] Therefore a declining functional status is an indicator to refer to a palliative care or hospice care team.

The symptom profile of the patient also assists in identifying those persons who may benefit from the expertise of a palliative care team. Dyspnea, dysphagia, xerostomia, anorexia, and cognitive impairment are consistently identified as being associated with decreased length of life.[16,17] Interestingly, pain is not predictive of poor survival, although increasing pain is reported to be more common in the last weeks of life.[17]

BOX 34-2   **Clinical Practice Guidelines for Quality Palliative Care**

1. Structure and Processes of Care

The plan of care is based on a comprehensive interdisciplinary assessment of the patient and family.

The care plan is based on the identified and expressed values, goals, and needs of patient and family, and is developed with professional guidance and support for decision making.

An interdisciplinary team provides services to the patient and family, consistent with the care plan.

The interdisciplinary team may include appropriately trained and supervised volunteers.

Support for education and training is available to the interdisciplinary team.

The palliative care program is committed to quality improvement in clinical and management practices.

The palliative care program recognizes the emotional impact on the palliative care team of providing care to patients with life-threatening illnesses and their families.

Palliative care programs should have a relationship with one or more hospices and other community resources to ensure continuity of the highest-quality palliative care across the illness trajectory.

The physical environment in which care is provided should meet the preferences, needs, and circumstances of the patient and family to the extent possible.

Physical Aspects of Care

Pain, other symptoms, and side effects are managed based on the best available evidence, which is skillfully and systematically applied.

Psychologic and Psychiatric Aspects of Care

Psychologic and psychiatric issues are assessed and managed based upon the best available evidence, which is skillfully and systematically applied.

A grief and bereavement program is available to patients and families, based on the assessed need for services.

Social Aspects of Care

Comprehensive interdisciplinary assessment identifies the social needs of patients and their families, and a care plan is developed to respond to these needs as effectively as possible.

Spiritual, Religious, and Existential Aspects of Care

Spiritual and existential dimensions are assessed and responded to based upon the best available evidence, which is skillfully and systematically applied.

Cultural Aspects of Care

The palliative care program assesses and attempts to meet the culture-specific needs of the patient and family.

Care of the Imminently Dying Patient

Signs and symptoms of impending death are recognized and communicated, and care appropriate for this phase of illness is provided to patient and family.

Ethical and Legal Aspects of Care

The patient's goals, preferences and choices are respected within the limits of acceptable state and federal law, and form the basis for the plan of care.

The palliative care program is aware of and addresses the complex ethical issues arising in the care of persons with life-threatening debilitating illness.

The palliative care program is knowledgeable about legal and regulatory aspects of palliative care.

From National Consensus Project for Quality Palliative Care: *Clinical practice guidelines for quality palliative care,* 2004, retrieved September 17, 2005, from http://www.nationalconsensusproject.org.

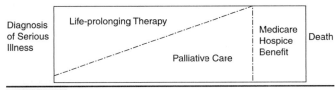

FIG. 34-1 Palliative care's place in the course of illness. (From National Consensus Project for Quality Palliative Care: *Clinical practice guidelines for quality palliative care,* 2004, retrieved September 17, 2005, from http://www.nationalconsensusproject.org.)

Physicians tend to be overly optimistic about patients' survival. There is a correlation between predicted and actual survival up to 6 months, with the most precise predictions being for those with less than 4 weeks to live. However, predictions beyond 6 months show no relationship to actual survival.[17] This helps explain why the median length of stay in hospice programs is only 22 days—physicians are most confident in estimating that a patient is in the last 6 months of life only about 4 weeks before the patient's death.

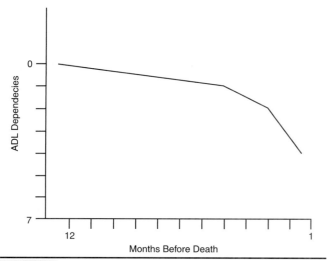

FIG. 34-2 Dependent activities for the cancer trajectory. *ADL,* Activities of daily living. (Adapted from Lunney JR, Lynn J, Foley DJ et al: Patterns of functional decline at the end of life, *JAMA* 289(18):2387-2392, 2003.)

In summary, all patients with advanced and progressing disease are at risk for uncomfortable physical symptoms and psychosocial, emotional, and spiritual challenges and should receive a palliative care consultation. Indicators of an advanced, progressive illness include a prognosis of less than 1 year, a tumor that progresses while on treatment or shortly after a course of treatment, a declining functional status, or the symptoms of dyspnea, dysphagia, xerostomia, anorexia and/or unintentional weight loss, or cognitive impairment.

Symptoms in Persons with Advanced Cancer

Common physical symptoms experienced by persons living with advanced cancer are pain, weakness and fatigue, anorexia and cachexia, constipation, nausea, and dyspnea.[18-20] Grieving, as well as social, spiritual, and existential concerns, may be issues for *both* patients and family members. Many of these symptoms and concerns are addressed elsewhere in this text. This chapter describes special considerations when selecting interventions for these symptoms with a focus on palliative care.

An appropriate intervention in palliative care is one that controls the symptom and improves overall quality of living. The patient's place on the "living-dying" trajectory is an important consideration when selecting interventions. Some interventions take days or weeks for maximal effectiveness (e.g., antidepressants; radiation therapy for pain) and therefore may not be appropriate in the final weeks of life. In addition, it is vital to consider the full impact of interventions on the overall quality of life when working with the patient, the family, and the interdisciplinary team to develop a plan of care. An "effective" intervention may be unacceptable because of social, cultural, or religious concerns, financial or physical burden, or impact on interpersonal interactions.

For example, consider a patient who needs pain medication, is unable to swallow, and does not have insurance coverage for most medications. The most common options for an alternate route of administration are parenteral, rectal, or transdermal. Suppositories cause the least financial burden, but around-the-clock administration of suppositories may be socially unacceptable to both the

patient and the family caregivers. The transdermal route is easy to manage if the patient has stable pain, but may be a financial burden. Insurance may actually cover the parenteral route, but the patient may feel "tied down" by the equipment or fearful of equipment failure. There is not one alternative route that is best for all patients and families. In this setting, the nurse should assess which of the effective alternative routes promotes the best overall quality of life for the individual patient and family and collaborate with the patient, the family, and the health care team to determine the best method to deliver medications.

PAIN

Pain is common with advanced cancer and usually worsens as the disease progresses. Persons with advanced cancers often have several different sites and types of pain, each requiring a comprehensive assessment and individualized interventions. Readers are referred to Chapter 39 for a detailed discussion of pain types, assessment, and interventions. A useful tool is a pain flow sheet to monitor each type of pain for the effectiveness of current interventions and to track the number of medication rescue doses required to manage break-through pain. The nurse can obtain orders to titrate medications to meet the patient's needs.

Chapter 39 also addresses the management of the common side effects of opioids: constipation, nausea, sedation, and pruritus. Anticipation and early recognition of side effects allows nurses to initiate treatments to prevent or minimize these side effects throughout the course of the disease, especially when opioid doses are increased.

Many patients with cancer pain require treatment with long-term opioids, increasing the potential for neuroexcitatory side effects. Myoclonus, the uncontrolled twitching and jerking of muscles or muscle groups, is typically the first neuroexcitatory effect seen. Patients with myoclonus sometimes report muscle jerking that awakes them from sleep. This side effect has been observed in patients receiving long-term therapy with morphine, hydromorphone, fentanyl, meperidine, sufentanil, and methadone.[19,21] The 3-glucuronide opioid metabolites are the most likely cause of this side effect. Because these are eliminated in urine, plasma levels of these metabolites increase in the presence of renal failure. Continued administration of the offending opioid makes the myoclonus worse and puts the patient at risk for hyperalgesia, delirium with hallucinations, and grand mal seizures.[21] The primary treatment for opioid-related myoclonus is opioid rotation.[22] Opioid rotation involves converting the patient to about 50% of the equianalgesic dose of different opioids (even less if the patient is on very high doses of the offending medication).[23] The nurse plays a critical role in assessing the adequacy of analgesia and side effects after opioid rotation to determine the need for further dose reductions or escalations.

WEAKNESS AND FATIGUE

Fatigue is a common symptom of advanced cancer, seen in 30% to 90% of persons in palliative care.[20,24-26] Fatigue has a profound negative impact on quality of living. Persons experiencing fatigue do not have the energy to participate in activities that are important to them, such as joining the family for dinner at a table, attending religious services, and performing ADLs. Mental fatigue makes it difficult for individuals to participate in conversations and make decisions. The combination of physical and mental fatigue puts patients at risk for isolation and loneliness.

Chapter 37 provides information on the definition, etiology, and interventions for fatigue. Evaluate these interventions for their appropriateness in the palliative care setting based on the patient's prognosis and functional status.

ANOREXIA AND CACHEXIA

The cancer cachexia syndrome is characterized by anorexia, involuntary weight loss, wasting of muscle and fat tissues, and poor performance status.[27,28] This syndrome is common with advanced cancer, affecting more than 80% of persons with cancer in palliative care settings.[28-30] Cachexia is associated with poor clinical outcomes, decreased survival, and compromised quality of life.[27]

Many factors contribute to cachexia. Cytokines (including tumor necrosis factor and several interleukins), produced either by the tumor or by the body in response to the tumor, and a chronic inflammatory response that involves C-reactive proteins are likely the cause of decreased appetite, increased metabolic rate, increased energy expenditures, interference with fat storage and muscle repair, loss of fat, and breakdown of muscle.[27,28,31-36] Some experts propose that cancer cachexia is more of a chronic inflammatory condition rather than a nutritional aberration.[37] Certainly, this is a complex syndrome that is different from starvation, during which energy expenditures are reduced and proteins are conserved.[28,36,38]

Some persons with cancer have the added burden of tumors that interfere with the ability to chew, swallow, or digest food, such as dysphagia with head and neck and esophageal cancers, and obstructions of ducts and lumens with pancreatic, bowel, and genitourinary cancers. The side effects of cancer treatments, such as mucositis, xerostomia, taste changes, nausea and vomiting, and diarrhea, also interfere with adequate intake of nutrients.

Depression may be both a result of and a contributing factor to cachexia.[39] The profound weakness associated with cachexia certainly interferes with persons being able to do the things that are important to them, contributing to feelings of worthlessness. The loss of self-worth may further contribute to loss of appetite.

Interventions for Cachexia. Simply providing high-calorie, high-protein feedings does not overcome the muscle and fat wasting of cancer cachexia. Indeed, many studies evaluating aggressive nutritional support of patients with malignancy show no impact on mortality and some increased risks.[40] Those whose weight loss is from disease processes interfering with their ability to ingest food, but who still feel hungry (e.g., head and neck or esophageal cancers), will benefit more from enteral nutrition than those persons with no appetite.

It is possible to improve the efficacy of nutritional support by using medications that alter the mechanisms leading to cachexia. Table 34-2 summarizes some of the medications showing promise in clinical trials that may become part of the palliative care plan for the management of cachexia in the future.

Despite evidence that increased intake alone does not reverse cachexia, nutritional intake is important to the extent to which it improves quality of life for the individual. For some patients, their nutritional intake makes a difference in their energy and activity level; for some patients, the act of eating is important; for others, eating is no longer important. Assessing the individual's desires and goals is essential to determine the best interventions in each situation.

Treatable factors contributing to decreased nutritional intake must be addressed.

TABLE 34-2 Promising Medications for the Management of Cachexia	
MEDICATION	**PROPOSED MECHANISM OF ACTION**
Omega-3 fatty acids	Inhibition of TNF, interleukins-1, -2, -4, and -6, and interferon-γ
Nonsteroidal antiinflammatory drugs (NSAIDs)	Decreases production of C-reactive protein
Melatonin	Inhibition of TNF
Thalidomide	Inhibition of TNF

TNF, Tumor necrosis factor.
Data from References 31, 36, 38, and 41.

- Early satiety and poor appetite:
  - Encourage small, frequent foods throughout the day instead of three larger meals, and keep snacks within reach.
  - Separate medication times from meals (except for medications that must be taken with food).
  - Make mealtime enjoyable by encouraging socialization; evaluate the pros and cons of sitting at a table with family for dinner (i.e., increased energy expenditure vs. improved socialization and nutritional intake).
  - Make the environment as pleasant as possible, paying attention to lighting, view, noise level, and odors.[29,31]
  - Consider use of a prokinetic agent, such as metoclopramide, to treat delayed gastric emptying. A prokinetic should be used before using an appetite stimulant.[29,31,35,42]
  - Consider use of an appetite stimulant:
    - Corticosteroids improve appetite and sense of well-being, but show no significant effect on body weight. In fact, corticosteroids increase muscle metabolism. Use for more than 2 months for appetite stimulation has not been evaluated, and there is concern about the side effects (muscle wasting, osteoporosis, spontaneous fractures, glaucoma, congestive heart failure) of long-term use of steroids.[29,35,38,42]
    - Progestational drugs such as megestrol acetate lead to weight gain and improve appetite and well-being. There is no difference in survival for patients treated with megestrol compared to those not receiving this medication.[29,42] Many untoward side effects are possible; those occurring in up to 10% of patients include peripheral edema, hypercoagulability, nausea, impotence, and diarrhea.[31,42,43]
    - Cannabinoids improve appetite and lead to weight gain, but many patients find the central nervous system (CNS) effects intolerable.[29,42]
- Taste changes:
  - Teach and encourage good mouth care before meals.
  - Persons who have received chemotherapy often report red meats have a metallic taste. Try marinating meats before cooking.
  - Sweet foods may taste "sickeningly" sweet. Try foods with tart flavors.
  - Serve foods at room temperature.
  - Encourage patient to try a variety of foods, even some that were not favorites in the past.

- Mucositis and xerostomia:
  - Teach and encourage good mouth care, including use of artificial saliva for xerostomia.
  - Treat any infections, such as oral candidiasis.
  - Encourage consumption of soft, moist, bland foods.
  - Avoid acidic or spicy foods and beverages.

Anorexia and weight loss are often distressing to patients and family members. The continued weight loss is a visible reminder of progressive disease. Often, family members believe that if they can just get their loved ones to eat, the patients will feel better and live longer. In the advanced stages of cancer, many patients do not feel like eating and actually feel worse when they do eat; when family members keep encouraging these persons to eat, everyone is frustrated. Explain to both patients and family members that the weight loss of advanced cancer is very different from starvation, and that eating more does not reverse this process. An honest, supportive discussion may avert the feelings of guilt for both patients and family members.[44] Sometimes the most important intervention is to make it "okay" for the patient to not eat, especially when eating causes discomfort.

CONSTIPATION

Constipation is a common problem in persons with advanced cancer and occurs in at least 32% to 55% of persons with advanced cancer.[20,45,46] This is a significantly higher rate than for the general population, but is still likely an underestimate of the incidence in advanced cancer.[47] Constipation is uncomfortable! Unmanaged constipation leads to impaction and symptoms of bowel obstruction.

Factors contributing to constipation with advanced cancer include immobility; dietary changes; medications, including opioids and anticholinergics; chemical imbalances, such as hypercalcemia; pressure on the bowel from tumors, ascites, or adhesions; changes to gastrointestinal (GI) tract innervation from spinal cord compression, surgical damage, or chemotherapy-induced neuropathies; and psychosocial concerns, including stress, anxiety, and embarrassment.[46,48,49]

Interventions for Constipation. Whenever possible, treat the underlying cause of constipation.

- Encourage activity (when fatigue or pain do not interfere) to stimulate the bowels. Isometric and range of motion exercises may be helpful for patients who are not able to get up out of bed.
- Assess dietary and fluid intake based the individual's goals and prognosis. Instruct patients with normal appetites to drink at least 8 glasses of fluids daily, encourage a diet high in fiber, and avoid constipating foods such as bananas, rice, cheese, and black tea.[50] Note, however, that the amount of fiber required to treat constipation is rarely tolerated by persons with advanced cancer.[47]
- Assist the patient to sit in an upright position for bowel movements to maximize the muscle strength required for defecation.
  - Use bedside commodes for patients unable to ambulate to the bathroom and allow for privacy during toileting.
- Evaluate the impact of discontinuing medications that cause constipation, keeping in mind that these medications are often required to control other symptoms (e.g., opioids, tricyclic antidepressants, and anticholinergics for pain control).

It is rare for the above prophylactic interventions alone to manage the constipation associated with advanced cancer.

Routine administration of stool softeners and laxatives is often necessary. The choice of laxative depends on the characteristics of the patient's stool and the individual's response to therapy. Hard, dry stool requires more softener; overly soft stool, causing fecal incontinence or leakage, requires less softener. Difficult-to-pass stool requires more stimulant; persons experiencing abdominal cramping may require less stimulant.[47,50] Many types of softeners and laxatives are available. Table 34-3 lists the most commonly used laxatives, their mechanisms of action, and comments about each.

Persons with advanced cancer, especially those on opioids, require combinations of softener and stimulant laxatives. Regularly assess amount and consistency of stools, as well as ease and frequency of defecation, to identify problems early and to adjust laxatives as necessary. Box 34-3 provides a guideline for managing constipation with laxatives.

Describing bowel movements to the health care team is often embarrassing to patients. Teach the importance of prevention and early management of constipation and allow for privacy during these conversations.

NAUSEA AND VOMITING

Nausea and vomiting unrelated to chemotherapy occur in 40% to 70% of persons with advanced cancer.[51-53] Nausea alone interferes with intake and causes emotional distress. When accompanied by vomiting, the impact on quality of life is even worse.

Figure 34-3 shows the mechanisms involved in nausea and vomiting. The vomiting center is located in the brain stem within the blood-brain barrier and receives stimulation from at least five areas: the chemoreceptive trigger zone (CTZ), midbrain afferents, vagal afferents, pharyngeal afferents, and the vestibular apparatus.[53,54] The CTZ lies outside the blood-brain barrier and is exposed to substances in the circulation. Emetogenic substances probably stimulate dopamine receptors in the CTZ.[55,56] Midbrain afferents stimulate the vomiting center in the presence of anxiety and stress and with increased intracranial pressure. Vagal afferents ending in the vomiting center are stimulated by irritation in the GI tract. Likewise, irritation of the glossopharyngeal nerves activates the vomiting center. Nausea and vomiting preceded by dizziness is often caused by stimulation of the vestibular apparatus that, in turn, stimulates the vomiting center. The common causes of nausea and vomiting in palliative care are identified in Box 34-4.

Interventions to Treat Nausea and Vomiting. Assess the cause of the nausea and work with the interdisciplinary team to choose interventions to eliminate the cause of nausea whenever possible.

- Consult with a clinical pharmacist to identify medications the patient is taking that stimulate the CTZ.
  - Medications that were previously well-tolerated, e.g., digoxin, may become toxic and cause nausea and vomiting as a result of declining renal and hepatic function.
- A high calcium or low sodium level also triggers the CTZ; assess for signs and symptoms of hypercalcemia and the syndrome of inappropriate antidiuretic hormone (SIADH) secretion.
- Determine whether emotional factors are contributing to this symptom. Listen to concerns, address fears, and treat pain.
  - Anxiolytics are used only when psychosocial and emotional support is not effective.

TABLE 34-3	Stool Softeners and Laxatives	
TYPE	**ACTION**	**COMMENTS**
Lubricant Softeners Mineral oil	Penetrates stool and prevents water absorption	Less palatable than others Avoided because of risk of aspiration pneumonia
Bulk-forming Laxatives Methylcellulose (e.g., Citrucel) Psyllium (e.g., Metamucil) Polycarbophil (e.g., Fibercon)	Resists bacterial breakdown, increasing bulk and shortening transit time Draws fluid from body to hydrate stool, causing dehydration	Must maintain fluid intake of 1.5 to 2 L of fluid per day Avoided in palliative care because of dehydrating effects and patient inability to tolerate required fluid intake
Saccharine Laxatives Lactulose Sorbitol Glycerin	Creates osmotic gradient in the intestine	High oral doses for effectiveness may cause bloating, cramping, and flatulence
Saline Laxatives Magnesium citrate Magnesium hydroxide (e.g., Milk of Magnesia) Sodium bisphosphate or sodium phosphate (e.g., Fleets enema)	Creates an immediate osmotic gradient in the intestine	Oral forms are effective in 0.5 to 3 hr Enemas often effective within 15 min
Polyethylene Glycol (e.g., MiraLax)	Hydrates stool with the oral fluids with which it is administered Does not draw water from the body	Taken with 125 ml of fluid Initial effect seen in 2 to 3 days; if taken regularly, bowel frequency tends to be daily Less flatulence, bloating, and cramping than saccharine laxative Does not dehydrate patient
Stimulant Laxatives Senna (e.g., Senokot) Bisacodyl (e.g., Dulcolax)	Stimulates submucosal nerve plexus to increase motility	May cause cramping Often used in combination with a softener
Emollient or Surfactant Softeners Docusate sodium (e.g., Colace)	Increases water penetration	Increased transit time caused by opioids negates action of these laxatives

Data from References 47, 49, and 50.

- Assess for the presence of poorly controlled pain. Although the side effects of opioids include nausea, sometimes the real problem of nausea is undertreated pain, resulting in continued nausea and vomiting and worsening of pain.
- Evaluate for signs and symptoms of increased intracranial pressure (ICP). If increased ICP is present, evaluation of the cause is necessary. Corticosteroids are helpful in controlling symptoms.
- Evaluate for signs and symptoms of gastric stasis and obstruction: nausea and vomiting, early satiety, and epigastric pain.[57]
  - Metoclopramide is a good medication to treat this problem since it promotes gastric peristalsis and shortens the gastric and upper intestinal transit time.[57,58] Patients with partial bowel obstruction may develop gastric colic from metoclopramide, so careful, ongoing evaluation is essential.[54]

- External pressure on the stomach from ascites or hepatomegaly can cause "squashed stomach syndrome." Patients who report feeling full and nauseous after eating meals may do better with small, frequent meals, with or without the addition of metoclopramide.
- Evaluate for thick sputum that is difficult to expectorate.
  - Inhalation therapy with saline or a commercial mucolytic such as acetylcysteine (Mucomyst) may be helpful.
  - Encourage the patient to drink more fluids to help thin secretions, when appropriate.
- Assess for prolonged coughing that stimulates pharyngeal afferents. Discuss antitussive interventions with the interdisciplinary team.
- Encourage good oral hygiene to eliminate unpleasant tastes.
- Treat any oral infections.

BOX 34-3 **Guidelines for Managing Constipation**

1. Rule out obstruction.
2. Manually remove an impaction in the bowel, if necessary.
3. Initiate bowel regimen using emollient softener alone or with a stimulant laxative (e.g., Senokot-S), depending on the assessment of the stool and ease of defecation.
4. If no bowel movement occurs over 2 to 3 days, add a stimulant (e.g., Dulcolax). If the extra stimulant works, evaluate the stool and increase the daily stimulant, the softener, or both.
5. If no bowel movement occurs after additional stimulant, use a saline enema (e.g., Fleets enema). If enema is effective, evaluate the stool and increase the daily stimulant, the softener, or both.
6. If enema is not effective, use an oral saline (e.g., magnesium citrate), saccharine laxative (e.g., lactulose), or polyethylene glycol (e.g., MiraLax). If this step is effective, evaluate the stool and increase the daily stimulant, the softener, or both. If this step is not effective, repeat unless the patient experienced cramping or bloating. Consider switching to polyethylene glycol as the daily laxative.

Data from References 48 and 49.

If the underlying cause is not treatable, or while the evaluation to determine cause is ongoing, administer antiemetics as ordered.

- Selection of the appropriate medication is based on the mechanism involved in transmitting the stimulus to vomit to the vomiting center.
  - Table 34-4 lists antiemetics based on their mechanism of action.
  - Metoclopramide or haloperidol are the preferred initial choices in palliative care.[53]
  - There is little information on the use of the serotonin antagonists except for the treatment of nausea related to highly emetogenic chemotherapy or refractory postoperative nausea. These medications are rarely more effective than other antiemetics for the nausea and vomiting seen in palliative care setting. Also, they are much more expensive than

BOX 34-4 **Common Causes of Nausea and Vomiting in Palliative Care**

Chemoreceptor Trigger Zone–Mediated
- Medications
  - Opioids
  - Antibiotics
  - Chemotherapy
  - Corticosteroids
  - Digoxin
  - Nonsteroidal antiinflammatory drugs (NSAIDs)
  - Iron
- Metabolic causes
  - Hypercalcemia
  - Hyponatremia
  - Uremia

Midbrain Afferents
- Emotional factors
  - Anxiety
  - Fear
  - Pain
- Increased intracranial pressure
- Primary or metastatic brain tumors
- Meningitis

Vagal Afferents
- Gastrointestinal (GI) distension, stasis, or obstruction
- Constipation
- Gastritis
- External pressure ("squashed stomach syndrome")

Pharyngeal Afferents
- Thick sputum
- Oral infection (e.g., candidiasis)
- Chronic cough
- Unpleasant tastes

Vestibular Apparatus
- Motion sickness
- Brain tumors
- Opioids

Data from References 51 and 54.

---

other antiemetics. Therefore serotonin antagonists are recommended only if other antiemetics are ineffective or if the side effects of these other medications preclude their use.

- The dose must be titrated to effectiveness while assessing for side effects.[53,54] If nausea persists, assess for other potential causes, such as the tumor itself causing partial or full obstruction. Consider switching medications, if a different cause is identified, or adding an antiemetic from a different class if no new cause is found.

DYSPNEA

Dyspnea is a subjective experience that includes difficulty breathing, an uncomfortable awareness of breathing, and shortness of breath. It may or may not be accompanied by tachypnea.[59]

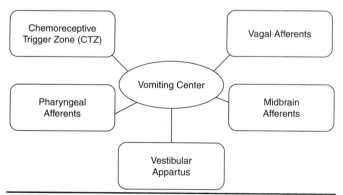

FIG. 34-3 Mechanisms leading to nausea and vomiting. (From Griffie J, McKinnon S: Nausea and vomiting. In Kuebler K, Berry P, Heidrich D, editors: *End of life care clinical practice guidelines*, St. Louis, 2002, W.B. Saunders.)

TABLE 34-4 Antiemetic Selection by Nausea and Vomiting Mechanism

MECHANISM	ACTION	EXAMPLES
CTZ Stimulation	Dopamine antagonist	Haloperidol Metoclopramide Prochlorperazine
	Serotonin antagonist	Ondansetron Granisetron Dolestron mesylate
Midbrain afferents		
Anxiety	Anxiolytic	Lorazepam
Increased intracranial pressure	Corticosteroid	Dexamethasone
Vagal afferents	Prokinetic	Metoclopramide
	Antisecretory	Octreotide
Vomiting center	Antihistamine	Diphenhydramine Hydroxyzine
	Anticholinergic	Scopolamine

CTZ, Chemoreceptive trigger zone.
Data from References 51 and 54.

The frequency of this symptom ranges from 21% to 90%, depending on the type of cancer, the stage of disease, and comorbid medical conditions.[20,60,61]

The respiratory center in the medulla controls breathing via stimuli from (1) chemoreceptors in the aorta, the carotid, and the medulla that primarily respond to the lowering of the pH that occurs with carbon dioxide retention; (2) mechanoreceptors in the diaphragm and chest wall that sense any increase in the work of breathing; (3) vagal stretch receptors in the pulmonary tissues that detect ventilatory impedance as may occur with narrowed airways or increased capillary pressure; and, (4) cortical areas of the brain where the sensation of dyspnea is perceived and where it is made worse by anxiety, fear, and depression.[59] The mechanisms involved in the dyspnea associated with advanced cancer are identified in Table 34-5.[62] Anxiety almost always accompanies dyspnea, causing a "snowball effect": increased anxiety makes dyspnea worse, which further increases anxiety, and so on.

Dyspnea is a warning sign of an underlying, and potentially treatable, problem. Identifying how suddenly the dyspnea appeared assists in determining the underlying cause. A sudden onset of dyspnea indicates a sudden process such as pulmonary embolus, cardiac dysrhythmia, or heart failure. Dyspnea that occurs over hours or days may be due to a pulmonary effusion or infection. A very gradual onset of dyspnea is caused by tumor growth, anemia, or weakness.

Interventions for Dyspnea. The goal of dyspnea management is to relieve the sensation of breathlessness.[19] Treatment of the underlying cause is the ideal therapy, when the interventions improve quality of living. However, as cancer progresses, some interventions may be too burdensome.[63,64] Consult with an interdisciplinary team to consider the patient's prognosis, the patient's goals, the likelihood of a positive outcome, the potential of adverse effects, and the cost of therapies to assist in determining appropriate interventions. For example, a transfusion to treat anemia may not relieve dyspnea if the patient is also cachectic and weak.

- Evaluate the patient's condition to determine the underlying cause of dyspnea, and work with the interdisciplinary team to treat these as appropriate:
  - *Anemia:* transfuse with packed red blood cells; administer erythropoietin agent
  - *Heart failure:* adjust cardiac medications, especially diuretics
  - *Tumor:* administer chemotherapy or radiation therapy for responsive tumors; administer corticosteroids for lymphangitic spread of tumors[64]
  - *Pleural effusion:* perform a thoracentesis or place a drainage catheter
  - *Pneumonia:* administer antibiotics
  - *Ascites:* perform a paracentesis
  - *Bronchospasm:* administer bronchodilators
- When the underlying cause cannot or should not be treated, use interventions to decrease the perception of dyspnea.
  - A cool sensation to the face is often very effective in easing dyspnea.[59] Place a small fan on the bedside table to blow air directly on the patient's face, or use cool, damp cloths.
  - Opioids also decrease the perception of dyspnea.[65] Consult with the interdisciplinary team about starting opioids.
    - Administer 2.5 to 5 mg of morphine by mouth (or, an equianalgesic dose of another opioid or via a different

TABLE 34-5 Causes of Dyspnea in Advanced Cancer

DISEASE OR CONDITION	BLOOD GAS ABNORMALITY (CHEMORECEPTOR)	INCREASED VENTILATORY DEMAND (MECHANORECEPTOR)	MUSCLE ABNORMALITY (MECHANORECEPTOR)	VENTILATORY IMPEDENCE (VAGAL RECEPTORS)
Pneumonia	X			X
Effusion	X	X		X
Tumor	X	X	X	X
Anemia	X			X
Superior vena cava syndrome	X			X
Generalized Weakness			X	

Adapted from Kuebler KK, Andry JM, Davis S: Dyspnea. In Kuebler K, Heidrich D, Esper P, editors: *Palliative and end of life care clinical practice guidelines*, St. Louis, 2007, Saunders.

route can be tried) every 3 to 4 hours as needed to the opioid-naive patient. The opioid dose can be titrated to effectiveness.

- Patients who are already on opioids for pain control may be given the equivalent of 10% to 15% of the 24-hour total of their opioid as an immediate-release, short-acting opioid to treat dyspnea. For example: a patient is receiving 60 mg of controlled-release morphine q 12 hours for pain control and is now experiencing dyspnea. The 24-hour total of morphine is 120 mg; 10% to 15% of that is 12 to 18 mg. Start with 15 mg of immediate-release oral morphine for the dyspnea, and assess for effectiveness.
    - Consider using a sustained-release opioid if frequent dosing is required.[63]
    - Opioids are sometimes given via a nebulizer when oral administration is no longer effective. Morphine 5 to 10 mg, hydromorphone 1 to 2 mg, or fentanyl 25 to 50 mcg in a nebulizer (add saline to make 3 to 5 ml) have been reported to be effective.[66,67] However, the studies on giving opioids via this route show conflicting results and usually involve small sample sizes.[59] Fentanyl may be a better choice for use in a nebulizer because of its lipophilic properties. As patients become weaker and take shallower breaths at end of life, the nebulizer may be less effective.
- Position the patient to maximize pulmonary function:
    - Sitting up and leaning slightly forward over a bedside table often improves breathing. This position can be exhausting to maintain and can put the patient at risk for pressure ulcers. Use wedge and other pillows to support the patient. Further, maintain a repositioning schedule to prevent pressure ulcers.
    - If the patient has a pleural effusion, position with the effusion side down so that the unaffected lung can expand fully.
    - Patients with ascites may find that having the head of the bed slightly elevated is more comfortable than sitting in a more upright position.
- Encourage patients to use their diaphragm to breathe. Many people do not know where their diaphragm is, so be prepared to teach deep-breathing techniques.
- Administer oxygen therapy as ordered.
    - Oxygen is most helpful if the oxygen saturation is less than 90%. However, even with higher oxygen saturations, some patients report feeling less dyspneic on oxygen.
    - Small studies show that some patients benefit from room air via a cannula. It may actually be the flow of cool air that helps those persons who are not hypoxic.[68]
    - Patients at the end of life who find cannulas or masks to be uncomfortable should not be forced to keep them in place. Use other measures like cool cloths and morphine to promote comfort in these patients.
    - When oxygen or supplemental air is used, be sure it is humidified.
- Treat the anxiety that often accompanies dyspnea.
    - Monitor the patient frequently, and be sure the patient has a mechanism to call for help, such as a call light, bell, or radio transmitter (i.e., "baby monitor"). Respond immediately when dyspneic patients call for assistance.
    - Although there are not a lot of data to support their use, administer ordered benzodiazepines as needed if other interventions are not effective or the patient is extremely anxious.[19,59,64]

Psychosocial and Spiritual Care

In palliative care, interventions to prevent or treat psychosocial and spiritual suffering are as important as interventions for controlling physical symptoms. Review the list of attributes that patients said were most important at the end of life presented in Table 34-2. Only 5 out of 34 of these attributes are related to physical symptoms or physical care. The rest of these attributes fall into one of these themes: (1) being able to discuss fears and concerns with physicians and nurses, (2) maintaining relationships with family and friends, (3) finding meaning in their lives, and (4) feeling prepared for death. Nurses play an important role in assisting patients and families to address their psychosocial and spiritual concerns. A death is never "good," but persons can "die well" by accomplishing meaningful tasks while living with dying.[69]

Establish a trusting relationship with the patient and family to encourage them to discuss their concerns about the illness and death. Simply asking, "How are you coping with what is happening to you?" gives the individual permission to discuss their concerns.[70] Be prepared to *listen* to their stories—not just hearing the words, but listening for the feelings. Be sensitive to the need for privacy for what may be an intensely emotional discussion. Avoid interruptions as much as possible during these discussions—turn off or silence beepers and cell phones when possible. Involve the interdisciplinary team to provide emotional support, including the physician, the social worker, the chaplain, aides, and volunteers. Make referrals to psychologists or psychiatrists as appropriate.

Maintaining relationships with family and friends can be very difficult for the person with advanced cancer, especially as functional status declines. Not only may the patient not be physically able to go out to meet friends, the friends may withdraw from the patient. For patients in inpatient setting, liberalize visitation policies to accommodate this need. When friends have withdrawn, volunteers with the hospice or palliative care program may help to fill this role. Family members also feel isolated as the physical care needs of the patient increase. They may need permission to take care of themselves by meeting with friends or attending a social activity. Discuss options to augment the family's support system by enlisting the assistance of extended family members, making referrals to appropriate community agencies, and using hospice and palliative care volunteers.

Patients need to find meaning in their lives and feel that life is complete. Ask patients about their personal accomplishments—these may be in work, family, or community. Encourage a life review. Some patients choose to share their life stories with their families in the form of letters, audiotapes, or videotapes. Ask if there is a religious or spiritual community that they are or would like to be connected with and make referrals to a chaplain or spiritual leader as appropriate, with the patient's permission.

Patients want to feel prepared for death. Encourage patients to complete advance directives so that they can name a health care proxy and put their preferences for care in writing. Achieving this outcome necessitates that patients receive accurate information about their condition so that they can anticipate the kinds of issues their proxy may face. Nurses serve as advocates for patients to get the information needed to make decisions truly consistent with their values.

Part of preparation for death includes getting financial affairs in order, resolving any unfinished business, and completing

TABLE 34-6 **Manifestations of Grief***

FEELINGS	PHYSICAL SENSATIONS	COGNITIONS	BEHAVIORS
Sadness	Hollowness in stomach	Disbelief	Sleep disturbances
Anger	Chest and throat tightness	Confusion	Appetite disturbances
Guilt or self-reproach	Over-sensitivity to noise	Preoccupation or obsessiveness	Avoiding reminders of the deceased
Anxiety	Sense of unreality	Sense the deceased person is	Social withdrawal
Loneliness	Feeling short of breath	close by	Searching and calling out
Fatigue	Muscle weakness	Visual or auditory hallucinations	Sighing
Helplessness	Lack of energy		Restless overactivity
Yearning	Dry mouth		Crying
Emancipation			Treasuring and carrying objects as reminders
Relief			Visiting places as reminders of the deceased
Numbness			

*NOTE: All of these are normal manifestations of grief. However, if any exist for long periods of time or at a high level of intensity, consider a consult to evaluate for a complicated grief reaction.
Adapted from Roberts KF, Berry PH: Grief and bereavement. In Kuebler K, Berry P, Heidrich D, editors: *End of life care clinical practice guidelines*, St. Louis, 2002, W.B. Saunders.

relationships. Byock discusses the "five things" of relationship completion: saying "I forgive you," "Forgive me," "Thank you," "I love you," and "Good-bye."[69] Introduce these five statements to patients and families to assist them in completing relationships with friends and family.

Bereavement Care

Bereavement care is an important component of any palliative care program.[14] Providing bereavement care requires an understanding of the normal grieving process and the tasks of grief work. Grief is a normal and expected reaction to a loss. Family members will grieve the loss of their loved ones. One role of the interdisciplinary team is to reinforce the understanding that

grieving is a healthy, necessary process that the family must go through to be able to move on in their lives. Nurses need to validate as normal the manifestations that the bereaved may be experiencing. Normal manifestations of grief are listed in Table 34-6.[71]

In addition to knowing the normal responses to grief, it is helpful for those working with the bereaved to understand the tasks of the grieving process. Four tasks of mourning must be accomplished in order for the bereavement to reach a satisfactory conclusion[7]:
- Accept the reality of the loss
- Work through the pain of grief
- Adjust to the environment in which the deceased is missing
- Emotionally relocate the deceased and move on with life

TABLE 34-7 **Interventions for Grieving Persons**

TASK	INTERVENTIONS
Accept reality of the loss	• Listen actively without judgment • Encourage gentle exploration of what the future may look like without the deceased • Assess and encourage the development of social support systems • Encourage time with the body of the deceased at the time of death • Offer ample opportunity to repeat the story of the death; listen patiently and attentively • Normalize feelings through personal contacts and written materials regarding grief and loss • Avoid the use of platitudes • Attend the funeral or visitation if possible; send a personal letter or card to the family • Respect survivor's feelings without judgment
Work through the pain of grief	• Assist in identifying manifestations of grief and normalize them • Assist the survivor in placing a meaning on the death
Adjust to the environment in which the deceased is missing	• Assist the survivor in further identifying the meaning of the loss in practical terms • Provide practical assistance with developing needed skills • Advise the survivor to minimize change and to grieve where things are familiar
Emotionally relocate the deceased and move on with life	• Provide a nonjudgmental and supportive ear as the survivor explores this task • Validate and normalize feeling associated with moving the thoughts and memories of the deceased to an effective place that allows for a reinvestment in life • Encourage attendance at grief and loss support or educational groups

Adapted from Roberts KF, Berry PH: Grief and bereavement. In Kuebler K, Berry P, Heidrich D, editors: *End of life care clinical practice guidelines*, St. Louis, 2002, W.B. Saunders.

This last task is the most difficult. It involves finding a place for the dead in the grievers' emotional lives that allow them to go on living effectively in the world. The grieving process takes time and energy. The first year of bereavement is the most intense—the first birthdays, holidays, and anniversaries without the deceased, as well as the anniversary of the death, can be very difficult. Hospice bereavement programs generally follow families for 13 months after a death to provide support through this time. Table 34-7 identifies interventions to assist persons with the grieving process.

Outcomes

Working in collaboration with the interdisciplinary team, nurses have a significant impact on patient outcomes in palliative and end-of-life care. Given and Sherwood identified 10 core nurse-sensitive outcomes across the continuum of oncology care that apply to palliative and end-of-life care: symptoms, physical function, role function, knowledge, emotional health, quality of life, self-care, cost, length of stay, and use of service.[75] In order to determine how well an agency is doing in providing palliative and end-of-life care, these outcomes must be measured using tools appropriate for palliative care.

Since the Joint Commission on Accreditation of Health Care Organizations (JCAHO) introduced pain standards in 2000, many agencies have developed tools to document patients' pain ratings and standards for addressing pain issues. Assuring quality pain care requires monitoring to see not only if pain assessments are being documented and standards followed, but if the desired outcomes are achieved—that is, are patients and families satisfied with the pain management? However, pain is only one of many symptoms common at the end of life. Assessment tools that include the measurements for other symptoms are also needed so the outcomes of interventions for them can be monitored. The Edmonton Symptom Assessment System is one example of a tool from a palliative care program that includes patient ratings of pain, fatigue, nausea, depression, anxiety, drowsiness, appetite, well-being, and dyspnea.[76] Again, the key to evaluating quality of care is not only documenting the presence of a symptom, but documenting improvement after implementing the treatment plan.

Depending on the setting and the priorities set by an organization, other measures of quality palliative care may include the following: an increase in the percentage of persons who receive palliative care or hospice services, an increase in the length of time between referral to the palliative service and patients' deaths, an increase in the percentage of persons who have documentation of advance care planning, a decrease in the number of patients with advanced cancer who are admitted to or die in an intensive care unit, and an increase in the percentage of patients and families who are satisfied with their care.

Two tools to measure the overall quality of palliative and end-of-life care that have demonstrated validity and reliability are the After-Death Bereaved Family Member Interview (available in versions for hospice, nursing home, and hospital settings) and the Family Evaluation of Hospice Care (FEHC) survey.[77,78] The FEHC is based on the After-Death Bereaved Family Member Interview and was developed by the NHPCO to provide individual agency and group data on quality of hospice care. Both of these tools are somewhat time-consuming to administer. The domains of these tools include physical and emotional comfort of the patient, informed decision making,

advance care planning, focus on the individual, emotional and spiritual needs of the family, and coordination of care.

Ethical Considerations

Autonomy, the right of individuals to choose their own course of action, is a highly valued ethical principle in our society, in health care, and in the nursing profession, and it is the basis for the Patient Self Determination Act passed by Congress in 1990. Nonetheless, the SUPPORT study showed that patients often received unwanted care at the end of life.[4] There are many potential reasons why patients may receive unwanted care, including the following: patients may not understand the consequences of treatment choices, health care providers may not ask patients about their preferences, undocumented discussions may be challenged by others (especially those related to refusal or withdrawal of treatment), written advance directives may be unclear or have limited application, and health care providers may disagree with the patient's decisions.

CONSIDERATIONS FOR OLDER ADULTS

- **Pain.** Older adults are more sensitive to both the therapeutic effects and the side effects of medications as a result of changes in absorption, distribution, metabolism, and elimination of medications.[64,72,73] This is no excuse for inadequate symptom management the elderly!

  Many experts avoid using nonsteroidal antiinflammatory drugs (NSAIDs) in the elderly because of increased toxicity, and prefer acetaminophen for mild pain or opioids for moderate to severe pain. The older adult may require a smaller dose and a longer dosing interval.[64,74] The adage "start low and go slow" is good advice when beginning opioid therapy.

  Because renal function declines with age, the elderly will be at higher risk for the neuroexcitatory toxicities of opioids due to accumulation of the 3-glucuonide metabolites of these drugs. Assess for myoclonus. If present, discuss opioid rotation with the prescribing physician or nurse practitioner.

- **Constipation.** The risk of electrolyte imbalances with osmotic laxatives that pull fluids from the body (e.g., magnesium citrate) is higher in the elderly.[64] Also, the elderly are at higher risk of aspirating mineral oil, leading to a lipid pneumonia. The use of mineral oil should be avoided in the elderly.

  Older, bedridden adults are more susceptible to fecal impaction. Monitor for bowel movements regularly. If liquid stool is present after a few days of no bowel movement, perform a rectal examination to rule out impaction before instituting therapy for diarrhea.

- **Nausea and Vomiting.** Older adults are at higher risk for adverse effects of antiemetics because of changes in how medications are absorbed, metabolized, distributed, and eliminated. Monitor for sedation, anticholinergic effects, and extrapyramidal effects.

- **Grieving.** Older adults may have experienced the deaths of a spouse, friends, and possibly children. Although life experience may assist persons in working through the grieving process, the loss of their networks of support can interfere with effective grieving and lead to isolation, loneliness, and depression.

Nurses have a duty to preserve, protect, and support patient autonomy by assessing patients' comprehension of both the information presented to them and the implications of decisions.[79] Nurses can promote patient autonomy in palliative care by encouraging advance care planning discussions and then being advocates to ensure that these plans are upheld. In agencies where extensive advance directive education programs exist, written advance directives are prevalent in medical records (85%) and effectively guide end-of-life decisions.[80]

Withholding or withdrawing medical treatment at a patient's request, including through a clearly written advance directive, is accepted as ethical based on the principle of autonomy. It is also ethical to withhold or withdraw life-sustaining treatments from patients who are not able to make the request and do not have advance directives, if the treatment is judged to be futile. A futile intervention may be defined as one that only prolongs the dying process, but there is no authoritative legal definition of medical futility.[81] It becomes complicated if there are disagreements among patients, families, and members of the health care team about the futility of an intervention. Some disagreements regarding withholding or withdrawing treatment are resolved when goals of care are clarified and outcomes data is objectively, but sensitively, reviewed. Other disagreements may require consultation with an ethics committee or other experts.

Assisted suicide is another frequently discussed ethical issue in end-of-life care. Some argue that providing appropriately screened terminally ill patients with prescriptions for medications that they may choose to use to end their own lives is ethically sound because it upholds the principle of self-determination. On the other side of the argument are those who feel there is a moral distinction allowing death to occur (e.g., withdrawing a life-sustaining treatment) and causing death to occur. Currently, Oregon is the only state that permits physicians to prescribe lethal medications that may be self-administered by the terminally ill patient who requests them. In some states, participation in assisted suicide is cause for loss of professional licensure or may be considered a criminal act. Some medical and nursing professional organizations have published position statements opposing assisted suicide. The Oncology Nursing Society's position statement on the nurse's responsibility to the patient requesting assisted suicide (1) emphasizes the nurse's responsibility to ensure patients receive care from compassionate, sensitive, and knowledgeable professionals, (2) acknowledges that only the patient can judge what is an acceptable level of personal suffering, (3) encourages frank discussion of the rationale for the request, (4) encourages the nurse to use nonjudgmental language when dealing with assisted suicide issues, (5) affirms the right of nurses in states where assisted suicide is legal to refuse to be involved if theses nurses arrange alternative sources of care, and (6) affirms the right of nurses in states where assisted suicide is legal to choose to continue to care for these patients if both the patient and nurse are comfortable with the arrangement.[82]

REVIEW QUESTIONS

✓ Case Study

George is a 79-year-old man who has stage IV non–small cell lung cancer (NSCLC). Since stage IV NSCLC is not considered curable, the palliative care consultation team was contacted and treatment options for his cancer were discussed with him. The palliative care team clarified what George knew about his disease—that he had incurable lung cancer, but with chemotherapy he had a potential of increased survival. The palliative care team discussed his fears and concerns about his disease and treatment. A plan of care to control side effects of this chemotherapy regimen was developed, and a discussion about advance care planning was facilitated among George, his wife, his minister, and the palliative care nurse. A power of attorney for health care, designating his wife as his proxy, was executed and placed in the medical record. In this advance directive, George stipulated that during the 2-month trial of chemotherapy, he wanted "everything" done to keep him alive, including cardiopulmonary resuscitation (CPR) and mechanical ventilation, in order to "give the chemotherapy a chance to work."

After the second cycle of chemotherapy, George is admitted to the hospital in severe distress with a respiratory rate of 38. A pulse oximeter indicates oxygen saturation is 85%. Lung auscultation reveals absence of breath sounds in the right middle and lower lobes, and lung sounds are dull to percussion over that area. Cool compresses are placed on George's face, and morphine 2.5 mg is administered by mouth (PO) for this dyspnea. His respiratory rate is now 24, and he rates his shortness of breath as a 4 on a 0-10 scale (reporting it had been a 10 earlier, but this rating was not requested while he was in acute distress). A chest x-ray exam reveals a pleural effusion. The pros and cons of a chest tube, a tunneled drainage catheter, and symptomatic treatment alone are presented to George and his wife. He opts for a tunneled drainage catheter so that he does not have to stay overnight in the hospital. The tunneled catheter is placed, and he is discharged home with a prescription and written instructions for morphine, 2.5 mg every 3 to 4 hours as needed for shortness of breath or pain; ibuprofen, 800 mg q4hr for 48 hours, then 400 mg q4hr as needed for pain at the chest tube insertion site; and Senokot-S, two tabs daily to prevent constipation from the opioid. Also, a home care program is notified to care for the pleural drainage catheter and to teach the patient's family how to care for the catheter and connect the catheter to the drainage canister.

Over his next two palliative care clinic visits, George's goals are identified: he wants to remain as active as possible for as long as possible, avoid hospitalization, be free of pain, and not be a burden to his family. His power of attorney for health care is changed to state that he does not want CPR, mechanical ventilation, or feeding tubes should he become unconscious and not able to refuse those interventions on his own. Hospice home care services are also discussed, and after noticing that he is losing weight and needing more naps (although he is still able to perform all self-care activities), he consents to hospice care, "as much for my wife as for me."

George's pleural catheter is no longer draining, and he has no shortness of breath. However, he is using the morphine, *Continued*

REVIEW QUESTIONS—CONT'D

2.5 mg PO, and ibuprofen, 400 mg PO, every 4 hours for "aches" in his hips and ribs. Metastatic disease to the bone is suspected, but diagnostic tests are not ordered since the combination of the diagnosis and relief obtained with opioid plus antiinflammatory are consistent with bone metastasis. Upon questioning, George reports he hasn't had a bowel movement for 3 days. He is instructed to take two Dulcolax tabs and then increase his daily dose of Senokot-S to three tablets.

Over the next 2 months, George becomes dependent in dressing, bathing, and transferring to the bedside commode. The hospice is providing a nurse case manager to assess and intervene for physical and emotional symptoms and coordinate the hospice team services, a certified home health aide to assist with personal care, a social worker and chaplain who alternate visits to provide emotional and spiritual support to George and his wife, and volunteers to sit with George 2 hours each week so that his wife can run errands or take a nap.

QUESTIONS

1. According to most surveys, the majority of Americans state they would prefer to die at home. Where do most Americans die, in fact?
   a. At home
   b. In a nursing home
   c. In a hospital
   d. In an emergency department
2. Which of the following is true regarding palliative care?
   a. Anyone who is eligible for palliative care is eligible for hospice care.
   b. Palliative care should be initiated at the time of diagnosis of a serious, life-threatening illness.
   c. Palliative care is the same as good symptom management.
   d. The emphasis on palliative is greatest at initial diagnosis and declines as the disease progresses.
3. Which of the following statements is true regarding patients who are most appropriate for a palliative team referral?
   a. All patients with a cancer diagnosis should have a palliative care referral.
   b. Any patient with stage IV cancer should have a palliative care referral.
   c. Only patients whose physicians identify them as having a prognosis 6 months or less should have a palliative care referral.
   d. A patient who has a local recurrence of cancer after a 3-year disease-free interval should have a palliative care referral.
4. Which of the following puts persons who have been on high doses of oral opioids and who have some renal dysfunction at risk for neurotoxicity?
   a. Euphoria that develops with high dose opioids
   b. Uremia due to renal failure
   c. Variations in how individuals metabolize opioids
   d. Accumulation of the 3-glucuronide metabolites of opioids
5. If myoclonus develops and opioid neurotoxicity is suspected, what is usually the first intervention?
   a. Discontinuation of all opioids

   b. Rotation to an equianalgesic dose of a different opioid
   c. Rotation to a different opioid at 50% of the equianalgesic dose
   d. Rotation to a different opioid at 50% more than the equianalgesic dose
6. Mrs. White has lost 85 pounds over the past year. She has no appetite. Her daughter states: "She just won't eat. You need to get her some tube or intravenous feedings or something. We can't just let her starve to death." What would be the most appropriate response?
   a. "Your mother is not dying from starvation. Her disease has changed both her appetite and how her body uses food. Artificial foods and fluid may actually make her feel worse."
   b. "When people give up, they often stop eating and allow themselves to starve to death. It is her choice: whatever makes her most comfortable."
   c. "Tube and intravenous feedings are not considered appropriate in hospice care."
   d. "You need to encourage her to eat more. Fix her favorite foods and offer her something every 2 hours."
7. The following laxative should be avoided in end-of-life care:
   a. Biscodyl (Dulcolax)
   b. Magnesium hydroxide (Milk of Magnesia)
   c. Psyllium (Metamucil)
   d. Senna, or docusate sodium (Senokot-S)
8. How does the mechanism operate by which medication and electrolyte disturbances lead to stimulation of the vomiting center of the brain?
   a. Via the chemoreceptive trigger zone (CTZ)
   b. Via the vagal nerve
   c. Via the cerebral cortex
   d. Via the labyrinth apparatus
9. Which of the following is an effective intervention for dyspnea in the palliative care setting?
   a. A fan at the bedside blowing cool are on the face
   b. Warm cloths applied to the face
   c. Oral morphine at an initial starting dose of 10 mg PO in an opioid naive patient
   d. Lying with the head of the bed flat
10. The widow of one of your recently deceased patients states: "Last night I thought I heard him say 'Good night, honey' just like he always had. Do you think I'm going crazy?" The best response would be to say:
    a. "You might want some extra support accepting your husband's death. I'll make a referral to our psychologist."
    b. "Many persons believe in ghosts or spirits who visit their loved ones. Do you believe in ghosts?"
    c. "Many persons have similar experiences of seeing or hearing the one who has died. You must miss him saying good night."
    d. "That must have been frightening for you. Do you have a friend or relative who can stay with you so you are not alone so much?"

ANSWERS:

1. **C.** *Rationale:* About 20% of deaths occur at home, 17% of deaths occur in nursing homes, and 57% of deaths occur in hospitals. Emergency department deaths are included in the statistics for hospitals.

2. **B.** *Rationale:* Hospice care is included in the continuum of palliative care but is limited in the United States according to the Medicare Hospice benefit to only the last 6 months of life. Palliative care should be initiated at the time of diagnosis of a serious, life-threatening illness. The management on physical, social, emotional, and spiritual symptoms of the patient *and* family differentiates palliative care from good symptom management. At diagnosis, the emphasis may be on curative interventions, but as the disease progresses, more and more emphasis is placed on palliative interventions.

3. **B.** *Rationale:* About 36% of persons will die from their cancer. Those who are diagnosed with early-stage disease are more likely to be cured and would not be referred to a palliative care program. Persons with stage IV disease will likely receive the most benefit from palliative care, because stage IV disease is often not curable. Interventions aimed at prolonging survival are consistent with good palliative care. Persons with a prognosis of 6 months or less will also benefit from palliative or hospice care, but this is likely a late referral since physicians tend to overestimate the time remaining to a patient. A person with a short disease-free survival is more likely to have a poor prognosis than one with a longer disease-free survival.

4. **D.** *Rationale:* Euphoria is a known side effect of opioids but is not a sign of neurotoxicity. Patients often develop tolerance to the euphoric side effects of opioids fairly quickly. Renal failure puts the patient at higher risk for neurotoxicity, but uremia does not cause the neurotoxicity. There are individual variations in how people metabolize medications. This may make some persons more prone to neurotoxicity, but this does not cause it. The 3-glucuronide metabolites of opioids may accumulate with decreased renal function, putting the patient at risk for myoclonus and, potentially, hyperalgesia.

5. **C.** *Rationale:* Discontinuation of opioids would lead to pain getting out of control and withdrawal. Opioids should never be stopped abruptly. An equianalgesic dose would likely be too high because (1) there is incomplete cross-tolerance between opioids, and (2) the opioid dose may have been increased to treat the hyperalgesia caused by the neurotoxicity. When the patient is rotated to a different opioid, the hyperalgesia may resolve, and the patient would need a lower dose of opioid. To treat myoclonus, obtain an order for a different opioid at 50% of the equianalgesic dose. This dose accounts for the factors just discussed. When the new (lower) dose is started, monitor for effectiveness and side effects, and titrate up or down as needed. Rotation to a different opioid at 50% higher than the equianalgesic dose would likely lead to

serious side effects since this dose would be too high, as explained.

6. **A.** *Rationale:* When patients feel worse when they eat toward the end of life, probably the most important intervention is to make it "okay" for them not to eat. Often the family needs much more support on this issue than the patient. The anorexia of advanced cancer is not a patient choice and is not a sign of giving up. The goal of hospice care is patient comfort. Some patients may benefit from artificial fluid and nutrition, and others may become more uncomfortable. Interventions must always be based on the specific individual's condition and goals. Focusing on eating often causes increased anxiety for both the patient and the family. Patients feel guilty and try to eat to please their family members, even though it makes them sick; family members focus on food and may become angry and frustrated with the patient for not eating.

7. **C.** *Rationale:* Biscodyl is an acceptable stimulant laxative. Magnesium hydroxide is an acceptable stimulant laxative. Bulk-forming laxatives like Metamucil are avoided in palliative care, because they are dehydrating and patients can rarely tolerate the large amounts of fluid intake these medications need to work effectively. Senna, or docusate sodium, is a good laxative to use in palliative care since it contains both a softener and a stimulant.

8. **A.** *Rationale:* The CTZ chemoreceptive trigger zone is where chemical changes that trigger nausea are detected. The vagal nerve stimulates the vomiting center when there is GI irritation, obstruction, or constipation. The cerebral cortex stimulates the vomiting center when there is stress, anxiety, or increase intracranial pressure. The labyrinth apparatus is the motion sensor of the body. If vomiting is associated with dizziness, the labyrinth apparatus may be involved.

9. **A.** *Rationale:* A fan blowing cool air to the face is an effective intervention for dyspnea. Cool, not warm, cloths applied to the face are often effective in treating dyspnea. The initial starting dose of oral morphine for dyspnea in the opioid-naive patient is 2.5 to 5 mg. Many patients find sitting up and leaning slightly forward to help with dyspnea. If the patient has significant ascites, having the head of the bed partially elevated may be more comfortable than a full upright position or lying down.

10. **C.** *Rationale:* The support of grief groups and counselors may be very helpful to the bereaved. However, this person's experience is a common manifestation of grief and does not indicated the need for a referral to a psychologist. The response in (b) does not acknowledge the grief experience and is not supportive. The (c) response both normalizes the common grief experience of visual or auditory hallucinations of the deceased and acknowledges her loss, allowing her the opportunity to express her grief. Although being with a friend or relative may, indeed, be helpful, this response (d) does not acknowledge that her experience is a normal manifestation of grief.

REFERENCES

1. American Cancer Society: *Cancer facts and figures 2006*, Atlanta, 2006, Author.
2. Ferrell B, Virani, R, Grant M: Analysis of end-of-life content in nursing textbooks, *Oncol Nurs Forum* 25(8):869-876, 1999.
3. SUPPORT Principal Investigators: A controlled trial to improve care for seriously ill hospitalized patients: the study to understand prognoses and preferences for outcomes and risks of treatments (SUPPORT), *J Am Med Assoc* 274(20):1591-1598, 1995.
4. Ferrell B, Virani R, Grant M et al: Evaluation of the End-of-Life Nursing Education Consortium undergraduate faculty training program, *J Palliat Med* 8(1), 107-114, 2005.
5. Kübler-Ross E: *On death and dying*, New York, 1969, McMillan.
6. Worden JW: *Grief counseling and grief therapy: a handbook for the mental health practitioner*, New York, 1982, Springer.
7. Centers for Medicare and Medicaid Services: *The hospice benefit*, CMS Publication No. 02154, Baltimore MD, 2005, Author.
8. National Hospice and Palliative Care Organization: *Hospice facts and figures,* retrieved September 17, 2005, from http://www.nhpco.org/files/public/Hospice_Facts_110104.pdf.
9. Last Acts: *Means to a better end: a report on dying in American today*, Washington, DC, 2002, Authors.
10. Friedman B, Harwood K, Shields M: Barriers and enablers to hospice referrals: an expert overview, *J Palliat Med* 5(1):73-81, 2002.
11. Steinhauser KE, Christakis NA, Clipp EC et al: Factors considered important at the end of life by patients, family, physicians, and other care providers, *J Am Med Assoc* 284(19):2476-2482, 2000.
12. Field MJ, Cassel CK, editors: *Approaching death: improving care at the end of life*, Washington, DC, 1997, National Academy Press.
13. National Consensus Project for Quality Palliative Care: *Clinical practice guidelines for quality palliative care,* 2004, retrieved September 17, 2005, from http://www.nationalconsensusproject.org.
14. Doyle D, Hanks G, Cherny NI et al: Introduction. In Doyle D, Hanks G, Cherney H et al, editors: *Oxford textbook of palliative medicine*, ed 3, New York, 2003, Oxford University Press.
15. Lunney JR, Lynn J, Foley DJ et al: Patterns of functional decline at the end of life, *J Am Med Assoc* 289(18):2387-2392, 2003.
16. Lamont EB, Christakis NA: Complexities in prognostication in advanced cancer, *J Am Med Assoc* 290(1):98-104, 2003.
17. Glare P: Clinical predictors of survival in advanced cancer, *J Support Oncol* 3(5):331-339, 2005.
18. Vainio A, Auvinen A: Prevalence of symptoms among patients with advanced cancer: an international collaborative study, *J Pain Symptom Manage* 12(1):3-10, 1996.
19. Von Roenn JH, Paice JA: Control of common, non-pain cancer symptoms, *Semin Oncol* 32(2):200-210, 2005.
20. Potter J, Hami F, Gryan T et al: Symptoms in 400 patients referred to palliative care services: prevalence and patterns, *Palliat Med* 17(4):310-314, 2003.
21. Wilson RK, Weissman DE: Neuroexcitatory effects of opioids: patient assessment #57, *J Palliat Med* 7(4):579, 2004.
22. Cherny N, Ripamonti C, Pereira J et al: Strategies to manage the adverse effects of oral morphine: an evidence-based report, *J Clin Oncol* 19(9):2542-2554, 2001.
23. Wilson RK, Weissman DE: Neuroexcitatory effects of opioids: treatment, *J Palliat Med* 7(4):580-581, 2004.
24. Sweeney C, Neuenschwander H, Bruera E: Fatigue and asthenia. In Doyle D, Hanks G, Cherney H et al, editors: *Oxford textbook of palliative medicine*, ed 3, New York, 2003, Oxford University Press.
25. Klinkenberg M, Willems D, Wal G et al: Symptom burden in the last week of life, *J Pain Symptom Manage* 27(1):5-13, 2004.
26. Stone P, Richardson A, Ream E et al: Cancer-related fatigue: inevitable, unimportant and untreatable? Results of a multi-centre patient survey, *Ann Oncol* 11(8):971-975, 2000.
27. Inui A: Cancer anorexia-cachexia syndrome: current issues in research and management, *CA Cancer J Clin* 52(2):72-91, 2002.
28. Strausser F: Pathophysiology of the anorexia/cachexia syndrome, In Doyle D, Hanks G, Cherney H et al, editors: *Oxford textbook of palliative medicine*, ed 3, New York, 2003, Oxford University Press.
29. Waller A, Caroline N: *Handbook of palliative care in cancer*, ed 2, Boston, 2000, Butterworth-Heinemann.
30. Bruera E: Anorexia, cachexia and nutrition, *Br Med J* 315(7117):1219-1222, 1997.
31. Davis MP, Dickerson D: Cachexia and anorexia: cancer's covert killer, *Support Care Cancer* 8(3):180-187, 2000.
32. Tisdale M: Metabolic abnormalities in cachexia and anorexia, *Nutrition* 16(10):1013-1014, 2000.
33. Tisdale M: Protein loss in cancer cachexia, *Science* 289(5488):2293-2366, 2000.
34. Martignoni M, Kunze P, Priess H: Cancer cachexia, *Mol Cancer* 2:36, 2003.
35. Barber M, Ross J, Voss A et al: The effect of an oral nutritional supplement enriched with fish oil on weight loss in patients with pancreatic cancer. *Br J Cancer* 81(1):80-86, 1999.
36. Davis MP: New drugs for the anorexia-cachexia syndrome, *Curr Oncol Rep* 4(3):264-274, 2002.
37. McCarthy, DO: Rethinking nutritional support for persons with cancer cachexia, *Biol Res Nurs* 5(1):3-17, 2003.
38. MacDonald N, Easson AM, Mazurak VC et al: Understanding and managing cancer cachexia, *J Am Coll Surg* 197(1):143-161, 2003.
39. Lanquillon S, Krieg JC, Bening-Abu-Sach U et al: Cytokine production and treatment response in major depressive disorder, *Neuropsychopharmacology* 22(4):370-379, 2000.
40. Klein S, Kinney J, Jeejeebhoy K et al: Nutrition support in clinical practice: review of published data and recommendations for future research directions, *Am J Clin Nutr* 66(3):683-706, 1997.
41. Bruera E, Sweeney C: Pharmacological interventions in cachexia and anorexia. In Doyle D, Hanks G, Cherney H et al, editors: *Oxford textbook of palliative medicine*, ed 3, New York, 2003, Oxford University Press.
42. Tyler L, Lipman A: Anorexia and cachexia in palliative care patients. In Lipman A, Jackson K, Tyler L, editors: *Evidence based symptom control in palliative care*, New York, 2000, Pharmaceutical Products Press.
43. Tomiska M, Tomiskova M, Salajka F et al: Palliative treatment of cancer cachexia with oral suspension of megestrol acetate, *Neoplasm* 50(3):227-233, 2003.
44. Fainsinger R, Pereira J: Clinical assessment and decision-making in cachexia and anorexia. In Doyle D, Hanks G, Cherney H et al, editors: *Oxford textbook of palliative medicine*, ed 3, New York, 2003, Oxford University Press.
45. Conill C, Verger E, Henriquez I et al: Symptom prevalence in the last week of life, *J Pain Symptom Manage* 46(6):328-331, 1997.
46. Bennett CJ, Cresswell H: Factors influencing constipation in advanced cancer patients: a prospective study of opioid dose, Dantron dose and physical functioning, *Palliat Med* 17(5):418-422, 2003.
47. Sykes N: Constipation and diarrhea. In Doyle D, Hanks G, Cherney H et al, editors: *Oxford textbook of palliative medicine*, ed 3, New York, 2003, Oxford University Press.
48. Heidrich D: Constipation. In Kuebler K, Berry P, Heidrich D, editors: *End of life care clinical practice guidelines*, St. Louis, 2002, W.B. Saunders.
49. Klaschik E, Nauck F, Ostgathe C: Constipation: modern laxative therapy, *Support Care Cancer* 11(11):679-685, 2003.
50. Beckwith M: Constipation in palliative care patients. In Lipman A, Jackson K, Tyler L, editors: *Evidence based symptom control in palliative care*, New York, 2000, Pharmaceutical Products Press.
51. Griffie J, McKinnon S: Nausea and vomiting. In Kuebler K, Berry P, Heidrich D, editors: *End of life care clinical practice guidelines*, St. Louis, 2002, W.B. Saunders.
52. Komurcu S, Nelson K, Walsh D: The gastrointestinal symptoms of advanced cancer, *Support Care Cancer* 9(1):32-39, 2001.
53. Davis MP, Walsh D: Treatment of nausea and vomiting in advanced cancer, *Support Care Cancer* 8(6):444-452, 2000.
54. Mannix K: Palliation of nausea and vomiting. In Doyle D, Hanks G, Cherney H et al, editors: *Oxford textbook of palliative medicine*, ed 3, New York, 2003, Oxford University Press.
55. Twycross R, Back O: Nausea and vomiting in advanced cancer, *Eur J Palliat Care* 5(1):39-45, 1998.
56. Hornby PJ: Central neurocircuitry associated with emesis, *Am J Med* 111(Suppl 8A):106S-112S.
57. Lacy BE, Weiser K: Gastric motility, gastroparesis, and gastric stimulation, *Surg Clin North Am* 85(5):967-987, 2005.

58. Jones MP: Management of diabetic gastroparesis, *Nutr Clin Pract* 19(2):145-153, 2004.
59. American Thoracic Society: Dyspnea mechanisms, assessment and management: a consensus statement, *Am J Respir Crit Care Med* 159(1):321-340, 1999.
60. Bruera E, Schmitz B, Pither J et al: The frequency and correlates of dyspnea in patients with advanced cancer, *J Pain Symptom Manage* 19(5):357-362, 2000.
61. Dudgeon DJ, Kristjanson L, Sloan JA et al: Dyspnea in cancer patients: prevalence and associated factors, *J Pain Symptom Manage* 21(2):95-102, 2001.
62. Kuebler KK, Andry JM, Davis S: Dyspnea. In Kuebler K, Heidrich D, Esper P, editors: *Palliative and end of life care clinical practice guidelines*, St. Louis, 2007, Saunders.
63. Lagman RL, Davis MP, LeGrand SB et al: Common symptoms in advanced cancer, *Surg Clin N Am* 85(2):237-255, 2005.
64. Brown JA, Von Roenn JH: Symptom management in the older adult, *Clin Geriatr Med* 20(4):621-640, 2004.
65. Jennings AL, Davies AN, Higgins JPT et al: Opioids for the palliation of breathlessness in terminal illness, *The Cochrane Database of Systematic Reviews* 2001, Issue 3, Art No: CD002066. DOI: 10.1002/14651858.CD002066.
66. Bruera E, Sala, R, Spruyt O et al: Nebulized versus subcutaneous morphine for patients with cancer dyspnea: a preliminary study, *J Pain Symptom Manage* 29(6):613-618, 2005.
67. Coyne PJ, Viswanathan R, Smith TJ: Nebulized fentanyl citrate improves patients' perception of breathing, respiratory rate, and oxygen saturation in dyspnea, *J Pain Symptom Manage* 23(2):157-160, 2002.
68. Bruera E, Sweeney C, Willey J et al: A randomized controlled trial of supplemental oxygen versus air in cancer patients with dyspnea, *Palliat Med* 17(8):659-663, 2003.
69. Byock I: *Dying well: the prospect for growth at the end of life*, New York, 1997, Riverhead Books.
70. Chochinov HM, Hack T, Hassard T et al: Dignity therapy: a novel psychotherapeutic intervention for patients near the end of life, *J Clin Oncol* 23(24):5520-5525, 2005.
71. Roberts KF, Berry PH: Grief and bereavement. In Kuebler K, Berry P, Heidrich D, editors: *End of life care clinical practice guidelines*, St. Louis, 2002, W.B. Saunders.
72. McCaffery M, Pasero C: *Pain: clinical manual*, ed 2, St. Louis, 1999, Mosby.
73. Yennurajalingam S, Braiteh F, Bruera E: Pain and terminal delirium research in the elderly, *Clin Geriatr Med* 21(1):93-119, 2005.
74. Ogle KS, Hopper K: End-of-life care for older adults, *Prim Care* 32(3):811-818, 2005.
75. Given BA, Sherwood PR: Nurse-sensitive patient outcomes—a white paper, *Oncol Nurs Forum* 32(4):773-784, 2005.
76. Edmonton Regional Palliative Care Program: Edmonton Symptom Assessment System, 2001, retrieved January 22, 2006, from http://www.palliative.org/PC/ClinicalInfo/AssessmentTools/esas.pdf.
77. Teno J: Center for Gerontology and Health Care Research. Toolkit of instruments to measure end of life care, 2004, retrieved January 22, 2006, from http://www.chcr.brown.edu/pcoc/linkstoinstrumhtm.htm.
78. Connor SR, Teno J, Spence C et al: Family evaluation of hospice care: results from voluntary submission of data via website, *J Pain Symptom Manage* 30(1):9-17, 2005.
79. American Nurses Association: Code of ethics for nurses with interpretive statements, Silver Springs, MD, 2001, American Nurses Publishing.
80. Hammes BJ, Rooney BL: Death and end-of-life planning in one midwestern community, *Arch Intern Med* 158(4):383-390, 1998.
81. American Medical Association: Medical futility in end-of-life care: report of the Council on Ethical and Judicial Affairs, *J Am Med Assoc* 281(10):937-941, 1999.
82. Oncology Nursing Society: The nurse's responsibility to the patient requesting assisted suicide, 2004, retrieved January 22, 2006, from http://www.ons.org/publications/positions/AssistedSuicide.shtml.

CHAPTER 35

Family Caregiving

Ellyn Matthews

Overview and Introduction

Cancer remains a major cause of morbidity and mortality in the United States, and treatment is often complex and expensive in financial and human terms. During the past few decades, rising health care costs and efforts to contain these costs resulted in a shift away from traditional inpatient hospital settings and an increased emphasis on home care and alternative care settings. Health care trends include accelerated use of home health care to provide postacute care services, increased use of home health care by patients aged 65 years or older, and increased percentages of the United States population enrolled in Medicare and Medicaid home care programs. A contributing factor in the exponential growth in home health care in the 1990s was an expectation that it could save health care dollars by preventing hospitalizations and placement in long-term care facilities. Demographic changes in America, technologic advances, and the fee-for-service payment system contributed to the rapid growth of home care before the Balanced Budget Act of 1997 (BBA).

Recent concerns about abuse and fraud prompted the federal government to make changes in policy and regulatory practices affecting the home health care industry.[1] Home health transformations can be traced back to the Tax Equity and Fiscal Responsibility Act of 1982 (TEFRA), which introduced the prospective payment system (PPS) to the inpatient setting, commonly called the diagnosis-related groups (DRG) method of payment. As a result of this system, Medicare paid hospitals according to predetermined inpatient length of stay and cost per case, reducing the number of inpatient days. The BBA extended the PPS across the continuum of care, and in 2000 phased in a PPS for Medicare home health services. Under the PPS, home health agencies conduct a comprehensive assessment of each patient and assign the patient to one of 80 home health resource groups (HHRGs). The home health agency receives a predetermined reimbursement based on the HHRG for each covered 60-day "episode of care," with some built-in adjustment for patients with greater-than-usual needs or changes in condition during the episode of care. Just as implementation of hospital-based PPS led to patients being discharged "quicker and sicker," the home health PPS creates the need for increasingly cost-effective delivery of quality of care with optimal patient outcomes in home care. The Outcomes and Assessment Information Set (OASIS), a tool currently mandated for home care, measures patient status, satisfaction, and outcomes at various specified points during an episode of care. It forms the foundation of the Centers for Medicare and Medicaid Services (CMS) (formerly the Health Care Financing Administration [HCFA]) Outcomes-Based Quality Improvement (OBQI) initiative as a part of every home care agency's quality management program.[2]

Now, well into the twenty-first century, family members and other informal caregivers such as friends and neighbors provide largely unpaid assistance to loved ones with cancer and other chronic illnesses. The economic value of this informal, unpaid caregiving is staggering and greatly surpasses the costs associated with home health care and nursing home care, since it comprises the majority of the long-term care delivered at home.[3-5] Only recently has federal public policy acknowledged and supported the service needs of families in the caregiving role. The Older Americans Act (OAA) Amendments of 2000 authorized the creation of the National Family Caregiver Support Program (NFCSP), which recognizes and encourages the caregiver role in the home and community. A national program that is designed and financed by individual states, the NFCSP includes five categories of support for the caregiver: (1) information about available services, (2) assistance in gaining access to supportive services, (3) individual counseling, support groups, and caregiver training, (4) respite care, and (5) limited supplemental services to complement the care provided by caregivers.[3,4]

Research indicates that a majority of Americans prefer receiving health care in the home over institutional care.[6-8] The identified advantages of home care include familiarity with surroundings and caregivers, increased sense of control, convenience for patients and families, less disruption in family life and related activities, less expense, reduction in infections, and overall improved quality of life. Although cost-effectiveness is a frequently mentioned justification, the best argument for home care is that it is a humane and compassionate way to provide needed health services and support. Home care enhances and supplements the care provided by families and friends and maintains the cancer patient's dignity and independence, qualities that are often lost in even the best institutions.[9-11]

Etiology and Risk Factors for Family Caregiving

Caregiving is a multifaceted role, and the demands placed on cancer caregivers are well documented. Jones first classified caregiver demands as objective (related to the actual performance of tasks) and subjective (related to the burden as perceived by the caregiver).[12] Objective burden is directly measurable (e.g., financial costs, symptom management, direct care, transportation). The less obvious, subjective feelings associated with caregiving—emotional stress, depression, hopelessness, loss of control, anger, guilt, resentment, and increased anxiety related to caretaking activities—are powerful predictors of distress.[5,13-17] The disadvantages of home care that must be considered include potential for increased out-of-pocket costs such as transportation and lost wages, increased stress and emotional strain related to caregiver burden, sleep disturbances, fatigue, relational deprivation, and competence of patients and caregivers in managing complications and emergencies. Significantly, cancer caregivers are more likely to provide "high burden" care—a level of help needed by an ill person with activities of daily living [ADLs] and instrumental activities of daily living [IADLs])—compared with non-cancer caregivers.[5,18-22]

Home care has increasingly included the use of technology, providing intravenous (IV) infusions, parenteral and enteral nutrition, supplemental oxygen, chemotherapy, and respirators in the home setting. Consequently, patients are discharged after only a short hospital stay, whereas in the past, they would have remained hospitalized for ongoing assessment and evaluation of their status and response to treatment. Many cancer therapies that were previously administered only in acute care settings are now given routinely in an outpatient or home care setting, including aspects of stem cell transplants and phase I clinical trials.[23] Advances in cancer treatments and the availability of improved technology have made outpatient and home cancer treatment both safe and effective, when appropriate standards of chemotherapy administration are adopted.[24,25]

Patients who are frequent visitors to the emergency department or who have frequent readmissions to the hospital because of exacerbations of chronic illnesses are often patients who could have benefited from home health care at an earlier time. As the trend for early inpatient discharge continues, nurses are expected to facilitate the transition between the acute care and community or convalescent settings. This transition is a complex and challenging task that requires timely, comprehensive data gathering, use of a variety of interventional options, and critical thinking skills. The health care professional must be able to gather and analyze pertinent information to develop a discharge plan that provides the least restrictive and most appropriate level of care. The early discharge process limits the time during hospitalization for health professionals to instruct the patient in the self-care practices necessary to enhance their recovery in the home. This health teaching, therefore, must be targeted to specific symptoms, include a clear reporting mechanism should symptoms occur, and be continued after hospital discharge to lessen the chance of illness exacerbation and rehospitalization. Thus, nursing care is needed to facilitate the patient's self-care practices, health teaching, continuation of skilled assessments, communication of changes in condition to the physician, and coordination of care.[23,25,26]

Economical, home-based, family-supported cancer care and treatment is on the increase. At the same time, demographic changes in U.S. society the decline of traditional extended family support systems necessitates use of additional community-based support services to maintain the patient in the home setting or alternative settings for care that are now more frequently available through managed care systems.[3,4,19,27] Little attention has been focused on the needs of lesbian, gay, bisexual, and transgender (LGBT) older adults and in particular, their caregivers; and it is important to recognize that nontraditional partnerships and families may have special needs when it comes to comfortable interactions with health care agency personnel and extended care placement.[28] It is essential that health care professionals accurately assess and identify the specific needs of the patient and the extent to which the family is willing and able to take on the caregiving role.[19,27]

Caregiving skill has been identified and categorized into nine processes: monitoring, interpreting, making decisions, taking action, making adjustments, providing hands-on care, accessing resources, working together with the ill person, and negotiating the health care system.[26] Recognition of the presence or absence of sufficient caregiving support is central to determining if home care or an alternative care setting is the best option. This is particularly important, because home care is essentially an intermittent and limited service that is not meant to substitute for long-term care. Patients and families need accurate information about home care to address their expectations of the services and ensure satisfaction with the care provided. The intent of home care is to promote independence in the management of health care needs. It is important that oncology nurses and other health care providers are cognizant of all the variables that will affect the patient's response to treatment at home or in an alternative care setting. The goal is to ensure the patient's safety and facilitate the transition throughout a coordinated system of health care delivery. This system includes various settings within a continuum of care in which comprehensive assessments of patient and family needs are communicated systematically to the health care providers involved in the patient's care. To accomplish this, the oncology nurse must thoroughly evaluate and accurately identify the patient's and the family's abilities and learning needs, as well as the environmental factors in the home that may interfere with the patient's safety and well-being.[5,25,29-32]

Research has demonstrated that supporting the caregiver in the caregiving role, particularly with the day-to-day management of care, and coaching for caregiving skill development is of paramount importance, particularly for caregivers of cancer patients. This assistance should be tailored to meet individual needs but must include information and skills relative to physical care, accessing resources, emotional support, and respite when possible.[5,26,32]

Hospital discharge planning, an essential component of quality patient-centered care, is supported by a federal law passed in December 1994 with a supplement in 1998 (42 U.S.C., Subchapter XVIII, Part D, Section 1395x,ee.1994, Supplement, January 26, 1998). The law requires that standards and guidelines for discharge planning contain the following eight key components:

1. The hospital must identify, at an early stage of hospitalization, patients who are likely to suffer adverse health consequences upon discharge in the absence of adequate discharge planning.
2. Hospitals must provide a discharge planning evaluation for patients identified under subparagraph (A) listed above and for other patients at the request of the patient, the patient's representative, or the patient's physician.
3. Any discharge planning evaluation must be made on a timely basis to ensure that appropriate arrangements for posthospital care will be made before discharge, and to avoid unnecessary delays in discharge.
4. This evaluation must include the patient's likely need for and availability of appropriate posthospital services, including hospice services and the availability of those services, such as the availability of home health services through individuals and entities that participate in the program and that serve the area in which the patient resides and that request to be listed by the hospital as available.
5. The discharge planning evaluation must be included in the patient's medical record for use in establishing an appropriate discharge plan, and the results of the evaluation must be discussed with the patient (or the patient's representative).

6. Upon the request of the patient's physician, the hospital must arrange for the development and initial implementation of a discharge plan for the patient.

7. Any discharge planning evaluation or discharge plan required must be developed by, or under the supervision of, a registered professional nurse, social worker, or other appropriate qualified personnel.

8. The discharge process will not specify or otherwise limit the qualified provider who may provide posthospital services, and will identify any entity to whom the individual is referred in which the hospital has a disclosable financial interest or which has such an interest in the hospital.

Previously, discharge planning often focused on the transition from the acute care setting; however, discharge planning or the more comprehensive term, transitional planning, is now needed throughout the cancer trajectory, and is not the sole responsibility of hospital-based care. Oncology patients move rapidly through the health care system and require various levels of services. The transitional care planning process used in the hospital setting can be applied to the outpatient setting, the emergency department, or any other health care setting in which a health care professional identifies discharge needs. The principles of transitional care planning include the following: (1) transitional planning begins at any entry point into the health care system; (2) any point on the health continuum can serve as a basis for entry into the health care system; (3) movement through the care continuum may be multidirectional; and (4) the complexity and intensity of care should be flexible and adaptable to the care needs of the patient.

TRANSITIONAL OR DISCHARGE PLANNING PROCESS

Transitional planning is a process that involves assessment, identification of continuing care needs, planning of outcomes and care, and implementation of a plan to meet the needs of patients and their caregivers during or after an episode or phase of illness. Transitional planning is a dynamic, interactive, collaborative, and interdisciplinary process. Expediting patient transfers to more cost-effective levels of care at the earliest possible time necessitates not only effective tools to facilitate the process, but also adherence to professional standards of practice for discharge planning. Transitional planning is performed by a variety of health care professionals, including nurses and social workers.[25] These professionals must have the basic skills necessary to assess, develop, and implement individualized continuing care plans. In recent years, the role of the hospital-based transitional planner has often expanded to a case coordination or case management role within a larger health care system. Therefore the need for standards of transitional planning applicable to all settings is important. The Case Management Society of America outlines the six essential components in the revised standards of practice related to transitional planning (Box 35-1).[33]

Adherence to standards of transitional planning and use of a systematic and dynamic approach is beneficial, because it helps to develop a comprehensive plan of care and provides a built-in mechanism for ongoing reevaluation and modification of the plan. Transitional planning is dynamic and must respond to changes in the practice such as growing numbers of people who receive "primary" care in emergency departments, high occupancy rates in hospitals, and the need to establish an "emergency preparedness" process to assess the marginally ready patient for potential discharge.[25,32,34]

Assessment and Common Problems, Issues, and Concerns

Hospital discharge referral decisions require time and skill for careful, thorough assessment, which is necessary to effectively determine patients' current needs, predict future requirements, make appropriate decisions, and coordinate follow-up services. Pressures to control costs from the PPS, truncated hospital stays, inconsistent criteria for assessment, and the tendency of hospital staff nurses to grossly overestimate patients' self-care abilities have combined to largely prevent today's health care climate from being conducive to such careful consideration.[35] The oncology nurse in the acute care setting has a unique opportunity to perform a comprehensive assessment of the patient's strengths and limitations over days and sometimes weeks, particularly in vulnerable older cancer patients. Frequently, when care is given over several days, the nurse is able to establish a therapeutic relationship and identify patient care needs that may not have been previously assessed. However, nursing care in the inpatient setting is frequently extremely hectic and priority-based; therefore oncology nurses are not consistently able to spend extended periods with patients exploring their transitional planning needs. In addition, cancer patients are frequently discharged before the full effect of treatment is evident and the patient and family understand the treatment plan, its side effects, and management strategies well enough to assume self-care. Assessments by hospital clinicians are often gathered and applied inconsistently; therefore it is important to understand that transitional planning cannot wait until the day the patient is leaving the hospital for home or for placement in an alternative care setting.[32,35,36]

The nursing process of clinical decision making consists of observations, gathering patient information, evaluating patient information, and taking action to achieve desired patient outcomes related to nursing care. Nurse-sensitive outcomes assessment in practice is important in acute care and discharge planning because outcomes measurement provides evidence of accountability. Five categories of nursing-sensitive outcomes relevant to the oncology population that have standardized assessment tools include functional status, symptom prevalence and distress (e.g., pain, nausea, dyspnea, fatigue), self-care (patients' readiness for discharge related to knowledge of medications and treatment), and the risk of falls and pressure ulcers.[29,32,37] See Table 27-1 for the Braden Scale for predicting pressure ulcer risk.

In the acute care setting, symptom assessment (i.e., presence, frequency, intensity) is assessed daily; functional status and risk of falls and pressure ulcers are assessed within 24 hours of admission and 24 hours before discharge, and self-care is assessed 24 hours before discharge.[29,32,37] Oncology nurses in outpatient clinics or alternative settings have the responsibility to assess for and identify the patient's specific health care needs related to living arrangements, home environment, self-care ability, and caregiver availability and skill. The oncology nurse can quickly and effectively assess, identify, and respond to patient and family needs as they surface, if the nurse is continuously cognizant of the importance of planning for continued care and has an appropriate method to facilitate the process.

Numerous factors are considered before discharge, and anticipatory planning is essential. Consultation with the designated

BOX 35-1   Standards of Practice and Discharge Planning

Standard One: Client Identification and Selection

This standard addresses the need to identify individuals who benefit the most from case management services, particularly those who would suffer adverse effects without discharge planning intervention.

A. Each clinical service unit or hospital establishes high-risk criteria for high-risk patient identification

B. Preset risk for adverse outcome without discharge planning (criteria sets for identification may be based on length of stay; review of criteria is an extension of utilization review)

Standard Two: Problem Identification

This standard includes using objective assessment data; specific problems are identified that require case management intervention. The assessment process is essential and requires time and experience.

A. Twofold assessment:
   1. Assessment of patient functional abilities and deficits
   2. Assessment of resources available to the patient

B. Assessment categories in discharge planning focus on functional patterns, including the activities of daily living (ADLs) and instrumental activities of daily living (IADLs)

C. After the twofold assessment, problems are identified

D. Problems can be ongoing diagnostic or therapeutic needs, newly identified or ongoing educational needs, or ways to monitor patient progress and response to therapy

E. Problem identification is a tool for planning and problems are stated as "goals," which sets up an expected outcome by which to evaluate the discharge plan

Standard Three: Planning

This standard involves collaboration with the individual and the health care team members. The individual and health care team develop immediate, short-term, and long-term strategies to address the individual's problems.

A. Discharge plans are based on "problem identification"

B. Problem identification leads to goals that drive the plan

C. Preliminary discharge plan with appropriate options is presented to the patient and family, who exercise their choice between options

D. Options are evaluated for appropriateness and availability before presenting them to the family (e.g., nursing home placement is matched to patient needs, and availability is ascertained)

E. There is a professional and legal responsibility to ensure appropriate and available options

F. Options reflect an accurate and thorough twofold assessment

G. There is no minimum or maximum number of choices to meet the plan of care

Standard Four: Monitoring

This standard involves an ongoing assessment of the identified problems.

A. Monitoring requires goal-oriented and ongoing problem identification based on the twofold assessment (patient functional status or resource availability can change)

B. Monitoring must be current and ongoing until the final plan is determined

Standard Five: Evaluating

This standard incorporates the application of a methodology designed to measure the processes used with a focus on patient response.

A. Evaluating the discharge plan is difficult if the patient is no longer in the health care system; however, there are some plans in which the patient is contacted after discharge

B. Evaluation of the plan crosses levels of care and is done in collaboration with quality assurance, quality improvement, or risk management department so that the overall process can be improved

C. Patient satisfaction surveys address a component of the "continuum of care" and the discharge plan, with survey results reviewed by discharge planners

Standard Six: Outcomes

This standard addresses the discharge end point, specifically patient-centered outcomes that are positive, measurable, and goal-oriented, such as readmissions or return visit to the emergency department.

A. Patient-sensitive outcomes examples are progressive rehabilitation to independence in ADLs and self-management of plan of care

Modified from Birmingham J: Discharge planning: the old/new wave. Part 2: the new wave of discharge planning, *Inside Case Manage* 10(9):1-5, 2003.

home care agency and/or hospice nursing staff facilitates an effective discharge planning transition from the acute care setting to the home setting. This process necessitates not only thorough assessment and evaluation, but also extensive planning, communication, and coordination. The medical record contains the patient admission data as an initial source of data for the discharge planner to screen and identify patients who may have continuing care planning needs. The oncology nurse, using the usual sources of data such as the patient's medical record, also relies on first-hand observations and assessment of the patient. Among several characteristics associated with the need for home or extended care, the likelihood of home care referral, and/or poor outcomes are the following:[32,35,38]

- Age (over age 70 or pediatric cases)
- Educational level below 12 years
- ADLs impairment, toileting problems, history of falls
- Two or more chronic conditions
- Fair or poor subjective health rating
- Cognitive impairment, mental status change
- Homebound, prior home care use
- Living alone, less social support
- Multiple hospital readmissions (more than two in past 6 months), long length of hospital stay, admission in the last 15 to 30 days
- Multiple IV medications or treatments, suspected noncompliance to medications, treatment complications
- Depression and/or psychiatric history
- Need for complex therapy or equipment (e.g., physical, occupational, or speech therapy; urinary catheter or bowel division; enteral or parenteral feedings; pain management; wound care; IV treatments; ventilator; new assistive device for mobility; specialized bed)

A typical example of a screening tool to detect the need for timely and appropriate referrals is the High Risk Discharge Assessment Instrument (HRDAI).[36,39] The HRDAI, originally developed for emergency department discharge screening, can be adapted to any patient population that is transitioning care. It consists of eight indicators that contribute to referral to home care: impaired mobility, living alone, mental status change, possible domestic violence, substance abuse, inadequate resources, noncompliance and repeated emergency department visits.

Regardless of the mechanism used in identifying patients for continuing care needs, the screening process should be followed by the patient interview, identification of the specific problems or needs, and development of a plan for solving patient problems or needs. These three major components of the discharge planning process (the patient interview, identification of problems and needs, and potential areas of concern and risk) have specific subcomponents that, when addressed, both clarify and simplify the continuing planning process.

The patient interview begins with an introduction (if necessary), then establishes the patient's relationships such as to a spouse, family including children, neighbors, church, and senior citizen support activities (if applicable). The interview focuses on how the patient's illness has affected roles and functions in the family, with special attention to financial support, shopping, meal preparation, transportation, living arrangements and prehospital daily routine. An assessment is made of the patient's learning and comprehension ability, interest in discharge planning services, and goals and expectations for the treatment and rehabilitation process.[13] During the assessment process, transitional care planners use multifaceted skills such as listening and formulating thoughtful questions, interpreting patient concerns and communicating this information to caregivers, using nonverbal communication skills to recognize patient responses to treatment, building relationships to manage social and cultural barriers to promote trust, observing abnormal functioning and subtle changes in patient responses, and setting both short- and long-term goals of care.

On completion of the patient interview, the oncology nurse or the designated transitional care planner determines the needs or potential problem areas that may exist and verifies the patient's interest in having continuing care planning services. Potential areas of concern that increase the risk of home care include the following: inadequate or no support system, inadequate financial resources, poor environmental conditions, inability to carry out treatment and medication regimen, inability to carry out ADLs, poor socialization, and potential problems related to disease progression or treatment.[32,35,38]

Transitional Planning

Planning is the next step after the patient's problems or needs are identified. It is a collaborative process involving the patient, the family or significant others, and health care professionals. At this time the oncology nurse assists the patient, the family, and significant others to look realistically at their goals and expectations and subsequently develop a plan for care. This may entail placement in an extended care facility or linkage with community-based agencies providing service in the home setting. With so many diverse services available, it is necessary to assist the patient or family with decision making by identifying the specific problem(s), the services needed, and available resources. In addition, the oncology nurse helps the patient and family to formally establish financial status, obtains consents to contact the resources on their behalf, and works out the details of the selected plan, including criteria to evaluate the plan's effectiveness.[25,32]

Nurses can use the resources available in their practice setting and establish a collaborative relationship with the continuing care team to facilitate the process for the benefit of the patient. Often, because of early discharge, there is not sufficient time to initiate all the appropriate referrals to community support services. In such cases the referrals may be made after the patient is home. The professional implementing the transition plan makes the initial contacts with the support services and then provides a family member with the name of the referred agency, the telephone number, and the name of agency contact person. A responsible family member may be willing to follow up on a referral made by the professional.[25,32]

If the patient needs skilled nursing care in the home setting, a referral to a skilled home care agency is made. Most hospitals have continuing patient care forms that must be completed when a referral is initiated. The nurse should include information about other identified needs and request that the home care agency's personnel assist the patient with the referral process. It is essential that all relevant patient information is communicated and documented clearly, concisely, and in a timely manner. In addition to information about identified support needs, the referral for continuing patient care in the home care setting includes information about significant factors related to this hospitalization, relevant past medical history, current medications and treatment orders, identified nursing problems, and results of recent diagnostic tests or blood work. Concise and comprehensive referrals are essential to facilitate the transition from one setting of care to another, and to promote continuity of care. The comprehensive information on the referral form is essential to make the home care nurse's job more efficient.

ASSESSMENT OF CAREGIVER AND INFORMAL SUPPORTS

In the majority of organizations, assessment of the support available from family, friends, and organized institutions is routinely done if it is determined that the patient needs assistance in the home setting. Frequently, a primary caregiver, usually the spouse, is identified, and some in-hospital teaching has been initiated by the nurses before discharge. As the trend for early discharge continues, the family support system is assuming greater responsibility for maintaining what is often a very aggressive posthospitalization treatment plan. The stress and anxieties associated with the caregiving responsibilities can be overwhelming. Often, caregivers are additionally burdened by unasked questions and feelings of inadequacy in their ability to care for their loved ones properly and safely. Teaching them not only the "what to do" but also the "what to expect" reduces stress and anxiety.

There are approximately 44.4 million unpaid caregivers in the United States, and family members or friends provide approximately 83% to 89% of in-home care (8% care for someone with cancer).[5,40] Often these individuals do not have the option of giving up this role because of a sense of responsibility, and because it is an expression of love and devotion to the patient. While the number of male caregivers is increasing, the majority of caregivers are women over 55 years of age. Compared with men caregivers, women provide more hours of care per week, give care at higher levels of burden, more often admit to having "no choice" in caregiving, and receive assistance from other family members. Older men with cancer are usually cared for by their spouses. Because of their longevity, older women with cancer are usually cared for by their adult children. Middle-aged cancer patients are cared for primarily by their spouses. Cancer affects the emotional well-being of both patient and family for years following diagnosis, particularly if cancer recurs and also at the end of life.[5,41,42] Caregivers have reported both negative and positive subjective feelings associated with caregiving. Negative feelings included emotional stress, depression, hopelessness, loss of control, anger, guilt, resentment, and anxiety.[14,16,43,44] Positive emotions related to providing care for seriously ill family members include feelings of satisfaction, improved self-esteem, and finding meaning.[10,45] Spousal caregivers are at particular risk for caregiver burden and illnesses associated with caregiver stress, because they maintain the caregiving role for longer periods and provide more extensive and comprehensive care. In addition to those who provide care for a long time, primary caregivers at high risk for caregiver burden and negative effects on their quality of life are individuals who are still working and those who live in a rural, isolated environment.[46] Additional patient and family risk factors for problems adjusting to cancer caregiving include increased symptom distress, uncertainty about the illness or treatment, additional demands on the family, and age.[5]

An important part of transitional planning is a comprehensive evaluation of the caregiver that includes the following areas of assessment:

1. Has the caregiver's age been considered as well as the patient's?
2. Does the caregiver's mental and physical condition allow that person to assume this responsibility?
3. Will the caregiver live in the patient's home? If the caregiver is not in the home, how accessible is that person?
4. Are family and/or friends available to provide respite or free time for the caregiver?
5. If the caregiver can no longer assume responsibility, who will be notified?
6. Is the caregiver aware of the patient's medical condition and the expected course of treatment?
7. Has the caregiver received suitable educational materials regarding the patient's diagnosis?
8. If there is to be a change in the patient's condition, does the caregiver know what problems and symptoms to watch for and whom to call?
9. If a home care agency will provide care at home, has the caregiver received the name and phone number of the physician directing the home care plan and the company or primary contact person?
10. If the patient will be using medical equipment in the home, has the caregiver been given the name and contact information of the company that supplies it?
11. Has the caregiver been helped to develop a list of emergency telephone numbers: community emergency numbers, rescue emergency numbers, physician, home care agency, equipment supplier, and other family members?
12. Does the caregiver know about any follow-up medical appointments scheduled for the patient, and is appropriate transportation available?
13. Has the caregiver been instructed regarding appropriate self-care activities for the patient (what to do for the patient and what the patient will do independently)?
14. Does the caregiver have medications for the patient's first 24 hours at home? If not, has a plan been developed to obtain these medications?
15. Are there immediate funds available to fill medication prescriptions? If a prescription is difficult to obtain at local pharmacies, does the caregiver know where it is available?
16. Has the caregiver received instructions on administering medications, observing for possible side effects, and managing them?
17. Have questions regarding financial matters related to the patient's home care needs been prearranged before discharge? Is the caregiver attending to financial matters?
18. Has the caregiver been made aware of any appropriate support groups available in the community?
19. Does the caregiver have the name and telephone number of the person who arranged for home care services and who can be called to clarify issues or further explain services to be expected?
20. Are there any remaining questions or problems concerning the discharge date and time, transportation home, or the services the caregiver and patient will be receiving?

The transitional planning process is an organized, systematic approach used primarily in the acute care setting to facilitate the move from hospital to home. As health care delivery systems attempt to control costs and avoid duplication of services while maintaining high-quality care, oncology nurses have become aware that the assessment and planning process characteristic of transitional planning should not be limited to the acute care setting. Oncology patients in outpatient oncology settings also have significant discharge planning needs because of the increase in outpatient cancer treatments. This process is ongoing and should continue as the patient moves through a variety of health care settings during the cancer trajectory. A patient-centered approach to provide continuity of care facilitates the delivery of holistic health services that serve the patient's best interests while assisting providers to plan services that are based on needs.[25,30,34,47]

THE ELECTRONIC AGE OF TRANSITIONAL PLANNING AND ELECTRONIC COMMUNICATION

The transition planning process is ideally suited to electronic applications. For example, case managers can access statewide comprehensive electronic lists of available home health agencies and other entities. Postacute providers can electronically report clinical services that are provided, the geographic area covered, and resource availability including currently vacant subacute beds. Nursing homes in a specific geographic region can be located by using the CMS program called Nursing Home Compare. This valuable website, *http://www.medicare.gov/nhcompare/home.asp*, is available to both health professionals and consumers. Mandatory patient assessment forms can be completed online using demographic data that is automatically downloaded to the form from existing admitting data. These legible, current, and complete forms supplied to the postacute provider take the place of inefficient phone calls and extensive faxing of documents and allow for more informed decisions about admitting the patient.[27,34,47]

The Internet allows immediate access to an abundance of health-related information and resources to enhance patient care services. The Internet is not only a source of empowerment for cancer patients and caregivers as they seek information, but it is also a source of online support from others. Caregivers participating in online support groups can tell their story. The opportunity to tell their story allows caregivers to meet the emotional and physical demands of care. However, further outcomes research is need to evaluate the effectiveness of this support venue as well as online nursing support interventions.[48-50] It is important to advise patients and families not to apply any recommendations of treatments from the Internet without first consulting their primary care provider. Oncology nurses and transitional care planners play a critical role in evaluating the quality of health care resources available on the Internet. Simple and standard evaluation of Internet-based health care information includes five components.[51] The five components are authority or source (i.e., author's credentials and expertise, reputation of the organization, contact information), purpose or objectivity (i.e., the sponsor, the purpose, and the intended audience are clearly stated), content (e.g., accurate, useful, relevant), currency (i.e., dates are given for posted information and any updates) and design (e.g., organized and uncluttered for easy navigation).

Cost and quality of care are inextricably woven together in today's health care system; therefore, oncology nurses find themselves managing and coordinating patient situations they once routinely encountered only in hospitals. The emphasis on short inpatient stays challenges oncology nurses to shape and implement adequate education and support programs for patients with cancer. Community health nurses and ambulatory care nurses now carry the responsibility of symptom management and education about self-care measures for patients with cancer and their families.

Settings for Care

Community care options include "informal" support networks involving the help of friends, family, religious communities, and others, information and referral resources, legal and financial counseling, transportation services, support groups, nutrition programs, extended care, and home care. In the past, the hospital was the primary setting for care. In recent years, hospitals, as well as other health care providers and payers, have created innovative alternative care sites that reduce the cost while maintaining quality care.

EXTENDED CARE

Family members may find the caregiving burden too overwhelming and may request information on and assistance with extended care placement. Community care programs and services vary in different states, counties, and communities; therefore it is wise to have a working knowledge about available resources in local areas. If it is determined that the patient's care needs necessitate placement in an extended care facility, the facility that will most effectively meet the patient's needs must then be identified. The following six basic types of extended care facilities vary according to the amount and type of care needed by the patient: subacute care facilities, skilled care facilities, intermediate care facilities, adult foster or sheltered care facilities, assisted living or residential care facilities, and adult day-care facilities.

Subacute care facilities, also known as long-term care hospitals, are cost-efficient settings that provide a variety of medical-surgical, oncologic, rehabilitation, and additional specialty care services in an alternative setting for those patients who no longer need acute care services but are too ill to send home. This alternative care setting offers outcomes-focused care as well as cost efficiency. Many hospitals and nursing homes have subacute facilities to enhance revenues, where appropriate care is provided to patients with specialized needs such as highly skilled nursing services. An added benefit to providing such a facility for care is that it separates the chronically ill patients from others. This enables health care providers to consider the underlying assumptions of care and the appropriateness of aggressive care measures while still providing care for chronically, critically ill patients in specialized "low-tech" units and without compromising prospects for recovery.

Skilled care facilities provide around-the-clock skilled nursing care and observation. In addition, there is frequent medical supervision. Intermediate care facilities provide around-the-clock basic nursing care for patients who are medically stable but unable to care for themselves. Adult foster care or sheltered care facilities are for individuals who require a protective living arrangement that provides general supervision and assistance with bathing, dressing, meals, and other personal needs. Assisted living or residential care facilities are for individuals who no longer want to live alone or have no place to live. At minimum, assisted living facilities provide 24-hour staff and two to three meals per day in a common dining area and occasionally, in times of illness, may provide intermediate care for the residents. These facilities often have various levels of living arrangements, ranging from independent to assisted living.

Adult day-care facilities provide various levels of care for cancer patients and much-needed respite for family caregivers. Adult day-care programs serve as a bridge between traditional care services and the home where there otherwise might be a gap in service delivery. Some adult day-care programs also provide services for the caregiver, ranging from counseling to caregiver support groups.

Supportive housing options vary widely in terms of size, cost, services offered, and facilities; therefore, selecting the best one can be an overwhelming task. The local area's agency on aging and long-term care ombudsman office in each state will provide a list of licensed extended care facilities in the area and information regarding reimbursement of these facilities by Medicare or Medicaid. Suggestions to assist in the search for a safe, comfortable and appropriate facility include the following: consider the resident's future needs when selecting a facility; visit each facility more than once, sometimes unannounced; visit at meal times and observe the quality of the food and service; talk to residents; and review state licensing reports. Table 35-1 outlines the settings for postacute care for cancer patients, examples of services, and appropriate types of patients.

HOME CARE

Home care is the provision of a variety of professional and paraprofessional services and equipment to patients and families in their homes for health maintenance, education, illness prevention and treatment, palliation, and rehabilitation. It has seen an increase in utilization because of the implementation of hospital-based PPS and, subsequently, earlier discharges. Increased momentum of consumerism and the desire to exercise more control over personal health care have also been influencing factors. In a time of increasing concern over federal health care expenditures, home care represents a humane, sensible alternative to institutionalized care for an increasing number of Americans. It also offers other benefits, including eliminating the risk of nosocomial infection, maintaining patients' and families' social and cultural patterns, and promoting patients' self-esteem, independence, and personal involvement in care.[25,32,34,47,52]

Home care combines health care and supportive services to help sick or disabled persons continue living at home as independently as possible. The hours, the level of care, and the types of services provided are dependent on the health care needs of the cancer patient and caregiver. The option of home care services is understandably attractive to cancer patients and their families, who face an illness that often diminishes their sense of personal control. The complex nature of cancer presents many challenges, because it is often not easily placed within the type of disease management pathway that many case managers are adopting to control home care costs. The reasons for this are the frequency and costs of treatments required for cancer patients, the constant reassessment required to manage changing health status, and the necessity for many treatments to be given during intermittent, short inpatient stays over an extended period of time. Case managers and oncology nurses have a critical role in identifying patient eligibility for clinical trials, coordinating monitoring and care needs that arise during participation in clinical trials, and discussing clinical information with health insurers. Home care agencies are challenged to develop strategies and relevant pathways

TABLE 35-1	Settings for Postacute Care for Cancer Patients	
SETTING	**EXAMPLES OF SERVICES**	**TYPES OF PATIENTS**
Subacute care	Around-the-clock skilled nursing care and observation with frequent medical supervision, physical, occupational, speech, and respiratory therapy, restorative care, social services	Patients needing IV therapy such as antibiotics, tube feedings, ventilator monitoring, complex or frequent wound care, management of total bladder or bowel incontinence, peritoneal dialysis, significant assistance with ADLs, and self-care management
Long-term care	Skilled nursing and custodial care, oxygen therapy, tube feedings, social services and activities, hospice care	Patients requiring 24-hour supervision, skilled nursing because of complex, chronic and/or deteriorating medical conditions, without capable or available caregiver, who cannot safely care for self, with cognitive or functional impairment
Residential care facilities	Various levels of living arrangements from independent to assisted Protective living arrangement that provides assistance with ADLs, medication supervision, social interaction, and activities In times of illness, may provide intermediate care	Patients needs vary from temporary stand-by assistance in ADLs, assistance with grocery shopping, or cooking, to skilled nursing, 24-hour supervision, incontinence management
Respite care	Custodial care, social services, activities for patient, and counseling and support groups for caregiver	Patients are appropriate for long-term care but are able to stay home or with family members, for caregivers who need a rest
Home care	Skilled nursing; physical, occupational, respiratory, intravenous infusion therapy; chemotherapy; home health aide; companion, hospice, and social services and activities; durable medical equipment	Homebound, needing assistance with ADLs, intermittent and skilled care including wound and ostomy care, Foley catheter, tube feeding, phlebotomy, vital signs' monitoring, medication supervision, patient teaching for self-care management, death and dying support

ADLs, Activities of daily living; *IV,* intravenous.

to address the unique requirements of cancer patients. This is accomplished best by using nurses with expertise in oncology as primary care nurses or case managers to coordinate the care of cancer patients in the home setting.[27]

The home care industry has four parts: home health, home medical equipment, home infusion therapy, and hospice. The home health segment can be subdivided into acute care (i.e., intermittent skilled care provided under the Medicare and Medicaid home care benefits) and long-term care (i.e., supportive services that assist patients with ADLs to maintain independence in the home). Four payer groups cover long-term home care: Medicaid waiver, government-funded supportive services, self-pay, and long-term care insurance.

Based on organizational and administrative functions, home health programs are categorized into the following general types: official, which are operated by state, county, city or other government units; private and voluntary (nonprofit), which are supported by charities, Medicare, Medicaid, third-party payers, and private-pay individuals; combination, a merged official and voluntary home health care; hospital-based home health care with access to the hospital's inpatient services; and proprietary (for-profit), which are ineligible for tax-exempt status, and reimbursement by third-party payers. Proprietary agencies outnumber all other types of Medicare-certified agencies.

Regardless of the type of home health agency, the primary goal is to provide health care based on needs in the community. Home care services available to health care consumers include both traditional and high-technology care. Traditional home care services generally provide skilled nursing care, including client's health status evaluation; provision of direct care (e.g., administer treatment and wound and colostomy care), patient and family education; development of coping skills; rehabilitative services such as physical, occupational, and speech and language therapies; social work intervention; and home health aide support. Rehabilitative services are especially important in ensuring quality care within the limits of home care services for patients with cancer. These patients often have significant fatigue associated with disease processes and treatments. Many treatments may also increase the risks for short- or long-term disabilities. Physical and occupational therapists can provide home exercise programs, and direct the implementation of assistive devices and home modification to maintain optimal independence. Speech and language therapists can initiate or continue programs to assist patients with both speech and dysphagia problems in the home setting. In addition, home health agencies often employ other specialists such as registered dietitians for nutrition consults, and certified enterostomal therapy nurses for wound and skin care and lymphedema management.[38,53]

Recent improvements in and the increasing availability of high technology in the home setting have made home care a viable option for cancer patients at all stages of treatment and illness. High-technology home care for patients with cancer generally refers to the home management of infusion therapies such as the following: analgesia, antiemetics, antifungals, antimicrobials, hydration, electrolyte replacement, chemotherapy, blood sampling for diagnostic tests, and enteral or parenteral nutrition.

Home IV therapy is one of the most rapidly growing trends in the home care industry. Cost containment and the growing threat of communicable disease transmission in hospitals are two major factors contributing to this trend. Not all patients with cancer are

good candidates for home infusion therapy. Cancer patients and their families must be carefully assessed before initiating such therapies in the home setting to ensure that the treatment will be both safe and efficacious. In addition, physician support and accessibility for clear, open communication must be present to ensure continuity of care and safe infusion therapy in the home setting.[54]

Criteria used by home health agencies to determine eligibility for services may include the guidelines established by Medicare regulations. To qualify for Medicare coverage of any home health services, the patient must meet each of the following criteria:

- The patient is homebound, except for infrequent, relatively short periods or for medical treatment.
- A physician initially certifies the patient's need for home health care and develops a care plan.
- The patient needs at least one qualifying service such as skilled nursing care, physical therapy, or speech therapy.
- Skilled care is needed part-time or intermittently. Medicare covers daily care (e.g., wound care) only for a limited time, and an end date must be established when the service is begun.
- The home health care agency that provides the service is Medicare-certified.

Generally speaking, a patient is considered "homebound" if he or she has a condition resulting from an illness or injury that restricts the ability to leave the place of residence except with the use of supportive devices (i.e., crutches, canes, wheelchairs) or the use of special transportation or the assistance of another person, or if medically contraindicated. Once qualified, a patient is also eligible for additional services including occupational therapy, medical social work services, limited home health aide services (e.g., assistance with ADLs), medical supplies and equipment, and prosthetic devices. Occupational therapy can be given only if the patient needs another qualifying service; but once started, it can be continued even if it remains the sole service provided. Prescribed services must be reasonable and necessary and must be provided in the patient's home. Patients who receive infusion therapy in the home must have a venous access device to ensure a reliable, safe, and patent access site. Venous access devices include the nontunneled subclavian catheters appropriate for acute care settings; devices commonly used in the subacute or the home care setting include Hickman, Broviac, Quinton, Raaf, and Groshong catheters, single- and dual-lumen implantable venous ports, and peripherally inserted single- and dual-lumen central catheters (PICC).

A variety of infusion pumps that are compact, reliable, and easy to manage are available for the home setting and help ensure that the prescribed medication is administered as ordered. A variety of central venous catheter types are available. Tables 35-2 to 35-5 present a general overview of tunneled central venous catheters and PICC lines and common complications, as well as guidelines for care and management. Detailed information regarding venous access devices is available in the Oncology Nursing Society's *Access Device Guideline: Recommendations for Nursing Practice and Education.*[55]

Total parenteral nutrition (TPN) and enteral therapy for cancer patients have been controversial issues from medical, ethical, and financial perspectives. Nevertheless, this form of treatment is frequently provided in the home setting when deemed safe and advantageous. It is generally believed that enhanced nutritional status improves the quality of life but does not necessarily prolong life. During the end stage of illness,

Text continued on page 636

TABLE 35-2   **Examples of Tunneled Central Venous Catheters Currently Marketed in the United States**

MODEL/MATERIAL (MANUFACTURER)	FRENCH SIZE	INNER DIAMETER	TOTAL LUMEN VOLUME (PRIMING VOLUME)
Single-Lumen Devices			
Hickman single-lumen catheter/silicone (Bard)	9	1.6 mm	1.8 ml
Groshong single-lumen catheter/silicone (Bard)	7 and 8	1.3–1.5 mm	0.7–1.2 ml
Quinton single-lumen central venous access catheter/silicone (Quinton)	3.9–9.7*	0.75–1.5 mm	0.9–2.0 ml
Harborin single-lumen central venous catheter/polyurethane (Harbor Medical Devices)	7	1.5 mm	0.9 ml
Double-Lumen Devices			
Hickman dual-lumen catheter/silicone (Bard)	7	0.8 mm/1.0 mm	0.6 ml/0.8 ml
	9	0.7 mm/1.3 mm	0.6 ml/1.3 ml
	12	1.6 mm each lumen	1.8 ml each lumen
Leonard dual-lumen catheter/silicone (Bard)	10	1.3 mm each lumen	1.3 ml each lumen
Groshong dual-lumen catheter/silicone (Bard)	9.5	1.1 mm/1.33 mm	0.5 ml/0.8 ml
Cook TPN double-lumen central venous catheters/silicone (Cook Critical Care)	5	0.5 mm each lumen	0.2 ml each lumen
	7	0.7 mm/1.0 mm	0.4 ml/0.6 ml
	9	1.0 mm/1.3 mm	0.6 ml/1.0 ml
	12	1.0 mm/1.6 mm	1.6 ml/2.3 ml
Quinton RAAF dual-lumen central venous catheters/silicone	9	1.1 mm each lumen	1.2 ml each lumen
	12	1.5 mm each lumen	2.2 ml each lumen
	13.5	2.0 mm each lumen	2.5 ml each lumen
Triple-Lumen Devices			
Nutritional support catheter/polyurethane (Arrow International)	7		0.7 ml/0.5 ml/0.5 ml
Hickman triple-lumen catheter/silicone (Bard)	12.5	1.0 mm/1.0/mm/1.5 mm	0.7 ml/0.7 ml/1.6 ml
Quinton triple-lumen central venous access catheter/silicone	11.7	1.0 mm/1.0 mm/1.25 mm	1.0 ml/1.1 ml/1.2 ml

*Size depends on model.
Modified from Finley RS: Drug-delivery systems: infusion and access devices, *Highlights Antineoplast Drugs* 13(2):15, 1995.

TABLE 35-3   **Examples of Peripherally Inserted Central Venous Catheters (PICCs) Currently Marketed in the United States**

MODEL OR TRADE NAME/MATERIAL (MANUFACTURER)	FRENCH SIZE	LUMEN DIAMETER	LENGTH	PRIMING VOLUME
Single-Lumen Devices				
Groshong PICC/silicone (Bard)	4	0.8 mm	56 cm	0.3 ml
C-PICS/silicone (Cook Critical Care)	5	0.91 mm	60 cm	0.6 ml
V-Cath/silicone (HDC Corporation)	2	0.3 mm	40 cm	0.1 ml
	4	0.9 mm	60 cm	0.4 ml
L-Cath PICCs/polyurethane (Luther Medical Products)	5	1.2 mm	56 cm	0.9 ml
	3.5	0.7 mm	56 cm	0.4 ml
	2.6	0.5 mm	56 cm	0.2 ml
Double-Lumen Devices				
D/L PICC/silicone (Bard)	5	0.8 mm/0.6 mm	53.9 cm	0.4 ml/0.3 ml
Double-lumen per-q-cath/silicone (Bard)	4	0.5 mm/0.3 mm	60 cm	0.1 ml/0.6 ml
	5	0.8 mm/0.4 mm	60 cm	0.3 ml/0.1 ml

Modified from Finley RS: Drug-delivery systems: infusion and access devices, *Highlights Antineoplast Drugs* 13(2):15, 1995.

TABLE 35-4 Central Venous Catheters: Recommended Nursing Management

TYPE	HEPARINIZATION*	DRESSING	BLOOD SAMPLING
Adult			
Central Venous Catheters, Short-Term Use, Subclavian Single-, dual-, triple-lumen	After each use, flush each lumen with 5 ml normal saline (N/S), and then heparinized saline, 2 ml (100 units/ml). For catheter *not* in use, flush each lumen with heparinized saline, 2 ml (100 units/ml) every 12 hours.	Daily sterile dressing change at the site for duration of catheter placement. Gauze dressing change every 24 hours Change Luer-Lok injection caps every 72 hours.	Shut off all intravenous (IV) lines for *1 to 3 minutes.* Withdraw 5 ml blood. Discard. Withdraw blood sample. Flush lumen with 5 ml N/S, then heparinize or resume IV line. *Total parenteral nutrition(TPN): shut off IV line 10 minutes.*
Peripherally Inserted Central Venous Catheters (PICCs) Long-line PICC† Single-, dual-lumen (Use gentle pressure on syringe plunger for PICCs.)	After each use, flush lumen with 2 ml N/S, then heparinized saline, 1 ml (100 units/ml). For catheter *not* in use, flush lumen with heparinized saline, 1 ml (100 units/ml) every 12 hours.	Sterile dressing change after first 24 hours, then every 72 hours Change Luer-Lok injection caps every 72 hours.	Shut off all IV lines for *1 to 3 minutes.* Withdraw 1.5 ml blood. Discard. Withdraw blood sample. Flush lumen with 2.5 ml N/S, then heparinize or resume IV line. *TPN: shut off IV line 10 minutes.*
Tunneled Catheters, Long-Term Use Hickman Quinton/Raaf Single-, dual-, triple-lumen	After each use, flush each lumen with 5 ml N/S, then heparinized saline 2 ml (100 units/ml). For catheter *not* in use, flush each lumen with heparinized saline 2 to 5 ml (100 units/ml) daily/biweekly.	Daily sterile dressing change at exit site for initial 14 days Gauze dressing change every 24 hours Thereafter, cleanse exit site daily (Betadine/alcohol). Optional daily clean dressing Change Luer-Lok injection caps *weekly.*	Shut off all IV lines for *1 to 3 minutes.* Withdraw 5 ml blood. Discard. Withdraw blood sample. Flush lumen with 5 ml N/S and then heparinize or resume IV line. *TPN: shut off IV lines 10 minutes.*
Groshong Single-, dual-lumen	Does not require heparin to maintain catheter patency. *Use force when flushing.* Flush *each* lumen with 5 ml N/S after each use, except for TPN, and then flush with 30 ml N/S. For catheter *not* in use, flush with 5 ml N/S weekly.‡	Daily sterile dressing change at exit site for initial 14 days. Gauze dressing change every 24 hours. Thereafter, cleanse exit site daily (Betadine/alcohol). Optional daily clean dressing. Change Luer-Lok injection caps weekly.	Shut off all IV lines for *1 to 3 minutes.* Withdraw 5 ml blood. Discard. Withdraw blood sample. Flush lumen with 30 ml N/S vigorously, and then resume IV line or apply injection cap.‡ *TPN: shut off IV line 10 minutes.*
Implantable Vascular Access Devices Davol Port Infuse-A-Port Port-A-Cath	After each use, flush *each* port with Huber needle: 10 ml N/S, followed by heparinized saline (100 units/ml).§ For port *not* in use, flush each port with 3 to 10 ml heparinized saline (100 units/ml) every *30 days* (venous placement). Intermittent flush > 1/day use N/S and/or low dose/low-volume heparin.||	Sterile bio-occlusive dressing when port accessed SteriStrips at new incision site for 3 days When incision site healed and port not accessed, no dressing required When port is accessed for continuous infusion, change needle and extension tubing every 5 to 7 days.	Shut off all IV lines for *1 to 3 minutes.* Withdraw 5 ml blood. Discard. Withdraw blood sample. Flush with 20 ml N/S, followed by 3 to 10 ml heparinized saline (100 units/ml)‡ or resume IV line. *TPN: shut off IV line 10 minutes.*
Pediatric			
Short-Term Use, Subclavian Single-lumen or multilumen	After each use, flush *each* lumen with 2 ml N/S, followed by 1 ml heparinized saline solution, 10 units/ml, after each use or at least twice a day.	Daily sterile dressing change at site for duration of catheter placement Gauze dressing change every 24 hours Change Luer-Lok injection caps every 24 hours.	Shut off all IV lines for *1 to 3 minutes.* Withdraw 3 ml blood. Discard. Withdraw blood sample. Flush lumen with 2 ml N/S, and then heparinize or resume IV line. *TPN: shut off IV line 10 minutes.*

Device	Flushing	Dressing/Care	Blood Sampling	
Peripherally Inserted Catheters Long-line PICC† Single-, dual lumen (Use gentle pressure on syringe plunger for PICCs.)	After each use, flush lumen: *Pediatrics:* 2 ml N/S in 5-ml syringe or larger, followed by 1 ml heparinized saline (10 units/ml) after each use or at least twice a day *Special care nursery (neonates):* 0.5 ml N/S, preservative free, in 5 ml syringe or larger, followed by 0.5 ml heparinized saline (4 units/ml) Intermittent flush schedule every 4 to 8 hours: consult with physician's orders.	Sterile dressing change after first 24 hours, then every 72 hours. Change Luer-Lok injection caps every 72 hours.	Shut off all IV lines for *1 to 3 minutes*. Withdraw 1.5 ml blood. Discard. Withdraw blood sample. Flush lumen with 2.5 ml N/S, and then heparinize or resume IV line. *TPN: shut off IV line.*	*10 minutes*
Tunneled Catheters, Long-Term Use Broviac	After each use, flush lumen with 2 ml N/S, then heparinized saline 1 ml (10 units/ml). For catheter *not* in use, flush lumen with heparinized saline, 1 ml (10 units/ml) daily.	Daily sterile dressing change at exit site for initial 14 days Gauze dressing change every 24 hours Thereafter, cleanse exit site daily with Betadine. Apply sterile 2 × 2. Change Luer-Lok injection caps *weekly.*	Shut off all IV lines for *1 to 3 minutes*. Withdraw 3 ml blood. Discard. Withdraw blood sample. Flush lumen with 2 ml N/S, and then heparinize or resume IV line. *TPN: shut off IV line 10 minutes.*	
Implantable Vascular Access Devices Port-A-Cath	After each use, flush the port with Huber needle, 5 ml N/S, followed by 2 ml heparinized saline (100 units/ml). For port *not* in use, flush port with 2 ml heparinized saline (100 units/ml) *every 30 days* (venous placement).	Sterile bio-occlusive dressing when port accessed SteriStrips at new incision site for 3 days When incision site healed and port not accessed, no dressing required When port is accessed for continuous infusion, change needle and extension tubing every 5 to 7 days.	Shut off all IV lines for *1 full minute*. Withdraw 3 to 5 ml blood (depending on size of child). Discard. Withdraw blood sample. Flush with 5 ml N/S, and then heparinize or resume IV line. *TPN: shut off IV line 10 minutes.*	

*Heparinization of central venous catheters varies in frequency, volume of solution, concentration of the heparin dilution, type of device, and patient's age and weight. Confirm with physician managing patient's care and agency/institution for nursing management protocol regarding heparinization of central venous catheters and implantable ports. Consider patient with an alteration in coagulation factors and/or heparin allergy or intolerance with frequency of use of intermittent device. Potentially these patients may require low-concentration (e.g., 10 units heparin/ml) and/or alternative flushing solution (e.g., sodium citrate, 1.4% solution).

†Use 5 ml or larger syringes when flushing and/or blood sampling from PICC.

‡Selected oncologists use 2 to 5 ml heparinized saline (100 units/ml).

§Check manufacturer's specific recommendations regarding volume. Oncologists use heparin, 10 ml (100 units/ml).

||Assess patient, disease, platelet count with frequency, volume, and concentration of heparinization schedule.

From Otto SE: *Mosby's Pocket Guide to infusion therapy,* ed 5, St. Louis, 2005, Mosby.

TABLE 35-5   Features of Ambulatory Infusion Devices

NAME/MODEL (MANUFACTURER)	PUMPING MECHANISM	DRUG RESERVOIR/ ACCESSORIES	BATTERY/ POWER SOURCE	RANGE OF INFUSION RATES	ALARMS/ SAFETY FEATURES	KEEP OPEN RATE	PROGRAM MODES	WEIGHT	SIZE
Ambulatory, Single Channel									
WalkMed 440 PIC (Medex, Division of Ivion)	Linear peristaltic	Disposable 65-, 150-, 250-ml bags; dedicated pump sets	9-V disposable battery (450-650 ml/ battery)	1-30 ml/hr (can also be programmed as mg/hr)	Near end of program; volume limit; occlusion; system malfunction; low battery; depleted battery; end of infusion; door open; programming error; lockout levels	0-9.9 ml/hr	PCA; intermittent; continuous	360 g	1.6 × 11.2 × 10.2 cm
WalkMed 350 (Medex Ambulatory Infusion Systems, Division of Ivion)	Linear peristaltic	Disposable 65-, 150-, 250-ml bags; dedicated pump sets	9-V alkaline battery (5-21 days)	0.1-19.99 ml/hr (increments of 0.01 ml)	Occlusion; system malfunction; low battery; depleted battery; prime; door open		Continuous	360 g	4.6 × 11.2 × 10.2 cm
WalkMed PCA (Medex Ambulatory Infusion Systems, Division of Ivion)	Linear peristaltic	Disposable 65-, 150-, 250-ml bags; dedicated pump sets	9-V alkaline battery (1-21 days depending on infusion rate)	0.1-19.99 ml/hr (increments of 0.01) or 0.1-30 ml/hr (increments of 0.1 ml)	Near end; volume limit; occlusion; system malfunction; low battery; depleted battery; end of infusion; total volume delivered; programming error		Continuous; continuous with patient-activated bolus bolus; only	360 g	4.6 × 11.2 × 10.2 cm
Provider One (Abbott)	Rotary peristaltic	Any collapsible IV bag; dedicated tubing	Two disposable 9-V lithium batteries (4800 ml); or 12-V rechargeable batteries (4000 ml)	1-400 ml/hr	Occlusion; cartridge improperly inserted; programming error; computer error; air in line; low battery; low reservoir; end of infusion	1 ml/hr	Continuous; tapering	400 g	132 × 86 × 33 cm
Provider 5500 (Pancretec/ Abbott)	Rotary peristaltic	Any collapsible IV bag	9-V alkaline battery	0.1-250 ml/hr	Occlusion; air in line; low reservoir; low battery; ending infusion; system problem; latch open	0.1 ml/hr	Continuous; PCA	400 g	

Pain Management Provider (Abbott)	Rotary peristaltic	Any collapsible IV bag		0.1-25 ml/hr in 0.1-ml increments; 0-10 ml/hr	Security lock box available	Continuous; loading dose; PCA (suitable for epidural injection)	425 g	2.8 × 8.9 × 16 cm
CADD-Plus (Pharmacia Deltec)	Linear peristaltic	50-, 100-, 250-ml custom cassettes or any collapsible IV bag with custom adapter	9-V disposable alkaline or lithium battery	0.1-75 ml/hr	High pressure; low reservoir; low battery; power-up failure; pump in stop mode; programmed volume depleted; high pressure; system error	Continuous; intermittent; delay start	425 g	2.8 × 8.9 × 16 cm
CADD-I (Pharmacia Deltec)	Linear peristaltic	50-, 100-, 250-ml custom cassettes or any collapsible IV bag with custom adapter	9-V disposable alkaline or lithium battery	0-299 ml every 24 h or 90 ml/hr in fixed high-flow mode	Power-up fault; pump in stop mode; low battery; low reservoir volume; programmed volume; depleted high pressure; system Error	Continuous		
CADD-PCA Ambulatory Infusion Pump Model 5800	Linear peristaltic	50-, 100-, 250-ml custom reservoir or any IV bag with remote adapter	9-V alkaline or lithium battery	0-20 ml/hr (may also be programmed in mg/hr)	Power-up failure; low battery; depleted battery; low reservoir; programmed volume depleted; high pressure; system error	Continuous; patient-activated bolus; continuous plus patient-activated bolus	425 g	2.8 × 3.5 × 6.4 cm
CADD TPN Ambulatory Infusion System Model 5700 (Pharmacia Deltec)	Linear peristaltic	Collapsible IV bag with dedicated adapter tubing	9-V alkaline (6-hr) or lithium (18-hr) battery, rechargeable battery pack (11-hr), or AC adapter	10-250 ml/hr with 9 V battery or 10-400 ml/hr with AC adapter	Low reservoir; programmed volume depleted; infusion period completed; low battery; depleted battery; invalid rate; high pressure; power up fault; system error	Continuous; continuous with tapering up or down	369 g	2.8 × 8.9 × 13.3 cm
EZ Flow Model 80-2 (Creative Medical Development)	Displacement chamber	Disposable 100- and 250-ml cassettes or large-volume adapter	Rechargeable NiCad battery or AC power adapter	0.6-250 ml/hr (16 incremental rates)	Infusion complete; occlusion; low battery	Continuous; intermittent	14 oz	6.75 × 3.5 × 1.27 inches

Continued

TABLE 35-5   Features of Ambulatory Infusion Devices—cont'd

NAME/MODEL (MANUFACTURER)	PUMPING MECHANISM	DRUG RESERVOIR/ ACCESSORIES	BATTERY/ POWER SOURCE	RANGE OF INFUSION RATES	ALARMS/ SAFETY FEATURES	KEEP OPEN RATE	PROGRAM MODES	WEIGHT	SIZE
MedMate 1100 (Patient Solutions)	Peristaltic	Custom cassettes or any IV bag	Two disposable 9-V alkaline or lithium batteries or external recharger	0.1-500 ml/hr	Programming error; system fault; low battery; dose due; air in line; door open; dose complete; low bag; bag end	0.1-9.9 ml/hr	Continuous; tapering; patient controlled anesthesia (PCA); intermittent; delay start	17 oz	4.4 × 3.3 × 1.4 inches
Vector MTI (Infusion Technology)		Any collapsible IV bag	Two 9-V alkaline batteries or AC power	0.1-400 ml/hr	Reservoir empty; infusion complete; over pressure; check cassette; dead battery; system malfunction; air in line; low battery; low reservoir	0-5 ml/hr	Continuous; intermittent; PCA; taper	14.5 oz	5.6 × 3.5 × 1.4 inches
MAXX 100 (Medication Delivery Devices)	Controlled-pressure technology	100-ml custom bag	9-V alkaline battery	50, 100, or 200 ml/hr	Pump malfunction; low battery; occlusion; end of infusion; overflow		Continuous	10.5 oz	6.7 × 4.7 × 1.4 inches
SideKick (I-Flow)	Spring-driven infusion	50- and 100-ml minibags; custom IV sets that determine flow rate	Self-contained Spring	50, 100, or 200 ml/hr	None		Continuous		
MEDFLO II (Secure Medical Products)	Elastomeric	Unit is disposable balloon reservoir: 100-, 200-, and -300 ml	None	50, 100,, 175 and 200 ml/hr	None	NA	Continuous		2.75 × 4.25 to 7.0 inches
ReadyMed (McGaw)	Elastomeric	50-, 100-, 250- ml reservoirs	None	50, 100, 167, and 200 ml/hr	None	NA	Continuous		
Intermate LV System (Baxter)	Elastomeric	Unit is disposable balloon reservoir: 105-, 275-ml	None	50, 100, 200, and 250 ml/hr	None	NA	Continuous		
PCA Infusor (Baxter)	Elastomeric	Unit is disposable balloon reservoir: 65-to 275-ml	None	0.5-10 ml/hr or 12-240 ml/d	With patient-controlled module attachment, lockout of 15 or 60 min		Continuous;		

Ambulatory, Multichannel

VIVUS 4000 Infuser (I-Flow Corporation), four channel	Positive displacement	Any IV bag; dedicated tubing; manifold line to connect up to four tubings to single IV line; programmer required for operation; communicator unit for remote programming	5 (5000 ml delivery) or 10 (10,000 ml delivery) AA disposable alkaline batteries; 1.5-V DC or external 110/120-V AC adapter	0.1–200 ml/hr	Low battery; dead battery; occlusion; empty reservoir; internal malfunction; runaway infusion; open door	Continuous; sequential; continuous bolus; intermittent	1.05 kg	19.7 × 11.43 × 5.1 cm
Intellject (Ivion), four channel	Rack and pinion drive (syringe driver)	Dedicated 30-ml syringes and manifold	Two 9-V disposable batteries	5.4–40 ml/hr/ channel	Occlusion; low battery; low reservoir; program error; electronic fault	Continuous; bolus; continuous plus bolus; sequential; alternating	1.54 kg	25.4 × 16.5 × 7.1 cm
Verifuse (Block Medical)	Linear peristaltic	Any IV container	Two 9-V alkaline batteries; rechargeable NiCad battery, or AC power adapter	0.1–300 ml/hr	Door open; barcode fault; change batteries; low batteries; pump interrupted; air in line; low reservoir; occlusion; bad batteries; pumping complete; overvoltage; end of program; malfunction	Continuous, tapering up or down; loading dose; delay start; PCA; intermittent	17 oz	6.4 × 3.1× 1.1 inches

Modified from Finley RS: Drug-delivery system: infusion and access devices, *Highlights Antineoplast Drugs* 13(2):15, 1995.

however, when vital organs begin to shut down, infusion therapies are not advised. This is particularly difficult for families to accept and understand, because they frequently believe that because the patient is not eating or drinking, the patient is suffering and thus that IV fluids are necessary. If the rationale for withholding, discontinuing, or decreasing fluids to keep a vein open (KVO) is not clearly explained to families at this time, they may be concerned that the patient is being denied vital treatment.

Cancer pain significantly affects the quality of life of patients and their families, particularly as the patient's disease progresses. The incidence of cancer pain in early and intermediate stages of the disease is 30% to 40%; and in advanced disease, the incidence of pain is 70% to 90%.[56,57] Fear and helplessness associated with inability to relieve pain and poor communication, and differences in perceptions of pain between patient and caregivers can influence assessment and management of pain. Caregivers may be reluctant to acknowledge the patient's pain to avoid facing the prospect of disease progression.[56,57] A great deal of this cancer-related pain can be effectively relieved with existing pain management techniques. Although the oral route of pain medication is the preferred method by pain experts, high-technology pain management is a reasonable option for patients whose pain cannot be effectively controlled otherwise. To optimize pain management in the home care setting, ongoing assistance with problem solving is needed to overcome the difficulties patients and caregivers face in putting a pain management regimen into practice. These difficulties include obtaining prescribed medication(s), accessing information, tailoring prescribed regimens to meet individual needs, managing side effects, cognitively processing information, managing new or unusual pain, and managing multiple symptoms. Empowering the caregiver with knowledge of pain assessment and management including nonpharmacologic techniques, validating feelings, and providing support throughout the disease progression can minimize the suffering of caregivers when a family member has pain.[58,59]

To meet the information needs of the general public and especially for people in pain, the American Pain Society (APS) developed the American Pain Foundation website, *http://www.painfoundation.org/*, an online resource for people with pain, their families, friends, and caregivers, and the general public. This site is devoted to patient information and advocacy and provides many links to additional resources.

With the advances in anticancer therapies and greater availability of portable infusion pumps, chemotherapy administration in the home setting has become both safe and effective when appropriate standards for administration of chemotherapy are met. Standards for safe chemotherapy administration include that the chemotherapy is administered by professional staff who are specifically trained in chemotherapy procedures and have current CPR training. Oncology specific certification is highly desirable.[24,60] Chemotherapy administration has become an increasingly common practice in the home setting. It is important that patients receive their first dose of chemotherapy in an inpatient or outpatient setting to facilitate expedient and proper treatment if any untoward reactions occur. To ensure safe administration and handling of chemotherapy agents, oncology nurses put into place a plan for properly disposing of all biohazardous waste in the home.[61]

Given the common myelosuppressive consequence of chemotherapy and because side effects typically occur with antibiotic and antifungal medications, these therapies are frequently initiated in the inpatient or outpatient setting. When considering the continuation of these two types of therapy in the home, it is important to consider the use of an infusion pump, especially if the medication must be infused more than once a day. An electronic pump that can be programmed for intermittent dosing will decrease the number of home nursing visits required and decrease the number of connections and disconnections of the IV line and thus reduce both the potential for infection and overall costs.

Once the patient's tolerance to the medication has been established, carrying out this treatment modality in the home setting is preferable to extended hospitalization, if the patient is medically stable. The patient is generally more comfortable at home, and the health care cost savings are considerable when such high-technology services are provided in the home setting. In addition, patient hospitalizations are reduced, there is increased quality of life for patients and their families, and patients have a sense of control and active participation in their treatment plan.

CONSIDERATIONS FOR THE OLDER ADULT WITH CANCER

Cancer occurs more frequently and causes more deaths in the older population. Environment and genetic predisposition contribute to the aging process, and older adults are more likely to have been exposed to carcinogens over a longer period of time. Immune function and reserve capacity decline, the number of comorbid conditions for which older adults take multiple drugs increases, and organ function declines with increasing age, particularly after age 70 years. Table 35-6 provides some of the main physiologic effects pertinent to older adults with cancer.[54,62-65] Physiologic changes, comorbidities, polypharmacy, fall risk, venous access considerations, and psychosocial concerns can make care of the geriatric-oncology patient population a challenging specialty. More than 80% of people over 65 years old have at least one chronic condition. In more than 50% of older adults with cancer, cancer only partially contributes to the cause of death. Hypertension, heart-related conditions, arthritis, gastrointestinal problems, hearing and eye impairments, diabetes, and anemia are some of the top chronic conditions affecting the older adult with cancer.[54,64] The high incidence of comorbid conditions and increased drug use leads to greater likelihood of an adverse drug reaction in older adults receiving cancer treatment and supportive care, compared with younger patients. An important consideration of the oncology nurse is evaluation of older patients at risk for falls due to orthostatic hypotension, mobility impairment, muscle fatigue, cognitive impairment, and polypharmacy. Falls in older adults can be very costly in terms of independent living, and may precipitate a move to a more supervised environment or an extended care facility. Age-related IV access considerations include reduced immune response, decreased sensory ability leading to delayed detection of phlebitis, and infiltration.

Ill older adults generally want to be home among family and familiar surroundings. Family members often feel inadequate in their abilities to care properly for their parent or spouse and may be reluctant to bring them home. This, in turn, may result in feelings of guilt and fears that they may be judged as uncaring. In addition, family members have feelings of guilt and helplessness associated with their parent or spouse's illness. The nurse must

TABLE 35-6	Physiologic Changes in Older Adults Related to Cancer Treatment	
BODY SYSTEM	**PHYSIOLOGIC CHANGES**	**ASSOCIATED RISK WITH CANCER TREATMENT**
Neurologic	• Decreased motor and mental responses • Decreased brain mass and functional neurons • Decreased sensory ability	• Decreased functional dependence • Decreased memory and capacity to understand instructions • Increased risk of delayed detection of phlebitis and infiltration with IV access
Respiratory	• Decreased vital capacity and lung compliance • Decreased cough reflex • Altered gas exchange	• Pneumonia
Cardiovascular	• Decreased cardiac output and reserve • Stiffer myocardium and heart valves • Decreased response to sympathetic stimulation • Fibrous and sclerosed veins	• Postural hypotension • Volume overload • Decreased peripheral access
Gastrointestinal	• Decreased intestinal motility • Decreased taste • Decreased absorption • Prolonged gastric emptying	• Constipation, ileus • Malnutrition • Altered drug absorption leading to increased toxicities or less-than-optimal dose
Hepatic	• Decreased hepatic flow • Decreased liver mass	• Increased risk of drug toxicities and interactions
Renal	• Decreased creatinine clearance • Decreased ability to concentrate urine and excrete water and electrolytes	• Increased risk of drug toxicities • Fluid volume excess • Electrolyte imbalances
Body Composition	• Decreased plasma volume and total body water • Decreased serum albumen levels	• Altered drug distribution leading to increased toxicities
Immune	• Decrease in bone marrow function • Decreased mechanical barriers	• Slow recovery of hematopoiesis • Prolonged myelosuppression resulting in treatment delay or dose reduction
Cutaneous	• Loss of dermal, subcutaneous mass, and elastic fibers • Decreased activity of sebaceous glands • Decreased circulation	• Thin, fragile, dry skin resulting in decreased barrier to infection • Reduced healing and increased pruritus

Adapted from Green JM, Hacker ED: Chemotherapy in the geriatric population, *Clin J Oncol* 8(6):591–597, 2004; and Colman EA, Hutchins L, Goodwin J: An overview of cancer in the older adult, *Medsurg Nurs* 13(2):75–80,109, 2004.

provide an opportunity for family members to discuss their fears, feelings, and concerns. Consideration should be given to how this illness is affecting the family's ability to meet their continuing needs.

Needs
1. What difficulties is the family experiencing with the medical treatment? (This would include management and changes in course of illness.)
2. What are the sources of financial strain from direct and indirect costs related to the illness?
3. What changes are required in ADLs for the family?
4. In what manner has the illness fostered social isolation?
5. How have relationships within the family been affected?
6. What impact has the illness or its management had on the ability to meet their continuing needs?

Coping Strategies
1. What is the level of knowledge and technical skill the family has gained concerning the illness and its treatment?
2. What strategies does the family use to help maintain a sense of normalcy in family life?
3. Who are identified supportive people or groups, and what do they provide for the family?

4. What activities do the family members use to enhance positive coping strategies?
5. Does this illness have any positive aspects or results as perceived by this family?

After the establishment of rapport with the family, it is expected that each of these areas can be explored in more depth. The nurse and the family can work together to identify and implement mutually acceptable interventions that will promote optimal family functioning. It is important to provide the family with education to enable them to care adequately for their parent or spouse and to provide the necessary resources to support their primary caregiving role and to foster optimal family functioning. Many community resources are available to aid and support families experiencing difficulties associated with caring for the older adult who has cancer. Table 35-7 presents an overview of recommendations related to the assessment and implementation of transitional planning for the older adult.[32]

HOSPICE

Hospice is family-centered care designed to allow patients to remain at home with comfort, independence, and dignity while managing the stress of terminal illness. The advent of

TABLE 35-7   Recommendation for Transitional Planning and Home Follow-up of Older Adults

Assessment	**General Principles:** • Plan is tailored to individual and family and caregiver needs. • Patient and family are involved throughout the process. • Assessment findings guide intervention strategies and educational requirements after discharge. • Assessment predicts patient-specific, measurable outcomes (yield to family wishes and preferences for optimal outcomes). • Planning begins at admission, is ongoing, and occurs before discharge.
Implementation	**The 4 "Cs" To Ensure Continuity Of Care:** *Communication* • Barriers to communication are identified and eliminated. • It occurs between multidisciplinary team and family and caregivers (formal and informal) throughout the • planning process and is multidirectional. • Medical care needs are communicated between acute care and community care providers. • Written communication is documented on the interdisciplinary record and includes hospital and/or acute care course summary, actual or potential sequelae, symptoms and symptom management, significant changes in status since admission, medication review and any difficulties for the patient, family, or caregiver, psychosocial adaptation to the illness, anticipated outcomes, and advance directives. • Verbal communication of health status and transitional plan occurs with the patient, family and/or caregiver, primary health care provider, multidisciplinary experts, and other providers of care. • Health teaching, guidance, and counseling is geared to the learning needs of the older adult. • Discussion takes place regarding special procedures (such as wound care, tube feedings, hydration), medication administration and ADLs, particularly in relation to mobility, transfers, and gait training. *Coordination* • Case manager or designated transitional planner coordinates the multidisciplinary team in the planning process and links the patient with the most appropriate services. • Communication between patient, family and/or caregiver and home health provider and/or community resources is clear. *Collaboration* • Multidisciplinary team is involved in specialized assessments, recommendations, and case conferences, including an advanced practice nurse expert in geriatrics and/or oncology. • Family and/or caregivers provide information about past experiences, potential barriers to care, and biopsychosocial needs of the patient. *Continual Reassessment* • The planning process is dynamic, not static; status of the older adult may change rapidly requiring frequent reassessment. • Functional and cognitive status are monitored continually. • Medication understanding, management capabilities, and side effects are ascertained regularly. • Family and/or caregiver abilities continually evaluated; caregiver support needs are met. • Transportation access and availability is assessed and ensured. • Change in condition is communicated to all team members. • Home care and/or extended care needs change as patient status changes.

ADLs, Activities of daily living.
Adapted from Zwicker D, Picariello G. Discharge planning for the older adult. In: Mezey M, Fulmer T, Abraham I et al, editors: *Geriatric nursing protocols for best practice,* ed 2, New York, 2003, Springer.

consumerism and the desire for greater control over the delivery and quality of care, particularly when all other treatment options have been exhausted or judged to be ineffective, have contributed to the increased public awareness of and interest in the hospice concept. Even though the term *hospice* is familiar to most, many do not understand the type of services provided under the umbrella of hospice.[66] (See Chapter 34 for further discussion of hospice, particularly its historical development the role it plays in the delivery of palliative care.)

Hospice is a philosophy of care that provides active, high-quality, comprehensive care to persons with a terminal disease and to their families. Hospice care is not exclusively terminal care. It is

sensitive and skilled care that addresses the physical, psychologic, and spiritual needs of the patient and family and is provided by an interdisciplinary team of professionals and volunteers. The setting for this care is usually in the home; however, hospice care may be provided by home health care agencies, freestanding programs, skilled nursing homes, and hospitals during acute medical crisis and impending death, or to give the family a short respite (2 to 5 days). Respite care may be provided in the home by respite care agencies or by home health care agencies; in the community by adult day care centers, respite care cooperatives, or freestanding respite facilities; or in a long-term care institution, in nursing homes, or in a hospital.

The duration of care may vary (e.g., respite care may be limited to 28 days in a calendar year). Medical crises may include uncontrolled pain, nausea and vomiting, or other situations that may warrant a brief hospitalization until the patient's symptoms are controlled.[53,66]

In hospice home care, an assessment of the family's ability to provide care and support for the patient is an essential part of the plan of care. The hospice team develops and coordinates an individualized care plan together with the patient and family members. Hospice nurses and physicians review the care plan, visit the patient regularly, prescribe drugs for palliative care, review the patient's condition and prognosis with hospice personnel, and sign the death certificate. Before choosing hospice care, patients and their family members are told that the hospice agency takes only limited action, if any, to prolong life. Hospice patients decide the number and kinds of treatment they will receive. Advance directives, including appointment of a health care proxy and durable power of attorney for health care, ensure that patients' choices are followed.

In the early 1980s, hospice treatment was formally acknowledged through reimbursement by Medicare and many other insurers, allowing people to die at home by providing financial and professional support, setting standards, and educating health care professionals about the hospice alternative. In Medicare-certified hospice programs, basic services include nursing and physician services (a physician must be a salaried member of the team); medical social work; counseling (including dietary and pastoral); physical, occupational, and speech therapy; home health aide and homemaker services; short-term inpatient care (including respite care and pain control or management); medical appliances and supplies; and drugs. Often, attorneys are available to provide legal aid to patients and their families if needed. Continuity is offered through bereavement counseling services for the patient's survivors with trained grief counselors for up to 13 months after the patient's death.

Patients who elect the Medicare hospice benefit must waive standard Medicare benefits for conditions related to the terminal illness. Eligibility to receive care for other, current problems is not affected (e.g., a hospice patient with lung cancer can be treated for injuries sustained in an automobile accident). The following five requirements must be met for a patient to qualify for the Medicare hospice benefit: [66]

1. The patient is qualified for Part A of Medicare Hospital Insurance.
2. The patient is certified by an attending physician and the hospice medical director to have a limited life expectancy with a poor prognosis.
3. The patient resides in an area where a Medicare-certified hospice program is available.
4. A written plan of care is established and regularly reviewed.
5. The patient formally elects the hospice benefit.

A purpose of hospice is to enhance the quality of life for the patient who is dying and for the family survivors. Most hospice facilities provide services that incorporate hospice guidelines developed by the National Hospice and Palliative Care Organization (NHPCO). The NHPCO is committed to hospice education and promoting beneficial legislation, regulation, and reimbursement for hospice care. Hospice programs enable terminally ill patients to receive supportive services and remain comfortable in their own homes. Pain control, frequently discussed in association with hospice care, is not exclusively physical pain and may be a sign of psychologic, social, or spiritual pain. Social pain may stem from troubled interpersonal relationships, unfinished business, and unsaid good-byes. Some hospice programs have expanded the range of services available to hospice including hospice day-care centers. These centers increase the continuity of care, provide additional support services such as individual counseling and support groups, and increase the patient's and family's sense of connectedness with others.[66,67]

Recently, in many areas of the United States, hospice programs have been particularly innovative in reaching out to the community at large by developing educational and bereavement programs that teach others not in hospice programs how to cope with loss and grief. These hospices also provide training programs and manuals to health care providers and teachers to enable them to form support groups in their community. Many hospice programs provide consultation services to other health care providers and institutions.

Volunteer support, staff support mechanisms, and the team concept all assist and support team members through the patient's death and beyond. Continuity and closure are also offered through bereavement counseling. The identification of overburdened caregivers who are at risk for long-term bereavement maladjustment is needed to facilitate timely interventions.

PRIVATE DUTY

One element of home health care that might potentially be expanded is private duty care. Many home care organizations provide this supplemental home care services on a fee-for-service basis. These additional services, such as nursing, nursing aides, companions, and housekeepers, can be used to supplement available caregiving resources or provide care when there is no available caregiver, thereby preventing or delaying institutionalization. Private-duty home care is not included in most health insurance policies as a benefit; therefore the patient or family is responsible for paying for this service. Responsibility for supervision, monitoring, government-mandated taxes, and workers' compensation coverage falls on the consumer. The private hire model can be a significant financial burden, risk, and liability, but when one considers the alternative of institutionalization, it may be worth the expense. In response to the increasing growth and the lack of standardized practice within this unregulated industry, the National Private Duty Association (NPDA) educates consumers about the risk and liabilities posed by using the private hire model, enhances the strength and professionalism of private duty home care providers through education, and supports legislative issues that protect consumers.[68,69]

If the cost of such services through an agency is prohibitive for the patient and family, the oncology nurse may suggest that they make arrangements with a friend or neighbor for light housekeeping, meal preparation, or sitter and companion services for nominal compensation. As the trend for managed care continues, some supplemental home care services will be included in the patient's health insurance plan. Third-party payers have noted that paying for additional support services to maintain the patient in the home or in nonhospital settings reduces the overall cost of long-term care.

REIMBURSEMENT ISSUES

In the United States, most health care has been provided through third-party payers, that is, private health insurance companies or government health care assistance at the state or the federal level. The inequity inherent in the growing numbers of uninsured and underinsured U.S. citizens is still a major component of discussions regarding health care reform on all levels. Economic assessments, analysis, and outcomes measures are being increasingly used to provide meaningful data regarding oncology studies, innovative treatments, and alternative care settings to health care providers, payers, and policy decision makers to facilitate identification of optimal treatment and care strategies. As third-party payers and health care institutions are attempting to control spiraling health care costs and implement health care reform proactively, such data will guide and direct the allocation of health care services and funding resources.

Currently the fastest growing coverage option in health care is the prepaid health plan, commonly known as health maintenance organization (HMO) and preferred provider organizations (PPOs). The HMO is an entity licensed by the state to provide comprehensive, coordinated medical services to an enrolled membership in a geographic area on a prepaid, capitated basis. There are four main HMO models that differ primarily in how and with whom the HMO contracts for provider services: group model, individual practice association (IPA), network model (health plan), and staff model. The PPO encourages the used of a more limited "panel of providers" and services within the network; however, patients can go outside the network for decreased reimbursement. To sum up, the spectrum of managed care options, used by HMOs and PPOs to improve delivery of services and contain costs, controls the means by which health care is delivered. Managed care is becoming the predominant health care delivery system and is likely to remain so in the future.[25,70]

As a result of health care changes, the number of subacute care facilities and the variety of alternative care facilities will probably increase dramatically to avoid high-cost nursing home placements and yet still provide the necessary services. To qualify for subacute care, there must be an expectation of a patient's continued recovery and a need for more interdisciplinary services than a skilled nursing facility or home care could provide. Subacute care facilities provide care that is outcomes focused, contributing to cost efficiency. Unlike acute care facilities, subacute care facilities are not bound by the PPS; long-term facilities generally have patients whose stay exceeds 25 days, and few short-stay, low-cost cases. Subacute care facilities can either be free-standing, long-term care institutions or housed within an existing acute care hospital as long as the federal guidelines and criteria for such facilities are met.[25]

Currently, most health care insurance policies cover home care and hospice services. All require that the service be ordered by a physician and that a medical plan of care be signed by the physician. The care provided must be intermittent, and the patient must also need skilled professional care provided by a nurse, physical therapist, or speech therapist and have a medical condition that warrants ongoing assessment and evaluation. Patients must also be homebound, that is, unable to leave home without assistance of others and assistive devices. If the patient or caregiver requires no additional instruction regarding the disease process or its management, and the patient is medically stable for more than 2 weeks, he or she is no longer considered in need of ongoing skilled nursing service unless specific treatments are ordered. With the advent of the PPS for home care patients covered under Medicare and the growth of managed care insurance, home health agencies will be asked to deliver more intensive services in a shorter number of visits.[25]

Insurance coverage for home care services and alternative care settings is based on a prospective nursing assessment completed at the time the patient was entered in home care services. In most cases, care is reimbursed for an episode of care, with a fixed dollar amount regardless of number of visits the patient receives. Insurance benefits are negotiated individually for group policies and benefit packages. More frequently now, health insurance providers are becoming more flexible regarding the services and benefits available to individuals, because the cost-saving benefits have been well documented. Prior approval usually is necessary. The medical plan of care must be reviewed and updated periodically (usually every 60 days) and again signed by the physician.

THE ROLE OF THE ONCOLOGY NURSE AS PATIENT ADVOCATE

In the role of a transitional care planner and liaison to the health care team, an important responsibility of oncology nurses and case managers is patient and family advocacy. Patient and family needs and wishes are communicated during case conferences, for the purposes of obtaining authorizations and certifications from third-party payers, and when negotiating with agencies for community services. Furthermore, as patient advocates, nurses can play an important role in clinical and community-based research that includes quality measures, patient outcomes, and access to care, in addition to economic assessments and analysis. Nurses are well positioned to take an active part in provider negotiations and in establishing new standards of care as part of their patient advocacy role. Greater numbers of clinical nurse specialists (CNSs) and nurse practitioners (NPs) have assumed the pivotal role of designated transitional care planner or case manager. With advanced education and specialized experience, oncology CNSs and NPs can effectively implement managed care and disease management strategies for the provision of cost-controlled, safe, quality care, and can act as change agents, ensuring a link in complex health systems between the cancer patient, the payer, and the provider.[25]

CULTURAL PERSPECTIVES

As the United States becomes increasingly multicultural, the need for oncology nurses and other health care providers who can provide culturally competent care to persons with cancer will also increase. For the individual with cancer, the native language and treasured traditions can become an obstacle, especially if the skills of the health care professionals are not tempered with cultural sensitivity. Oncology nurses must engage in cultural self-assessment to discover biases and prejudices that sometimes lead to insensitive care and cultural imposition. One result of the absence of culturally sensitive care is the breakdown of communication and trust, often leading to the reluctance of minorities to access health resources. For instance, all cultures emphasize the importance of truth-telling and consider deception as wrong; however, definitions of truth and deception vary widely. To some cultures, truth is what corresponds to reality; whereas to other cultures, truth is what brings the greatest benefit to the group. Deception is considered a loss of advantage, prestige, or favor. The implications of truth as an ingrained cultural value must be considered when deciding whether to inform patients about their impending death. Some cultures believe in the power of words to create reality, such that talking about impending death and creating advance directives may actually cause death to happen.[71]

Issues related to availability and acceptability of care and services have also contributed to cultural barriers to cancer care in America. Many organizations have made significant efforts to reduce cultural barriers to cancer care.[71] Innovations include the following:

- Establishing a minority and/or cultural group: a task force can be composed of members of the target group to identify specific barriers and create a plan to reduce these obstacles
- Establishing a community speakers bureau that uses members of the targeted minority or cultural group
- Involving culturally specific minority media in outreach and education efforts
- Involving culturally specific spiritual and religious institutions in the spectrum of care services and delivery
- Forming culturally specific minority support groups
- Recruiting diverse health care workers through employment advertising in publications aimed at ethnic groups
- Forming an informal "language bank" of bilingual employees
- Using available technology, such as the AT&T Language Line, to facilitate communication through an over-the-phone interpretation service

As community-based and home-based health care continues to grow, health care providers will encounter individuals from more and more diverse cultures and ethnic groups. Although an important first step is to improve communication with these groups, it is imperative that health care providers be knowledgeable in issues related to cultural diversity and conceptual differences between cultures. These providers must be proficient in modifying cancer care accordingly to make this care culturally sensitive.

Interventions

In addition to observation and evaluation of physical and emotional status, interventions for patients and their families with altered self-care management needs in the home or extended care facility generally fall into five main categories: (1) direct care, (2) medication management, (3) education, (4) coordination of care, and (5) referrals and surveillance.[25,52]

Direct care refers to the actual physical aspects of nursing in the home or the extended care facility, including administering treatments and medications, providing rehabilitative exercises, and performing catheter insertion, colostomy irrigation, and wound care.[25,27,58] Direct care interventions are individualized to the patient's health status and patient/family abilities and goals.

The goal of medication management is to assist the patient and family to safely take medications, as prescribed by the primary care provider (PCP) or obtained over the counter. Nursing actions include obtaining orders for medication prescriptions, updating the medication list, and teaching the patient and family about the medication regimen and possible side effects, and giving instructions about the criteria and the process for contacting health care providers if necessary.[30,44,54,72] Additional interventions include providing assistance in obtaining medications from the pharmacy and filling medication and/or pill boxes.[25]

The goals of education of the patient and caregiver are frequently that they demonstrate understanding of the disease process and complications, signs and symptoms to expect and report to a health care provider, medication administration, treatment measures, safety in the home, and specific areas unique to the patient, the family or health status.[23,30,31,54,70] In addition to teaching patients and families to carry out treatments and medication administration as prescribed, individualized instructions may include a variety of topics such as proper handwashing; symptom and pain management; skin and wound care; diet and hydration; activity limits, exercise, and energy conservation; and additional self-care activities.[25,72,73]

To reduce or eliminate identified barriers to learning, nursing interventions include delaying the teaching until the individual is ready to learn, acknowledging cultural practices, and incorporating health beliefs and past experiences in the teaching materials. Patient and family learning is most effective in a quiet, nonstressful environment; with active participation in the learning process through question-and-answer sessions and with sufficient time to discuss the planned topics.[25,30,44,54,70]

Coordinating and facilitating a plan of care for home or extended care requires thorough and ongoing communication with the patient, the family, and the multidisciplinary team. In a time of ill health and high stress for patient and caregiver, the oncology nurse must establish a level of mutual understanding of the patient and caregiver needs, the available care options, the likely consequences of each choice, and requisite self-care education.[25] It is at this point that the patient and the family caregiver reach a level of awareness and motivation, and the plan can be implemented. For example, with transitional planning, the oncology nurse or transition planner implements three steps to ensure the plan's success: (1) clarify the responsibilities of care, (2) review the plan with the patient, the family, and the multidisciplinary team to ensure that nothing has been overlooked, and (3) make last-minute adjustments to the plan as needed.[15,25,27,31,35]

Oncology nurses and transition planners regularly coordinate the involvement of specialists in the care of cancer patients and family caregivers. Specialty health care providers include nutritionists, social workers, physical therapists, home care service providers, pain management specialists, and pharmacists. Nutrition teaching may include suggestions to freeze complete meals that require only heating (e.g., small containers of soup, stew, casseroles) or teach patient and family about foods that are easily prepared and nutritious. Nurses may intervene or initiate appropriate referrals to assist patients and families to develop appropriate strategies based on personal strengths and previous experience with constructive problem-solving techniques and coping skills. Other interventions include helping patients and families identify outlets that foster feelings of personal achievement and self-esteem, reduce social isolation by facilitating contact with supportive others, and assist with managing new roles and responsibilities.[15,25,27,31,35]

In the community, patients and families may be referred to a local nursing agency, support groups (e.g., American Cancer Society [ACS], Encore, Y-Me), and community agencies (e.g., volunteer visitors, meal programs, homemakers, adult day care). Nursing home care agencies provide needed equipment or aids and teach care and maintenance of supplies that increase their durability. If the patient and family has insufficient funds, oncology nurses can contact local social services and service organizations for assistance (e.g., Lung Association, ACS). When transportation is needed, nurses may suggest that patients request rides with neighbors to places they drive to routinely, or consult transportation resources in the community.[15,25,31,52]

Surveillance or follow-up care of the patient and the caregiver consists of anticipatory guidance related to emotional and social needs of the family and alternatives to home care as appropriate.[44] Oncology nurses can share alternatives to reduce strain and fatigue of caregiving, such as obtaining relief from responsibilities each week for short periods (e.g., engage a sitter, neighbors, or relatives), enlisting the aid of others to meet some of the patient's needs (e.g., transportation to treatments), and maintaining contact with friends and relatives even if only by telephone or from Internet support groups.[44,49] Additional nursing interventions consist of providing patients and caregivers the opportunity to share problems and feelings, reducing stress through the use of humor, and commending caregivers for their diligence in caring for the patient.[10,18,21,25,30,44,45]

Nursing-Sensitive Patient Outcomes

Given the chronic and potentially devastating nature of cancer and the significant burden it places on patients, family caregivers, and society, it is essential that oncology nurses describe and measure the impact of nursing care on patient outcomes. The ability to clearly communicate the relationship between nursing interventions and patient outcomes is crucial to ensure quality care in an environment of rising health care costs and the diminishing nursing workforce. The effect of nursing interventions on outcomes can be viewed from the provider, administrator or patient perspective. Nursing-sensitive patient outcomes (NSPOs) such as quality of life, symptom management, physical functioning, performance status, patient and family satisfaction, resource utilization, and cost are amenable to the interventions of oncology nurses across many settings.[73]

For patients with advanced disease or those receiving palliative care, appropriate outcomes are related to symptom relief, optimal functioning, health-related quality of life, quality of death, and quality of patient and family care. For example, outcomes for the patient or caregiver in the home setting include the ability to do the following:
- Identify factors that restrict self-care and home management
- Demonstrate the ability to perform skills necessary for care of patient at home
- Express satisfaction with home situation
- Experience less anxiety and stress related to caregiving role
- Identify personal strengths and receive support through the nursing relationship and community resources

PATIENT AND FAMILY TEACHING

Educating the patient and family is an essential part of successful transitional planning. Patients need to know what to do when they get home, how to do it, what to observe for when problems develop, and how to contact an appropriate health care provider. A critical part of the oncology nurse role is patient and family education that uses understandable language and gives consideration to cultural and health care beliefs. The trend of consumerism, shortened hospital stays, and the complex nature of cancer, combined with current, often aggressive treatment modalities necessitates improved, comprehensive patient and family education. Documented evidence supports the idea that

patients and families with increased knowledge of their illness and treatment plan experience significantly less anxiety and stress. The oncology nurse must consider internal and external factors influencing patient, family, and caregiver ability to learn. Individual internal factors include literacy, coping style, emotions, stress and anxiety, fatigue, and culture of origin. External factors include knowledge and skill of the educator, educational media, environmental factors, and timing of the instruction. Important areas to evaluate are readiness, motivation, past experiences, physical and intellectual abilities, preferred methods of teaching e.g., (verbal, written words or pictures, audio, video), and physical and psychologic comfort. Asking patients and families if they are interested in obtaining additional information helps in determining what the patient or the family member already knows, thus reducing boredom and "tuning out." Oncology nurses in acute, community, clinic, and outpatient settings need to emphasize more the psychosocial and informational needs of family home caregivers. Because of shorter hospitalizations, nurses must begin this educational process early, and continue the counseling process through the discharge process and into the home setting. Linking families to volunteer and professional community agencies with appropriate services will provide additional resources to meet a variety of needs. Regulatory and accreditation agencies require compliance with standards of patient and family education.[25,71,74,75]

Low literacy is a significant problem in the United States today, particularly as it relates to health care education. Frequently, the reading level of patient education materials exceeds the abilities of patients and families or caregivers. Functional illiteracy is defined as reading at or below the fifth-grade level, and marginal literacy is between the sixth- and eighth-grade levels. As many as 44 million Americans are functionally illiterate, and 50 million are marginally literate. Illiteracy is more endemic among the elderly and poor persons. It is important for the oncology nurse to carefully and sensitively determine the patient's reading capabilities. Low literacy is associated with feelings of shame, higher health care costs, and increased use of the health care system. Many adults are embarrassed about the inability to read, and over the years they become very skillful in covering up this deficit, typically using statements such as: "I don't have my glasses with me now; can you read it to me?" or "I'll read it later." Additional indicators of low literacy that require additional assessment include lack of interest in the material, expressions of frustration, lack of reading speed, and inability to answer questions about the content of the text.[25,74,75]

Many patients with cancer want as much information about their illness as possible, preferably through discussion with a physician or nurse. Written materials are helpful in reinforcing information learned through discussion. Patients and families tend to prefer a variety of media. It is important that the oncology nurse realize the importance of a multifaceted, creative approach to patient and family education. The oncology nurse must be aware of the limitations of these materials and individualize the teaching plan to meet the unique needs of each patient. The nurse must also assess for the appropriate instructional method for the individual, using all available educational resources and modalities such as audiovisual, pictorial, as well as written, material. These can only enhance and facilitate the learning process.[25,72]

Contract learning, an alternative way of structuring a learning experience, is an agreement between educator and learner that specifies what is to be learned, how it is to be learned, and how learning is verified. Researchers have found that contract learning has had good results when used with adult learners, because it includes concepts of independent, individualized, and self-directed learning. The education process, as with the nursing process, includes the steps of assessing, planning, implementing, and evaluating. Ongoing assessments are needed, because educational needs vary throughout the cancer experience. The primary learner in the family must be identified and learning needs assessed. After this assessment, a mutually acceptable plan to meet the identified educational needs is developed by the nurse-teacher and the patient-learner. Appropriate teaching strategies are used to implement the plan and are jointly evaluated, with the evaluation serving as a basis for further decision making. Addressing the educational wants and needs of the family caregiver is a top priority if the patient is to receive proper care and be able to remain in the home.[25,72,74,75]

ADVANCE DIRECTIVES

Recent studies have reported fewer than 15% of Americans have prepared an advance directive (AD), and only 27% of cancer patients admitted to an intensive care unit had an AD.[57,76] Legal, ethical, and professional issues arise from decision making on life-prolonging procedures when death is inevitable. The Patient Self-Determination Act (PSDA) under which the durable power of attorney for health care (DPAHC), the living will, and the advance directive are subsumed, was created by the U.S. Congress in 1990 and implemented in all states in December 1991. The PSDA is based on the belief in the preservation of individual rights in decision making related to personal survival. Since 1991, hospitals have responded to the mandate by creating pamphlets and educational materials regarding advance directives.[37] These are usually presented to patients on admission to the acute care facility, which is not ideal because at that time patients are usually either ill, anxious, or under great stress. This poor timing does not facilitate a well-reasoned health care decision. It is preferable that patients and their families collaborate with their primary health care provider well before an acute episode of care and revise the AD regularly as needed.[77]

Many people have misconceptions regarding advance directives, believing that these are only for elderly or terminally ill patients and that if one does have an advance directive, it will result in limited or denied care in the future. The oncology nurse must address these misconceptions, serve as a resource person, and overcome any barriers to education created by illiteracy and cultural differences. For most people diagnosed with cancer, death is a well-known but uncomfortable topic. When people with cancer understand that everyone should have an AD, regardless of current health status, they feel less targeted because of having cancer and more comfortable with the subject.[77]

DISCHARGE INSTRUCTIONS

To help facilitate the transition to the home or the alternative care setting and ensure continuity of care and medical follow-up, it is important to clearly convey specific discharge instructions to the patient and family members at discharge. The time of discharge is particularly hectic, and often instructions given at this time may not be remembered accurately or at all. Consequently, it is advisable to have specific written instructions to review with and give the patient and family at discharge.

ACCESSING THE HEALTH CARE SYSTEM

Many institutions have discharge instruction sheets that are completed by the nurse and include instructions regarding follow-up appointments and medications. Patients and their families need to know how to access the health care system after discharge. The following questions can be used by the nurse as prompts to ensure the patient and family understand issues concerning home or office care.

- Whom should I call when questions arise that cannot wait until the next appointment?
- What should I expect?
- When do I worry?
- When should I call?
- How can I reach these professionals?
- What about after hours? Who is the contact person then?

In addition, in all settings the experienced oncology nurse should anticipate potential problems that may arise as a result of treatment or disease progression, such as side effects specific to the chemotherapy and other medications. The nurse can provide the patient or the responsible caregiver with information regarding anticipated problems and self-care measures to manage these problems. Consider the patient's reading ability, and assess the readability of the written material provided. If the reading skills of the patient or the family member are limited, it may be more appropriate and more effective to write out very simple instructions or information specifically tailored for the individual. Alternative teaching modalities such as audiotapes or videotapes may also be effective teaching tools to augment any teaching plan.[32]

FOLLOW-UP APPOINTMENTS AND PHONE CALLS

Essential to an effective treatment of any cancer is consistent medical follow-up. Ongoing assessment, evaluation, and subsequent modification of the treatment plan are critical. Follow-up appointments are important, but are often a difficult undertaking for patients and their families. The nurse can implement several actions to facilitate keeping follow-up appointments.

Patients may not have transportation resources available to them, and frequently this issue is disregarded when setting up the follow-up appointment. It is important to ask the patient or family member if appropriate transportation is available. If necessary, they may be referred to local agencies that provide transportation services at no charge or at a minimal cost. Many private companies provide transportation services for disabled persons for a fee.[32]

In addition to information about transportation resources, patients need to know what assistance is available when they arrive for their follow-up appointment. If a wheelchair is needed, how do they arrange to have one available? Most hospitals and clinics have wheelchairs available for such purposes. This should be determined before the appointment. If a wheelchair is not available, the patient should be advised to arrange for the use of one.

At busy oncology clinics, follow-up appointments can become an exhausting, all-day effort. Patients frequently are scheduled for blood work before their appointment with the physician, and later may receive chemotherapy or be scheduled for other tests. Patients and their families should be advised to bring the medications that they may need to take while still at the clinic, especially pain medications. Patients and their families should be told what to expect at the follow-up appointment, especially if the patient is going to receive a treatment or particular diagnostic test for the first time. Knowing what to expect greatly reduces fears and anxieties associated with the unknown.

Ideally, a follow-up telephone call to patients and their families should be made within 24 to 48 hours after discharge. It is helpful for the nurse to have a copy of the continuing patient care form and discharge instruction sheets so they can ask appropriate questions and obtain accurate information about the patient's status. Initial questions, such as, "How are things going since you came home?" or "Have any problems occurred?" or "Do you have any questions that I can answer for you?" allow the patient to express concerns. These questions can open communication, but the nurse must ask specific questions related to the patient's illness and treatment plan to ensure receiving an accurate assessment of the home situation. If it becomes apparent that activities are not going well in the home, the nurse may recommend that the patient be brought in to see the physician. Often, home care needs are not easily identified before discharge, but once the patient is at home, this need becomes apparent. If a home care referral has not been made, the nurse may determine at this time that a referral is warranted and initiate this process.

DURABLE MEDICAL AND ADAPTIVE EQUIPMENT

Durable medical equipment (DME) is equipment patients need for a medical purpose to maintain self-care. It withstands repeated use and is appropriate in the home setting. DME includes hospital beds, wheelchairs, and much more. Many assistive devices are available to patients and their families that enhance home care management and promote home safety. Essential equipment such as hospital beds, wheelchairs, and bedside commodes should be in the home at discharge, but some equipment and adaptive devices should not be ordered until a home evaluation is completed. Although an experienced nurse can assess and evaluate home equipment needs, a physical or occupational therapist is consulted. These therapists have an extensive knowledge of available equipment and may be able to meet the patient's equipment needs more effectively. Most insurance policies provide coverage for some DME; however, a physician's order is usually required, accompanied by a related neuromusculoskeletal diagnosis. Some insurance companies require prior approval before the equipment can be delivered to the patient. DME companies can help with this process.

COMMUNITY RESOURCES

Patient and family use of available community resources varies, but generally is minimal even when these services are needed. The reasons are not clear, but contributing factors may include the following:
- Service cost
- Access and availability
- Lack of awareness of available resources
- Lack of flexibility in services
- Inappropriate use of limited resources
- Consumer dissatisfaction
- Labeling of services

Further exploration into these factors is warranted to provide appropriate, well-coordinated community resources in a cost-efficient manner. Many national and local community resources are available to cancer patients and their families, ranging from personal services to informational services, social services, and support services. A telephone call to the Cancer Information Service (1-800-4-CANCER) and the local ACS chapter is a good starting point when first attempting to identify resources available in the community. Local community services often include agencies that provide or assist with housekeeping services, adult day care, socialization services (e.g., Friendly Visitor, In-Home Companion), nutritional services (e.g., Meals on Wheels, nutrition sites, food supplements, food banks or cupboards), financial savings and grant programs, transportation services, support groups, and counseling services.

Ethical Considerations

Transitional care planners face ethical dilemmas and challenges in their role as patient, family, and caregiver advocates. Trends in health care and today's managed care environment have generated ethical problems such as lack of access to care and denial of services. These ethical dilemmas are best resolved through shared decision making with an ethicist and/or organizational ethics committee. In dealing with ethical issues, the principles of autonomy, beneficence, justice, truth-telling and nonmaleficence are applied. Codes of professional ethics also guide the process of ethical decision making and problem solving. It is important to remember that when transitional care planners function within a quality-based managed care environment to limit costs, this is serving the interests of both payers of health care services and consumers. Some principles and strategies for approaching an ethical dilemma include the following:
- Maintain patient confidentiality and privacy
- Affirm the dignity and worth of each party, and promote trust
- Project a commitment to truthfulness and thorough gathering of information
- Respect diversity of values and opinions
- Allow sufficient time to discuss the issues
- Involve others in a shared decision making, but assume responsibility and accountability for one's own actions
- Distinguish ethical issues from other general patient care issues
- Apply institutional policies and procedures to support practice
- Document pertinent information in the patient's medical record

Summary

Patients with cancer move through a number of health care settings during the course of their illnesses. A successful transition through these settings depends on the collaborative efforts of a variety of health care providers and a systematic, coordinated transitional plan. Ongoing communication is the key to the effectiveness of these efforts.

In addition to collaboration, a thorough assessment and evaluation of the unique and specific care requirements of the cancer patient must be performed to identify the appropriate community support services and facilitate the transition of care. Ongoing reassessment and adjustment of the care plan must be done periodically to ensure attainment of expected outcomes and to avoid inappropriate use of limited services. To ensure the delivery of high-quality cancer care, it is important for oncology nurses to champion their role in quality cancer care through measurable nursing-sensitive patient outcomes. It is a challenge to meet the increasingly complex, multidimensional needs of patients with cancer and their families. Nurses must be competent, caring, and knowledgeable to successfully achieve these goals.

REVIEW QUESTIONS

✓ Case Study

Mrs. S., a 68 year-old woman whose mobility is impaired from rheumatoid arthritis, was diagnosed with stage III colon cancer. She underwent surgery at an urban academic medical center, located approximately 3 hours from home. She received chemotherapy with 5-flourouracil and leucovorin at the local community hospital. Two months after the bowel resection and chemotherapy, a small bowel obstruction necessitated hospitalization and placement of a gastrostomy tube. Over the next 8 months, she was admitted to the hospital several times for respiratory tract infection, gastrostomy tube infection, mucositis, diarrhea, and vomiting and dehydration.

Before the diagnosis of colon cancer, Mrs. S. lived at home with her husband of 51 years and worked part-time in the grocery store that the couple opened in 1964, now managed by a daughter, Ms. T., who lived in the same small town with her teenaged son and daughter. An older son, a computer programmer, lived far away but visited every few weeks; the younger son had been estranged from the family for many years. The older son and daughter were active caregivers in the course of their mother's illness. Despite Mr. S.'s congestive heart failure and other health problems, he was determined to care for his wife at home with the assistance of a home care nurse and a housekeeper to assist with daily chores.

As Mrs. S.'s health deteriorated, the home care nurse advised the family about a local in-hospital palliative care unit. When Mrs. S.'s pain and nausea could not be managed adequately at home, she was admitted to the palliative care unit. At the time of admission, Mrs. S. was alert and oriented but too weak get out of bed or participate in activities of daily living. As the family hoped, the symptoms were brought under control in a few days, and discussions began about the transition home with the support of hospice care. The family struggled with the desire to honor Mrs. S.'s request to die at home and the complex level of nursing care provided in the palliative care unit. Following a bedbath, on the morning she was to be transported home, Mrs. S.'s breathing became irregular with long periods of apnea. The transfer home was cancelled, and she died with her family at the bedside in the palliative care unit.

DISCUSSION

The story of a person who has cancer and dies is also the story of the impact on family members of this illness and death. Cancer death is often preceded by many months of family caregiving, including informal support and medical care provided by family members, partners, and friends. Informal support includes help with transportation, shopping, emotional support, nutritional care, nursing care, personal care, and financial management. There are financial costs, as well: caregiving creates an uncompensated financial burden for family members, including outright expenses and lost income.

Priority interventions before Mrs. S.'s health status deteriorated included nutritional support, including central venous access (CVA) for fluids and gastrostomy tube, symptom and pain management, and infection prevention. Later in the progression of Mrs. S.'s illness, palliative care interventions also included symptom management and supportive care. Interventions for the family included education related to the process of dying, support for the decision making regarding the transition to the inpatient palliative care unit, and enhancement of coping strategies and strategies to reduce caregiver strain, particularly the physical burden of care for Mr. S.

QUESTIONS

1. What should the hospital-based oncology nurse understand to be one factor influencing increased emphasis on home care and alternative care settings?
   a. Demographic changes such as steady growth of the elderly ill population
   b. Disbanding of the Prospective Payment System (PPS)
   c. Decrease in the availability of extended care facilities
   d. Joint Commission on Accreditation of Healthcare Organizations (JCAHO) definition of alternative care settings

2. What are some of the patient characteristics associated with the need for home care or extended care?
   a. Adequate family support at home, rehabilitation, first-time home care use
   b. Weight loss, nutrition deficits, adult 40 to 55 years old
   c. New cancer diagnosis, new diabetes diagnosis, educational level below 12 years
   d. New cancer diagnosis, ADLs impairment, age over 70 years

3. In the United States, family members and friends provide approximately what percentage of in-home care?
   a. 50% to 75%
   b. 65% to 70%
   c. 83% to 89%
   d. 90% to 100%

4. What is the primary reason more people do not have an advance directive?
   a. Fear that having an advance directive will increase care received in the future
   b. Belief that advance directives are for elderly and terminally ill patients
   c. Consistently optimal timing of health care provider in offering information to patient
   d. No advance directive information is provided to patients on admission to acute care facilities.

5. The Medicare definition regarding "homebound status" includes which of the following?
   a. Confined to home only on occasion because of chemotherapy side effects
   b. Confined to home because of illness and injury except with the use of supportive devices or special transportation
   c. Confined to home on intermittent basis because of illness
   d. Confined to home because of an intravenous device that restricts the ability to drive

6. The oncology nurse determines that patient and family education about hospice is successful when the patient states that which of the following is a major goal of hospice?
   a. Hospice aims to completely eliminate all physical pain regardless of the patient's desire to remain alert.

Continued

REVIEW QUESTIONS—CONT'D

b. Hospice provides a setting for care that is supportive of both the terminally ill individual and the family.

c. Hospice enhances the quality of life for the surviving family through many years of bereavement services.

d. Hospice provides a solely medical approach to terminal and palliative care.

7. What is an external factor that influences patient and family or caregiver ability to learn?
   a. Literacy level
   b. Timing of the instruction
   c. Stress and anxiety
   d. Culture of origin

8. During a discussion with a patient's family regarding evaluation of Internet-based health care information, the oncology nurse understands that the family needs further teaching when they make the following statement:
   a. "I like to check the author's credentials and expertise on the website."
   b. "The first thing I look for is when the website was last updated."
   c. "I look for websites that are well organized and easy to navigate."
   d. "I don't worry about who sponsors the website; I just like to look at a lot of different information."

9. What is included among the basic elements for the standards of practice for transitional planning?
   a. Client identification and selection, problem identification, planning, monitoring, evaluating, and outcomes development
   b. Assessment, communication, documentation, implementation, and patient and program education
   c. Assessment, needs identification, communication, patient evaluation, and program education
   d. Assessment, communication, documentation, patient education, and program presentation

10. An 82-year-old woman with multiple myeloma is preparing to go home with supervised care from her daughters. Which of the following reflects a possible drawback of home care for this patient and family?
    a. Sense of control and dignity
    b. Caregiver infections
    c. Familiarity with surroundings
    d. Out-of-pocket costs and lost wages for the caregivers

ANSWERS

1. **A.** *Rationale:* A contributing factor in the growth of home health care are demographic changes, particularly the rapidly growing population of older adults with chronic illness. The PPS has expanded into home health services, not disbanded; extended care facilities are increasing, and the JCAHO definition of alternative care settings is unrelated to the increased emphasis on home care and alternative care settings.

2. **C.** *Rationale:* Characteristics associated with the need for home or extended care include age over 70 years or pediatric cases, education level below 12 years, and impairment in ADLs. Weight loss, nutritional deficits, and middle age are not associated with greater need for home or extended care.

A new cancer diagnosis is not necessarily associated with the need for home or extended care.

3. **C.** *Rationale:* The percentage of in-home care provided by family members or friends is approximately 83% to 89% percent. Options (a) and (b) indicate percentages that are too low, and option (d) one that is too high. There are 44.4 million unpaid caregivers in the U.S., and often caregivers take on the role because of a sense of responsibility or expression of love.

4. **B.** *Rationale:* Misconceptions regarding advance directives include the belief they are for elderly and terminally ill patient and that having an advance directive will *limit* care, not increase it in the future (a). Optimal timing in offering advance directive information facilitates a well-reasoned decision rather than impeding one (c). Since 1991, under the directive of the Patient Self-Determination Act, acute care facilities present advance directive information upon admission to the facility (d).

5. **B.** *Rationale:* A patient is considered "homebound" by Medicare regulations if he or she has a condition due to illness or injury that restricts the ability to leave the residence except with the use of supportive devices (e.g., crutches, canes, wheelchairs) or with the use of special transportation. The homebound patient' absences in options (a) and (c) from the home are rare, of short duration, and attributable to the need to receive medical treatments. The presence of an intravenous device that restricts driving does not necessarily restrict the ability to leave the home by other transportation means (c).

6. **B.** *Rationale:* The goal of hospice is to provide supportive, multidisciplinary, and comprehensive care to the patient, family and friends. Option (a) can be eliminated because it indicates the patient is not allowed independence and control over the delivery of care, which is an important goal of hospice care. Bereavement counseling services for patient's survivors with trained grief counselors are typically offered for up to 13 months after the patient's death (c). Option (d) inaccurately indicates that a hospice has a medical focus of care, when it is interdisciplinary in approach.

7. **B.** *Rationale:* External factors influencing patient and family caregiver ability to learn include knowledge and skill of the educator, educational media, environmental factors, and timing of the instruction. Options (a), (c), and (d) are individual internal factors.

8. **D.** *Rationale:* The family's statement "I don't worry about who sponsors the website; I just want to look at a lot of information" indicates the family needs additional teaching regarding how to evaluate the quality of health care resources on websites. The remaining options are family responses that indicate teaching regarding the evaluation of Internet-based health care information has been successful and no further teaching is needed.

9. **A.** *Rationale:* The six standards of practice and discharge planning include (1) client identification and selection, (2) problem identification, (3) planning, (4) monitoring, (5) evaluating, (6) outcomes development (see Box 35-1), which are outlined in option (a), but not in options (b-d).

10. D. *Rationale:* Disadvantages of home care include potentially increased out-of-pocket costs and lost wages, increased physical and emotional strain for the caregiver, and lack of patients' and families' competence to manage complications and emergencies. Many family caregivers are middle-aged, female children who work outside of the home and care for their elderly parents. Advantages of home care include familiarity with surroundings and caregivers, increased sense of control, convenience for patients and families, less disruption of family life, reduced cost of care, reduction in infections, and improved quality of life. Option (d) is a disadvantage of home care, and options (a-c) are advantages of home care and can be eliminated.

REFERENCES

1. Murkofsky RL, Phillips RS, McCarthy EP et al: Length of stay in home care before and after the 1997 Balanced Budget Act, *JAMA* 289(21):2841-2848, 2003.
2. Yadgood MC, Miller, PJ: Solving the mystery the role of competency assessment in OASIS documentation, *Home Healthcare Nurse* 23(4):224-232, 2005.
3. Fernberg LF, Newman SL, Gray L et al: *The state of the states in family caregiver support: a 50 state study*, San Francisco, CA, 2004, Family Caregiver Alliance.
4. Fernberg LF, Newman SL, Van Steenberg C: *Family caregiver support: policies, perceptions and practices in 10 states since passage of the national family caregiver support program*, San Francisco, CA, 2002, Family Caregiver Alliance.
5. Northouse LL: Helping families of patients with cancer, *Oncol Nurs Forum* 32(4):743-750, 2005.
6. Higginson IJ, Sen-Gupta GJ: Place of care in advanced cancer: a qualitative systematic literature review of patient preferences, *J Palliat Med*, 3(3):287-300, 2000.
7. Sung, L, Feldman, BM, Schwamborn G et al: Inpatient versus outpatient management of low-risk pediatric febrile neutropenia: measuring parents' and healthcare professionals' preference, *J Clin Oncol* 22(19):3922-3929, 2004.
8. Thomas C, Morris SM, Clark D: Place of death: preferences among cancer patients and their careers, *Soc Sci Med* 58(12):2431-2444, 2004.
9. Baine WB, Yu W, Summe JP: The epidemiology of hospitalization of elderly Americans for septicemia or bacteremia in 1991-1998: application of Medicare claims data, *Ann Epidemiol* 11(2):118-126, 2001.
10. Cohen CA, Colantonio A, Vernich L: Positive aspects of caregiving: rounding out the caregiver experience, *Int J Geriatr Psychiatr* 17(2):184-188, 2002.
11. Loeser C, von Herz U, Huchler T et al: Quality of life and nutritional state in patients on home enteral tube feeding, *Nutrition* 19:605, 2003.
12. Jones SL: The association between objective and subjective caregiver burden, *Arch Psych Nurs* 10(2):77-84, 1996.
13. Edwards B, Clark V: The psychological impact of cancer diagnosis on families: the influence of family functioning and patient illness characteristics on depression and anxiety, *Psychooncology* 13:562-576, 2004.
14. Flaskerud JH, Carter PA, Lee P: Distressing emotions in female caregivers of people with AIDS, age-related dementias, and advanced-stage cancers *Perspect Psychiatr Care* 36(4):121-130, 2000.
15. Fink JLW: Long-term care: helping families make the best decision, *Nursing 2004* 34(6):18-20, 2004.
16. Gaston-Johnsson F, Lachica EM, Fall-Dickson JM et al: Psychological distress, fatigue, burden of care, and quality of life in primary caregivers of patients with breast cancer undergoing autologous bone marrow transplantation, *Oncol Nurs Forum* 31(6):1161-1169, 2004.
17. Navaie-Waliser M, Feldman PH, Gould DA et al: When the caregiver needs care: the plight of vulnerable caregivers, *Am J Pub Health* 92(3):409-413, 2002.
18. Carter PA, Chang BL: Sleep and depression in cancer caregivers, *Cancer Nurs* 23(6):410-415, 2000.
19. Donelan K, Falik M, DesRoches CM: Caregiving: challenges and implications for women's health, *Women's Health Issues* 11(3):185-200, 2001.
20. Hayman JA, Langa KM, Kabeto MU et al: Estimating the cost of informal caregiving for elderly patients with cancer, *J Clin Oncol* 19(13):3219-3225, 2001.
21. Matthews BA, Baker F, Spillers RL: Family caregivers and indicators of cancer-related distress, *Psychol Health Medicine* 8(1):45-56, 2003.

22. Northouse LL, Walker L, Schafenakcker A et al: A family-based program of care for women with recurrent breast cancer and their family members, *Oncol Nurs Forum* 29(10):1411-1419, 2002.
23. Grant M, Cook L, Bhatia S et al: Discharge and unscheduled readmissions of adult patients undergoing hematopoietic stem cell transplantation: implications for developing nursing interventions, *Oncol Nurs Forum* 32:E1-E8, 2005.
24. American Society of Clinical Oncology: American Society of Clinical Oncology statement regarding the use of outside services to prepare and administer chemotherapy drugs, *J Clin Oncol* 21(9):9,1882-1883, 2003.
25. Cesta TG, Tahan HA: *The case manager's survival guide*, St. Louis, 2003, Mosby.
26. Schumacher KL, Steward BJ, Archbold PG et al: Family caregiving skill: development of a concept, *Res Nurs Health* 23(3):191-203,, 2004.
27. Jones LS: Case management across settings. In Fieler VK, Hanson PA, editors: *Oncology nursing in the home*, Pittsburgh, 2000, Oncology Nursing Press.
28. Family Caregivers Association. Family caregiving statistics, retrieved November 14, 2006, from http://www.nfcacares.org/who/stats.cfm#1.
29. Cranley L, Doran DM: Nurses' integration of outcomes assessment data into practice, *Outcomes Manage* 8(1):13-18, 2004.
30. Duhamel F, Dupuis F: Guaranteed returns: investing in conversations with families of patients with cancer, *Clin J Oncol Nurs* 8(1):68-712004.
31. Fieler VK, Hanson PA: *Oncology nursing in the home*, Pittsburgh, 2000, Oncology Nursing Press.
32. Zwicker D, Picariello G: Discharge planning for the older adult. In Mezey M, Fulmer T, Abraham I et al, editors: *Geriatric nursing protocols for best practice*, ed 2, New York, 2003, Springer.
33. Case Management Society of America: *Standards of practice for case management*, Little Rock, Ark, 2002, Author.
34. Birmingham J: Discharge planning: the old/new wave. Part 2: the new wave of discharge planning, *Inside Case Manage* 10(9):1-5, 2003.
35. Bowles KH, Naylor MD, Foust JB: Patient characteristics at hospital discharge and a comparison of home care referral decisions, *J Am Geriatr Soc*, 50:336-342, 2002.
36. Yeaw EM, Burlingame PA: Identifying high-risk patients from the emergency department to the home, *Home Healthcare Nurse* 21(7):473-480, 2003.
37. Doran DM: *Nurse-sensitive outcomes: state of the science*, Sudbury, Mass, 2003, Jones & Bartlett.
38. Lueckenotte A: *Gerontologic nursing*, ed 2, St. Louis, 2000, Mosby.
39. Burlingame PA: *Assessment instrument for high-risk emergency department discharges*, Unpublished manuscript, 1999, University of Rhode Island.
40. National Alliance for Caregiving, American Association of Retired Persons: Caregiving in the U.S, retrieved November 14, 2006, from http://www.caregiving.org/data/04finalreport.pdf.
41. Given B, Wyatt G, Given C et al.: Burden and depression among caregivers of patients with cancer at the end of life, *Oncol Nurs Forum* 31(6):1105-1117, 2004.
42. Lethborg CE, Kissane D, Burns WI: 'It's not the easy part': the experience of significant others of women with early stage breast cancer, at treatment completion, *Soc Work Health Care* 37(1):63-85, 2003.
43. Carter P: Caregivers' descriptions of sleep changes and depressive symptoms, *Oncol Nurs Forum* 29(9):1277-1283, 2002.
44. Grbich C, Parker D, Maddocks I: The emotions and coping strategies of caregivers of family members with terminal cancer, *J Palliat Care* 17():30-36, 2001.
45. Ayers L: Narratives of family caregiving: the process of making meaning, *Res Nurs Health* 23(6):424-434, 2000.

46. Meyers JL, Gray LN: The relationship between family primary caregiver characteristics and satisfaction with hospice care, quality of life, and burden, *Oncol Nurs Forum* 28(1):73-82, 2001.

47. Birmingham J: Discharge planning: the old/new wave. Part 1, *Inside Case Manage* 10(5):1-5, 2003.

48. Klemm P, Bunnell D, Cullen M et al: Online cancer support groups: a review of the research literature, *Comput Nurs* 21(3):136-142, 2003.

49. Klemm P, Wheeler E: Cancer caregivers online, *Comput Informatics Nurs* 23(1):38-45, 2005.

50. Monnier J, Laken M, Carter C: Patient and caregiver interest in Internet-based cancer services, *Cancer Pract* 10(6):305-310, 2002.

51. Romano C, Hinegardner P, Phyillaier C: Some guidelines for browsing the Internet. In Fitzpatrick J, Montgomery K, editors: *Internet resources for nurses*, New York, 2000, Springer.

52. Stanhope M: Community health nurse in home health and hospice care. In Stanhope M, Lancaster J, editors: *Community health nursing: process and practice for promoting health*, ed 5, St Louis, 2000, Mosby.

53. Potter PA, Perry AG: *Fundamentals of nursing*, St. Louis, 2005, Mosby.

54. Green JM, Hacker ED: Chemotherapy in the geriatric population, *Clin J Oncol* 8(6):591-597, 2004.

55. Camp-Sorrell D: *Access device guidelines: recommendations for nursing practice and education*, Pittsburgh, 2004, Oncology Nursing Society.

56. Mazanec P, Bartel J: Family caregiver perspective of pain management, *Cancer Pract* 10(1): S66-S69, 2002.

57. Rosenbaum EH, Rosenbaum IR, Addison T et al: Decisions for life: advance directives. In Rosenbaum EH, Rosenbaum IR: *Supportive cancer care*, Naperville, Ill, 2001, Sourcebooks.

58. Schumacker KL, Koresawa S, West C et al: Putting pain management regimens into practice at home, *J Pain Symptom Manage* 23(5):369-382, 2002.

59. Yates P, Aranda S, Edwards H et al: Family caregivers' experiences and involvement with cancer pain management, *J Palliat Care* 20(4):287-296, 2004.

60. Polovich M, White JM, Kelleher LO: *Chemotherapy and biotherapy guideline and recommendations for practice*, Pittsburgh, 2005, Oncology Nursing Society.

61. Polovich M: *Safe handling of hazardous drugs*, Pittsburgh, 2003, Oncology Nursing Society.

62. Colman EA, Hutchins L, Goodwin J: An overview of cancer in the older adult, *Medsurg Nurs* 13(2):75-80,109, 2004.

63. Goodwin JA, Coleman EA: Exploring measures of functional dependence in the older adult with cancer, *Medsurg Nurs* 12(6):359-366, 2003.

64. Hodgson NA: Epidemiological trends of cancer in older adults: implications for gerontological nursing practice and research, *Gerontol Nurs* 27(4):34-43, 2002.

65. Kagan SH: Gero-oncology nursing research, *Oncol Nurs Forum* 31(2):293-299, 2004.

66. Marrelli TM: *Hospice and palliative care handbook*, ed 2, St. Louis, 2005, Mosby.

67. Hess P: End-of-life issues *Toward healthy aging*, ed 6, St. Louis, 2004, Mosby.

68. McMackin S: Setting the standard for private duty home care, *Home Healthcare Nurse* 22(12):851-853, 2004.

69. Tweed SC: The five most frequently answered questions about private duty home care, *Home Healthcare Nurse* 21(7):467-472, 2003.

70. Kongstvedt P: *Essential of managed health care*, Gaithersburg, Md, 2001, Aspen.

71. Andrews MM: Cultural perspective. In Fieler VK, Hanson PA, editors: *Oncology nursing in the home*, Pittsburgh, 2000, Oncology Nursing Press.

72. Chelf JH, Agre P, Axelrod A et al.: Cancer-related patient education: an overview of the last decade of evaluation and research, *Oncol Nurs Forum* 28(7):1139-1147, 2001.

73. Given B, Sherwood P: Nursing-sensitive patient outcomes—a white paper, *Oncol Nurs Forum* 32(4):773-783, 2005.

74. Treacy JT, Mayer DK: Perspectives on cancer patient education, *Semin Oncol Nurs* 16:47-56, 2000.

75. Hayes KS: Literacy for health information of adult patients and caregivers in a rural emergency department, *Clin Excellence Nurse Pract* 4(1):35-40, 2000.

76. Kish SK, Martin CG, Price KJ: Advance directives in critically ill cancer patients, *Crit Care Nurs Clin North Am* 12:373-383, 2000.

77. Stearns L, Butler S, Hollander J: Patients' and families' receptivity to discussions about future healthcare, *Community Oncol* 2(5):446-451, 2005.

CHAPTER 36

Ethical Considerations

Paula Nelson-Marten and
Jacqueline Glover

Introduction and Overview

WHY ETHICS?

Ethical decision making is part of every nurse's professional life. Knowledge of key concepts, skill in identifying and analyzing ethical issues, and professional attitudes and behaviors are part of core competencies for the nurse in training. But what is ethics, and why does one have to "study" it? Isn't it enough to be a good person?

It is important that students enter the nursing profession with strong personal values and a desire to care for and about patients. However, personal morality is not sufficient. Personal morality is different from ethics. Although most people use the terms interchangeably, when a distinction is made, it is that "morality" refers to one's own personal moral choices on the basis of one's upbringing, culture, and beliefs, and "ethics" refers to the formal process of analyzing the basis for one's moral judgments for clarity and consistency. There is potential conflict between personal values and professional values, between one's personal values and the personal values of one's patients, and among professional values; ethics is what is needed to help resolve such conflicts. Ethics provides a formal way to step back from the conflict, search for reasons to support one choice over another, and apply this reasoning in the future.

This process of stepping back to formally analyze values is necessary because the nurse is accountable for his or her actions as a professional, not just personally. What a nurse does reflects on the profession of nursing as a whole. Patients, other professionals, and the general public do not know a nurse's personal values. But they do have expectations for the nurse's professional conduct. Standards arise from the trust that the public places in the nurse. Ethics is particularly important for oncology nursing and for the challenging ethical issues that are raised across the continuum of care for cancer patients.

ANA Code of Ethics

The nursing profession has had "a distinguished history of concern for the welfare of the sick, injured, and vulnerable and for social justice," as articulated from the earliest "Nightingale Pledge" in 1893 through the newest version of the American Nurses Association (ANA) Code of Ethics for Nurses in 2001 (Box 36-1).[1] "Whatever the version of the Code, it has always been fundamentally concerned with the principles of doing no harm, of benefiting others, of loyalty, and of truthfulness. As well, the Code has been concerned with social justice and, in later versions, with the changing context of health care as well as the autonomy of the patient and the nurse."[1]

The Oncology Nursing Society (ONS) endorses the ANA Code for Nurses. In an article in the *Oncology Nursing Forum*, written by two members of a past ONS Ethics Advisory Council,

there is further discussion of five core values that speak from the shared experience of oncology nurses and provide a context for applying the Code of Nurses in oncology nursing practice.[2] These core values include respectful care, quality of life, competence, collegiality, and fairness. But how does one translate the core professional values into the clinical context?

TOOLS FOR ETHICAL DECISION MAKING

The implementation of a code of ethics depends on both the reinforcement of strong moral character and on the development and refinement of critical analysis skills. Nurses must be taught to make reliable moral judgments, just as they are taught to make reliable clinical judgments. However, what is meant by a reliable moral judgment? A judgment is based on adequate information and sound reasoning. Ethics may not involve determining with certainty an absolute right or wrong, but it does involve disciplined and sustained reflection on moral judgments about which actions are better or worse.

Tools for ethical decision making are necessary to apply these fundamental values and the codes of ethics in specific clinical situations. Still, even these tools do not provide mechanical rules or unambiguous instruction. There is no "cookbook" that can replace ongoing reflection and dialogue.

Various models for ethical decision making are available in the literature, but all share some of the basic components or steps, that are proposed here and illustrated later in this chapter.[3-5]

EIGHT-STEP PROCESS FOR ETHICAL ANALYSIS[6]

Step 1: What are the Ethical Questions? These are the "should" questions, such as, "Who should speak for the patient? Should we respect that family's wishes? What should be done for this patient?"

Step 2: What is One's First Reaction to this Case? What is one's "gut" saying, on an emotive level, that one should do? Ethical issues often involve deeply held value commitments and are emotionally charged. Attunement to personal emotions and the emotions of others is a necessary part of moral life. Many philosophers have come to identify well-educated emotions as necessary to the process of identifying when one is confronting an ethical issue.[7] However, nurses cannot practice professionally and remain only on the level of emotion. The nurse must be able to describe the ethical issue clearly so that it can be addressed by all parties, even those with different sensibilities.

Step 3: What are the Clinically Relevant Facts, and What Facts Does One Need to Gather? Just like a reliable clinical judgment, a reliable moral judgment is based on adequate information. In real clinical situations, one must determine what facts are known and what facts need to be gathered. In the classroom, it is always tempting to avoid a discussion of ethics by claiming that not enough information is available to make a decision.

BOX 36-1 ANA Code of Ethics for Nurses

Nine General Provisions

1. The nurse in all professional relationships practices with compassion and respect for the inherent dignity, worth, and uniqueness of every individual, unrestricted by considerations of social or economic status, personal attributes, or the nature of the health care problem.
2. The nurse's primary commitment is to the patient, whether an individual, family group, or community.
3. The nurse promotes, advocates for, and strives to protect the health, safety, and rights of the patient.
4. The nurse is responsible and accountable for individual nursing practice and determines the appropriate delegation of tasks consistent with the nurse's obligation to provide optimal patient care.
5. The nurse owes the same duties to self as to others, including the responsibility to preserve integrity and safety, to maintain competence, and to continue personal and professional growth.
6. The nurse participates in establishing, maintaining, and improving health care environments and conditions of employment conducive to the provision of quality health care and consistent with the values of the professional through individual and collective action.
7. The nurse participates in the advancement of the profession through contributions to practice, education, administration, and knowledge development.
8. The nurse collaborates with other health care professionals and the public in promoting community, national, and international efforts to meet health needs.
9. The profession of nursing, as represented by associations and their members, is responsible for articulating nursing values, maintaining the integrity of the profession, and shaping social policy.

From American Nurses Association: *Code of ethics for nurses with interpretive statements,* Silver Spring, MD, 2001, American Nurses Publishing, retrieved January 10, 2007, from www.nursingworld.org/ethics/chcode.htm.

Although facts are very important—good ethics begins with good facts—the discussion can proceed if one considers why one wants to know something and how it might affect or change the analysis.

Step 4: What are the Values at Stake for All Relevant Parties? It is important to consider the values from various perspectives—the patient, the family, health care professionals, the hospital administration, and the broader society, if appropriate. In the previous discussion of the ANA Code for Nurses, key nursing values were described.

Step 5: What Could be Done? Identify a range of options. There almost never is only one right answer. There is almost always a range of ethically acceptable choices that respect or balance the values of each party. Although several options may be available, each probably has desirable and less-desirable aspects. Some choices may even be outside the range of ethical acceptability because they involve compromising an important value.

Step 6: What Should be Done? Make a choice with the information and understanding available at the time. Sometimes, choices will be less than satisfactory, and ambiguity remains. Just like clinical judgments and the ongoing evaluation of them, one can always identify things that could have been done differently and/or celebrate things that were done well.

Step 7: What Justifies the Choice? Provide reasons to support a choice based on the values at stake. Why did the nurse choose these options? Anticipate objections to these reasons, and respond to them. What are the most powerful arguments against a choice, and what are counterarguments? Most would acknowledge that a major difficulty in ethical analysis comes in articulating what reasons count as adequate justification for a particular choice. There is broad consensus concerning many ethical issues in practice. But even when an accepted ethical and legal consensus exists, team members may not be aware of them or may show resistance to accepting them. It is important to identify the possible sources of disagreement. People can have disagreements about each of the steps in the process. They can disagree about facts, the values involved, or the application of moral reasoning. Although a comprehensive and clear process of ethical reasoning usually results in consensus, there can still be deep disagreement. Disagreement is part of moral life because people do hold markedly different values, and conscientious objection (withdrawing from participation in certain situations because of personal moral beliefs) is an essential ethical concept. One must help build moral consensus when possible, and respect moral freedom when it is not.

Step 8: How Could Confrontation with this Ethical Issue Have Been Prevented? Each discussion of an ethical issue provides an opportunity to reflect on how organizational and professional structures, policies, and practices have contributed to the issue or how they can be changed to address it.

ETHICAL THEORIES AND APPROACHES

Ethical standards and analysis depend on the systematic application of key ethical concepts. This process of ethical reasoning is very complex. One does not just memorize a few ethical theories and then apply them to problems that arise. Rather than being a kind of special "truth" about the moral life that one can learn and apply, **ethical theories** are organizing structures that help one to identify important language and key concepts and provide systematic reflection and dialogue. Philosophers develop ethical theories in their search for an ordered set of ethical standards that can be used to assess what is right and wrong in certain circumstances. In recent years, many philosophers have come to doubt that there is one "correct" theory. They believe that it would be a mistake to view the various theories and approaches as mutually exclusive claims to moral truth. Arras and Steinbock suggest, "Instead, we should view them as important but partial contributions to a comprehensive, although necessarily fragmented, moral vision."[8] What follows is a brief overview of major theories and approaches that can guide and direct the nurse's ethical reasoning as he or she strives to make reliable moral judgments.

ANALYZING PRINCIPLES

A principle is a basic truth, assumption, or source that is meant to inform, guide, and shape the behavior and decisions of health care professionals. Four major principles in the bioethics literature and many codes of professional ethics are the following: respect for **autonomy** (autonomy means "self-rule"—respecting the choices of people), **beneficence** (doing good), **nonmaleficence** (not harming), and **justice** (treating people fairly).

Values. Many people use the terms values and principles interchangeably. "Values" are used in the eight-step process of ethical decision making to broaden the scope of ethical "content" to include other actions or traits of character that promote the good, are good, or are otherwise meant to describe actions that are right. In addition to the four principles above, other values include veracity (truth-telling), fidelity (keeping promises), respect for life (life having intrinsic value), respect for persons (not just their decisions, but their privacy, their identity, or physical boundaries), confidentiality (not disclosing patient information to others who do not need to know); respect for family relationships; and respect for colleagues.

Virtue Ethics. Virtue ethics is characterized by an emphasis on the moral character of the person; it is presumed that morally appropriate decisions occur as a result of being decided by morally sensitive people. Virtue theorists focus primarily on the education and development of the person making the decision. Common virtues are integrity, fairness, compassion, kindness, openness, and honesty.

Deontology or Formalism. Deontologic (from the Greek word "deon" for duty) or formalist theories begin with the assumption that what makes an action right or wrong is some intrinsic property of the action itself, not the person choosing the action. From a Judeo-Christian perspective, for example, an action con*forms* (the source of the word formalism) with one of the 10 Commandments or 10 duties. From another point of view, an action conforms with the golden rule: "Treat others as one would wish to be treated oneself." Notice that two of the four main principles mentioned above are formalistic—respect for autonomy and justice.

Consequentialism and Utilitarianism. Consequentialist theories focus on what a person seeks to accomplish with an action. Actions that are likely to produce good consequences are good actions, and actions that are likely to produce bad consequences are bad actions. Notice that two of the main principles are consequentialist in nature—beneficence and nonmaleficence. The most prevalent form of consequentialist theory is that theory known as utilitarianism—a theory that instructs people to act so as to cause the greatest amount of utility or happiness for the greatest number of people.

Analysis of Rights. Much moral discussion, especially in the United States, uses the language of rights. A right is an especially powerful moral claim that others are obligated to respect. In the United States, people speak of such basic human rights as life, liberty (freedom) and the pursuit of happiness. In health care ethics, scholars debate a right to die, a right to life, a right to choose, and a right to health care.

Ethics of Care. Proponents of this approach to ethical analysis emphasize the importance of relationships.[9] An ethic of care considers the emotional commitment and a willingness of individuals in relationships to act unselfishly for the benefit of others. An ethic of care emphasizes sympathy, compassion, fidelity, discernment, and love. The origins of the ethics-of-care approach are predominantly in theology and in some feminist writings.[10] Nursing literature has also emphasized the importance of caring and its role as a central and defining feature of professional nursing and nursing ethics.[11]

MORAL DISTRESS

Sometimes in professional practice, the ethical issue is not determining what the right thing to do is, but rather how to do it, given the practice environment. This type of ethical issue has been labeled **moral distress.**[12] The greatest challenge to implementing a code of ethics remains how to create a moral community where nurses are expected to raise and address ethical issues and are supported for such practices. Too often, deciding what ought to be done is less difficult than speaking up and advocating for what is known to be right. Health care organizations play a vital role in creating environments to sustain relationships, settle conflicts, establish goals based on chosen values, and support ethical practice.[13] Nurses also have responsibilities to shape the organizational climate and integrate ethical review into professional life.[14]

ETHICS RESOURCES

Nurses who are facing ethical issues in their practice have many sources of assistance. They can look in the nursing literature for information about current ethical problems and their resolution. They can also talk with their professional colleagues about the ANA Code for Nurses or directly contact the ANA's Center for Ethics and Human Rights at *ethics@ana.org*. Ethics resources also are available in individual health care organizations, including patient care ethics committees and ethics consult services. The Joint Commission on the Accreditation of Health Care Organizations (JCAHO) includes standards that require an "ethics mechanism" to help patients, families, and staff to address ethical issues in clinical care. Ethics committees are multidisciplinary committees and almost always include nurses, whose members have training and experience in identifying and addressing ethical issues. Most committees also educate staff about ethical issues and write policies that address institutional practices. The JCAHO also requires consideration of the ethical issues that arise in the business practices of health care organizations. These standards have prompted many institutions to develop organizational ethics committees in addition to their patient care ethics committees.[15]

Ethical Issues throughout the Continuum of Cancer Care

TAKING THE ETHICAL JOURNEY

Ethical issues can be found in every aspect of oncology nursing. Cancer nurses need to remember that it is an honor to join a cancer patient on his or her cancer journey, being present for the good times as well as for the tough times. Being an advocate is the most important role for the nurse in relation to ethics. The role of advocate will take various shapes during different aspects of the journey. The ANA Code of Ethics for Nurses with Interpretative Statements should be the nurse's ethical guide for his or her journey with patients in our complex health care environment.[1] The ANA Code of Ethics has nine general provisions (see Box 36-1); each of the provisions has interpretative statements (*www.nursingworld.org*).

ETHICAL ISSUES AT TIME OF DIAGNOSIS

When a patient is first diagnosed, communication is very important. An important role for the oncology nurse is to be an effective communicator. To be an effective communicator, the nurse must be aware of the knowledge that needs to be communicated to the patient and family, and then must pay close attention to the communication going on between the nurse, the health care team, and the patient and family. For communication to be two-way, the nurse must also be a good listener. A good listener knows when the patient needs more information, time to talk, or a chance to be listened to, and when the patient may feel afraid and/or is overwhelmed by all that is taking place in the "new role of patient." Shared decision making is an important concept for the oncology nurse to use with the cancer patient. Shared decision making requires "open and ongoing communication about all aspects of client care from the most mundane aspects of hospital or clinic policies and procedures to diagnosis and prognosis, treatment alternatives, and the effects of illness on the lives of clients and their families."[16] The ethical value of veracity (truth-telling) should be employed early on with the patient and family. This value requires the nurse to consider whether communication is honest. Telling the truth can be difficult for the nurse, a time investment for the health care team, and distressing for the patient and family. In general, it is assumed that the patient has the right to full and accurate information about his or her medical condition. If the patient is not accurately informed, he or she may envision a situation that is far worse than reality. The patient has the right to refuse to be informed and/or may request that the family not be told. In the current era of concentration on privacy issues, the family may or may not have the right to be told what is going on with the patient, depending on their role and what the patient has said. Privacy of information issues also extend to the health care team. The nurse must be savvy about what he or she shares about patient information and with whom.[17]

ETHICAL ISSUES AT TIME OF TREATMENT

Before the beginning of treatment, the patient and family must have all possible treatment alternatives presented to them so that they can assist in making the best possible decisions in choosing cancer treatment. In the oncology nurse's role as advocate for the patient and family, he or she must be aware of what treatment options are possible for the diagnosis the patient has, know what treatment options are usually available at the institution where the care is happening, and be aware of the treatment options that have been presented to the patient and family. An important ethical consideration at this time is to determine if the patient has decision-making capacity.[18] Is the patient able to understand information, communicate, and reason and deliberate about his or her choices? It is important to determine if the patient has decision-making capacity because the patient will need to give informed consent before the beginning of treatment. Helpful questions to determine if a patient has decision-making capacity include the following:[19]

1. Can the patient understand what is wrong with him or her and what the proposed procedures and treatments are?
2. Can the patient understand the benefits and risks of the proposed procedures or treatment and the benefits and risks of the alternative procedures and treatments, including nontreatment?
3. Is the patient able to reason and make a decision using the clinical information that has been disclosed to him or her and to incorporate his or her personal values and wishes?

4. Is the patient able to explain why he or she made the health care decision that he or she did, and is the explanation consistent with his or her stated values and wishes?

If the patient lacks capacity, he or she will need someone to speak on his or her behalf. This could be a family member or friend with medical power of attorney authority or someone who has been appointed to be a proxy. Informed consent is an important ethical and legal consideration. Informed consent is an "ethical and legal concept that requires health care professionals to provide sufficient information about the client's condition and the recommended treatments—its benefits, risks, and alternatives—to enable the patient to make a responsible decision to accept or reject the recommendations."[16] Informed consent involves the ethical principles of autonomy and beneficence. The cancer nurse and the health care team must ensure that the patient has access to a sufficient amount of information and that the information is understood. The patient must understand that he or she can request to withdraw from treatment at any time and that this will not affect either the medical or the nursing care the patient is receiving. The oncology nurse's role in informed consent is to be an advocate. The following issues are important in the role of advocate: (1) inquire about and understand the patient's goals for care and value system; (2) respect the patient's right to choose; (3) encourage the patient to ask questions and to actively participate in decision making; (4) access and report the patient's response to treatment; (5) ensure the privacy and confidentiality of the patient; (6) be willing to intercede on behalf of the patient with the health care team; and (7) the nurse must be aware of his or her own biases and prevent them from interfering with patient care. If this is not possible, the nurse should ask to be removed from the care of the patient.[16]

CLINICAL TRIALS

During the course of treatment, the health care team may decide to offer the patient a clinical trial. Clinical trials are research studies with patients who volunteer to take part. Clinical trials are frequently used in both inpatient and outpatient cancer settings. There are many potential ethical issues in cancer clinical trials.[20] Potential ethical issues can relate to the following:

1. Exclusion criteria that may bar the patient from participation
2. Inclusion of minorities; often clinical trials are not representative of minorities
3. Patient perspective; the patient may feel that the trial is the only hope for a cure. In this case, the patient, family, and health care team should discuss all issues openly so that the best decision can be made for the particular individual
4. Ethics of randomization; clinical trials may create a conflict of interest for the physician, related to the dual roles of physician and researcher
5. Cost issues; drugs may not be covered by the trial or by the patient's insurance or drug costs may be covered while tests and visits necessary for the protocol are not covered[16,20]

The role of the nurse in clinical trials is that of advocate for the patient and family. If the nurse is caring directly for the patient during the clinical trial, other important roles of the nurse include the following: ensuring that informed consent is obtained; monitoring symptoms that occur; obtaining interventions as appropriate for symptoms; ensuring confidentiality and patient privacy; and monitoring documentation for completeness and timeliness.[16]

ETHICAL ISSUES DURING MAINTENANCE THERAPY

Once the patient has survived initial cancer therapy and moved into the period of time known as maintenance, there may be more drugs and/or protocols for patient participation. It is important that the nurse continue open communication with the patient and family and advocate for their best interests. Sometimes this role falls to the cancer nurse in the clinic. Communication between the nurse from the inpatient setting and the nurse from the clinic setting is important so that the patient and family continues to have someone who is aware of what is happening to them. An ethical issue during this time period for the patient and family can be the experience of isolation and/or abandonment, especially if they have been discharged from care by both the inpatient and outpatient clinical settings. In this case, the clinic nurse should take on the responsibility of informing the patient's primary care practitioner (physician or nurse practitioner) as to the patient's cancer care, as well as any special needs.

ETHICAL ISSUES IN SURVIVORSHIP

As the cancer patient moves into the role of survivor, the clinic nurse or office nurse must assume the role of advocate. Several ethical issues and concerns can arise in the survivorship period. These include (1) employment concerns, (2) insurance concerns, and (3) privacy issues. The cancer nurse in the clinic or the office needs to be familiar with the current public policies on these issues in his or her community to be able to be an advocate for the cancer survivor in job seeking, managing insurance needs, and for other related issues as they arise.

ETHICAL ISSUES IN DISEASE REOCCURRENCE

If the patient's original cancer recurs, and/or if a second cancer occurs, the patient will once again need the cancer nurse to serve as an advocate. Several important ethical issues might arise at this time including the need for confidentiality, the need for open and honest communication between patient and nurse and between patient and health care team, and the need to consider writing or revising advance directives.[18]

ETHICAL ISSUES IN END-OF-LIFE CARE

Ethical issues at end of life can be many.[18] Every oncology nurse needs to be aware of possible end-of-life ethical issues so that he or she is able to detect them as early as possible. Often patients and families are asked their goals for care neither at any point along the continuum nor at end of life. The result can be a mismatch between the care that is desired and the care that is given. This may result in angry patients and families, but it may also result in a poor end-of-life experience for the patient and family. Other common end-of-life ethical issues include lack of advance directives and/or clarity of directives, quality of life issues, issues related to nutrition and hydration, withdrawal or withholding of care, and requests for help in dying. The ANA has published several position statements on end-of-life issues dealing with ethical issues and end-of-life care; every cancer nurse needs to be familiar with these statements (*www.nursingworld.org*). Communication can be difficult at this time.[21] Issues in end-of-life care can be very stressful for the health care team; individuals on the team may not agree with one another and/or may not agree with patient or family requests. The nurse may need to take the lead and consult with the rest of the health care team about having a family conference and/or requesting either a palliative care consult and/or ethics consult.[21]

ETHICAL CONSIDERATIONS IN CARING FOR THE FAMILY

The family or significant other is usually the patient's major source of support. Because of privacy rights, the adult patient should be approached and asked if sharing information with the family is okay. If the patient says okay, then the nurse can share with the family (individuals as noted) what is going on with the patient and include the family in care. The ethical responsibility of the nurse is to be an advocate for the patient first and for the family second. Often, family members need a listening ear, a question answered, and to be included as appropriate in a family meeting or in a decision regarding treatment modalities. Many times, one of the family members can be appointed by the family as a spokesperson for the family.

ETHICAL ISSUES IN GRIEF AND BEREAVEMENT

When a patient dies, the cancer nurse continues to have an ethical responsibility to the patient-family unit. The patient is gone, but the family remains. The ethical value of respect for personhood encourages the nurse to assist the family in grief and bereavement. This aspect can occur in several ways: sending a sympathy card; meeting with the family; attending a memorial service; and providing resources for support. The concept of caring for the family and significant others after the death of the patient is not routinely done by inpatient or outpatient cancer settings. However, this is an important task and is becoming more common.

ETHICAL ISSUES IN CARING FOR ONESELF

Oncology nurses do not routinely take the time to care for themselves. A patient dies, and the bed is cleaned and assigned to another patient. The nurse starts all over with caring for another cancer patient, but has not taken time to acknowledge the death and/or his or her own feelings related to this experience of care. The oncology nurse has the duty to care for her- or himself. To care effectively for patients, the oncology nurse must first care for her- or himself. The nurse has the obligation to remind others that he or she needs some space and needs time for self-care.[17] Sometimes oncology units set up policies to this effect and can change workload assignments for a few days, honor a vacation day, and so on. Nurses need to learn to be effective advocates for themselves and each other.

ETHICAL ISSUES IN CARING FOR OLDER ADULTS

Caring for the older adult may involve the ethical concepts of informed consent and disclosure. The older adult may not have decision-making capacity and may need to have a designated decision maker and/or an appointed proxy. Determination of decision-making capacity can be made by the health care team. It is important to communicate with the patient in terms that can be understood, and share all that is being done. Sometimes decision-making ability and understanding comes and goes in an older patient. If the cancer nurse has spent some time with the older patient and is alert to the patient, he or she can determine when it might be a good time to talk with the patient and share what is going on in relation to diagnosis and care, and elicit patient wishes in these regards. Many myths exist about the older patient and end-of-life care.[22] The oncology nurse needs to be familiar with these myths (e.g., the elderly are less damaged by cumulative loss; older people don't feel much pain; advance directives drive care) so that he or she can educate others.[22]

ETHICAL ISSUES AND CULTURE

The ethical value of respect for persons encourages the cancer nurse to pay close attention to issues of culture in caring for the cancer patient and family. Developing cultural competence is a step every cancer nurse and nursing unit needs to take. Barriers to cultural competence related to providers and to systems must be sought out and worked on as a nursing team.[23] Cultural issues to be considered include importance of the culture in the patient's and/or the family's way of life, special beliefs about illness and death, language needs, and certain cultural or religious customs that require observation and/or adherence. Many cultures outside of the Western world revere the family or group as more important than the individual. Consequently, the family may want to receive health care information and then decide what will be shared with the patient. The family may expect to be the decision maker rather than the patient. Caring for children with cancer may elicit varying cultural needs. Some families will desire for the child to be included in discussion and decision making. The child, depending upon the age, may wish to give assent (a child's version of consent). Many of the above-noted issues may intersect with the ethical concepts of informed consent and full disclosure. The oncology unit should develop procedures for working with patients and families of different ages and cultures that meet the patient and the family's needs in their cultural aspects as well as the meet the ethical/legal requirements of the unit for informed consent and disclosure.

Summary

There were three main purposes for writing this chapter. One purpose was to provide the oncology nurse with a basic review of bioethics. A second purpose was to apply basic bioethics to oncology nursing practice and discuss ethical issues that can arise throughout the continuum of cancer care. The third purpose for the chapter was to provide a framework for resolving ethical dilemmas. Two examples of case studies (one adult and one child) and suggested resolutions using an eight-step framework have been included.

Cancer is a chronic illness, and patients can go through periods of time when they are very ill and involved in a whirlwind of therapies, and other times when they are in a steady state and doing well. Ethical dilemmas, however, can occur at any time. Oncology nurses should understand ethics related to oncology care, practice identifying ethical issues and dilemmas, and spend time practicing case study resolution, because ethical dilemmas tend to occur often in every aspect of cancer care. The more an oncology nurse knows about ethics and about identifying ethical issues and dilemmas, the better he or she will be at applying this knowledge when it is needed in the clinical setting.

REVIEW QUESTIONS

✓ Case Study

ADULT ETHICS: BREAST CANCER

Mrs. Garcia, a 30-year-old Hispanic woman, has just had her third child at the local City Hospital. She is married and has two young children, ages 2 and 4. The Garcia's only source of health insurance is through the state Medicaid program, and thus they obtain most of their medical care through the City Hospital and its clinics. At breastfeeding class, the post partum nurse notices that Mrs. Garcia's left breast looks larger than her right breast and appears to be red and somewhat inflamed. The nurse brings this to the attention of the unit nurse manager, and they discuss whether the inflammation may be due to the recent birth and attempts at breast feeding. They agree that the nurse should document the finding, since Mrs. Garcia is to be discharged home today. Mrs. Garcia is discharged, and 6 weeks later at her post partum visit, the clinic nurse notices that her left breast is swollen and red. She inquires about this and Mrs. Garcia says that she too noticed this, and that it began sometime during her pregnancy. The nurse proceeds to do a breast exam and upon palpation feels several small, lumpy areas. She alerts the obstetrics doctor, he repeats the exam, and they set up an appointment for Mrs. Garcia to be seen in surgery clinic for a work-up and biopsy. Two weeks later, Mrs. Garcia is seen and a biopsy is done. The pathology report reveals an aggressive stage II infiltrating breast cancer. Mrs. Garcia is referred to the cancer clinic. Two weeks later, Mrs. Garcia keeps her appointment in cancer clinic. She is very scared about the diagnoses and worries that maybe she should not be breastfeeding her baby.

Mrs. Garcia's referral to cancer clinic is a dilemma for the cancer clinic staff. They have been through similar scenarios many times with patients from the state Medicaid program. They are able to provide surgical intervention and chemotherapy but not radiation therapy, since the City Hospital does not have a radiation therapy department. All patients who require radiation therapy are referred to other local hospitals. However, most of the other local hospitals are not very willing to serve the state Medicaid patients, since they are not fully compensated for care and lose money. Radiation therapy is very expensive, and the private hospitals are not willing to lose money on this therapy.

The dilemma for the cancer clinic staff lies in the fact that they are not able to offer standard-of-care therapy. It has been well documented that the standard of care for this type of aggressive cancer in a young woman is to have all three therapies and as promptly as possible.

Questions to consider: What is the obligation of the cancer clinic staff to Mrs. Garcia? Is it better to offer part of a standard plan of care than no care?

CASE RESOLUTION

Step 1: *Questions:*

Should the cancer center do just the surgery and chemotherapy? Should staff tell Mrs. Garcia about all of the options, not just the ones that they provide? Should Mrs. Garcia take her story to the newspapers to raise money for standard-of-care therapy?

Step 2: *Feelings* range from a sense that the nurse should do everything it takes to advocate for the standard-of-care therapy (three therapies), since Mrs. Garcia is so young and has young children, to the sense that it takes a lot of energy to fight for every patient and that the two-therapies care is probably okay for Mrs. Garcia and she should take her chances.

Step 3: *Facts:* Mrs. Garcia has stage II breast cancer. She needs triple therapy—surgery, chemotherapy, and radiation therapy. She is 30 years old, with a newborn and two other young children. She is on the state Medicaid program. None of the other hospitals in town are willing to offer radiation therapy for state Medicaid program patients, because they have busy radiation therapy schedules and lose money with the Medicaid plan. The city hospital does not offer radiation therapy.

Facts to be gathered: Does Mrs. Garcia have any other means of financial support? Do we know how much less effective getting two out of the three therapies will be? Are two therapies better than no therapy? What is the prognoses for stage II infiltrating breast cancer with and without standard-of-care treatment (all three therapies)? Can Mrs. Garcia qualify for a research protocol?

Step 4: *Values:*

Mrs. Garcia: Beneficence and nonmaleficence—needs standard therapy to potentially save her life; needs some therapy rather than no therapy. Respect for autonomy—respect her wishes to receive treatment. Justice—access to the standard of care. Fidelity—she is a patient and should not be abandoned.

Cancer team: Beneficence and nonmaleficence—providing the standard of care to maximize Mrs. Garcia's chance of survival or providing some treatment rather than no treatment. Truth-telling—providing all of the information about all options, not just what the city hospital can offer. Respect the patient's autonomy—respect the patient's wishes for treatment. Justice—providing access to the standard of care, but making wise allocation decisions; consider what other care will be foregone to provide Mrs. Garcia the standard of care; going to the press will not solve the problem for anyone but Mrs. Garcia. Fidelity—a patient-professional relationship has been established with the clinic, and this patient should not be abandoned. Advocacy—the nurse has an obligation to secure the best care possible for his or her patients.

Society: Justice—allocating resources wisely and fairly; consider the benefits of health care and also the burdens (costs).

Step 5: *Options:*

Full disclosure of all options; Partial disclosure (two therapies instead of three; offer surgery and chemotherapy; or say, "Go to the media.")

Step 6: *Choice:*

Partial disclosure is not an option; truth-telling, respect for Mrs. Garcia and her autonomy, and informed consent demand full disclosure.

Do what you can (two therapies). Something is better than nothing, and you cannot secure her more therapy in the city hospital system.

Step 7: *Justification:*

The ethical principles of beneficence and nonmaleficence require the nurse to do what he or she can even if it is not all of the care that is offered at other hospitals. This also shows respect for Mrs. Garcia's decisions. Encouraging justice or the

seeking of media attention would only solve the case of Mrs. Garcia and would not solve the systemic problem of lack of availability of radiation therapy at the city hospital. Serving only one individual through allocation based on the media is not a fair principle of allocation.

A counterargument would be that the principle of justice demands that Mrs. Garcia receive the standard of care, and to be a patient advocate as the nurse means that the nurse should do all he or she can to correct the system and to get the care for Mrs. Garcia that she needs—so go to the media!

A response to the counterargument would be—are you going to do this for all of your patients? You can't possibly do this, so why do it for Mrs. Garcia? Wouldn't it be more effective to work on a plan to find radiation therapy for all cancer patients who need it?

The nurse should consider the American Nurses' Association Code of Ethics in his or her justification. Provision number 8 of the ANA Code notes that the nurse should collaborate with other health care professionals and the public in promoting community, national, and international efforts to meet health care needs.

Step 8: *Prevention:*

Secure greater funding for city hospitals—acquire radiation therapy services.

Work for better charity care policies of the other local (private) hospitals—each hospital helping to share the burden.

Achieve universal access to health care.

PEDIATRICS ETHICS

Jason is a 16-year-old boy who has recently been admitted to the hospital for a third relapse of his leukemia. Jason had a spinal sarcoma at age 5 that was successfully treated with chemotherapy and radiation. As is not uncommonly the case, he then developed acute leukemia about 5 years later. He relapsed twice after standard chemotherapy and then started on a round of bone marrow transplants. His older sister, Katherine, was able to donate bone marrow. Jason had two bone marrow transplants over a period of several years but was constantly in and out of the hospital. He has relapsed a third time, and he and his family have been offered the option of a cord blood transplant of stem cells. Jason has confided to his nurses that he really doesn't want to go ahead with another treatment. He is tired, and he feels that it is not worth going through all the misery for a very small chance of success. He believes that it will not be successful, and he would just rather go home to be in his own room with his guitar and his dog. However, Jason seems unwilling to share this information with his doctors or his parents. Jason's parents, Mark and Marilyn, are very controlling of the situation and very demanding of staff time and energy. Jason's mother is especially determined to pursue the cord blood transplant. She is very emotional and needy and depends on Jason to be the strong one. Jason's father, Mark, is more distant and deals with the situation by being at work for longer hours.

PEDIATRIC ETHICAL FRAMEWORK

The ethical framework for adults centers on respect for patient autonomy and the patient's ability to make informed

Continued

choices about treatment options that support the patient's unique assessment of his or her own well-being. A pediatric framework depends on loving parents or guardians who work with health care professionals to make treatment choices based on the infant or child's "best interests." The term "best interest" is used to describe the obligations of both parents and professionals to promote the well-being of infants and children. It is assumed that this well-being includes a concrete assessment of what health care benefits are possible, how likely they are, and what risks are associated. But parents and guardians are not completely free to choose according to their unique values and preferences. Health care professionals are independent advocates for the well-being of their pediatric patients. Children do not only belong to their families, but also to the larger community, which values the protection of vulnerable members. When parental choices seem to constitute medical neglect, health care professionals must advocate for treatment of their patients. It is a matter of justice that all infants and children receive adequate access to health care, regardless of the family to which they belong. It is an essential part of pediatric nursing to help build trust between a child, his or her family, and the health care team.[24]

Another challenging aspect of pediatric care is that children's needs change as they grow and develop. As children grow older and mature, health care professional's obligations also change. Insofar as older children and adolescents are capable of being involved in health care decision making, they should be, as a matter of respect.[25]

A final challenge is the "unnaturalness" of the possible death of a child and the unique needs of dying children, their families, and the community.[26] Death in childhood may result from a sudden illness or injury or a chronic condition leading to irreversible damage. According to the Institute of Medicine's recent report, *When Children Die,* approximately 55,000 children up to age 19 years die in the United States annually.[27] Yet fewer than 1% of children who need hospice care in the United States receive it, according to the Children's Hospice International.[28]

CASE RESOLUTION

Step 1: *Questions:*

What should Jason's nurses do? Should they talk with Jason's family? His doctors? Should they respect Jason's confidentiality and encourage Jason to speak up for himself?

Step 2: *Feelings* range from the sense that Jason should have a say to sympathy for his family and the impact on them. There is a concern that conflict in this family be avoided, since Jason is still a child and his parents are very important at this time.

Step 3: *Facts:* Jason is 15 and has relapsed. Jason has a history of chemotherapy and bone marrow transplants. A cord blood stem cell transplant is recommended. Jason confides in his nurses that he really doesn't want this treatment but won't speak up. Jason parents want the transplant.

Facts to be gathered: How mature is Jason—does he understand his condition and the risks and benefits of the proposed treatment? What are the risks and benefits of the proposed stem cell treatment? Why doesn't he want to talk with his physicians or his parents?

Step 4: *Values:*

Jason: respect for his needs and values and preferences; promoting his well-being as he understands it; avoiding harm in the form of treatments with side effects and little chance of

effectiveness, or the harm of not receiving a treatment with a reasonable chance of effectiveness; respecting his confidentiality; building a trusting relationship; having a supportive, loving relationship with his family

Jason's parents: promoting their child's well-being by maximizing his chances for survival and avoiding the harms associated with nontreatment; maintaining a supportive, loving relationship with their child; the well-being of their family

Jason's nurses: respecting Jason's needs and unique values and preferences; promoting his well-being as he understands it; avoiding harm in the form of treatments with side effects and little chance of effectiveness, or the harm of not receiving a reasonable chance of effectiveness; advocating for Jason and his needs and values; respecting his confidentiality; building a trusting relationship; nurturing a supportive, loving relationship with his family; maintaining a good working relationship with colleagues in the health care team

Jason's physicians: respecting Jason's needs and unique values and preferences; promoting his well-being as he understands it; avoiding harm in the form of treatments with side effects and little chance of effectiveness, or the harm of not receiving a reasonable chance of effectiveness; building a trusting relationship; nurturing a supportive, loving relationship with his family; maintaining a good working relationship with colleagues in the health care team

Step 5: *Options:*

Don't mention anything to anyone: encourage Jason to speak up; talk with Jason's physicians; talk with Jason's parents

Step 6: *Choice:*

Talk with Jason and learn why he is reluctant to speak up; encourage and help him express himself with his physicians and parents: only speak to his physicians or his parents with his permission

Step 7: *Justification:*

To do nothing is to violate your obligation to advocate for your patients, and to go directly to his parents or his physicians is to risk escalating a possible conflict and lose Jason's trust. Talking with Jason and encouraging him to speak up supports the most values while avoiding possible harms from escalating the conflict.

Possible counterargument: Being an advocate requires you to speak up for your patient; as his nurse, you are a central member of the team, and your information is vital to the team's care of Jason. It is not a violation of confidentiality, because you are a member of the team and the team needs to know. Why did he tell you in the first place, if he didn't want help in making the others aware of how he feels?

Response: You don't know why he told you—you should ask him and not simply assume you know the answer. He might just want someone to talk with and try out ideas, without really wanting you to speak up for him. Even if it is not technically a violation of confidentiality, Jason may not expect you to tell others—especially his parents. It is a serious breach of his trusting relationship.

Step 8: *Prevention:*

Talk with Jason and his parents about Jason's role in decision making before big questions have to be decided. Have care conferences where the team is expected to share information on a regular basis—and make Jason aware of this team concept.

REFERENCES

1. American Nurses Association: *Code of ethics for nurses with interpretive statements*, 2001, Silver Spring, MD, 2001, American Nurses Publishing, retrieved January 10, 2007, from www.nursingworld.org/ethics/chcode.htm.
2. Scanlon C, Glover J: A professional code of ethics: providing a moral compass for turbulent times, *Oncol Nurs Forum* 22(10):1515-521, 1995.
3. Glover JJ: Ethical decision-making guidelines and tools. In Harman L, editor: *Ethical challenges in the management of health information*, 2001, Aspen.
4. Jonsen AR, Siegler M, Winslade WJ: *Clinical ethics: a practical approach to ethical decisions in clinical medicine*, ed 5, 2002, McGraw-Hill.
5. Purtilo R: *Ethical dimensions in the health professions*, Philadelphia, 1999, W.B. Saunders.
6. Glover JJ: Course Material: *Ethics in the health professions*, Center for Bioethics and Humanities, UCD-HSC, Fall, 2005.
7. Carse A: The voice of care: implications for bioethical education. *J Med Philos* 16(1):5-28, 1991.
8. Arras J, Steinbock B: *Ethical issues in modern medicine*, Mountain View, CA, 1995, Mayfield.
9. Gilligan C: *In a different voice: psychological theory and women's moral development*, Cambridge MA, 1982, Harvard University Press.
10. Larrabee M: *An ethic of care: feminist and interdisciplinary perspectives*, New York, 1993, Routledge.
11. Watson J: *Nursing: the philosophy and science of caring*, Boston, 1979, Little, Brown.
12. Jameton A: *Nursing practice: the ethical issues*, Upper Saddle River, NJ, 1984, Prentice Hall.
13. Reiser S: The ethical life of health care organizations, *Hastings Center Rep* 24(6):28-35, 1994.
14. Corley M, Raines D: An ethical practice environment as a caring environment, *Nurs Admin Q* 17:68-74, 1993.
15. Worthley J: *Organizational ethics in the compliance context*, Chicago IL, 1999, Health Administration Press.
16. Nelson-Marten P, Glover JJ: Selected ethical issues in cancer care. In Itano JK, Taoka KN, editors: *Core curriculum for oncology nursing*, ed 4, 2004, Elsevier.
17. Nelson-Marten P, Braaten, JS: Common ethical dilemmas. In Gates RA, Fink RM, editors: *Oncology nursing secrets*, ed 2, 2001, Hanley & Belfus.
18. Scanlon C: Ethical concerns in end-of-life care, *Am J Nurs* 103(1):48-55, 2003.
19. Moss AH: *Course book for health care ethics*, Morgantown, WV, 2003, West Virginia University Center for Health Care Ethics and Law.
20. Works C: Principles of treatment planning and clinical research. In Yarbro CH, Frogge MH, Goodman M et al, editors: *Cancer nursing: principles and practice*, 2000, Jones & Bartlett.
21. Griffie J, Nelson-Marten P, Muchka S: Acknowledging the "elephant": communication in palliative care, *Am J Nurs* 104(1):48-58, 2004.
22. Sheehan DK, Schirm V: End-of-life care of older adults: debunking some misconceptions about dying in old age, *Am J Nurs* 103(11):48-58, 2003.
23. Mazanec P, Tyler MK: Cultural considerations in end-of-life care: how ethnicity, age, and spirituality affect decisions when death is imminent, *Am J Nurs* 103(3):50-58, 2003.
24. Rushton CH, Glover JJ: Involving parents in decisions to forego life-sustaining treatment for critically ill infants and children, *AACN Clin Issues Crit Care Nurs* 1:206-14, 1990.
25. American Academy of Pediatrics Committee on Bioethics: Informed consent, parental permission and assent in pediatric practice, *Pediatrics* 95:314-317, 1995.
26. Rushton CH: Ethics and palliative care in pediatrics, *Am J Nurs* 104(8):54-63, 2004.
27. Institute of Medicine: Patterns of childhood death in America. In *When children die: improving palliative and end-of-life care for children and their families*, Washington, DC, 2003, National Academy Press.
28. Children's Hospice International: *About children's hospice, palliative and end-of-life care*, 2003, retrieved January 11, 2007, from http://www.chionline.org/resources/about.phtml.

UNIT FIVE

Symptom Management

Fatigue

Sarah Wilson

Definition

The concept of fatigue, although widely recognized and experienced, is one that has been defined in many different ways. The effects of fatigue on a healthy individual are both objective and subjective; however, the intrinsic implications on quality of life are unique to the person experiencing it. Cancer-related fatigue (CRF) is different from fatigue experienced by otherwise healthy individuals in its onset, its duration, its etiology, and, most strikingly, in how it is best managed. When a person without a malignancy experiences fatigue, he or she is often able to attribute it to a specific cause which, when remedied, eliminates the fatigue. By contrast, CRF is often unexpected and remains unrelieved by sleep, or by a change in routine, and is caused not only by the malignancy but also by the treatments for that malignancy. CRF is also exacerbated by some of the activities that would normally relieve fatigue in a healthy person, such as a decrease in physical activity. This chapter is by no means intended to be a comprehensive compilation of the many different works on CRF, but rather is an overview designed to provide the oncology nurse with improved understanding of how the current body of literature and evidence affects clinical interventions. It should be recognized that the little we know about CRF will hopefully be eclipsed by all we have yet to learn, as more research is done, and more is discovered regarding ways to successfully manage CRF.[1]

For the purpose of a standardized oncology-specific definition, CRF is particularly difficult to elucidate since no one definition can completely describe the degree to which CRF is experienced by each individual. Additional difficulties are noted because often CRF overlaps with depression, pain, sleep deprivation, and anxiety. A variety of descriptions by researchers characterize CRF as a subjective feeling of increased discomfort with decreased functional status related to a decrease in energy.[2] Other explanations include those which depict CRF as an unrelenting overall condition that interferes with individuals' ability to function in their normal capacity. Although patients do not have any trouble explaining their particular experience with CRF, one universal definition of CRF remains elusive.[2,3]

It was not until the late 1980s and the 1990s that literature began to reflect CRF as an emerging priority in terms of patient issues to be studied and addressed. Pain and CRF have similar evolutions of care in a variety of ways; specifically, in the relation to the heightened awareness of the issue's severity on the part of both the public and the health care profession, the focus on both pharmacologic and nonpharmacologic interventions, and the slow emerging of research studies to provide an evidence base on which to build standardized treatment recommendations, specific patient interventions, and future research studies. The delay in recognizing CRF as an issue was partly due to the failure of early trials to include an assessment for CRF, as well as

CRF being subsumed under nausea and the underlying assumption that CRF was an unavoidable and untreatable part of the cancer experience.[4] Once CRF was recognized as a pervasive problem, little was done on the clinical side even though research was mounting, largely because CRF was poorly understood in terms of both mechanisms and interventions.

In 2000, the National Comprehensive Cancer Network (NCCN) developed the first national practice guidelines for CRF.[5] Revised in 2003, the NCCN guidelines characterize CRF as a persistent subjective sense of tiredness related to cancer or cancer treatment.[6] CRF, like pain—and as is true for many patient symptoms—is best described or defined by the person experiencing it.[6] CRF has also been described in affective, cognitive, and physical terms by grouping patients' specific descriptions into categories.[7] Researchers have often focused on the quantifiable attributes of CRF, such as intensity, duration, outcomes, and its objective association with other factors.[7] Cancer-related fatigue has also been conceptualized as a response to continual stress inflicted by multiple physiologic, psychologic, and situational factors related to disease and treatment and depleting energy reserves.[8] Due to the multicausal, multidimensional nature of CRF, multiple theories and models were developed and subsequently revised, as researchers recognized the need for increased clarity and gained a better understanding of CRF.

Prevalence

The prevalence of CRF during diagnosis and treatment and in the year immediately following completion of treatment is reported as being as high as 61% to 100%. Patients consistently describe it as the most common and distressing symptom experienced during treatment.[9] Despite the high prevalence of CRF, it is the symptom most frequently reported as unmanaged by patients who are receiving chemotherapy, radiation therapy, or biologic response modifiers.[10] The physiologic etiology, and the cause for the varying levels of the severity of CRF, are less understood because of the many possible factors involved in antineoplastic treatment such as anemia, cachexia, metabolic disturbances, sleep deprivation, and infection. CRF may be a presenting symptom when the patient is diagnosed with cancer. Subsequent treatment of the cancer with surgery or chemotherapy, radiation, or biotherapy can induce or exacerbate the CRF.[11]

Cancer survivors have reported CRF as a persistent disruptive symptom at time of diagnosis, at pretreatment, and during treatment, as well as months to years after completing treatment.[9] More than 75% of patients with metastatic disease have reported increasing levels of CRF irrespective of whether or not they continued to aggressively pursue treatment or are under palliative care for their advancing disease.[9,12] Several studies have demonstrated that many people consider CRF to be an inevitable and unmanageable consequence of cancer and its treatments. These perceptions contribute to patients' reluctance to discuss CRF with their health care provider.[13] Literature has shown that CRF is experienced by 75% to 99% of patients with cancer currently undergoing chemotherapy treatment, and that it increases with each cycle.[14]

Never assume that because patients have not complained of CRF, or because the patient is capable of self-care, that there is no need to assess for CRF. Routine assessments of CRF will allow for early intervention and better management than relying on patients to self-report when CRF becomes troublesome enough to warrant a complaint. Patients often believe there is little or nothing that can be done about CRF and have been discouraged from voicing concerns by interactions in the past with health care professionals who dismissed their complaints. Patients who are at any stage of treatment are at risk for CRF.

Risk Factors

The one assumption underlying CRF, and its single risk factor, is the diagnosis of cancer itself. The correlative to a malignant diagnosis is the single modality treatment or the combined treatments of surgery, chemotherapy, radiotherapy, and biotherapy. Conflicting data exist on whether demographic factors influence the level of CRF.[10] Some studies show that female patients' total CRF scores were higher than those of male patients while undergoing biotherapy.[15] One comparison study showed that patients with ovarian cancer experienced greater levels of CRF than patients with breast cancer.[2] Another study showed that patients with newly diagnosed lung cancer had reported greater CRF than newly diagnosed breast cancer patients.[16] Patients with various tumor types such as melanoma and lung and uterine cancers, and those with leukemia or lymphoma, have also been studied but not in a comparison study. Because of the difference in the definitions of CRF used in the different studies and the variety of assessment tools, there is not yet enough research to stratify risk for CRF based solely on the patient's diagnosis.

Because fatigue in otherwise healthy individuals is a sign of depression, and because it may also be a component of CRF, those oncology patients with a history of depression may be at greater risk for CRF. Patients with other preexisting psychiatric illnesses may also be at greater risk.

Although nutritional deficiency is a risk factor for general fatigue in healthy individuals, one recent study failed to show a relationship between CRF and caloric intake or specific nutrients such as protein, carbohydrates, or fat.[11] A traditional theory suggests that energy taken in is highly related to the level of CRF. However, the sample size in this study included a substantial number of obese patients, and researchers speculated that nutrition could be more important in relationship to CRF when the patient is underweight and intake is depleted.[11] No study to date has shown that nutritional deficiencies, when isolated from other factors (such as severe electrolyte imbalances), are related to CRF.

Sleep deprivation, electrolyte imbalances, rapid metabolic shifts, fever, pain, infection, and dehydration may also be risk factors, as well as potential root causes of CRF. Combination treatments such as concurrent radiation and chemotherapy are considered to pose a cumulative risk, particularly as patients progress through treatments.[8]

Etiology

Because of the multidimensionality of CRF, it is highly unlikely that a core etiology, single definition, or gold standard of measurement will be established.[3,17] Instead, interventions aimed at specific contributing factors have been incorporated into guidelines for assessment and treatment of CRF.

The major contributing factors for CRF can be divided into five separate categories: disease-related, treatment-related, psychologic, environmental, and symptom patterns.[15] While more studies are beginning to look at symptom cohorts and extrapolate for various factors, the multiple facets of CRF make it a challenge to design a study in which all the factors can be simultaneously studied and measured. The nurse's job is to assess each patient and identify those factors that can be addressed, while recognizing that each patient's experience of CRF is specific and individual.

Disease-related factors include tumor growth, metastatic spread, and the side effects from each malignancy-specific presentation. For example, lung cancer patients often experience CRF before diagnosis as a result of changes in oxygenation patterns, location of tumors, and chronic persistent cough. Patients who have difficulty breathing and wake up several times a night with a productive or nonproductive cough have CRF as a result of the disease process itself.[8] Similar symptoms related to the site of malignancy are noted.

Treatment-related factors can be further subdivided into surgery, chemotherapy, radiation, and biotherapy or immunotherapy. The hazards of surgery are well documented and well known to nursing—particularly those that arise from the lack of mobility and failure to heal. It is not uncommon for situations to occur in which oncology patients have undergone a surgical procedure and go on to develop many of the common complications, resulting in increased CRF. Some patients may not recognize CRF following surgery, since they expect to be more tired after surgery.

Studies of several different types of cancer have been done looking specifically at the effects of various chemotherapy agents, comparing both the effects of doses and drugs. Throughout the trajectory of chemotherapy-induced side effects, anemia and neutropenia were associated with higher reports of CRF.[13] With the advent of medications such as Procrit, Neulasta, Aranesp, and other colony-stimulating factors, there is better management of the hematologic side effects of chemotherapy. Anemia is a well known and easily identified contributing factor of CRF. Several quality of life studies have shown that the use of Procrit and subsequent rise in hemoglobin levels can slightly improve quality of life (QOL) assessments.[2] Nausea, vomiting, diarrhea, fevers, chills, night sweats, pain, sleep deprivation, malaise, and electrolyte imbalances are all commonly expected occurrences that can both exacerbate and/or overshadow CRF. Interestingly, some patients have reported CRF as being more distressing than any of the aforementioned symptoms.[7]

Radiation-induced CRF is a common and debilitating side effect for oncology patients that occurs both during and after treatment.[8,10] CRF associated with radiation therapy may be cumulative, increasing during the course of therapy and most severe during the last week of treatment; or CRF may rise, plateau, and then rise again.[8] The physiologic mechanism behind radiation-induced CRF is not completely understood. Impairment is thought to occur in multiple ways. Various theories include that the CRF is caused by toxic metabolite accumulation caused by cellular destruction, and changes in energy and energy substrate patterns that allow for fibroblastic proliferation and reepithelialization to repair affected tissue.[8] Radiation may also cause nutritional problems such as malnutrition, dehydration, and electrolyte imbalance, as well as negative changes in activity and rest patterns, altered oxygenation patterns caused by destruction of radiosensitive hematopoietic cells resulting in anemia, and impaired aerobic metabolism. Increasing requirements for cellular repair may precipitate CRF by increasing the body's need for resources.[10] Additional psychosocial factors associated with CRF in relation to radiation therapy include the role of anxiety and depression, coping resources, and the patient's overall functional status. The incidence and severity of radiation-induced CRF is dependent on the radiation dose, the area being radiated, and the length of radiation treatment.[10]

Biotherapy, or treatment with biologic response modifiers, and immunotherapy, which is given with or without standard chemotherapy, can result in toxicities such as myelosuppression, nausea, vomiting, chills, fever, malaise, and capillary leak syndrome (shift of intravascular fluid to extravascular spaces, resulting in significant hypotension and generalized edema). Medical literature acknowledges CRF as one of the pharmacologic biotherapy toxicities, although limited studies have been done on this specific patient population.[15]

Psychologic distress (anxiety and depression) causing CRF may be experienced by patients at diagnosis, during treatment, following completion of treatment, or as they experience adjustment to life as a survivor. A significant association between CRF and anxiety has been shown, as well as between CRF and depression. Emotional aspects of CRF include "attentional CRF"—a specific deficit in the ability to direct attention, maintain mental focus, and concentrate.[4] Much has been published in recent years regarding attentional CRF, often referred to as "chemo brain." However, despite the increasing literature documenting the occurrence, few chemotherapy patient teaching sheets warn patients about this possible side effect. Attentional fatigue is an aspect of CRF that may one day warrant a chapter all of its own.

Inactivity is a substantial risk factor—as well as a result of—CRF. In 1987, Aistars published one of the earliest models of CRF, in which exercise was conceptualized as an energy-conservation strategy based on the idea that physiologic and psychologic adaptations occur in response to exercise and improve activity tolerance.[18] Rest had been the dominant recommendation before that time for patients with cancer, because both clinicians and families assumed that even if the cancer patient was able to tolerate exercise, it would increase rather than decrease CRF. Since 1987, many other models, including those by Victoria Mock and the NCCN guidelines, reinforce the use of exercise not only as a conservation strategy, but also as a management tool. Physiologic deconditioning occurs with rest, which can lead to decreased activity tolerance, leading to even further inactivity and, ultimately, functional disability. Winningham's CRF inertia spiral model used well-established concepts from exercise physiology to explain how rehabilitative efforts with exercise might ameliorate CRF.[17] Exercise is the main nonpharmacologic intervention recommended by the NCCN guidelines.[5,17]

Effects and Consequences

Just as each cancer patient's experience of CRF is unique, so are the effects and consequences of CRF. CRF has mental and physical consequences, and many patients report that CRF is more limiting than nausea and vomiting or pain and is not as well controlled.[16,19]

During treatment for malignancy, CRF has multiple consequences in a patient's life—many of which are functional deficits. Barsevick used the Common Sense Model (CSM) to categorize information from patients in their own words of how the CRF limited their lives. The CSM is an information-processing model built on the proposition that individuals create their own "common sense" interpretations of symptoms to guide their coping efforts.[7] This allowed patients to provide concrete examples of the ways that CRF had everyday effects on their lives. See Box 37-1 for specific consequences of CRF.

Barsevick classified the comments of patients regarding the effect of CRF into four categories: consequences, pattern, identity, and cause. Quotes from patients may help to further illuminate the magnitude of the problem as it relates to how patients' lives are affected. The quotes in Box 37-2 are taken from the four different categories.[7]

For a majority of patients, the consequences of CRF were substantial, and they were what distinguished CRF from the kind of fatigue they experienced before their illness. Most described CRF in relation to the inability to function, loss of functioning, or inability to engage in a wide variety of usual activities.[7]

Psychologically, the uncontrolled symptom of CRF can lead to depression in patients who have not previously struggled with depression over time, and can also interfere with a patient's overall mindset regarding cancer. Patients described the presence of CRF as a factor in eroding their hope for long term recovery—partly because they were uncertain if the persistence of CRF indicated occult disease, but also because it kept them from returning to what they considered "normal" life even when they had completed treatment. CRF has been found to negatively affect QOL, pain tolerance, mood, cognition, and sleep, and even to increase caregiving hours.[14]

Assessment and Measurement

Because of the many different definitions, theoretical frameworks, and conceptual models of CRF, researchers have had to

---

BOX 37-1 **Specific Consequences of CRF— Things That Patients Cannot Do**

- Cook dinner
- Pick my head up
- Get out of the house
- Concentrate
- Stand up
- Work
- Answer the phone
- Get up the steps to go to bed
- Anything I used to do
- Barely lift my arms
- Turn the pages of the newspaper
- Walk to the bus (it's not far)
- Prepare a meal
- Wash a sink full of dishes
- Be productive
- Half the things I did before

BOX 37-2 **Representations of the Consequences, Pattern, Identity, and Cause of CRF**

Consequences

"When I think about fatigue… to me, at least, it's not only physical; [it's] that I want to do things, that I want to plan my day, that I want to do something productive—and you can't, and the frustration level is enormous. You might start the task and run out of gas halfway into it, and that's it for the day."

"I was the kind of person that never missed a day of work. I never stayed at home, never got the flu. I've had the ordinary things. It was my selling point. I never missed work. And now, 2 1/2 years later I became a liability instead of an asset. I feel that way, anyhow."

Pattern

"And I believe that was the beginning of the fatigue… but I find that fatigue is erratic, not predictable; that is really frightening. I can be in the supermarket doing fine, pushing my cart, picking groceries, and all of a sudden my body seems to shut down. And all I want to do is lie down on the floor, and I wouldn't care if the entire world walked all over me like I was a carpet and I would sleep for hours. I have walked out of the supermarket with the cart just sitting there, just knowing I could not do it."

"And I think you are more accepting when you are going through chemo. Everybody says you can expect that. It's this chronic fatigue, 3 years posttreatment—and I still have this problem and it doesn't go away."

Identity

"Fatigue is a mental and physical thing, and one feeds the other. And I think the combination brings you mighty low at times."

"Okay, let me start: because fatigue was my first symptom when I had cancer, and I didn't realize that was one of the symptoms… and I kept saying, I was tired, and this is not me. [The doctor] said, "You know, you are getting older." And then I got a second opinion and that was the two things I told him. When I come home nights, I sit down and I have to think about getting out of my chair and going across my living room into the kitchen to do my dishes. I said I'm not just tired. I'm sick tired. That is how tired I felt."

Cause

"As I said, fatigue didn't hit me until the radiation started taking its effect."

"With chemo, you kind of knew when you were going to be tired because you knew about the blood count."

---

define in each study what exactly they were assessing for and how they would quantify those specific factors. Consequently many different assessment and measurement tools have been developed—each with advantages, disadvantages, and limitations. None of the major tools used in research studies have been adopted by the NCCN, but several are widely endorsed, recognized, and easy to use. This text is by no means exhaustive, nor is it designed to give an in-depth analysis of which tool is best in

---

BOX 37-3 **Assessment Tools for CRF**

- Brief CRF Inventory (BFI)
- The Functional Assessment of Cancer Therapy-Anemia. (FACT-G)
- The Functional Assessment of Cancer Therapy-CRF (FACT- F)
- Piper Fatigue Self-Report Scale (PFS)
- The Schwartz Cancer Fatigue Scale (SCFS)
- Fatigue Symptom Inventory (FSI)
- The Profile of Mood States Fatigue-Inertia Subscale (POMS)
- Lee's Visual Analogue Scale for Fatigue (LVASF)
- Cancer Fatigue Scale (CFS)
- Quick Fatigue Assessment Survey (QFAS)

---

which setting. A brief overview is given to some of the tools endorsed by the National Cancer Institute (NCI) and by the Oncology Nursing Society (ONS) that are listed in Box 37-3.[20]

BRIEF FATIGUE INVENTORY (BFI)

The Brief Fatigue Inventory (BFI) was designed to measure the intensity and interference of CRF. The BFI uses a scale from 0 (none) to 10 (severe). Three of the nine items in the BFI assess the intensity of CRF, and six of the nine measure the effects of CRF.

Advantages: The BFI is very easy to use in clinical practice and easy to translate into other languages.

Disadvantages: Although well validated, the single-dimension aspect of the BFI does not measure the multiple dimensions that longer instruments represent, such as the cognitive, affective, and somatic components of CRF. [21]

THE FUNCTIONAL ASSESSMENT OF CANCER THERAPY (FACT-F)

Consisting of 41 items, the Functional Assessment of Cancer Therapy (FACT-F) consists of 28 questions regarding QOL and health-related issues, and 13 questions about CRF in patients with cancer. The 13 fatigue questions have been separated out as a fatigue subscale and cover five points, measuring presence and intensity of CRF, affective aspects of CRF, and interference with functional performance 7 days before the test.

Advantages: FACT-F addresses not only the effects or consequences of CRF but also the symptomatic expressions.

Disadvantages: FACT-F has only been tested in limited patient populations with certain treatments. Wider testing is needed.[21]

PIPER CRF SCALE (PFS) AND REVISED PFS

The Piper CRF Scale (PFS)[3] contains 22 items that measure four dimensions of subjective CRF: behavioral severity (six items), sensory(five items), cognitive or mood (six items), and affective meaning (five items). Each item is anchored by two words (strong vs weak), and subjects circle a number from 0 to 10 that best describes their current CRF experience. Five open-ended questions regarding the temporal dimension of CRF, perceived cause, effects, and additional symptoms are also part of the PFS.

Advantages: The PFS was the first validated and best-developed multidimensional measure of CRF, developed according to a strong theoretic model and using a comprehensive approach to assess CRF.

Disadvantage: The first PFS was so lengthy that it was difficult for patients to complete, and patients sometimes could not understand all of the complex wording of the questions. The revised version, although shorter, has a complex scaling system and was primarily tested on female breast cancer patient survivors.[21]

MULTIDIMENSIONAL CRF INVENTORY (MFI-20)

The Multidimensional CRF Inventory (MFI-20)[10] is a tool consisting of 20 statements that assess five dimensions of CRF based on different modes of expressing CRF: (a) general fatigue, including general statements concerning a person's function, such as "I feel rested"; (b) physical fatigue, referring to the physical sensation related to the feeling of tiredness; (c) reduced activities; (d) lack of motivation to start any activity; and (e) mental CRF—which covers cognitive symptoms such as difficulty concentrating. Each dimension contains four items with two indicative of CRF and two contradicting CRF. The response consists of five squares and ranges from agreement with the accompanying statement ("Yes, that is true") to disagreement ("No that is not true").

Advantages: The tool can be presented to patient as a written questionnaire in the absence of a researcher, and has demonstrated high reliability and validity, and good internal consistency.

Disadvantage: MFI-20 limits patients' experience of CRF to fit into one of the five different dimensions—few of which fully address the emotional or psychosocial components of CRF.

SCHWARTZ CANCER FATIGUE SCALE (SCFS)

Consisting of 28 single-word items, the Schwartz Cancer Fatigue Scale (SCFS) is based on an extensive literature review and various self-report instruments. Four dimensions are conceptualized in this scale: physical, emotional, cognitive, and temporal aspects of CRF.

Advantage: SCFS was the first instrument to measure perceptual dimensions of CRF. It is the shortest multidimensional instrument—useful in both clinical and research settings; it showed good construct validity and internal consistency.

Disadvantages: Some patients may find it difficult to describe their feelings of CRF if they experienced change in the past 3 days since the SCFS measures in 3-day time segments. It had limited generalizability since it was developed with primarily male patients, and test-retest reliability must be further examined. Some aspects of this tool are possibly redundant and repetitive.[21]

PROFILE OF MOOD STATES (POMS)

The Profile of Mood States (POMS) contains 65 5-point, adjective rating scales, and measures six identifiable mood states. The POMS-CRF subscale form shows good reliability when compared with other tools. POMS include several physical items that overlap with either disease-related or treatment-related symptoms experienced by patients.

Advantages: POMS is short and easy to use.

Disadvantages: A single-dimension measure, POMS was developed for use as a mood scale for psychiatric outpatients and not specifically designed to measure CRF.[21]

QUICK CRF ASSESSMENT SCALE (QFAS)

The Quick CRF Assessment Scale (QFAS) is based on five primary symptoms: sleep disturbance, pain, anxiety, nausea and vomiting, and depression. It is a 17-item assessment technique designed to provide an efficient method for obtaining descriptive data about a patient's CRF. Similar to standard pain assessment techniques, the QFAS offers a choice of three scales to determine intensity: (1) a numerical rating of 0 to 10, (2) a mild to severe visual analogue scale, and (3) the ONS CRF rating scale. The ONS CRF rating scale shows a graphic image of an individual with various levels of CRF, accompanied by a scale to indicate level of intensity.

Advantages: Easy to use, this tool also includes a section to assess other possible contributing factors such as electrolyte panel abnormalities, hemoglobin levels, and thyroid function. It is simple for patients to understand and easy to read, and provides information that can be measured against repeat assessments.

Disadvantages: The wording of some of the open-ended questions, such as "Is there anything that makes your fatigue better or worse?" allows for confusion in the patient's answer. Revisions of this tool should either clarify separate questions, or solicit information on only one factor at a time.[22]

Interventions and Outcomes

NCCN guidelines divide treatment interventions for CRF into two major categories: pharmacologic and nonpharmacologic.[4,23] In addition to the website, *www.nccn.org*, patients and professionals can order hard copies of the published guidelines. Although many of the recommendations may seem to be redundant, obvious, or mere common sense, practical suggestions are important to help direct patients and to educate them in specific ways to possibly prevent CRF, identify it early, and be proactive in managing their care.

Erythropoietin is by far the most researched pharmacologic agent used in treatment of chemotherapy-induced anemia and, consistently, studies show that improved hemoglobin levels are accompanied by improved self-reported energy levels.[4,5] However, all of the studies focus on correcting chemotherapy-induced anemia, not on preventing it, and each study applied a specific hemoglobin level as a cutoff point, rather than examining the relative change of the hemoglobin in relation to changes in individual patients. Because each study withdrew erythropoietin after the hemoglobin reached a designated level, there are no data on the degree to which CRF might be affected if the hemoglobin cutoff point was set at normal or the patient's pretreatment level. This is an area which requires further research.[4]

Psychostimulants such as methylphenidate have been tested in certain patient populations, such as those with malignant melanoma, as well as in patients with advanced cancer.[24] Patients reported improvement in symptoms of CRF with use of methylphenidate, but it remains an area where more research is needed.

Antidepressants have been used in some patient populations with mixed results. One study of breast cancer patients showed that an antidepressant improved mood without improving CRF.[4] However, despite different patterns of CRF and depression in oncology patients as compared to the general population, the thought persists that CRF is a symptom of depression. The wide acceptance of CRF as an indicator of depression can have a negative effect, particularly for nondepressed patients who have CRF and potentially treatable physiologic problems such as anemia, or those who may be candidates for nonpharmacologic interventions (such as exercise). Ongoing research is needed to provide more data regarding patients in both categories.[4]

Nonpharmacologic interventions include exercise, energy conservation, sleep and rest, restorative activities, stress management, and psychosocial support, as well as nutritional support and supplements.[4,5] Not all caregivers are aware of the current knowledge or evidence supporting management of CRF. Information about CRF and available interventions must be included in patient and family education.

Exercise has been shown to improve QOL and reduce reported CRF in multiple studies. Individuals in these studies preformed aerobic interval training for 15 to 30 minutes for various numbers of days per week. Dr. Victoria Mock, the lead author of the NCCN guidelines on CRF, reviewed nine different studies using exercise an intervention, and all nine showed both increased energy, and a decreased level of CRF. Each of the studies reviewed used different formats for exercise—walking was the main activity, and some of the studies used cycle ergometers and stationary bicycles.[9] One study showed that even during the hematologic nadir, a program of bed- or chair-based bicycle ergometer pedaling was found to be safe and effective in reducing CRF in hospital patients undergoing peripheral blood and stem cell transplants.[25] Although physicians and nurses are aware of the evidence showing that inactivity exacerbates or causes CRF, they often are guilty of giving contradictory advice to patients regarding how much rest as opposed to exercise or activity the patient should be doing.

"'Try to get some exercise, but don't overdo it, and rest when you are tired'; but how much is too much? And if you are always tired, and rest doesn't help, does that mean you should never exercise?" Patient questions such as these are part of the reason that cancer rehabilitation programs are beginning to be developed across the nation. "Strides to Strength" is an exercise-based, comprehensive fatigue management and wellness program based in Charlotte, NC. Patients who enroll in the 12-week program not only meet twice a week with an exercise physiologist, but they are monitored by an oncology-certified RN, a registered dietitian,

and a psychosocial counselor. Specific instructions, with careful assessment of other underlying root factors, have resulted in tremendous changes in patient-reported quality of life measures. Patients who are alumni of the program repeatedly return to share the advances they have made in battling CRF.[26]

Energy conservation includes priority-setting, delegation of tasks, scheduling of activities around times when energy peaks, and planning daily routines. Nurses can help patients to identify which activities are most taxing, and which ones can be postponed. Patients who are overwhelmed often don't have the presence of mind to think through simple ways to conserve energy, and should be encouraged to do one activity at a time.

Sleep and rest are others areas where patients may need education and support in terms of how to have good sleep hygiene. Once treatments are underway or completed, patients should be encouraged to maintain the patterns they had before diagnosis, such as going to bed at the same time every night.

Survivors have many options to reduce their stress levels; psychosocial support is provided through many support groups, through individual counseling, and through recreational activities. Identifying for each individual what has been helpful in managing stress prior to their diagnosis may help the patient recognize what option to explore first in dealing with his or her emotions regarding the malignancy. Relaxation techniques, meditation, and distractions such as games, music, reading, or seeing visitors are all ways that patients can reduce the level of attentional CRF, which can be draining. Other restorative ideas include journaling, gardening, volunteer activities, and visiting with family.[5]

Assessment of CRF in any patient should include attention to possible physiologic, psychosocial, and environmental factors, with interventions geared toward correcting the abnormalities that are discovered. Patients should be educated in advance regarding what to expect by way of CRF as they approach and undergo treatment. Validation that their experiences and the struggle with CRF are real can be reassuring and provide the opportunity for more in-depth assessment of which intervention is best for that particular patient.

REVIEW QUESTIONS

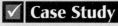 **Case Study**

Ruth is a 52-year-old breast cancer patient who underwent a radical right mastectomy 7 weeks ago and is currently undergoing chemotherapy. She is receiving dose-dense Adriamycin and Cytoxan and is coming in for her third cycle. She will receive chest wall radiation once she completes chemotherapy. While taking her vital signs, you casually ask how she is doing. Ruth replies "Worn out from doing nothing!! I am so exhausted, and I've become so lazy. I can't seem to ever get myself out of this slump. I go to bed every night and wake up feeling more tired and nauseated than when I went to bed. I can't concentrate, and just taking a shower makes me short of breath. I know it has to be this chemo, and I guess there is nothing I can do. I felt better after the blood transfusion on Tuesday, but here it is Friday and I am still dragging. I am actually looking forward to moving to the next step. At least radiation doesn't make you tired or throw up!"

QUESTIONS

1. What would your correct response be?
   a. "That's right, once you are done with chemo, you won't feel tired during radiation, and you'll be back to your usual self."
   b. "You are tired because the chemo is killing all your cancer cells, and that is a good sign! Remember, your body is fighting for you, so take it easy."
   c. "I think you're depressed. Let's talk to the doctor today about choosing an antidepressant that won't interact with your other medications."
   d. **"We can** do something about your fatigue!! It sounds like this is really affecting your quality of life. Tell me what you mean when you say you are 'worn out from doing nothing.' What is your typical day like?"

2. Based on the information you've been given, which of the following concerns should you address as the primary culprit for Ruth's fatigue?
   a. Anemia
   b. Nausea and electrolyte imbalance
   c. Insomnia and inactivity
   d. All of the factors which can cause fatigue should be addressed including – but not limited to disease process, medications, abnormal hematological and chemistry levels, and activity status, as well as psychosocial/emotional state of mind.

3. Ruth tells you the surgeon told her to take things easy, and to be very careful not to overdo it. She thinks this means she should not do any exercise, should take frequent naps during the day, and should avoid any activity that makes her feel tired. What do you say to her to explain what regular exercise would do to help her to have more energy?
   a. Her cancer cells are sucking all the oxygen out of the healthy cells, and exercise forces the oxygen back into the good cells.
   b. Being overweight causes her body to have to work harder at everything, even fighting cancer, so exercise would help her lose weight and then have less work.
   c. Inertia and inactivity lead to physiologic deconditioning, which can create even lower tolerance levels for activity.
   d. Regular activity helps your body to maintain its ability to respond to the various treatments and builds your immune system. While rest is important, getting too much rest, or not enough activity, can actually increase your fatigue levels.

4. Breast cancer is the solid tumor which causes the highest levels of fatigue in patients—more than colon cancer, lung cancer, or ovarian cancer.
   a. True
   b. False

5. Patients who eat a healthy diet and have no nutritional deficiency are less likely to have CRF than obese or underweight patients who do not eat a balanced diet.
   a. True
   b. False

6. Ruth is *most* likely to experience her highest levels of fatigue at which time:
   a. During chemotherapy
   b. After chemotherapy, before radiation
   c. During radiation
   d. Immediately after radiation
   e. Three to 6 months after completing radiation

7. Which of the following medications is most likely to be used to help prevent Ruth from experiencing chemotherapy-induced anemia and anemia-related CRF?
   a. Aranesp or Procrit
   b. Neupogen or Neulasta
   c. Zofran
   d. Vitamin B

8. Which of the following nonpharmacologic interventions would be appropriate to discuss with Ruth?
   a. Regular exercise program and energy conservation techniques

   b. Breast cancer support group
   c. Meditation and relaxation exercises
   d. Adequate sleep evaluation, consistent activity, stress reduction, psychosocial support, and journaling to track which intervention provides best outcome.

9. Upon reviewing Ruth's case, you realize part of her insomnia is due to her medication regimen. Which of the following changes would hinder Ruth from getting the best sleep possible?
   a. Changing daily Decadron to be taken every AM instead of PM
   b. Instructing Ruth to take a Zofran or Kytril before going to bed to prevent early AM nausea
   c. Drinking a glass of red wine to help unwind before bed
   d. Prescription for Lunesta

10. Ruth returns for her fourth treatment and informs you she is sleeping better, and that she is able to walk for 1 mile 4 days a week. She is experiencing less nausea, and although discouraged about her alopecia, is excited that she is nearing the end of her chemotherapy treatments. When filling out routine hospital paperwork, however, she becomes frustrated at her inability to focus or concentrate, and throws down the pen and clipboard. "I cannot fill out any more forms!!" she exclaims. What is Ruth is experiencing?
    a. CRF exacerbated by hospital paperwork
    b. Emotional fatigue
    c. Attentional fatigue AKA "chemo brain"
    d. Attention deficit disorder induced by chemotherapy

ANSWERS

1. **D.** *Rationale:* Investigating Ruth's activity level will give you more information to begin formulating a plan to address each specific factor that contributes to her fatigue. Radiation causes fatigue and has a progressive, cumulative effect, but it is not an indicator of the efficacy of chemotherapy or radiation. Fatigue may be exacerbated by treatment but is not a prognostic indicator. Although depression may contribute to fatigue, Ruth has many other easily identified factors for fatigue, which should be investigated before adding another medication. Her feelings of hopelessness may be triggered by frustration over her circumstance.

2. **D.** *Rationale:* This answer is the most comprehensive because it recognizes that while the other answers are correct, they are incomplete. All of Ruth's case history should be reviewed.

3. **C.** *Rationale:* Exercise has benefit for patients with CRF of all sizes: those who are underweight, those of correct weight, and those who are overweight. Although losing excess body weight does reduce the stress on the body, there has been no study showing a correlation between reduction in CRF and loss of excess body fat. No study has shown that exercise forces oxygen away from cancer and into healthy cells.

4. **B.** *Rationale:* Although no study has been done to compare and contrast which solid tumor cancer causes the single highest levels of fatigue, there have been studies showing that lung cancer is associated with higher levels of fatigue than breast cancer.

Continued

REVIEW QUESTIONS—CONT'D

5. B. *Rationale:* No study has shown any correlation between nutritional deficiencies and CRF. A healthy diet is good for any patient, but the benefit in terms of reducing fatigue is only found in otherwise healthy individuals.

6. E. *Rationale:* Studies have repeatedly shown that patients report their highest levels of fatigue 3 to 6 months after completing radiation.

7. A. *Rationale:* Aranesp or Procrit are indicated for use of preventing and treating chemotherapy-induced anemia and anemia-related CRF. Neupogen and Neulasta are used to improve white blood cell counts. Zofran is an antiemetic, and Vitamin B does not prevent anemia.

8. D. *Rationale:* Exercise, support groups, stress relaxation, and energy conservation are all appropriate nonpharmacologic methods for helping to manage CRF and provide a more comprehensive answer than the other choices.

9. C. *Rationale:* Alcohol acts initially as a depressant on the nervous system but can cause diuresis, as well as waking throughout the night, and should be avoided by patients with insomnia.

10. C. *Rationale:* Attentional fatigue is noted partly by inability to complete tasks that require concentration, focus and/or recall of detail.

REFERENCES

1. Berger AM, Von Essen S, Kuhn BR et al: Adherence, sleep and CRF outcomes after adjuvant breast cancer chemotherapy: results of a feasibility intervention study, *Oncol Nurs Forum* 30(3):513-522, 2003.
2. Payne JK: The trajectory of CRF in adult patients with breast and ovarian cancer receiving chemotherapy, *Oncol Nurs Forum* 29(9):1334-1339, 2002.
3. Piper B, Dibble S, Weiss M et al: The revised Piper Fatigue Scale: psychometric evaluation in women with breast cancer, *Oncol Nurs Forum* 25(4):677-684, 1998.
4. Nail LM: CRF in patients with cancer, *Oncol Nurs Forum* 29(3):537-543, 2002.
5. Mock V, Atkinson A, Barsevick A et al: National Comprehensive Cancer Network oncology practice guideline for cancer related CRF, *Oncology,* 14(11A):151-161, 2000.
6. Mock V: Clinical excellence through evidence-based practice: CRF management as a model, *Oncol Nurs Forum* 30(5):790-796, 2003.
7. Barsevick AM, Whitmer K, Walker L: In their own words: using the Common Sense Model to analyze patient descriptions of cancer-related CRF, *Oncol Nurs Forum* 28(9):1363-1369, 2001.
8. Beach P, Siebeneck B, Buderer NF et al: Relationship between CRF and Nutritional status in patients receiving radiation therapy to treat lung cancer, *Oncol Nurs Forum* 28(6):1027-1031, 2001.
9. Stricker C, Drake D, Hoyer K et al: Evidence-based practice for CRF management in adults with cancer: exercise as an intervention, *Oncol Nurs Forum* 31(5):963-973, 2004.
10. Ahlberg K, Ekman T, Gaston-Johansson F: CRF, psychological distress, Coping resources, and functional status during radiotherapy for uterine cancer, *Oncol Nurs Forum* 32(3):633-639, 2005.
11. Porock D, Behears B, Hinton P et al: Nutritional, functional, and emotional characteristics related to CRF in patients during and after biochemotherapy, *Oncol Nurs Forum* 32(3):661-667, 2005.
12. Gibson F, Mulhall AB, Richardson A et al: A phenomenological study of CRF in adolescents receiving treatment for cancer, *Oncol Nurs Forum* 32(3):651-660, 2005.
13. Donovan HS, Ward S: Representations of CRF in women receiving chemotherapy for gynecologic cancers, *Oncol Nurs Forum* 32(1):113-116, 2005.
14. Headley JA, Ownby KK, John LD: The effect of seated exercise on CRF and quality of life in women with advanced breast cancer, *Oncol Nurs Forum* 31(5):977-983, 2004.
15. Fu MR, Anderson CM, McDaniel R et al: Patients perceptions of CRF in response to biochemotherapy for metastatic melanoma: a preliminary study, *Oncol Nurs Forum* 29(6):961-966, 2002.
16. Wilmoth MC, Coleman EA, Smith SC et al: CRF, Weight gain, and altered sexuality in patients with breast cancer: exploration of a symptom cluster, *Oncol Nurs Forum* 31(6):1069-1073, 2004.
17. Coon SK, Coleman EA: Keep moving: Patients with myeloma talk about exercise and CRF, *Oncol Nurs Forum* 31(6):1127-1135, 2004.
18. Aistairs J: CRF In the cancer patient: a conceptual approach to a clinical problem, *Oncol Nurs Forum* 14(6):25-30, 1987.
19. Stone P: The measurement, causes and effective management of cancer-related CRF, *Int J Palliat Nurs* 8(3):120-128, 2002.
20. National Cancer Institute: *Assessment of CRF*, 2005, retrieved August, 2005, from www.nci.nih.cancer.gov.
21. Wu HS, McSweeney M: Measurement of CRF in people with cancer, *Oncol Nurs Forum* 28(9):1371-1386, 2001.
22. Quick M, Fonteyn M: Development and implementation of a clinical survey for cancer-related CRF assessment, *Clin J Oncol Nurs* 9(4):435-446, 2005.
23. National Coalition Cancer Network: *Cancer Related fatigue and anemia,* 2003, retrieved July 2005 from www.nccn.org.
24. Homsi J, Walsh D, Nelson KA: Psychostimulants in supportive care, *Support Care Cancer* 8(5):385-397, 2000.
25. Dimeo FC: Effects of exercise on cancer-related CRF, *Cancer* 92(6 Suppl):1689-1693, 2001.
26. Ballard TM: *Cancer rehabilitation: strides to strength,* 2005, retrieved August, 2005, from www. novanthealth.org.

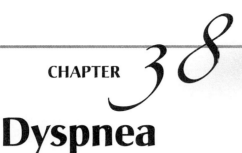

Dyspnea

Audrey Gift and Amy Hoffman

Dyspnea is one of the most devastating symptoms experienced by patients with cancer. This symptom does not only occur in patients with lung cancer but rather can occur in patients with any kind of the disease, especially at its more advanced stages. The inability to get one's breath, a feeling of not being able to take in enough air, and/or the feeling of suffocating produces a level of anxiety in patients that results in them seeking the attention of a health care provider. It is important that health care providers have an understanding of this distressing symptom and focus care not only on the physical needs of the patient, but on the psychologic and social needs as well. The strategies that have been identified as effective in alleviating or eliminating dyspnea focus on the underlying disease and its treatment, and/or the palliation of the symptom to provide temporary comfort. Attention also must focus on the psychologic and cognitive aspects of care. Thus it is important to select a way to measure dyspnea that will provide information about the aspect of the symptom that is being targeted in a given intervention. Relieving shortness of breath can be one of the most rewarding aspects of nursing care of the patient with cancer.

Definition

Dyspnea is subjectively perceived breathing difficulty or distress that encompasses a variety of unpleasant respiratory sensations and includes the cognitive, affective, and behavioral responses to those sensations. Dyspnea consists of qualitatively distinct sensations that vary in intensity. The dyspneic experience derives from interactions among multiple physiologic, psychologic, social, and environmental factors, and may induce secondary physiologic and behavioral responses."[1]

Dyspnea is characterized by its duration. Acute dyspnea has a sudden onset, whereas chronic dyspnea lasts for weeks. In addition to duration, dyspnea can be described like other symptoms according to frequency, intensity, distress, and quality.[2] The cognitive response to dyspnea is also important, because the meaning or interpretation of the symptom that patients put to the sensation influences how they respond to it.[3] The affective aspect of dyspnea is highly correlated with the presence of anxiety; however, dyspnea can be differentiated from anxiety.[4] In addition, patients have a wide variety of behavioral responses to the sensation of dyspnea such as altering activities to avoid the sensation, positioning to enhance diaphragmatic excursion (such as leaning forward and raising elbows to shoulder level), and engaging in pursed-lip breathing.

The qualitatively different sensations are manifested by the different descriptors used to report dyspnea. Descriptions used by persons who are experiencing dyspnea include the following: I feel I am suffocating; my chest feels tight; my breathing is heavy; I feel I am smothering; my breath does not go in all the way; my breath does not go out all the way; I feel that I am breathing more; I feel my breathing is rapid; my breathing requires effort; I cannot get enough air; I feel a hunger for air; my breathing is shallow; I feel out of breath; my chest is constricted; and, my breathing requires work.[5] These descriptors have been identified as clustering together to form three dimensions of dyspnea: (1) depth and frequency of breathing, (2) perceived need or urge to breathe, and (3) difficulty breathing and phase of respiration.[6]

Prevalence

In patients with cancer, dyspnea occurs at varying rates depending on the type of cancer, the treatment selected for their cancer and the severity of the disease. The prevalence of dyspnea is also related to the number of risk factors.[7]

Dyspnea is most commonly associated with breast, lung, and colorectal cancers. The prevalence of dyspnea in patients with lung cancer is reported to range from 46% to 73% and even 87%.[7-9] In a study of patients newly diagnosed with lung cancer, 58% of them reported experiencing dyspnea; however, an examination of symptom clusters in these patients did not include dyspnea in the cluster.[10] Severe dyspnea has only been reported in 32% of patients with lung cancer.[11]

Dyspnea occurs with almost all types of cancer therapy. It can occur after surgery, during and after chemotherapy, and after radiation therapy. Dyspnea is reported by patients in all stages of cancer but is more prevalent in the later stages of disease. Patients with cancer experience a more rapid onset of dyspnea than other patients who experience dyspnea.[12] Dyspnea is at the moderate to severe level in 10% to 63% of patients with advanced cancer.[13] Dyspnea has been shown by some to increase as the disease progresses, whereas others, studying symptoms over time, have shown them to decrease as the disease progressed.[14,15] Children with advanced cancer have been shown to be very distressed by dyspnea.[16]

Risk Factors

Among persons with cancer, the risk factors for dyspnea include comorbid respiratory disease (e.g., chronic obstructive pulmonary disease [COPD] or asthma) or cardiac disease (e.g., heart failure). The exposure to the risk factors for these diseases, such as a history of smoking or exposure to toxic substances—asbestos, coal dust, cotton dust or grain dust—also increases the risk for dyspnea.[7]

The risk for dyspnea may be a direct result of a tumor or an indirect result of having cancer and the debilitating nature of the disease. Direct causes of cancer-related dyspnea include bronchial or airway obstruction, superior vena cava syndrome, tumor invasion of lung tissue, pleural effusion, ascites, hepatomegaly, or the like. Indirect causes of cancer-related dyspnea are those resulting from the debilitating nature of the disease, such as anemia, cachexia, pneumonia, electrolyte imbalance, infection, pulmonary embolism, or pulmonary aspiration, to name those most relevant. Psychologic factors may also increase the risk for dyspnea. Dyspnea is more likely to occur in the presence of anxiety. Dyspnea may also be accompanied by feelings of fear, extreme fatigue, loss of memory, inability to concentrate, and decreased appetite.

Cancer treatment may increase the risk of dyspnea or may relieve dyspnea. Chemotherapy may result in destruction of lung parenchyma, and/or cardiomyopathy, and thus increase the risk for dyspnea. Surgery, especially in the immediate postoperative phase is likely to result in dyspnea. However, reduction in tumor size, especially if it is in the abdomen or thorax and is impeding diaphragmatic excursion, will often result in dyspnea relief. Radiation therapy, especially radiation of the chest, puts a patient at risk for pulmonary pneumonitis and fibrosis and the resulting dyspnea. The area of lung involved in the radiation therapy and the dose of the radiation contribute to the risk. Age, histologic type, number of nodal sites involved, and radiotherapy duration affect the risk of dyspnea, which may occur immediately or may not appear until long after the completion of the radiation. Radiation therapy can also be effective in palliation of respiratory symptoms such as dyspnea.[17] Radiation therapy can reduce the size of a tumor and facilitate better diaphragmatic excursion and the relief of dyspnea; thus relief is a result of decreased compression.[18]

Patients with severe respiratory involvement requiring mechanical support often report experiencing dyspnea while on the ventilator, even when arterial blood gas levels are normal and the ventilator supplies a large portion of their minute ventilation requirement. In this situation, the perception of dyspnea is believed to result from a mismatch between the patient's ventilatory drive and the ventilator settings, such as a flow rate that is too slow, a respiratory rate that is too fast, and/or a V_T that is too large.[19]

The presence of other symptoms have been noted along with reports of dyspnea. Pain and dyspnea have been shown to be related in patients with lung cancer.[9] Cough, pain, psychologic distress, and organic factors (such as tumor growth) predict 33% of dyspnea in patients with lung cancer.[20] Pollution or other respiratory irritants can also exacerbate dyspnea.

Etiology

PHYSIOLOGICAL MECHANISMS OF DYSPNEA

Neuromechanical or the efferent-reafferent dissociation theory of dyspnea states that dyspnea is caused by a dissociation or mismatch between central respiratory motor activity and incoming afferent information from receptors in airways, lungs, and the chest wall. Therefore dyspnea is intensified when changes in airflow, respiratory pressure, or respiratory movement are not appropriate for the outgoing motor command.[1] Dyspnea can be caused by heightened ventilatory demand, respiratory muscle abnormalities, abnormal ventilatory impedance, and abnormal breathing patterns.

A second mechanism producing dyspnea is when neurochemical changes in blood gases result in hypoxemia and hypercapnia stimulating the chemoreceptors. This stimulation results in respiratory motor activity that produces dyspnea. Chemoreceptors may also have a direct dyspneogenic effect, since dyspnea can occur even without ventilatory changes. Hypoxia also contributes to the sensation of dyspnea.

In addition to the disease of cancer resulting directly in dyspnea are the effects of treatment. Radiation therapy results in destruction of the lung parenchyma and thus in dyspnea.[21] The clinical pathologic course is biphasic and is dependent upon the dose and volume of lung exposed to the radiation as well as the patient's preexisting pulmonary reserves. The process involves changes in the surfactant system, leading to alterations in alveolar surface tension and low compliance, which are the direct result of the radiation and become evident within weeks to months after exposure to radiation. These changes usually resolve with in few weeks or months but may lead to acute radiation pneumonitis. The late lung injury is characterized by progressive fibrosis. The mechanisms of chronic complications are believed by some to be related to the effects of radiation on the vascular tissue and may be evident months to years following treatment.[22]

After surgery, dyspnea is prevalent in the immediate postoperative period and may decline as the patient recovers from the surgery. Dyspnea is also commonly seen in those receiving chemotherapy. Patients often confuse the feeling of shortness of breath with their feelings of fatigue. Dyspnea is triggered by activity such as walking, climbing stairs, washing, bending, talking, and the like.[23]

PSYCHOLOGIC MECHANISMS OF DYSPNEA

There are affective influences on dyspnea perception. The correlation between dyspnea and anxiety has been demonstrated in a number of studies.[4,9] Although the two are related, there are no studies demonstrating a cause-and-effect relationship between dyspnea and anxiety. In fact, dyspnea and anxiety are separate dimensions.[4] Research supports the relationship of dyspnea and emotional status.[24] Dyspnea is accompanied by panic, fear, and a feeling of impending death, but it is not certain if these emotions are the cause or the result of dyspnea.[23]

Cognition, judgment, and attention have also influenced the perception of dyspnea. The interpretation or meaning of dyspnea influences the patient's perception of severity.[25] There have not been any studies in cancer patients to determine if a diagnosis of cancer or advanced cancer enhances the perception of dyspnea intensity. Dyspnea severity is influenced by perception. An adaptive response occurs with long-standing dyspnea and influences the patient's interpretation of dyspnea severity.[25]

Effects and Consequences

The presence of dyspnea results in a reduced quality of life that includes a reduction in social, work, and personal care activities. Often patients reduce their own activities in an effort to alleviate their dyspnea. Functional status is the consequence of dyspnea that is measured most often. When asked about the limitation on their activities, over 75% of lung cancer patients reported significant shortness of breath interfering with their functioning and overall quality of life.[9] Patients have also reported that dyspnea interferes with their psychologic functioning, such as mood and enjoyment.[26] This interference occurs even with mild dyspnea.[26]

Unrelieved dyspnea is very frightening for both the patient and family and is one of the main factors leading to hospitalization of cancer patients. Unrelieved symptoms requiring emergency department treatment have been shown to be predictive of the need for hospitalization.[27] Even without emergency department treatment, the presence of dyspnea is of deep concern because it is associated not only with loss of function but also with increased mortality.

Furthermore, those who reported respiratory symptoms were 39% more likely to complain of other symptoms than patients with no shortness of breath, and were 55% more likely to report other symptoms as being severe.[28] Symptom severity, including dyspnea, has also been found to be one of the factors, in addition to stage of cancer and age, to be predictive of death.[14]

There are also consequences for the person caring for the patient with dyspnea. Caring for a person experiencing dyspnea has been shown to have a negative influence on the caregiver, especially when the dyspnea is unrelieved. Caregivers may experience severe anxiety and helplessness as they witness the suffering and feel powerless to reduce it.[12] Caregiver distress is further complicated by the lack of an understanding of strategies to relieve symptoms on the part of health care providers.

Dyspnea Measurement and Patient Assessment

Dyspnea is a subjective symptom and is evaluated by patient self-report. It is also a multidimensional experience; however, the valid and reliable measures that are available focus mostly on the intensity of the sensation, not its many dimensions. There is no single measure of dyspnea that takes into account all the components such as duration, frequency, rate of onset, quality of the sensation, and the like.[1] In obtaining a patient's history, it is important to determine the onset of dyspnea, whether sudden or gradual. Acute dyspnea is characterized by rapid onset, whereas chronic dyspnea is characterized by persistence over time and a changing intensity.[29] Dyspnea is also contextual and is, therefore, rated along with activities or situations provoking it. Strategies used by the patient in coping with dyspnea, such as decreasing activities, pursed-lip breathing, avoiding emotional conflict, and the like, will influence patient report of dyspnea and are to be considered when evaluating dyspnea.[30] Dyspnea occurs along with other symptoms and changes over time, so it is measured along with other symptoms and monitored over time.[14]

The best way to measure dyspnea is determined by the purpose for the measurement. Disease-specific measures are most valuable when assessing changes in an individual patient after therapeutic interventions. Patient subjective report measures will be discussed first, followed by measures that include multiple symptoms, and then more global measures, such as quality of life measures. Finally, a full assessment of the patient will be discussed.

PATIENT REPORT MEASURES

Numeric Rating Scale (NRS). A numeric rating scale (NRS) has patients rate the intensity of their shortness of breath by choosing a number on a scale from 0 to 10 that represents the shortness of breath they are feeling right now (Fig. 38-1). Zero represents no shortness of breath, and 10 is shortness of breath as bad as can be. The NRS can be administered either in a written or verbal form and is extremely easy to administer and score. This scale is used clinically as a measure of dyspnea and was shown to be a valid measure of dyspnea in the patient with COPD.[31]

Graphic or Verbal Rating Scale (GRS). A graphic or verbal rating scale (GRS) is similar to the NRS but uses words instead of numbers, usually with choices for a rating. Scores on a verbal rating scale—with none, mild, moderate, severe, and horrible as the ratings—correlate highly with dyspnea ratings obtained using the visual analogue scale.[7]

Visual Analogue Dyspnea Scale (VADS). A visual analogue dyspnea scale (VADS) is another valid measure of dyspnea intensity. It consists of a 100-mm vertical visual analogue scale with anchors of "shortness of breath as bad as can be" at the top and "no shortness of breath" at the bottom (Fig. 38-2). Concurrent validity of this scale was established using both a horizontal visual analogue scale and a measure of airway obstruction. The correlation between the two analogue scales was 0.97, whereas those between the VADS and peak expiratory flow rate was −0.85.[32] Construct validity was established using the contrasted groups approach between those expected to have dyspnea and those not expected to have dyspnea. Differences between the two groups were significant for patients with COPD ($t = 9.73$, $p < 0.01$), as they were for asthmatic subjects ($t = 12.35$, $p < 0.01$).[33] Another anchor used is breathing distress. Distress, how much the patient is bothered by his or her breathing difficulty, is a different sensation from shortness of breath; thus it is suggested that two visual analogue scales be used, one for dyspnea intensity and another for dyspnea distress.[4] Breathing effort has also been used as an anchor for the VADS and produces ratings that are stabile and sensitive.[34] A change of 21 mm in the VADS would be clinically meaningful, showing the effectiveness of an intervention.[35]

DYSPNEA DESCRIPTORS

In addition to the intensity and distress of dyspnea, the quality of the dyspnea experience is measured by the descriptors patients use to characterize it. The words used to describe dyspnea have been shown to vary according to the disease state or cause of dyspnea. The words have also been shown to be stable over time, demonstrating their reliability as a measure of dyspnea.[34] Patients with lung cancer were compared in the descriptors they used to patients with asthma, COPD, interstitial lung disease, and cardiac failure. The patients with lung cancer were found to use "I cannot get enough air," "I feel out of breath," and

---

NUMERICAL RATING SCALE

On a scale from 0 to 10, indicate how much shortness of breath you have had in the past week where 0 = no shortness of breath and 10 = shortness of breath as the worst possible. Circle the number.

0   1   2   3   4   5   6   7   8   9   10

No shortness of breath   Worst possible

FIG. 38-1   Numeric rating scale.

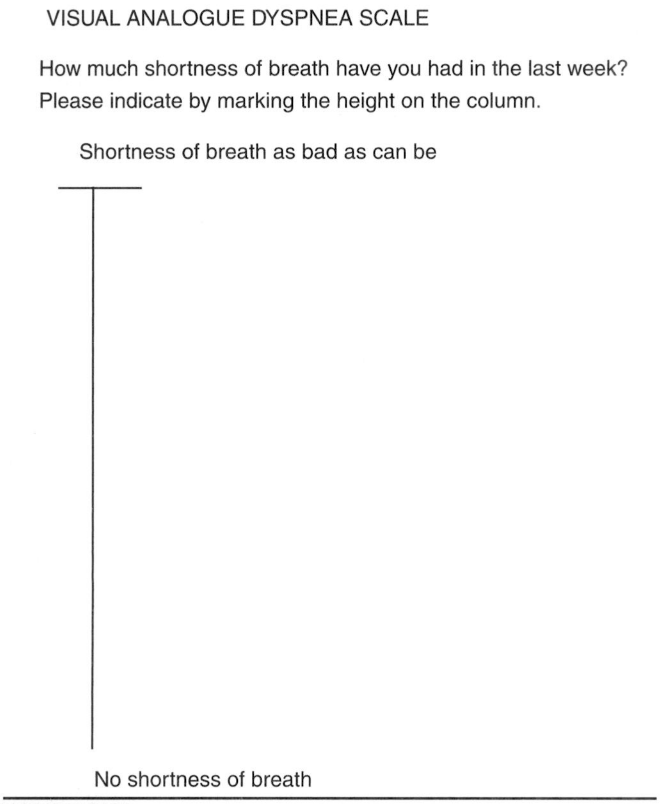

VISUAL ANALOGUE DYSPNEA SCALE

How much shortness of breath have you had in the last week?
Please indicate by marking the height on the column.

Shortness of breath as bad as can be

No shortness of breath

FIG. 38-2 Visual analogue dyspnea scale.

"My breathing requires effort" more than those with other diseases. Those with metastases were more likely to use descriptors such as "My chest feels tight," and "I feel that I am breathing more," than those without metastasis.[36] The study of patient descriptors has shown that different clusters of descriptors describe qualitatively different experiences of breathlessness. These analyses have differentiated feelings of the following: rapid, heaving breathing, exhalation and/or inhalation difficulty, work and/or effort, suffocating and/or smothering, air hunger, tightness and/or constriction, as well as not getting enough air and feeling out of breath.[36] Others have characterized the different dimensions or constructs of dyspnea to be "depth and frequency of breathing," "perceived need or urge to breathe" and "difficulty breathing and phase of respiration."[37] They propose that the different grouping of descriptors represent different underlying mechanisms of dyspnea, but further work is needed to determine the usefulness of these descriptor groupings in patient diagnosis and management.[37]

MEASURES THAT INCLUDE MULTIPLE SYMPTOMS

Dyspnea has also been found to occur with other symptoms such as fatigue, cough, and pain.[10] Thus, it is often included in a complete inventory of symptoms, such as with the **Memorial Symptom Assessment Scale.**[38] This scale consists of 24 symptoms in which respondents are asked to rate the frequency (how often it occurs), severity (intensity), and the distress (bother) dimension of each reported symptom on a range from 0 (not at all) to 4 (very much). In addition, there are 8 symptoms (such as hair loss and changes in appearance) for which frequency is not relevant, so respondents are only asked to rate severity and distress.

This scale was tested for validity on 246 patients with a variety of cancers. A factor analysis found three factors that were labeled as psychologic, high-prevalence physical, and low-prevalence physical. High correlations with the clinical status and quality of life measures give further support for the validity of the scale. Reliability was established using Cronbach's alpha with coefficients of 0.83 to 0.88.[38]

Symptom Distress Scale (SDS). The symptom distress scale (SDS) is another example of a measure that includes multiple symptoms, dyspnea being one of them. In this scale, patients are asked to rate each symptom on a 5-point response format ranging from 1 (normal or no distress) to 5 (extensive distress). Evidence for validity and Cronbach's alpha reliability (0.82 for the total scale) have been reported.[39,40]

Cancer Dyspnea Scale. The cancer dyspnea scale is a 12-item scale that records a sense of effort, a sense of anxiety, and a sense of discomfort related to dyspnea. These factors were developed using a factor analysis. The scale has construct and convergent validity as well as internal consistency and test-retest reliability.[41]

Breathlessness, Cough, and Sputum Scale. The breathlessness, cough, and sputum scale is a new scale that evaluates two symptoms (dyspnea and cough) and one sign commonly seen in patients with respiratory disease: sputum.[42] Patients are asked to rate the severity of the two symptoms and the one sign on a 5-point Likert scale. Higher scores indicate more severe symptoms and are summed to yield a total score. Internal consistency for the scale was established using the Cronbach's alpha and found to range from 0.70 for daily measures to 0.95 over time.[42] Reproducibility of the scores was found to range from 0.77 to 0.88. Validity was established by comparing scale scores with pulmonary function measures and quality of life measures. Pearson product-moment correlations ranged from −0.36 for FEV_1 to −0.44 for quality of life (using the St. George's Respiratory Questionnaire) to 0.59 for the SF-36 Physical Functioning subscale. It was also found to be sensitive to changes in patient disease severity.[42]

MEASUREMENT OF SYMPTOMS FROM RADIATION THERAPY

Symptoms resulting from radiation therapy are often evaluated by the grading system developed by the Radiation Therapy Oncology Group and the European Organization for Research in the Treatment of Cancer (RTOG/EORTC). This system for evaluation of acute lung injury proposes four grades. Grade 0 is no change; grade 1 is mild symptoms of dry cough or dyspnea on exertion; grade 2 is persistent cough requiring narcotic antitussive agents and/or dyspnea with minimal effort; grade 3 includes severe cough, unresponsive to narcotic antitussive agents, dyspnea at rest, clinical or radiographic evidence of acute pneumonitis, intermittent oxygen requirements, or requirements for steroids; and grade 4 is severe respiratory insufficiency that is unresponsive to treatment.[22] This grading system has not been demonstrated to be linear and is not related to the dose of radiation.

QUALITY OF LIFE MEASURES

There are also quality of life measures that include shortness of breath as a dimension of quality of life. An example would be the **EORTC QLQ-LC13,** which includes many of the symptoms experienced by cancer patients as well as the side effects from conventional chemotherapy and radiation therapy. This is a valid measure of quality of life because of its ability to discriminate between patients having different performance levels. The dyspnea subscale is reliable with a Cronbach's alpha of 0.70.[43]

A quality of life scale that includes a measure of dyspnea and was developed specifically to measure quality of life in lung cancer patients is the **Lung Cancer Symptom Scale.** Although this scale is described as measuring the physical and functional dimensions of quality of life, patients rate six symptoms (loss of appetite, fatigue, cough, dyspnea, hemoptysis, and pain) using a visual analogue scale or a numeric rating scale.[8] Patients rate their symptoms using five descriptors with clarifying sentences. In the case of dyspnea, the clarifying sentences relate to the level of exercise needed to provoke dyspnea. The descriptors are none (scored as 100), mild (scored as 75), moderate (scored as 50), marked (scored as 25), and severe (scored as 0). Patients also rate their overall symptom distress but not the distress of each symptom separately. The reliability of the scale (internal consistency) yielded a Cronbach's alpha of 0.89. Convergent validity was established for the NRS form of the scale with an intraclass correlation coefficient of 0.90.[44] This scale was found to be sensitive to the effects of palliative radiation therapy resulting in a significant reduction in dyspnea (p = 0.0003).[45]

Monitoring dyspnea in the clinical setting is an important but complex issue. The best measure to use depends on the purpose for the measurement, the patient's level of disease, the patient's reading level and the setting in which the measurement is occurring. Since dyspnea is defined as a subjective sensation, the most accurate measure is one that measures it directly from the patient. However, all direct-report dyspnea measures are currently one-dimensional, usually assessing the severity or intensity of the symptom. Among these measures the one that is most often selected in the emergency or critical care situation, is the NRS. It is a useful way to assess dyspnea quickly and easily. In most settings it also matches the measure used to assess pain, making it easier for patients to report. There are situations where symptom alleviation must be balanced with a desire to maintain physical and social functioning, such as in patients with advanced disease. In this situation a more comprehensive quality of life measure, such as the EORTC QLQ-LC13, or the Lung Cancer Symptom Scale would be more desirable.

DYSPNEA IN CHILDREN

Although symptom management has been placed at the top of the list of nursing research priorities in the area of childhood cancer, surprisingly little research has focused on this problem. Age-appropriate measures are needed to monitor symptoms in children and adolescents. Dyspnea is one of the most commonly experienced symptoms in children at the end of life.[16] To assess dyspnea in children, a word descriptor scale, using language commonly used by children, has been found to be appropriate: a 4-point scale using "rotten," "just okay," "good" and "great." Colors have also been used to have children rate dyspnea.[46] For adolescents, Hinds and colleagues found that McCorkle and Young's Symptom Distress Scale was easy for them to use and produced Cronbach's alphas of 0.82 and 0.85, demonstrating internal consistency for the scale in this population.[39,47] More research is needed to develop age-appropriate scales for assessing symptoms in children. It is important to understand how children and adolescents experience, create meanings about, and respond to their symptoms, as well as how they communicate these experiences to the adults in their world.

Comprehensive Patient Assessment

The assessment of the patient is comprehensive and includes an assessment of the patient's history and physical, pulmonary function, and comorbid conditions, or other factors that may contribute to respiratory compromise.

HISTORY

Patient history is important in dyspnea assessment to determine the onset of dyspnea, its duration, and the circumstances under which it occurs, as well as the patient's prior experience with dyspnea. Prior exposure to dyspnea influences the patient's sensitivity to the sensation.[25] In addition, risk factors are assessed, such as the type, the location, the size, and the stage of the cancer. Cancer treatment the patient has received or is receiving is also important. Comorbidities that the patient may have must be determined, such as respiratory disease, cardiac disease, and anemia.

PULMONARY FUNCTION TESTS (PFTs)

Pulmonary function tests (PFTs) are not useful in determining dyspnea; dyspnea can only be determined by self-report. Dyspnea can occur in a person without lung involvement and with normal or near normal PFTs; however, 93% of cancer patients with dyspnea were found to have abnormal PFTs.[48] Assessment of respiratory muscle function is also important in determining the patient's potential for dyspnea, since diminished maximum inspiratory pressure (MIP) is present in those cancer patients with severe dyspnea.[48] PFTs are used to rule out respiratory disease. The ratio of forced expiratory volume to forced vital capacity (FEV_1/FVC%) is the accepted standard measure of obstructive lung disease when compared with the predicted normal values. In radiation pneumonitis, abnormalities relate to the volume of irradiated lung tissue and will consist of decreases in the vital capacity, the residual volume, and the FEV_1. Decreases in lung compliance will also be noted. The diffusion capacity appears to be the most sensitive parameter in this situation.[22]

ARTERIAL BLOOD GASES

ABGs are important in the assessment of dyspnea and should be taken at rest without supplemental oxygen, if possible. The parameters should include partial pressure of oxygen and carbon dioxide, as well as oxygen saturation. Since dyspnea is contextual and related to exercise, oxygen saturation during graded exercise may be useful for some patients.

PHYSICAL EXAM

The physical exam should assess for accessory muscle use for breathing. In a clinical setting, accessory muscle use can be determined by placing the subject in a sitting position and observing for the rise of the clavicle during inspiration. If it is not detected, it can be described as absent; if it is seen to rise but it is barely perceptible, it can be described as mild; and if it is pronounced, it can be described as severe. In a study of 20 patients with COPD measured at a time of high, medium, and low dyspnea, the only clinical sign found to be significantly increased as dyspnea increased was the retraction of the sternomastoid muscle.[32] Sternomastoid muscle use was also found to be greater during high dyspnea compared to low dyspnea. The use of accessory muscles such as the sternomastoid muscle, and not the primary muscle of respiration, the diaphragm, is associated with dyspnea. Thus, accessory muscle is the most appropriate clinical sign of dyspnea. However, it is also important to observe the positioning chosen by the patient for breathing comfort, such as being unable to lie flat, needing support, and so on.

Interventions

The first step in alleviating dyspnea is to ensure that the patient is receiving adequate ventilation. Checking that the patient has a patent airway and adequate level of ventilation and oxygenation are the first step. For those with hypoxemia, one of the most widely used therapies is the use of **supplemental oxygen.** In an emergency department, oxygen therapy was found to be the most common treatment for dyspnea, being prescribed for 34% of cancer patients there.[27] The benefits of oxygen therapy in relieving dyspnea are clear for the patient with hypoxemia. However, the benefits of supplemental oxygen for those without hypoxemia are mixed, with some finding oxygen to be of benefit and others not finding such a benefit over compressed air.[49] It is thought that perhaps the flow of air at the nose and across airway receptors may be more important than oxygen concentration in the relief of dyspnea.

In patients with cancer who have adequate ventilation and oxygenation, some have recommended using this finding and having oxygen blow through a nasal cannula for its placebo effect. This finding led to the recommendation of using a **fan blowing** on the patient's cheek for the relief of dyspnea. Although there is little empirical evidence documenting the effectiveness of this as a dyspnea-relieving strategy, it is something that patients have reported using and that hospital nurses have recommended for dyspnea relief. The first well-designed study exploring this therapy was done by Schwartzstein and colleagues in which they studied 16 normal subjects in whom dyspnea was induced by having them breath air containing 55 torr of CO_2 through an inspiratory resistive load.[50] Dyspnea was recorded using a modified Borg scale, comparing times when cold air was blown on the cheek to times when there was no flow and to times when cold air was blown on the leg. Dyspnea was rated as significantly lower when cold air was blown on the cheek.

There are a variety of other nonpharmacologic interventions that have been shown to be effective in relieving dyspnea. Many take advantage of the high correlation observed between respiratory distress and anxiety. **Relaxation techniques** have been shown to be effective in reducing dyspnea and anxiety. Patients have reported using self-taught relaxation techniques for the relief of dyspnea as an adjunct to other therapies. Others have found that these self-management strategies are different for patients with different diseases and from different ethnic backgrounds.[51] Patients can be taught progressive muscle relaxation techniques that they can initiate themselves periodically to help reduce their dyspnea. These techniques will also result in a decrease in anxiety, an emotion that is often associated with increased dyspnea. During progressive muscle relaxation, respiratory rate is decreased and tidal volume is increased, changes that are often associated with a decrease in dyspnea.[52]

Guided imagery in which the patient plays a tape guiding them to visualize a scene that the patient finds relaxing has also been proposed as a technique to reduce dyspnea. Distraction techniques, such as the playing of music the patient finds relaxing, have been shown to alleviate dyspnea.[52] Reflexology has shown some positive, but short-lasting effects.[53] Acupuncture has also been shown to be effective in reducing respiratory rate, in relieving dyspnea, and reducing anxiety.

Slowing the breathing to increase the expiratory phase of respiration reduces dyspnea. **Pursed-lip breathing** slows expiratory flow and maintains back pressure to avoid airway collapse during expiration. It also improves the pattern of respiratory muscle recruitment, thus alleviating the sensation of dyspnea.[52] Pursed-lip breathing techniques are helpful for most patients, but they are especially helpful in those with a pattern of obstructive respiratory impairment.

Positioning the patient for comfort and adequate ventilation and perfusion is one strategy that patients may find helpful. Using a semi-Fowler's position maximizes the strength of the diaphragm in expiration. Leaning forward over a table or chair and using the elbows to brace the patient by forming a tripod with the body can be of help to some. If the patient has a tumor of the lung and is lying down in bed, positioning the patient has to be planned. Both perfusion and lung expansion have to be considered. Perfusion is better in the dependent part of the lung, which would advocate having the good lung on the down side. However, if the tumor is large or for some other reason impairs lung expansion, then the patient would achieve better oxygenation with the good lung positioned in the up position, where it is free to expand. Having the patient lie prone is not often used, but patients often find it helpful.

Modification of activity is another recommended intervention. Often patients will make individual modifications. This involves having patients slow or pace their activity to fit their limitations. Techniques such as reducing the number of steps necessary to complete a task or scheduling tasks for peak energy periods have been found to be helpful. Eliminating activities that require unsupported arm-lifting activities have been found to be helpful, because arm lifting competes for the use of respiratory accessory muscles and can produce dyspnea.[54]

Exercise has also been recommended for dyspnea alleviation. Patients who are able are encouraged to participate in exercise programs to provide graded exercises in a structured, safe environment to desensitize the patient to dyspnea. Exercise training substantially improves the impact of a dyspnea self-management program with a home walking prescription.[55] It also improves aerobic capacity, increases neuromuscular coupling, and improves tolerance to dyspnogenic stimuli.[56]

For those patients who are producing mucus and are having difficulty expelling it, it is important to teach effective cough technique for airway clearance and removal of mucus plugs. Chest physiotherapy is also recommended in this situation since it assists in mobilizing secretions and using gravity to assist in removal. Encouragement of adequate fluid intake (if no cardiac contradictions are present) is thought by some to aid in thinning respiratory secretions. Promotion of health via smoking cessation support and education is important to reduce the risk of further respiratory compromise.

A **comprehensive nursing intervention** has also been shown to be effective in improving dyspnea in lung cancer patients.

In a multicenter randomized controlled trial comparing a nursing clinic offering interventions for breathlessness with best supportive care, the intervention group improved significantly at 8 weeks in breathlessness, performance, depression, and physical symptom distress. The nursing interventions combined breathing control, activity pacing, relaxation techniques, and psychosocial support. Others have suggested that such a comprehensive approach include an assessment of the factors ameliorating and exacerbating dyspnea, the meaning of breathlessness for the individual, goal setting, and patient and family education to alert them to recognize problems warranting pharmacologic or medical intervention. Teaching patients coping and adaptation strategies, along with a comprehensive nursing intervention, has been shown to improve breathlessness and functional capacity.[53] However, it is not known what components of the intervention are most critical to include, or if certain aspects are more effective and essential to dyspnea relief than others. Symptom relief is best achieved by working with patients in their home rather than requiring them to come to an office.

Education in symptom management is advocated by nurses, yet few patients with lung cancer reported receiving any education by health care professionals in relation to their shortness of breath. This may be because patients rarely report the presence of dyspnea unless they are asked. When asked, between 21% and 90% of cancer patients have indicated they experienced dyspnea, depending upon the stage and type of cancer.[49] Yet dyspnea is rarely assessed or noted in the patient's chart. Patients report feeling isolated and being left to cope with their dyspnea in their own manner. Nurses must assess for the presence of dyspnea and if needed teach patients effective coping strategies such as pacing activities, medication use, and dyspnea self-management.

Furthermore, symptom management at the end of life is crucial for both patients and their family. It is important to prepare a patient's family for serious dyspnea to be able to provide comfort in the final phase of life. Comfort strategies such as use of opiates and benzodiazepines to relieve dyspnea and promote comfort are discussed and incorporated as part of the plan of care. It is important to evaluate whether a patient wants to be more alert to participate in family interaction or more sedated for symptom relief.

PHARMACOLOGIC THERAPIES

Opiates have been recommended in the treatment of dyspnea because of their respiratory depressant effect on the central process of neural signals within the central nervous system. They have been shown to decrease expiratory volume (V_E) at rest and during submaximal levels of exercise. The danger with the use of these drugs is the concomitant increase in CO_2. Opioids have been described as alleviating dyspnea by blunting perceptual responses and decreasing the intensity of the respiratory sensation. They have been recommended for acute dyspnea, but there is little to recommend their use in long-term, progressive dyspnea such as occurs with cancer.[1] There is some evidence to indicate that nebulized morphine is effective in the relief of dyspnea, but the evidence is minimal and this is not recommended for practice.[1] Another nebulized medication, although not an opiate, is lidocaine; however, its effectiveness is reported to be much weaker.

Diuretic medication may be recommended to decrease the demand on the heart, if fluid overload is found. Bronchodilator administration by nebulizer or metered dose inhaler may be prescribed to relieve brochospasm. The goal of nebulizer treatments is to deliver a therapeutic dose to reduce dyspnea and cough.

Steroids and nonsteroidal antiinflammatory drugs (NSAIDs) have been used in the treatment of dyspnea resulting from an inflammatory process such as radiation-induced pneumonitis. The effectiveness of steroid treatment has been questioned, but steroids continue to be used, mostly because of their documented effectiveness in controlling inflammation, and also because there is little else to offer the patient. In addition to their antiinflammatory effect is the effect of steroids on general well-being. NSAIDs are recommended to reduce airway inflammation and create more patent airways. They are used in palliative care.

Benzodiazepines are recommended for use in the relief of dyspnea only when there is accompanying anxiety. The studies, however, involved large doses and much sedation of the patient.[57]

Palliative radiotherapy can reduce a tumor and decrease dyspnea for a period of time. On the other hand, radiation therapy can also result in dyspnea when it produces radiation pneumonitis.

Assessment and Teaching of Caregivers

In addition to the care of the patient with dyspnea is the care of the person providing this care. Oftentimes provided in the home by family members, this caregiving is a taxing experience. The caregiver becomes increasingly stressed and reports an increase in physical and emotional symptoms during this time. Family members who are competent to care for chronically ill individuals report the need for more information about providing care that will relieve the stress of the illness on themselves and their loved ones. It is not enough that interventions be effective in relieving dyspnea; they must also meet the needs and acceptance of the family caregivers who are to put them to use. In addition to providing information is the need to encourage patients and caregivers to build social support networks and to provide for respite care to relieve the burden on the caregiver.

There are a variety of therapies possible for the relief of dyspnea. The most appropriate intervention to use to alleviate dyspnea depends on the factors contributing to the symptom, such as the presence of underlying respiratory disease or the level of oxygenation, the stage of the cancer, the availability of assistance from health professionals or family, and the desires of the patient and family members. It may also depend on the cultural preferences of the patient and family. For instance, African American patients have been found to cope with dyspnea using traditional medical care, self-care wisdom, self-care action, and self-care resources.[54] (See Chapter 35 for more discussion on caring for the caregiver and cultural variations in family adaptations to caregiving.)

Outcomes of Nursing Interventions

The main outcome desired is the reduction or the elimination of dyspnea. Thus to evaluate outcomes and monitor the effectiveness of interventions implies that the symptoms will be assessed on a regular basis. Since dyspnea is exacerbated by the presence of other symptoms, assessment is not limited to dyspnea but rather includes a full inventory of symptoms. It is reasonable to expect that dyspnea interventions, if effective, will result in a reduction or the elimination of other symptoms, in addition to dyspnea.

The reduction of symptoms has to be balanced against the patient's response to the therapy. For instance, if morphine is needed to alleviate dyspnea, the patient may not be fully alert and able to interact with his or her family. The patient may feel it is more desirable to have some level of dyspnea but be able to interact with family and friends, rather than achieve full relief from dyspnea. Meeting the desires of the patient is thus another outcomes indicator of a successful dyspnea intervention.

Considerations for Older Adults

Elderly persons experience changes in lung function and respiratory muscle function that results in increased air trapping and enhanced likelihood of dyspnea. Indeed, some researchers have found that older patients report more dyspnea than younger patients.[24,20] However, other researchers have not found age of the patient to be predictive of the extent of symptoms experienced, or of the time to appearance of symptoms.

It must be noted, however, that elderly patients do have difficulty using the visual analogue scale. It is recommended in these patients that a numeric rating scale be used to assess for dyspnea.

End of Life

Not all patients at the end of life are elderly, but it is important to recognize that dyspnea is frequently experienced by those at end of life, and patients and caregivers have reported it to be the most frightening and upsetting symptom. It is accompanied by feelings of fear, extreme fatigue, and loss of memory, concentration, and appetite. A study of terminally ill patients with cancer showed them to be troubled by dyspnea and pain, with the dyspnea increasing until the time of death. It is thus recommended that dyspnea be assessed in the patient along with other symptoms.[58] However, it is important to assess symptoms directly from patient report, because use of a proxy, such as the caregiver in end of life, may not provide adequate assessment of a patient's dyspnea.[59]

REVIEW QUESTIONS

✓ Case Study

Mr. Jones was newly diagnosed with advanced-stage lung cancer with a mediastinal tumor. He was a male in his early 60s. He was admitted to the hospital because of his complaints of shortness of breath and fatigue. Mr. Jones had a family history of lung cancer. His father had died of it when he was in his early 60s. Mr. Jones had tried to stop smoking on several occasions using a variety of techniques, including hypnosis, but had not been successful. He had been having what he referred to as a "smoker's cough" for several years, but had assumed that it was a normal occurrence because of his smoking. He then noticed that he gradually was having more and more difficulty with mild exertion, such as climbing the stairs. So he limited the times he climbed the stairs each day. He then began to have more and more difficulty with his breathing and became more and more fatigued. This is what led him to seek medical attention.

The goal of his care was the relief of symptoms. This was accomplished by nebulized bronchodilation to expand the airways and allow for better oxygen flow to the alveoli. Morphine was used to ease the breathing discomfort. Chemotherapy was explored to decrease the tumor size and relieve some of the pressure on the bronchioles. The challenge for nursing was to talk with the family of this newly diagnosed man and discuss the use of hospice in his home. The family was surprised by the diagnosis and, although they had been having difficulty with his steadily decreasing activity level, they were not prepared to deal with the notion of him only having 6 months to live. They wanted to be sure he would be free of symptoms. They needed much teaching about symptom management and to learn to become comfortable with the hospice nurses.

QUESTIONS

1. Which of the following best describes dyspnea?
   a. Dyspnea can be determined by evaluating the patient's level of functioning compared to his or her peers.
   b. Dyspnea can be evaluated by observing or asking the patient about the effort required to breathe.
   c. Dyspnea is a subjective experience that is inadequately characterized as related to physiologic changes.
   d. Dyspnea is caused by emotions.
2. Patients at high risk for dyspnea include which of the following?
   a. Patients with lung cancer and patients on a ventilator
   b. Patients at end of life and patients who smoke
   c. Patients with cancer of the liver and respiratory patients
   d. Patients who exercise vigorously and those with angina
3. Dyspnea has been shown to occur when the patient is on a ventilator. What is one rationale proposed for this?
   a. There is inadequate oxygenation.
   b. There is an imbalance in the information coming from the chest wall and the central respiratory sensory activity.
   c. The patient is anxious and is fighting the ventilator.
   d. The tidal volume is too large.
4. What can be said about the visual analogue scale used for patient self-report of dyspnea?
   a. This scale is not recommended for older adults.
   b. This scale is to be used for all patients at risk for developing dyspnea.
   c. This scale is not as valuable in dyspnea assessment as is patient report of activities.
   d. This scale is not a valid measure of dyspnea.

5. Which of the following is most important to be included in patient assessment for dyspnea?
   a. Pulmonary function tests
   b. An assessment of all symptoms experienced by the patient and the factors precipitating dyspnea
   c. A review of the patient's activities of daily living
   d. Examination of chest distention

6. A patient with late-stage lung cancer comes into the office and does not appear to be having difficulty breathing. What does the provider proceed to do?
   a. Focuses assessment on the stage of cancer and the response to therapy
   b. Does a thorough assessment of the patient including pulmonary function tests
   c. Has the patient complete an inventory of his or her symptoms including frequency, severity, and how much the patient is bothered by the symptom
   d. Draws a blood gas to determine the patient's level of oxygenation

7. Dyspnea is relieved by which of the following?
   a. Placing the patient in a room without distractions
   b. Having the patient lie supine to fully perfuse the patient's lungs
   c. Having a fan blow on the patient's arm
   d. Regular visits to the pulmonologist

8. Relaxation reduces dyspnea. Which of the following statements is also true?
   a. This should be a recommended technique for all patients complaining of dyspnea.
   b. Relaxation should only be used after the patient has received a full pulmonary workup to be sure the dyspnea does not have an organic cause.
   c. This technique is effective only through the reduction of anxiety.
   d. Relaxation is used as an adjunct to other dyspnea-reduction techniques.

9. At the end of life, how is dyspnea relief best achieved?
   a. Using deep breathing techniques
   b. Using morphine to dull the sensation of dyspnea
   c. Using a variety of techniques that match the wishes of the patient
   d. Careful assessment of the patient's symptoms

10. The numeric rating scale for assessment of dyspnea is a self-report measure. What else is true about the NRS?
    a. It is not as good to use as the visual analogue scale.
    b. It is more difficult for older patients to use.
    c. It provides a wide range of scores for patients to indicate their dyspnea.
    d. It is recommended for measurement of dyspnea in children.

ANSWERS

1. **C.** *Rationale:* Dyspnea is a subjective experience of the patient best evaluated by self-report, not by physiologic measures. Functioning is the result of dyspnea, not dyspnea itself. Effort is different from dyspnea, which is sensation of difficulty with breathing. Dyspnea is related to emotions but not caused by them.

2. **A.** *Rationale:* Lung cancer is one of the cancers with a high rate of patients experiencing dyspnea. Patients on a ventilator are also at risk for dyspnea. Although patients at end of life are at high risk for dyspnea, smoking is only indirectly related to dyspnea. Patients with cancer of the liver are not at high risk for dyspnea. Although exercise will produce an increase in respiratory rate, it does not result in dyspnea.

3. **D.** *Rationale:* The size of the tidal volume, the respiratory rate, and the flow rate all influence the patient's perception of dyspnea. On a ventilator the patient's oxygen levels are monitored and unlikely to be inadequate. Dyspnea is not related to central respiratory sensory activity. Anxiety, although related to dyspnea, is not a cause of dyspnea.

4. **A.** *Rationale:* The visual analogue scale is not recommended for older adults. It is therefore not recommended for use with all patients at risk for dyspnea. It is also not recommended for use with children. Assessing patient activities does not assess dyspnea, but rather the consequences of dyspnea.

5. **D.** *Rationale:* Dyspnea assessment should include the other symptoms experienced along with dyspnea, as well as the precipitating factors. Pulmonary function tests are not diagnostic of dyspnea. Limitation in the patient's activities of daily living may or may not be a consequence of dyspnea. Chest distension is not diagnostic of dyspnea.

6. **C.** *Rationale:* It is important to ask patients about their symptoms even if they do not report them when they come in for a checkup. The practitioner does need to focus on the patient's cancer and treatment, but symptom assessment is also required. Dyspnea is not directly related to the patient's level of oxygenation.

7. **D.** *Rationale:* Lying supine has been shown to reduce dyspnea. For a fan to be effective it would need to blow on the patient's face, not on the patient's arm. Avoiding distractions is more likely to exacerbate dyspnea rather than relieve it. Pulmonologists focus on the underlying respiratory disease rather than dyspnea itself.

8. **D.** *Rationale:* Relaxation is a complementary technique and should be used along with other measures, such as pharmacologic interventions. Although relaxation has the potential to help all patients, some do not want to use the technique or respond better to other techniques. A full pulmonary workup is not needed in all patients, especially those who already have a diagnosis, such as lung cancer. Relaxation works directly on dyspnea as well as through the reduction of anxiety.

9. **C.** *Rationale:* The wishes of the patient are most important in planning care at end of life. Although morphine is effective in relieving dyspnea, the patient may not want to experience the side effects of morphine, such as sleeping. Deep breathing can relieve dyspnea, but it is unlikely to alleviate it completely. Assessment alone is not effective in dyspnea relief.

10. **C.** *Rationale:* The NRS provides a range of scores for patients to indicate their dyspnea. It is easier to use than the visual analogue scale, and is less difficult for older people to use. This scale has not been evaluated for use in children.

REFERENCES

1. Meek PM, Schwartzstein RM, Adams L et al: Dyspnea: mechanisms, assessment, and management: A consensus statement, *Am J Respir Crit Care Med* 159(1):321-340, 1999.
2. Lenz E, Pugh LC, Milligan RA et al: The middle range theory of unpleasant symptoms: an update, *ANS Adv in Nurs Sci* 19(3):14-27, 1997.
3. Armstrong TS: Symptoms experience: a concept analysis, *Oncol Nurs Forum* 30(4):601-606, 2003.
4. Carrieri-Kohlman V, Gormley JM, Eiser S et al: Dyspnea and the affective response during exercise training in obstructive pulmonary disease, *Nurs Res* 50(3):136-146, 2001.
5. Schwartzstein RM: The language of dyspnea. In Mahler DA, editor: *Dyspnea*, New York, 1998, Marcel Dekker.
6. Harver A, Mahler DA, Schwartzstein RM et al: Descriptors of breathlessness in healthy individuals, *Chest* 118(3):679-690, 2000.
7. Dudgeon DJ, Krisjanson L, Sloan JA et al: Dyspnea in cancer patients: prevalence and associated factors, *J Pain Symptom Manage* 21(2):95-102, 2001.
8. Lutz S, Norrell R, Bertucio C et al: Symptom frequency and severity in patients with metastatic or locally recurrent lung cancer: a prospective study using the lung cancer symptom scale in a community hospital, *J Palliat Med* 4(2):157-165, 2001.
9. Smith EL, Hann DM, Ahles TA et al. Dyspnea, anxiety, body consciousness and quality of life in patient with lung cancer, *J Pain Symptom Manage* 21(4):323-329, 2001.
10. Gift AG, Jablonski A, Stommel M et al: Symptom clusters in patients with lung cancer, *Oncol Nurs Forum* 31(2):203-210, 2004.
11. Claessens MT, Lynn J, Zhong Z et al: Dying with lung cancer or chronic obstructive pulmonary disease: insight from support, *J Amer Ger Soc* 48(5):S146-S153, 2000.
12. Booth S, Silvester ST, Todd C: Breathlessness in cancer and chronic obstructive pulmonary disease: using a qualitative approach to describe the experience of patients and careers, *Pall Supp Care* 1:337-344, 2003.
13. Ripamonti C: Management of dyspnea in advanced cancer patients, *Support Care Cancer* 7(4):133-143, 1999.
14. Gift AG, Stommel M, Jablonski A et al: Symptoms over time in patients with lung cancer, *Nurs Res* 52(6):393-399, 2003.
15. McCarthy EP, Phillips RS, Zhong Z et al: Dying with cancer: patients' function, symptoms and care preferences as death approaches, *J Am Geriatr Soc* 48(Suppl):S110-S121, 2000.
16. Wolfe J, Grier HE, Klar N et al: Symptoms and suffering at the end of life in children with cancer, *N Engl J Med* 342(5):326-333, 2000.
17. Lutz ST, Huang DT, Ferguson CL et al. A retrospective quality of life analysis using the Lung Cancer Symptom Scale in patients treated with palliative radiotherapy for advanced nonsmall cell lung cancer, *Int J Radiat Oncol Biol Phys* 37(1):117-122, 1997.
18. Kirova YM, Chen J, Rabarijaona LI et al: Radiotherapy as palliative treatment for metastatic melanoma, *Melanoma Res* 9(6):611-613, 1999.
19. Knebel A, Strider VC, Wood C: The art and science of caring for ventilator-assisted patients: learning from our clinical experience, *Crit Care Nurs Clin North Am* 6(4):819-829, 1994.
20. Tanaka K, Akechi T, Okuyama T et al: Factors correlated with dyspnea in advanced lung cancer patients: organic causes and what else? *J Pain Symptom Manage* 23(6):490-500, 2002.
21. Beinert T, Binder D, Stuschke M et al: Oxidant-induced lung injury in anticancer therapy, *Eur J Med Res* 4(2):43-53, 1999.
22. McDonald S, Rubin P, Phillips TL et al: Injury to the lung from cancer therapy: clinical syndromes, measurable endpoints, and potential scoring systems, *Int J Radiat Oncol Biol Phys* 31(5):1187-1203, 1995.
23. O'Driscoll M, Corner J, Bailey C: The experience of breathlessness in lung cancer, *Eur J Cancer Care* 8:37-43, 1999.
24. Martinez-Moragon E, Perpina Belloch M, de Diego A et al: Determinants of dyspnea in patients with different grades of stable asthma, *J Asthma* 40(4):375-382, 2003.
25. Meek PM: Influence of attention and judgment on perception of breathlessness in healthy individuals and patients with chronic obstructive pulmonary disease, *Nurs Res* 49(1):11-19, 2000.
26. Tanaka K, Akechi T, Okuyama T et al: Prevalence and screening of dyspnea interfering with daily life activities in ambulatory patients with advanced lung cancer, *J Pain Symptom Manage* 23(6):484-489, 2002.
27. Parshall, MB, Welsh, JD, Brockopp et al: Dyspnea duration, distress and intensity in emergency department visits for heart failure, *Heart Lung* 30(1):47-56, 2001.
28. Farncombe M: Dyspnea. Assessment and treatment, *Support Care Cancer* 5(2):94-99, 1997.
29. McCarley C: A model of chronic dyspnea, *Image J Nurs Schol* 31(3):231-236, 1999.
30. Tanaka K, Akechi T, Okayama T et al: Factors correlated with dyspnea in advanced lung cancer patients: organic causes and what else? *J Pain Symptom Manage* 23(6):490-500, 2002.
31. Gift AG, Narsavage G: Validation of the numeric rating scale as a measure of dyspnea, *Am J Crit Care* 7(3):200-204, 1998.
32. Gift AG, Plaut SM, Jacox AK: Psychologic and physiologic factors related to dyspnea in subjects with chronic obstructive pulmonary disease, *Heart Lung* 15:595-60l, 1986.
33. Gift AG: Validation of a vertical visual analogue scale as a measure of clinical dyspnea, *Rehabil Nurs* 14(6):323-325, 1989.
34. Meek PM, Lareau SC, Hu J: Are self-reports of breathing effort and breathing distress stable and valid measures among persons with asthma, persons with COPD and healthy persons? *Heart Lung* 32(5):335-346, 2003.
35. Ander DS, Aisiku IP, Ratcliff JJ et al: Measuring the dyspnea of decompensated heart failure with a visual analog scale: how much improvement is meaningful? *Congest Heart Failure* 10(July/August):188-191, 2004.
36. Wilcock A, Crosby V, Hughes A et al: Descriptors of breathing in patients with cancer and other cardiorespiratory diseases, *J Pain Symptom Manage* 23(3):182-189, 2002.
37. Harver A, Mahler DA, Schwartzstein RM Et al: Descriptors of breathlessness in healthy individuals, *Chest* 118:679-690, 2000.
38. Portenoy RK, Thaler HT, Kornblith AB: et al: The memorial symptom assessment scale: an instrument for the evaluation of symptom prevalence, characteristics and distress, *Eur J Cancer* 30A(9):1326-1336, 1994.
39. McCorkle R, Young K: Development of a symptom distress scale, *Cancer Nurs* 1(5):373-378, 1978.
40. McCorkle R, Benoliel JQ: A randomized clinical trial of home nursing care for lung cancer patients *Cancer* 64(6):1375-1382, 1989.
41. Tanaka K, Akechi T, Okuyama T et al: Development and validation of the cancer dyspnea scale: a multidimensional, brief, self-rating scale, *Br J Cancer* 82(4):800-805, 2000.
42. Leidy NK, Schmier JK, Jones MK et al: Evaluating symptoms in chronic obstructive pulmonary disease: validation of the breathlessness, cough and sputum scale, *Respir Med* 97(Suppl A):S59- S70, 2003.
43. Bergman B, Aaronson NK, Ahmedzai S et al: The EORTC QLQ-LC13: A modular supplement to the EORTC Core Quality of Life Questionnaire (QLQ-C30) for use in lung cancer clinical trials. EORTC Study Group on Quality of Life, *Eur J Cancer* 30A(5):635-642, 1994.
44. Hollen PJ, Gralla RJ, Kris MG et al: A comparison of visual analogue and numerical rating scale formats for the lung cancer symptom scale (LCSS): does format affect patient ratings of symptoms and quality of life? *Qual Life Res* 14:837-847, 2005.
45. Lutz ST, Huang DT, Ferguson CL et al: A retrospective quality of life analysis using the lung cancer symptom scale in patients treated with palliative radiotherapy for advanced nonsmall cell lung cancer, *Int J Radiat Oncol Biol Phys* 37(1):117-122, 1997.
46. Kohlman-Carrieri V, Kieckhefer G, Janson-Bjerklie S et al: The sensation of pulmonary dyspnea in school-age children, *Nurs Res* 40(2):81-85, 1991.
47. Hinds PS, Quargnenti A, Bush AJ et al: An evaluation of the impact of a self-care coping intervention on psychological and clinical outcomes in adolescents with newly diagnosed cancer, *Eur J Oncol Nurs* 4(1):6-17, 2000.
48. Dudgeon DJ, Lertzman M: Dyspnea in the advanced cancer patient, *J Pain Symptom Manage* 16(4):212-219, 1998.
49. Thomas JR, von Gunten CF: Management of dyspnea, *J Support Oncol* 1(1):23-34, 2003.
50. Schwartzstein RM, Lahive K, Pope A et al: Cold facial stimulation reduces breathlessness induced in normal subjects, *Am Rev Respir Dis* 136(1):56-61, 1987.
51. Nield M: Dyspnea self-management in African Americans with chronic lung disease, *Heart Lung* 29(1):50-55, 2000.

52. Carrieri-Kohlman V, Janson S: Managing dyspnea. In Hinshaw AS, Feetham SL, Shaver JLF, editors: *Handbook of clinical nursing research*, Thousand Oaks, Calif, 1999, Sage.

53. Sola I, Thompson E, Subirana M et al: Non-invasive interventions for improving well-being and quality of life in patients with lung cancer, *Cochrane Database Syst Rev*, 2004, Issue 4. Art No:CD004282.pub2. DOI:10.1002/14651858.CD004282.pub2.

54. Lareau SC, Meek PM, Press D et al: Dyspnea in patients with chronic obstructive pulmonary disease: does dyspnea worsen longitudinally in the presence of declining lung function? *Heart Lung* 28(1):65-73, 1999.

55. Stulbarg MS, Carrieri-Kohlman V, Demir-Deviren S et al: Exercise training improves outcomes of a dyspnea self management program, *J Cardiopulm Rehabil* 22:109-121, 2002.

56. Gigliotti F, Coli C, Bianchi R et al: Exercise training improves exertional dyspnea in patients with COPD, *Chest* 123(6):1794-1802, 2003.

57. Greene JG, Pucino F, Carlson JD et al: Effects of aprazolam on respiratory drive, anxiety, and dyspnea in chronic airflow obstruction, a case study. *Pharmacotherapy*, 9(1):34-38, 1989.

58. Tranmer JE, Heyland D, Dudgeon D et al: Measuring the symptom experience of seriously ill cancer and noncancer hospitalized patients near the end of life with the Memorial Symptom Assessment Scale, *J Pain Symptom Manage* 25(5):420-429, 2003.

59. Klingenberg M, Smit JH, Deeg DJ et al: Proxy reporting in after-death interviews: the use of proxy respondents in retrospective assessment of chronic diseases and symptom burden in the terminal phase of life, *Palliat Med* 17:191-201, 2003.

CHAPTER 39

Pain

Mary Pat Johnston

Unrelieved cancer pain continues to be a common problem and the most feared, distressing symptom that people living with cancer and families experience.[1] An estimated 20% to 50% of patients with early-stage cancer experience pain requiring analgesics, and patients with advanced cancer experience pain at estimated rates of 55% to 95%.[2] Despite more than 30 years of advancing the science of pain management, together with education initiatives for health care clinicians and the public about pain management and its treatment, undertreatment of pain persists.[3]

Definition

Pain is an unpleasant sensory and emotional experience associated with actual or potential tissue damage.[4] This definition implies both physical and emotional facets to the pain experience.[5] McCaffery defined pain as "whatever the experiencing person says that it is, existing whenever he or she says that it does," emphasizing the subjective nature of pain.[6] The most reliable indicator of pain is the patient's self-report.[6,7] Based on the consensus definitions developed by the American Academy of Pain Medicine, the American Pain Society, and the American Society of Addiction Medicine, **addiction** is "a primary, chronic, neurobiologic disease, with genetic, psychosocial, and environmental factors influencing its development and manifestations. It is a pattern characterized by behaviors that include one or more of the following: impaired control of over drug use, compulsive use, continued use despite harm, and craving."[8] The addicted person has a continued craving for an opioid and the need for the use of the opioid for effects other than pain relief. **Pseudoaddiction** is a term that has been used to describe patient behaviors, such as "clock watching" and "drug seeking," occurring when pain is undertreated. It differs from a true addiction because these behaviors resolve when pain is relieved. In contrast to addiction, **physical dependence** is "a state of adaptation that is manifested by a drug class–specific withdrawal syndrome that can be produced by abrupt cessation, rapid dose reduction, decreasing blood levels of the drug, and/or administration of an antagonist."[8] It is an expected response to chronic opioid therapy, occurring within 2 weeks of initiation.[7] If the pain medication is abruptly stopped, the patient will experience a withdrawal syndrome including flu-like symptoms. **Tolerance** is "a state of adaptation in which exposure to a drug induces changes that result in diminution of one or more of the drug's effects over time."[8] After repeated administration of the same opioid, the same dose produces a decreased effect, decreased analgesia, and decreased side effects such as sedation, respiratory depression, nausea, and pruritus.[9] Tolerance develops so as to limit many side effects of opioids within 1 to 2 weeks.[2] However, misunderstandings about these terms may lead to treatment delays, withholding opioids and, subsequently, poor pain outcomes.

Distress is an unpleasant feeling of a physical, psychological, social, or spiritual nature that interferes with one's ability to cope.[10] **Suffering,** which is severe distress associated with events that threaten the individual's perception of wholeness, is identified within the spiritual dimension of quality of life, but it transcends all dimensions, often occurring when health care providers fail to attend to the symptoms of cancer and its treatment.[11] Kuppelomaki and Lauri described suffering as a negative, undesirable experience with a physical foundation in the cancer itself and its treatment, identifying pain as one of the worst symptoms of physical suffering.[12]

Of concern to health care providers, the principle of **double effect** differentiates between providing analgesic medications with the *intent* to relieve pain that might inadvertently hasten death versus providing medications to **intentionally** cause death. While often a concern of nurses managing cancer pain and pain at end of life, opioid increases in dosage at end of life are not associated with shorter survival.[13] According to the American Nurses Association and the Hospice and Palliative Care Nurses Association, nurses have a responsibility to be aware of the potential risks of treating pain with opioids and other analgesics. Although the risk is present that opioid doses might hasten death, it is quite small and ethically acceptable.[14,15] Most patients stated that suffering had meaning in their lives; however, the emphasis for nurses and other health care providers is to identify and treat to alleviate pain and suffering. Nurses should consult with more experienced team members when increasing opioids beyond a range that is comfortable for them.[12,13]

Prevalence

The Study to Understand Prognoses and Preferences for Outcomes and Risks of Treatments (SUPPORT) concluded that "more proactive and forceful measures may be needed" to improve the care of seriously ill and dying patients.[16] The Joint Commission for the Accreditation of Healthcare Organizations (JCAHO) changed standards to incorporate pain assessment and management, mandating health care organizations to create the infrastructure to develop, implement, and evaluate improvements in pain assessment and management.[3] Yet, one third of persons receiving treatment for cancer and two thirds of those with advanced malignant disease experience pain.[7] People with cancer suffer because of inadequate pain and symptom management, and their treatment preferences are often ignored.[17] The management of pain and other symptoms related to cancer and its treatment is pivotal to oncology nursing practice since oncology nurses sustain contact with patients across the cancer illness trajectory and are in the best position to identify untreated pain and advocate for its relief.[1]

Risk Factors

For people with cancer pain, risk factors can be categorized as disease-related, treatment-related, health care provider–related, and patient- and family-related.[18] Disease-related factors include bone metastasis, abdominal visceral pain, and nerve compression or injury. Because of bone destruction or compression of the bone on nerves and soft tissue, bone metastasis is a common source of cancer pain, with the greatest incidence in patients with breast, prostate, and lung cancer and multiple myeloma. Abdominal visceral pain may be caused by tumor obstruction of the bowel, liver metastasis, and occlusion of blood flow to visceral organs such as liver and spleen. Nerve compression or injury to peripheral, sympathetic, or central nerves may cause pain due to spinal cord compression, plexopathies, and peripheral neuropathies.

Treatment-related factors may include pain from chemotherapy, radiation therapy, and surgery. Chemotherapy may induce pain through symptoms, like mucositis, peripheral neuropathies, and herpetic neuralgia.[19] Patients receiving radiation therapy for head and neck cancer may experience pain from mucositis. Radiation may cause pain through skin reactions and peripheral nerve tumors in previously treated areas.[20] Some patients may experience chronic pain following surgeries like mastectomy, thoracotomy, radical neck dissection, nephrectomy, or limb amputation.[21]

There are also patient-related factors and health care provider–related factors that are barriers for effective pain relief.[5,22,23] Despite the JCAHO pain standards and other cancer pain practice guidelines, health care systems are challenged by assigning a low priority to pain management, restrictive regulation of controlled substances, insufficient availability or access to treatment, and inadequate reimbursement.[5] Often, pain medications such as opioids are not available in inner-city or rural pharmacies. Oncology nurses should advocate for the availability of necessary medications for their patients, regardless of their environment.[24]

Health care provider–related factors include inadequate knowledge of pain, poor pain assessment; lack of responsibility, fear of patient addiction, concerns of adverse side effects of analgesics, and concerns about patients becoming tolerant to analgesics.[5,9] Lack of knowledge and negative attitudes have resulted in the undertreatment of cancer pain despite the development of standards and practice guidelines.[25] Poor pain assessment is the greatest barrier for health care providers.[26] In addition, poor verbal and written documentation of assessment findings creates a communication barrier among health care providers.[5] Finally, lack of accountability is a barrier since health care providers do not consistently integrate thorough assessments and documentation of assessments, interventions, and evaluations into practice.

Similarly, patients and families have fears of addiction or being thought of as an addict, worries about unmanageable adverse side effects, and concerns about becoming tolerant to the analgesic regimen.[5,9] As a result, patients have a reluctance to take pain medications and do not adhere to the analgesic regimen.[27] Patients are concerned about distracting the physician from treatment of the underlying disease, and they desire to be a "good" patient. Therefore many patients have a reluctance to report pain. Because pain is identified primarily through patient self-report, patients who have problems communicating are at high risk for undertreatment, including older patients, children, and cognitively impaired patients.[7] Older adults may have multiple chronic and painful conditions, be more sensitive to analgesic affects of opioids,

experience more drug to drug-or-drug-to-disease interactions, and harbor fears about pain and pain medications, especially opioids.[28] They may consider pain to be a normal part of aging, and therefore, they do not report pain to their physician.[29] Other patients at risk include unresponsive or unconscious patients; patients who deny pain; non-English speaking patients; persons of cultures different from that of the health care professional; patients with a history of an addictive disease; and underinsured or unemployed persons.[5,9] These special needs may exist as a result of limited verbal communication, physical and emotional dependence, lack of an advocate, differences from health care providers, and stigmatization. Patients have identified cost as a significant barrier to good pain relief, especially for older adults.[28]

Despite the prevalence of cancer and its impact on patients and their families, little has been accomplished to change patients', families, and caregivers' knowledge, attitudes, and behaviors toward cancer pain management.[25] Patients' beliefs have been identified as important barriers to effective pain management, and nursing interventions that assess and manage these patient barriers will strengthen the patient's knowledge, improve pain-related behaviors, and empower patients, families, and caregivers to assert themselves, especially when they encounter less knowledgeable health care providers.[30]

Etiology

Cancer pain is a complex symptom also because it may be characterized as acute, chronic, or intermittent.[7] It includes both acute cancer-related pain, caused by cancer or cancer therapy, and chronic cancer-related pain. Frequently, cancer pain has a definable etiology, usually related to tumor recurrence or treatment.[31] Cancer pain differs from acute pain in that it is rarely accompanied by signs of arousal of the sympathetic nervous system, such as tachycardia, tachypnea, and elevated blood pressure.[7] For a patient with cancer, increased pain may trigger fears of disease progression, anxiety, hopelessness, depression, and fatalism.[32]

TYPES OF PAIN

Nociceptive pain is damage to bones, soft tissues, or internal organs, resulting from activation of nociceptors or pain fibers in deep and cutaneous tissues.[18] It is inclusive of somatic and visceral pain. Somatic pain arises from bones, joints, muscle, skin, and connective tissue. It is well localized and aching, gnawing, or throbbing in quality. Some examples of somatic pain are bone metastasis, mucositis, and skin lesions. Visceral pain arises from the viscera, such as pancreas, liver, spleen, and gastrointestinal (GI) tract, as a result of nociceptor activation in the thoracic or abdominal tissue. Visceral pain is poorly localized, intermittent, cramping, squeezing, or sharp in quality. Neuropathic pain is damage to the peripheral, sympathetic, and/or central nervous system, which may be described as sharp, burning, tingling, electrical, or shooting in quality. Some examples of neuropathic pain include postherpetic neuropathy, diabetic neuropathy, and peripheral neuropathy associated with human immunodeficiency virus (HIV) or chemotherapy.[33,34] The patient may experience hyperalgesia, a severe pain from a stimulus that is usually mild (e.g., pin prick) or allodynia, pain from light touch or stimulus that is not usually painful (e.g., inability to tolerate clothing touching their skin or the movement of air from a fan or air-conditioning).[34] Taxanes, vinca alkaloids, and platinol-based chemotherapy agents are more likely to cause peripheral neuropathies in people receiving cancer treatments for tumors such as breast and lung cancers.[19,34]

PHYSIOLOGY OF PAIN

Nociception is the process by which the individual becomes aware or conscious of pain. The pain message is processed in four basic steps (Fig. 39-1).[5] Transduction is initiated by a mechanical, thermal, or chemical noxious stimulus, which sensitizes or activates nociceptors, primary afferent fibers or free nerve endings that identify noxious stimuli in the periphery.[2,5] C fibers and A delta fibers are the primary nociceptors responsible for the transmission of pain impulses from the site of transduction to the spinal cord. C fibers are unmyelinated, small-diameter, slow-conducting fibers, transmitting poorly localized, dull, aching pain and sensitive to mechanical, thermal, and chemical stimuli. In contrast, A delta fibers are sparsely myelinated, large-diameter, fast-conducting fibers, transmitting well-localized, sharp pain and sensitive to mechanical and thermal stimuli. Mechanical stimuli include incisions or tumor growth; thermal stimuli may be related to burns; and a chemical stimulus refers to a toxic substance. After cell damage occurs from these noxious stimuli, neurotransmitters, prostaglandins (PG), bradykinin (BK), serotonin (5-HT), substance P (SP), and histamine (H) are released, generating an action potential along the neuron when sodium moves into a cell and calcium moves out of the cell.[18] The pain message begins traveling from the site of injury to the central nervous system. Transmission is movement of the action potential or impulses to the dorsal horn of the spinal cord, where nociceptors end. Neurotransmitters, such as SP, continue the pain impulse across the synaptic cleft between the nociceptive neurons and the dorsal horn neurons,.[5,18] From the dorsal horn of the spinal cord, neurons ascend pathways, like the spinothalamic tract to the thalamus, and other neurons carry the message to various centers in the brain. The thalamus transmits the message to central structures of the brain, like the cerebral cortex.

Perception is the end result of pain transmission, but the exact location of where pain is perceived is unclear.[5] The reticular system is involved in the autonomic response to pain and provides a warning signal to the individual to attend to it. The limbic system is considered the source of an individual's emotional and behavioral response to pain, and the cerebral cortex processes the experience of pain. Finally, modulation occurs as descending neurons, originating in the brainstem, travel to the dorsal horn and release neuromodulators, such as endogenous opioids, norepinephrine, and serotonin, γ-aminobutyric acid, and neurotensin, that inhibit the transmission of noxious stimuli and produce analgesia.[2,5]

Effects and Consequences

Unrelieved pain has several consequences, such a depressed immune system, impaired cardiac and respiratory systems, decreased gastric and bowel motility, muscle spasms, immobility, which may lead to deep vein thrombosis or pneumonia, and poor quality of life.[5] In addition, Liebeskind identified cancer-promoting consequences of unrelieved pain.[35] Pain intensity scores of 4 to 5 out of 10 have demonstrated interference with activities and enjoyment.[36] According to National Comprehensive Cancer Network (NCCN) Cancer Pain Guideline, "Unrelieved pain denies them comfort and greatly affects their activities, affect, motivation, interactions with family and friends, and overall quality of life."[37]

Pain Assessment

As the foundation for pain management, a comprehensive pain assessment contains the following key components: location, intensity, quality, pattern, precipitating factors, pain history, medication history, and meaning of the pain (Fig. 39-2).[5] Assess pain on admission to the hospital or during each outpatient clinic and home visit.[9]

The first component is location: where is the pain located. Often, for patients with cancer, **locations** of pain may be multiple.[5] Patients may experience referred pain or pain "all over," which may be due to myalgias or may be total pain, meaning more than just physical pain but the encompassing of psychologic, social, and spiritual distress. Of importance with older adults, assess the patient's emotional state for depression, fear, anxiety, and hopelessness.

Quantify pain with a standard **pain intensity** scale.[38] A numerical rating scale that asks patients to rate their pain on a 0-10 scale, with 0 representing no pain and 10 the worst pain imaginable, is the simplest and most common to use for both clinicians and patients (Figs. 39-3 and 39-4).[5] When using the numerical pain scale with a patient, show and describe the purpose and components of the scale, discuss pain as a broad concept, such as discomfort anywhere in the body, and identify what words the patient uses for pain.[39] If the patient is having difficulty using the numerical pain scale, ask the patient to practice by rating some common pain examples on the scale such as toothache, backache, or labor. When patients continue having difficulties conceptualizing a number, an alternative pain scale can be useful, such as simple word descriptors like mild, moderate, or severe pain. Pain scales with faces or smaller numerical ratings may be more helpful for children and cognitively impaired adults.[40] For unconscious or unresponsive patients, a behavioral pain scale may be used.[41,42]

Quality of pain can be broadly divided into nociceptive pain—somatic and visceral—and neuropathic pain.[5] Patients will often describe a universal experience that will likely be familiar to the clinician to increase the clinician's understanding of what living with that pain feels like. For example, a patient may state that his or her pain feels like a toothache, describing somatic pain. It is important to seek the patient's own words or description of the quality of the pain since it guides selection of pain medications.

Pattern refers to the persistent nature of the pain or breakthrough pain. Persistent pain has duration of longer than 12 hours per day or may always be present. It may also be labeled as constant, baseline, or basal pain. In contrast, breakthrough pain is additional pain with rapid onset, greater severity, and intermittently occurs. Breakthrough pain can be triggered by incident pain related to various activities or involving movement, or may be idiopathic pain that is unpredictable and often, has an unknown etiology. It can also be attributed to end-of-dose failure related to an increase in pain before the next scheduled dose. For patients with controlled, persistent pain, breakthrough pain occurs suddenly, frequently reaches maximum intensity in 3 minutes of moderate to severe pain, and has duration of 30 minutes with episodes occurring 1 to 4 times per day.

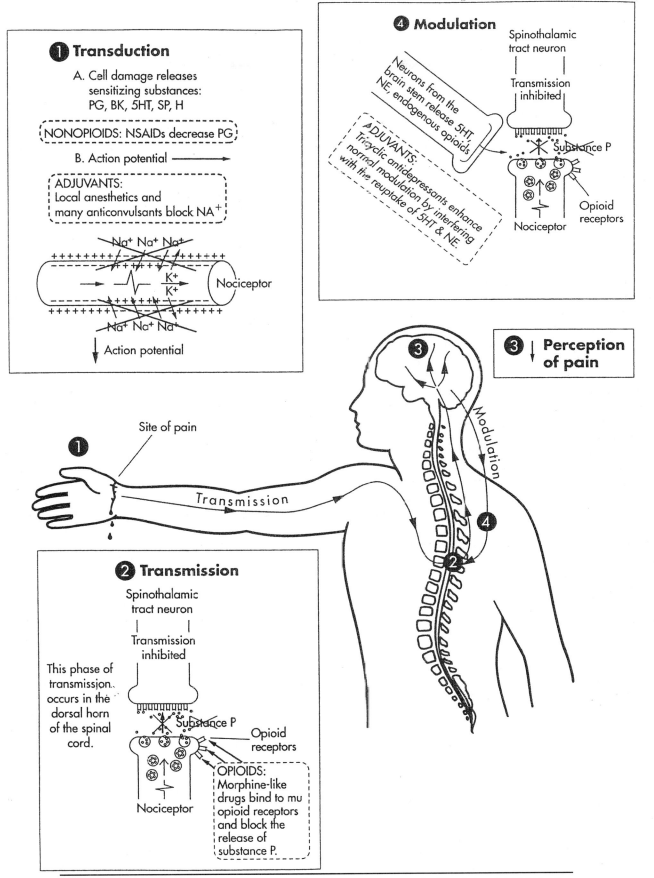

FIG. 39-1   Mechanism of pain transmission. *BK*, bradykinin; *5-HT*, serotonin; *SP*, substance P; *H*, histamine; *NSAIDs*, nonsteroidal antiinflammatory drugs; *PG*, prostaglandins. (From McCaffery M, Pasero C: *Pain: clinical manual*, ed 2, St. Louis, 1999, Mosby.)

FORM 3.1 **Initial Pain Assessment Tool**

Date _____

Patient's Name _____   Age _____   Room _____

Diagnosis _____   Physician _____

Nurse _____

1. LOCATION: Patient or nurse mark drawing.

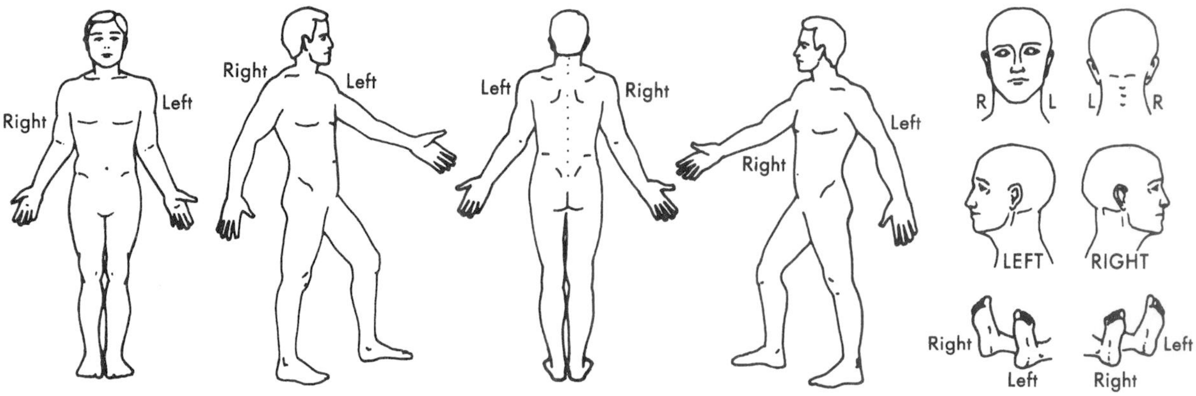

2. INTENSITY: Patient rates the pain. Scale used _____

   Present: _____
   Worst pain gets: _____
   Best pain gets: _____
   Acceptable level of pain: _____
3. QUALITY: (Use patient's own words, e.g., prick, ache, burn, throb, pull, sharp) _____
   _____
4. ONSET, DURATION, VARIATIONS, RHYTHMS: _____
   _____
5. MANNER OF EXPRESSING PAIN: _____
   _____
   _____
6. WHAT RELIEVES THE PAIN? _____
   _____
   _____
7. WHAT CAUSES OR INCREASES THE PAIN? _____
   _____
   _____
8. EFFECTS OF PAIN: (Note decreased function, decreased quality of life.)
   Accompanying symptoms (e.g., nausea) _____
   Sleep _____
   Appetite _____
   Physical activity _____
   Relationship with others (e.g., irritability) _____
   Emotions (e.g., anger, suicidal, crying) _____
   Concentration _____
   Other _____
9. OTHER COMMENTS: _____
   _____
10. PLAN: _____
    _____
    _____

FIG. 39-2   Pain intensity scales. (From McCaffery M, Pasero C: *Pain: Clinical manual*, ed 2, St. Louis, 1999, Mosby.)

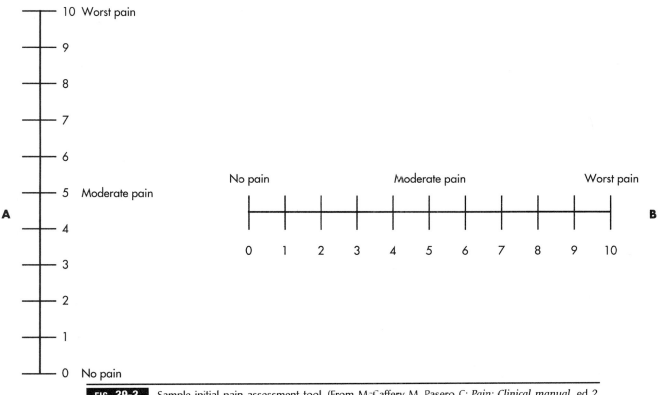

FIG. 39-3   Sample initial pain assessment tool. (From McCaffery M, Pasero C: *Pain: Clinical manual,* ed 2, St. Louis, 1999, Mosby.)

Poorly understood by health care providers, breakthrough pain is often inadequately assessed and managed.[43] Approximately 52% to 67% of patients with cancer pain experience breakthrough pain.[44]

Precipitating factors are aggravating or alleviating factors—descriptions of circumstances that make the pain worse and of what makes the pain better. Assess the impact of pain on function, such as how pain interferes with activities of daily living, work, leisure, and social interactions. In addition, ask about changes in gait, frequent falls, or bruises, which may be an indicator for decreased sensation due to neuropathic pain and lead to identification of patient safety issues.[34] These assessment findings guide the nurse toward the selection of non-pharmacologic strategies for managing the patient's pain.

Pain history includes words that are used by the patient to indicate pain, descriptions of the patient's significant prior pain experiences; and agents or actions that have been effective in relieving the patient's pain. Instead of using the word pain, patients may use other words like discomfort, hurt, or ache. Asking about prior pain experiences, the nurse will gain insights into the patient's worst experiences of pain and expectations about the current pain experience. Determine interventions that have been effective in relieving pain in the past. Past history assists in planning pharmacologic and non-pharmacologic strategies that might be useful in managing the current pain experience. To explore cultural considerations in pain, this question may be expanded: how did your grandmother or mother manage pain, and do you continue to use these strategies?

In addition, a **medication history** provides key information regarding what medications the patient has already tried, as does determining their effectiveness or adverse effects. It is important to ask the patient how they are actually taking the medication and compare that to what was prescribed. If a disparity is noted, the nurse may inquire about the disparity to identify unmet patient education needs. As part of the medication history, use of and experience with over-the-counter medications, recreational drugs, and herbal products are also explored.

Finally, psychosocial issues, such as the meaning of the pain, cultural considerations, and spiritual or religious beliefs may affect the patient's perception of the pain. **Meaning of the pain** significantly influences the patient's perception of the pain experience and, subsequently, pain relief. Patients may, for example, view pain as a punishment for prior indiscretions or a challenge for building character or faith. In addition, the meaning of the pain will be influenced by the individual's culture and spiritual or religious beliefs. The nurse explores these beliefs to understand their impact on pain and reframe these beliefs to provide better pain relief.[45] For example, for a patient who believes that pain is a punishment, it may be helpful to teach about the source of the pain and demonstrate that pain can be relieved. It may also be necessary to include clergy in planning interventions to relieve spiritual distress associated with the meaning of the pain.

Reassessment of pain occurs regularly with any new report of pain or increase in pain and with changes in the analgesic regimen.[9] Pain is reassessed after appropriate intervals following pain interventions. For patients with rapidly progressing disease, more frequent pain assessments are required. It is important for nurses to instruct patients and their families or caregivers to report any changes in pain. To evaluate the effectiveness of an analgesic regimen, assessment questions may include

TRANSLATIONS OF WONG-BAKER FACES PAIN RATING SCALE*

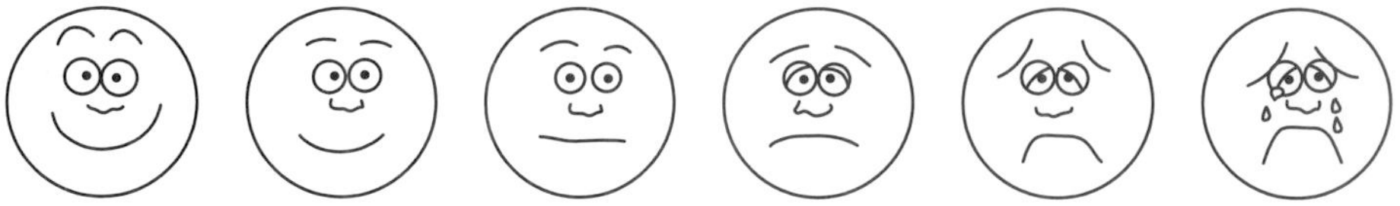

0–5 coding	0	1	2	3	4	5
0-10 coding	0	2	4	6	8	10
ENGLISH	No hurt	Hurts little bit	Hurts little more	Hurts even more	Hurts whole lot	Hurts worst
SPANISH	No duele	Duele un poco	Duele un poco más	Duele mucho	Duele mucho más	Duele el máximo
FRENCH	Pas mal	Un petit peu mal	Un peu plus mal	Encore plus mal	Très mal	Très très mal
ITALIAN	Non fa male	Fa male un poco	Fa male un po di piu	Fa male ancora di piu	Fa molto male	Fa maggiormente male
PORTUGUESE	Não doi	Doi um pouco	Doi um pouco mais	Doi muito	Doi muito mais	Doi o máximo
BOSNIAN	Ne boli	Boli samo malo	Boli malo više	Boli još više	Boli puno	Boli najviše
VIETNAMESE	Không dau	Hỏi dau	Dau hỏn chút	Dau nhiêu hỏn	Dau thât nhiêu	Dau qúa dô
CHINESE †	無痛	微痛	較痛	更痛	很痛	劇痛
GREEK	Δεν Πoναï	Πoναï Λιγo	Πoναï Λιγo Πιo Πoλν	Πoναï Πoλν	Πoναï Πιo Πoλν	Πoναï Παρα Πoλν
ROMANIAN	No doare	Doare puţin	Doare un pic mai mult	Doare şi mai mult	Doare foarte tare	Doare cel mai mult

FIG. 39-4 Wong-Baker FACES Pain Rating Scale. (From Hockenberry MJ, Wilson D, Winkelstein ML: Wong's essentials of pediatric nursing, ed 7, St. Louis, 2005, Mosby. Used with permission. Copyright, Mosby.)

the following: how much pain relief did the pain medication provide, and for how long did you get relief? One strategy for reassessment is for patients to maintain a pain diary to record intensity scores, times and doses of breakthrough medications given, and comments about activities. Schumacher and colleagues found that the pain diary heightened awareness of pain, guided pain management behaviors, enhanced a sense of control, and facilitated communication, all of which promoted self-care.[23] Pain diaries may be beneficial for patients in outpatient and home care settings, where nurses have intermittent contact with patients.

The next step is to **communicate assessment findings** to the health care team, including all disciplines involved in the care of the patient. One communication strategy is to state the problem, using the objective data obtained; describe the consequences of pain on function; list the current medications, including what has the patient taken in the last 24 hours and how long the pain medication is effective; and collaborate with a pharmacist, and then make recommendations to the physician.[5] For written communication of assessment findings, document at regular

intervals, with each new report of pain, and after each pharmacologic and non-pharmacologic intervention.[9] The components to be documented are pain intensity, how pain interferes with function, and the degree to which pain is relieved.[9] If the patient has both persistent and breakthrough pain, these components are documented for each type of pain in reassessment.

Pharmacologic Interventions for Pain Management

"The success of opioid therapy often depends on achieving a balance between analgesic effectiveness and side effects."[46] Key pharmacologic management principles include the following: match the initial drug choice to the intensity and the type of pain; give pain medications orally whenever possible; avoid intramuscular injections; provide pain medications around the clock when pain is continuous, along with breakthrough pain medications; use equianalgesic dosing principles and conversion tables as a guide when changing from one opioid to another or one route to another route; implement strategies to minimize side effects; and assess response to analgesic regimen.[7,9,18,21,37,47] Historically, the World Health Organization (WHO) Ladder has provided a guide for the initial selection of an analgesic. However, although the model was effective for educational purposes, the complexities of cancer pain make the WHO Ladder too simplistic for clinical practice.[9,37] Clinical practice guidelines, like the NCCN Adult Cancer Pain Guidelines, provide direction for managing mild, moderate, and severe pain in opioid naive and opioid tolerant patients, based on pain intensity ratings.[37]

For mild pain (pain intensity of 1 to 3 on a scale of 0-10, where 0 equals no pain and 10 equals the worst possible pain), nonopioids are recommended. Acetaminophen, possessing antipyretic and analgesic properties, inhibits prostaglandin and provides relief of bone pain, dysmenorrhea, and other pain syndromes.[9,37] The maximum daily dose is 4000 mg—higher doses may cause renal and liver dysfunction. Acetaminophen is present in many over-the-counter products and prescription medications, another reason why it is so important to obtain an accurate, current medication list from the patient. Other examples of nonopioid analgesics include aspirin and nonsteroidal antiinflammatory drugs (NSAIDs) such as ibuprofen and naproxen, possessing antiinflammatory, antipyretic, and analgesic properties. Adverse effects include GI bleeding, renal dysfunction, and decreased platelet aggregation. These medications all have a ceiling effect, meaning that increasing the dose beyond a certain point will only increase the adverse effects and will not promote further analgesia.[5] Cox-2 inhibitors also belong to this class of drugs. Although associated with a lower incidence of GI side effects and altered platelets, they continue to have renal toxicities as well as recently noted adverse cardiovascular effects. NSAIDs are most effective in providing relief from inflammation related to bone metastasis. Patients who may be at risk for adverse effects of NSAIDs are older adults, patients with history of GI disorders, dehydration, or renal impairment, those who are neutropenic or thrombocytopenic, and those who concurrently use corticosteroids.[9] In addition, coanalgesics or adjuvant medications may be warranted, if patient experiences mild neuropathic pain.

For moderate pain (pain intensity of 4 to 6 on a scale of 0-10, where 0 equals no pain and 10 equals the worst possible pain), slow titration of short-acting oral or intravenous opioids is recommended.[9,37] Examples of pain medications for moderate pain include hydrocodone and oxycodone in fixed combinations with acetaminophen or aspirin, and lower doses of short-acting opioids, like morphine or oxycodone. Remember, opioids with acetaminophen combinations have a ceiling dose of 4000 mg per day. Because of the potential for metabolite accumulation of norpropoxyphene, causing central nervous system (CNS) toxicity, avoid propoxyphene (Darvon). In addition, agonist-antagonists, like pentazocine (Talwin) and butorphanol (Stadol) may cause confusion and hallucinations in older adults and patients with renal impairment.[7] Mixed agonists-antagonists have ceiling effects that limit the ability to titrate doses as pain increases. Therefore they are not recommended for cancer pain management. Nonopioids and coanalgesics may also be continued if the patient experiences moderate inflammatory or neuropathic pain.

For severe pain (pain intensity of 7 to 10 on a scale of 0-10, where 0 equals no pain and 10 equals the worst possible pain), rapid titration of short-acting oral or intravenous opioids is recommended.[9,37] Pharmacologic principles for long-acting and breakthrough opioids are the following: begin with immediate-release formulations for 24 to 48 hours; calculate the 24-hour dose of the opioid, convert to a long-acting formulation, and add breakthrough medication with immediate-release formulation, usually 10% to 20% of the total 24-hour dose every 1 to 2 hours.[9] For upward titration of an opioid, general guidelines are based on the pain intensity scale, increasing 50% to 100% for severe pain (7 to 10 on a 10-point scale); 25% to 50% for moderate pain (4 to 6 on a 10-point scale), or 25% for mild pain (1 to 3 on a 10-point scale).[37] However, other considerations in titration are based on patient's goals, comorbid illnesses, the severity of undesirable side effects such as sedation, requirements for supplemental analgesics, and the effect of pain on quality of life.[5] If one opioid is ineffective after an adequate upward titration of the dose, or it produces adverse effects, switch to another opioid.[48] For the older adult, special considerations should be given to assessment and management of pain (See Considerations for Older Adults box).[49]

The opioids most frequently prescribed for cancer pain include morphine, oxycodone, hydromorphone, and transdermal fentanyl. Because of the accumulation of the metabolite normeperidine, causing CNS toxicity as demonstrated by tremors and seizures, meperidine (Demerol) is not recommended for cancer pain treatment. Because of individual pharmacokinetic variation, long half-life, and high potency, methadone is difficult to utilize in persons with cancer pain.[37] However, for persons experiencing neuropathic pain, methadone may have some benefit. For these patients, methadone should be started at lower doses and titrated upward slowly with appropriate breakthrough pain medications with consultation of a pain management specialist.[9,37] With opioid therapy, nonopioids and coanalgesic medications may also be continued for the treatment of severe neuropathic pain.

MANAGING OPIOID SIDE EFFECTS

Opioids have predictable, manageable side effects, but there are many myths that create barriers to patients taking them, as well as to health care providers prescribing and administering them. **Allergic reactions** to opioids are extremely rare. More often, patients will state that they have an allergy, but after further assessment, a side effect, like nausea, vomiting, or pruritus, is identified as poorly controlled and opioid therapy is discontinued. **Respiratory depression** is also rare and is more likely to occur in the opioid-naive patient—a patient who is receiving opioids for the first time. It is almost always preceded by sedation that health care clinicians should heed as a warning. In addition, respiratory depression may also occur after a change in the dose of an opioid. True respiratory depression occurs when the patient is unarousable, has a low respiratory rate less than 8 per minute, and poor oxygenation. The opioid can be reversed by administering an antagonist, naloxone or Narcan, which may induce a withdrawal syndrome and reverse all the analgesic effect of the opioid. However, be cautious in using naloxone to patients who have been receiving opioids and are physically dependent. Naloxone can precipitate withdrawal symptoms that are extremely painful and distressing.

To reverse the sedation and respiratory depression without reversing the analgesia, mix one ampule of naloxone (0.4 mg) in a 10-ml sterile syringe with 9 ml of normal saline and administer slowly in 0.5 to 1.0 ml increments over 2 minutes.[50] If no response is obtained, continue administration until a total dose of 0.8 mg or 20 ml of diluted naloxone is given. Discontinue naloxone when the patient opens his or her eyes, responds to physical stimulation, or has a respiratory rate greater than 12 per minute. Monitor the patient for sedation, respiratory status, and analgesia. Recognize that the duration of naloxone is 30 to 60 minutes, whereas the duration of the opioids may be longer. Several doses of naloxone may be necessary. Continue to reassess the patient. Provide nonopioid pain relief, such as NSAIDs. Resume opioid administration at one half the original dose when the patient is easily aroused.[7]

Although **sedation** can occur, tolerance generally develops to this side effect. Since patients may be exhausted from unrelieved pain, once the patient is able to get pain relief, he or she is likely to rest. Strategies for managing sedation include initiating opioids at recommended starting doses, starting lower doses for the older patient, and slowly titrating the opioid dose by 25% to 50%. Another option is to administer a stimulant, like methylphenidate (Ritalin), 5 to 10 mg in the morning and at noon.[51] Other stimulants include caffeine, 100 to 200 mg orally every 6 hours, or dextroamphetamine, 5 to 10 mg orally every day.[37] If sedation persists longer than 1 week, consider other causes of sedation. CNS pathology, medications with sedative effects, hypercalcemia, dehydration, hypoxia, and sepsis are all causes of sedation to be investigated in cancer patients. Also consider adding a coanalgesic to decrease the dose of opioid, or change the opioid. **Constipation** is the most common side effect of opioid therapy, leading to decreased usage or discontinuation of opioids if not managed. Constipation may worsen other symptoms, such as nausea and vomiting and anorexia, and lead to the development of hemorrhoids and anal fissures, which are painful as well as being potential sites of infection. Tolerance does not develop to opioid-induced constipation. Therefore, a laxative–stool softener combination is needed to counteract this effect, beginning with the first dose of an opioid.[9] A minimum goal for a bowel movement is at least one every 72 hours regardless of intake. Encourage patients to drink plenty of fluids as tolerated, increase their physical activity as appropriate, and consume high-fiber foods, if fluid intake is adequate. Urinary retention is more common in opioid-naive patients and with spinal analgesia. **Nausea and vomiting** may also occur, but antiemetics for 2 to 3 days will manage these symptoms until tolerance is developed. Possible antiemetics are prochlorperizine, 10 mg orally every 6 hours as needed, or metoclopramide, 10 to 20 mg orally every 6 hours as needed.[37] **Pruritus** (itching) occurs more commonly with spinal analgesia. Antihistamines may be helpful in managing this side effect; however, they may contribute to sedation. **Myoclonus,** a side effect of high-dose opioid therapy, is described as jerky motion, related to the accumulation of metabolites.[9] Often, myoclonus occurs in patients receiving meperidine as a result of normeperidine accumulation, or from high doses of morphine with subsequent morphine-6-glucuronide (M6G) and morphine-3-glucuronide (M3G) accumulation. To treat myoclonus, switch the opioid.[52] In summary, the nurse anticipates, prevents, and treats opioid-induced side effects to support the analgesic regimen and promote optimal pain relief.

ROUTES OF ADMINISTRATION

Oral is the preferred route of administration as it is the least invasive for chronic pain treatment because of its convenience, flexibility, and maintenance of steady blood levels.[7,9,37] For patients, who cannot swallow capsules or tablets, many opioids

are available in liquid formulations. Sustained-release medications, like MS Contin or OxyContin, should never be crushed, because this makes them into them immediate-release forms, causing severe and potentially lethal toxicities. Oral morphine medications, like Kadian or Avinza, can be opened and sprinkled on soft food for patients with swallowing difficulties. Onset of action for oral medications is typically 45 minutes, with peak drug effect in 1 to 2 hours after administering immediate-release opioids.[7] Therefore patients may take a second opioid dose of an immediate-release medication safely 2 hours after the first dose. However, with sustained-release medication, a second dose may produce a serious overdose, because the sustained-release medications are still releasing the medication slowly over time. It is important that patients, families, and caregivers understand these key points. When **oral medications** are given **sublingually,** little drug is actually absorbed through oral mucosa. The majority of the drug trickles to the back of throat and into the GI tract. Although it does not have a faster onset of action, it does provide convenience for patients with difficulty swallowing. **Intravenous (IV)** bolus administration provides the most rapid onset of action, with peak effect occurring at 1 to 5 minutes for fentanyl and 15 to 30 minutes for morphine.[7] For patients with intensifying cancer pain, repeated IV boluses may be titrated to provide effective pain relief, and a maintenance infusion may be necessary. Patient-controlled analgesia (PCA) delivers small doses of drug through an infusion pump on demand by the patient. It is rapidly administered when needed, reduces delays in obtaining pain medication, and gives the patient control over his or her pain medicines and experience. Subcutaneous continuous opioid infusion is an alternative to an intravenous infusion, producing equivalent blood levels. Often, it is used as an alternative when IV access is limited and for patients at end of life. Continuous infusions are better tolerated by opioid-tolerant patients, whereas caution is necessary when caring for the opioid-naive patient. The **transdermal** route is appropriate for lipophilic opioids, which are readily absorbed through the skin, like fentanyl (Duragesic patch), providing continuous administration of an opioid over 48 to 72 hours. The advantage of this route is that it bypasses the GI tract, potentially causing less constipation. Body mass and temperature extremes (e.g., fever) may accelerate or decelerate distribution. **Oral transmucosal** fentanyl citrate (Actiq) is indicated for breakthrough cancer pain. This medication is composed of a fentanyl on an applicator that the patient rubs on the oral mucosa for 5 to 15 minutes. Since the baseline opioid dose does not guide appropriate dose, careful titration is necessary. The **intramuscular route** is not recommended for cancer pain treatment since it is a painful administration, absorption from muscle is unpredictable, and it has a 30 to 60 minute onset of action and a rapid decline of action compared to oral administration. The **rectal route** is an alternative for patients who are unable to take oral medications and provides rapid systemic absorption. However, the rectal route may be contraindicated if the patient has neutropenia or thrombocytopenia.

Since most opioids are hydrophilic or water-based, **topical** opioids are controversial. For neuropathic pain, topical capsaicin may be used, although studies are at odds regarding its benefits. For postherpetic neuralgia, Lidoderm, a patch with 5% lidocaine, may be helpful. EMLA cream, a local anesthetic, has been used for brief painful procedures, such as bone marrow biopsy and implanted port needle access. For the treatment of neuropathic pain such as Pancoast syndrome or lumbosacral plexopathy, or visceral pain including thoracic or abdominal regions, nerve blocks, neurolytic blocks, or spinal analgesia may be necessary.[34,53] **Spinal analgesia** includes epidural and intrathecal administration of opioids, like fentanyl and morphine, and local anesthetics directly to the dorsal horn of the spinal cord, producing analgesia.[7] The epidural route may be appropriate for neuropathic pain relief, and the intraspinal route may be necessary when adverse systemic effects of these opioids are no longer tolerable to the patient.[53] These routes allow for increased titration of the opioid with decreased side effects such as fatigue, confusion, sedation, constipation, vomiting, pruritus, and mood changes. Other coanalgesics may be administered in conjunction with epidural or intrathecal analgesia. Nerve blocks disrupt nerve signals, may be temporary or permanent, and are used for diagnostic, prognostic, and therapeutic purposes. One indication for a nerve block may be neuropathic pain associated with herpes zoster.[54] The most highly effective neurolytic block is the celiac plexus block to relieve upper abdominal and referred back pain due to pancreatic cancer.[34] Unfortunately, many patients are not offered this therapeutic intervention as an option because of lack of knowledge about this intervention.[53]

COANALGESICS

Coanalgesics were historically known as adjuvant medications, describing medications with a primary indication other than pain relief, but whose analgesic properties were discovered in some chronic nonmalignant pain conditions.[54] Even though they can be administered alone, more often, coanalgesics such as antidepressants, anticonvulsants, or corticosteroids are given with acetaminophen, NSAIDs, and/or opioids to treat cancer pain. Traditionally, opioids have been a first-line therapy in managing cancer pain, and coanalgesics were added after opioid doses were maximized. Although it is considered best practice to initiate one medication at a time to evaluate response and adverse side effects, more consideration of coanalgesics is warranted. As new classes of analgesics are developed, Miaskowski and others recommend that the broad classification of opioids and coanalgesics are revised to a more informative classification, based on drug class and physiologic effect.[9]

Carbamazepine (Tegretol) and phenytoin (Dilantin) are **anticonvulsants** that have been used to treat painful diabetic neuropathy; however, the usage has declined as a result of the intolerable adverse reactions such as confusion, ataxia, and nausea, and the need to monitor hematology profiles and liver function tests. Carbamazepine is contraindicated in patients with low leukocyte counts (below 4000/mm³) or an absolute neutrophil count less than 1500/mm³, and for patients at risk for bone marrow failure, making it a poor choice for cancer patients.[9] Gabapentin (Neurontin) is appropriate for the management of neuropathic pain. It is generally well tolerated, with the most common side effects of sedation, dizziness, nausea, confusion, and lower-extremity edema. When the dose is initiated at a low dose and titrated slowly to optimal efficacy, these side effects are more easily monitored. Randomized clinical trials have not demonstrated a benefit at dosages above 1800 mg per day, administered in 3 divided doses.[9] McQuay found that there was no difference between gabapentin and older anticonvulsants in effectiveness, providing no clear recommendations for first-line treatment for neuropathic pain.[55] However, because of efficacy and limited adverse effects, gabapentin has become the first-line

treatment for many neuropathic pain conditions with improved outcomes for pain, sleep, and mood.[34]

For patients with cancer, **tricyclic antidepressants,** like amitriptyline (Elavil), nortriptyline (Pamelor), and desipramine (Norpramin, Pertofrane), have been used to treat neuropathic pain related to cancer treatments or malignant nerve infiltration. The most common side effects are sedation, dry mouth, constipation, confusion, and orthostatic hypotension. Because amitriptyline produces more sedation and other anticholinergic effects, clinicians prefer nortriptyline or desipramine. It is important to take amitriptyline at bedtime to promote sleep and reduce daytime side effects, whereas nortriptyline and desipramine should be taken during the day since they may cause insomnia.[7] Tricyclic antidepressants are contraindicated for patients with cardiac dysrhythmias, conduction abnormalities, glaucoma, and prostatic hyperplasia.

Corticosteroids are useful in the treatment of cancer plexopathies, metastatic bone pain, spinal cord compression, and liver pain due to metastasis and stretching of the liver capsule. Dexamethasone is the preferred corticosteroid because it has the least mineralocorticoid effect, meaning the least change in sodium and potassium excretion due to the drug affect on the adrenal gland.[7] The standard dose of dexamethasone is 16 to 24 mg per day. Corticosteroids are also useful in managing other side effects such as nausea, anorexia, malaise, and increased intracranial pressure, and improve overall quality of life.[54] With chronic use, patients are at risk for weight gain, osteoporosis, Cushing syndrome, myopathy, and psychosis. If taken concurrently with NSAIDs, the risk for GI bleeding and peptic ulcer disease increases. If the corticosteroid is rapidly withdrawn, the pain may exacerbate.

Local anesthetics may be given through epidural and intravenous infusions. They may be useful in management of acute pain associated with cancer, but long-term use does not seem appropriate. Other local anesthetics are **topical agents,** such as a lidocaine 5% patch and capsaicin; they are directly applied to the painful area to treat the skin and peripheral tissues. These agents are useful in the treatment of neuropathies, stump pain, and complex regional pain syndrome. Generally, the lidocaine 5% patch (Lidoderm) is worn 12 hours on and 12 hours off, and may be cut to the appropriate size to cover the affected area, making it ideal for small, localized areas of neuropathic pain.[7] Capsaicin (Zostrix), an enzyme found in hot chili peppers, decreases pain perception by depleting SP from nociceptive neurons. It has been beneficial in the treatment of postsurgical pain such as postmastectomy pain. Capsaicin is available in two concentrations (0.025% and 0.075%) and is applied 3 to 4 times a day to the affected area. For some patients, it may cause a localized burning sensation, which generally diminishes after a few days, but some patients may find it intolerable. Instruct patients to wash hands well after application and to keep it away from eyes and mucous membranes.

Baclofen, a potent **antispasmodic agent,** is useful in treating spasm-associated muscle pain, with doses initiated at 10 to 20 mg per day and titrated gradually based on the patient's analgesic response and adverse reactions.[54] With higher doses, weakness and confusion may occur. Patients may experience a withdrawal syndrome if it is suddenly stopped; gradually taper doses.

OTHER PAIN-RELIEVING THERAPIES

Bisphosphonates inhibit osteoclast activity and subsequently reduce bone resorption.[18] Zoledronic acid (Zometa) is the newest,

690   UNIT FIVE   Symptom Management

most potent bisphosphonate and has effectiveness in treating both osteoblastic and osteolytic lesions, reducing pain and skeletal complications for patients with a variety of solid tumors including breast, prostate, and lung cancers, as well as multiple myeloma.[56] It is administered intravenously over 15 minutes at a dose of 4 mg every 3 weeks. The side effects for bisphosphonates include bone pain, elevated serum creatinine, and hypocalcemia, and adverse reactions are renal toxicity and osteonecrosis of the jaw.

Radiopharmaceuticals may also be utilized to treat pain in combination with radiation therapy. Strontium-89 and samarium-153 are the radionuclides that are available in the United States.[18] Because of the myelosuppression associated with them, the radiopharmaceuticals are not considered until other treatment modalities are exhausted.[53]

Non-Pharmacologic Interventions

Non-pharmacologic interventions are a beneficial adjuvant to analgesics. These interventions are not a substitute for the pain medication, but are especially useful when managing breakthrough pain or a delay in onset of action and response to the pain medication.[9] Key principles for non-pharmacologic interventions include the following: assess the patient's willingness to utilize non-pharmacologic interventions, including attitude toward these interventions; assess the level of fatigue and cognitive status, considering factors such as the presence of other symptoms, co-morbid conditions, and disease progression; review aggravating and alleviating factors from the comprehensive assessment to determine what the patient has successfully used in the past to obtain pain relief; and include the family and the caregiver in discussion, selection, and teaching on a non-pharmacologic intervention.[5] Through the integration of these interventions into the pain management plan, patients reduce their distress, increase a sense of control, improve mood, and increase positive coping behaviors.[34] In addition, family members and caregivers may learn a new skill that will allow them to contribute to the care of their loved one. Physical techniques include heat, cold, massage, positioning, acupuncture, acupressure, and assistive devices to increase function and independence.[5] Smith and colleagues reported findings that supported massage as a nursing intervention for hospitalized cancer patients receiving chemotherapy and radiation therapy.[57] Cognitive-behavioral strategies include relaxation techniques, such as music therapy, breathing exercises, guided imagery, distraction, cognitive reframing, support groups, pastoral counseling, and prayer.[5] Lewandowski and co-workers identified changes in verbal descriptions of pain when guided imagery was used over a consecutive 4-day period.[58] Within the intervention group, patients described their pain as changeable rather than as never-ending following use of guided imagery. Some strategies for managing pain may require the expertise of other team members to implement, such as physical therapists, occupational therapists, medical social workers, chaplains, and psychiatrists. Clearly, several of the interventions, such as breathing exercises, heat, cold, and massage, are easily implemented by the nurse.

Outcomes

Although JCAHO and other governing bodies have focused on measuring how well pain management is integrated throughout an institution, the measurement of pain outcomes tends to be system-focused rather than patient-oriented. Although subjective symptoms, like cancer pain, are difficult to measure and evaluate, nurses individualize the pain management plan of care, based on the comprehensive pain assessment findings, and emphasize patient outcomes daily in providing care to patients and their families. According to the Oncology Nursing Society's *Core Curriculum for Oncology Nursing*, there are several patient pain outcomes:

- Patient verbalizes the importance of preventing and controlling pain.
- Patient communicates pain intensity using standardized measures.
- Patient states that pain is reduced or relieved to his or her satisfaction.
- Patient uses pharmacologic and non-pharmacologic interventions.
- Patient participates in the usual daily activities with appropriate medications.
- Patient reports adequate amounts of sleep and feels rested.

To achieve these outcomes, the patient and family should be provided verbal and written instructions about the pain

CONSIDERATIONS FOR OLDER ADULTS

1. On initial presentation and with each subsequent contact, assess for persistent pain.
2. Select an alternative pain scale if unable to utilize numerical pain intensity scale.
3. Identify patient's own words used to describe pain (e.g., discomfort, hurt, ache, pressure).
4. Assess impact of persistent pain on physical function (e.g., impact on daily activities), psychosocial function (e.g., mood, anxiety, depression) and other aspects of quality of life (e.g., social support and coping skills).
5. Consider use of acetaminophen for mild to moderate musculoskeletal persistent pain in patients with normal renal and liver function and without history of alcohol abuse, to a maximum of 4000 mg per day. Traditional nonsteroidal antiinflammatory drugs (NSAIDs) should be avoided in treating older adults with cancer who requiring daily medications for chronic analgesic therapy. A selective NSAID or fixed combination of an opioid with acetaminophen may be more beneficial.
6. Even though older adults are more susceptible to adverse drug reactions, opioids are effective. For moderate to severe pain, initiate opioid therapy at lowest anticipated effective dose, and titrate slowly.
7. Conduct a medication history to identify any new medications in use, including over-the-counter medications and herbal products, because of the dangers of drug-to-drug interactions, drug-to-disease interactions, and comorbid illnesses in the older adult.
8. Frequent evaluation is necessary to determine response to analgesia and adverse reactions.
9. Outcomes are decreased pain, increased function, and improvements in mood and sleep.

From American Geriatrics Society Panel on Chronic Pain in Older Persons: The management of persistent pain in older persons, *J Am Geriatr Soc* 50(6 Suppl):S205-224, 2002.

management plan. Miaskowski and colleagues identified the key components of cancer pain education as the following[9]:

- The types of and rationale for pain medications
- How to get prescriptions filled, how to take the pain medication and safely titrate the dose, if needed, how to store the medication, and how to manage side effects
- How and when to incorporate non-pharmacologic interventions
- Who to call if pain is not relieved, increases in pain intensity, or produces side effects

Patient education is the cornerstone of cancer pain management, and patient education clarifies the myths and misconceptions that arise as barriers to effective pain management.[9] Through conversations with patients and their families, the fear of addiction and other barriers have been seen to interfere with adherence to the pain management plan.[45] In outpatient settings, cancer patients take only 50% to 60% of their prescribed analgesics as a result of these myths and misconceptions.[27] With a focus on patient safety issues, nurses will need to assess and educate patients and families or caregivers on signs and symptoms of spinal cord compression for patients at high risk for bone metastasis and decreased sensation related to peripheral neuropathies or neuropathic pain, increasing safety risks in home environment.[18] Finally, nurses should instruct patients and their families or caregivers when to call and who to call for help. When to call includes the following circumstances: problems are encountered in obtaining prescriptions; a new pain is experienced; a change in pain occurs; pain is not relieved with medication; no bowel movement occurs for 3 days; there is difficulty in awakening the patient from sleep during the day; and setting or clarifying the date of next appointment or telephone contact.

Summary

Despite the advancement of pain as a science, as well as the development of education and training for health care providers and of practice guidelines, cancer pain remains under-treated. The oncology nurse has a pivotal role in the assessment, management, and evaluation of this complex symptom. Nurses need to cultivate their knowledge, skills, and expertise in pain assessment and management to apply what they have learned to the care of individual patients. The oncology nurses' role as patient advocate and educator will be paramount to educating patients and families, evaluating the patient's progress toward pain outcomes, and rallying the interdisciplinary team toward achieving optimal pain relief for each person experiencing cancer pain.

REVIEW QUESTIONS

✓ Case Study

Mrs. G., a 55-year-old woman diagnosed 2 years ago with small cell lung cancer with metastasis to brain, spine, and liver, receives her third cycle of her fourth chemotherapy regimen, and recently completed a course of palliative radiation therapy for metastasis to her brain. Her performance status is Eastern Cooperative Oncology Group (ECOG) 3. Her pain medications are the following: OxyContin, 200 mg every 12 hours, with oxycodone, 15 to 30 mg orally every 4 hours as needed for breakthrough pain; she has taken 4 doses a day of her oxycodone. She reports dull, aching back pain and sharp pain in her legs, radiating down her legs to a burning pain in her feet, rating her pain at an 8 to 10 out of 10 and states, "I do not really understand that number scale. She describes her pain as severe "all over" and expresses frustration about how the pain is good one day and bad the next day. Accompanying symptoms are anxiety, fatigue, and a decubitus ulcer on her coccyx. Over the weekend, she called the telephone triage nurse because a friend told her that people who are dying sleep a lot, and she finds herself sleeping a lot. She is a widow, has one adult son, and two sisters, all living nearby. In the past, there were concerns noted in the chart regarding "drug-seeking behaviors" and "slightly" impaired judgment or insights. Because of poorly controlled pain, 6 weeks ago, patient-controlled analgesia with morphine was set up with home care nurses to monitor, but Mrs. G. experienced more severe pain and nausea, and this delivery method was discontinued within 3 days of initiation. She says, "People don't take care of me because I am dying."

QUESTIONS

1. Who is the most reliable source of information on Mrs. G's pain?
   a. Mrs. G
   b. Nurse
   c. Family member or caregiver
   d. Physician
2. To assess pain in a cognitively impaired person, what does the nurse do?
   a. Obtains the pain rating from a family member or caregiver
   b. Observes the patient for pain behaviors (e.g., grimacing or restlessness)
   c. Utilizes a small numerical scale (e.g., 0 to 3 or simple word descriptors)
   d. Does not assess pain with a numerical scale
3. For a comprehensive assessment of Mrs.'s pain, what other assessment component requires further exploration?
   a. Quality of pain
   b. Meaning of the pain
   c. Medication history
   d. Pain history
4. When communicating these assessment findings to the physician, what should the nurse include?
   a. Impact on daily function
   b. Concerns about dying
   c. Drug-seeking behaviors
   d. Anxiety and fatigue

Continued

REVIEW QUESTIONS—CONT'D

5. When Mrs. G. was given morphine by patient-controlled analgesia at home, she experienced more severe pain and nausea. For Mrs. G., 3 days was not a sufficient amount of time for her to develop tolerance to morphine. What is the most likely rationale for her experience of more severe pain?
   a. Insufficient education on how to use the patient-controlled analgesia delivery method
   b. Noncompliance related to side effects, like nausea
   c. Inadequate equianalgesic dose conversion from oral OxyContin to IV morphine
   d. Patient too anxious

6. Based on Mrs. G.'s description of her pain and because escalating the doses of her opioids was not effective, what would be the *best* coanalgesic to add to her pain management plan?
   a. Baclofen
   b. Neurontin
   c. Zometa
   d. Nortriptyline

7. The nurse will monitor Mrs. G. for which of the following side effects when Neurontin is initiated?
   a. Constipation, nausea, itching, tremors, and hallucinations
   b. Sedation, dizziness, nausea, confusion, and lower-extremity edema
   c. Ataxia, nausea, alterations in liver enzymes, and weight gain
   d. Stomatitis, nausea, vomiting, and diarrhea

8. What is an appropriate intervention for Mrs. G.'s opioid therapy?
   a. Discontinue OxyContin and initiate Dilaudid subcutaneous continuous infusion
   b. Switch from OxyContin to MS Contin
   c. Administer OxyContin, 200 mg every 8 hours, rather than every 12 hours
   d. Change dose of oxycodone to 10% to 20% of total 24-hour dose every 1 to 2 hours

9. What nonpharmacologic strategies are the most appropriate to suggest to Mrs. G.?
   a. Breathing exercises, music therapy
   b. Hypnosis, guided imagery
   c. Support groups, heat and/or cold
   d. Massages, music therapy

10. What is the most appropriate pain outcome for Mrs. G.?
    a. Patient communicates pain intensity using standardized scales.
    b. Patient states the pain is reduced or relieved.
    c. Patient participates in usual daily activities.
    d. Patient reports adequate amounts of relief and feels rested.

ANSWERS

1. **A.** *Rationale:* Patient self-report is the most reliable indicator of pain.

2. **C.** *Rationale:* Cognitively impaired patients are capable of using pain scales, such as small numerical scales or simple word descriptors. Other responses are not appropriate or not appropriate on their own.

3. **B.** *Rationale:* The case study suggests but does not provide sufficient assessment of the meaning of the pain related to increasing pain, concerns about death and dying, and cultural or spiritual concerns.

4. **A.** *Rationale:* When communicating assessment findings to a physician, state the problem, using objective data, describe the impact on function, and describe current medications, including what has been taken in the past 24 hours and how long the pain medication is effective. Also, collaborate with the pharmacist on recommendations for pharmacologic strategies to discuss with the physician.

5. **C.** *Rationale:* Equianalgesic dosing principles and conversion guides are necessary when changing from one opioid to another, or from one route to another. For Mrs. G., both the opioid and the route were changed, but her pain increased. Other responses were not identified as issues in the case study. Effective pain management relies on analgesics selected, based on pharmacology management principles.

6. **B.** *Rationale:* Mrs. G. described sharp pain in her legs, radiating down her legs to a burning pain in her feet, indicating neuropathic pain. Neurontin has demonstrated efficacy and limited adverse effects, making it the first-line treatment for neuropathic pain.

7. **B.** *Rationale:* Neurontin is generally well tolerated, with the most common side effects of sedation, dizziness, nausea, confusion, and lower-extremity edema. The other responses include side effects of other medications.

8. **D.** *Rationale:* After reviewing pain medications, Mrs. G.'s oxycodone dose for breakthrough pain is not based on pharmacologic management principles. The sustained-release dose of OxyContin may not be maximized, making it premature to switch to another opioid. The patient has experienced nausea with IV PCA morphine, making MS Contin a less likely option. The sustained-release dose of OxyContin may have to be increased for improved analgesia, but not necessarily the time interval.

9. **A.** *Rationale:* With Mrs. G's anxiety, brain metastasis, and types of pain, relaxation techniques such as breathing exercises and music therapy may be most appropriate. Hypnosis and support groups may be difficult for her with brain metastasis. Massages may not be appropriate with bone pain and metastasis.

10. **B.** *Rationale:* Although all of these responses are pain outcomes, only "patient states pain is reduced or relieved" is appropriate for the patient in this case study. Mrs. G. indicated that she has difficulty with the numerical pain intensity scale. She is sleeping a lot (i.e., no insomnia) and has a decubitus ulcer on her coccyx, suggesting decreased mobility at home.

REFERENCES

1. Oncology Nursing Society: *Position Paper: cancer pain management*, Pittsburgh, 2004, Author; retrieved June 6, 2005, from http://www.ons.org.
2. Cady J: Understanding opioid tolerance in cancer pain, *Oncol Nurs Forum* 28(10):1561-1568, 2001.
3. Berry P, Dahl J: The new JCAHO pain standards: implications for pain management nurses, *Pain Manage Nurs* 1(1):3-12, 2000.
4. Merskey H: Classification of chronic pain: description of chronic pain syndromes and definitions of pain terms, *Pain* 3(Suppl):S217, 1979.
5. McCaffery M, Pasero C: *Pain: a clinical manual*, ed 2, St. Louis, 1999, Mosby.
6. McCaffery M. *Nursing practice theories related to cognition, bodily pain, and man-environment interactions*, Los Angeles, 1968, UCLA Student Store.
7. American Pain Society: *Principles of analgesic use in the treatment of acute pain and cancer pain*, ed 5, Glenview, IL, 2003, Author.
8. American Academy of Pain Medicine: *Definitions related to the use of opioids for the treatment of pain* (Joint consensus statement American Academy of Pain Medicine, American Pain Society, American Society for Addiction Medicine), 2001, retrieved June 6, 2005, from http://www.painmed.org/productpub/statements.
9. Miaskowski C, Cleary J, Burney R et al: *Guideline for the management of cancer pain in adults and children*, APS clinical practice guide series no. 3, Glenview, IL, 2005, American Pain Society.
10. Holland J: Psychosocial distress in the patient with cancer: standards of care and treatment guidelines, oncology symptom management: symptom management for the cancer patient: team approach part II, *Oncology Issues* 15(4 Suppl):19-24, 2000.
11. Ferrell BR: To know suffering, *Oncol Nurs Forum* 20(10):1471-1477, 1993.
12. Kuuppelomaki M, Lauri S: Cancer patients' reported experiences of suffering, *Cancer Nurs* 21(5):364-369, 1998.
13. Thorns A, Sykes N: Opioid use in the last week of life and implications for end-of-life decision-making, *Lancet* 356(9227):398-399, 2000.
14. American Nurses Association: *Position statements: pain management and control of distressing symptoms in dying patients*, Washington, DC, 2003, Author; retrieved July 22, 2005, from http://www.ana.org.
15. Hospice and Palliative Nursing Association: HPNA position paper: pain, *J Hospice Palliat Care Nurs* 6(1):62-64, 2004.
16. SUPPORT Principal Investigators: A controlled trial to improve care for seriously ill hospitalized patients: the study to understand prognoses and preferences for outcomes and risks of treatments, *JAMA* 274(20):1591-1598, 1995.
17. Institute of Medicine: *Enhancing data systems to improve the quality of cancer care*, Washington, DC, 2000, National Academy Press.
18. Brant J: Comfort. In Itano J and Taoka K, editors: *ONS Core curriculum for oncology nursing*, St. Louis, 2005, Elsevier.
19. Polovich M, White J, Kelleher L: *Chemotherapy and biotherapy guidelines: recommendations for practice*, ed 2, Pittsburgh, 2005, Oncology Nursing Society.
20. Shih A, Miakowski C, Dodd M et al: A research review of the current treatments for radiation-induced oral mucositis in patients with head and neck cancer, *Oncol Nurs Forum* 29(7):1063-1080, 2002.
21. Jacox A, Carr DB, Payne R et al: *Management of cancer pain*, clinical practice guideline no. 9, Agency for Health publication no. 94-0592, Rockville, MD, 1994, Department of Health and Human Services.
22. Davis GC, Hiemenz ML, White TL: Barriers to managing chronic pain of older adults with arthritis, *J Nurs Schol* 34(1):121-126, 2002.
23. Schumacher KL, West C, Dodd M et al: Pain management autobiographies and reluctance to use opioids for cancer pain management, *Cancer Nurs* 25(2):125-133, 2002.
24. Morrison RS, Wallenstein S, Natale D et al: "We don't carry that"—failure of pharmacies in predominately non-white neighborhoods to stock opioid analgesics, *New Engl J Med* 342(14):1023-1026, 2000.
25. West CM, Dodd MJ, Paul S et al: Pro-Self©: pain control program-an effective approach for cancer pain management, *Oncol Nurs Forum* 30(1):65-73, 2003.
26. Vega-Stromberg T, Holmes S, Gorski L et al: Road to excellence in pain management: research, outcomes, and direction (ROAD), *J Nurs Qual* 17(1):15-26, 2002.
27. Miaskowski C, Dodd M, West C et al: Lack of adherence with analgesic regimen: a significant barrier to effective cancer pain management, *J Clin Oncol* 19(23):4275-4279, 2001.

28. Luggen AS: Cancer pain in the older adult. In Luggen, SA, Meiner, SE, editors: *Handbook of care for the older adult with cancer*, Pittsburgh, 2000, Oncology Nursing Society.
29. Mitty EL: Ethnicity and end of life decision-making, *Reflect Nurs Leadership* 27(1):28-31, 46, 2001.
30. Dawson R, Sellars DE, Spross J et al: Do patients' beliefs act as barriers to effective pain management behaviors and outcomes in patients with cancer-related or non-cancer-related pain, *Oncol Nurs Forum* 32(2): 363-381, 2005.
31. Portenoy, R, Lesage, P: Management of cancer pain, *Lancet* 353(9165):1695-1700, 1999.
32. Zaza C, Baine N: Cancer pain and psychosocial factors: a critical review of the literature, *J Pain Symptom Manage* 24(5):526-542, 2002.
33. Dworkin RH: An overview of neuropathic pain: syndromes, symptoms, signs, and several mechanisms, *Clin J Pain*, 18, 343-349, 2002.
34. Paice J: Mechanisms and management of neuropathic pain in cancer, *J Support Oncol* 1(2):107-120, 2003.
35. Liebeskind JC: Pain can kill, *Pain* 44(1):3-4, 1991.
36. Serlin RC, Mendoza TR, Nakamura Y et al: When is cancer pain mild, moderate, or severe? Grading pain severity by its interference with function, *Pain* 61(2):277-284, 1995.
37. National Comprehensive Cancer Network Practice Guidelines, *Adult Cancer Pain* v. 2, 2005, retrieved July 6, 2005, from http://www.nccn.org.
38. McCaffrey M: Using the 0-10 Pain Rating Scale, *Am J Nurs* 101(10): 81-82, 2001.
39. Pasero C: Teaching patients to use a numerical pain rating scale, *Am J Nurs* 99(12):22, 1999.
40. Soscia J: Assessing pain in cognitively impaired older adults with cancer, *Clin J Oncol Nurs* 7(2):174-177, 2004.
41. Lane P, Kuntupis M, MacDonald S et al: A pain assessment tool for people with advanced Alzheimer's disease and other progressive dementias (PAINAD), *Home Health Nurse* 21(1):32-37, 2003.
42. Salmore R: Development of a new pain scale: Colorado behavioral numerical pain scale for sedated adult patients undergoing gastrointestinal procedures, *Gastroenterol Nurs* 25(6):257-62, 2002.
43. Rhiner M, Palos G, Termini M: Managing breakthrough pain: a clinical review with three case studies using oral transmucosal fentanyl citrate, *Clin J Oncol Nurs* 8(5):507-512, 2004.
44. Caraceni A, Porteno, RK, An international survey of cancer pain characteristics and syndromes. IASP task force on cancer pain, *Pain* 82(3): 263-274, 1999.
45. Ferrell B, Dean G: The meaning of cancer pain, *Semin Oncol Nurs* 11(1):17-22, 1995.
46. Ersek M, Cherrier MM, Overman SS et al: The cognitive effects of opioids, *Pain Manage Nurs* 5(2):75-93, 2004.
47. Levy M: Pharmacologic treatment of cancer pain, *New Engl J Med* 335(15):1124-1132, 1996.
48. Indelicato R, Portenoy RK: Opioid rotation in the management of refractory cancer pain, *J Clin Oncol* 21(Suppl 9):81s-91s, 2003.
49. American Geriatrics Society Panel on Chronic Pain in Older Persons: the management of persistent pain in older persons, *J Am Geriatr Soc* 50(6 Suppl):S205-224, 2002.
50. Sargent C: Naloxone: How well do you know this drug, *Clin J Oncol Nurs* 6(1):17-18, 2002.
51. Rozans M, Dreisbach A, Lertora JL, et al: Palliative uses of methylphenidate in patients with cancer: a review, *J Clin Oncol* 20(1):335-339, 2002.
52. Cherny N, Ripamonti C, Pereira J et al: Strategies to manage the adverse effects of oral morphine: an evidence-based report, *J Clin Oncol* 19(9):2542-2554, 2001.
53. Coyne P: When the world health organization analgesic therapies ladder fails: the role of invasive analgesic therapies, *Oncol Nurs Forum* 30(5):777-783, 2003.
54. Lusser D, Huskey AG, Portenoy RK: Adjuvant analgesics in cancer pain management, *Oncologist* 9(5):571-591, 2004.
55. McQuay HJ: Neuropathic pain: evidence matters, *Eur J Pain* 6(A Suppl):11-18, 2002.
56. Berenson JR: Recommendations for zoledronic acid treatment of patients with bone metastases, *Oncologist* 10(1):52-62, 2005.
57. Smith M, Kemp J, Hemphill L et al: Outcomes of therapeutic massage for hospitalized cancer patients, *J Nurs Schol* 34(3):257-262, 2002.
58. Lewandowski W, Good M, Draucker C: Changes in the meaning of pain with the use of guided imagery, *Pain Manage Nurs* 6(2):58-67, 2005.

CHAPTER 40

Sleep Disturbance

Patricia A. Carter

Definition

Sleep is a complex highly structured activity that is regulated by internal biologic processes such as melatonin, and environmental factors such as amount of daylight. Normal sleep consists of five stages, four episodes of non–rapid eye movement (NREM) sleep plus one episode of rapid eye movement (REM) sleep. Each sleep cycle is approximately 90 minutes in duration and is generally repeated 4 or 5 times throughout the night. The last third of the night is mostly characterized by REM sleep, whereas delta (slow-wave) sleep is predominant at the beginning of the night.[1,2]

Adult sleep disturbances (disorders) include narcolepsy, sleep apnea, periodic leg movements, restless leg syndrome, and insomnia. Insomnia is by far the most common of these disorders. Insomnia can be diagnosed as primary (not the result of another medical or psychologic condition) or secondary (resulting from a comorbidity). Diagnosis of insomnia is made through a series of self-report and objective assessments. Diagnostic criteria include (1) difficulty initiating and/or maintaining sleep that (2) occurs at least 3 nights per week and (3) causes significant impairment of daytime functioning (e.g., fatigue) or marked distress. The duration of these three symptoms determines the diagnosis of transient or situational insomnia (1 month or less), short-term or subacute (1 to 6 months), or chronic insomnia (6 months or more).[2]

Prevalence

Sleep is an area of functioning that is frequently impaired in cancer patients.[1,3] Studies conducted among mixed samples of cancer patients suggest that between 30% and 50% of newly diagnosed or recently treated cancer patients report sleep difficulties.[4-6] Most patients reported the onset of insomnia was highly correlated with the time of cancer diagnosis.[7,8] Insomnia symptoms were found 2 to 5 years after initiation of cancer therapy in 25% to 45% of patients, suggesting that insomnia develops a chronic course in a substantial proportion of cancer patients.[6] The National Cancer Institute (NCI) estimates that sleep disturbances are twice as prevalent in cancer patients as in the general population.[9]

Differences in prevalence rates of sleep-wake disturbances exist according to site-specific cancers with ranges from 30% to 88% in women with breast cancer, 25% to 52% in patients with lung cancer, and 52% to 62% in patients with solid tumors.[6,10]

The most prevalent sleep-wake problems reported by cancer patients (mixed diagnoses) were excessive daytime fatigue (44%), insomnia (31%), and excessive daytime sleepiness (28%). Insomnia commonly involved multiple awakenings (76% of cases) and had lasted longer than 6 months (75% of cases).[6]

Women with breast cancer reported sleeping an average of 6 hours per night and 1 hour during the day before beginning chemotherapy.[11] Men with prostate cancer and benign prostatic hypertrophy (BPH) reported significantly more fatigue and sleeping difficulties than men in the general population. Sleep difficulties and fatigue were most frequently associated with micturition problems.[12]

Risk Factors

PREDISPOSING FACTORS

Women report more difficulty sleeping than men across populations.[13-15] In the general population,[16] sleep tends to decline with age; however, in cancer patients, the reverse was observed. That is, younger cancer patients reported more sleep disturbances than older cancer patients.[6,17] For those patients diagnosed before the age of 55 the chances of having sleep problems was increased by 26% over those diagnosed after 55 years of age.[6]

Additional predisposing factors for insomnia in cancer patients include hyperarousability trait, family and/or personal history of insomnia, and presence of depression and/or anxiety.[1] Although gender, age, history, and personality traits are less modifiable predisposing factors to insomnia, depression and anxiety are conditions that can be addressed in the cancer patient. Anxiety and depression are reported by approximately half of all cancer patients at some time during their illness.[1] The relationship between psychologic conditions and insomnia is only beginning to be explored in cancer patients. Redeker and colleagues found a positive correlation between depression and insomnia in 263 cancer patients with mixed diagnoses.[17] Similarly, Koopman and colleagues found that problems falling asleep, and waking during the night were significantly correlated with depression in a sample of breast cancer patients.[18]

Etiology

PRECIPITATING FACTORS

Precipitating factors for insomnia in cancer patients include the variety of stressful life events experienced from the point of diagnosis throughout treatment.[1] Specific stressful points in the cancer process are initial diagnosis, surgery, treatment, and recurrence, as well as the period of the palliative and terminal stages of the disease.[19] Appraisal of stressors and perceived lack of control are strong predictors of insomnia in noncancer populations.[20]

Cancer treatments may increase the risk for insomnia. One example is surgery; particularly those interventions involving disfigurement or a functional loss may produce psychologic distress, which in turn, might increase the risk for insomnia.[21] Although, it is important to consider the psychologic impact of surgery, the influence on insomnia symptoms may not occur until after discharge. A more immediate risk factor to consider is that surgery often requires hospitalization. Hospitalization in itself can trigger sleep disturbance, because of environmental factors (e.g., noise, bed discomfort), as well as psychologic and behavioral factors (e.g., anxiety, loneliness, modification of sleep routine).[22] In a study with cancer patients, those with a recent surgery had higher odds of reporting insomnia symptoms than those with distant surgeries or no surgical intervention.[6]

Radiotherapy (RT) is strongly associated with insomnia. Miaskowski and Lee observed increased latency (time to fall asleep after lights out) and nocturnal awakenings, and decreased sleep efficiency, in a sample of outpatients receiving RT for bone metastasis.[23] Similarly, women with uterine cancer experienced sleep difficulties during treatment, with a peak in symptoms during the last week of treatment and a return to baseline levels at the 3-month follow-up.[24] Insomnia was a commonly reported symptom experienced by bone marrow transplant patients.[14] Antiemetics used for chemotherapy-related nausea and vomiting correlated with higher rates of insomnia.[25] Insomnia is a well-known side effect of dexamethasone, but prochlorperazine, metoclopramide, and granisetron, a serotonin (5-HT$_3$)–receptor antagonist, have also been found to disturb sleep in some cancer patients.

In women, the estrogen deficiency produced by surgical menopause, chemotherapy, and hormonal therapy (e.g., tamoxifen) caused the occurrence of premature menopause or the aggravation of menopausal symptoms that can interfere with sleep.[10] Of particular importance are vasomotor symptoms such as nocturnal hot flashes and sweating, reported by at least half of all women treated with tamoxifen and frequently reported by men with prostate cancer treated with androgen-deprivation therapy.[26,27,28] Some studies have demonstrated that objectively assessed hot flashes were strongly associated with more frequent and longer nocturnal awakenings in healthy postmenopausal women.[29,30] Similarly, researchers have found a relationship between severity of hot flashes and prevalence of sleeping difficulty among women treated for breast cancer.[31,32] Women receiving chemotherapy for breast cancer reported increased duration, latency, and frequency of nighttime awakenings.[33]

Further evidence of the relationship between climacteric symptoms and sleep disturbance is provided by data showing that estrogen therapy among cancer-free postmenopausal women significantly improves sleep, and that this improvement is mostly explained by the alleviation of hot flashes and sweating.[31] Weitzner and colleagues found that treating hot flashes in breast cancer patients improved sleep quality and depression.[34] Dorsey and colleagues found that zolpidem (Ambien) was effective in treating sleep difficulties in perimenopausal and postmenopausal insomnia.[35]

Insomnia can also be precipitated by cancer pain. It has been estimated that 30% to 50% of cancer patients receiving treatment and 60% to 80% of advanced cancer patients experience pain.[36] In addition, approximately 10% to 25% of cancer patients have pain unrelated to their cancer.[36] In a mixed sample of cancer patients, 45% of patients with all diagnoses and 55% of lung cancer patients reported that sleep was significantly impaired because of pain.[6] Slightly lower percentages of nonmetastatic breast cancer patients (35%) reported that sleep problems were a result of pain.[4] Of cancer patients with pain, 37% reported difficulties initiating sleep, whereas 58% and 60% reported nocturnal awakenings because of pain.[4] In addition, researchers have found that poor sleep quality reduces pain thresholds.[37]

Cancer related fatigue (CRF) has been strongly associated with insomnia.[38] The relationship between CRF and insomnia is complex. Cancer treatments, such as chemotherapy and radiation therapy, have been shown to precipitate CRF.[17,33] Fatigued breast cancer patients reported more sleep difficulties than less fatigued patients.[39] Specific sleep difficulties expressed by patients with CRF include sleep initiation and maintenance problems, lower overall sleep adequacy, and increased daytime sleepiness.[39]

In order of prevalence, cancer patients identified the following factors as precipitating their insomnia: thoughts (52%), pain (45%), concerns about their health (40%), concerns about family and friends (33%), cancer diagnosis (32%), physical effects of cancer (27%), and concerns about finances (23%). Lung cancer patients reported a different order of priorities. Cancer diagnosis was the first precipitating factor, followed in order by concerns about their health, pain, thoughts, and the physical effects of cancer.[6]

PERPETUATING FACTORS

In many cases, insomnia is situational, and sleep returns to normal after the precipitating factors have been removed or adapted to. The individual responses to insomnia contribute to whether the sleep disturbance will cease or become chronic. According to cognitive-behavioral theory, maladaptive sleep habits and dysfunctional thoughts in reaction to sleep disturbance serve to maintain insomnia. Both exert negative effects by increasing arousal (physiologic, cognitive, and emotional) and performance anxiety (the pressure to sleep), which are in direct opposition to the relaxation state required for sleep.

To make up for lost sleep, chronic insomnia sufferers tend to spend more time in bed, nap during the day, and have an irregular sleep-wake schedule. These sleep habits can desynchronize the sleep-wake cycle. Unfortunately, these maladaptive sleep habits are common in cancer patients, who are encouraged to get rest and sleep to recuperate from their cancer treatments.[40] In addition, persons with chronic insomnia, including those with cancer, may participate in sleep-interfering activities in their bedroom. Sleep-interfering behaviors may include watching TV, listening to music, eating, working, or reading in bed or the bedroom. These habits tend to weaken the association (deconditioning) between certain normally sleep-inducing stimuli (bed, bedtime, and bedroom) and sleep.[41]

Faulty beliefs and attitudes about sleep and sleeplessness may contribute to insomnia.[41] Common beliefs and attitudes that can contribute to insomnia include the following: (1) unrealistic sleep expectations (I have to sleep 8 hours each night); (2) inaccurate assessment of sleep problems (I don't sleep); (3) attributing all daytime difficulties to poor sleep (bad days always follow bad nights); and (4) misunderstanding of the causes of insomnia (my sleep problems are caused by age and hormones). Breast cancer patients participating in a clinical trial of a cognitive-behavioral sleep intervention reported faulty beliefs and attitudes specific to cancer that may have contributed to their sleep problems. These ruminating thoughts included the following: If I don't sleep well, my cancer will come back. My doctor told me to rest, and I can't do it. I have to do everything possible to cure my cancer, so I must sleep well. If I have a recurrence, it will be because I can't sleep.

The literature suggests that many factors are implicated in the development and persistence of insomnia in cancer patients.

Some of these factors are more cancer-specific (precipitating factors), whereas others are more generalizable to all insomnia sufferers (perpetuating factors). It is important to note that there is a paucity of systematic studies exploring these factors and their interrelationships in cancer patient populations.

Effects and Consequences

PSYCHOLOGIC AND BEHAVIORAL CONSEQUENCES OF INSOMNIA

Fatigue, impaired daytime functioning, and mood disturbances often coexist in cancer patients and are all potential psychologic and behavioral consequences of insomnia. One of the most common complaints of insomnia patients is fatigue.[42] Fatigue is also a common complaint of cancer patients, particularly after chemotherapy and/or radiotherapy.[43-45] Cancer-related fatigue has traditionally been viewed as a temporary reaction to cancer treatments; however, more recent findings suggest that fatigue persists several months after treatment is completed.[45] Therefore, insomnia adds an additional risk for intense and persistent fatigue after cancer treatment. Sarna and Brecht found that 31% of lung cancer patients with fatigue also experienced insomnia.[46]

Sleep loss leads to decreased daytime functioning, including impaired concentration and motor skills.[47] Similarly, cancer patients indicated that sleep problems negatively affected physical and emotional well being, coping ability, and daytime functioning.[6,23,46] As mentioned earlier, sleep disturbance often coexists with depression and anxiety. Although anxiety and depression precipitate insomnia, there are also instances when anxiety and depression are consequences of insomnia. For example, individuals with insomnia can worry about the consequences of their sleep disorder and feel anxiety and depression about their inability to overcome this problem.[41] In fact, researchers found that chronic insomnia contributed to the development of subsequent depression, anxiety, and substance abuse up to 5 years later.[13] Interestingly, the risk of developing depression is decreased following resolution of insomnia symptoms, supporting the hypothesis that insomnia is a key risk factor for mood disorders.[13]

PHYSIOLOGIC CONSEQUENCES OF INSOMNIA

Health problems, medical consultations, and hospitalizations are more common in poor sleepers than in good sleepers.[48] The most common complaints in patients with insomnia include headache, diarrhea, gastrointestinal distress, palpitations, and nonspecific pain.[5]

Recent studies indicate sleep disturbance is associated with increased mortality. Sleeping 5, 6, or 7 hours was found to increase mortality in women by 1.8, 1.3, and 1.1 times respectively at a 10-year follow up as compared to women who reported sleeping 8 hours each night.[49] At a 12-year follow-up, difficulties initiating sleep were related to coronary artery disease deaths in men, but not in women.[50] Degner, in a study with newly diagnosed lung cancer patients, found that high symptom distress predicted lower 5-year survival, even when disease stage was held constant.[51]

There is growing evidence that suggests prolonged sleep deprivation may impair innate immunity and that restorative sleep enhances immune competence.[42] A number of laboratory-based studies have shown a detrimental effect of sleep deprivation on immune functioning; however, studies of this relationship in naturalistic settings are much more limited.[52,53] In laboratory settings, total sleep duration, efficiency, and non–REM duration have been positively correlated with natural killer cell activity.[54,55] In a study with cervical cancer patients, higher satisfaction with sleep duration was associated with a higher concentration of helper T cells in circulating blood.[56]

Insomnia appears to have a number of consequences, although several of these effects must be examined more rigorously in longitudinal studies. Regardless of the role of sleep in recovery from cancer, it is likely that improved sleep will enhance the patient's quality of life, tolerance to treatment, and mood.

Assessment and Measurement

Approximately 50% of patients reported that sleep problems occurred most nights.[6] Although patients expressed concern regarding the impact that not getting enough rest might have on their overall health and well-being, most did not report their sleep difficulties to their health care provider. Some patients stated that their sleep problems were not important enough to risk distracting their physician from the work of "curing" their cancer.[10] These findings suggest that health care providers must take a proactive role in assessing for sleep disturbances. One of the most commonly used insomnia assessment instruments is the sleep diary. This is a 1- to 2-week prospective diary that the patient fills in each day and night. Areas assessed are time to bed, time to fall asleep, duration of sleep, number, duration, and cause of nighttime awakenings, and daytime functioning (i.e., fatigue, cognitive, motor skills). The information collected with the sleep diary helps to identify areas of sleep problems as well as suggest potential treatment options that would be most effective in treating the identified sleep disturbance.

Interventions

Interventions for sleep can be classified into the following categories: pharmacologic and cognitive-behavioral. In the following section, a brief overview of interventions that can be useful in the cancer patient is presented.

PHARMACOLOGIC THERAPIES

Hypnotic medications are by far the most commonly used treatment for insomnia. One quarter of cancer patients in Davidson's study reported using tranquilizers to promote sleep.[6] New compounds (e.g., eszopiclone [Lunesta], zaleplon [Sonata], zolpidem) are showing promise for treatment of transient and chronic insomnia in noncancer populations. However, empiric evidence of the effectiveness of and the side effects associated with use of hypnotics in cancer patients is severely limited, and the studies that have been conducted are outdated.[10] That said, cancer patients who complain of insomnia to their health care provider are likely to receive a prescription for a hypnotic medication. Therefore, it is important to be aware that the use of hypnotic medications is associated with a number of risks and limitations. Individuals using hypnotic medications often experience residual effects the next day (e.g., daytime drowsiness, dizziness or lightheadedness, and cognitive and motor skill impairments).[41] Elderly people are more vulnerable to experience these effects as a result of having a slower drug metabolism. Another potential side effect is respiratory suppression when hypnotics are used in conjunction with opioids.

CONSIDERATIONS FOR OLDER ADULTS

- Older adults are more likely to report somatic symptoms when experiencing sleep difficulties.
- Older adults are more likely to attribute sleep difficulties to "normal changes with age" and consider them untreatable.
- Older adults are more susceptible to toxicity and thus side effects from hypnotics than younger patients because of slower drug metabolism. Pharmacologic agents with a long half-life, such as flurazepam (Dalmane) or other benzodiazepines, should be avoided in older adults.

General rules for treatment with hypnotics are to start with low dosages, increase slowly, and treat for a maximum of 4 weeks to limit dependency, although it must be noted that these recommendations lack empirical support. Finally, it is important to remember that many patients treat their insomnia with over-the-counter medications and herbal therapies. Most of the over-the-counter drugs contain diphenhydramine, which does not enhance sleep architecture, but causes some of same negative side effects as prescriptions including dry mouth, oversedation, and tolerance. Herbal sedatives such as valerian and kava have only recently been empirically investigated. A recent literature review found that studies revealed the relative safety and efficacy of valerian, whereas they showed disturbing toxicity concerns for kava when used by cancer patients.[57] There is limited and inconclusive evidence on the effectiveness and relative safety of other commonly used herbal sedatives (e.g., chamomile, lavender) and nutritional supplements (e.g., melatonin) for cancer patients.

Given these limitations and recommendations, if insomnia is recurrent or persistent, as seen in cancer patients, the first-line intervention should be cognitive-behavioral therapies (CBT) with the use of hypnotics as an adjuvant therapy. With time and further research, however, perhaps even that use of hypnotics in cancer patients will be superceded by the use of the newer compounds that are having success in the general population.

COGNITIVE-BEHAVIORAL THERAPIES (CBT)

Cognitive-behavioral therapies (CBT) have been found to be efficacious in the treatment of insomnia in the general population.[58] Sleep quality, total duration, efficiency, latency, and duration of awakenings were all significantly improved with the use of these therapies. In fact, the magnitude of improvement seen is comparable to those measured with the use of hypnotic medications, although without the side effects seen with medications.[59]

Stimulus control, sleep restriction, and multimodal treatments (combining several approaches) have generally been found to be the most effective nondrug interventions.[60] Relaxation therapies have been found to be effective in reducing cognitive arousal, a major contributor to sleep latency problems.[60] Cognitive therapy, focused on reframing the individual's thoughts about sleep, has not been tested as a single-mode treatment for insomnia; however, it is commonly used as part of a multimodal treatment plan. Use of CBT for cancer patients'

insomnia is gaining popularity. Studies have used a variety of combinations of commonly used therapies to effectively treat insomnia in cancer patient populations. Breast cancer patients have been the most frequently studied cancer population.[61,62] However, prostate and mixed cancer patient samples have also benefited from multimodal CBT interventions for insomnia.[63,64] Most common outcomes reported by participants across studies were increased duration and efficiency, with decreased latency and nighttime awakenings.

For those patients who do not achieve a satisfying improvement of their sleep pattern with these simple strategies or who meet diagnostic criteria for an insomnia syndrome, a referral to a sleep specialist should be considered.

Outcomes

The outcomes of all interventions, either pharmacologic or CBT, used to treat insomnia are focused on reducing the negative physical and/or emotional impacts of sleep disturbances. The goals of treatment are to bring the patient's sleep patterns closer to the recommendations for quality sleep. Those recommendations include at least 8 hours' duration (time asleep), at least 85% efficiency (time asleep/time in bed $\times$ 100), and less than 15 minutes latency. Not all patients will be able to obtain these recommended levels; however, findings from recent studies suggest that even small improvements in these sleep parameters result in significant clinical improvements in physiologic and emotional well being.[58]

Summary

Sleep disturbances are common problems in cancer patient populations. These symptoms continue to persist even after successful treatment for cancer.[4-6] Etiologies of insomnia in cancer patients are complex and far from well understood. Predisposing, precipitating, and perpetuating factors must be evaluated individually for each patient in order to understand the potential cause for the insomnia.

Treatment options are somewhat clearer. It is important to note that when patients with cancer report only one symptom (e.g., pain or fatigue), it is likely that other symptoms may also be present. Therefore, treatment for the symptom cluster is most appropriate. Ignoring one symptom while focusing on others may not be as efficacious as designing a treatment that would consider the effects on all symptoms. For example, treating sleep disturbances with hypnotics that may increase the feelings of daytime sleepiness in a patient already complaining of daytime fatigue will be less effective than using nonpharmacologic therapies. As part of the plan of care, it would also be prudent to include patient and family education regarding available counseling and/or therapy services and support groups that might be helpful in decreasing anxiety and/or depressive symptoms. Patients report higher overall quality of life when their symptoms are treated holistically.

Health care providers have to be aware of the frequency of which patients suffer from sleep disturbances. Patients are reluctant to share these symptoms with their health care providers; therefore providers must seek the information and provide options for treatment. Good sleep allows for restoration of the body and mind, and without it patients experience decreased quality of life and overall well-being, and may be at higher risk for negative physical and psychologic outcomes.

REVIEW QUESTIONS

✓ Case Study

Mrs. P. is a 50-year-old woman diagnosed 6 weeks ago with nonmetastatic breast cancer. She underwent a surgical resection and nodal biopsy and started chemotherapy. Mrs. P. filled out a 2-week sleep diary and is here to meet with the advanced practice nurse (APN) to discuss her sleep quality. The sleep diary reveals that Mrs. P. is sleeping an average of 4 hours per night and 2 hours during the day; she has an efficiency of 62% and an average latency of 50 minutes. To assess the etiology of the sleep problems, the APN asks Mrs. P. about when her sleep problems began. Mrs. P. says, "When I was in the hospital I just couldn't get comfortable away from home. I would sleep 1 to 2 hours at a time throughout the day and night. Now that I am at home, I still can't sleep." The nurse asks Mrs. P. to describe her typical night. She responds, "I go to bed at 8 pm, watch TV for about 1 hour, then turn out the lights. I lie in bed until I fall asleep (30 to 60 minutes). My mind just starts working; I worry a lot about what this cancer diagnosis will do to my marriage. My husband says he loves me, but I am not whole anymore after the surgery. In the morning, I force myself to stay in bed long enough so that I will get the 8 hours I need to get well." A short-term hypnotic agent is prescribed by the physician in conjunction with a nurse-initiated CBT prescription including sleep restriction, relaxation, stimulus control, and sleep hygiene.

QUESTIONS

1. Predisposing factors to Mrs. P.'s sleep problems include which of the following?
   a. Surgery
   b. Being female
   c. Chemotherapy
   d. Watching TV in bed
2. What is the recommended length of time for patients to assess their sleep with a sleep diary?
   a. Three days
   b. Seven days
   c. Four weeks
   d. Two weeks
3. By "forcing" herself to stay in bed while awake, Mrs. P. is affecting what aspect of her sleep profile?
   a. Duration
   b. Efficiency
   c. Latency
   d. Efficacy
4. Recommended pharmacotherapy for Mrs. P. should include which of the following directions?
   a. Start with the largest dose possible for quick symptom relief
   b. Increase dosage regularly to maintain effectiveness
   c. Treat for as long as necessary
   d. Educate the patient about daytime side effects
5. Mrs. P.'s statement "My husband says he loves me, but I am not whole anymore after the surgery" would indicate a need for further assessment for which common comorbidity of insomnia?
   a. Anxiety
   b. Depression
   c. Pain
   d. Immune deficiency
6. Which of the following is a precipitating factor to Mrs. P.'s insomnia?
   a. Gender
   b. Chemotherapy
   c. napping during the day
   d. Watching TV in bed
7. By prescribing relaxation therapy as part of a multimodal CBT, the nurse is addressing which aspect of Mrs. P's insomnia?
   a. Latency
   b. Efficiency
   c. Duration
   d. Nighttime awakenings
8. A physiologic consequence of insomnia is which of the following?
   a. Impaired concentration
   b. Hot flashes
   c. Anxiety
   d. Mortality
9. One of the criteria for an insomnia diagnosis is which of the following?
   a. Time to fall asleep
   b. Number of awakenings during the night
   c. Daytime dysfunction
   d. Sleeping less than 8 hours per night
10. What is the average percentage of newly diagnosed cancer patients who report sleep difficulties?
    a. 10%-20%
    b. 30%-50%
    c. 80%-90%
    d. 50%-60%

ANSWERS

1. **B.** *Rationale:* Women are at higher risk of experiencing sleep disturbances. Surgery and chemotherapy are precipitating factors, and watching TV in bed is a perpetuating factor.
2. **D.** *Rationale:* Two weeks allows for a representative presentation of sleep that is not affected by day-to-day changes. Timeframes of 3 and 7 days may not allow for a representative presentation of sleep. The timeframe of 4 weeks is often too burdensome for the patient, leading to nonadherence with the data recording.
3. **B.** *Rationale:* Sleep efficiency is time asleep/time in bed × 100. When Mrs. P. forces herself to lie in bed even though awake, she decreases her sleep efficiency. Duration is the total amount of time spent asleep during a single sleep period, and latency is the total amount of time required to fall asleep at the beginning of a sleep period. The option of "efficacy" is meant to serve as a distracter.
4. **D.** *Rationale:* All patients need to be educated about possible daytime effects (e.g., drowsiness, dizziness, and cognitive and motor skill impairment). Additionally, the general rules for hypnotic use are the following: start low, increase slowly, and treat for a maximum of 4 weeks.

5. B. *Rationale:* Depression may be secondary to surgery. The symptoms of anxiety, pain, and immune deficiency may each result from cancer therapy; however, the patient's statement is indicative of depressive symptoms.

6. B. *Rationale:* Chemotherapy is a precipitating factor for insomnia in cancer patients. Gender is a predisposing factor, while napping during the day and watching TV are perpetuating factors to insomnia.

7. A. *Rationale:* Relaxation therapy reduces cognitive arousal, the primary cause of sleep latency. Sleep dysfunction in efficiency, duration, and nighttime awakenings are most frequently treated with psychoeducational therapies (e.g., sleep hygiene, sleep restriction, etc).

8. D. *Rationale:* Mortality is the only physical outcome listed. Hot flashes are a precipitating factor of insomnia, not a physiologic consequence. Impaired concentration and increased anxiety are considered emotional responses rather than physical outcomes.

9. C. *Rationale:* The criteria for insomnia diagnosis include a difficulty initiating and/or maintaining sleep that occurs at least 3 nights a week and causes significant impairment of daytime functioning. Specific numbers (e.g., sleep duration, awakenings, minutes to fall asleep) are not part of the insomnia diagnosis.

10. B. *Rationale:* Recent studies report 30% to 50% of newly diagnosed or recently treated patients report sleep difficulties.

REFERENCES

1. Savard J, Morin CM: Insomnia in the context of cancer: a review of neglected problem, *J Clin Oncol* 19(3):895-908, 2001.
2. Hauri P, Sateia M, editors: *International classification of sleep disorders: diagnostic and coding manual,* ed 2, Westchester IL, 2005, American Academy of Sleep Medicine.
3. Chen ML, Chang HK: Physical symptom profiles of depressed and nondepressed patients with cancer, *Palliat Med* 18(8):712-718, 2004.
4. Savard J, Simard S, Blanchet J et al: Prevalence, clinical characteristics, and risk factors for insomnia in the context of breast cancer, *Sleep* 24(5):583-590, 2001.
5. Sateia MJ, Doghramji K, Hauri PJ et al: Evaluation of chronic insomnia: an American academy of sleep medicine review, *Sleep* 23(2):243-308, 2000.
6. Davidson JR, MacLean AW, Brundage MD et al: Sleep disturbances in cancer patients, *Soc Sci Med* 54(9):1309-1321, 2002.
7. Vena C, Parker K, Cunningham M et al: Sleep-wake disturbances in people with cancer, part I: an overview of sleep, sleep regulation, and effects of disease and treatment, *Oncol Nurs Forum* 31(4):735-746, 2004.
8. Savard J, Simard S, Hervouet S et al: Insomnia in men treated with radical prostatectomy for prostate cancer, *Psychooncology* 14(2):147-156, 2005.
9. National Cancer Institute: *Sleep disorders (PDQ) Health Professional Version.* Washington DC, 2002, US National Institutes of Health.
10. Clark J, Cunningham M, McMillan S et al: Sleep-wake disturbances in people with cancer, part II: evaluating the evidence for clinical decision making, *Oncol Nurs Forum* 31(4):747-771, 2004.
11. Ancoli-Israel S, Liu L, Marler MR et al: Fatigue, sleep, and circadian rhythms prior to chemotherapy for breast cancer, *Support Care Cancer* 14(3):201-209;2006
12. Jakobsson L, Loven L, Hallberg IR: Micturition problems in relation to quality of life in men with prostate cancer of benign prostatic hyperplasia: comparison with men from the general population, *Cancer Nurs* 27(3):218-229, 2004.
13. Ford DE, Cooper-Patrick L: Sleep disturbances and mood disorders: an epidemiologic perspective, *Depress Anxiety* 14(1):3-6, 2001.
14. Heinonen H, Volin L, Uutela A et al: Gender-associated differences in the quality of life after allogeneic BMT, *Bone Marrow Transplant* 28(5):503-509, 2001.
15. Mercadante S, Girelli D, Casuccio A: Sleep disorders in advanced cancer patients: prevalence and factors associated, *Support Care Cancer* 12(5):355-359, 2004.
16. Bliwise DL: Normal aging. In Kryger MH, Roth T, Dement WC, editors: *Principles and practice of sleep medicine,* ed 3, Philadelphia, 2000, Saunders.
17. Redeker NS, Lev EL, Ruggiero J: Insomnia, fatigue, anxiety, depression, and quality of life of cancer patients undergoing chemotherapy, *Schol Inq Nurs Pract* 14(4):275-290, 2000.
18. Koopman C, Nouriani B, Erickson Y et al: Sleep disturbances in women with metastatic breast cancer, *Breast J* 8(6):362-370, 2002.
19. Edwards B, Clark V: The psychological impact of a cancer diagnosis on families: the influence of family functioning and patients' illness characteristics on depression and anxiety, *Psychooncology* 13(8):562-576, 2004.
20. Morin CM, Rodrigue S, Ivers H: Role of stress, arousal, and coping skills in primary insomnia, *Psychosom Med* 65(2):259-267, 2003.
21. Pandey M, Singh SP, Behere PB et al: Quality of life in patients with early and advanced carcinoma of the breast, *Euro J Surg Oncol* 26(1):20-24, 2000.
22. Griffiths MF, Peerson A: Risk factors for chronic insomnia following hospitalization, *J Adv Nurs* 49(3):245-253, 2004.
23. Miaskowski C, Lee KA: Pain, fatigue, and sleep disturbances in oncology outpatients receiving radiation therapy for bone metastasis: a pilot study, *J Pain Symptom Manage* 17(5):320-332, 1999.
24. Ahlberg K, Ekman T, Gaston-Johansson F: The experience of fatigue, other symptoms and global quality of life during radiotherapy for uterine cancer, *Int J Nurs Stud* 42(3):377-386, 2005.
25. Poli-Bigelli S, Rodrigues-Pereira J, Carides AD et al: Addition of the neurokinin 1 receptor antagonist aprepitant to standard antiemetic therapy improves control of chemotherapy-induced nausea and vomiting: results from a randomized, double-blind, placebo-controlled trial in Latin America, *Cancer* 97(12):3090-3098, 2003.
26. Knobf MT: The menopausal symptom experiences in young mid-life women with breast cancer, *Cancer Nurs* 24(3):201-210, 2001.
27. Love RR, Hutson PR, Havighurst TC et al: Endocrine effects of tamoxifen plus exemestane in postmenopausal women with breast cancer, *Clin Cancer Res* 11(4):1500-1503, 2005.
28. Sharifi N, Gulley JL, Dahut WL: Androgen deprivation therapy for prostate cancer, *JAMA* 294(2):238-244, 2005.
29. Levine DW, Dailey ME, Rockhill B et al: Validation of the women's health initiative insomnia rating scale in a multicenter controlled clinical trial, *Psychosom Med* 67(1):98-104, 2005.
30. Eichling PS, Sahni J: Menopause related sleep disorders, *J Clin Sleep Med* 1(3):291-300, 2005.
31. Schultz PN, Klein MJ, Beck ML et al: Breast cancer: relationship between menopausal symptoms, physiologic health effects of cancer treatment and physical constraints on quality of life in long-term survivors, *J Clin Nurs* 14(2):204-211, 2005.
32. Savard J, Davidson JR, Ivers H et al: The association between nocturnal hot flashes and sleep in breast cancer survivors, *J Pain Symptom Manage* 27(6):513-522, 2004.
33. Berger AM, Higginbotham P: Correlates of fatigue during and following adjuvant breast cancer chemotherapy: a pilot study, *Oncol Nurs Forum* 27(9):1443-1448, 2000.
34. Weitzner MA, Moncello J, Jacobsen PB et al: A pilot trial of paroxetine for the treatment of hot flashes and associated symptoms in women with breast cancer, *J Pain Symptom Manage* 23(4):337-345, 2002.
35. Dorsey CM, Lee KA, Scharf MB: Effect of zolpidem on sleep in women with perimenopausal and postmenopausal insomnia: a 4-week, randomized, multicenter, double-blind placebo-controlled study, *Clin Ther* 26(10):1578-1586, 2004.

36. Miaskowski C, Cleary J, Burney R et al: *Guideline for the management of cancer pain in adults and children. APS Clinical Practice Guidelines Series, no. 3*, Glenview IL, 2005, American Pain Society.

37. Chiu YH, Silman AJ, Macfarlane GJ et al: Poor sleep and depression are independently associated with a reduced pain threshold. Results of a population based study, *Pain* 115(3):316-321, 2005.

38. Anderson KO, Getto CJ, Mendoza TR et al: Fatigue and sleep disturbance in patients with cancer, patients with clinical depression, and community-dwelling adults, *J Pain Symptom Manage* 25(4):307-318, 2003.

39. Bower JE, Ganz PA, Desmond KA et al: Fatigue in breast cancer survivors: occurrence, correlates, and impact on quality of life, *J Clin Oncol* 18(4):743-753, 2000.

40. Theobald DE: Cancer pain, fatigue, distress, and insomnia in cancer patients, *Clin Cornerstone* 6(Suppl 1D):S15-S21, 2004.

41. Morin CM: *Insomnia: psychological assessment and management*, New York, 1993, Guilford Press.

42. Krueger JM, Majde JA, Obal Jr F: Sleep in host defense, *Brain Behav Immun* 17(Suppl 1):S41-S47, 2003.

43. Lipman AJ, Lawrence DP: The management of fatigue in cancer patients, *Oncology* 18(12):1527-1533, 2004.

44. Greenberg DB: Clinical dimensions of fatigue, *Prim Care Companion J Clin Psychiatry* 4(3):90-93, 2002.

45. Stone P, Richards M, Alhern R et al: A study to investigate the prevalence, severity and correlates of fatigue among patients with cancer in comparison with a control group of volunteers without cancer, *Ann Oncol* 11(5):561-567, 2000.

46. Sarna L, Brecht ML: Dimensions of symptom distress in women with advanced lung cancer: a factor analysis, *Heart Lung* 26(1):23-30, 1997.

47. Metlaine A, Leger D, Choudat D: Socioeconomic impact of insomnia in working populations, *Ind Health* 43(1):11-19, 2005.

48. Novak M, Mucsi I, Shapiro CM et al: Increased utilization of health services by insomniacs—an epidemiological perspective, *J Psychosom Res* 56(5):527-536, 2004.

49. Ayas NT, White DP, Manson JE et al: A prospective study of sleep duration and coronary heart disease in women, *Arch Intern Med* 163(2):205-209, 2005.

50. Mallon L, Broman JE, Hetta J: Sleep complaints predict coronary artery disease mortality in males: a 12-year follow-up study of a middle-aged Swedish population, *J Intern Med* 251(3):207-216, 2002.

51. Degner LF, Sloan JA: Symptom distress in newly diagnosed ambulatory cancer patients and as a predictor of survival in lung cancer, *J Pain Symptom Manage* 10(6):423-432, 1995.

52. Irwin M: Effects of sleep and sleep loss on immunity and cytokines, *Brain Behav Immun* 16(5):503-512, 2002.

53. Pollmacher T, Schuld A, Kraus T et al: Experimental immunomodulation, sleep, and sleepiness in humans, *Ann NY Acad Sci* 917:488-499, 2000.

54. Dinges DF, Douglas SD, Hamarman S et al: Sleep deprivation and human immune function, *Adv Neuroimmunol* 5(2):97-110, 1995.

55. Irwin M, Miller C: Decreased natural killer cell responses and altered interleukin-6 and interleukin-10 production in alcoholism: an interaction between alcohol dependence and African-American ethnicity, *Alcohol Clin Exp Res* 24(4):560-569, 2000.

56. Irwin M, Smith TL, Gillin JC: Electroencephalographic sleep and natural killer activity in depressed patients and control subjects, *Psychosom Med* 54(1):10-21, 1992.

57. Block KI, Gyllenhaal C, Mead MN: Safety and efficacy of herbal sedatives in cancer care, *Integr Cancer Ther* 3(2):128-148, 2004.

58. Smith MT, Neubauer DN: Cognitive behavior therapy for chronic insomnia, *Clin Cornerstone* 5:28-40, 2003.

59. Smith MT, Perlis ML, Park A et al: Comparative meta-analysis of pharmacotherapy and behavior therapy for persistent insomnia, *Am J Psychiatry* 159(1):5-11, 2002.

60. Lichstein KL, Riedel BW, Wilson NM, et al: Relaxation and sleep compression for late-life insomnia: a placebo-controlled trial *J Consult Clin Psychol* 69(2):227-239,2001.

61. Quesnel C, Savard J, Simard S et al: Efficacy of cognitive-behavioral therapy for insomnia in women treated for non-metastatic breast cancer, *J Consult Clin Psychol* 71(1):189-200, 2003.

62. Berger AM, VonEssen S, Kuhn BR et al: Adherence, sleep, and fatigue outcomes after adjuvant breast cancer chemotherapy: results of a feasibility intervention study, *Oncol Nurs Forum* 30(3):513-522, 2003.

63. Kim Y, Roscoe JA, Morrow GR: The effects of information and negative affect on severity of side effects from radiation therapy for prostate cancer, *Support Care Cancer* 10(5):416-421, 2002.

64. Simeit R, Deck R, Conta-Marx B: Sleep management training for cancer patients with insomnia, *Support Care Cancer* 12(3):176-183, 2004.

INTERNET RESOURCES:

The American Sleep Disorders Foundation can be contacted at
http://www.asda.org
The Sleep Home Pages can be accessed at
http://bisleep.metsch.ucla.edu
The National Sleep Foundation can be contacted at
www.sleepfoundation.org
Educational site for professionals and laypersons can be accessed at
www.sleepeducation.com

CHAPTER 41

Nausea

Mei R. Fu, Roxanne W. McDaniel, and Verna A. Rhodes

Definition

Vomiting or emesis is the forceful expulsion of gastric, duodenal, or jejunal contents through the oral cavity caused by powerful contraction of the abdominal and chest wall muscles.[1] Nausea is a person's conscious awareness of potential vomiting, characterized by a subjective unpleasant wavelike sensation at the back of the throat, in the epigastrium, or in the abdomen that may or may not culminate in vomiting.[2,3] Nausea may be accompanied by physiologic responses such as hot or cold feelings, diaphoresis, increased salivation, pallor, tachycardia, light-headedness, dizziness and weakness.[4,5] Retching is the physical effort to vomit without expulsion of gastric contents.[1] Although nausea, vomiting, and retching are separate phenomena, they usually occur together as a cluster. The terms "vomiting" and "retching" usually capture the notion of the worst possible nausea.[1,3] Thus, these three symptoms, the unpleasant sensations created by nausea followed by the physical effort of vomiting or actual expulsion of gastric, duodenal, or jejunal contents, are frequently recognized as a symptom cluster of nausea, vomiting, retching (NVR).[1,3] For decades, this symptom cluster of NVR has been studied, evaluated, and treated as a single entity in practice and research.[2,3,6,7] Very few researchers have studied nausea, vomiting, and retching as a separate entity.[8]

Chemotherapy-induced nausea and vomiting can be classified as acute, delayed, and anticipatory. Acute nausea and vomiting occur within 24 hours of chemotherapy administration.[7] Delayed nausea and vomiting generally occur 24 hours after administration of chemotherapy and may persist for 6 to 7 days.[7,8] Anticipatory nausea and vomiting occur before the administration of the scheduled subsequent chemotherapy.[9]

Prevalence

Despite advances in pharmacologic antiemetic treatment, nausea and vomiting remains one of the most feared and distressing symptoms in patients with cancer.[13] The incidence of nausea and vomiting related to cancer and its treatment ranges from 30% to over 80%.[8,10-14] In a study of 320 cancer patients with thoracic or head and neck, gastrointestinal (GI), and hematologic cancer, 41% of the patients were admitted to a palliative care inpatient service for the symptom of nausea.[12] Clark and colleagues reported that 34% of 188 patients treated for metastatic prostate cancer experienced nausea and vomiting.[10] The postoperative symptoms of nausea and vomiting continue to be a concern with patients who undergo surgical treatment for cancer. A study of 68 patients following breast cancer surgery revealed that 72% of the patients experienced postoperative nausea and vomiting; furthermore, the patients judged the problem of nausea and vomiting to be worse than postoperative pain.[11]

Radiation-induced nausea and vomiting continue to be distressing for patients with cancer. High rates of acute nausea and vomiting were reported in a study of 243 patients with non–small cell lung cancer who received hyperfractionated radiation therapy in conjunction with chemotherapy of paclitaxel and carboplatin.[15] A study of 111 colorectal cancer patients who received radiation therapy revealed that patients experienced higher rates of nausea and vomiting.[14]

Chemotherapy remains the major causal factor to the development of nausea and vomiting in patients with cancer. A review of literature that showed 70% to 80% of all patients receiving chemotherapy experienced nausea and vomiting, with inadequate antiemetic therapy; 10% to 60% of patients still experienced nausea following chemotherapy, even with aggressive antiemetic therapy.[9] Hickok and colleagues conducted a study on 360 patients receiving doxorubicin, cisplatin, or carboplatin and all patients received 5-hydroxytryptamine-3 (5-HT$_3$)–receptor antagonist (ondansetron) with dexamethasone.[13] The results of the study showed that 76% of the patients developed nausea, and the patients reported the intensity of nausea as moderate or great.

The advent of 5-HT$_3$–receptor antagonists shows effectiveness in treating acute nausea and vomiting induced by chemotherapeutic agents with moderate emetogenicity. Despite the use of 5-HT$_3$–receptor antagonists, the incidence of delayed nausea and vomiting ranged from 22% to 89% in patients receiving chemotherapy.[6,16] Chemotherapy regimens for breast cancer are considered to have lower to moderate emetogenicity; these consist of standard regimens such as cyclophosphamide, methotrexate, and 5-fluorouracil (CMF), cyclophosphamide and doxorubicin with or without fluorouracil (CA or CAF) and with or without paclitaxel (CAT, CAFT). However, significant incidence of delayed nausea and vomiting still occurs with such regimens. In a study of 303 patients who underwent chemotherapy for breast cancer, despite antiemetic treatment, 82% of the patients reported delayed nausea during chemotherapy and approximately one fifth of the patients experienced the worst vomiting 2 days after chemotherapy administration.[8,17] A study of 33 Chinese breast cancer patients receiving doxorubicin and cyclophosphamide showed that the worst delayed nausea occurred in 87.9% of patients and vomiting in 63.6% of the patients on the third day following chemotherapy administration.[18]

Approximately one third of patients receiving chemotherapy for cancer have experienced anticipatory nausea. In a study of 63 female cancer patients receiving chemotherapy, anticipatory nausea developed in 40% of patients who expected nausea.[19] In another study of 60 women with breast cancer receiving adjuvant chemotherapy of cyclophosphamide, methotrexate, 5-fluorouracil, Adriamycin, or Taxol, Montgomery and colleagues found that 53% of the patients developed anticipatory nausea before the second chemotherapy administration, and 63% before the third administration.[20]

Risk Factors

Incidence and severity of nausea and vomiting in patients with cancer are affected by multiple factors, including (1) patient-specific factors, (2) treatment-specific factors, (3) disease-specific factors, and (4) environmental factors.

PATIENT-SPECIFIC FACTORS

Patient-specific factors that increase the risk of nausea and vomiting include age, gender, weight, previous experience of nausea and vomiting, and alcohol use. Patients younger than 50 years have a higher risk for nausea and vomiting than older patients.[8,9,17] This was first explained as being due to higher doses of more emetogenic drugs being received by younger patients; however, older patients frequently receive similarly aggressive therapy, and still have less nausea and vomiting than younger patients.[8,17] Since women, especially younger women, are more likely to experience nausea and vomiting, they are more prone to anticipatory nausea and delayed nausea and vomiting.[8,9,17] Women are 2 to 3 times more likely to experience nausea and vomiting and have distressing symptom experiences postoperatively than are men.[21] Body weight and body mass index (BMI = ratio of weight to height) are associated with the risk for nausea and vomiting. Dibble and colleagues found that women with higher BMI had significantly more nausea.[8] Previous experience of motion sickness, car sickness, or pregnancy-induced nausea and vomiting predispose patients to nausea and vomiting associated with cancer and its treatment; such patients reported significantly more frequent, more severe, and longer episodes of nausea and vomiting after cancer treatment.[7,9,17] Patients who chronically and regularly consume one to five drinks of alcohol per day or more than 10 units of alcohol per week have a reduced risk for nausea and vomiting, and such patients reported less nausea and vomiting during cancer treatment.[7] Prior experience of chemotherapy predisposes patients to both anticipatory nausea and postchemotherapy nausea and vomiting.[20,22]

TREATMENT-SPECIFIC FACTORS

Treatment-related risk factors include types of treatment, site, emetic potential, schedule, dose, route, and rate of administration. There is an approximately 75% incidence of postoperative nausea and vomiting after breast surgery under general anesthesia.[11] The site of radiation therapy is the primary factor that affects the risk for nausea and vomiting in patients receiving radiation therapy. Patients who receive larger field site irradiation such as total body, upper-body, and abdominal irradiation have the greatest likelihood of developing nausea and vomiting.[14,15] Additional factors that affect radiation-induced nausea and vomiting include dose and dose rate. The risk for nausea and vomiting is greater if radiation is delivered as a single high dose than fractionated smaller doses.[23] Patients receiving radiation with combined chemotherapy therapy have higher rates of nausea and vomiting.[15]

The intrinsic emetogenicity of antineoplastic chemotherapeutic agents is the most important cause of nausea and vomiting in patients receiving chemotherapy. Chemotherapeutic agents differ in the time-to-onset and duration of the emetic response. The incidence, onset, duration, and severity of nausea and vomiting

depend primarily on the emetogenic potential of chemotherapeutic agents. Chemotherapeutic agents are commonly classified into five levels: level 1, minimal emetogenicity (fewer than 10% of patients experience acute nausea and vomiting even with no antiemetic prophylaxis); level 2, low emetogenicity (10% to 30%); level 3, moderate emetogenicity (30% to 60%); level 4, high emetogenicity (60% to 90%); level 5, very high emetogenicity (more than 90%) (Table 41-1).[5,24,25] For example, cisplatin, one of the most highly emetogenic agents, at doses greater than 50 mg/m^2 usually induces acute nausea and vomiting in more than 90% of patients without administration of antiemetic prophylaxis. Even with appropriate antiemetic prophylaxis, the risk for nausea and vomiting associated with cisplatin is still 20% higher than with non–cisplatin-based chemotherapy protocols.[7] Cisplatin has a primary peak for nausea and vomiting on day 1 for acute nausea and vomiting, and a second peak during the 48 to 72 hours afterwards for delayed nausea and vomiting. Whereas mechlorethamine can stimulate nausea and vomiting within 30 minutes of intravenous administration, cyclophosphamide has a latency period of about 10 hours before the onset of nausea and vomiting, which then continues for up to 3 days. Studies support that cyclophosphamide and carboplatin increase the risk for delayed nausea and vomiting.[17,18] In a study on the incidence of delayed nausea in 303 patients with breast cancer who mostly received doxorubicin and cyclophosphamide, 67% of the patients experienced delayed nausea despite antiemetic therapy.[8] Other factors that affect the severity of chemotherapy-induced nausea and vomiting include dose and rate of administration. For most chemotherapeutic agents, higher doses increase the risk for nausea and vomiting. Slowing the infusion rate (e.g., with cisplatin or cytarabine) may decrease the risk of nausea and vomiting.[23]

DISEASE-RELATED FACTORS

The symptom experience (symptom occurrence and symptom distress) of patients with cancer may vary at different phases throughout their illness trajectory. The disease itself, its treatment, or concurrent disorders may contribute to the additional symptoms of nausea and vomiting. Seriously ill patients with cancer have a high symptom burden: they frequently experience a variety of additional severe concomitant symptoms associated with nausea and vomiting, including constipation, pain, bowel obstruction, metabolic abnormality (e.g., hypercalcemia, hyponatremia, hyperglycemia, uremia,) and increased intracranial pressure.[12,26]

Constipation or increased intraabdominal pressure may stimulate the peripheral pathways to the vomiting center (VC) and trigger vomiting. Constipation is one of the most common causes of nausea and vomiting in patients with end-stage cancer. Multiple factors contribute to constipation, including decreased fluid intake, tumor compression and invasion of the bowel and abdomen, or opioid use.[26] Tumor enlargement that impinges upon bowel and abdomen may cause severe nausea and vomiting by activating mechanoreceptors in the bowel wall.[4] Inadequate pain control may be a contributing factor for the symptoms of nausea and vomiting. Some of the medications that are used to manage cancer-related pain may also contribute to nausea and vomiting. To control pain, patients after cancer surgery and in the advanced stages of cancer often take several medications concurrently, including opioids, nonsteroidal antiinflammatory drugs (NSAIDs), and steroids, which are examples of medications that

TABLE 41-1 Chemotherapeutic Agents: Potential Emetogenicity and Emesis Prevention*

LEVEL OF EMETOGENIC POTENTIAL + EMETIC FREQUENCY	LEVEL	CHEMOTHERAPEUTIC AGENTS	ONSET AND DURATION OF RESPONSE (HOURS)	EMESIS PREVENTION
Minimal (<10%)	Level 1	Asparaginase	1-12	No routine prophylaxis. If N&V occur, use the regimen for level 2 chemotherapeutic agents. Start before chemotherapy:
		Bleomycin	3.5-24	▪ Dexamethasone
		Chlorambucil (oral)	48-72	▪ Prochlorperazine
		Hydroxyurea	8-48	▪ Metoclopramide
		Melphalan	6-12	▪ Lorazepam as needed
		Methotrexate ≤50mg/m²	4-12	
		Tamoxifen	12-36	
		Vinblastine	3.5-34	
		Vincristine	4-8	
Low (10%-30%)	Level 2	Amifostine <300 mg/m²	—	Start before chemotherapy:
		Cytarabine 100-200 mg/m²	1-48	▪ Dexamethasone
		Docetaxel	—	▪ Prochlorperazine
		Doxorubicin	4-6	▪ Metoclopramide
		Etoposide	3.5-34	▪ Lorazepam as needed
		5-Fluorouracil	3-10	
		Gemcitabine	—	
		Methotrexate <250mg/m²	4-12	
		Paclitaxel	4-8	
		Topotecan	6-72	
Moderately (30%-60%)	Level 3	Amifostine 300-500 mg/m²	—	**Day 1** Start before chemotherapy
		Cyclophosphamide (oral)	9-28	▪ Dexamethasone
		Cyclophosphamide <750 mg/m²	9-28	▪ 5-HT₃ antagonist
		Doxorubicin 20 to <60 mg/m²	3.5-34	

N&V, Nausea and vomiting.

†Emetic frequency: proportion (%) of patients experiencing N&V in the absence of antiemetic prophylaxis.

*Data from Hesketh PJ, Kris MG, Grunberg SM et al: Proposal for classifying the acute emetogenicity of cancer chemotherapy, *J Clin Oncol* 15(1):103-109, 1997; Antonarakis ES, Hain RD: Nausea and vomiting associated with cancer chemotherapy: drug management in theory and in practice, *Arch Dis Child* 89(9):877-880, 2004; and National Comprehensive Cancer Network: *Antiemesis: clinical practice guidelines in oncology: v.* 1. 2005, retrieved July 10, 2006, from http://www.nccn.org/professionals/physician_gls/PDF/antiemesis.pdf.

Continued

TABLE 41-1 Chemotherapeutic Agents: Potential Emetogenicity and Emesis Prevention—cont'd

LEVEL OF EMETOGENIC POTENTIAL

+ EMETIC FREQUENCY	LEVEL	CHEMOTHERAPEUTIC AGENTS	ONSET AND DURATION OF RESPONSE (HOURS)	EMESIS PREVENTION
High (60%–90%)		Ifosfamide	3–72	▪ Lorazepam as needed
		Interleukin II >12–15 million units/m²	–	▪ Add aprepitant for patients receiving carboplatin, cyclophosphamide, doxorubicin, epirubicin, ifosfamide, irinotecan, or methotrexate
		Irinotecan	6–24	
		Methotrexate 250–1,000 mg/m²	4–12	
	Level 4	Amifostine >500 mg/m²	–	
		Busulfan >4mg/m²	–	**Days 2–4**
		Carboplatin	6–46	▪ Dexamethasone
		Carmustine ≤250 mg/m²	–	▪ 5-HT₃ antagonist
		Cisplatin <50mg/ m2	1.5–56	▪ Metoclopramide or diphenhydramine
		Cyclophosphamide 750–1,000 mg/ m²	9–28	▪ Aprepitant for days 2–3 if used on day 1
		Doxorubicin ≥60 mg/m²	3.5–34	▪ Lorazepam as needed
		Epirubicin >90 mg/m²	6–24	
		Methotrexate >1,000 mg/m²	4–12	
		Melphalan >50 mg/m²	6–12	
		Procarbazine (oral)	24–27	
Very high (90%)	Level 5	Carmustine >250 mg/m²	2–24	Start before chemotherapy
		Cisplatin >50mg/m²	1.5–56	▪ Aprepitant
		Cyclophosphamide >1,000 mg/m²	9–28	▪ Dexamethasone
		Dacarbazine >500mg/ m²	4–24	▪ 5-HT₃ antagonist
		Mechlorethamine	0.5–24	▪ Lorazepam as needed
		Streptozocin	1–24	

may induce nausea and vomiting. NSAIDs and steroids may cause nausea and vomiting by irritating gastric lining. Opioids decrease peristalsis, resulting in delayed gastric emptying and constipation. Opioids activate the chemotherapy trigger zone (CTZ) in the area postrema and may cause nausea and vomiting with gastric stasis. The area postrema has one of the highest densities of opioid receptors.[26] Accumulation of plasma morphine, morphine-3-glucuronide (M3G), and morphine-6-glucuronide (M6G) concentrations may be a causal or aggravating factor for nausea and vomiting. Increased intracranial pressure from primary and metastatic brain cancer induces nausea and vomiting by triggering pressure receptors in the brain.[26]

ENVIRONMENTAL FACTORS

Individuals who suffer from motion sickness and carsickness are more prone to the nausea and vomiting induced by cancer treatments.[7,17] In a study, researchers employed two different strategies for exploring virtual environments and found that nausea increased steadily both when the head was kept still and when head movement was encouraged while exploring the virtual world; however, head movement appeared to further accentuate the symptom.[27] This study provided support for maintaining a quiet position and atmosphere during cancer treatments. In a randomized clinical trial using virtual reality of the bedside wellness system for patients with cancer, Oyama found that the virtual reality intervention was effective to relieve emesis and fatigue.[27]

The effect of changes in family relationships on patients' physical adjustment to chemotherapy has been explored. In a study of 233 cancer patients, Kim and Morrow found that the prevalence of nausea was related to the degree of conflict in the family; an increase in family conflict was associated with an increased duration of postchemotherapy nausea and greater severity of anticipatory nausea for younger patients, but not for older patients.[30] Furthermore, the study also revealed that an increase in family conflict was associated with a greater severity of anticipatory nausea for female patients, but not for male patients. Future study is needed to further explore this relationship.

As learned responses, anticipatory nausea and vomiting are conditioned responses to the environment during chemotherapy. Conditioned stimuli that may trigger anticipatory nausea and vomiting include a neutral stimulus (such as the chemotherapy nurse), a smell, or the clinic environment. Over time, reexposure to certain conditioned stimuli (such as the sight of the chemotherapy nurse, smells, sounds, or the clinic setting) during treatment can produce nausea and vomiting before chemotherapy administration.[9,20] Despite recent pharmacologic advances in the management of acute and delayed nausea and vomiting, pharmacologic interventions are less effective for controlling anticipatory nausea and vomiting. This highlights the need for research on interventions that focus on the modification of the conditioned stimuli (clinical stimuli) and alternative treatment (such as psychologic and behavioral interventions) to prevent anticipatory nausea and vomiting and to enhance the patient's quality of life throughout the illness trajectory.

Etiology

PHYSIOLOGY OF NAUSEA AND VOMITING

Vomiting or emesis is a complicated process that involves coordination of the emetic or vomiting center (VC) in the lateral reticular formation of the medulla. Activation of the VC is stimulated by afferent impulses transmitted to the VC through one of the following pathways: (1) the cerebral cortex and the limbic system, which are stimulated by senses and learned associations; (2) the CTZ, located in the area postrema of the medulla oblongata, which is outside of the blood-brain barrier and is sensitive to chemical stimuli from the cerebrospinal fluid and systemic circulation of blood; (3) the vestibular apparatus of the middle ear, which activates the VC via body positional changes; and (4) the peripheral pathway, which is activated by neurotransmitter receptors in the GI tract and vagus and spinal sympathetic nerves and responds to chemical stimuli in the visceral and blood.[26] Vomiting occurs when afferent impulses activate the VC via one or more of the four pathways, and efferent impulses from the VC are sent to the salivation center, the abdominal muscles, the respiratory center, and the cranial nerves (Fig. 41-1). Although the mechanisms leading to vomiting have been elucidated, there is very limited knowledge about nausea. Nausea might be mediated by the autonomic nervous system, since nausea is usually accompanied by such symptoms as hot or cold feelings, diaphoresis, increased salivation, pallor, tachycardia, light-headedness, dizziness, and weakness. Nausea might also be mediated by the pathway of cerebral cortex and limbic system, since nausea occurs more commonly than vomiting by the stimulation of this pathway. For example, anticipatory nausea occurs much more frequently than vomiting. Research has shown that anticipatory and delayed nausea have been difficult to manage, whereas the occurrence and frequency of vomiting has been controlled by the use of 5-HT$_3$–receptor antagonists combined with other antiemetics.[6,31] Such a lack of knowledge regarding the cause and mechanism of nausea has hindered the progress in developing effective interventions to manage nausea. In addition, although it is important to study nausea and vomiting as a symptom cluster in terms of symptom experience and even possible causative combinations, additional research is needed to reveal the mystery of nausea so as to develop more effective interventions to manage each entity of the symptom triad.

PATHOPHYSIOLOGY OF NAUSEA AND VOMITING

Nausea and vomiting in patients with cancer are most commonly caused by administration of chemotherapy, radiation therapy, and other, disease-related conditions. Chemotherapy-induced nausea and vomiting is a complex interaction between neurotransmitters and receptors in the central and peripheral nervous system. Chemotherapy induces nausea and vomiting through direct or indirect stimulation of the CTZ and the VC. The CTZ and VC contain numerous receptors sites for neurotransmitters such as dopamine, 5-HT$_3$), neurokinin-1, acetylcholine, and histamine. The CTZ is exposed to both cerebrospinal fluid and the systemic circulation; therefore, cytotoxic chemotherapeutic agents circulating in the bloodstream or cerebrospinal fluid can stimulate directly the area postrema to release neurotransmitters. The CTZ activates the VC through key receptors: 5-HT$_3$, dopamine, and neurokinin.[32] The GI tract, the CTZ, and the VC have abundant receptors for these neurotransmitters. 5-HT$_3$ is stored and released from platelets, form neurons, and from high concentrations of enterochromaffin cells in the GI tract. The serotonin or 5-HT$_3$ receptors are in peripheral tissues, the nucleus of the solitary tract, and the CTZ, where the majority of vagal afferents enter the brain. Peripherally, the CTZ can also be

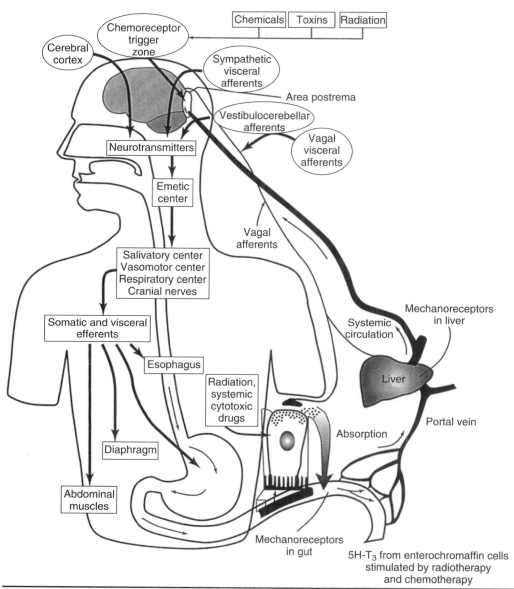

FIG. 41-1 Neuropathophysiology of vomiting. (Carrieri-Kohlman V, Lindsey AM, West CM, eds: *Pathophysiological phenomena in nursing: human responses to illness*, ed 3, St. Louis, 2003, Saunders. Data from Andrews PRL, Davis CJ: The mechanism of emesis induced by anticancer therapies. In Andrews PRL, Sanger GJ, editors: *Emesis in anticancer therapy: mechanisms and treatment*, New York, 1993, Chapman & Hall Medical; and Grundberg SM: Nausea and vomiting. In Haskel CM, editor: *Cancer treatment*, ed 5, Philadelphia, 2001, Saunders.)

stimulated indirectly by enterochromaffin cells in the GI mucosa, which are rich in 5-HT$_3$ and dopamine receptors. The damage of enterochromaffin cells from chemotherapy causes release of massive 5-HT$_3$, which binds to receptors along the vagus nerve and in the CTZ, and ultimately sends impulses to the VC, causing vomiting.[25,26] The simulation of enterochromaffin cells and resultant of release of serotonin largely is responsible for acute chemotherapy-induced nausea and vomiting.[33] The use of 5-HT$_3$–receptor antagonists has decreased the frequency of vomiting, but delayed nausea is more common.[6,31] The pathways mediating chemotherapy-induced delayed nausea are less understood.[8,17] Studies have showed that ondansetron, a 5-HT$_3$–receptor antagonist, is less effective in preventing delayed nausea than preventing acute nausea and vomiting; this suggests that serotonin is not the primary mediator of delayed nausea.[23] Chemotherapy-induced anticipatory nausea and vomiting are

conditioned and learned responses to the environment resulting from stimulation of the cerebral cortex and the limbic system of the brain where memories reside.[9,34] Anticipatory nausea and vomiting develop when the patient pairs unconditioned response of nausea and vomiting to unconditioned stimulus (chemotherapeutic agent) with the conditioned stimuli such as smells, sights, sounds, clinic settings, or the clinic staff). The occurrence of anticipatory nausea and vomiting are usually associated with unsuccessful control of nausea and vomiting during previous cycles of chemotherapy, and nausea is more common than vomiting.[8,35] Patients with the greatest amount of nausea after previous chemotherapy are more likely to develop anticipatory nausea. As learned responses, anticipatory nausea and vomiting may be a result of the distressing experience with uncontrolled nausea and vomiting during previous chemotherapy. Reexposure to the conditioned stimuli associated with the distressing experience may help the patient develop particular cues (the smell of the clinic or sight of the chemotherapy nurse) by pairing certain conditioned stimuli with the unconditioned nausea and vomiting. Such cues may trigger nausea and vomiting before the subsequent chemotherapy treatment. It is usually difficult to control anticipatory nausea and vomiting that are mediated by the pathway of cerebral cortex and the limbic system through pharmacologic antiemetic agents that target on blocking the neurotransmitters.

Radiation-induced nausea and vomiting most commonly occur in patients receiving whole body, upper body, or abdominal radiation therapy.[14,15] The GI tract contains rapidly dividing cells that are sensitive to radiation. Radiation damages the enterochromaffin cells in the GI tract, causing serotonin release; serotonin binds to vagal afferent receptors, which stimulates the VC through the CTZ. Radiation may also stimulate the VC directly or indirectly through chemical mediators, including beta-endorphin, prostaglandins, histamine, methionine, encephalin, and catecholamines.[23]

In addition to chemotherapy and radiation therapy, nausea and vomiting in patients with cancer can be the result of other, disease-related conditions. As constipation slows down intestinal peristalsis and increases abdominal pressure and bowel distension, the GI tract releases neurotransmitters (serotonin) that stimulate the peripheral pathways along the vagus nerve to the VC and trigger vomiting.[12,25] GI compression or stasis from tumor growth, bowel obstruction, hepatomegaly, or splenomegaly may stimulate the vagus and other visceral nerves, which triggers vomiting. Medications for pain management such as opioids, NSAIDs, aspirin, and steroids, may cause nausea and vomiting. NSAIDs and steroids may induce nausea and vomiting by irritating the gastric lining, stimulating the VC through the peripheral pathway of the vagus or another visceral nerve. Although the vestibular apparatus is responsible largely for nausea and vomiting caused by motion sickness, medications such as aspirin and opioids also directly stimulate the vestibular apparatus and may induce nausea and vomiting through the same pathway.[26] High levels of plasma opioids can stimulate the CTZ in the area postrema that has higher densities of opioid receptors, causing nausea and vomiting.[26] Increased intracranial pressure from primary and metastatic brain cancer can stimulate the cerebral cortex through pressure receptors, then communicate with the VC, inducing nausea and vomiting.[26] Nausea and vomiting in patients with cancer may also be caused by metabolic abnormalities from cancer or treatment, such as uremia, hypercalcemia, hyperglycemia, hyponatremia, and ketoacidosis.

PSYCHOSOCIAL CONTRIBUTING FACTORS

Anxiety, stress, fear, and pretreatment expectations may trigger or aggravate nausea and vomiting in patients with cancer. These psychologic conditions enhance nausea and vomiting by stimulating pituitary and adrenal glands to release hormones that mediate the stress response, causing nausea and vomiting.[9] Nausea and vomiting are often a physical reaction to stress. Patients with a history of nausea with stress had significantly more severe and higher rates of delayed nausea during chemotherapy for breast cancer.[8] Highly anxious patients may be more prone to the development of anticipatory nausea because they may be more aware of their environment and pay more attention to clinical stimuli, which enhances the pairing of the neutral conditioned stimuli with the unconditioned response of nausea and vomiting.[9] The effect of patients' pretreatment expectations on anticipatory

nausea and vomiting has been studied. Patients with greater expectation of being nauseated after chemotherapy were more likely to develop anticipatory nausea.[31,32] The expectation of nausea and vomiting may exacerbate the intensity of the subsequent experience of nausea and vomiting during chemotherapy.[35]

Dibble and colleagues[17] found that a significantly greater number of minority women who underwent chemotherapy for breast cancer were affected by delayed vomiting than their white counterparts, although there was no difference in antiemetics ordered for or taken by whites and minority women. The researchers pointed out two potential contributing factors to such a difference. First, health care providers and researchers are currently trained to address the needs of the cultural majority, whites. Often minority clients (African American, Asian, or Hispanic or Latino) are assumed to be like white clients, who will report symptoms and seek appropriate medications and interventions, but they may not, in fact, exhibit this behavior. Secondly, the effectiveness of medications may largely rely on findings from the white population. Minority patients may metabolize medications differently and different foods and lifestyle may affect symptom manifestation and the effectiveness of antiemetics. This highlights the need for more studies that focus on the effectiveness of antiemetics with culturally diverse populations.

Effects and Consequences

Nausea and vomiting can be devastating for patients with cancer in fact, this symptom cluster has been consistently rated by patients with cancer as one of the most distressing, debilitating, and feared symptoms they suffer.[36,37] The distress from nausea and vomiting refers to the degree of physical or mental suffering, discomfort, or bothersomeness perceived by individuals in relation to their experience of nausea and vomiting. Although 5-HT$_3$ antagonists are effective to reduce the incidence of nausea and vomiting induced by chemotherapy, patients who experienced nausea and vomiting still ranked the symptom cluster as highly distressing.[36] The distress from inadequately controlled nausea and vomiting can affect patients' quality of life, functional status, and withdrawal from or interruption of potentially curable treatment.[37] A study of 136 patients having chemotherapy for breast cancer showed that patients' perceived satisfaction with antiemetic treatment was related to all the domains of quality of life assessed by the Rotterdam Symptom Checklist ($p = 0.002$): psychologic distress, physical symptom distress, and activity level.[39] Research has documented that nausea contributed to patients' reluctance to begin chemotherapy and could result in the discontinuation of potentially effective treatment.[40] Passik and colleagues examined cancer patients' fear of chemotherapy following treatment and their findings revealed that nausea and vomiting were the most feared side effects of chemotherapy.[37] The fear of nausea and vomiting may cause 10% to 50% of patients to refuse or delay chemotherapy.[40] The distress from nausea also affected patients' perceived regrets concerning cancer treatment decisions. A study of 188 patients treated for metastatic prostate cancer revealed that 52% of the patients who experienced nausea in the preceding week expressed regrets of their treatment choices.[10] In addition, nausea and vomiting may affect patients' perception of total treatment burden. A study of 249 patients who underwent chemotherapy for breast and lung cancer revealed a substantial correlation ($r = 0.58$) between patients' perceived burden of nausea and vomiting and total treatment burden.[38]

Nausea and vomiting also affect cancer patients' daily functional status. Nausea and vomiting have a measurable negative impact on patients' functional status, including the ability to enjoy meals and liquid, to maintain usual leisure and recreational activities, the desire to enjoy family and friends, and the ability to maintain daily functioning.[41,42] In a study of 115 patients who underwent chemotherapy for cancer, Farley and colleagues examined patients' self-reported functional status in relation to chemotherapy-induced nausea and vomiting and antiemetic therapy.[42] Findings of the study revealed that the patients perceived their functional status as impaired if they experienced nausea and vomiting.

Nausea and vomiting can precipitate potential life-threatening medical complications such as dehydration, electrolyte imbalances, anorexia, nutritional deficit, wound dehiscence, and esophageal tears. The need for hydration, repletion of electrolytes, or hospitalization may increase the costs for health care in patients with cancer.[7,43]

Assessment and Measurement

Whereas nausea is a subjective phenomenon that can only be assessed and measured subjectively, vomiting can be objectively observed and measured. As a symptom cluster, nausea and vomiting can be assessed through key measurable indicators of symptom occurrence, symptom distress, and symptom experience.[44] Symptom occurrence of nausea and vomiting includes the frequency (i.e., number of times nausea and vomiting is experienced by an individual within a given time frame) and duration of nausea and vomiting (i.e., the persistence of the subjective experience of nausea and vomiting). Symptom distress from nausea and vomiting is the degree of physical or mental suffering, discomfort, or bothersomeness experienced by individuals in relation to their perception of nausea and vomiting. Symptom experience of nausea and vomiting is an individual's perception and response to the occurrence of and distress from nausea and vomiting.

Effective management of nausea and vomiting in patients with cancer starts with accurate and thorough assessment. Assessment is an ongoing process that should begin with the initial patient contact and continue through treatment or illness trajectory. The initial assessment of nausea and vomiting should be conducted before cancer treatment, focusing on a careful history describing the pattern of emetic history and identifying the risk factors contributing to the occurrence of nausea and vomiting. The efficacy of managing nausea and vomiting is influenced by individual risk factors; thus patients should be treated according to their individual unique risk profile (Table 41-2).[7] An accurate and thorough initial assessment is essential for planning effective preventive interventions for nausea and vomiting. Subsequent assessment following initial treatment should focus on the identification of the pattern, onset, duration, intensity of, and distress from nausea and vomiting, as well as exploration of factors that exacerbate or alleviate it. Assessment should also include nutritional intake, changes in appetite and weight, and psychologic factors.

A complete history obtained from the patient and family is essential to determine the best approaches for the individualized management of nausea and vomiting. A medical history should include concurrent health problems, current medications, and treatment history, as well as other associated side effects or conditions. The history and physical examination should be used to differentiate causal factors for nausea and vomiting, rather than taking a global or synonymous approach when assessing nausea and vomiting. For example, conditions such as tumor enlargement or bowel obstruction require pain control; hence careful assessment is critical to determine if the nausea and vomiting is due to pharmacologic agents.

Information obtained by interviews, questionnaires, or self-report instruments should use words that have the same meaning to patients, family members, and caregivers. A balance between obtaining accurate data about the specific symptom and patient or family burden must be maintained. Assessment tools that can be completed quickly and reviewed can expedite less expenditure of patient energy and nursing time. These are important criteria to consider when choosing an instrument to measure the individual symptoms, determining symptom patterns, and making comparisons.

Many cancer patients have had the experience of nausea and vomiting during earlier surgery, chemotherapy, radiation, or other conditions associated with nausea and vomiting; therefore, nurses or researchers must avoid directing suggestive attention to the symptom. During the initial contact, the patient's prior symptom experience, management methods, and anticipated expectations must be assessed. Nurses and researchers should pay special attention to family members' and/or significant others' suggestions, evaluations, and possible assistance in recording observations and patients' description of symptom experience of nausea and vomiting in a daily diary or journal. Patient journals, logs, or daily diaries that are completed by the patient or caregiver provide useful assessment information. As a result of these reflective self-report tools, family caregivers and patients frequently have developed increased experience in problem solving, a greater sense of control, and improved self-care management.[4] From patient journals, logs, or daily diaries, nurses are often able to recognize patterns of symptom occurrence; self-care management strategies, including individualized pharmacologic and nonpharmacologic interventions; and situational or concomitant circumstances.

Instruments that specifically measure symptom onset, frequency, and amount of nausea and vomiting are available such as the Index of Nausea, Vomiting, and Retching (INVR). The INVR has eight statements that measure the three symptoms over a 12-hour time frame. It measures the duration, frequency, distress of nausea, and amount of vomiting. The INVR has strong internal consistency with Cronbach's alpha of 0.98.[45] An accurate and effective research-based instrument for assessing nausea, vomiting, and retching, the INVR has been translated into many languages. The reported reliability of the Chinese and the Korean INVR is very high, with Cronbach's alphas of 0.952 and 0.90, respectively.[46,47]

Several comprehensive instruments that include one or more of the components of nausea and vomiting are available to help assess concomitant symptomatology. An example of this type of instrument is the Adapted Symptom Distress Scale (ASDS), a 31-item, 5-point self-report instrument that measures patients' perception of the occurrence and distress of 14 symptoms.[48] This instrument yields a total score for symptom experience, scores for symptom occurrence and distress, and subscale scores for six symptom categories. The ASDS is a highly reliable instrument with an internal consistency of 0.91 for the total occurrence, and reliability for the subscales ranging from 0.38 for the appearance

TABLE 41-2	Risk Factors for the Development of Nausea and Vomiting in Patients with Cancer	
RISK FACTORS	**HIGHER RISK**	**LOWER RISK**
Patient-Specific Factors		
Age	Younger than 50 years	Older than 50 years
Gender	Female	Male
Weight	Heavy weight/higher BMI	
Previous experience	Motion sickness	
	Carsickness	
	N&V during pregnancy	
Alcohol consumption		Chronic and regular consumer
Anxiety	High anxiety	
Stress	Nausea with stress	
Responses to chemotherapy	Pretreatment expectation of more and severe N&V	
	Uncontrolled N&V in the previous chemotherapy	
	Severe N&V postchemotherapy	
	Ability to associate conditioned stimuli to N&V	
Treatment-Specific Factors		
Emetogenicity of chemotherapeutic agents	Very high	
	High	
	Moderate or low	
Radiation	Total body	
	Upper body	
	Abdomen	
	Single high dose	
	Combined with chemotherapy	
Other Disease-Related Factors		
GI conditions	Constipation	
	Partial or complete bowel obstruction	
	Tumor compression and invasion to the bowel and abdomen	
Intracranial pressure	Increased: primary brain tumor	
	Increased: brain metastases	
Metabolic imbalance	Hypercalcemia	
	Hyperglycemia	
	Hyponatremia	
	Uremia	
Environmental-Factors		
Clinic atmosphere		Quiet and soothing
Family Relationship	Conflict	

BMI, Body mass index; *N&V,* nausea and vomiting.

subscale to 0.84 for the concentration subscale.[45] Others, such as the Symptom Distress Scale (SDS) and The Memorial Symptom Assessment Scale measure either a single component or provide global measures of the concepts.[49,50] The SDS is a 13-item instrument with an internal consistency (Cronbach's alpha) of 0.84. Internal consistency for physical symptoms on the Memorial Assessment Scale is 0.88.

Interventions

Nausea and vomiting in patients with cancer have multiple potential causative factors that may work alone or together to produce overwhelming and distressing nausea and vomiting that affect cancer patients' quality of life. Prevention of nausea and vomiting is the key to the effective management of nausea and vomiting. A single intervention (e.g., administration of 5-ET₃–receptor antagonists) is unlikely to be the one solution that offers complete control of nausea and vomiting. A variety of management interventions have been identified and recommended, including pharmacologic, psychologic, and behavioral interventions. Nursing interventions include independent and collaborative nursing interventions. The goal of nursing interventions is to minimize and eliminate nausea and vomiting in patients with cancer. To achieve optimal prevention and effective management of nausea and vomiting, nursing interventions must meet the psychologic and physical needs of the patient, and must consider the causes of nausea and vomiting.

PREVENTION

Prevention is the optimal intervention for nausea and vomiting in patients with cancer. Prevention should aim at minimizing or eliminating the stimulation of the VC that potentially elicits nausea and vomiting, as well as at providing preparatory information about the sensory experience to come. Pharmacologic intervention is effective for the prevention of chemotherapy-induced and radiation-induced nausea and vomiting. Prevention of nausea and vomiting includes prechemotherapy and postchemotherapy intervention.[5] Prechemotherapy intervention starts antiemetic medications before the administration of chemotherapy in patients receiving levels 5 (very high emetogenicity), 4 (high emetogenicity), 3 (moderate emetogenicity), and 2 (low emetogenicity) agents. Delayed nausea and vomiting is managed through postchemotherapy intervention, in which antiemetic medications are continued through the period after chemotherapy administration when delayed nausea and vomiting may occur in patients receiving chemotherapeutic agents of emetogenic levels 5, 4, or 3. To effectively prevent anticipatory nausea and vomiting, optimal antiemetic therapy is used to prevent the occurrence of nausea and vomiting during each cycle of chemotherapy.[5,7,35]

Nurses play an important, independent role in providing preparatory education. Teaching should incorporate sensory and procedural information that reflects the experience of the upcoming event from the patient's point of view. Although accurate ongoing assessments are always essential for the recognition and monitoring the progress of nausea and vomiting, it is essential that the patient's expectations about nausea and vomiting be included in the initial assessment. Information conveyed in a positive, nonthreatening manner and given before the treatment allows the patient to formulate a more effective mental image about the pending experience. An accurate mental image also decreases ambiguity about the event, activates innate coping strategies, and permits effective cognitive management of the experience of nausea and vomiting. The goals and behaviors of patients with cancer are largely determined by their perceptions of the illness. Therefore it is important to understand an individual's perception and its potential influence on actual experience and self-care and coping behaviors. For example, the individual's expectations about the experience of nausea and vomiting and the actual experience have been shown to be related.[8,19,35] Roscoe and colleagues found a significant relationship (p < 0.05) between patients' pretreatment expectations for nausea development in two studies: a group of 29 female cancer patients as inpatients (study 1), and 81 female cancer patients as outpatients (study 2).[36] Often, nausea and vomiting is referred to as a side effect that may convey a sense of secondary importance to the disease process and treatment. Yet nausea and vomiting is often a chief concern of individuals receiving chemotherapy.[36,37] Studies have demonstrated that preparatory information and realistic expectations reduce symptom experience and improve coping behaviors used to manage nausea and vomiting.[51] Information that clearly describes what patients can expect before, during, and after treatment is crucial for effective patient education. Williams and Schreier tested the effectiveness of informational audiotapes on the use of self-care behaviors regarding symptoms such as nausea and vomiting in 70 female patients receiving their first chemotherapy treatment.[51] The study revealed that audiotapes were effective in managing side effects of chemotherapy such as nausea and vomiting and in teaching self-care behaviors. Information about nausea and vomiting, including neutral descriptions of specific sensations to be experienced and realistic expectations, helps the patient cope and develop self-care behaviors more easily. For example, if an individual is starting a treatment regimen whose participants have experienced little or no nausea and vomiting, then it is appropriate to give this factual information to prepare the patient. The amount of factual information provided will depend on what individuals want to know and what they need to know to safely live with their treatment and its side effects. Therefore, preparatory information and early management of the symptoms of nausea and vomiting enable patients to develop effective coping mechanisms and lead to improved quality of life. Individualized educational strategies are considered to be the most effective preventive interventions; however, definitive research is needed.

PHARMACOLOGIC INTERVENTIONS

Pharmacologic interventions are independent and collaborative nursing interventions. The symptoms of nausea and vomiting induced by chemotherapy and radiation therapy can be frequently managed with antiemetic drugs (See Table 41-1 and Table 41-3). Antiemetics are chosen based on the causes of

TABLE 41-3	Prevention for Anticipatory and Radiation-Induced Nausea and Vomiting*
Emesis Prevention	
Type of Radiation Therapy	
Upper abdomen irradiation	Start pretreatment for each day of radiation • Ondansetron *or* • Dexamethasone *or* • Granisetron
Total body irradiation	Start pretreatment each day of radiation • Ondansetron *or* • Granisetron
Chemotherapy and radiation	Follow emesis prevention for chemotherapy
Radiation of other sites	No routine prophylaxis

Anticipatory Nausea and Vomiting
Optimal control of N&V during every cycle of treatment
Behavioral therapy
- Progressive muscle relaxation
- Music therapy and guided imagery
- Hypnosis
- Massage

N&V, Nausea and vomiting.
Data from National Comprehensive Cancer Network: *Antiemesis: clinical practice guidelines in oncology*, v. 1. 2005, retrieved July 10, 2006, from http://www.nccn.org/professionals/physician_gls/PDF/antiemesis.pdf.

nausea and vomiting, the pharmacologic action, the receptor, the site, the appropriate route of administration, and the appropriate dose. Adequate management may require combination drug therapy. The cost/benefit of various drug combinations also has to be considered. A variety of antiemetics and other drugs available to manage and even prevent nausea and vomiting allows individualized symptom management; however, currently available pharmacologic agents are still unable to provide complete protection for every patient.[6] Several classes of antiemetics are available in the management of nausea and vomiting (Table 41-4).

Serotonin 5-HT$_3$–Receptor Antagonists. The serotonin 5-HT$_3$–receptor antagonists (e.g., ondansetron, granisetron, dolasetron mesylate, and palonosetron) represent a major improvement in the management of chemotherapy-induced nausea and vomiting. Serotonin antagonists are effective in controlling acute nausea and vomiting by blocking the action of serotonin centrally and peripherally.[34,52] 5-HT$_3$–receptor antagonists such as ondansetron are effective to relieve the nausea and vomiting induced by radiation therapy in patients with total body irradiation and radiation to the upper abdomen.[5] 5-HT$_3$ antagonists combined with dexamethasone provide the most effective control of acute nausea and vomiting induced by chemotherapy.[7,53] Several large, randomized studies have shown that the use of a 5-HT$_3$ antagonist with dexamethasone produced effective prevention for acute emesis in 60% to 70% of patients receiving highly emetogenic chemotherapeutic agents; however, they are less effective for delayed emesis.[6,52] Palonosetron is a newer 5-HT$_3$–receptor antagonist with an approximately 100-fold higher 5-HT$_3$–receptor binding affinity compared to other serotonin antagonists.[54,55] Its half life is about 40 hours. Studies have shown that palonosetron is as effective as other serotonin antagonists in preventing acute nausea and vomiting, but palonosetron is more effective in preventing delayed nausea and vomiting in patients receiving moderately emetogenic chemotherapeutic agents.[54,55] Patients who receive 5-HT$_3$ antagonists experience few side effects except for headache and constipation in some patients.

NK-1–Receptor Antagonists. Aprepitant represents the first substance P neurokinin-1 (NK-1)–receptor antagonist. Substance P, a tachykinin found in the vagal afferent neurons, can induce nausea and vomiting by binding to NK-1 receptors. Aprepitant reduces nausea and vomiting induced by chemotherapy and radiation by blocking the NK-1 receptors and can cross the blood-brain barrier, penetrating into the central nervous system.[53,56] In a large multicenter randomized double-blind placebo-controlled phase III study, 260 patients received cisplatin, 70 mg/m^2 or more, and were given either standard therapy (ondansetron on day 1and dexamethasone on days 2 to 4) or the aprepitant regimen (aprepitant plus dexamethasone and ondansetron on day 1; aprepitant and dexamethasone on days 2 to 3, and dexamethasone on day 4).[56] The results showed that added aprepitant produced higher complete response (no emesis and no rescue therapy) from days 1 to 5 (72.7% versus 53.3%, p < 0.001) in comparison with the standard therapy; the aprepitant regimen was well tolerated and provided consistently higher protection against nausea and vomiting induced by cisplatin. Warr and colleagues conducted a phase III randomized study of 866 patients who were naïve to chemotherapy and treated with moderately emetogenic chemotherapy of cyclophosphamide and doxorubicin or epirubicin.[30] The study showed that an aprepitant regimen (aprepitant, ondansetron, and dexamethasone) and a control regimen (ondansetron and dexamethasone) produced greater complete response (no vomiting and no rescue therapy) during 120 hours after initiation of chemotherapy in cycle 1 (50.8% versus 42.5%; p = 0.015), and more patients in the aprepitant regimen arm reported minimal or no impact of nausea and vomiting on daily life (63.5% versus 55.6%; p = 0.019). Aprepitant, a substrate, an inhibitor, and inducer of CYP3A4, is metabolized by cytochrome P450 enzyme 3A4 (CYP3A4) in the liver; thus caution is recommended with concomitant use of other agents metabolized by the same enzyme. The following chemotherapeutic agents should not be used concurrently with aprepitant: docetaxel, paclitaxel, etoposide, irinotecan, ifosfamide, imatinib, vinorelbine, and vincristine.[56] Other side effects of aprepitant include hiccups or asthenia.[34]

Dopamine-Receptor Antagonists. The dopamine-receptor antagonists prevent nausea and vomiting by binding to the dopamine receptors to block impulses to the VC. Dopamine antagonists are useful in treating postoperative nausea and vomiting.[34] Examples of this class include prochlorperazine, promethazine, metoclopramide, and the butyrophenones. Although side effects from dopamine antagonists such as sedation and extrapyramidal effects (e.g., akathesia and oculogyric crisis) can be resolved by administering diphenhydramine, such side effects can be distressing for patients.[34]

Benzodiazepines. Benzodiazepines are antianxiety agents. Medications in this class, such as lorazepam and alprazolam, reduce anxiety, a risk factor for anticipatory nausea and vomiting; thus they can be effective in preventing nausea and vomiting, when used in conjunction with other antiemetics.[5] Side effects include sedation and possible loss of short-term memory.

Other Antiemetic Medications. Other medications that have antiemetic effects include antihistamines, corticosteroids, and cannabinoids. Antihistamines, such as cyclizine and promethazine, and anticholinergics, particularly hyoscine, also exhibit an antiemetic effect. Corticosteroids are useful in heightening the effects of other antiemetics.[34]

NONPHARMACOLOGIC INTERVENTIONS

Nonpharmacologic interventions are usually used in conjunction with pharmaceutical agents to manage nausea and vomiting.

TABLE 41-4	Commonly Used Antiemetic Agents
CLASSIFICATIONS	**DRUGS**
5-HT$_3$–receptor antagonists	Ondansetron
	Granisetron
	Dolasetron
	Palonosetron
Neurokinin (NK)-1–receptor antagonists	Aprepitant
Dopamine receptor antagonists	Prochlorperazine
	Promethazine
	Metoclopramide
	Butyrophenones
Benzodiazepines	Lorazepam
	Alprazolam
Corticosteroids	Dexamethasone
Antihistamines	Diphenhydramine
Cannabinoids	Dronabinol

Nurses play an independent and essential role in nonpharmacologic interventions. Most nonpharmacologic interventions are based on biologic understanding to enhance pharmacologic interventions and psychologic understanding to assist in developing more effective behavioral interventions.[57] Behavioral therapy may be helpful to prevent anticipatory nausea and vomiting.[5] Although research is limited, there are studies that support the effectiveness of a variety of nonpharmacologic interventions. In addition, nonpharmacologic interventions are often noninvasive and can frequently be performed by the patient alone, thus enhancing patients' feelings of control.

Diet and Environment. Limited research has been conducted to determine the effectiveness of the impact of diet and environment on nausea and vomiting in patients with cancer. Ginger (*Zingiber officinale*) has traditionally been used in China for GI symptoms such as nausea and vomiting.[58,59] Studies demonstrated mixed results concerning the effectiveness of ginger for treating nausea and vomiting in postoperative patients and chemotherapy patients. In a systematic review of six studies, Ernst and Pittler concluded that ginger is a promising antiemetic herbal remedy, but the clinical data were insufficient to draw firm conclusion.[58] In a randomized study of 81 patients who underwent outpatient gynecologic laparoscopy, significant difference was found in the occurrence of nausea in patients in the interventional group who received two ginger capsules (1 g of ginger powder) and patients in the placebo group (30% versus 57.5%, p < 0.05).[60] In another randomized study of 48 gynecologic cancer patents receiving cisplatin-based chemotherapy, Manusirivithaya and colleagues found that the addition of 1g of ginger root powder to the antiemetic regimen made no significant reduction of the nausea and vomiting induced by chemotherapy.[61]

Peppermint oil has a long history as a folk remedy for relieving GI symptoms. The primary active chemical constituents include menthol, pulegone, and menthofuran. Menthol is the main therapeutic agent, and therefore high concentrations are desirable, whereas pulegone and menthofuran are toxic chemicals and it is suggested that for the purposes of aromatherapy low concentrations of these components are desirable. The desirable range for pulegone is less than 2% and for menthofuran less than 3%.[62] Orally administered peppermint oil has been studied for relief of flatulence, colic pain, and symptoms of irritable bowel syndrome.[63-65] Physiologic effects of peppermint oil on animals include decreasing the gut contractile response to histamine, serotonin, acetylcholine, and substance P.[65] Limited research has been conducted on the effect of olfactory administration of peppermint oil to relieve nausea and vomiting. Tate conducted a placebo-controlled study (n = 18) in patients undergoing gynecologic surgery; a finding of the study suggested that peppermint oil might have a role in reducing postoperative nausea.[62] However, more studies are needed to establish the therapeutic effect of peppermint oil on the relief of nausea.

Although there is no study on the effect of food on nausea and vomiting in patients with cancer, anecdotal clinical experience shows that small amounts of attractively prepared food, bland foods, cool, carbonated beverages, and sour foods (such as lemons, sour pickles, or sour hard candy) are generally more desirable, whereas sweet, fatty, highly salted, and spicy foods may exacerbate nausea and vomiting. The patient's preference or desire not to eat must be recognized, since ingestion of food may cause nausea and vomiting with concomitant abdominal symptoms such as pain, abdominal distention, constipation, or diarrhea.

Theoretically, modification of environment factors should be a helpful strategy to prevent anticipatory nausea and vomiting, a learned and conditioned response to environment. Before antiemetics are prescribed, the stimuli for nausea in the environment should be reduced or eliminated. This may include minimizing sights, sounds, or smells that can initiate nausea. Unpleasant odors and smells from cooking should be eliminated. Future research should explore the impact of environment on anticipatory nausea and vomiting.

Acupressure. Acupressure is based on the ancient oriental concept that chi (or qi) energy travels through pathways known as meridians. Along the meridians are points known as acupoints in Chinese, that is, the controlling points for chi energy flow. Applying pressure with fingers or bands, or acustimulation to the acupoints where chi energy is supposed to be blocked, slowed, or overstimulated, can reestablish the balance of chi energy. Two acupoints are known for relieving nausea and vomiting: the P6 point (Nei-Guan point) and the Joksamly (ST36 point). The P6 point is located on the anterior surface of forearm, 3 finger-widths up from the first wrist crease and between the tendons of flexor carpiradialis and palmaris longus.[47,66] ST36 point is located 4 finger-breadths below the knee depression, lateral to the tibia.[47,66] The use of acupressure to relieve nausea and vomiting has been found to be effective in chemotherapy-induced nausea and vomiting. In a single-cycle, randomized clinical trail for women receiving chemotherapy for breast cancer, Dibble reported significant differences in the experience of nausea (p < 0.01) and nausea intensity (p < 0.04) between women receiving usual care plus acupressure training and treatment, and those receiving only usual care.[66] Patients in the acupressure group also reported less intensity and symptom experience of nausea. In an interventional study of 40 postoperative gastric cancer patients receiving chemotherapy of cisplatin and 5-flurouracil, acupressure at the P6 point was found effective in reducing the severity of nausea and vomiting, the duration of nausea, and the frequency of vomiting.[47] This study showed that acupressure on P6 point appears to be an effective adjunct strategy for the control of nausea and vomiting. Roscoe and colleagues conducted a three-arm clinical trial (active acustimulation, sham acustimulation, and no acustimulation), using an acustimulation band for the relief of chemotherapy-induced nausea and vomiting in 96 women with breast cancer in addition to antiemetic treatment.[67] The researchers found no significant differences among the three groups and concluded that acustimulation bands were not effective in relieving chemotherapy-induced nausea and vomiting in patients with breast cancer. Comparing the acupressure band and the acustimulation band, Roscoe and colleagues found that acupressure was effective in reducing nausea and vomiting in the first day of chemotherapy in a randomized study of 739 patients who underwent chemotherapy. However, the acustimulation band was found not effective in controlling nausea and vomiting in this study.[67]

Progressive Muscle Relaxation Training (PMRT). In PMRT, patients are taught to actively tense and relax major muscle groups to allow complete relaxation. PMRT has been used with the intent to reduce chemotherapy-induced nausea and vomiting and to prevent anticipatory nausea and vomiting. PMRT is complementary intervention that can be used with pharmacologic and other nonpharmacologic interventions such as guided imagery and systematic desensitization.[68,69] Studies have shown that PMRT is a useful adjunct strategy to complement antiemetics for chemotherapy-induced nausea and vomiting. In a randomized clinical trial of 71 breast cancer patients with chemotherapy, the use of PMRT significantly decreased the duration of nausea and vomiting in the experimental group.[68]

Music Therapy and Guided Imagery. Music therapy is an intervention to promote relaxation or distraction. Music therapy serves as an adjunct to medication and other comfort measures, such as guided imagery. Guided imagery has been found to be effective in decreasing nausea and vomiting and can be used alone or with combination with music therapy and PMRT.[69] In guided imagery, the individual visualizes pleasant, soothing images or scenes while relaxing or listening to soothing music.[69] In a study, patients who received 5 minutes of guided imagery and PMRT had significantly decreased duration of nausea and vomiting than the patients in the control group, who received only antiemetics. More studies are needed to establish the effectiveness of this intervention.[70]

Hypnosis. Hypnosis or suggestive therapy is a self-control technique in which individual learn to invoke a physiologic state incompatible with nausea and vomiting.[69] Usually, induction of total body relaxation is followed by presentation of restful imagery. Hypnosis may be effective in controlling nausea and vomiting by relaxing the patient, which, when used in conjunction with antiemetics, may result in a reduction of the dose and frequency required. In a study of 16 cancer patients who were affected by anticipatory nausea and vomiting, patients were induced to relaxation followed by hypnosis. The study showed that anticipatory nausea and vomiting disappeared in all the patients, and patients reported more control of chemotherapy-induced nausea and vomiting.[70]

Massage. Massage is an important way that nurses use touch to communicate caring to patients. Massage can also be used to relieve symptoms in patients with cancer. In a large cancer center, over a 3-year period, 1290 patients with cancer were treated with massage to relieve symptoms such as nausea, pain, fatigue, stress and anxiety, and depression.[71] Patients reported perceived reduction in symptom severity after each massage treatment. In a study of 87 patients with cancer, Grealish and colleagues found a significant immediate effect of a 10-minute foot massage on the patients' perception of nausea, pain, and relaxation as measured by a visual analogue scale.[72] Foot massage as a complementary strategy is a relative simple nursing intervention that can be used to relieve nausea and pain in patients with cancer.

Outcomes

Outcomes of symptom management encompass symptom status, quality of life (QOL), and performance.[44] The expected outcomes of nursing interventions for managing the symptom cluster of nausea and vomiting should also include these three measurable dimensions. Symptom status is a direct outcome of symptom management. Effective management of nausea and vomiting should lead to an optimal symptom status in which there is relief of nausea and vomiting, a decreased degree of distress from nausea and vomiting, or prevention of and decrease in occurrence of nausea and vomiting. QOL is also an expected outcome of symptom management. Research findings show that an increase in number and distress of symptoms is associated with decreased QOL.[44] Performance is conceptualized as an outcome of symptom management. Performance includes functional (e.g., physical activities, activities of daily living, social activities and interactions, role performance) and cognitive (e.g., concentrating, thinking, and problem-solving) dimensions. Less effective role performance and lower cognitive functioning are related to greater numbers of symptoms and more severe symptom experience.[44]

The expected outcome of nursing interventions for nausea and vomiting is manifested by complete relief from nausea and vomiting in terms of symptom status, improved QOL, and improved functional and cognitive performance. Despite continuous progress in pharmacologic treatment for nausea and vomiting and aggressive pharmacologic interventions, approximately 30% to 80% patients with cancer still suffer from nausea and vomiting.[8,10,13,14] To achieve the expected outcomes of nursing interventions, an integrative approach is needed. Such an integrative approach should encompass a variety of interventions, for example, a combination of pharmacologic, behavioral, psychologic, and environmental approaches. Currently, pharmacologic intervention is the mainstay of the management of nausea and vomiting. More studies are needed to test the effectiveness of the combination of pharmacologic and nonpharmacologic interventions to ensure an integrative approach. As future research documents the effectiveness of such integrative approaches to the management of nausea and vomiting, the QOL in patients with cancer will be improved.

CONSIDERATIONS FOR OLDER ADULTS

- Fortunately, older adults more than 50 years old usually have less risk for nausea and vomiting (N&V), especially chemotherapy-induced N&V. Older adults usually also experience less distress from N&V. Although the pharmacologic approach has been effective to control the frequency of vomiting, anticipatory and delayed nausea remain especially distressing for patients who receive chemotherapy. However, older adults seem to also have less risk for both anticipatory and delayed nausea. For the symptoms of N&V, being an older adult seems to a beneficial factor that may prevent the patient from these distressing symptoms.
- Although older adults seems to have less risk for and experience of N&V, it is of critical important to conduct thorough nursing assessment to formulize individualized interventions based each older adult's personal risk profile of N&V.

REVIEW QUESTIONS

✓ Case Study

The following case study illustrates a patient's experiences of the symptom cluster of nausea and vomiting associated with chemotherapy treatment for ovarian cancer. Mrs. Kady, a 48-year-old female, was diagnosed with stage II ovarian cancer. Her height is 5'2" and her weight is 153 pounds with a body mass index (BMI) of 29. She is married and has two daughters who are in their late 20s. With both of her pregnancies, she had slight nausea and vomiting during the first trimester. The year before her diagnosis of ovarian cancer, Mrs. Kady began a job at the chamber of commerce for her community. Because this was a new position, she felt it was important for her to be able to continue to work if at all possible.

Mrs. Kady had a total hysterectomy, bilateral salpingoophorectomy, peritoneal cytology studies, omentectomy, and biopsies with debulking. Following her surgery she was scheduled to receive six cycles of chemotherapy. The chemotherapy consisted of carboplatin, 350 mg/m^2, and paclitaxel. This cycle was scheduled for every 21 days. Mrs. Kady was very concerned about managing the side effects associated with chemotherapy to continue working. For the first cycle of chemotherapy, Mrs. Kady was given dexamethasone (Decadron), 20 mg orally, and granisetron (Kytril), 2 mg administered before chemotherapy. The evening following her first chemotherapy, she took Decadron, 10 mg orally. The day following chemotherapy she took Decadron, 8 mg, twice a day; the second day she took Decadron, 4 mg, twice a day; and the third day she took Decadron, 2 mg, twice a day. In addition to Decadron she took ondansetron (Zofran), 8 mg orally for 3 days. Mrs. Kady had nausea the first week following chemotherapy, but did not have any episodes of vomiting. She was able to work following chemotherapy, but felt that the nausea interfered with her ability to do her usual quality of work.

For the second cycle of chemotherapy the medications to control nausea and vomiting remained the same. Mrs. Kady reported that she had seven episodes of vomiting 24 hours after the chemotherapy administration and persistent nausea for 1 week following chemotherapy. She reported that she did miss 2 days of work because of the nausea and vomiting. She did manage to work for other days, but it had been a "real effort" to make it through the week.

Mrs. Kady came to the clinic for her third cycle of chemotherapy. She started to report severe nausea once she was seated in an armchair in the treatment room. The nurse instructed Mrs. Kady in using relaxation and provided guided imagery with music therapy. She reported that her nausea was relieved a lot with guided imagery and music therapy. The premedications were changed before the third cycle of chemotherapy, to control nausea and vomiting immediately following chemotherapy. Mrs. Kady received Decadron, 20 mg, along with Zofran, 32 mg intravenously, before her chemotherapy. Following chemotherapy she took Decadron, 10 mg every 8 hours for four doses; then Decadron, 8 mg twice a day for 1 day; then 4 mg twice `a day for 1 day; and then 2 mg twice a day for 1 day; along with Zofran 8 mg orally for 3 days. Compazine and Ativan were ordered to be taken as needed for nausea and vomiting. Following this cycle,

Mrs. Kady reported moderate nausea and three episodes of vomiting following chemotherapy. She also continued relaxation exercises daily. She had persistent nausea again for 1 week following chemotherapy. Although the vomiting was less severe, she found the persistent nausea to be more distressful.

For her fourth cycle of chemotherapy, Mrs. Kady started to have nausea again once she was in the treatment room. She asked the nurse to give her guided imagery treatment with the music therapy since she felt less nauseated with the behavioral treatment. The antiemetic regimens were changed to replace ondansetron with palonosetron for the fourth cycle of chemotherapy. She continued relaxation exercise daily. Mrs. Kady's nausea and vomiting were controlled following chemotherapy, and she did not have persistent nausea following chemotherapy.

The fifth cycle premedications were the same as for the fourth cycle, since immediate postchemotherapy vomiting and delayed nausea had been controlled. She was able to continue her work. The final cycle of chemotherapy, Mrs. Kady received the same premedications she had received for the fourth and fifth cycles. She experienced some nausea and no vomiting. She was able to function both at work and at home. Although she felt her energy level was decreased somewhat, she felt alert and was able to concentrate at work.

Although Mrs. Kady reported nausea and vomiting with the chemotherapy she felt that the symptoms had been managed. Her main concern had been continuing with work, and the antiemetic therapy allowed her to do so.

QUESTIONS

1. Upon assessment, the nurse recognized several risk factors that may predispose Mrs. Kady to the symptoms of nausea and vomiting. The risk factors that Mrs. Kady presented include being female younger than 50 years old, history of nausea and vomiting during pregnancy, possible stress from work, and highly emetogenic chemotherapeutic agent. The nurse correctly categorized the risk factors into the following:
   a. Patient-specific and treatment-specific factors
   b. Treatment-specific and environmental factors
   c. Patient-specific and environmental factors
   d. Treatment-specific and other disease-specific factors

2. Mrs. Kady had granisetron (Kytril) to manage nausea and vomiting for her first cycle of chemotherapy. Which of the following did the nurse say to her to explain how granisetron controls nausea and vomiting?
   a. Granisetron, a dopamine-receptor antagonist, controls nausea and vomiting by blocking the action of dopamine receptors that usually trigger nausea and vomiting during chemotherapy.
   b. Granisetron, a 5-HT$_3$ receptor antagonist, controls nausea and vomiting by blocking the action of serotonin receptors that usually trigger nausea and vomiting during chemotherapy.
   c. Granisetron, a NK-1–receptor antagonist, controls nausea and vomiting by blocking the action of NK-1 receptors that usually trigger nausea and vomiting during chemotherapy.

d. Granisetron, an antihistamine, controls nausea and vomiting by blocking the action of histamines that usually trigger nausea and vomiting during chemotherapy.

3. Mrs. Kady had seven episodes of vomiting 24 hours after she received her second cycle of chemotherapy. She also experienced persistent nausea for 1week following chemotherapy. Which of the following best describes Mrs. Kady's experience of nausea and vomiting?
   a. Acute nausea and vomiting
   b. Anticipatory nausea and vomiting
   c. Delayed nausea and vomiting
   d. Recurrent nausea and vomiting

4. Which of the following patients has the most risk for delayed nausea and vomiting during chemotherapy?
   a. A female patient of 45, with BMI of 30, who often suffers nausea from stress
   b. A male patient of 45, BMI of 32, consuming alcohol daily
   c. A female patient of 65, BMI of 22, no experience of nausea and vomiting during pregnancy
   d. A male patient of 65, BMI of 23, no experience of nausea and vomiting

5. What is the reason that Mrs. Kady did not receive aprepitant (NK-1–receptor antagonist) for her nausea and vomiting?
   a. Carboplatin and aprepitant are not metabolized by liver enzyme CYP3A4.
   b. Paclitaxel and aprepitant are both metabolized by liver enzyme CYP3A4.
   c. Aprepitant is ineffective for ovarian cancer.
   d. Aprepitant and dexamethasone are contraindicated.

6. Mrs. Kady came to the clinic for her third cycle of chemotherapy. She started to report severe nausea once she was seated in a large armchair in the treatment room. For Mrs. Kady, the treatment room was serving as which of the following?
   a. Conditioned stimulus
   b. Conditioned response
   c. Unconditioned stimulus
   d. Unconditioned response

7. The use of pharmacologic agents is less effective to control anticipatory nausea and vomiting, because as learned and conditioned responses, anticipatory nausea and vomiting are mediated by which of the following?
   a. The pathway of cerebral cortex and the limbic system where memory resides
   b. The vestibular apparatus of the middle ear
   c. The chemoreceptor trigger zone (CTZ)
   d. The peripheral pathway activated by neurotransmitter receptors in the GI tract

8. Why is palonosetron, a 5-HT$_3$–receptor antagonist, effective for both acute and delayed nausea and vomiting?
   a. It has a 100-fold higher 5-HT$_3$–receptor binding affinity compared to other serotonin antagonists.
   b. Its half-life is approximately 40 hours.
   c. Both (a) & (b) are correct.
   d. Both (a) & (b) are incorrect.

9. During her chemotherapy treatment, Mrs. Kady's major concern was her ability to continue work. Although Mrs. Kady reported nausea and vomiting with her chemotherapy, she felt that the symptom of nausea and vomiting had been managed because the antiemetic therapy (pharmacologic and behavioral intervention) allowed her to do so. Which expected outcomes of nursing interventions helped Mrs. Kady to have such a perceived success regarding the management of nausea and vomiting?
   a. Improved symptom status, quality of life, functional and cognitive performance
   b. No complaints of nausea and vomiting, changes in antiemetic regimens
   c. Decreased symptom status, changes in antiemetic agents, ability to work
   d. Improved quality of life, performance, and ability to work

10. What might one way be to decrease the occurrence of anticipatory nausea and vomiting?
    a. Better control acute and delayed nausea and vomiting during each course of chemotherapy
    b. Develop more sophisticated chemotherapy regimens
    c. Ignore anticipatory nausea and vomiting, because it will go away once the treatment is finished
    d. Minimal control of nausea and vomiting during each course of chemotherapy

ANSWERS

1. A. Rationale: Patient-specific factors include being female younger than 50 years old, history of nausea and vomiting during pregnancy, and possible stress from work; and treatment-specific factors include chemotherapy.

2. B. Rationale: The serotonin 5-HT$_3$ antagonists such as oncasetron, granisetron, dolasetron mesylate, and palonosetron are effective in controlling nausea and vomiting by blocking the action of serotonin centrally and peripherally.

3. C. Rationale: Delayed nausea and vomiting generally occur 24 hours after chemotherapy administration and may persist for 6 to 7 days, whereas acute nausea and vomiting occur within 24 hours of chemotherapy administration and anticipatory nausea and vomiting occur before the administration of the scheduled subsequent chemotherapy.

4. A. Rationale: Research shows that young, female patients with higher BMI, those who are heavyweight, and those who experience nausea with stress are at great risk for delayed nausea and vomiting during chemotherapy.

5. B. Rationale: Aprepitant is metabolized by liver enzyme CYP3A4. Caution is recommended with concomitant use of other agents metabolized by the same enzyme. The following chemotherapeutic agents should not be used concurrently with aprepitant: paclitaxel, docetaxel, etoposide, irinotecan, ifosfamide, imatinib, vinorelbine, and vincristine.

6. A. Rationale: Anticipatory nausea and vomiting are conditioned responses to the environment during chemotherapy. Conditioned stimuli that may trigger anticipatory nausea and vomiting include a neutral stimulus (such as the chemotherapy nurse), a smell, or the clinic environment.

7. A. Rationale: Pharmacologic antiemetic agents that target on blocking the neurotransmitters are usually effective for nausea and vomiting mediated though peripheral pathway.

Continued

REVIEW QUESTIONS—CONT'D

8. C. *Rationale:* Palonosetron, a 5-HT$_3$–receptor antagonist, is effective for both acute and delayed nausea and vomiting because it has a 100-fold higher 5-HT$_3$–receptor binding affinity compared to other serotonin antagonists, and its half-life is approximately 40 hours.

9. A. *Rationale:* The expected outcomes of nursing interventions for symptom management such as nausea and vomiting include symptom status, quality of life, and performance. Over the course of Mrs. Kady's chemotherapy, integrative approach of pharmacologic and behavioral interventions had helped her to improve the symptom status by controlling symptom occurrence, decreasing symptom distress, and preventing nausea and vomiting; thus her quality of life was also improved, and she was able to function at home and work, which was her major concern.

10. A. *Rationale:* Patients with the greatest amount of nausea after previous chemotherapy are more likely to develop anticipatory nausea and vomiting. As learned responses, anticipatory nausea and vomiting may be a result of negative experience with uncontrolled nausea and vomiting during previous chemotherapy. Reexposure to the conditioned stimuli associated with the negative experience may help the patient develop particular cues (the smell of the clinic or the sight of the chemotherapy nurse) by pairing certain conditioned stimuli with the unconditioned nausea and vomiting. Such cues may trigger nausea and vomiting before the subsequent chemotherapy treatment.

REFERENCES

1. Rhodes VA: Criteria for assessment of nausea, vomiting, and retching, *Oncol Nurs Forum-Suppl* 24(7):13-19, 1997.
2. Rhodes VA, Watson PM, Johnson MH et al: Patterns of nausea, vomiting, and distress in patients receiving antineoplastic drug protocols, *Oncol Nurs Forum* 14(4):3544, 1987.
3. Dodd MJ, Onishi K, Dibble S et al: Differences in nausea, vomiting, and retching between younger and older outpatients receiving cancer chemotherapy, *Cancer Nurs* 19(3):155-161, 1996.
4. Rhodes VA, McDaniel RW: Nausea, vomiting, and retching: complex problems in palliative care, *CA A Cancer J Clin* 51(5):232-248, (2001).
5. National Comprehensive Cancer Network: *Antiemesis: clinical practice guidelines in oncology,* v. 1. 2005, retrieved July 10, 2006, from http://www.nccn.org/professionals/physician_gls/PDF/antiemesis.pdf.
6. de Wit R, Herrstedt J, Rapoport B et al: Addition of the oral NK1 antagonist aprepitant to standard antiemetics provides protection against nausea and vomiting during multiple cycles of cisplatin-based chemotherapy, *J Clin Oncol* 21(22):4105-4111, 2003.
7. Schnell FM: Chemotherapy-induced nausea and vomiting: the importance of acute antiemetic control, *Oncologist* 8(2):187-198, 2003.
8. Dibble SL, Israel J, Nussey B et al.: Delayed chemotherapy-induced nausea in women treated for breast cancer, *Oncol Nurs Forum* 30(2):40-47, 2003.
9. Eckert RM: Understanding anticipatory nausea, *Oncol Nurs Forum* 28(10):1553-1560, 2001.
10. Clark JA, Wray NP, Ashton CM: Living with treatment decisions: regrets and quality of life among men treated for metastatic prostate cancer, *J Clin Oncol* 19(1):72-80, 2001.
11. Oddby-Muhrbeck E, Eksborg S, Bergendahl HTG et al: Effects of clonidine on postoperative nausea and vomiting in breast cancer surgery, *Anesthesiology* 96(5):1109-1114, 2002.
12. Elsayem A, Swint K, Fisch MJ et al: Palliative care inpatient service in a comprehensive cancer center: clinical and financial outcomes, *J Clin Oncol* 22(10):2008-2014, 2004.
13. Hickok JT, Roscoe JA, Morrow GR et al: Nausea and emesis remain significant problems of chemotherapy despite prophylaxis with 5-hydroxytryptamine-3 antiemetics: a University of Rochester James P. Wilmot Cancer Center Community Clinical Oncology Program study of 360 cancer patients treated in the community, *Cancer* 97(11):2880-2886, 2003.
14. Ravasco P, Monteiro-Grillo I, Vidal PM et al: Dietary counseling improves patient outcomes: a prospective, randomized, controlled trial in colorectal cancer patients undergoing radiotherapy, *J Clin Oncol* 23(7):1431-1438, 2005.
15. Movsas B, Scott C, Langer C et al: Randomized trial of amifostine in locally advanced non-small-cell lung cancer patients receiving chemotherapy and hyperfractionated radiation: radiation therapy oncology group trial 98-01, *J Clin Oncol* 23(10):2145-2154, 2005.
16. Italian Group for Antiemetic Research: Dexamethasone alone or in combination with ondansetron for the prevention of delayed nausea and vomiting induced by chemotherapy, *N Engl J Med* 342(21):1554-1559, 2000.
17. Dibble SL, Casey K, Nussey B: Chemotherapy-induced vomiting in women treated for breast cancer, *Oncol Nurs Forum* 31(1):Online Exclusive:E1-8, 2004.
18. Molassiotis A, Mok TSK, Yam BMC et al: An analysis of the antiemetic protection of metoclopramide plus dexamethasone in Chinese patients receiving moderately high emetogenic chemotherapy, *Eur J Cancer Care* 11(2):108-113, 2002.
19. Hickok JT, Roscoe JA, Morrow GR: The role of patients' expectations in the development of anticipatory nausea related to chemotherapy for cancer, *J Pain Symptom Manage* 22(4):843-850, 2001.
20. Montgomery GH, Bovbjerg DH: Specific response expectancies predict anticipatory nausea during chemotherapy for breast cancer, *J Consult Clin Psychol* 69(5):831-835, 2001.
21. Alon E, Buchser E, Herrera E et al: Tropisetron for treating established postoperative nausea and vomiting: a randomized, double-blind, placebo-controlled study, *Anesth Analg* 86(3):617-623, 1998.
22. Montgomery GH. Bovbjerg DH: Expectations of chemotherapy-related nausea: emotional and experiential predictors, *Ann Behav Med* 25(1):48-54, 2003.
23. American Society of Health-System Pharmacists: ASHP therapeutic guidelines on the pharmacologic management of nausea and vomiting in adult and pediatric patients receiving chemotherapy or radiation therapy or undergoing surgery, *Am J Health-Syst Pharm* 56(8):729-64, 1999.
24. Hesketh PJ, Kris MG, Grunberg SM et al: Proposal for classifying the acute emetogenicity of cancer chemotherapy, *J Clin Oncol* 15(1):103-109, 1997.
25. Antonarakis ES, Hain RD: Nausea and vomiting associated with cancer chemotherapy: drug management in theory and in practice, *Arch Dis Child* 89(9):877-880, 2004.
26. Haughney A: Nausea and vomiting in end-stage cancer, *Am J Nurs* 104(11):40-48; 2004.
27. Howarth PA, Finch M: The nauseogenicity of two methods of navigating within a virtual environment, *Appl Ergonomics* 30(1):39-45, 1999.
28. Oyama H, Kaneda M, Katsumata N et al: Using the bedside wellness system during chemotherapy decreases fatigue and emesis in cancer patients, *J Med Syst* 24(3):173-182, 2000.
29. Kim Y, Morrow GR: Changes in family relationships affect the development of chemotherapy-related nausea symptoms, *Support Care Cancer* 11(3):171-177, 2003.
30. Warr DG, Hesketh PJ, Gralla RJ et al: Efficacy and tolerability of aprepitant for the prevention of chemotherapy-induced nausea and vomiting in patients with breast cancer after moderately emetogenic chemotherapy, *J Clin Oncol* 23(12):2822-2830, 2005.
31. Oettle H, Riess H: Treatment of chemotherapy-induced nausea and vomiting, *J Cancer Res Clin Oncol* 127(6):340-345, 2001.
32. Maisano R, Spadaro P, Toscano G et al: Cisapride and dexamethasone in the prevention of delayed emesis after cisplatin administration, *Support Care Cancer* 9(1):61-64, 2001.

33. Viale PH: Integrating aprepitant and palonosetron into clinical practice: a role for the new antiemetics, *Clin J Oncol Nurs* 9(1):77-84, 91-93, 2005.

34. Roscoe JA, Bushunow P, Morrow GR et al: Patient expectation is a strong predictor of severe nausea after chemotherapy: a University of Rochester Community Clinical Oncology Program study of patients with breast carcinoma, *Cancer* 101(11):2701-2708, 2004.

35. Roscoe JA, Hickok JT, Morrow GR: Patient expectations as predictor of chemotherapy-induced nausea, *Ann Behav Med* 22(2):121-126, 2000.

36. Passik SD, Kirsh KL, Rosenfeld B: The changeable nature of patients' fears regarding chemotherapy: implications for palliative care, *J Pain Symptom Manage* 21(2):113-120, 2001.

37. Bernhard J, Maibach R, Thurlimann B et al: Patients' estimation of overall treatment burden: why not ask the obvious? *J Clin Oncol* 20(1):65-72, 2002.

38. Bosnjak S, Radulovic S, Neskovic-Konstantinovic Z et al: Patient statement of satisfaction with antiemetic treatment is related to quality of life, *Am J Clin Oncol* 23(6):575-578, 2000.

39. Pendergrass KB: Options in the treatment of chemotherapy-induced emesis, *Cancer Pract* 6(5):276-281, 1998.

40. Noonan KA: The impact of chemotherapy-induced nausea and vomiting on the daily function and quality of life of patients, *Advanced Studies Nurs* 3(1):16-21, 32-34, 2005.

41. Farley PA, Dempsey CL, Shillington AA et al: Patients' self-reported functional status after granisetron or ondansetron therapy to prevent chemotherapy-induced nausea and vomiting at six cancer centers, *Am J Health Syst Pharm* 54(21):2478-2482, 1997.

42. Ihbe-Heffinger A, Ehlken B, Bernard R et al: The impact of delayed chemotherapy-induced nausea and vomiting on patients, health resource utilization and costs in German cancer centers, *Ann Oncol* 15(3):526-536, 2004.

43. Fu MR, LeMone P, McDaniel RW: An integrated approach to an analysis of symptom management in patients with cancer, *Oncol Nurs Forum* 31(1):65-70, 2004.

44. Rhodes VA, McDaniel RW: The Index of Nausea, Vomiting, and Retching: a new format of the Index of Nausea and Vomiting, *Oncol Nurs Forum* 26(5):889-894, 1999.

45. Fu MR, Rhodes V, Xu B: The Chinese translation of the Index of Nausea, Vomiting, and Retching, *Cancer Nurs* 25(2):134-140, 2002.

46. Shin YH, Kim TI, Shin MS et al: Effect of acupressure on nausea and vomiting during chemotherapy cycle for Korean postoperative stomach cancer patients, *Cancer Nurs* 27(4):267-274, 2004.

47. Rhodes VA, McDaniel RW, Homan SS et al: An instrument to measure symptom experience: symptom occurrence and symptom distress, *Cancer Nurs* 23(1):49-54, 2000.

48. McCorkle R, Young K: Development of a symptom distress scale, *Cancer Nurs* 1(5):373-378, 1978.

49. Portenoy RK, Thaler HT, Kornblith AB et al: The Memorial Symptom Assessment Scale: an instrument for the evaluation of symptom prevalence, characteristics and distress, *E J Cancer* 30A(9):1326-1336, 1998.

50. Williams SA, Schreier AM: The effect of education in managing side effects in women receiving chemotherapy for treatment of breast cancer, *Oncol Nurs Forum Online* 31(1):E16-23, 2004.

51. Italian Group For Antiemetic Research: Randomized, double-blind, dose-finding study of dexamethasone in preventing acute emesis induced by anthracyclines, carboplatin, or cyclophosphamide, *J Clin Oncol* 22(4):725-729, 2004.

52. Navari RM: Role of neurokinin-1 receptor antagonists in chemotherapy-induced emesis: summary of clinical trials, *Cancer Invest* 22(4):569-576, 2004.

53. Gralla R, Lichinitser M, Van Der Vegt S et al: Palonosetron improves prevention of chemotherapy-induced nausea and vomiting following moderately emetogenic chemotherapy: results of a double-blind randomized phase III trial comparing single doses of palonosetron with ondansetron, *Ann Oncol* 14(10):1570-1577, 2003.

54. Grunberg SM, Koeller JM: Palonosetron: a unique 5-HT3-receptor antagonist for the prevention of chemotherapy-induced emesis, *Expert Opin Pharmacother* 4(12):2297-2303, 2003.

55. Hesketh PJ, Grunberg SM, Gralla RJ: et al: Aprepitant Protocol 052 Study Group. The oral neurokinin-1 antagonist aprepitant for the prevention of chemotherapy-induced nausea and vomiting: a multinational, randomized, double-blind, placebo-controlled trial in patients receiving high-dose cisplatin—the Aprepitant Protocol 052 Study Group, *J Clin Oncol* 21(22):4112-4119 2003.

56. Morrow GR, Roscoe JA, Hickok JT: Nausea and emesis: evidence for a biobehavioral perspective, *Support Care Cancer* 10(2):96-105, 2002.

57. Ernst E, Pittler MH: Efficacy of ginger for nausea and vomiting: a systematic review of randomized clinical trials, *Br J Anaesth* 84(3):367-371, 2000.

58. Golembiewski J, Chernin E, Chopra T: Prevention and treatment of postoperative nausea and vomiting, *Am J Health Syst Pharm* 62(12):1247-1260, 2005.

59. Pongrojpaw D, Chiamchanya C: The efficacy of ginger in prevention of post-operative nausea and vomiting after outpatient gynecological laparoscopy, *J Med Assoc Thai* 86(3):244-250, 2003.

60. Manusirivithaya S, Sripramote M, Tangjitgamol S et al: Antiemetic effect of ginger in gynecologic oncology patients receiving cisplatin, *Int J Gynecol Cancer* 14(6):1063-1069, 2004.

61. Tate S: Peppermint oil: A treatment for postoperative nausea, *J Adv Nurs* 26(3):543-549, 1997.

62. Sommerville KW, Richmond CR, Bell GD: Delayed release peppermint oil capsules (Colpermin) for the spastic colon syndrome: a pharmacokinetic study, *Br J Clin Pharmacol* 18:638-640, 1984;

63. Dew MJ, Evans BJ, Rhodes J: Peppermint oil for the irritable bowel: a multicentre trial, *Br J Clin Pract* 38:397-398, 1984.

64. Hills JM, Aaronson PI: The mechanism of action of peppermint oil on gastrointestinal smooth muscle. *Gastroenterology* 101(1):55-65, 1991.

65. Dibble SL, Chapman J, Mack KA et al: Acupressure for nausea: results of a pilot study, *Oncol Nurs Forum* 27(1):41-47, 2000.

66. Roscoe JA, Matteson SE, Morrow GR et al: Acustimulation wrist bands are not effective for the control of chemotherapy-induced nausea in women with breast cancer, *J Pain Symptom Manage* 29(4):376-384, 2005.

67. Molassiotis A, Yung HP, Yam EM et al: The effectiveness of progressive muscle relaxation training in managing chemotherapy-induced nausea and vomiting in Chinese breast cancer patients: a randomised controlled trial, *Support Care Cancer* 10(3):237-246, 2002.

68. Matteson S, Roscoe J, Hickok J et al: The role of behavioral conditioning in the development of nausea, *Am J Obstet Gynecol* 186(5 Suppl Understanding):S239-S243, 2002.

69. Marchioro G, Azzarello G, Viviani F et al: Hypnosis in the treatment of anticipatory nausea and vomiting in patients receiving cancer chemotherapy *Oncology* 59(2):100-104, 2000.

70. Cassileth BR, Vickers AJ: Massage therapy for symptom control: outcome study at a major cancer center, *J Pain Symptom Manage* 28(3):244-249, 2004.

71. Grealish L, Lomasney A, Whiteman B: Foot massage: a nursing intervention to modify the distressing symptoms of pain and nausea in patients hospitalized with cancer, *Cancer Nurs* 23(3):237-243, 2000.

CHAPTER 42

Hot Flashes

Debra Barton

Definition

Hot flashes are one of the most common symptoms associated with hormone depletion in both men and women. Also called vasomotor hot flushes, they can manifest as night sweats. They may be preceded or followed by chills. A hot flash is defined as a sudden sensation of intense warmth that begins in the chest area and may rise to the neck and face as well as down to the toes.[1-3] Hot flashes can be accompanied by red blotches on the skin, profuse sweating, palpitations, anxiety, and embarrassment. A hot flash can last for 1 minute or as long as 10 to 20 minutes.[1,4]

Prevalence

Hot flashes are experienced by up to 75% (but generally fewer) of women in the general population as they travel through the menopause transition.[4,5] For most women, hot flashes persist for up to 2 years and then subside. A minority of women can experience hot flashes for as many as 15 or more years.[5] The median age of menopause is 51 years. However, hot flashes can begin in the perimenopausal phase up to 8 years earlier.[5]

For women with a history of cancer, the overall prevalence of hot flashes is more commonly 65% to 75%.[6,7] However, because of treatment, menopause can come prematurely, with hot flashes beginning long before others in her peer group.[8] Likewise, hormone therapies for breast cancer are associated with hot flashes in over 50% of women.[3] In general, studies have shown that women with a history of breast cancer who are also experiencing menopause are more likely to experience symptoms than the noncancer population and experience more severe symptoms.[6,9-11]

Men do not normally experience a menopause as do women. Testosterone, the male sex hormone, does decrease throughout a man's lifetime (a process termed andropause). However, the decline is not precipitous as it is in female menopause. Men receiving androgen ablation therapy for prostate cancer do experience a sudden and severe decrease in testosterone. Both surgical and medical castration puts men at risk for experiencing hot flashes. About 40% to 80% of men undergoing androgen ablation therapy will experience hot flashes.[4,12,13] The trajectory and severity of these hot flashes is not well elucidated in the literature.

Risk Factors

In studies with the general population, risk factors for hot flashes include being postmenopausal, advanced age, increased body mass index (BMI), and currently smoking.[14,15] Other identified risk factors for symptoms include ethnicity (African American), low socioeconomic status, and lack of physical activity.[4,5] Receiving treatment for breast cancer is also a risk factor leading to increased incidence and severity of hot flashes. Chemotherapy treatment can induce a premature menopause for those women over 40 years of age who have not yet reached menopause.[8,16] Alkylating agents,

anthracyclines, antimetabolites, and plant alkaloids can cause ovarian dysfunction and lead to premature menopause.[17] Treatment with tamoxifen, raloxifene, or an aromatase inhibitor can also induce hot flashes.[18-20] Tamoxifen has the highest incidence of hot flashes, at 46% to 50% depending on whether a woman is premenopausal or postmenopausal, with postmenopausal women having more hot flashes with tamoxifen.[19] The combination of chemotherapy and tamoxifen seems to cause the greatest risk of having menopausal symptoms.[21]

Women on raloxifene are more likely to experience hot flashes if they are closer to the menopause transition or have experienced a surgical menopause.[20] Radiation therapy to the ovary can also cause cessation of menstruation, thus precipitating hot flashes.[8] Surgery to remove the ovaries, used to prevent or treat cancer, results in a surgical menopause, which can also precipitate hot flashes.

Men who have had surgical castration will develop hot flashes, with more hot flashes being experienced by younger men than by older men.[13] Men receiving luteinizing hormone–releasing hormone (LHRH) analogues have an even higher incidence of hot flashes (around 70% to 80%).[12,13]

Etiology

The pathophysiology of a hot flash has not been definitively determined.[22] Animal models of natural menopause are lacking because few species live beyond their reproductive years. Without a relevant animal model, precise determination of hot flash physiology must be determined through more indirect methods that take longer for discovery. Nevertheless, advances in knowledge are occurring, and the following information is now known about hot flash physiology.

Primarily, in order for hot flashes to develop, estrogen deprivation must occur. Women who have had diseases such as hypogonadism do not experience hot flashes unless they have received treatment with estrogen that was then stopped. Second, as a result of estrogen loss, there is a narrowed zone in which the body is able to regulate its temperature. Thus, small increases in core body temperature that once would have been easily accommodated are now a cause of vasodilatation, increased skin temperature, decreased skin resistance, and sweating—a hot flash. Core body temperature has been shown to increase as much as 20 minutes before the beginning of a hot flash.[23] Thirdly, it is thought that hot flashes are centrally mediated, as opposed to peripherally mediated, and that neurotransmitters such as serotonin may play an important role.[22,24] In fact, it may well be an imbalance in serotonin and norepinephrine that is responsible for precipitating a hot flash.[22]

There has been very limited research in small numbers of women that has attempted to describe the pattern of hot flashes in terms of circadian rhythm. To date, no conclusions can be drawn from this literature, since it is too sparse and too varied. There are no data to suggest that the pathophysiology of hot flashes differs by whether a woman has had a surgical, natural, or chemotherapy- or radiation therapy–induced menopause. The only data available suggest that symptoms are more frequent and severe in sympto- matic women who are cancer survivors. Furthermore, intervention studies have not shown a difference in efficacy between women taking tamoxifen and not taking tamoxifen.[25]

In the case of hot flashes in men, the withdrawal of andro- gens, specifically testosterone, causes a similar change in the thermoregulatory zone, making body temperature more difficult to control. In addition, men undoubtedly have similar centrally mediated events related to neurotransmitters. Evidence for this is demonstrated by the fact that antidepressants work similarly for both men and women (to be discussed later in this chapter).

Effects and Consequences

Hot flashes are not just a physiologic phenomenon but are accompanied by both emotional and behavioral responses. When asked to record what factors led to a designation of mild, moder- ate, severe, or very severe hot flashes, women listed several nega- tive emotions that accompanied their hot flashes. These emotions included panic, irritation, and being embarrassed or annoyed and distressed.[1] The more negative the emotion, the more severe the hot flash. Behaviors were also undertaken as a result of the hot flash experience. Again, the more drastic behaviors were associ- ated with more severe hot flashes: major sleep disturbance, bed linen changes, and cold showers.[1]

In addition, hot flashes can be a source of bother and distress and negatively affect the quality of life. In one study, hot flashes were associated with more interference in terms of work, social life, leisure, sleep, concentration, relationships, sex, and mood than was found for those postmenopausal women who were not having hot flashes.[26] This sample included women who were breast cancer survivors as well as those who were not. In another report, data were analyzed across several identically designed pilot studies evaluating treatments for hot flashes. Authors found that distress from hot flashes was correlated with concomitant symptoms such as difficulty sleeping, fatigue, interference with sex, nervousness, and negative mood.[27] In a study of 300 women without breast cancer, investigators looked at the relationship between vasomotor symptoms and psychologic symptoms.[28] These investigators report that premenopausal women who experi- ence vasomotor symptoms have an increased risk of negative emotions (such as anxiety and depression) and somatic symptoms. This finding was not true for women who were postmenopausal. Perhaps the increased incidence of premature menopause in women being treated for cancer (making them experience vasomotor symp- toms at an earlier, usually premenopausal, age) predisposes them for increased negative emotions and makes the experience of hot flashes more distressing than it would have normally been.

In men with prostate cancer, hot flashes are also associated with interfering with daily activities, sleep, and the ability to get as much enjoyment from life.[4] A study done in Japan with 55 men experiencing hot flashes as a result of prostate cancer treatment found a statistically significant decrease in several quality of life parameters, compared to men who were not expe- riencing hot flashes.[29] Some of the measures that found quality of life to be worse in men experiencing hot flashes include the general Functional Assessment of Cancer Therapy (FACT-G) as

well as the prostate-specific version (FACT-P), and the physical and social or family well-being subscale of the FACT.

In a study asking men to describe how they came to rate their hot flashes as mild, moderate, severe, or very severe, negative emotions were included as being associated with their hot flashes. These negative emotions included anxiety, irritability, restlessness, and feeling out of control.[30]

Assessment

Initial assessment for hot flashes should include several phys- ical as well as psychologic parameters. These parameters apply to both men and women experiencing hot flashes. Assessment begins with obtaining information about the frequency, the sever- ity, and the duration of the hot flashes. The incidence and frequency of nighttime flashes or night sweats is also important to determine. The degree to which interruptions in sleep and work activities occurs is another critical element. It may be helpful for men or women to keep a diary for a week noting the frequency, the severity, and the times of hot flashes. This process can help to identify peak hot flash occurrence, may help in identifying possible hot flash triggers, and may provide a more real-time picture of the person's actual experience with hot flashes. Sometimes, in recollecting from the past, people can underesti- mate their hot flash experience and the negative impact it is having on their lives.

The next part of assessment is to determine what behaviors or other interventions the person has tried previously for hot flash management. How meticulously did the person implement the intervention, and what were their results? How did the person evaluate the results?

This assessment helps to match the level of intervention to the degree of severity of the hot flash experience.

Measurement

The measurement of hot flashes is important for both research and clinical practice purposes. The question arises as to what the best method for measuring hot flashes is. Most symptoms (be it for research or practice) are measured with self-report question- naires that are validated, reliable tools developed for symptom assessment (Schwartz Cancer Fatigue Scale, Brief Pain Inventory, Pittsburgh Sleep Quality Index).[31,32,33] These measures generally have time, duration, and severity components as well as interference or impact questions. It is intriguing that a similar scale has not been created for hot flashes.

There is one specific hot flash scale that has been developed called the Hot Flash Related Daily Interference Scale.[26] This tool consists of 10 items on a 0- to 10-point scale asking the person to rate the degree of interference hot flashes pose on various aspects of life; work, social, leisure, sleep, mood, concentration, relationship, sex, enjoyment, and overall quality of life. The initial study that used it for psychometric evaluation was good, with 134 female participants. However, use of this tool has not been widely published and although this scale would provide the clinician or researcher with an assessment of the degree to which hot flashes made an impact on a patient's life, it does not specif- ically measure the number or severity of hot flashes. This tool has not been evaluated in men. Several general menopausal scales exist that include a question on hot flashes and/or night sweats. Many of these scales have not been well validated (e.g., Kupperman Index) and many of them measure degree of bother related to the menopausal symptoms and don't directly measure the frequency or severity of the symptom itself (e.g., Menopausal Quality of Life).[34,35,36] These scales would be helpful in assessing the impact of hot flashes and help better understand the level of intervention necessary. However, these scales are not as helpful in evaluating the efficacy of an intervention directly on hot flashes. The general menopausal scales are not used, and would not be appropriate, for men.

There is a current debate with respect to hot flash measurement for research purposes revolving around subjective (self-report) versus objective (mechanical) measurement of hot flash frequency and severity. Hot flashes can be measured with various objective measures: core and finger temperature skin conductance, body temperature, and sternal conductance monitoring.[4,37,38]

Many of these devices have not been tested and may not be practical for use in ambulatory settings, and, in studies to date, measurements had to be done in a laboratory setting; thus the ability to capture hot flashes in the natural environment is lost. Devices that can objectively and accurately measure hot flashes in an ambulatory subject are being developed but have not been validated on large samples. Furthermore, it has yet to be shown how these objective and subjective measures correlate, and what precisely is gained with an objective measure of a symptom that is experienced subjectively and would be treated (presumably) according to that subjective experience. It is also not yet clear how these measures differentiate skin conductance changes as a result of more vigorous activity (i.e., climbing stairs) and a hot flash.

To date, most studies evaluating hot flash interventions use a prospective diary that is either kept electronically or with pen and paper.[4,25,26] The daily diary requires that people keep track of their hot flashes in real time, for every 24-hour period within each week. The number of hot flashes as well as the severity of each hot flash are recorded on a 1- to 4-point scale (1—mild hot flash to 4—very severe). Researchers at various institutions have used this diary and the hot flash score as the primary endpoint in clinical trials. The hot flash score is defined by multiplying the daily frequency times the average hot flash severity.[4,25] This diary and endpoint have been used in well over 10 prospective randomized clinical trials involving over 1,000 people (men and women) with hot flashes and has shown good reliability and validity.[39-49] Results have been replicated using this instrument. For clinical assessment purposes, the diary can be expanded to include times and environmental and behavioral factors, so people can more easily identify the patterns and triggers that are associated with their hot flashes. In addition, adding questions about the impact of hot flashes on various aspects of daily life (as in the Hot Flash Related Daily Interference Scale) may be helpful in determining interventions and evaluating responses to those interventions.[26]

Interventions

HORMONAL-RELATED THERAPIES

Estrogen. Historically, hot flashes have been effectively treated with hormonal therapy. The gold standard of therapy for hot flashes has been estrogen-based therapy. Review of studies using estrogen showed that it reduced both the frequency and severity of hot flashes by 90%. Estrogen therapy can be delivered orally, transdermally, or intravaginally and can be given with progesterone (where the patient has a uterus) or even with testosterone. Given the new information published by the Women's Health Initiative (WHI), many women are not willing to take the risks associated with estrogen-progesterone therapy.[50,51] In the aftermath of the WHI publications, some health care providers advocate very–low dose, short-term, transdermal estrogen-based hormone therapy for those patients whose quality of life is so compromised that effective treatment is imperative. However, the efficacy of this treatment is not well documented. Earlier studies with estrogen-based therapy clearly indicate a dose response.[52,53] Aside from risks associated with breast cancer, stroke, and thrombosis, estrogen is not without side effects. Side effects include nausea, water retention, headache, irritability, withdrawal vaginal bleeding, breast tenderness, and increased risk of clots.[54] Therefore, in this new era, evidence-based therapy is still critical. Even before the WHI, women with a history of hormone-sensitive cancers were not likely to be offered any options with estrogen-based therapies. The challenge for health care providers is to offer a therapy with a better risk and toxicity profile, while delivering the same level of efficacy as estrogen based therapy.

For the most part, estrogen-related hormonal therapies do not apply to men, since there is not a recognized need to replace estrogen in men. However, there is a study in progress looking at treating men who are receiving androgen ablation therapy with risedronate, calcium, vitamin D, and estrogen for prevention of osteoporosis. A secondary endpoint if this trial is to look at how estrogen therapy affects hot flashes in men.

Progesterone. Both megestrol acetate (Megace) and depot medroxyprogesterone acetate (Depo-Provera [DMPA]) have been shown to be effective in relieving hot flashes in prospective randomized clinical trials and pilot trials.[46,55,56] Megestrol acetate, 40 mg/day, was used for hot flash control in both men and women, and then titrated down to 20 mg/day or 20 mg every other day, and was shown to be both effective (decreasing hot flashes by about 85%) and well tolerated for 4 or more years.[46,57] The only side effect seen in the 4-week trial was withdrawal vaginal bleeding.[46] In a 6-week study of oral megestrol acetate, side effects reported included appetite increase, fluid retention, dizziness, and dry mouth.[56]

A few studies have evaluated the use of intramuscular DMPA for hot flashes.[55,56] An abstract was published that described using 400 mg DMPA intramuscularly for hot flash control in men with prostate cancer.[58] Men were followed up to 3 years. Hot flashes were controlled (although this was not defined) in 51% of men after just one injection, and the duration of this response was up to 1 year.[58] A pilot clinical experience was undertaken with men and women giving three injections of 500 mg DMPA, one every 2 weeks. Hot flashes decreased an average of 90%, and the duration of response lasted several months.[55] A larger randomized trial in women comparing oral megestrol acetate to injections of DMPA found both forms of progesterone to be very effective in reducing hot flashes and very well tolerated.[56] Yet another study comparing one injection of 400 mg DMPA with venlafaxine (Effexor) in women reported a 79% decrease in hot flash scores with a single injection of DMPA compared to a 55% reduction with venlafaxine. The DMPA, overall, was also better tolerated than venlafaxine.[44] The randomized study confirms the efficacy of DMPA injections seen in the pilot studies.

Currently a controversy exists as to whether it is safe to use progesterone alone for hot flashes in women with hormone-sensitive cancers or in those at risk for developing cancer. The answer is not definitively known, and there are pros and cons on either side. High-dose progesterone is used to treat cancer in Europe. Some epidemiologic studies have shown that progesterone alone has not increased the risk of breast cancer.[59] Studies looking at endogenous hormone levels have hypothesized that progesterone may be protective for breast cancer.[60] Further, there is speculation that the progesterone receptor is inhibitory with respect to breast cancer. The risk/benefit of any hormone-related treatment must be carefully evaluated for individual women, particularly those who are at increased risk for developing breast cancer or for breast cancer recurrence.

Other Hormonal Agents. Finally, androgens have been used to assist with hot flash reduction. Androgenic agents have shown efficacy on their own against hot flashes; also, hot flash reduction was improved with the addition of androgens to estrogenic compounds.[61-63] Again, the safety of the use of androgens in a population of women with hormone-sensitive tumors or those at risk for breast cancer is not fully known. Androgens can be aromatized into active estrogens; however, as with progesterone, there exists the hypothesis that the androgen receptor is inhibitory with respect to breast cancer, and androgens have also been used to treat breast cancer.[64] Androgens are not an option for men with prostate cancer.

NONHORMONAL THERAPIES

One of the most effective nonhormonal alternatives for hot flash management appears to be the newer antidepressants. Research has been completed looking at a selective serotonin/norepinephrine reuptake inhibitors such as venlafaxine (SNRIs), as well as selective serotonin reuptake inhibitors(SSRIs) (e.g., fluoxetine [Prozac], paroxetine [Paxil], sertraline [Zoloft], citalopram [Celexa], and mirtazapine [Remeron]). For most of these agents, the dosage used for hot flashes is lower than that used for depression, and therefore the agents are associated with very little toxicity as evidenced by placebo-controlled trials. Most of these agents provide a 50% to 60% reduction in hot flashes.

Venlafaxine has had the most research and appears to consistently deliver a 55% to 60% reduction in hot flashes.[39] The venlafaxine tested in hot flash studies is the extended-release formulation. Patients are started at 37.5 mg daily, and the dosage is titrated up after 1 week to 75 mg if sufficient relief is not obtained at the 37.5-mg level. Side effects seen in placebo-controlled trial included transient nausea that resolved in 2 weeks, some dry mouth, and decreased appetite.[39] Studies have not shown any additional benefit in using more than 75 mg daily. When a decision is made to discontinue the drug, patients should be titrated off of the medication over a week. There is some concern about sexual dysfunction with the use of venlafaxine. Literature on venlafaxine used for depression includes the side effect of the inability to reach orgasm. Health care providers have reported that patients comment about decreased libido while taking the drug. The short-term study with venlafaxine actually showed an increase in libido. There are no long- term randomized prospective placebo-controlled trials using low-dose venlafaxine to evaluate the effect on sexuality. Venlafaxine has also been studied in a pilot study with men and showed similar efficacy.[65]

Paroxetine has been studied in more than one placebo-controlled trial for hot flashes in women. Dosages of 12.5 mg and 25 mg[42] of controlled-release paroxetine have been evaluated, as well as 10-mg and 20-mg dosages[66] of short-acting drug.

Both studies reported significant reductions in hot flash scores and frequencies. In the trial with long-acting paroxetine, which included 165 menopausal women, reductions in hot flash scores were 62% for the 12.5-mg dosage and 65% in the 25-mg dosage, with the placebo group reporting a decrease of 38%.[42] There were no statistically significant differences in toxicities reported between the active and the placebo arms, although there was a trend for more nausea in the 25-mg arm.[42] In the short-acting paroxetine study, which accrued 151 women who were mostly breast cancer survivors, hot flash score was reduced by 46% in the 10-mg group and 56% in the 20-mg group.[66] However, because of the fact that more women withdrew from the study on the 20-mg arm, the authors recommend using the 10-mg dosage. Furthermore, sleep was significantly improved in the 10-mg arm over the placebo arm. Paroxetine, 37.5 mg, was studied in a small pilot trial in 18 men with prostate cancer. Hot flash scores were reduced by 50%, and the medication was well tolerated.[67] There have not been placebo-controlled trials of this agent in men.

The other antidepressant medications, fluoxetine[40] (20 mg per day) and sertraline (50 mg per day)[68] have also been studied in larger, placebo controlled trials, but with slightly lower levels of hot flash reduction. Fluoxetine reduced the mean hot flash score by 50%, without any significant differences in toxicities between the active and the placebo arms. Sertraline reduced the mean hot flash score by about 25%, but in 36% of the sample, hot flashes were reduced by 50%.[68] In contrast to the studies with venlafaxine and paroxetine, neither study with fluoxetine or sertraline evaluated different dosages. This fact alone could account for the varying results.

It should be noted that neither paroxetine, sertraline, nor fluoxetine should be used if a woman is taking tamoxifen. It is known that these medications inhibit the CYP2D6 pathway in cytochrome P450 metabolism. Alterations in this pathway have been found to interfere with the metabolism of tamoxifen to endoxifen. Women with genetic variations in CYP2D6 had worse relapse-free time and disease-free survival on tamoxifen, suggesting endoxifen is an important metabolite clinically.[69]

Smaller pilot studies have been done with citalopram (20 mg daily) and show similar positive results without significant side effects.[70] One pilot study was done with mirtazapine, since sleep disturbances can accompany hot flashes despite not being related to them.[71] Mirtazapine has sleepiness as its main side effect; therefore, it was thought that this antidepressant may be helpful in both areas: controlling hot flashes and resolving sleep disturbances.[71] Mirtazapine was shown to reduce hot flashes by about 55%, but did have substantial sleepiness as a side effect, which was not acceptable to most women.

Since many of the serotonergic antidepressants seem to work similarly against hot flashes, it is reasonable to wonder if there is cross-resistance between them with respect to hot flashes. In other words, if a woman tries venlafaxine and it doesn't work, can she try citalopram, or is it to be assumed that none of these agents will work? That question was studied by the Mayo Clinic in a pilot fashion after positive clinical experience with switching between antidepressants. A study was done with 22 women who had not gotten adequate relief with venlafaxine.[72] These women were switched to citalopram. By the end of 4 weeks of active treatment, these women experienced a 53% reduction in their hot flash score.[72] Citalopram was well tolerated, with over 60% of patients wishing to stay on the agent after completing the study.

Therefore, if one antidepressant does not work, it is reasonable to try another. Hot flash activity on these agents is experienced relatively quickly. In 2 weeks, a person should be able to tell what type of response the medication can provide. Therefore time is not wasted trying an unsuccessful agent for a month or more. Again, it is important to titrate up and down in dosage when using these medications. It is also important to note that since the physiology of hot flashes is not definitively known, practitioners cannot assume that all antidepressants will work equally to reduce hot flashes. Antidepressants that target only norepinephrine or dopamine may not have activity against hot flashes. Each agent must be studied.

Another novel, effective nonhormonal treatment for hot flashes is gabapentin (Neurontin). This agent has been studied by different groups of investigators in women experiencing natural menopause and surgical menopause and those with a history of breast cancer.[41,73,74] In randomized placebo-controlled trials, gabapentin is effective in reducing hot flashes by 46% to 54%. Gabapentin is an anticonvulsant and is also used for neuropathic pain. How it works to relieve hot flashes is not well understood since the exact mechanism of action of gabapentin is not known. The dosage studied for hot flashes is 300 mg 3 times per day, starting with 300 mg once daily and titrating up to 3 times per day over a week. Gabapentin has a short half-life, which necessitates 3-times-per-day dosing. When used to manage hot flashes, side effects of gabapentin include somnolence, dizziness, rash, and peripheral edema.[41] Over time, patients may develop generalized edema, due to changes in serum albumin. Some patients report an increase in clothing size. It is important that patients be aware of the symptom if it occurs, because the gabapentin will have to be discontinued. A study has recently been completed that added gabapentin to the current use of an antidepressant to see if there is an additive benefit. Such benefit has been seen in clinical practice, but was not seen in the randomized trial as reported at the American Society of Clinical Oncology 2006.[75] However, negative mood effects occurred when patients stopped their antidepressant. Further, a large randomized placebo-controlled trial of gabapentin is underway to evaluate this treatment for men receiving androgen ablation therapy.

Older treatments for hot flashes include clonidine (Catapres) and Bellergal; there are also some older data on propanolol. Clonidine has had the most evidence and is available in different delivery systems; oral or transdermal. Both delivery systems appear to be effective. In a study using a transdermal patch, a dose equal to an oral dose of 0.1 mg was used.[49] Hot flashes were reduced significantly more than placebo, with a 56% reduction. Side effects included dry mouth, constipation, itchiness associated with the patch, and drowsiness.[49] A more recent study evaluating 0.1 mg per day of oral clonidine found a 37% reduction in hot flash frequency; the only side effect that was different from placebo was difficulty sleeping.[48] Bellergal, a combination of ergotamine tartrate, levorotatory alkaloids, and phenobarbital, has also been used to treat hot flashes and, in very early studies, a reduction up to 75% was seen.[76,77] However, in a study by Bergmans, Merkus, Corbey, and colleagues, the placebo group experienced a reduction in hot flashes of 68%. In this particular study, there was a very large dropout rate (12 out of 33 in the active treatment group and 16 out of 33 in the placebo group), a result of either adverse events (dry mouth, dizziness, sleepiness, headache, and nausea) or ineffectiveness.[77]

The older medications were not evaluated in men with prostate cancer. However, at least one study has shown that clonidine is not equally effective in men as in women.[78]

NUTRACEUTICAL THERAPIES

Given the negative press hormone therapy has received with respect to breast cancer risk, cognition, and cardiovascular health, and answering to the desire to avoid costs and side effects associated with pharmacologic interventions, the search is on for "natural" remedies for hot flashes. Because of the popularity of herbal and food supplement products, evidence is starting to mount to help clarify the efficacy, or lack thereof, of many of these products with respect to hot flashes. Randomized placebo-controlled trials have been completed with vitamin E, soy, and black cohosh.

Vitamin E had been touted in women's health books and journals as a remedy for hot flashes, yet had not had any formal, prospective research associated with it until the 1990s. A randomized placebo-controlled study was done in the mid 1990s that showed that vitamin E, 400 international units twice a day, did decrease hot flashes significantly more than a placebo did, statistically; but clinically, this resulted in only about 1 more hot flash per day over placebo (an overall reduction of 25%).[45] There were no side effects in this trial.[45] For milder hot flashes that do not limit the quality of life, vitamin E has been a reasonable suggestion. However, in light of the more recent research suggesting that 400 international units of daily vitamin E may increase heart failure in people with diabetes or vascular disease, caution should be used and care taken to assess patients' histories before this intervention is suggested.

Debate has been long as to the beneficial effects of soy in menopausal symptoms and, in particular, in hot flashes. There have been numerous placebo-controlled studies with various amounts and types of soy over the past decade.[47,79-82] Most of these studies are negative, with a few showing some positive, but inconsistent results. To date, there is no compelling evidence to recommend soy for hot flash control.[82]

Black cohosh is another herb popularly thought to decrease hot flashes. There are several positive studies in Germany, but until recently, no studies had been done in the United States. To date, there are two published studies in the United States, and one recent study from Germany, evaluating black cohosh for hot flashes.[43,83,84] Two of them are negative studies, and one is positive. All three of these studies are placebo-controlled randomized trials over various lengths of time: 4, 8, and 12 weeks. The 12-week study was the only one that yielded positive results.[84] Does that imply that black cohosh works if you take it long enough? More research would have to be done. There is a major weakness in the one positive study. Instead of measuring the number and severity of hot flashes as the main outcome, this study looked at a combination of hot flashes, night sweats, and sleep problems (including falling asleep and waking up early).[84] It was this combined outcome that was positively affected by the black cohosh at week 12. Therefore, it is not possible to know whether hot flashes were actually affected and to what degree. At this time, the evidence for the use of black cohosh for hot flashes is very weak.

There are some herbal products that have not yet been evaluated in clinical trials in the United States for hot flashes, but are popularly thought to positively influence menopausal symptoms. These agents are dong quai, red clover, hops, chasteberry, and licorice. There is some evidence that all of these agents have estrogenic properties, either binding weakly (dong quai, licorice) or strongly and competitively with estrogen receptors (red clover, chasteberry, hops).[85] Therefore, if estrogen is to be avoided, these herbs should also be avoided. None of these products have been evaluated in men.

BEHAVIORAL INTERVENTIONS

There are a few behavioral interventions that either have some evidence base through prospective trials or have merit based on scientific rationale. The first of these revolves around keeping the environment cool with moving air. There is some published data that ambient temperatures can affect frequency and severity of hot flashes.[86,87] Also, since scientists know that core body temperature rises as much as 20 minutes before a hot flash is experienced, it makes scientific sense to try to keep the body cool. Ways in which one can help the body from overheating is to be in cool temperatures (e.g., use air conditioning), keep air exchange going around the skin (e.g., with a fan, wind) and to wear open-weave cottons that allow the passage of air over the skin. Dressing in layers so as to be able to regulate how many clothes are on the body as air temperature changes is also important. Other behaviors that can increase the body temperature include drinking warm—rather than cold—drinks, eating spicy foods, and drinking alcohol.

Behaviors that have been tested in clinical trials include paced respirations and applied relaxation. Two of the studies involved a randomization to deep, diaphragmatic, slowed breathing versus control groups. In both studies, the paced respirations and relaxation response significantly decreased either hot flash frequency or intensity. Although both studies were very small, it provides some evidence that attention to slow, diaphragmatic breathing, practiced daily, may afford some relief of hot flashes (as much as 40% reduction).[87,88] Another study, using a case study series with 6 women, found significant reductions in hot flashes through the learning and practice of applied relaxation.[89]

Another behavioral intervention that has received mixed outcomes with respect to hot flashes is exercise. The most rigorous prospective clinical trial evaluating moderate-intensity exercise versus a stretch control group for hot flashes showed no effect of the exercise on hot flash frequency or severity.[90] What is not known is whether a history of consistent exercise influences the incidence or severity of hot flash symptoms during the menopause transition. There is no information on men regarding any of these interventions.

A new behavioral, complementary intervention that has promising pilot data and is being studied in larger randomized controlled trials is hypnosis. Two manuscripts discussing case study reports and one small pilot trial provide encouraging data regarding the potential of hypnosis to reduce hot flashes.[91-93] Evidence from larger, more definitive trials must be obtained before the role of hypnosis in treatment of hot flashes is clearly defined.

Outcomes

In order to obtain positive outcomes with respect to hot flashes, what is the best way to proceed when working with a patient? The first thing is to do a comprehensive assessment, evaluating the degree to which the hot flashes interfere with the person's life. Secondly, determine what and how many interventions the person has already tried to gain control of the hot flashes, how long she or he tried it, and how well it worked. Both of these elements will help with decisions about interventions and target outcomes. If patients have hot flashes that strongly interfere with the ability to function in their jobs and they have already tried one or more interventions unsuccessfully, being sure to use an effective intervention will be critical to minimize any further frustration and enhance coping. A reasonable first-line treatment for someone with significant hot flashes that interfere with daily activities or sleep is to use one of the antidepressants that have been studied in a placebo-controlled trial (e.g., venlafaxine, paroxetine) (Table 42-1).

Paroxetine, fluoxetine, and sertraline should not be used in women taking tamoxifen. If satisfactory relief is not obtained with

---

TABLE 42-1   **Effective Interventions for Hot Flashes**

HOT FLASH CHARACTERISTICS	INTERVENTION	CONTRAINDICATIONS
Mild to moderate, not interfering with sleep or daily activities	Behavioral strategies: Air movement, breathing, identifying and controlling triggers	None
	Vitamin E	Diabetes, vascular disease, radiation therapy
Moderate to severe, interferes with sleep and/or daily activities	Venlafaxine or paroxetine or other serotonergic antidepressant therapy, or gabapentin	Do not use paroxetine, fluoxetine or sertraline if woman is taking tamoxifen
Severe to very severe, patient unable to sleep and unable to fulfill daily obligations	Antidepressant or gabapentin therapy combined with a behavioral therapy such as paced respirations or hypnosis (no evidence base) *OR*	If currently taking tamoxifen, do not use paroxetine, fluoxetine, or sertraline
	DMPA injection 400 mg, repeat 1 time in 1 month if hot flash relief not sufficient	Unknowns, risk/benefit ratio of progesterone therapy in breast cancer survivors well discussed between provider and patient

DMPA, Depot medroxyprogesterone acetate.

CONSIDERATIONS FOR OLDER ADULTS

- In many people, hot flashes do get better over time. If older women have been on hot flash treatment for some time, it is reasonable to titrate the dosage down and then stop the medication to see if their hot flashes have resolved.
- Gabapentin may be less well tolerated in older individuals. Starting with 100 mg daily and titrating up to 300 mg 3 times a day may be better tolerated in terms of dizziness (in particular).
- When treating older individuals, be sure to assess for comorbidities and concomitant medications, including dietary supplements. For example, St. John's wort should be avoided while taking many other prescription medications because of cytochrome P450 pathway interference.

one antidepressant, it is reasonable to switch to a different antidepressant (e.g., venlafaxine to citalopram) and determine if that antidepressant works better for the individual, or switch to gabapentin. Adding a behavioral intervention, such as paced respirations, to a pharmacologic one may provide additive effects, although this has not been formally studied. For those patients who have not had success from therapy with an antidepressant or gabapentin and who are unable to sleep or function well during the day, an injection of DMPA may be required if the health care provider and patient agree on the risk/benefit ratio of using a progestational agent.

As mentioned earlier in this chapter, for both men and women, hot flashes are accompanied by both emotions and behaviors that interrupt life's activities and can decrease the quality of life. Therefore, when choosing an intervention for hot flashes, in addition to monitoring the frequency and severity of hot flashes, it is important to monitor other hot flash–related quality of life outcomes. Does the intervention help the person sleep through the night and feel more rested in the morning? Does the intervention affect mood in a positive way? Does it improve general well-being or overall quality of life?

Studies evaluating the treatment of hot flashes with the newer antidepressants have revealed several additional beneficial outcomes. Effective hot flash treatments have improved mood (specifically anxiety), sleep, fatigue, and overall quality of life.[39, 63-65] Therefore nurses who use evidence-based interventions to help their patients diminish hot flashes and their effects will be helping to improve the overall function and quality of their patients' lives.

REVIEW QUESTIONS

✓ Case Study

AJ was diagnosed with breast cancer of the right breast at age 42. She completed surgery and chemotherapy. AJ has been coping well with the help of her supportive husband and young teenage daughter, as well as citalopram, 20 mg daily. AJ stopped getting her periods during treatment and began experiencing hot flashes. AJ is now taking tamoxifen. AJ estimates her hot flashes at about one per hour during the day and every 90 minutes at night. She can not sleep in the same room as her husband since she gets up 5 times at night, changes her sheets because of sweat, and faces the day with utter exhaustion. She runs two fans at night. She brings a fan to work and wears a thin, sleeveless top always so she can remove layers to cool down. AJ is unable to concentrate and gets irritable very easily, despite the citalopram use. She and her husband have not been intimate since she completed chemotherapy. AJ is frustrated and disappointed since she thought life would return to normal.

The health care provider starts AJ on gabapentin, 300 mg daily, titrating up to 300 mg tid every 3 days. AJ comes back in 3 weeks, stating her hot flashes are now 4 per day and she gets up once at night. AJ has moved back into her bedroom with her husband. She no longer sweats profusely and feels sharper cognitively and emotionally. The health care provider gives instructions for tapering and then stopping the citalopram, and checks to make sure the hot flashes haven't increased.

QUESTIONS

1. What are the risk factors AJ has with respect to hot flashes?
   a. AJ doesn't have any risk factors.
   b. Chemotherapy, tamoxifen, stress
   c. Chemotherapy, tamoxifen, citalopram
   d. Age 42, taking citalopram, stress of breast cancer

2. What is the scientific, physiologic rationale behind the use of fans and the tank top under AJ's work clothes?
   a. Air movement and layering helps AJ psychologically feel she is doing something for her hot flashes.
   b. There is no scientific rationale for the use of these.
   c. Air movement and layering helps AJ keep her core body temperature down, thus possibly preventing some hot flashes.
   d. Air movement and layering helps cool AJ after sweating.

3. What impact are AJ's hot flashes having on her personal and professional life at the beginning of this case study?
   a. The hot flashes are responsible for ruining all current quality of life.
   b. The hot flashes are not affecting AJ's life; it is the stress of the diagnosis of breast cancer. Focus should be on managing her stress.
   c. The hot flashes are having a moderate effect on AJ's life; they warrant some mild attention.
   d. The hot flashes are having a significant effect on AJ's life and warrant immediate attention with an effective, strong treatment.

4. If AJ was on citalopram and this SSRI has been shown to help hot flashes, why was AJ having such interfering hot flashes?
   a. Citalopram does not work for everyone.
   b. The cause of this phenomenon is not known.
   c. Citalopram is known to cause hot flashes.
   d. Citalopram only works for natural menopause, not chemotherapy-induced menopause.

5. What is the rationale for choosing to try gabapentin?
   a. Since citalopram didn't work, there is no point in trying another antidepressant.
   b. Gabapentin is the most effective agent for hot flashes.

c. Gabapentin can be added to AJ's current medication, citalopram, without negative interactions, for possible additive effects against hot flashes.

d. The first step should have been to switch her to a different antidepressant.

6. Besides gabapentin, what other options are available for this patient?

a. Nurses could have taught AJ relaxation and paced respirations, which would have been equally as helpful as medications.

b. The patient could have tried venlafaxine.

c. The patient could have started using black cohosh.

d. The patient could have tried paroxetine.

7. What might have been suggested for this patient if the hot flashes started to increase while tapering or being off the citalopram?

a. Keep AJ on the citalopram, and see how they both work together.

b. Finish tapering off the citalopram, and add venlafaxine.

c. Finish tapering off the citalopram, taper off the gabapentin, and try another antidepressant.

d. Finish tapering off the citalopram, taper off the gabapentin, and give DMPA.

8. What side effects must the nurse assess for with gabapentin?

a. Dizziness, fluid retention, somnolence, and rash

b. Dizziness, weight gain, and nausea

c. Nausea, dry mouth, and pruritus

d. Dizziness, dry mouth, nausea, and rash

9. What would a reasonable second-line intervention if AJ's hot flashes increase while she is on gabapentin alone?

a. Refer her to a therapist for stress management therapy since this must be a critical etiology in AJ's case.

b. There are no other options for AJ if gabapentin doesn't work, since she has already been on an SSRI.

c. Try a different antidepressant, add paced respirations, or try DMPA, depending on the degree of interference with her life.

d. Increase gabapentin to 1800 mg per day.

10. How will gabapentin affect AJ's sexual relationship with her husband?

a. Gabapentin directly improves sex drive, so the sexual relationship will get better

b. Gabapentin decreases sex drive, so despite improvement in hot flashes, the relationship will get worse.

c. Gabapentin decreases ability to have an orgasm; the relationship will get worse.

d. Gabapentin has no direct effect on sex drive; however, improvement in hot flashes could improve the sexual relationship.

ANSWERS

1. **B.** *Rationale:* Chemotherapy, tamoxifen, and stress are all risk factors for hot flashes. Citalopram and an age of 42 are not risk factors for hot flashes.

2. **C.** *Rationale:* Studies have shown core body temperature rises before a hot flash—environmental conditions (heat) can precipitate a hot flash. Although air movement and layering *may* help AF feel she is doing something for her hot flashes, such as making her cold and/or shiver, this is not the scientific rationale for the behavioral intervention, nor is it related to the management of the hot flash.

3. **D.** *Rationale:* The hot flashes are interfering with sleep. This interference has multiple negative effects and necessitates effective treatment. Although the hot flashes have a significant impact, they are not ruining her life; they are affecting her ability to sleep with her husband as well as sleep at all. Because of the lack of sleep, exhaustion, and inability to sleep with her husband, the hot flashes call for considerable attention and an effective solution.

4. **B.** *Rationale:* Definitive data about this phenomenon is not known. However, our clinical practice demonstrates that antidepressants do not appear to be "protective" in preventing the start of hot flashes if women are already taking them when the menopause transition occurs. The incidence of sweating with citalopram is 2%, but if this were the reason for AJ's hot flashes, she would have experienced them when starting or shortly after starting citalopram. Citalopram has been demonstrated to be effective in breast cancer survivors in a pilot trial, and there are no data to demonstrate that hot flashes that are due to natural menopause respond differently to treatment than hot flashes that are due to premature menopause that arises from cancer treatment.

5. **C.** *Rationale:* Although the research evidence is not available to support the statement that gabapentin is the *most* effective agent for hot flashes, gabapentin can be added to an antidepressant for better overall symptom control. If the patient's mood was being controlled with her current antidepressant, changing her regimen for hot flashes may not be the best thing to do. There is no absolute right or wrong sequence for introducing medication management of hot flashes.

6. **B.** *Rationale:* A different antidepressant (venlafaxine) could have been tried. Although relaxation and paced respirations can be valuable interventions, current scientific evidence does not suggest that these interventions are equal to medication management. In randomized trials, black cohosh has not been shown to be effective for hot flashes. Paroxetine cannot be taken with tamoxifen.

7. **A.** *Rationale:* Having AJ continue with both medications is the best response. Changing the antidepressant is not optimal; changing many medications at once is likely to cause uncontrolled symptoms during the transition. Too many drastic changes and not giving the medications enough time to be effective is likely to result in uncontrolled symptoms and increase the patient's fatigue.

8. **A.** *Rationale:* Dizziness, fluid retention, somnolence, and rash are the most common side effects of gabapentin.

9. **C.** *Rationale:* If initial treatment has failed, then it would be time to consider switching to a different antidepressant,

Continued

REVIEW QUESTIONS—CONT'D

adding a behavioral intervention or trying a nonestrogenic hormone if acceptable to provider and patient. There are always other options to try, both pharmacologic and nonpharmacologic. Studies have only suggested, but not shown, a clear dose response; increased dosages of gabapentin would increase side effects. Stress management may help as an adjunct therapy, but to say that stress is the main reason for AJ's hot flashes is not correct. The evidence supports that

premature menopause is associated with more frequent and more severe hot flashes than natural menopause. A new small, randomized clinical trial does provide evidence of a dose effect with gabapentin.[94]

10. **D.** *Rationale:* Evidence does suggest that hot flashes negatively affect sexual health; the randomized venlafaxine trial found that those women with fewer hot flashes reported an improved sex drive.

REFERENCES

1. Finck G, Barton DL, Loprinzi CL et al: Definitions of hot flashes in breast cancer survivors, *J Pain Symptom Manage* 16(5):327-333, 1998.
2. Loprinzi CL, Barton DL, Rhodes D: Management of hot flashes in breast cancer survivors, *Lancet Oncol* 2(4):199-203, 2001.
3. Molina JR, Barton DL, Loprinzi CL: Chemotherapy induced ovarian failure, *Drug Safety* 28(5):401-416, 2005.
4. Stearns V, Ullmer L, Lopez JF et al: Hot flushes, *Lancet* 360(9348):1851-1861, 2002.
5. Gracia CR, Freeman EW: Acute consequences of the menopausal transition: the rise of common menopausal symptoms, *Endocrinol Metabol Clin North Am* 33(4):675-689, 2004.
6. Crandall C, Peterson L, Ganz P et al: Association of breast cancer and its therapy with menopause related symptoms, *Menopause* 11(5):519-530, 2004.
7. Carpenter JS, Andrykowski MA, Cordova M et al: Hot flashes in postmenopausal women treated for breast carcinoma, *Cancer* 82(9):1682-1691, 1998.
8. Poniatowski BC, Grimm P, Cohen G: Chemotherapy induced menopause: a literature review, *Cancer Invest* 19(6):641-648, 2001.
9. Harris PF, Remington PL, Trentham-Dietz A et al: Prevalence and treatment of menopausal symptoms among breast cancer survivors, *J Pain Symptom Manage* 23(6):501-509, 2002.
10. Carpenter JS, Johnson DH, Wagner LJ et al: Hot flashes and related outcomes in breast cancer survivors and matched comparison women, *Oncol Nurs Forum* 29:2002. Retrieved August 15, 2005, from http://www.ons.org/publications/journals/onf.
11. McPhail G, Smith LN: Acute menopause symptoms during adjuvant systemic treatment for breast cancer, *Cancer Nurs* 23(6):430-443, 2000.
12. Holzbeierlein JM, McLaughlin MD, Thrasher JB: Complications of androgen deprivation therapy for prostate cancer, *Curr Opin Urol* 14(3):177-183, 2004.
13. Kouriefs C, Georgiou M, Ravi R: Hot flushes and prostate cancer: pathogenesis and treatment, *Br J Urol Int* 89(4):379-383, 2002.
14. Ford K, Sowers M, Crutchfield M et al: A longitudinal study of the predictors of prevalence and severity of symptoms commonly associated with menopause, *Menopause* 12(3):308-317, 2005.
15. Windham GC, Elkin EP, Swan SH et al: Cigarette smoking and effects on menstrual function, *Obstet Gynecol* 93(1):59-65, 1999.
16. Lower EE, Blau R, Gazder P et al: The risk of premature menopause induced by chemotherapy for early breast cancer, *J Women's Health Gender Based Med* 8(7):949-953, 1999.
17. Ireland AM: Alterations in sexuality and reproductive function. In Polovich M, White JM and Kelleher LO, editors: *Chemotherapy and biotherapy guidelines and recommendations for practice*, Pittsburgh, PA 2005, ONS.
18. Morales L, Neven P, Timmerman D et al: Acute effects of tamoxifen and third-generation aromatase inhibitors on menopausal symptoms of breast cancer patients, *Anti-Cancer Drugs* 15(8):753-760, 2004.
19. Loprinzi CL, Zahasky KM, Sloan JA et al: Tamoxifen induced hot flashes, *Clin Breast Cancer* 1(1):52-56, 2000.
20. Aldrighi JM, Quail DC, Levy-Frebault J et al: Predictors of hot flushes in postmenopausal women who receive raloxifene therapy, *Am J Obstet Gynecol* 191(6):1979-1988, 2004.
21. Ganz PA, Rowland JH, Desmond K et al: Life after breast cancer: understanding women's health-related quality of life and sexual functioning, *J Clin Oncol* 16(2):501-514, 1998.
22. Shanafelt TD, Barton DL, Adjei AA et al: Pathophysiology and treatment of hot flashes, *Mayo Clin Proc* 77(11):1207-1218, 2002.
23. Carpenter JS, Gilchrist JM, Chen K et al: Hot flashes, core body temperature, and metabolic parameters in breast cancer survivors, *Menopause* 11(4):375-381, 2004.
24. Berendsen HG: Hot flushes and serotonin, *J Br Menopause Soc* 8:30-34, 2002.
25. Sloan JA, Loprinzi CL, Novotny PJ et al: Methodologic lessons learned from hot flash studies, *J Clin Oncol* 19(23):4280-4290, 2001.
26. Carpenter JS: The hot flash related daily interference scale: a tool for assessing the impact of hot flashes on quality of life following breast cancer, *J Pain Symptom Manage* 22(6):979-989, 2001.
27. Barton D, Loprinzi CL: Making sense of the evidence regarding nonhormonal treatments for hot flashes, *Clin J Oncol Nurs* 8(1):39-42, 2004.
28. Blumel JE, Castelo-Branco C, Cancelo MJ et al: Relationship between psychological complaints and vasomotor symptoms during climacteric, *Maturitas* 49(3):205-210, 2004.
29. Nishiyama T, Kanazawa S, Watanabe R et al: Influence of hot flashes on quality of life in patients with prostate cancer treated with androgen deprivation therapy, *Int J Urol* 11(9):735-741, 2004.
30. Quella S, Loprinzi CL, Dose AM: A qualitative approach to defining hot flashes in men, *Urol Nurs* 14(4):155-158, 1994.
31. Schwartz AL: The Schwartz Cancer Fatigue Scale: testing reliability and validity, *Oncol Nurs Forum* 25(4):711-717, 1998.
32. Selin RC, Mendoza TR, Nakamura Y et al: When is cancer pain mild, moderate or severe? Grading pain severity by its interference with function, *Pain* 61:277-284, 1995.
33. Buysse DJ, Reynolds CF, Monk TH et al: The Pittsburgh Sleep Quality Index: a new instrument for psychiatric practice and research, *Psychiatry Res* 28(2):193-213, 1989.
34. Alder E: The Blatt-Kupperman menopausal index: a critique, *Maturitas* 29(1):19-24, 1998.
35. Greene JG: Constructing a standard climacteric scale, *Maturitas* 29(1):25-31, 1998.
36. Heinemann K, Ruebig A, Potthoff P et al: The Menopause Rating Scale: a methodological review, *Health Qual Life Outcomes*, retrieved August 15, 2005, from http://www.hqlo.com/content/2/1/45.
37. Carpenter JS, Andrykowsk MA, Freedman RR et al: Feasibility and psychometrics of an ambulatory hot flush monitoring device, *Menopause* 6(3):209-215, 1999.
38. Freedman RR, Norton D, Woodward S et al: Core body temperature and circadian rhythm of hot flashes in menopausal women, *J Clin Endocrinol Metabol* 80(8):2354-2358, 1995.
39. Loprinzi CL, Kugler JW, Sloan JA et al: Venlafaxine in management of hot flashes in survivors of breast cancer: a randomized controlled trial, *Lancet* 356(9247):2059-2063, 2000.
40. Loprinzi CL, Sloan JA, Perez EA et al: Phase III Evaluation of fluoxetine for treatment of hot flashes, *J Clin Oncol* 20(6):1578-1583, 2002.
41. Guttuso T, Kurlan R, McDermott M et al: Gabapentin's effects on hot flashes in postmenopausal women: a randomized controlled trial, *Obstet Gynecol* 101(2):337-345, 2003.
42. Stearns V, Beebe K, Malini I et al: Paroxetine controlled release in the treatment of menopausal hot flashes: a randomized controlled trial, *JAMA* 289(21):2827-2834, 2003.
43. Pockaj BA, Gallagher J, Loprinzi CL et al: Phase III double blinded randomized trial to evaluate the use of black cohosh in the treatment of hot flashes: a NCCTG study, *J Clin Oncol* 23(16S):732s, 2005.
44. Loprinzi CL, Levitt, R, Barton DL et al: Phase III comparison of depomedroxyprogesterone acetate to venlafaxine for managing hot flashes: NCCTG trial N99C7, *J Clin Oncol* 24(9):1409-1414, 2006.

45. Barton DL, Loprinzi CL, Quella SK et al: Prospective evaluation of vitamin E for hot flashes in breast cancer survivors, *J Clin Oncol* 16(2):495-500, 1998.

46. Loprinzi CL, Michalak JC, Quella SK et al: Megestrol acetate for the prevention of hot flashes, *N Engl J Med* 331(6):347-352, 1994.

47. Loprinzi CL, Quella SK, Barton D et al: Evaluation of soy phytoestrogens for the treatment of hot flashes in breast cancer survivors: an NCCTG Trial, *J Clin Oncol* 16(2):495-500, 1999.

48. Pandya K, Rauberta R, Flynn P et al: Oral clonidine in postmenopausal patients with breast cancer experiencing tamoxifen induced hot flashes: a University of Rochester Cancer Center Community Clinical Oncology Program study, *Ann Intern Med* 132(10):788-793, 2000.

49. Goldberg RM, Loprinzi CL, O'Fallon JR et al: Transdermal clonidine for ameliorating tamoxifen induced hot flashes, *J Clin Oncol* 12(1):155-158, 1994.

50. Rossouw JE, Women's Health Initiative Investigators: Risks and benefits of estrogen plus progestin in healthy postmenopausal women: principal results from the Women's Health Initiative Randomized Controlled Trial, *JAMA* 288(3):321-333, 2002.

51. Espeland MA, Rapp SR, Shumaker SA et al: Conjugated equine estrogens and global cognitive function in postmenopausal women. Women's Health Initiative Memory Study, *JAMA* 291(24):2959-2968, 2004.

52. Greendale GA, Reboussin BA, Hogan P et al: Symptom relief and side effects of postmenopausal hormones: results from the postmenopausal estrogen/progestin interventions trial, *Obstet Gynecol* 92(6):982-988, 1998.

53. Bachmann G: Vasomotor flushes in menopausal women, *Am J Obstet Gynecol* 180(3 pt 2):S312-316, 1999.

54. Barton D, Loprinzi C, Wahner-Roedler D: Hot flashes: aetiology and management, *Drugs Aging* 18(8):597-606, 2001.

55. Barton D, Loprinzi C, Quella S et al: Depomedroxyprogesterone for the management of hot flashes, *J Pain Symptom Manage* 24(6):603-607, 2002.

56. Bertelli G, Venturini M, DelMastro L et al: Intramuscular depot medroxyprogesterone versus oral megestrol for the control of postmenopausal hot flashes in breast cancer patients: a randomized study, *Ann Oncol* 13(6):883-888, 2002.

57. Quella SK, Loprinzi CL, Sloan JA et al: Long term use of megestrol acetate by cancer survivors for the treatment of hot flashes, *Cancer* 82(9):1784-1788, 1998.

58. Brosman S: Depo-Provera as a treatment for hot flashes in men on androgen ablation therapy, *J Urol* 153(4 suppl):448A, 1995.

59. Schairer C, Lubin J, Troisi R et al: Menopausal estrogen and estrogen-progestin replacement therapy and breast cancer risk, *JAMA* 283(4):485-491, 2000.

60. Missmer SA, Eliassen AH, Barbierie RL et al: Endogenous estrogen, androgen, and progesterone concentrations and breast cancer risk among postmenopausal women, *J Natl Cancer Inst* 96(24):1856-1865, 2004.

61. Foster GV, Zacur HA, Rock JA: Hot flashes in postmenopausal women ameliorated by danazol, *Fertil Steril* 43(3):401-404, 1985.

62. Simon J, Klaiber E, Wijta B et al: Differential effects of estrogen-androgen and estrogen-only therapy on vasomotor symptoms, gonadotropin secretion, and endogenous bioavailability in postmenopausal women, *Menopause* 6(2):138-146, 1999.

63. Notelovitz M: Hot flashes and androgens: a biologic rationale for clinical practice, *Mayo Clin Proc* 78(Suppl):S8-S13, 2004.

64. Labrie F, Luu-The V, Labrie C et al: Endocrine and intracrine sources of androgens in women: inhibition of breast cancer and other roles of androgens and their precursor dehydropeiandrosterone, *Endocrine Rev* 24(2):152-182, 2003.

65. Loprinzi CL, Pisansky TM, Fonseca R et al: Pilot Evaluation of venlafaxine hydrochloride for the therapy of hot flashes in cancer survivors, *J Clin Oncol* 16(7):2377-2381, 1998.

66. Stearns V, Slack R, Greep N et al: Paroxetine is an effective treatment for hot flashes: results from a prospective randomized clinical trial, *J Clin Oncol* 23(28):6919-6930, 2005.

67. Loprinzi CL, Barton DL, Carpenter LA et al: Pilot evaluation of paroxetine for treating hot flashes in men, *Mayo Clin Proc* 79(10):1247-1251, 2004.

68. Kimmick GG, Lovato J, McQuellon R et al: Randomized, double-blind, placebo-controlled, crossover study of sertraline (Zoloft) for the treatment of hot flashes in women with early stage breast cancer taking tamoxifen, *Breast J* 12(2):114-122, 2006.

69. Goetz MP, Rae JM, Suman VJ et al: Pharmacogenetics of tamoxifen biotransformation is associated with clinical outcomes of efficacy and hot flashes, *J Clin Oncol* 23(36):9312-9318, 2005.

70. Barton DL, Loprinzi C, Novotny P et al: Pilot evaluation of citalopram for the relief of hot flashes, *J Support Oncol* 1(1):47-51, 2003.

71. Perez D, Loprinzi C, Barton D et al: Pilot evaluation of mirtazapine for the treatment of hot flashes, *J Support Oncol* 2(1):50-56, 2004.

72. Loprinzi CL, Flynn PJ, Carpenter LA et al: Pilot evaluation of citalopram for the treatment of hot flashes in women with inadequate benefit from venlafaxine, *J Palliat Med* 8(5):924-930, 2005.

73. Loprinzi CL, Barton DL, Sloan JA et al: Pilot evaluation of gabapentin for treating hot flashes, *Mayo Clin Proc* 77:1159-1163, 2002.

74. Pandya KJ, Morrow GR, Roscoe JA et al: Gabapentin for hot flashes in 420 women with breast cancer: a randomized double-blind placebo-controlled trial, *Lancet* 366(9488):818-824, 2005.

75. Loprinzi CL, Kugler JW, Barton DL et al: A phase III randomized trial of gabapentin alone or in conjunction with an antidepressant in the management of hot flashes in women who have inadequate control with an antidepressant alone, *J Clin Oncol* (in press).

76. Lebharz TB, French L: Nonhormonal treatment of the menopausal syndrome: a double blind evaluation of an autonomic system stabilizer, *Obstet Gynecol* 33(6):795-799, 1969.

77. Bergmans MGM, Merkus JMWM, Corbey RS et al: Effect of Bellergal retard on climacteric complaints: a double-blind, placebo-controlled study, *Maturitas* 9(3):227-234, 1987.

78. Loprinzi CL, Goldberg RM, O'Fallon J et al: Transdermal clonidine for ameliorating post-orchiectomy hot flashes, *J Urol* 151(3):634-636, 1994.

79. Nikander E, Kilkkinen A, Metsa-Heikkila M et al: A randomized placebo-controlled crossover trial with phytoestrogens in treatment of menopause in breast cancer patients, *Obstet Gynecol* 101(6):1213-1220, 2003.

80. St. Germain A, Peterson C, Robinson JG et al: Isoflavone-rich or isoflavone-poor soy protein does not reduce menopausal symptoms during 24 weeks of treatment, *Menopause* 8(1):17-26, 2001.

81. Van Patten CL, Olivotto IA, Chambers GK et al: Effect of soy phytoestrogens on hot flashes in postmenopausal women with breast cancer: a randomized controlled clinical trial, *J Clin Oncol* 20(6):1449-1455, 2002.

82. North American Menopause Society: The role of isoflavones in menopausal health: consensus opinion of the North American Menopause Society, *Menopause* 7(4):215-229, 2000.

83. Jacobson JS, Troxel AB, Evans J et al: Randomized trial of black cohosh for the treatment of hot flashes among women with a history of breast cancer, *J Clin Oncol* 19(10):2739-2745, 2001.

84. Osmers R, Friede M, Liske E et al: Efficacy and safety of isopropanolic black cohosh extract for climacteric symptoms, *Obstet Gynecol* 105 (5 part 1):1074-1083, 2005.

85. Liu J, Burdette JE, Xu H et al: Evaluation of estrogenic activity of plant extracts for the potential treatment of menopausal symptoms, *J Agricult Food Chem* 49(5):2472-2479, 2001.

86. Kronenberg F: Hot flashes: Epidemiology and physiology. In Flint M, Kronenberg F, Utian W, editors: *Annals of the New York Academy of Sciences*, NY, 1990, New York Academy of Sciences.

87. Freedman RR, Woodward S: Behavioral treatment of menopausal hot flushes: evaluation by ambulatory monitoring, *Am J Obstet Gynecol* 167(2):436-439, 1992.

88. Irvin JH, Domar AD, Clark C et al: The effects of relaxation response training on menopausal symptoms, *J Psychosom Obstet Gynecol* 17(4):202-207, 1996.

89. Wijma K, Melin A, Nedstrand E et al: Treatment of menopausal symptoms with applied relaxation: a pilot study, *J Behav Ther Exp Psychiatry* 28(4):251-261, 1997.

90. Aiello EJ, Yasui Y, Tworoger SS et al: Effect of a year long, moderate-intensity exercise intervention on the occurrence and severity of menopause symptoms in postmenopausal women, *Menopause* 11(4):382-388, 2004.

91. Elkins G, Marcus J, Palamara L et al: Can hypnosis reduce hot flashes in breast cancer survivors? A literature review, *Am J Clin Hypnosis* 47(1):29-41, 2004.

92. Stevenson DW, Delprato D: Multiple component self-control program for menopausal hot flashes, *J Behav Ther Exp Psychiatry* 14(2):137-140, 1983.

93. Younus J, Simpson I, Collins A et al: Mind control of menopause, *Women's Health Iss* 13(2):74-78, 2003.

94. Reddy SY, Warner H, Guthso T et al: Gabapentin, estrogen, and placebo for treating hot flushes: a randomized controlled trial. *Obstet Gynecol* 108(1):41-48, 2006.

APPENDIX A

Glossary

Ablation destruction of, as in myeloablation, which refers to destruction of the bone marrow in conjunction with high-dose chemotherapy in preparation for bone marrow transplantation.

ABO compatibility testing is required for whole blood; red blood cells; testing is preferred for fresh-frozen plasma.

absolute neutrophil count (ANC) the actual count of the neutrophils in the blood.

$$\frac{\text{Total WBC count} \times (\%\ \text{segmented neutrophils} + \text{band neutrophils})}{100} = \text{absolute neutrophil count}$$

absolute risk the number of specific cancer cases (e.g., breast) in a given population divided by the number of people (e.g., women) in the population—may be expressed as an average risk for every woman in that group.

acquired immunity specific and depends on the recognition of self and nonself.

active immunotherapy the administration of biologic or chemical products that stimulate the immune system of the host.

adenocarcinoma a malignant neoplasm of epithelial cells arising from glandular tissue or in which the cancer cells form recognizable glandular structures.

adjuvant chemotherapy chemotherapy designed to eradicate microscopic foci of metastatic disease after local control with surgery, radiation therapy, or both.

adoptive immunotherapy (passive immunotherapy) the direct transfer of cells or products of the immune system to a host.

ageism prejudice or discrimination against a person because of his or her age.

allogenic having cell types that are antigenically distinct.

allograft a graft of tissue between individuals of the same species but of different genotype, called also allogenic graft.

alopecia lack or loss of hair from skin areas where it is normally present. Results from chemotherapy, radiation therapy, or endocrine disorders. May be transient or permanent, depending on the type of cancer treatment received.

anaphase a stage of mitosis in which the chromosomes begin to move apart toward opposite poles of the spindle.

anaplasia the loss of structural organization and useful function of a cell.

anemia below normal concentration of circulating red blood cells or hemoglobin, measured by volume of red blood cells per 100 ml of blood. Symptomatic anemia occurs when the oxygen-carrying demands of the body are not met. Anemia is not a disease; it is a symptom of illness.

aneuploid having more or less than the normal diploid number of chromosomes.

angiogenesis in relation to tumor angiogenesis, the induction of the growth of blood vessels from surrounding tissues into the tumor by a diffusible protein factor released by the tumor cells.

anorexia loss of appetite.

antibody an immunoglobulin protein produced by plasma cells and B cells in response to antigen, which has the ability to combine with the antigen that stimulated its production.

anticipatory nausea the inclination or desire to vomit because of the sight or odor of a substance that stimulates a mental image of a distressing situation that has occurred previously; occurs in cancer patients as a result of classic operant conditioning from stimuli associated with chemotherapy, most commonly when efforts to control vomiting related to the therapy have been unsuccessful.

antigen a molecule that is specifically recognized by antibody and by cells of the adaptive immune system.

anti-oncogenes genes that inhibit tumor cell growth; also referred to as tumor suppressor genes.

attributable risk the number of cancer cases in a population that are associated with a given risk factor and that could potentially be prevented by alteration or removal of that factor.

autologous related to self, designating products or components of the same individual organism.

azotemia an excess of urea or other nitrogenous bodies in the blood.

B cells (B lymphocytes) cells derived from bone marrow stem cells in humans, capable of responding to antigen by the production of antibody.

beneficence a person has the duty to take active positive steps to help others; prevent or remove harm.

benign non-malignant; favorable for recovery.

biological response modifier (BRM) an agent that can modify host reactions against disease, with resultant potential to prevent progression of cancer or metastatic spread; includes, but not limited to, immunotherapy.

biotherapy treatment with agents derived from biologic sources or affecting biologic response.

blast cell an immature form of a blood cell or a normal embryonic cell.

blast crisis a sudden, severe change in the course of chronic myelocytic leukemia in which the clinical picture resembles that seen in acute myelogenous leukemia; that is, the proportion of myeloblasts increases.

blocks devices used in radiation therapy to prevent radiation beams from striking areas of the body that require shielding from treatment, such as the heart.

brachytherapy treatment with ionizing radiation, the source of which may be placed within the body or on the surface of the body.

breast self-examination (BSE) visual and manual examination of the breast. A physician should be contacted if any lump in the breast can be felt.

cachexia malnutrition with overall general poor health.

cancer control a term including the entire spectrum of cancer care: prevention, screening, early detection, diagnosis, treatment, rehab, and palliation.

cancer in situ early stage cancer; before the invasion of surrounding tissue; usually implies total cancer removal with surgical incision or biopsy.

capillary leak syndrome shift of fluid from the intravascular space resulting in accumulation of fluid in the extravascular space; symptoms include hypotension, tachycardia, and weight gain.

carcinoembryonic antigen (CEA) a glycoprotein found in increased amounts in the blood of patients with cancers of the colon, breast, stomach, lung, pancreas, thyroid, liver, bladder, and cervix. It is also increased in other diseases and in heavy smokers. Used to monitor the effectiveness of treatment for colorectal cancer.

carcinogen a substance that causes cancer or increases the risk of developing cancer.

carcinogenesis the production or origin of cancer.

CD4 cell cell expressing the CD4 protein on its surface, primarily cells of the immune system, particularly T helper cells (T4 cells) and monocytes/macrophages.

CD8 cell cell expressing the CD8 protein on its surface, primarily a subpopulation of T cells, particularly cytotoxic T cells (T8 cells) and suppressor T cells.

cell cycle sequence of steps through which cells grow and replicate. Consists of 5 phases: the Go phase, the resting or dormant phase in which cells are out of the cycle but have the potential to reenter at any time; the G1 phase, in which RNA and protein synthesis occur; the G2 phase, the time after cells complete DNA synthesis and are preparing to enter mitosis; the S phase, in which DNA is synthesized; and the M phase, which includes the four phases of mitosis.

cellularity the ratio of hematopoietic (blood-forming) tissue to adipose tissue in the marrow.

cell-mediated immunity specifically involves immune T cells and cells of the natural immune system (natural killer [NK] cells and monocytes/macrophages), particularly important to the body's defense against viral-infected cells and malignant cells.

chemotactic the movement of an organism or an individual cell, such as a leukocyte, in response to a chemical concentration gradient.

chemotherapy the systemic treatment of illness by medication. The term was first applied to the treatment of infectious diseases, but it is now used primarily in the context of cancer treatment. Also referred to as antineoplastic drugs.

clinical trial rigorous evaluation to determine the effectiveness and safety of a specific intervention; the procedure by which new cancer treatments are tested in humans

co-carcinogen an agent that becomes carcinogenic when it interacts with a cancer-causing agent.

cognitive function includes all aspects of thinking, perceiving, and remembering; the operation of the mind by which an individual becomes aware of objects by means of thought or perception.

colony-stimulating factor (hematopoietic growth factor) a group of hormone-like glycoproteins that are secreted by a wide range of cells in the body and on which the processes of hemopoiesis depend; substances that stimulate growth or orderly maturation of cells of the hematopoietic system; commitment process by which components of the hemopoietic hierarchy increasingly lose the potential to differentiate into alternative cell lines.

colopscopy the process of examining the vagina and cervix by means of a speculum and a magnifying lens; procedure used for the early detection of malignant changes on the cervix/vaginal cuff.

complete carcinogens carcinogens that have initiating and promoting properties; exposure to a complete carcinogen can cause malignant transformation without additional exposure to an additional promoter.

computed tomography a radiologic imaging technique that produces images of "slices" 1 cm thick through the patient's body; also referred to as computerized axial tomography, CAT scan, or CT scan.

confidentiality handling of information in a way that contributes to patient care and does not disclose information.

consolidation chemotherapy a phase of treatment in leukemia consisting of one to three intensive cycles of chemotherapy designed to bring together the gains made during remission-induction therapy. The therapy begins as soon as a complete remission is documented to ensure that any remaining leukemic cells are eradicated; typically, doses of chemotherapy are administered to induce an anticipated marrow hypoplasia, from which the patient recovers within 7-14 days.

contact inhibition the growth and movement of a normal cell stops when it comes in contact with another cell.

culture a set of values, beliefs, and rules for behavior; provides structure for meaning and decision-making.

cytokine a protein hormone of the immune system that is responsible for communication with other cells of the immune system or with cells outside this system.

cytokinesis the changes that occur in the cytoplasm during mitosis, meiosis, and fertilization.

cytoreduction decrease in the number of cells, such as in a cancerous tumor after chemotherapy.

cytostatic suppresses cell proliferation.

cytotoxic able to kill cells.

debulking surgery to reduce tumor size/burden; improves the response to postoperative chemotherapy; also called cytoreductive surgery.

deafferentation the elimination or interruption of afferent nerve impulses, as by destruction of the afferent pathways.

detection finding or discovering the existence of disease. In relation to cancer, this can occur via screening methods or tests such as mammography, colonoscopy, situation, or problem.

diaphanoscopy examination with the diaphanoscope; transillumination.

differentiation development of a specialized shape, character, or function that differs from that of other cells or tissues; usually implies a loss of malignant nature.

diploid an individual or cell having two full sets of homologous chromosomes.

DNA a complex protein of high molecular weight, consisting of deoxyribose, phosphoric acid, and four bases (two purines, adenine and guanine, and two pyrimidines, thymine and cytosine). These are arranged as two long chains that twist around each other to form a double helix joined by bonds between the complementary system. Nucleic acid is present in chromosomes of the nuclei of cells and is the chemical basis of heredity and the carrier of genetic information for all organisms except the RNA viruses.

doubling the period of time required for a tumor mass to double in size.

Duke's staging a system of staging colorectal tumors based on an assessment of the depth of invasion of the carcinoma and the absence or presence of metastasis.

dysphagia difficulty swallowing.

dysphonia difficulty or pain in speaking.

dysplasia disturbance in the size, shape, and organization of cells and tissues.

dyspnea shortness of breath, difficulty breathing

effector cells cells of the immune system that mediate an immune response.

ELISA (enzyme-linked immunosorbent assay) assay capable of detecting either antibody or antigen by the binding of an enzyme coupled to either anti-Ig or antibody specific to the antigen; used to detect HIV antibodies.

emetogenic an agent or stimulus with the propensity to cause vomiting.

enzymes proteins that act as a catalyst to induce or speed up chemical reactions inside or outside the cell.

epidemiology the science concerned with the study of factors determining and influencing the frequency and distribution of disease, injury, and other health-related events.

epidemiologic approach an approach that examines the frequency of a disease among relatives.

equianalgesic having equal pain relief potential: morphine sulfate, 10 mg intramuscularly is generally used for opioid comparisons.

estrogen/progesterone receptor status (ER/PR status) use of a biomarker to determine whether the tumor is sensitive to estrogen and/or progesterone. Tumors lacking estrogen and progesterone receptors are not sensitive to these hormones. Tumors that are estrogen receptor negative but progesterone receptor positive still respond to an anti-estrogen such as Tamoxifen. In general, tumors that are ER/PR positive grow slightly slower and have a slightly better prognosis.

extravasation an inadvertent leakage of blood or drug, from a vessel into the tissues.

fecal occult blood test test of a stool sample to determine the presence of hidden (occult) blood. This test is indicated when intestinal bleeding is suspected but the stool does not appear to contain blood on gross examination.

fractions (fractionation) division of the total dose of radiation into small doses given at intervals, usually causing less biologic destruction than the same total dose given at once.

gene therapy insertion of a functioning gene into a human cell to direct the natural antiviral human cell response; provides a new function to the cell.

genetic approach the study of the pattern of disease expression among relatives.

genetics the study of heredity and possible genetic factors influencing the occurrence of a pathologic condition.

genome the complete set of hereditary factors, as contained in the haploid assortment of chromosomes.

genotype the entire set of genes one inherits from both parents.

Gleason score score used in prostate cancer to determine the tumor grade through microscopic examination of the biopsied tissue. A scale of 2-10 is used; the higher the number, the faster the cancer is likely to grow and the likelier it is to spread beyond the prostate.

glycoprotein any of a class of conjugated proteins consisting of a compound of protein with a carbohydrate group.

grade a qualitative assessment of the differentiation of tumor cells to the extent that tumor cells resemble the normal tissue at the site; expressed in numeric grades of differentiation from most differentiated (grade 1) to least differentiated (grade 3).

graft-versus-host disease (GVHD) a frequent complication of allogeneic bone marrow transplantation. Immunocompetent T lymphocytes derived from the donor tissue recognize the recipient's tissue as foreign and react to it, producing clinical manifestations that include skin disease ranging from maculopapular eruption to epidermal necrosis; intestinal disease marked by diarrhea, malabsorption, and abdominal pain; venoocclusive disease; loss of hair; and heart and joint lesions similar to those that occur in connective tissue disorders.

granulocytopenia a decrease in white blood cells.

gray the S1 (Systeme Internationale d'Unites) unit of absorbed radiation dose, defined as a transfer of 1 joule of energy per kilogram of absorbing material. 1 gray = 100 rads.

haplotype the group of alleles of linked genes contributed by either parent.

hematopoiesis the process by which blood cells are produced in the bone marrow.

hematopoietic pertaining to or affecting the formation of blood cells.

hemolytic destruction of blood cells, resulting in liberation of hemoglobin from the red blood cell.

heterogeneous derived from a different source or species; xenograft.

heterogeneity cancer cells that are different cells within the tumor and have different characteristics.

histology examination of tissue dealing with the minute structure, composition, and function of tissues as seen through a microscope.

homeostasis the condition in which the external and internal environment of a cell remains relatively constant.

homogeneous composed of similar elements or ingredients; of a uniform quality throughout.

humoral immunity specific immunity activated by antibody found in blood and lymph; particularly important in trapping viral and bacterial organisms that have not yet invaded cells of the body.

hybridoma technological process by which fusion cells, produced by myeloma plasma cells, are introduced into an immunized mouse.

hyperbaric characterized by greater than normal pressure or weight; applied to gases under greater than atmospheric pressure; as hyperbaric oxygen.

hyperplasia an increase in the number of cells in a tissue or organ.

hypertrophy enlargement or overgrowth of an organ or body part due to an increase in size of its constituent cells.

hypoguesia abnormally diminished acuteness of the sense of taste.

idiotype an antigenic determinant present on and characteristic of a certain antibody molecule, usually located in the variable region.

immunity a protective mechanism that serves to maintain the integrity of the body against foreign substances or agents.

immunogenic capable of stimulating an immune response.

immunoglobulin a glycoprotein composed of heavy and light chains that functions as antibody; in humans, the five classes are designated as IgG, IgA, IgM, IgD, and IgE.

immunomodulation alteration of the immune response to induce up-regulation, suppression, or tolerance.

immunosuppression blocking or diminishing the functioning of the immune system.

immunosurveillance a theory that postulates that the immune system plays an important role in the prevention of development of detectable cancer.

incidence the number of newly diagnosed cases of cancer in a specified period of time (e.g., calendar year) in a defined population.

incidence rate the number of new cases of cancer divided by the number of people in the population during a given period of time (usually 1 year). The results are usually multiplied by 100,000 to express the rate more conveniently.

indolent slow-growing tumor.

informed consent a person's agreement to allow something to happen (e.g., surgery); 5 basic steps: explanation of medical condition; purpose of the procedure/treatment; treatment/procedure process; known risks, benefits, alternatives, and consequences of not accepting treatment; and the right to refuse consent or withdraw consent at any time.

initiation the first step in turning a normal cell cancerous as by drugs, chemicals, or other agents.

in situ confined to the site of origin.

interferon (IFN) a class of cytokines originally identified for their ability to inhibit growth of viruses within cells; selectively inhibit the synthesis of viral RNA in infected cells; immunoregulatory functions, including enhancing the activities of macrophages and natural killer cells.

interleukin (IL) a class of cytokines produced by lymphocytes or macrophages in response to antigenic or mitogenic stimulation that mediate communication among cells of the immune system.

interphase initial phase of mitosis; cells grow in size; chromosomes elongate; replication of DNA.

intraoperative radiation (IORT) specialized radiation technique used during surgery to treat cancers deep in the body with large, single doses while avoiding irradiation of normal tissues; it can be used alone or can be given as a boost to fractionated external-beam radiation

intraperitoneal implanted port a hollow housing containing a septum over a portal chamber that is connected via a tube of silicone or a polyurethane catheter that is inserted into the peritoneal cavity; peritoneal ports usually have catheters with larger lumens and multiple exit sites to allow for rapid infusion of fluids; usually placed on the lower rib cage but could be in a pocket of the lower abdomen; used to administer intermittent intraperitoneal chemotherapy for colon or ovarian cancer.

intrathecal chemotherapy cytotoxic drugs injected into the cerebrospinal fluid, thereby bypassing the blood brain barrier.

in vitro within a glass; observable in a test tube; in an artificial environment.

in vivo within the living body.

ionizing radiation a type of radiation that involves gamma rays that penetrate deeply into tissues; this form of radiation may have an enhanced biologic effect on tumors by degrading tumor DNA.

ipsilateral on the same side.

justice a basic ethical principle that describes the duty to give others what is due or owed to them.

karyotype the chromosomal constitution of the nucleus of a cell.

lentivirus any of a group of retroviruses, including those that cause maedi and visna in sheep.

leukoagglutinin an agglutinin directed against leukocytes.

leukocytosis a transient increase in the number of leukocytes in the blood, resulting from various causes such as hemorrhage, fever, or infection.

lymphadenectomy surgical excision of one or more lymph nodes.

lymphocyte any of the mononuclear, nonphagocytic leukocytes found in the blood, lymph, and lymphoid tissue. Divided into two classes, B and T lymphocytes, which are responsible for humoral and cellular immunity, respectively.

lymphocytapheresis the selective removal of lymphocytes from withdrawn blood, which is then retransfused into the donor.

lymphokine activated killer cell; effector cell capable of killing tumor cells; activated by cytokines derived from lymphocytes (lymphokine), particularly interleukin-2; has broad activity.

lymphotoxin a product of lymphocytes; lymphotoxin is toxic for certain tumor cells and shares several properties with tumor necrosis factor.

magnetic resonance imaging (MRI) a type of diagnostic radiography that visualizes soft tissues of the body by applying an external magnetic field that distinguishes between hydrogen atoms in different environments, producing an image. Provides information that allows the distinction between normal tissues and cancerous, atherosclerotic, or traumatized tissues.

malignant having the properties of anaplasia, invasiveness, and metastatsis; referring to cancerous growths and tumors.

metaphase the stage of mitosis in which the chromosome becomes aligned between the centrioles.

metaplasia one adult cell type is substituted for another type not usually found in the involved tissue (e.g., glandular for squamous).

metastasis the spread of cells from a primary tumor via the lymphatic system or venous system to distant body parts where such cells give rise to tumor mass.

micrometastases formation of microscopic secondary tumors created by cancerous cells escaping into the lymphatic or vascular flow, where they can travel to distant sites.

monoclonal antibody (MoAb) antibody formed through a special process of immunizing mice with a desired antigen, removing immunized lymphocytes from the mice, and fusing the lymphocytes with mouse myeloma cells to form a hybridoma, which is capable of unlimited cell division. Cells that produce the desired antibody are selected, and those are cloned to produce large amounts of uniform antibodies specific to the target antigen. These antibodies are still being tested in an attempt to find antibodies that are tumor cell specific for various cancers.

monocytosis increase in the proportion of monocytes in the blood.

monokines cytokines such as tumor necrosis factor released by mononuclear phagocytes.

morbidity the condition of being diseased or morbid; the sick rate; the ratio of sick to well persons in a community.

morphology the science of the forms and structures of organisms.

mortality the number of deaths attributed to cancer in a specified time period in a defined population.

mucositis inflammation of a mucous membrane. Oral mucositis is a common side effect of some types of chemotherapy.

multipotent progenitor cell an early component of the hematopoietic hierarchy that has undergone some degree of differentiation but still has the potential to develop into any of several of the cell lines and has limited self-replicative ability.

murine pertaining to or affecting mice or rats.

mutagen a substance that alters DNA in a cell.

mutation a change in genetic material; usually occurs in one gene; the change is transmissible.

myelophthisis invasion of the bone marrow by neoplastic elements.

myeloproliferative pertaining to or characterized by medullary and extramedullary proliferation of bone marrow constituents.

myelosuppression a reduction in bone marrow function, resulting in a reduced release of erythrocytes, leukocytes, and platelets into the peripheral circulation and/or release of immature cells into the circulating blood.

nadir the period of time when antineoplastic therapy has its most profound effects on the bone marrow; when the blood counts reach their lowest point.

natural killer cells a group of large, granular lymphocytes that have the intrinsic ability to recognize and destroy some virally infected cells and some tumor cells.

neoadjuvant chemotherapy chemotherapy administered before other therapies.

neoplasm an abnormal mass of cells typically exhibiting progressive and uncontrolled growth; classified by the cell type from which they originate and their biologic behavior.

neuropathic functional disturbances or pathologic changes in the peripheral nervous system.

neutropenia abnormally low number of white blood cells (neutrophils) in the blood.

nonmaleficence a basic ethical principal that purports the duty of avoiding intentional conflict or harm.

nociceptive receiving injury.

odynophagia painful swallowing.

Ommaya reservoir a subcutaneous cerebrospinal fluid (CSF) reservoir that is implanted surgically under the scalp and provides access to the CSF through a burr hole in the skull. Drugs are injected into the reservoir with a syringe, and the domed reservoir is then depressed manually to mix the drug within the CSF. This device eliminates the need for multiple lumbar punctures during repeated administration of intrathecal chemotherapy.

oncogene a gene involved in the transformation of a normal cell into a malignant cell, or a gene that increases neoplastic properties of a cell.

opioids natural, semisynthetic, and synthetic drugs that relieve pain by binding to opioid receptors in the nervous system.

Opioids include all agonists and antagonists with morphine-like activity, as well as naturally occurring and synthetic opioid peptides.

osteoradionecrosis necrosis of the bone, most commonly the mandible, resulting from high-dose radiation, occurs in treatment of head and neck cancer.

paraneoplastic syndrome a collective term for disorders arising from metabolic effects of cancer on tissues remote from the tumor. These disorders may appear as primary endocrine, hematologic, or neuromuscular problems.

passive immunotherapy the direct transfer of cells or products of the immune system to a host.

phenotype the entire physical, biochemical, and physiologic makeup of an individual as determined both genetically and environmentally, as opposed to genotype.

pleiotropic the quality of a gene to manifest itself in multiple ways.

plexopathy any disorder of a plexus, especially of nerves.

ploidy the determination of the aggressiveness of a neoplasm by analyzing the cellular DNA content.

pluripotent stem cell the most primitive of the blood cells in the hematopoietic hierarchy; these cells, as yet unidentified in humans, are the forerunners of all of the cell lineages; the pluripotent stem cell is characterized by infrequent cell cycling and the ability to self-replicate.

precursor cell a nucleated cell that is morphologically recognizable as belonging to a specific lineage and that gives rise immediately to the mature components of the circulating blood.

prevalence measurement of all the cancer cases, both old and new, at a designated point in time.

primary prevention measures taken to ensure that cancer never develops (e.g., decreasing the number of new smokers).

progenitor cells an early ancestor of the mature components of the blood; pluripotent stem cells are called also common progenitor cells.

prophase the second phase of mitosis, in which the DNA coils and the centrioles move to opposite poles.

prospective in advance; usually with respect to utilization: admissions and/or payment.

provirus the genome of an animal virus integrated into the genetic material of a host cell.

radiobiology the branch of science that is concerned with the effect of light and ultraviolet and ionizing radiations on living tissue or organisms.

randomized to make random for scientific experimentation.

recombinant DNA technology process by which there is identification of a gene for a specific substance; the gene is then cloned and inserted into a bacterium that then serves as a factory to produce the desired substances (IL-2, TNF, IL-1).

refractory not readily yielding to treatment.

relative risk the incidence of cancer (e.g., breast) in a population (e.g., women) with a known or suspected risk factor (e.g., genetic) divided by the incidence rate of cancer (e.g., breast) in a population (e.g., women) without that risk factor (e.g., genetic).

reticuloendothelial pertaining to tissues having both reticular and endothelial attributes.

retinoid any derivative of retinol, whether naturally occurring or synthetic.

retrovirus a large group of RNA viruses that carry reverse transcriptase.

reverse transcriptase an enzyme that catalyzes RNA-directed polymerization of DNA.

risk factor an element of personal behavior, genetic make-up, or exposure to a known cancer-causing agent that increases a person's chances of developing a particular form of cancer.

RNA (ribonucleic acid) a part of the messenger system through which DNA controls protein production within the cell.

secondary prevention measures used for detecting and treating early diagnosed cancer while in its most curable stage.

sensitivity the probability that a screening test will correctly classify an individual as positive for cancer when the individual has the disease.

sequestration isolation of a patient; the net increase in the quantity of blood within a limited vascular area.

seroconversion the change of serologic test from negative to positive, indicating the production of detectable, circulating antibodies.

specificity the probability that a person not having a disease will be correctly identified by a clinical/diagnostic test; the number of true negatives divided by the number of true negatives and false positives

specific immunity antigen response that is recognized by lymphocytes, triggering a cascade of events to destroy the invader.

somatic growth factors substances that regulate growth of nonblood cells in the body; this is a more diverse and less well understood system, with positive and negative regulation (insulin-like, epidermal, and platelet-derived growth factors).

staging the classification of the severity of disease in distinct stages on the basis of established criteria.

stem cell a cell with unlimited reproductive capacity; daughter cells may differentiate into other cells.

stereotactic pertaining to or characterized by precise positioning in space, said especially of discrete areas of the brain that control specific functions.

stereotactic radiosurgery using a stereotactic frame to accurately deliver a high dose of ionizing radiation to a relatively small target area in one fraction; known as stereotactic radiotherapy when delivered in a fractionated manner. These methods offer patients with brain tumors and arteriovenous malformations an alternative to surgery.

stratification the art or process of stratifying; developing different levels.

suppressor T cells a subset of T lymphocytes that reduces the activity of other T and B cells.

survival rate percentage of people with no trace of disease within a specific time frame after diagnosis or treatments; for example, a 5-year survival rate.

survivorship the state of living with cancer.

syndrome of inappropriate secretion of antidiuretic hormone (SIADH) a disorder in which antidiuretic hormone (e.g., ADH, vasopressin) is continually released, resulting in a persistent hyponatremia, hypovolemia, and elevated urine osmolality, leading to weakness, confusion, nausea, and vomiting. Causes include ADH-secreting tumor cells (especially pancreatic carcinoma or oat-cell lung carcinoma). Treatment aims to remove the underlying cause (the tumor), restrict fluid intake/output, and protect patients from injury.

syngeneic having identical matched cell type.

tachyphylaxis a rapidly decreasing response to a drug or physiologically active agent after administration of a few doses.

targeted therapy new drugs that affect the cancer cells by inhibiting either angiogenesis or certain growth factors and their receptors.

T cells (T lymphocytes) thymus-dependent cells that are involved in a variety of cell-mediated immune responses.

telangiectasis the spot formed most commonly on the skin by a dilated capillary or terminal artery.

telophase the final phase of mitosis, in which migration of chromosomes to cells is complete.

tenesmus straining, especially ineffectual and painful straining at stool or in urination.

teratogen a substance causing mutation in a developing fetus.

tertiary prevention interventions aimed at limitation of disability and rehabilitation of those with disability.

thermography a technique wherein an infrared camera is used to photographically portray the surface temperatures of the body, based on the self-emanating infrared radiation.

threshold (for evaluation) a preestablished level or pattern of performance related to an indicator at which further evaluation of the quality and appropriateness of an important aspect of care is initiated.

thrombocytopenia an abnormally low quantity of platelets in the circulating blood.

TNM staging classification a system of cancer staging (determining how much and where cancer is present) in which T stands for the extent of the primary tumor, N stands for the presence or absence and extent of regional lymph node metastasis, and M stands for the presence or absence of distant metastasis. This is the staging system recommended by the American Joint Committee on Cancer.

transcription the normal cellular response of turning a DNA gene copy into messenger RNA (mRNA).

translocation an interchange in which one segment of a chromosome is transferred to another chromosome, generally the result of breakage and abnormal reattachment.

trending analyzing the results of numerous studies on the same indicator to identify patterns that may influence the quality of outcomes related to the important aspect of care or service being monitored.

tumor neoplasm; a new growth of tissue in which cell growth is uncontrolled and progressive.

tumor marker a product produced by a cancer cell or in response to the presence of cancer, which may be released into the circulation or may remain associated with the cancer cell.

tumor necrosis factor (TNF) produced primarily by activated macrophages; TNF is cytostatic or cytotoxic for some neoplastic cells, induces hemorrhagic necrosis of some tumors, and has a range of activities similar to lymphotoxin.

undifferentiated or anaplastic characterized by a loss of differentiation of cells, an irreversible alteration in adult cells toward more primitive cell types; a characteristic of cancer cells.

unipotent progenitor cell early component of the hematopoietic hierarchy that has undergone further differentiation and is committed to one or two cell lines.

vascular access device (VAD) a device that provides intravascular access.

veracity telling the truth; giving information regarding the nature and prognosis of illness/treatment.

Western blot an immunoassay used for measuring antiviral antibody responses, useful for distinguishing antibody responses to specific viral proteins; frequently used as a confirmatory test for HIV status.

window phase the time between the dates of actual exposure leading to infection and development of detectable serum antibodies.

xerostomia dryness of mouth from salivary gland dysfunction.

Oral Grading Scale

A. Cancer Focused Assessment Scales

TABLE B-1	Grading Scale: Western Consortium for Cancer Nursing Research		
STAGE	**LESIONS**	**COLOR**	**BLEEDING**
0	None	Pink	None
1	1–4	Slightly red	None
2	More than 4	Moderately red	With eating and oral hygiene
3	Coalescing	Very red	Spontaneous

Stage 0: Health Status
The mouth appears healthy. The color is normal pink. There are no lesions present. There is no bleeding. The mucosa is moist. There is no edema or infection present. There are no oral limitations to eating or drinking. The patient experiences no oral discomfort.

Stage 1
The mouth has evidence of slightly increased redness in one or more areas. There are 1 to 4 lesions (may be small ulcers or canker sores) somewhere in the oral cavity. The mucosa may appear to be thinning in several areas. There is no bleeding or infection present. The mucosa is moist. There is mild edema in one to several areas. The patient tends to avoid harsh, hot or spicy foods because the mouth is sensitive to such irritation. The patient experiences mild discomfort that may be described as burning sensation.

Stage 2
There is moderate increase in redness throughout most of the mucosal surfaces. There are more than 4 lesions (may be ulcers, canker sores) somewhere in oral cavity, but they still are discretely separate and not coalescing with adjacent lesions. The mucosa tends to bleed upon probing or manipulating. The mucosa appears slightly direr than normal. The saliva may be slightly thicker than normal. Most areas are moderately edematous. There may be evidence suggesting that infection is present in the mouth manifested by white or yellow patches. The patient is unable to eat except for very bland soft foods, but is able to drink liquids that are not hot, spicy, or acidic. The patient experiences moderate, continual pain and requires intermittent (usually topical) analgesics.

Stage 3
The oral mucosa is severely red throughout all of the oral cavity. There are multiple confluent ulcers which may be to the point of total denudation of the oral cavity. Bleeding is occurring spontaneously without any particular stimulation. There is marked xerostomia. Edema is severe throughout the entire mouth. There are white, yellow, or purulent patches present in the mouth, suggesting infection. The patient is unable to eat or drink, or even to swallow own saliva. With persuasion, the patient may be able to take oral medications. The patient has severe constant pain requiring systemic analgesia.

From the Western Consortium for Cancer Nursing Research (WCCNR): Assessing stomatitis: refinement of the WCCNR stomatitis staging system, *Can Oncol Nurs J* 8(3):1605, 1998.

TABLE B-2	Oral Assessment Guide				
	TOOLS FOR	METHOD OF	NUMERICAL AND DESCRIPTIVE RATINGS		
CATEGORY	ASSESSMENT	MEASUREMENT	1	2	3
Voice	Auditory	Converse with patient.	Normal	Deeper or raspy	Difficulty talking or painful
Swallow	Observation	Ask patient to swallow. To test gag reflex, gently place blade on back of tongue and depress.	Normal swallow	Some pain on swallow	Unable to swallow
Lips	Visual/palpatory	Observe and feel tissue.	Smooth, pink, moist	Dry or cracked	Ulcerated or bleeding
Tongue	Visual/palpatory	Feel and observe appearance of tissue.	Pink and moist. Papillae present	Coated or loss of papillae with a shiny appearance with or without redness	Blistered or cracked
Saliva	Tongue blade	Insert blade into mouth touching the center of the tongue and the floor of mouth.	Watery	Thick or ropy	Absent
Mucous membranes	Visual	Observe appearance of tissue.	Pink and moist	Reddened or coated (increased whiteness) without ulcerations	Ulcerations with or without bleeding
Gingival	Tongue blade and visual	Gently press tissue with tip of blade.	Pink and stippled and firm	Edematous with or without redness	Spontaneous bleeding or bleeding with pressure
Teeth or dentures (or denture bearing area)	Visual	Observe appearance of teeth or denture bearing areas.	Clean and no debris	Plaque or debris in localized areas (between teeth if present)	Plaque or debris generalized along gum line or denture bearing area

From Eilers J, Berger AM et al. Development, testing, and application of the oral assessment guide. *Oncol Nurs Forum* 15(3): 325–330, 1988.

TABLE B-3	Oral Mucositis Index-20									
	LABIAL MUCOSA		BUCCAL MUCOSA		TONGUE			FLOOR OF	SOFT	
	LOWER	UPPER	RIGHT	LEFT	DORSAL	LATERAL	VENTRAL	MOUTH	PALATE	
Atrophy										
Erythema										
Edema										
Ulcer/ Pseudomembrane										
Comments										
Total Score										

Instructions for grading: Each box must have a number

Record 00 to 03 in each box based on the following criteria:

Dorsal tongue atrophy: scored from *normal* length of filiform papilla to grade 3 (total loss of normal architecture [i.e. bald tongue])
00 = normal; 01 = mild atrophy; 02 = moderate atrophy; 03 = severe atrophy

Erythema: scored from *normal* redness for a site to grade 3 (color of fresh oxygenated red blood) 00 = normal; 01 = mild erythema; 02 = moderate erythema; 03 = severe erythema

Lateral tongue edema: scored from *normal* to grade 03 (tongue indented s/p pressure of teeth, ad *fills* the oral cavity to palate)
00 = normal; 01 = mild edema; 02 = moderate edema; 03 = severe edema

Ulceration/Pseudomembrane: Surface area of involvement for each site. 00 = no ulceration/pseudomembrane; 01 = >0 cm^2 but <1 cm^2; 02 = ≥1 cm^2 but <2 cm^2; 03 = ≥2 cm^2

OMI-20 Grading Rules

I. If there are no changes in erythema, ulceration/pseudomembrane, or edema for any areas, all elements to be scored as grade 0.

II. Any alterations from normal in erythema or edema for any area must be scored as follows:

A. If there are only mild changes, no matter what the total surface area of involvement, the change must be scored as 1.

B. If there are any grade 2 or 3 level changes for erythema or edema for any areas, you must first estimate the total surface area involved for EACH grade of change for EACH quality (i.e. erythema, edema). The following decision tree is then followed:

1. If the total estimated surface area for a site has only one grade of change and it is less than 25%, enter a score as one grade lower.

Examples: Right buccal erythema is a 2 for only 20% of the area, enter a score of 1. Lower labial erythema is a series of spots of grade 3, but adding surface areas for all spots together give a total surface area of involvement of 15%, enter a score of 2.
(Remember rule II.A.—if upper labial mucosa has grade 1 erythema of 21% of the surface area, it is still scored as a grade 1 change).

2. If an area has one grade change and the total estimated surface area for the grade is a change of ≥25%, then enter that grade.

Example: Lateral tongue has a grade 2 edema for about 33% of the area, enter score of 2 for that area.

3. If an area has two or more different grades of change for a quantity (i.e. erythema or edema) estimate the total surface for EACH grade. Use the following scale:

a. If each grade of change is <25% of the surface area, score as one grade lower than the higher of the grades

Example: Soft palate erythema is a mixture of 10% grade 3, and 24% grade 1, then score as grade 2

b. If an area has two or more different grades of change with one change ≥25% of surface area, and the other <25%, enter the score for the larger/largest surface area.

Example: Lower labial mucosa is 40% grade 2 and 15% grade 3, score as grade 3

4. If an area has two or more different grades of change with all the changes >25%, enter the score for that area that is highest score.

Example: Soft palate erythema is 30% grade 3, 50% grade 2, score as grade 3.

Oral Mucositis Index – 20 (OMI-20) from McGuire DB, Peterson DE et al: The 20 item oral mucositis index: reliability and validity in bone marrow and stem cell transplant patients, *Cancer Invest* 20(7-8):893-903, 2002.

TABLE B-4   **Oral Mucositis Assessment Scale (OMAS)**

LOCATION/SITE	OBJECTIVE SCORING						
	ULCERATION/ PSEUDOMEMBRANE				ERYTHEMA		
	0	1	2	3	0	1	2
Upper lip							
Lower lip							
Right cheek							
Left cheek							
Right ventral & lateral tongue							
Left ventral & lateral tongue							
Floor of mouth							
Soft palate/ fauces							
Hard palate							

Scoring

0 = no lesion
1 = <1cm^2
2 = 1 cm^2 – 3 cm^2
3 = >3 cm^2

0 = none
1 = not severe
2 = severe

<u>Extent of mucositis score</u>: Number of sites of with either ulceration = 3 or erythema = 2. Range = 0 to 27
<u>Worst site score</u>: The maximum erythema (range = 0 to 18) plus the maximum ulceration (0 to 27) across all sites. Range = 0 to 45

SUBJECTIVE SCORING

Mouth Pain	Please indicate by a vertical line on the scale below how severe the pain in your mouth is NOW.
	No pain Most Severe Pain
Impact on Swallowing	Please indicate by a vertical line on the scale below how severe the pain in your mouth is NOW.
	No pain Most Severe Pain
Function	Please indicate how well you can swallow foods or liquids by checking below:

Normal ___
Only soft, solid foods ___
Only liquids ___
No foods or liquids ___

From Sonis ST, Eilers JP et al: Validation of a new scoring system for the assessment of clinical trial research of oral mucositis induced by radiation or chemotherapy. Mucositis Study Group, *Cancer* 85(10): 2103-2013, 1999.

B. Clinical Toxicity Assessment Scales

TABLE B-5 World Health Organization (WHO) Oral Toxicity Scale

| | ORAL MUCOSITIS | | | |
GRADE 0	GRADE 1	GRADE 2	GRADE 3	GRADE 4
None	Erythema and soreness. May include buccal scalloping with or without erythema. No ulcers.	Ulcers, erythema, able to eat solids. Ulcers with or without erythema. Patient can swallow a diet.	Ulcers, requires a liquid diet. Ulcers with or without extensive erythema. Patient is able to swallow liquid but not solid diet.	Alimentation not possible. Mucositis to the extent that alimentation is not possible. Patients may use fluids for medications only.

Data from Table 1: Recommendations for Grading of Acute and Subacute Toxic Effects in the WHO Handbook. *Handbook for reporting results of cancer treatment,* Geneva, 1979, Author.

TABLE B-6 National Cancer Institute (NCI) Common Toxicity Criteria for Oral Mucositis

| | ORAL MUCOSITIS: CHEMOTHERAPY INDUCED | | | | |
	GRADE 1	GRADE 2	GRADE 3	GRADE 4	GRADE 5
Clinical Exam	Erythema of mucosa	Patchy ulceration/ pseudomembrane	Confluent ulcerations or pseudomembrane; bleeding with minor trauma	Tissue necrosis; significant spontaneous bleeding; life-threatening consequences	Death related to toxicity
Functional/ Symptomatic	Minimal symptoms, normal diet; minimal respiratory symptoms but not interfering with function	Symptomatic but can eat and swallow modified diet; respiratory symptoms interfering with function but not interfering with function.	Symptomatic and unable to adequately aliment or hydrate orally; respiratory symptoms interfering with ADL	Symptoms associated with life-threatening consequences	
	ORAL MUCOSITIS: RADIATION INDUCED				
	GRADE 1	GRADE 2	GRADE 3	GRADE 4	GRADE 5
	Erythema of the mucosa	Patchy pseudomembranous reactions (patches <1.5 cm in greatest dimension)	Pseudomembranous reaction (contiguous patches general >1.5 cm in greatest dimension)	Ulceration and occasional bleeding not induced by minor trauma or abrasion	Death related to toxicity
	XEROSTOMIA (DRY MOUTH) *SUBJECTIVE MEASURES*				
	GRADE 1	GRADE 2	GRADE 3		
	Symptomatic (dry or thick saliva) without significant dietary alteration.	Symptomatic and significant oral intake alteration (e.g. copious water, other lubricants, diet limited to purees and/or soft, moist foods).	Symptoms leading to inability to adequately aliment orally; IV fluids, tube feedings, or TPN indicated.	—	—

From National Cancer Institute: *Common terminology criteria for adverse events,* v.3.0, 2006, retrieved October 11, 2006, from http://ctep.cancer.gov/forms/CTC.

Cancer Internet Resources

Nursing Organizations

American Nurses Association: www.ana.org
American Radiological Nurses Association: www.arna.net
American Society of Pain Management Nurses: www.aspmn.org
Association of Nurses in AIDS Care: www.anacnet.org
Association of Pediatric Oncology Nurses: www.apon.org
Association of Rehabilitation Nurses: www.rehabnurse.org
Case Management Society of America: www.cmsa.org
Home Healthcare Nurses Association: www.nahc.org/hhna
Hospice and Palliative Nurses Association: www.hpna.org
International Transplant Nurses Society (ITNS): www.itns.org
Infusion Nurses Society: www.ins1.org
National Association of Nurse Massage Therapists:
    www.nanmt.org
National Council of State Boards of Nursing: www.ncsbn.org
National Gerontological Nursing Association: www.ngna.org
National League for Nursing: www.nln.org
Oncology Nursing Society: www.ons.org
Society for Vascular Nursing: www.svnnet.org
Wound, Ostomy, & Continence Nurses Society: www.wocn.org

Professional Organizations

Alliance of State Pain Initiatives: http://aspi.wisc.edu/
Alternative Medicine Foundation: www.amfoundation.org
American Academy of Family Physicians: www.aafp.org
American Association of Blood Banks: www.aabb.org
American Cancer Society: www.cancer.org
American Cancer Society: Tobacco and Cancer:
    www.cancer.org/quittobacco
American Cancer Society Complementary & Alternative
    Methods: http://www.cancer.org/docroot/ETO/ETO_5.asp
The American Geriatrics Society: www.americangeriatrics.org
American Health Decisions: www.ahd.org
American Hospital Association:
    http://www.aha.org/aha_app/index.jsp
American Medical Association: www.ama-assn.org
Americans for Better Care of the Dying: www.abcd-caring.org
American Red Cross: www.redcross.org
American Society for Bioethics and Humanities: www.asbh.org
American Society for Enteral and Parenteral Nutrition:
    www.clinnutr.org
American Society of Clinical Oncology (ASCO):
    www.asco.org
American Pain Society: www.ampain.org
Cancer Centers Program: www.cancer.gov/cancercenters
Cancer Hope Network: www.cancerhopenetwork.org
Cancer Research Institute: www.cancerresearch.org
Clinical Trials Listings: www.cancer.gov/clinicaltrials
Candlelighters Childhood Cancer Foundation:
    www.candlelighters.org

Caring Connections: www.caringinfo.org
Hospice Association of America: www.hospice-america.org
International Myeloma Foundation: www.myeloma.org
The Joint Commission (formerly Joint Commission on
    Accreditation of Healthcare Organizations):
    www.jointcommission.org
Leukemia and Lymphoma Society:
    www.leukemia-lymphoma.org
Look Good ... Feel Better: www.lookgoodfeelbetter.org
Lung Cancer Alliance: www.lungcanceralliance.org
Make-A-Wish Foundation: www.wish.org
National Association for Home Care & Hospice: www.nahc.org
National Brain Tumor Foundation: www.braintumor.org
National Breast Cancer Coalition: www.natlbcc.org
National Cancer Survivors Day (NCSD): www.ncsdf.org
National Coalition for Cancer Survivorship:
    www.canceradvocacy.org
National Family Caregivers Association: www.nfcacares.org
National Foundation for Cancer Research: www.nfcr.org
National Hospice and Palliative Care Organization:
    www.nho.org
National Lymphedema Network: www.lymphnet.org
National Marrow Donor Program (NMDP): www.marrow.org
Neuropathy Association: www.neuropathy.org
Robert Wood Johnson Foundation: www.rwjf.org
Susan G. Komen Breast Cancer Foundation: www.komen.org
Y-Me National Breast Cancer Organization: www.y-me.org

Government and Regulatory Websites

Agency for Healthcare Research and Quality (AHRQ):
    www.ahrq.gov
Centers for Disease Control and Prevention (CDC):
    www.cdc.gov
Food and Drug Administration: www.fda.gov
FDA MedWatch Program: www.fda.gov/medwatch
National Institutes of Health: www.nih.gov
National Center for Complementary and Alternative Medicine:
    www.nccam.nih.gov
Occupational Safety and Health Administration (OSHA):
    www.osha.gov
Office of Minority Health Resource Center (OMH-RC):
    www.omhrc.gov/omhrc
PDQ (Physician Data Query) Cancer:
    www.nci.nih.gov/cancerinfo/pdq
World Health Organization: www.who.int

Pharmaceutical and Infusion Therapy Products and Sources

3M Healthcare (United States): http://solutions.3m.com/en_US/
Abbott Laboratories: www.abbott.com

ALARIS Medical System: www.alarismed.com
Amgen, Inc.: www.amgen.com or www.immunex.com
Arrow International: www.arrowintl.com
AstraZeneca: www.astrazeneca.com
Axcan Scandipharm: www.axcanscandipharm.com
B. Braun: www.bbraunusa.com
Bard Access Systems: www.bardaccess.com
Bayer Corporation: www.bayer.com
Baxter Healthcare Corporation: www.baxter.com
BD (Becton, Dickinson, and Company): www.bd.com
Berlex: www.berlex.com
Best Glove Manufacturing Company: www.bestglove.com
Biogen Idec: www.biogenidec.com
Bioject: www.bioject.com
Braintree Laboratories: www.braintreelabs.com
Bristol-Myers Squibb: www.bms.com
Celgene: www.celgene.com
Cell Therapeutics: www.cticseattle.com
Centocor: www.centocor.com
Cephalon: www.cephalon.com
Chiron: www.chiron.com
ConMed Corporation: www.conmed.com
Cook Group Incorporated: www.cookgroup.com
Eli Lilly and Company: www.lilly.com
Genentech BioOncology: www.gene.com
GlaxoSmithKline: www.gsk.com
Grifols (formerly Alpha Therapeutics): www.grifols.com
RITA Medical Systems: www.hmpvascular.com
ICU Medical: www.icumed.com
Imclone Systems: www.imclone.com
IMPAC Medical Systems: www.impac.com
Infusystem: www.infusystem.com
Ivax Pharmaceuticals: www.ivax.com
Kendall: www.kendallhq.com
Ladies First: www.ladiesfirst.com
Ligand Pharmaceuticals Inc.: www.ligand.com
Maxim Pharmaceuticals: www.maximonline.com
Mead Johnson Nutritionals: www.meadjohnson.com
Med-Derm Pharmaceuticals: https://host3.thehostgroup.com/crownlaboratories/medderm.asp
Medi-Flex Hospital Products: www.medi-flex.com
MedImmune: www.medimmune.com
Medtronic: www.medtronic.com
Merck Human Health: www.merck.com
Myriad Genetic Laboratories: www.myriad.com
Nabi Pharmaceuticals: www.nabi.com
Novartis Pharmaceutical Corporation
Now Medical: www.now-med.com
Pall Corporation: www.pall.com
Oncology Supply: www.oncologysupply.com
Ortho Biotech Oncology: www.orthobiotech.com
Pfizer: www.pfizer.com
Partners Against Pain: www.partnersagainstpain.com
Priority Healthcare Corporation: www.priorityhealthcare.com
Purdue Pharma LP: www.pharma.com
Roche Laboratories: www.roche.com
Ross Products Division: www.ross.com
Roxane Laboratories: www.roxane.com
Sanofi-Aventis: www.sanofi-aventis.us
Scale-Tronix: www.scale-tronix.com

Schering-Plough Corporation: www.schering-plough.com
Smiths Medical (formerly Deltec): www.smiths-medical.com
Solvay Pharmaceuticals: www.solvaypharmaceuticals.com
SuperGen: www.supergen.com
Tap Pharmaceuticals: www.tap.com
Tyco Healthcare/Kendall-LTP: www.kendall-ltp.com
US Labs: www.uslabs.net
US Oncology: www.usoncology.com
Vata: www.vatainc.com
Viasys Healthcare: www.viasyshealthcare.com
Wyeth Pharmaceuticals: www.wyeth.com
Zila Pharmaceuticals: www.zila.com

Complementary and Alternative Medicine

American Holistic Nurses Association: www.ahna.org
Cancer Consultants: www.cancerconsultants.com
MD Anderson's Complementary/Integrative Education Resource: www.mdanderson.org/departments/cimer
Memorial Sloan-Kettering Cancer Center: www.mskcc.org
National Center for Complementary and Alternative Medicine: www.nccam.nih.gov
NCI's Office of Cancer and Complementary and Alternative Medicine: www.cancer.gov/cam
Rosenthal Center for Complementary and Alternative Medicine: www.rosenthal.hs.columbia.edu

Ethics

Center for Clinical Ethics and Humanities in Healthcare: http //wings.buffalo.edu/faculty/research/bioethics/
Ethics Committee of the Society of Critical Care: www.sccm.org
Ethics in Medicine—University of Washington School of Medicine: http://depts.washington.edu/bioethx/
European Association for Palliative Care: www.eapcnet.org
Institute of Medicine: www.iom.edu
Medical College of Wisconsin: Center for the Study of Bioethics: www.mcw.edu/bioethics

Evidence-Based Practice

BioMed Central/Palliative Care: www.biomedcentral.com
Centre for Evidence-Based Medicine: www.cebm.utoronto.ca
Cochrane Library: www.cochrane.org
Critical Care Workgroup: http://www.mywhatever.com/cifwriter/library/41/pe1208.html
Evidence-Based Nursing: http://ebn.bmjjournals.com
National Guidelines Clearinghouse: www.guidelines.gov
Graduate Research in Nursing: www.graduateresearch.com
International Medical Volunteers Association: www.imva.org
Oncology Nursing Society Evidence-Based Practice: www.ons.org/ceCentral/
Online Journal of Clinical Innovations: www.cinahl.com/cexpress/ojcionline3
Quality of Life Care: www.cddc.vt.edu

Oncology Patient Information

American Institute for Cancer Research: www.aicr.org
American Lung Association: www.lungusa.org
American Society of Clinical Oncology: www.asco.org
Association of Pediatric Oncology Nurses: www.apon.org
Cancer Care, Inc.: www.cancercare.org
Cancer Index: www.cancerindex.org

Colorectal Cancer Network: www.colorectal-cancer.net
Conversations! The International Newsletter for Those Fighting
    Ovarian Cancer: www.ovarian-news.org
FertileHope: www.fertilehope.org
Gilda Radner Familial Ovarian Cancer Registry:
    www.ovariancancer.com
Gilda's Club Worldwide: www.gildasclub.org
Gynecologic Cancer Foundation: www.wcn.org/gcf
Harvard's Center for Cancer Prevention:
    www.yourdiseaserisk.harvard.edu
International Association for the Study of Lung Cancer (IASLC):
    www.iaslc.org
Intercultural Cancer Council: www.iccnetwork.org
Lance Armstrong Foundation: www.livestrong.org
Living Beyond Breast Cancer: www.lbbc.org
Lung Cancer Online Foundation (LCOF):
    www.lungcanceronline.org/foundation
Lymphoma Research Foundation: www.lymphoma.org
National Breast Cancer Coalition: www.natlbcc.org
National Cancer Institute: www.nci.nih.gov
National Cancer Institute Genetics of Breast and Ovarian Cancer:
    www.cancer.gov/cancertopics/pdq/genetics/breast-and-ovarian
National Coalition for Cancer Survivorship:
    www.canceradvocacy.org
National Comprehensive Cancer Network: www.nccn.org
National Directory of Trained Genetics Professionals:
    www.cancer.gov/search/genetics_services
National Familial Lung Cancer Registry (NFLCR):
    www.path.jhu.edu/nfltr
National Lung Cancer Partnership: www.4walc.org
National Ovarian Cancer Association (NOCA):
    www.ovariancanada.org
National Ovarian Cancer Coalition (NOCC): www.ovarian.org
Native American Cancer Research: www.natamcancer.org
Oncolink: www.oncolink.upenn.edu
Ovarian Cancer National Alliance (OCNA):
    www.ovariancancer.org
Ovarian Cancer Research Fund, Inc. (OCRF): www.ocrf.org
People Living with Cancer: www.peoplelivingwithcancer.org
SHARE: Self-help for Women with Breast or Ovarian Cancer:
    www.sharecancersupport.org
Society of Gynecologic Oncologists: www.sgo.org
Young Survival Coalition: www.youngsurvival.org

Pain

Alliance of State Pain Initiatives: http://aspi.wisc.edu
American Chronic Pain Association: www.theacpa.org
American Pain Foundation: www.painfoundation.org
American Pain Society: www.ampainsoc.org
American Society of Addiction Medicine: www.asam.org
American Society of Pain Management Nurses: www.aspmn.org
British Medical Journal Pain Articles:
    www.bmj.com/cgi/collection/pain
City of Hope Pain/Palliative Care Resource Center:
    http://cityofhope.org/prc
International Association for the Study of Pain (IASP):
    www.iasp-pain.org
Mayday Pain Project: www.painandhealth.org

MD Anderson Cancer Center Pain Management:
    www.mdacc.tmc.edu
Pain Medicine and Palliative Care: www.stoppain.org
Partners Against Pain: www.partnersagainstpain.com
World Institute of Pain: www.worldinstituteofpain.org

Palliative Care Resources

Aging with Dignity: www.agingwithdignity.org
American Academy of Hospice and Palliative Medicine:
    www.aahpm.org
Americans for Better Care of the Dying: www.abcd-caring.org
Association for Multicultural Counseling and Development:
    www.bgsu.edu/colleges/edhd/programs/AMCD
Association of Oncology Social Work: www.aosw.org
Caregiver Survival Resources: www.caregiver911.com
Caring Connections: www.partnershipforcaring.org
Center for Practical Bioethics: www.practicalbioethics.org
Center to Advance Palliative Care: www.capcmssm.org
Australian Centre for Grief and Bereavement: www.grief.org.au
Cleveland Clinic Palliative Medicine:
    www.clevelandclinic.org/palliative
Compassion & Choices: www.compassionandchoices.org
Dying Well: www.dyingwell.com
Edmonton Palliative Care Service: www.palliative.org
Education for Physicians on End-of-Life Care: www.epec.net
End-of-Life Nursing Education Consortium:
    www.aacn.nche.edu/elnec
Family Caregiver Alliance: www.caregiver.org
Family Care Research Program:
    www.cancercare.msu.edu/default.htm
Growth House, Inc.: www.growthhouse.org
Hospice Association of America: www.hospice-america.org
Hospice Foundation of America: www.hospicefoundation.org
Hospice and Palliative Nurses Association: www.hpna.org
Innovations in End-of-Life Care: www.edc.org/lastacts
International Association for Hospice and Palliative Care
    (IAHPC): www.hospicecare.com
    International Association for Hospice and Palliative Care
        access to palliative care journals:
        www.palliativecarejournals.com
    International Association for Hospice and Palliative Care
        access to palliative care texts: www.pallcarebooks.com;
        www.palliativebooks.com
MD Anderson Cancer Center Palliative Care and Rehabilitation
    Medicine: www.mdanderson.org/departments/palliative
National Association of Social Workers: www.socialworkers.org
National Hospice and Palliative Care Organization:
    www.nhpco.org
National Prison Hospice Association: www.npha.org
Oncology Nursing Society: www.ons.org
Palliative Care Policy Center: www.medicaring.org
Promoting Excellence in End-of-Life Care:
    www.promotingexcellence.org
San Diego Hospice and Palliative Care: www.sdhospice.org
Shaare Zedek Cancer Pain and Palliative Care Reference
    Database: www.chernydatabase.org
Social Work Resources: www.clinicalsocialwork.com
Supportive Care Coalition: www.careofdying.org

Patient Advocacy

Hospice Network: www.hospicenet.org
Hospice Patients Alliance: www.hospicepatients.org
National Academies, Office of New and Public Information:
www.nationalacademies.org/news.nsf

National Institute on Aging: www.nia.nih.gov
National Public Radio: The End of Life:
www.npr.org/programs/death

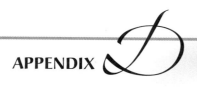
Laboratory Values

TEST	PURPOSE	NORMAL VALUES (ADULT)
Arterial blood gases (ABGs)	Assess respiratory status, acid–base balance. Include respiratory rate and O_2 therapy status when reporting ABG results to physician	pH, 7.35–7.45; $Paco_2$, 35–45 mm Hg; Pao_2, >70 mm Hg; Hco_3^-, 23–28; BE, 0 ± 3 mEq/L; Sao_2, >93% Fio_2

CHEMISTRY
Electrolytes

TEST	PURPOSE	NORMAL VALUES (ADULT)
Calcium (Ca++)	Renal, neuromuscular bone status; parathyroid, thyroid function; increase levels with bone metastasis. Increased or decreased neuromuscular activity with Ca++ level <7 mg/dL or >13 mg/dL	8.5–10.5 mg/dL
Serum ionized calcium	*Not* affected by changes in serum protein/albumin concentrations; more accurate reflection of calcium metabolism than total calcium values	4.4–5.9 mg/dL 2.2–2.5 mEq/L 1.1–1.24 mmol/L
Chloride (Cl–)	Renal status, acid–base balance. Potassium replacement therapy should be accompanied by a 1:1 ratio of potassium to chloride	95–100 mEq/L
Magnesium (Mg++)	Renal, metabolic, neuromuscular status, GI losses, alcoholism. Check antacid ingestion. Increased levels = seizure precautions	1.4–2.3 mEq/L
Phosphorus (P)	Renal, parathyroid function, bone status, metabolism, starvation	2.5–4.5 mg/dL
Potassium (K+)	Renal status, endocrine, cardiac function, acid–base balance. High levels, possible metabolic acidosis; high or low levels potentiate cardiac toxicity	3.5–5.0 mEq/L
Sodium (Na+)	Monitor fluid intake/output; <120 mEq/L. Implement safety precautions; lower levels with metabolic acidosis	135–145 mEq/L
Albumin serum	Renal and nutritional status	3.5–5.0 g/dL (20-d half-life)
Prealbumin	Nutritional status and protein status within past 48 hrs	17–42 mg/dL (short half-life)
Bilirubin	Hepatic, biliary tract, or hemolytic function; hemorrhage, drug toxicities, blood transfusion	Total: 0.2–1.2 mg/dL Direct: 0.1–0.4 mg/dL Indirect: 0.1–0.8 mg/dL
Calcitonin serum	Malignancy of thyroid	50–500 pg/mL
High-density lipoproteins (HDLs)		High-risk: Male: 25, Female: 35 Moderate-risk: Male/female: 45–55 Moderate-risk: Male/female: 45–55
Cholesterol	Hepatic, pancreatic, biliary tract, thyroid function, risk of CAD. 12-14 hr fast required. High-fat/sugar diet may alter results	Age 40+: 150–300 mg/dL Age 30–39: 140–270 mg/dL Age 20–29: 120–240 mg/dL
Copper serum	Hepatic function	70–165 µg/dL
Creatinine serum	Renal and urinary tract function, bone status; ARF profile: increased BUN, creatinine, potassium; decreased sodium	0.7–1.4 mg/dL

TEST	PURPOSE	NORMAL VALUES (ADULT)
CHEMISTRY—cont'd		
Glucose serum	Pancreatic, liver, or endocrine status, diabetes mellitus, hypoglycemia, malabsorption, Cushing's syndrome	Fasting (FBS) 65-110 mg/dL NPO past midnight prior to test Call levels of <40 mg/dL or >400 mg/dL immediately; post pyrandial (2-h PP) glucose level should be within normal limits
Glycohemoglobulin (Hemoglobin A_{1c})	Assess pancreatic, liver, or endocrine status, diabetes mellitus Reveals steady-state blood glucose over prior 4-6 wks	4.3-6.1%
Urea nitrogen blood (BUN)	Assess renal function, hydration status Bun/creatinine ration >1:10 = decreased cardiac output, dehydration or GI bleed	10-20 mg/dL
Uric acid serum	Renal function; hypercalcemia related to chemotherapy; monitor I&O	Female: 2.2-7.7 mg/dL Male: 3.9-9.0 mg/dL
Lipid profile	Risk of coronary and vascular disease	Adult/elderly: Female: 35-135 mg/dL or 0.40-1.52 mmol/L (SI units) Male: 40-160 mg/dL or 0.45-1.81 mmol/L (SI units)
Guaiac (fecal); occult blood; Hemoccult	Determine presence of blood that is not visible No red meats or vitamin C 48–72 h before test	Negative
HEMATOLOGY		
Complete blood count (CBC)	**Do not draw blood sample from same extremity as IV infusion**	RBC, WBC, platelets
Red blood cells (RBC)	Anemia, hydration, oxygen transport; RBC fragmentation, acute leukemia/myelodysplasia	Female: 4.2-5.5 mil/mm³ Male: 4.4–6.0 mil/mm³ Older adult: 3.5 mil/mm³
Hematocrit (Hct)	Blood loss, hydration, hematologic disorders	Female: 37–47% Male: 42-52%
Hemoglobin (Hgb)	Blood loss, anemias, dehydration	Female: 12-16 g/dL Male: 14-18 g/dL
RBC indices	Anemia and polycythemia	
Mean corpuscular hemoglobin (MCH) (normal color)	Chronic blood loss, lead poisoning	28-34 pg Older adult: 28-32 pg
Mean corpuscular hemoglobin concentration (MCHC)		30-40% Older adult: 29-33%
Mean corpuscular volume (MCV) (size of RBC)		82-101 µg³ Older adult: 90.5–105 µg³
Reticulocyte count	Anemia; bone marrow function	Female: 0.5-1.5% of erythrocytes Male: 0.5-2.5% of erythrocytes
White blood cell count (WBC)	Infection, inflammation, and healing Can be decreased with steroids	4,000-11,000/mm³
Neutrophils	Determine presence of infection, inflammation, and stress	42-66% or 3000-7000/µL Older adult: 43-79%
Granulocytes–neutrophils, basophils: (polymorpho-nuclears [polys] or segmentals [segs])	Monitor for neutropenia; measures to prevent or minimize infectious process	
Band cells (stabs)	Presence of recent infection	3%
Basophils	Status of polycythemia vera, leukemia, Hodgkin's disease, allergic reactions, and stress	0.4-1.0% or 40-100/µL
Eosinophils	Response to ACTH, epinephrine or status of allergy, leukemia, Hodgkin's disease	1-3% or 50-400/µL Older adult: 0-0.3%
Lymphocytes	Status of infection, especially viral, and stress.	25-33% or 1000-4000/µL Older adult: 11-48%
Monocytes	Status of bacterial phagocytosis and healing	0-9% or 100-600/µL Older adult: 1-5%

TEST	PURPOSE	NORMAL VALUES (ADULT)
HEMATOLOGY—cont'd		
Erythrocyte sedimentation rate (ESR)	Nonspecific inflammation and tissue injury; malignancy, rheumatic fever, and arthritis; acute and/or chronic infections	Female: 0–30 mm/h Male: 0–20 mm/h
Platelets	Bone marrow, clotting status; increases in advanced malignancy Thrombocytopenia, bleeding precautions.	150,000–450,000/mm^3
Platelet adhesion	Platelet function	5,000–18,000/mm^3 Moderate risk <50,000
Platelet aggregation	Platelet function	Visible <5 min Severe risk <20,000 for CNS hemorrhage
Platelet volume	Determine platelet size; assess purpura, DIC, anemias	8–10 fl 2.5 μm in diameter
Ferritin serum	Hematopoietic status; increased levels with neuroblastoma	Female: 50–100 ng/mL Male: 10–270 ng/mL
Folic acid serum	Anemia	4–16 ng/mL
Iron serum	Anemia	50–100 μg/dL
Total iron-binding capacity (TIBC)	Amount of available iron if transferrin were completely saturated: anemia, chronic blood loss, and liver disease	250–400 μg/dL
Ham (acid serum test)	Paroxysmal nocturnal hemoglobinuria Of no value if recently transfused	10–50% hemolysis of RBCs
Coagulation factors	Clotting status, hemophilia	
Factor I: fibrinogen		60–100 mg/mL
Factor II: prothrombin	Assess vitamin K deficiency	10–15 mg/dL
Factor V: proaccelerin		5–10 mg/dL
Factor VII: proconvertin		5–20 mg/dL
Factor VIII: antihemophilic globin	Von Willebrand hemophilia A	30–35 mg/dL
Factor IX: thromboplastin	Assess hemophilia B (Christmas disease)	30 mg/dL
Factor X: Stuart-Prower		8–10 mg/dL
Factor XI: morphilic		20–30 mg/dL
Factor XII: Hageman	DIC	0 mg/dL
Factor XIII: fibrin stabilizing	Bleeding tendency	1 mg/dL
Coagulation time (Lee-White, clotting time) D–dimer	Assess coagulation; potential bleeding, monitor heparin therapy and bleeding sites DIC	5–15 min Negative (no D–dimer fragments present); <250 ng/mL or 250 μg/L (SI units)
Fibrin split products (FSPs)	Degree of coagulation. Report elevated levels of FSP	<4 μg/ml
Fibrin degradation products (FDPs)	DIC Report elevated levels of FDP	<10
Fibrinogen	Clotting ability. Leukemia, liver damage, DIC DIC profile: Call stat: decreased platelets, fibrinogen, plasminogen; increased PT, PTT, FDPs	160–300 mg/dL Older adult: 470–485 mg/100 mL
Prothrombin time (pro time PT)	Coagulant activity of the "extrinsic" system including factors V, VII, X, fibrinogen, and prothrombin Potential for bleeding Pressure puncture site 5 min Results—ratio of patient to control rather than seconds	100%; also reported in seconds, approximately 11–15; varies with laboratory
Plasminogen	DIC	73–122%
Protamine sulfate	Coagulation, DIC	Negative
Activated partial thrombo-plastin time (APTT) or partial thromboplastin time (PTT)	Plasma coagulation factors except VII and XII (e.g., stage II clotting disorders such as hemophilia)	APTT: 30–45 sec PTT: 16–25 sec
Template B time (bleeding time)	Coagulation, monitor heparin therapy	1–8 min.
Thrombin clotting time (thrombin time; TT)	Factor III clotting	10–20 sec or within 3 sec of control

TEST	PURPOSE	NORMAL VALUES (ADULT)
HEMATOLOGY—cont'd		
Agglutin febrile	Infectious disease, e.g., salmonella	No agglutination titers <1:80
Agglutin cold	Diagnose pneumonia, influenza, mononucleosis	No agglutination titers <1:15
Immunoglobulins	Immune system status	Levels vary with age
IgA	Autoimmune disease	65-650 mg/dL
IgD	Multiple myeloma	0-30 mg/dL
IgE	Allergies	0-200 ng/mL
IgG	Multiple myeloma	600-1700 mg/dL
IgM	Hepatitis, mononucleosis, autoimmune disease, sarcoidosis	50-300 mg/dL
ISOENZYMES		
Acid phosphatase serum	Prostate status, multiple myeloma, parathyroid, or renal function Drawn 3 consecutive days Elevated in bone metastases	<4 ng/mL
Alkaline phosphatase (ALP) serum	Bone, renal, hepatic, intestinal, and biliary tract Indicates GVHD, osteogenic sarcoma NPO 8 h prior-may raise levels up to 25%	30-115 mU/mL
Amylase serum CPK serum	Pancreatic, renal, or salivary gland Myocardial, muscle, brain damage, HIV, hepatitis Elevation 3-6 h after acute MI; peaks in 24 h	20-110 mU/mL CPK: total Female: <51 mU/mL Male: <82 mU/mL CPK-MB bands 3% indicate cardiac damage CPK-MM bands 97-100% indicate muscle damage CPK-BB bands 0% indicate brain damage
Lactic dehydrogenase (LDH) serum	Hepatic, cardiac, renal, muscular, or RBC status Elevation seen 12-24 h after onset of acute myocardial infarction; peaks in 2-6 days; can indicate high-risk leukemia, lymphoma, or relapse of either	100-205 mU/mL
LDH_1 cardiac	A flipped LDH_1/LDH_2 ratio with LDH_1 the highest indicates a myocardial infarction	14-26%
Lipase serum	Pancreatic function	0-190 U/L
Aspartate aminotransferase (AST) (former SGOT)	Liver, heart; cellular death- chemotherapy and radiotherapy Elevated 8-12 h after onset of acute MI; peaks in 48 h	1-36 U/L 5-35 IU/L
Alanine aminotransferase (ALT) (former SGPT)	Liver; cellular death (chemotherapy and radiotherapy); hepatitis, cirrhosis, mononucleosis	8-20 U/L 5-40 IU/L
OTHER TESTS		
Cerebrospinal fluid values CSF	Cerebrospinal system—brain tumor, CVA, meningitis Sterile procedure, specimen to laboratory immediately *Do not* refrigerate	Albumin mean: 29.5 mg/dL + 112 SD: 11-48 mg/dL Bilirubin: 0 Cell count: 0-5 mononuclear cell per mm³ Chloride: 120-130 mEq/L Glucose: 50-75 mg/dL IgG mean: 4.3 mg/dL + 112 SD: 0-8.6 mg/dL Protein Lumbar: 15-45 mg/dL Cisternal: 15-25 mg/dL Ventricular: 5-15 mg/dL
Estrogen receptor assay	Prognosis & treatment of breast cancer	Negative: <10 fmol/mg of protein Positive: >10 fmol/mg of protein
Progesterone receptor assay	Prognosis and treatment of breast cancer	Negative: <10 fmol/g of tissue Positive: >10 fmol/g of tissue
Prostate specific antigen (PSA)	Prostate disease	Normal: 0-4 ng/mL BPH: 4-19 ng/mL Prostate cancer: 10-120 ng/mL

TEST	PURPOSE	NORMAL VALUES (ADULT)
OTHER TESTS—cont'd		
Helicobacter pylori	*H. pylori* infection in gastric mucosa, gastric function; gastric carcinoma, pernicious anemia, gastric atrophy NPO 8 h before, NG tube, check gag reflex afterward	Negative, Basal-Female: 2.0 + 1.8 mEq/h Male: 3.0 + 2.0 mEq/h; Maximal (after histalog or gastrin) Female: 16 + 5 mEq/h Male: 23 + 5 mEq/h
Papanicolaou smear (Pap) Cervical tissue	Collected on three separate slides; determine presence of disease	Negative
Creatinine clearance—urine	Renal status, collected over 24 h; container kept on ice	75-125 mL/min Female: 0.8-1.8 g/24 h Male: 1.0-2.0 g/24 h
TUMOR MARKERS		
Alpha-fetoprotein	Response to treatment for hepatocellular carcinoma, cancer, increases with size of tumor >500 ng/ml Higher in embryonal cell, endodermal sinus types of testicular cancer; ovarian yolk sac tumors	Normal = 20 ng/ml
Bence-Jones urine protein	Multiple myeloma	Negative
Beta-2 microglobulin (B2M)	Elevated in multiple myeloma, CLL, and some lymphomas, estimate of long term survival in some of these cancers	Normal levels <2.5 µg/ml
Beta-HCG		
Bladder Tumor Antigen (BTA)	In urine of many patients with bladder cancer; used with NMP22 to test for recurrence	Either present—positive or not present—negative
Ca 15-3	Used to monitor breast cancer; elevated levels found in 10% of patients with early disease and 70% of patients with advanced disease Levels usually drop following effective treatment	Normal: 25 U/ml; can be as high as 100 U/ml in women who do not have cancer, noncancerous conditions, and hepatitis
Ca 27.29	Follow-up of patients with breast cancer during or after treatment; can be positive in people without cancer—replaced by Ca 15-3	Normal levels <38-40 U/ml
Ca 125	Standard tumor marker during or after treatment for epithelial ovarian cancer; levels may be elevated in 50% of patients with disease confined to ovary; endometriosis, uterine fibroids; lung cancer; or previous cancer	Normal blood levels <30-35 U/ml
Ca 72-4	Investigational for ovarian cancer and cancers arising from the GI tract; stomach	Studies in progress
Ca 19-9	Initially developed for colorectal cancer, used to monitor colorectal, less sensitive than CEA; more sensitive for pancreatic for follow-up; bile duct carcinoma; pancreatitis	Normal blood levels <37 U/ml; high level at diagnosis = advanced disease
Calcitonin Thyroid gland hormone (parafollicular C cells)	Medullary thyroid carcinoma (MTC); does detect early disease; drawn in family members; may be elevated in lung cancer	Adult male <10 pg/ml Adult female <5 mg/ml
Carcinembryonic antigen (CEA)	Used in colorectal cancer follow-up; higher the level at diagnosis more advanced the disease; may be elevated in lung, breast, thyroid, pancreas, liver, stomach, bladder, ovary cancers; noncancer diseases and heavy smokers	Normal blood levels vary lab to lab Levels >5 ng/ml considered abnormal
Chromogranin A (CgA)	Carcinoid tumors, including neuroblastoma, small cell lung cancer; will be elevated in 1/3 with local disease; 2/3 with advanced disease	Normal blood levels <76 ng/ml (men) <51 ng/ml (women)
Estrogen receptors/ progesterone receptors	Breast tissue tested in women or men with breast cancer; 7/10 patients test positive for one of these; more likely to respond to hormonal therapy	ER positive: contains estrogen receptors PR positive: contains progesterone receptors ER negative: does not contain estrogen receptors; PR negative: does not contain progesterone receptors

TEST	PURPOSE	NORMAL VALUES (ADULT)
TUMOR MARKERS—cont'd		
HER-2/neu (c-erb-2)	Tested on breast tissue; predicts prognosis; 1/3 will be positive for HER-2 neu; not as responsive to chemotherapy; may be responsive to Herceptin, an antibody which works against HER-2 neu	Positive for HER-2 neu Negative for HER-2 neu
Human chorionic gonadatropin (HCG; beta HCG)	Elevated in some types of testicular and ovarian cancer; gestational trophoblastic disease; males with mediastinal germ cell cancers; used in diagnosis, monitoring and recurrence	Normal levels hard to define Various methods of testing for this marker and each has its own value
Immunoglobulins IgA, IgG, IgD, and IgM	Antibodies, blood proteins Multiple myeloma, Waldenstrom Macroglobulinemia; diagnosis must be confirmed with bone marrow biopsy	Normally many different immunoglobulins in the blood, each one varying slightly; myeloma or Waldenstrom macroglobulinemia: excess immunoglobulins in the blood and urine; will be seen as identical in protein electrophoresis, will not separate: monoclonal spike or M spike; level of the spike important; elderly may have low levels
Lactic dehydrogenase (LDH) serum	Hepatic, cardiac, renal, muscular, or RBC status Elevation seen 12-24 h after onset of acute myocardial infarction; peaks in 2-6 days; can indicate high-risk leukemia, lymphoma, or relapse of either	100-205 mU/mL
Lipid associated sialic acid in plasma (LASA-P)	Investigational for ovarian cancer; not specific for a particular cancer; can be elevated in noncancerous conditions; used along with other markers to monitor treatment	
Neuron-specific enolase (NSE)	Marker for neuroendocrine tumors such as small cell lung, neuroblastoma, carcinoid tumors; can be elevated in non-neuroendocrine tumors	Normal <9 µg/ml
NMP22	Protein; elevated in urine of patients with bladder cancer; used to detect recurrence; less invasive than cystoscopy, less accurate	Normal <10 U/ml
Protate-specific antigen (PSA)	Blood levels can be elevated in men with prostate cancer, but also in men with BPH, older men, or those with large prostate glands For screening along with DRE; valuable in follow-up In patients who had curative radiation or chemo: PSA should be undetectable; PSA returning indicates recurrence Reduced levels with effective treatment, increased levels as cancer grows	PSA <4 ng/ml: cancer unlikely Levels >10 ng/ml: cancer likely Levels >4 and < 10 ng/ml: "gray zone"; recommend prostate biopsy; draw free FSA (or percent-free PSA); when free FSA makes up more than 25% of the total PSA, prostate cancer unlikely; if free PSA less than 10%, chance of prostate cancer higher (about 50%)
Prostatic acid phosphatase-PAP (not to be confused with Pap smear for women)	Prostate cancer Predates the PSA, is rarely used today	
Prostate-specific membrane antigen (PSMA)	Substance found in all prostate cells, blood levels increase with age and with prostate cancer PSMA is a very sensitive marker but has not as yet been proven more effective than PSA	Currently used as part of nuclear scan to detect metastatic disease
S-100	Protein found in *most* melanoma cells Blood levels of S-100 are elevated in most patients with metastatic melanoma	Tissues suspected for melanoma are often tested for this marker for diagnosis; test is then used to detect spread before, during, or after treatment
TA-90	Protein found on the outer surface of melanoma cells Its value in following melanoma is investigational It is also being evaluated for colon and breast cancer	Test's value in following the treatment course in melanoma is investigational It is also being evaluated for colon and breast cancer

TEST	PURPOSE	NORMAL VALUES (ADULT)
TUMOR MARKERS—cont'd		
Thyroglobulin	Protein substance made by thyroid gland Elevated in some common forms of thyroid cancer Some people will produce antibodies against thyroglobulin, which can affect test results	Normal levels depend upon age and gender Treatment for thyroid cancer is often surgery and/or radiation; thyroglobulin should fall to undetectable levels after treatment
	Anti-thyroidglobulin antibodies are often followed	A rise in thyroglobulin suggests the cancer may have returned In metastatic disease, levels can be followed to evaluate effect of treatment
Tissue polypeptide antigen (TPA)	Protein marker present in high levels where cells are rapidly dividing (cancer cells)	Sometimes used with other markers to follow patients with lung or bladder cancer as well as noncancerous diagnoses

Tumor marker data from American Cancer Society: *Prevention and early detection—What are tumor markers?* From http://www.cancer.org/docroot/PED/content/PED_2_3X_Tumor_Markers.asp?sitearea=PED. Accessed February, 4, 2007.

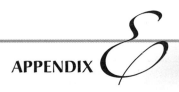

Selected Diagnostic Tests

DIAGNOSTIC TEST	PURPOSE	PROCEDURE/PREPARATION	AFTER PROCEDURE
Angiography	Used in various segments of the arterial system to determine vessel patency or the presence of an aneurysm, embolism, or arterial/venous malformations.	Assess for allergy to iodine preparation; NPO past midnight, sedation before procedure, local anesthesia before catheter insertion via fluoroscopy; contrast medium is infused via catheter; serial-timed radiographs are obtained.	A pressure dressing or sandbag may be applied to the entry site; monitor vital signs as ordered.
Barium studies	Assess for evidence of disease, anatomic abnormalities, malabsorption syndrome.	NPO status before test varies; 300-600 mL of contrast medium swallowed by patient for upper GI; lower GI preparation may include clear liquids, bowel prep of laxatives, suppositories, or enemas.	Large fluid intake is encouraged to promote barium excretion and minimize fluid loss.
Bone densitometry	Determine bone mineral content and density, diagnose osteoporosis, osteopenia, multiple myeloma, and/or unexplained fractures.	Should NOT be performed within 10 days of barium studies because barium may falsely increase bone density in the lumbar spine. Remove all metallic objects (belt buckles, zippers, keys, coins,) that might be in the scanning path. Procedure takes about 30–45 min to perform.	Data are interpreted by radiologist.
Bone marrow biopsy	Examine the bone marrow for number, size, and shape of RBCs, WBCs, and megakaryocytes, estimation of cellularity, and determination of the presence of fibrotic tissue.	Aspiration of the marrow from the sternum, iliac crest, anterior and/or posterior iliac spine; proximal tibia in children; local anesthesia.	Apply pressure to puncture site; observe site for bleeding.
Bronchoscopy	Assess strictures, inflammation, or bleeding. Examine or remove pooled secretions and foreign bodies. Perform biopsy for analysis; place radiation beads for unresectable lung tumors.	NPO past midnight, sedation and atropine before procedure; fiberoptic bronchoscope inserted through nares.	Monitor vital signs; NPO status maintained until return of gag reflex.
Chest tomography	Allows visualization of a section ("slice") of lung at any vertical plane, shows characteristics of border, central area, and/or presence of calcification of a lung nodule, lung lesion, cavitation and/or metastasis.	No fasting is required. No special care required. Remove all metal objects.	Data are interpreted by radiologist.
Chest x-ray	Visualization of heart, lung, mediastinum, pulmonary vessels, trachea, bronchi, pleura, and diaphragm; assess response to therapy, location of catheters, pacemaker wires, etc., pleural effusions, neoplasms.	Optimal visualization requires that patient take in and hold a deep breath.	Data are interpreted by radiologist.

Continued

DIAGNOSTIC TEST	PURPOSE	PROCEDURE/PREPARATION	AFTER PROCEDURE
Cholangiogram IV	Visualization of the biliary ductal system; assess inflammation; presence of stones and/or obstruction.	NPO past midnight; bowel preparation; IV infusion of iodine dye. Bilirubin level <3.5 mg/dL for visualization. If >3.5, procedure may be cancelled.	Observe for allergic reaction from dye.
Colonoscopy	Examine the left, transverse, and right colon and sigmoid.	Clear liquid diet 1–3 days before; sedation and cathartics before exam, NPO past midnight; colonoscope inserted through anus.	Observe for unexpected bleeding, severe pain, i.e., colon perforation.
Colposcopy	Direct visualization of vagina, vulva, and cervical epithelium; to biopsy cervical tissue.	Colposcope is inserted into the vagina and advanced toward the cervix.	Monitor vital signs; observe for vaginal bleeding.
Computed axial tomography (CT scan)	Noninvasive procedure to analyze tissue for density, assess for evidence of disease, inflammation, displacement, or enlargement.	May require NPO status. Performed with or without a dye injection; provides a cross-sectional image.	Data are interpreted by radiologist.
Computed tomography portogram	Evaluate presence of disease in the chest, e.g., tumor, pneumonia, atelectasis, abscess, and/or pleural effusion.	Verify NON-allergy to iodinated dyes. NPO 4 h before test.	Evaluate response to test.
Culdoscopy	Permit observation of the uterus, fallopian tubes, ovaries, broad ligaments, rectal wall, and sigmoid colon from inside the cul-de-sac.	NPO past midnight; local, regional, or general anesthesia; surgical incision is made in the posterior vaginal wall; culdoscope is inserted into the vagina and passed through the incision into the cul-de-sac.	Monitor vital signs; observe for vaginal bleeding.
Cystoscopy	Permit direct examination of the urethra and bladder for strictures or bleeding sites; remove biopsy specimens of the prostate, bladder, and urethra; place ureteral catheters.	May require sedation or anesthesia before examination; cystoscope is inserted into the urethra and advanced into the bladder.	Monitor for urinary retention or bleeding and monitor vital signs.
Echocardiography	Congenital ischemic or acquired heart disease, presence of pericardial effusion, structure and mobility of heart.	Gel is applied to the skin, and the transducer is moved along the skin with some pressure. Heart valves and pericardial sac examined.	Monitor vital signs.
Electrocardiography (12–lead ECG)	Record electrical activity within the heart.	Electrodes are attached to patient's chest and to each of the four extremities.	Observe patient status.
Electroencephalography (EEG)	Intracranial pathophysiology, organic brain syndrome, and determines presence and type of epilepsy.	From 16 to 32 electrodes are applied to the head with electrode paste.	Assist with hair washing.
Endoscopic retrograde cholangiopancreato-graphy (ERCP)	Assess suspected biliary duct pathology and pancreatic disease. Percutaneous transhepatic cholangiog-raphy (PTC) and ERCP are the only methods available to visualize the biliary tree in jaundiced patients.	NPO, sedative before procedure; IV access for medication administration; fiberoptic scope inserted for visualization.	Monitor vital signs; observe for bleeding; NPO status maintained until return of gag reflex.
Esophagoscopy with gastroscopy	Permit direct visualization of esophagus and stomach. Biopsy specimens, brushings, or washings may be obtained.	NPO, sedative before procedure; local anesthesia. Fiberoptic scope is inserted through the mouth.	Monitor vital signs; NPO status maintained until return of gag reflex.
I-125 fibrinogen uptake	Noninvasive test to identify suspected thrombus formation in the deep veins.	IV access for medication administration.	Monitor vital signs.
Immunoscintigraphy	Detect recurrent metastatic colorectal or ovarian cancer.	No fasting required; injection with radiolabeled monoclonal antibody (radionuclide indium chloride-111). Images are obtained in 48–72 hours; the procedure takes approximately 1 h each day for at least 1–4 d.	Same as nuclear scans. Encourage fluids.

DIAGNOSTIC TEST	PURPOSE	PROCEDURE/PREPARATION	AFTER PROCEDURE
Intravenous pyelogram (IVP)	Visualization of the kidneys, ureters, and bladder to determine abnormalities, obstruction, and/or hematoma.	Assess for allergy to iodine preparation; contrast medium is injected IV and concentrates in the urine; NPO for 12 h before examination; bowel prep may be required.	Monitor vital signs; encourage fluid intake.
Laparoscopy	Permit visualization of pelvis and intestines; ovarian biopsy or other surgical procedures may be performed as part of laparoscopy (e.g., lysis of adhesions, tubal ligation).	NPO past midnight; general anesthesia; a surgical incision is made and a trocar is inserted and then aspirated to ensure that intestine or large vessels have not been perforated; nitrous oxide or carbon dioxide may be inserted to create a pneumoperitoneum.	Monitor vital signs; observe for abdominal discomfort and bleeding.
Liver biopsy	Assess liver malfunction or disease.	NPO 6-8 h before; sedative before procedure; local anesthetic; needle insertion to obtain specimen.	Apply pressure to biopsy site; turn patient on right side; observe for bleeding; give vitamin K injection; monitor vital signs.
Lumbar puncture	Assess diagnosis of brain or spinal cord neoplasm, hemorrhage, meningitis, encephalitis, autoimmune disorders of CNS, and/or degenerative brain disease.	Sterile procedure; place patient in lateral decubitus (fetal) position; local anesthetic; obtain 3 sterile specimens.	Explain to the patient that he or she MUST lie still during the procedure; rest in bed (flat position) for 1 h after procedure.
Lymphangiography	Performed for staging purposes with lymphoma or to detect metastasis; to examine lymph vessels for obstruction.	Assess for allergy to iodine preparation: dye injected intradermally to test for allergy. If no apparent reaction, then give dye intravenously; serial-timed radiographs obtained.	Monitor vital signs; observe for respiratory distress.
Magnetic resonance imaging (MRI)	Noninvasive method for assessing tissue function and chemical composition of the body.	May require NPO status; contraindicated for patients with aneurysm clips or pacemakers because of magnetic field.	Ensure return of personal items (e.g., jewelry).
Mammography	Determine presence of benign or malignant breast disease, cysts, and to guide needle biopsy.	Breast is placed between the camera and film and compressed for a clear image.	Data are interpreted by radiologist.
Mediastinoscopy	Visualization of mediastinum; potential biopsy of lymph nodes; to permit diagnosis and staging of cancer, infection, and sarcoidosis.	NPO past midnight; sedation before procedure; local or general anesthesia before insertion of mediastinoscope via incision at suprasternal notch.	Monitor vital signs; potential for bleeding and dyspnea; NPO status until return of gag reflex.
Myelography	Permit visualization of the subarachnoid space to detect abnormalities of the spinal cord and vertebrae and locate obstruction in the flow of cerebrospinal fluid (CSF).	NPO for 4 h before procedure; local anesthetic; needle inserted into lumbar space; contrast medium injected with timed serial radiographs.	Monitor vital signs and neurologic status; follow postprocedure body position orders.
Nuclear medicine scans			
Bone	Detect focal defects in the bone, infection, fractures; to assess disease process.	Assess for previous reaction to contrast media; requires IV access for injection of dye; serial radiographs are obtained; NPO and sedation may be required.	Encourage fluid intake to aid in urinary excretion of radionuclide.

Continued

DIAGNOSTIC TEST	PURPOSE	PROCEDURE/PREPARATION	AFTER PROCEDURE
Nuclear medicine scans—cont'd			
Brain	Delineate subdural hematoma, arteriovenous malformation, thrombosis, abscess, neoplasms, glioma, or other metastatic tumors.	Assess for previous reaction to contrast media; requires IV access for injection of dye; serial radiographs are obtained; NPO and sedation may be required.	Encourage fluid intake to aid in urinary excretion of radionuclide.
Gallium	Determine presence of neoplasms, lymphoma, bronchogenic cancer, Hodgkin's disease, or inflammation.	Assess for previous reaction to contrast media; requires IV access for injection of dye; serial radiographs are obtained; NPO and sedation may be required.	Encourage fluid intake to aid in urinary excretion of radionuclide.
Gastric emptying scan	Assess obstruction, (e.g., ulcer, malignancy); patency of surgical anastomosis.	Patient to ingest "test meal" containing a radionuclide technetium; stomach is scanned until gastric emptying is complete.	Encourage fluid intake to aid in urinary excretion of radionuclide.
Liver and spleen	Detect lesions (e.g., cysts, hematomas, abscesses, adenomas, lacerations, metastasis).	Assess for previous reaction to contrast media; requires IV access for injection of dye; serial radiographs are obtained; NPO and sedation may be required.	Encourage fluid intake to aid in urinary excretion of radionuclide.
Lung	Examine pulmonary vascular circulation, locates pulmonary emboli.	Assess for previous reaction to contrast media; requires IV access for injection of dye; serial radiographs obtained; NPO and sedation may be required.	Encourage fluid intake to aid in urinary excretion of radionuclide.
Multiple gated acquisition (MUGA)	Assess indices of ventricular effectiveness, ejection fraction, and ventricular volume of heart.	Assess for previous reaction to contrast media; requires IV access for injection of dye; serial radiographs obtained; NPO and sedation may be required.	Encourage fluid intake to aid in urinary excretion of radionuclide.
Positron emission tomography (PET)	A unique technique that combines nuclear medicine with precise localization to penetrate body's metabolism by recording traces of nuclear annihilations in body tissue. Designed to measure blood flow and volume, protein metabolism.	Requires multiple IV sites (infusion of radioisotope and serial blood samples); no restriction on diet or fluids; no sedatives or tranquilizers should be taken.	Encourage fluid intake to aid in urinary excretion of radionuclide.
Renal	Provide data on kidney size, shape, location, and perfusion.	Assess for previous reaction to contrast media; requires IV access for injection of dye; serial radiographs are obtained; NPO and sedation may be required.	Encourage fluid intake to aid in urinary excretion of radionuclide.
Thallium	Identify myocardial fibrosis and ischemia; perfusion imaging.	Assess for previous reaction to contrast media; requires IV access for injection of dye; serial radiographs are obtained; NPO and sedation may be required.	Encourage fluid intake to aid in urinary excretion of radionuclide.
Thyroid	Assess location, size, shape, and anatomic function of the substernal or enlarged thyroid glands.	Assess for previous reaction to contrast media; requires IV access for injection of dye; serial radiographs are obtained; NPO and sedation may be required.	Encourage fluid intake to aid in urinary excretion of radionuclide.

DIAGNOSTIC TEST	PURPOSE	PROCEDURE/PREPARATION	AFTER PROCEDURE
Nuclear medicine scans—cont'd			
Oximetry	Assess arterial oxygen saturation (Sao_2); shock lung, pneumonia, asthma, mechanical ventilation status.	Place monitoring probe or sensor on the earlobe/fingertip.	Noninvasive.
Paracentesis	Confirm presence of ascites; specimen analyzed for protein, amylase, RBC, WBC, fat, specific gravity, and cancer cells; fluid may be removed for palliative measures.	Local anesthetic; insertion of trocar, then catheter for drainage; may be continuous flow set-up.	Monitor vital signs; observe and record fluid loss.
Pericardiocentesis	Needle aspiration of fluid from pericardial sac; used for diagnostic or therapeutic purposes; ECG monitoring for localization and position of needle tip.	IV access, KVO rate; supine position with HOB elevated 60 degrees.	Observe and monitor vital signs, potential bleeding, and dyspnea.
Proctoscopy	Explore anus, rectum, and sigmoid colon.	Clear liquid diet, laxatives, NPO, enemas till clear before examination.	Observe for unexpected bleeding or sharp pain.
Sella turcica radiography	Screen for pituitary adenomas.	All objects above the neck must be removed.	No special aftercare.
Sialography	Assess salivary ducts (parotid, submaxillary, submandibular, sublingual) and related glandular structures.	Ingestion of contrast medium; x-ray films are taken with the patient in various positions; patient is given a sour substance to stimulate salivary excretion.	Provide fluids or food upon return from exams.
Sigmoidoscopy (flexible)	Visualizes rectum and lower colon using thin lighted tube. Tissue samples may be collected, and removal of polyps may be performed at this time.	Clear liquid diet 1-3 days before, NPO 6-8 h before; cathartics before examination; fiberoptic endoscope inserted via anus.	Observe for unexpected bleeding or sharp pain.
Spinal radiography patient positioning (cervical, thoracic, lumbar, test sacral, or coccygeal)	Determine traumatic or pathologic fractures, degenerative arthritis changes.	Remove all metal objects. Immoblize patient if spinal fracture is suspected. Patient positioning depends on results.	Data are interpreted by radiologist.
Thermography	Technique by which differences in heat energy emanating from the skin of the breast are photographed using an infrared detector; hot spots may be a tumor, fibrocystic changes, or infection.	Thermoscope is placed over a small area of the breast to determine normal breast temperature; then both breasts scanned with infrared device; no discomfort is associated with the test.	Data are interpreted by radiologist.
Thoracentesis	Obtain pleural fluid for analysis; performed to relieve intrathoracic pressure associated with excess fluid in the lung.	Local anesthesia before insertion of trocar, then chest tubes; needle insertion for biopsy may be guided by fluoroscopy.	Monitor vital signs; observe for respiratory distress, bleeding at entry site, and excessive blood in sputum.
Tomography	Assess nodules or calcification in pulmonary mass or infiltrate.	Radiographic imaging through a pre-determined cross section of the body; optimal visualization requires that patient take in and hold a deep breath.	Data interpreted by radiologist.
Ultrasonography Doppler	Noninvasive procedure using sound waves to assess tissue function, abscess, trauma; determine blood flow velocity.	Gel is placed on the patient and the transducer is moved along the skin with some pressure.	Provide shin cleansing items.

Continued

DIAGNOSTIC TEST	PURPOSE	PROCEDURE/PREPARATION	AFTER PROCEDURE
Nuclear medicine scans—cont'd			
Venography	Demonstrate nonfilling of a vessel; assess for abnormal valves, thrombophlebitis, or hematoma.	Assess for allergy to contrast medium; inject contrast medium; serial-timed radiographs are obtained.	Monitor vital signs; observe for bleeding at entry site.
Ventriculography	Observe size, shape, and filling of ventricles; detect lesions and/or cerebral anomalies.	Serial x-ray of the skull after air or contrast material is injected via burr holes in the skull. Requires general/local anesthesia, NPO status past midnight; monitor vital signs after procedure every 15-30 min for the initial 24 h; head of bed elevated 10-15 degrees for 24 h.	Observe scalp dressing; monitor pain and administer analgesics. Monitor vitals and return of gag reflex.

BIBLIOGRAPHY

1. Becker D, Mihm M, Hewitt S et al: Markers and tissue resources for melanoma: meeting report, *Caner Res* 66(22):10652-10657, 2006.
2. Buc E, Kwiatkowski F, Alves A et al: Tobacco smoking: a factor of early onset colorectal cancer, *Dis Col Rectum* 49(12):1893-1896, 2006.
3. Chak A, Faulx A, Eng C et al: Gastroesophageal reflux symptoms in patients with adenocarcinoma of the esophagus or cardia, *Cancer* 107(9):2160-2166, 2006.
4. Chan J, Meyerhardt J, Chan A et al: Hormone replacement therapy and survival after colorectal cancer diagnosis, *J Clin Oncol* 24(36): 5680-5686, 2006.
5. Chang H, Lee S, Goodman S et al: Assessment of plasma DNA levels, allelic imbalance, and Ca-125 as diagnostic tests for cancer, *J Natl Can Inst* 94(22):1697-1703, 2002.
6. Fischer B, Olsen M, Minna W et al: How few cancer cells can be detected by positron emission tomography? A frequent question asked by an in vitro study, *Eur J Nucl Med Mol Imaging* 33(6):697-702, 2006.
7. Gross C, Andersen M, Krumholz H et al: Relation between Medicare screening reimbursement and stage at diagnosis for older patients with colon cancer, *JAMA.* 296(23):2815-2822, 2006.
8. Horan A: Cystectomy delay more than 3 months from initial bladder cancer diagnosis results in decreased disease specific and overall survival, *J Urol* 175(4):1262-1267, 2006.
9. Issa M, Zasada W, Ward K et al: The value of digital rectal examination (DRE) as a predictor for prostate cancer diagnosis among United States veterans referred for prostate biopsy, *Cancer Detect Prev* 30(3):269-275, 2006.
10. Mathelin C, Cromer A, Wendling C et al: Serum biomarkers for detection of breast cancers: a prospective study, *Breast Cancer Res Treat* 96(1):83-90, 2006.
11. Muira NN, Nakamura H, Sato R et al: Clinical usefulness of serum telomerase reverse transcriptase (hTERT) mRNA and epidermal growth factor receptor (EGFR) mRNA as a novel tumor marker for lung cancer, *Cancer Sci* 97(12):1366-1373, 2006.
12. Polednak A: Co-morbid diabetes mellitus and risk of death after diagnosis of colorectal cancer: a population based study, *Cancer Detect Prev* 30(5):466-472, 2006.
13. Raab S, Hornberger J, Raffin T: The importance of sputum cytology in the diagnosis of lung cancer: a cost effective analysis, *Chest* 112(4): 937-945, 1997.
14. Warren J, Klabunde C, Schrag D et al: Overview of SEER-Medicare data: content, research applications, and generalizability to the United States elderly population, *Med Care* 40(8 Suppl):IV-3-18, 2002.

Index

Note: Page numbers followed by f indicate figure(s); t, table(s); b, box(es) and boxed material.